Fourth Edition

ADVANCED PRACTICE NURSING

An Integrative Approach

Ann B. Hamric, PhD, RN, FAAN
Associate Professor, School of Nursing
Faculty Affiliate, Center for Biomedical Ethics
University of Virginia
Charlottesville, Virginia

Judith A. Spross, PhD, RN, FAAN
Professor
University of Southern Maine
College of Nursing and Health Professions
Portland, Maine

Charlene M. Hanson, EdD, RN, FNP-BC, FAAN
Professor Emerita
Georgia Southern University
Statesboro, Georgia

SAUNDERS

ELSEVIER

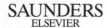

SAUNDERS
ELSEVIER

11830 Westline Industrial Drive
St. Louis, Missouri 63146

Notice

Neither the Publisher nor the Authors assume any responsibility for any loss or injury and/or damage to persons or property arising out of or related to any use of the material contained in this book. It is the responsibility of the treating practitioner, relying on independent expertise and knowledge of the patient, to determine the best treatment and method of application for the patient.

The Publisher

Previous editions copyrighted 2005, 2000, 1996

Library of Congress Cataloging-in-Publication Data
Advanced practice nursing: an integrative approach/ [edited by] Ann B. Hamric, Judith A. Spross, and Charlene M. Hanson. —4th ed.
 p. ; cm.
Rev. ed. of: Advanced practice nursing: an integrative approach/ Ann B. Hamric, Judith A. Spross, and Charlene M. Hanson. 3rd ed. c2005.
Includes bibliographical references and index.
ISBN 978-1-4160-4392-8 (hardcover: alk. paper) 1. Nurse practitioners. 2. Midwives. 3. Nurse anesthetists. I. Hamric, Ann B. II. Spross, Judith A. III. Hanson, Charlene M. IV. Hamric, Ann B. Advanced practice nursing. [DNLM: 1. Specialties, Nursing—methods. 2. Nurse Anesthetists. 3. Nurse Clinicians. 4. Nurse Midwives. 5. Nurse Practitioners. WY 101 A2447 2009]

RT82. 8. A384 2009
610. 73—dc22

2008020336

Senior Editor: Sandra Clark
Senior Developmental Editor: Cindi Anderson
Publishing Services Manager: Deborah L. Vogel
Project Manager: Jodi M. Willard
Design Direction: Maggie Reid

Printed in United States of America

Last digit is the print number: 9 8 7 6 5 4 3 2

We dedicate this book to our advanced practice nursing students, past and future, and to our author contributors (you are the best!), who have shaped our understanding of advanced practice nursing.

To my co-editors, with admiration, respect, and great affection.
ABH

With gratitude to Mom, Dad, Nan Solomons, Timi Iddings (nurse practitioner), Tawnya Adkisson (clinical nurse specialist), and the Maine Beacon community.
JS

To my wonderful family, who make it possible for me to do this work.
CH

Contributors

Ann Reid Anderson, MSN, RNC, ANP
Nurse Practitioner
Student Health Services
Virginia Commonwealth University
Richmond, Virginia
Chapter 13. The Primary Care Nurse Practitioner

Anne-Marie Barron, PhD, RN, CS
Associate Professor and Associate Chair for
    Undergraduate Nursing
Simmons College;
Clinical Nurse Specialist and Faculty Nurse
    Scientist
Massachusetts General Hospital
Boston, Massachusetts
Chapter 7. Consultation

Sally D. Bennett, MSN, ACNP-BC, FNP
Owner and Clinician
Camden Healthcare Associates, Inc.
Kingsland, Georgia
*Chapter 19. Business Planning and Reimbursement
    Mechanisms*

Karen A. Brykczynski, DNSc, RN, FNP, FAANP
Professor
UTMB School of Nursing
Galveston, Texas
*Chapter 4. Role Development of the Advanced
    Practice Nurse*

Cathy C. Cartwright, RN, MSN, PCNS
Pediatric Clinical Nurse Specialist
Division of Neurosurgery
University of Missouri Health Care
Columbia, Missouri
Chapter 12. The Clinical Nurse Specialist

Sarah A. Delgado, RN, MSN, ACNP-BC
Assistant Professor, Nurse Practitioner
School of Nursing
University of Virginia
Charlottesville, Virginia
Chapter 11. Ethical Decision Making

Judith A. DePalma, PhD, RN
Chair and Associate Professor
Department of Nursing
Slippery Rock University
Slippery Rock, Pennsylvania;
Professor
Rocky Mountain University of Health Professions
Provo, Utah
Chapter 8. Research

Margaret Faut-Callahan, CRNA, PhD, FAAN
Chair, Adult Health Nursing
Director, Nurse Anesthesia Program
College of Nursing
Rush University
Chicago, Illinois
*Chapter 17. The Certified Registered Nurse
    Anesthetist*

**Jane Guttendorf, RN, MSN, CRNP, ACNP-BC,
    CCRN**
Acute Care Nurse Practitioner
Department of Critical Care Medicine
Cardiothoracic Intensive Care Unit
University of Pittsburgh Medical Center
    Presbyterian
Pittsburgh, Pennsylvania
Chapter 14. The Acute Care Nurse Practitioner

Ann B. Hamric, PhD, RN, FAAN
Associate Professor, School of Nursing
Faculty Affiliate, Center for Biomedical Ethics
University of Virginia
Charlottesville, Virginia
*Chapter 3. A Definition of Advanced Practice
    Nursing; Chapter 11. Ethical Decision Making;
    Chapter 15. The Blended Role of the Clinical Nurse
    Specialist and the Nurse Practitioner; Chapter 18.
    Evolving and Innovative Opportunities for
    Advanced Practice Nursing*

Charlene M. Hanson, EdD, RN, FNP-BC, FAAN
Professor Emerita
Georgia Southern University
Statesboro, Georgia
*Chapter 9. Clinical, Professional, and Systems
    Leadership; Chapter 10. Collaboration; Chapter 19.
    Business Planning and Reimbursement
    Mechanisms; Chapter 21. Understanding
    Regulatory, Legal, and Credentialing
    Requirements*

Patricia M. Hentz, EdD, CS, CRNP
Associate Professor
Associate Dean of Undergraduate Nursing Programs
Jefferson School of Nursing
Thomas Jefferson University
Philadelphia, Pennsylvania
*Chapter 15. The Blended Role of the Clinical Nurse
    Specialist and the Nurse Practitioner*

**Donna R. Hodnicki, PhD, FNP-BC, FAAN,
    CLNC**
Professor, Graduate Program Director
Georgia Southern University
Statesboro, Georgia
*Chapter 20. Marketing and Contracting
    Considerations*

**Marilyn Hravnak, RN, PhD, ACNP-BC, FCCM,
    FAAN**
Associate Professor
School of Nursing
University of Pittsburgh
Pittsburgh, Pennsylvania
Chapter 14. The Acute Care Nurse Practitioner

Gail L. Ingersoll, EdD, RN, FAAN, FNAP
Director, Clinical Nursing Research Center
Loretta Ford Professor of Nursing
University of Rochester Medical Center
Rochester, New York
*Chapter 24. Outcomes Evaluation and Performance
    Improvement: An Integrative Review of Research
    on Advanced Practice Nursing*

Jean E. Johnson, PhD, RN, FAAN
Senior Associate Dean and Professor
Health Care Sciences
The George Washington University
Washington, DC
*Chapter 22. Health Policy Issues in Changing
    Environments*

Arlene W. Keeling, PhD, RN
The Centennial Distinguished Professor of
    Nursing
Director, The Center for Nursing Historical Inquiry
University of Virginia School of Nursing
Charlottesville, Virginia
*Chapter 1. A Brief History of Advanced Practice
    Nursing in the United States*

Maureen A. Kelley, CNM, PhD
Clinical Associate Professor
Nell Hodgson Woodruff School of Nursing
Emory University
Atlanta, Georgia
Chapter 16. The Certified Nurse-Midwife

Ruth M. Kleinpell, PhD, RN, FAAN
Professor
Rush University College of Nursing
Nurse Practitioner
Our Lady of the Resurrection Medical Center
Chicago, Illinois
Chapter 14. The Acute Care Nurse Practitioner

Michael J. Kremer, PhD, CRNA, FAAN
Associate Professor and Chair
Nurse Anesthesia Department
Rosalind Franklin University
North Chicago, Illinois
*Chapter 17. The Certified Registered Nurse
    Anesthetist*

Marjorie Thomas Lawson, PhD, FNP-BC
Associate Professor of Nursing
Coordinator, Graduate Nursing Programs
College of Nursing and Health Professions
University of Southern Maine
Portland, Maine
*Chapter 2. Conceptualizations of Advanced
    Practice Nursing*

Kathy S. Magdic, MSN, RN, ACNP-BC, FAANP
Program Coordinator
Acute Care Nurse Practitioner Program
University of Pittsburgh
Pittsburgh, Pennsylvania
Chapter 14. The Acute Care Nurse Practitioner

Vicky A. Mahn-DiNicola, RN, MS, CPHQ
Vice President
Clinical Decision Support Services
ACS MIDAS+
Tucson, Arizona
*Chapter 25. Outcomes Evaluation and Performance
    Improvement: Using Data and Information
    Technology to Improve Practice*

Brenda M. Nevidjon, MSN, RN, FAAN
Clinical Professor
Nursing and Health Leadership;
Chair, Master's Program
Duke University
Durham, North Carolina
*Chapter 23. Strengthening Advanced Practice Nursing
    in Organizational Structures: Administrative
    Considerations*

Eileen T. O'Grady, PhD, RN, NP
Policy Editor
The American Journal of Nurse Practitioners and
    Nurse Practitioner World News
McLean, Virginia
*Chapter 13. The Primary Care Nurse Practitioner;
    Chapter 22. Health Policy Issues in Changing
    Environments*

Jeanne Salyer, PhD, RN
Associate Professor
Adult Health and Nursing Systems
Virginia Commonwealth University
Richmond, Virginia
*Chapter 18. Evolving and Innovative Opportunities
    for Advanced Practice Nursing*

Cheryl A. Sarton, PhD, CNM
Assistant Professor
College of Nursing and Health Professions
University of Southern Maine
Portland, Maine
Chapter 16. The Certified Nurse-Midwife

Cynthia J. Simonson, MS, ANP, AOCN®
Adult Nurse Practitioner
Division of Medical Oncology
Duke Comprehensive Cancer Center
Duke University Health System
*Chapter 23. Strengthening Advanced Practice Nursing
    in Organizational Structures: Administrative
    Considerations*

Patricia S. A. Sparacino, RN, PhD, FAAN
Vice Chair and Clinical Professor
Family Health Care Nursing
School of Nursing
University of California, San Francisco
San Francisco, California
Chapter 12. The Clinical Nurse Specialist

Judith A. Spross, PhD, RN, FAAN
Professor
University of Southern Maine
College of Nursing and Health Professions
Portland, Maine
*Chapter 2. Conceptualizations of Advanced Practice
    Nursing; Chapter 6. Expert Coaching and Guid-
    ance; Chapter 9. Clinical, Professional, and Systems
    Leadership; Chapter 10. Collaboration*

Mary Fran Tracy, PhD, RN, CCRN, CCNS, FAAN
Critical Care Clinical Nurse Specialist
University of Minnesota Medical Center, Fairview;
Adjunct Assistant Professor
School of Nursing and School of Medicine
University of Minnesota
Minneapolis, Minnesota
Chapter 5. Direct Clinical Practice

Patricia A. White, PhD, NP-BC, ANP
Clinical Assistant Professor
School for Health Studies, Nursing Programs
Simmons College
Boston, Massachusetts
Chapter 7. Consultation

Reviewers

Catherine Dearman, RN, PhD, CNS
Professor and Chair, Maternal Child Health
College of Nursing
University of South Alabama
Mobile, Alabama

Loretta Brush Normile, PhD, MSN, BSN, RN
Coordinator, Advanced Practice Nursing
Assistant Professor
College of Nursing and Health Science
George Mason University
Fairfax, Virginia

Preface

Advanced practice nursing has continued its rapid evolution since 1996, when the first edition of this text was published. Although there continue to be divergent perspectives, we are heartened to see a unified and integrative understanding of advanced practice nursing and its core competencies emerging both within and outside of the profession. Advanced practice nursing has continued to develop and flourish as evidence mounts that the advanced practice of nursing is good for patients/consumers. Indeed, the number of advanced practice nurses (APNs) in the United States increased 52% between 1996 and 2004, with sustained growth in all APN groups, particularly nurse practitioners (NPs) (USDHHS, 2006).

These increases have occurred against a backdrop of continuing cost containment pressures and patient safety concerns. Market and social forces have fostered competition among providers, notably physicians and APNs, even as the national and global nursing shortage continues. The expanding populations of elderly persons and those with chronic diseases, an increasing volume of information and regulation, new technologies, and other innovations have increased the complexity of care delivery and clinical decision making. Some of these trends have created favorable conditions for APNs. Physician-dominated primary care is being reexamined, and primary and specialty care provided by APNs has achieved significant gains in the health care marketplace. The clinical nurse specialist (CNS) role is experiencing a resurgence as hospitals recognize the need for expert subspecialty care, strong mentoring of nursing staff, and clinical leadership for systems issues that affect patient care. Acute care nurse practitioners (ACNPs) and blended roles are finding strong markets as changes continue within institutional structures. Two major national initiatives, the Doctor of Nursing Practice (DNP) degree spearheaded by the American Association of Colleges of Nursing (AACN, 2006) and the Consensus Model for APN regulation developed by the National Council of State Boards of Nursing (NCSBN) Advisory Committee and the Advanced Practice Registered Nurse (APRN) Consensus Work Group (2008), have significant implications for the future of advanced practice nursing. These two initiatives provided the major impetus for this latest revision.

PURPOSE

Our goal remains to describe an integrated understanding of advanced practice nursing that provides clarity and structure for students, practicing APNs, and the profession at large. We believe this fourth edition defines and strengthens our understanding of advanced practice nursing—the competencies, roles, and the issues facing APNs—with more clarity and authority than our earlier efforts. We have woven DNP competencies and expectations throughout the book *as they apply to and support this core understanding of advanced practice nursing*. However, the book is equally useful for both MSN- and DNP-level APN educational programs.

UNDERLYING PREMISES

Our work is grounded in the conviction that advanced practice nursing must have a defined core that provides a framework for standardizing the profession's understanding of this level of practice. At the same time, the core must be flexible enough to accommodate the differing roles necessary to enact the varied practices of all APNs. As new roles evolve, this advanced practice core becomes even more important. Several premises underlie this conviction:

- For certain patient populations, APNs are the best providers for delivering quality care at a reasonable cost.
- A uniform definition of advanced practice nursing and standards for educating and credentialing that are consistent across APN groups are essential for continued legitimacy of APN roles and regulatory parity with other providers. In the absence of a consistent definition, the instability of the health care system and increased competition among providers pose a threat to the legitimacy of all APNs as

providers. Such threats may lead to the loss of hard-won legal and regulatory battles.

- A consistent definition of core competencies for APNs is essential in order to standardize APN education and regulation and to evaluate the outcomes of APN care across roles. It is also imperative that APNs practice these competencies in order to demonstrate the value-added component they bring to care delivery and to ensure that advanced practice nursing is not confused with physician substitution.
- A uniform definition is essential for interdisciplinary teamwork. Administrators, physicians, and other providers must be able to rely on a core set of role expectations to design and implement cost-effective health care delivery systems that fully utilize all APN roles.
- We remain convinced that advanced practice nursing is good for patients. However, a higher level of standardization of the definition and expectations of advanced practice nursing, in addition to internal cohesion within the nursing profession regarding the worth and focus of advanced practice, are necessary for the larger health care establishment to agree with this claim.

ORGANIZATION

As is our practice, this fourth edition of *Advanced Practice Nursing: An Integrative Approach* has been extensively updated and revised to reflect current literature and trends. We have increased the number of exemplars throughout the text to better demonstrate advanced practice nursing in action. In addition, we have made a number of major revisions to this latest edition.

In Part I, "Historical and Developmental Aspects of Advanced Practice Nursing," Chapter 1 has been revised to incorporate the author's research on the history of prescriptive authority. Chapter 2 considers the work of the APRN Joint Dialogue Group (2008) as it relates to conceptualization of advanced practice nursing. Chapter 3 has been revised to contrast the definition of advanced practice nursing with the more expansive definition of advanced practice that includes non-APN roles put forward in the DNP Essentials (AACN, 2006).

In Part II, "Competencies of Advanced Practice Nursing," the seven core competencies are examined. The stability of the seven core APN competen-

cies throughout the four editions of this text is noteworthy, even though elements of various competencies continue to be refined. Chapter 5 has been extensively revamped to reflect current APN practice. In Chapter 6, the increasing emphasis on chronic disease management as it relates to coaching by APNs is considered. The chapters describing the competencies of research, leadership, and ethical decision making (Chapters 8, 9 and 11) have been extensively revised to incorporate DNP competencies as applicable.

The chapters in Part III, "Advanced Practice Roles: The Operational Definitions of Advanced Practice Nursing," continue to explicitly incorporate the core competencies and demonstrate how these competencies are played out in current APN practices. Features unique to each APN role, as well as the latest professional and policy changes relevant to the specific role, are described. The blended CNS/NP role chapter (Chapter 15) now more strongly incorporates the psychiatric–mental health APN specialty, which has moved quickly toward blended role practice. Chapter 18 now includes forensic nursing and new ACNP hospitalist roles. The reader will note that this chapter describes a new Stage 4 in the evolution of specialties to advanced practice nursing. This provocative chapter opens new vistas for APNs and at the same time presents a standardized framework for assessing the potential of evolving roles and specialties to become advanced practice nursing.

Part IV, "Critical Elements in Managing Advanced Nursing Practice Environments," continues to explore key environmental factors affecting APN practice. Each chapter incorporates the social, political, and organizational contexts that APNs must manage for success. Chapter 21 has been updated to review the recent work of the APRN Joint Dialogue Group (2008), which is promulgating national guidelines for APN regulation, certification, accreditation, and education. Chapter 22 on health policy is essentially a new chapter in this edition. It provides a primer on the policy process and trends shaping health care policy decisions and provides strategies for APNs to develop competence in the health policy arena. For this edition, we have divided the previous final chapter on outcome evaluation into two chapters that explore this critical element in depth. Chapter 24 presents a thorough integrative review of existing APN outcome research and suggests strategies for individual APNs to demonstrate their impact through performance evaluation. Chapter 25 integrates and updates information that appeared in the APN Case Manager chapter in earlier editions. In addition, this chapter describes the landscape of health information technology and pay-for-performance initiatives as they will affect APN practice. The author gives APNs the tools needed to use data and information technology to improve practice so they are prepared to meet agency expectations for achieving clinical and institutional outcomes.

AUDIENCE

This book is intended for graduate students, practicing APNs in all roles, educators, administrators, and leaders in the nursing profession. For students in any APN graduate program, whether master's or doctorate, this text provides a comprehensive resource useful throughout their program of study. Initial clarity about the definition and competencies of advanced practice nursing can guide students as they enter their clinical coursework. We strongly recommend the book's use early in the program of study—in theory, research, policy, and APN role courses. This text is a valuable tool for use throughout clinical courses as students see the various APN roles and related competencies in action and as they begin practicing their chosen APN role. Students who are nearing graduation, in role transition or capstone courses, will appreciate the role development chapter, the in-depth information on evidence-based practice, and the content in Part IV that explores business practices and environmental issues that they must be prepared to manage in the workplace.

For practicing APNs, the book updates both theoretical and practical content to guide role implementation. Individuals interested in strengthening or changing their roles will find many strategies for accomplishing these changes. The exploration of current issues in the health care environment makes the book particularly useful to practicing clinicians who face challenges within a marketplace that changes daily. The interdisciplinary, collaborative focus in many chapters may be useful to clinicians and educators in other fields. For example, interdisciplinary teams could benefit from discussions of the chapters that address expert coaching and guidance, collaboration, ethical decision-making skills, and health care policy. Administrators will appreciate the descriptions of various APN roles and the strategies for justifying and supporting APN positions.

For educators, the book will serve as a comprehensive curricular resource in preparing APNs for practice. It also serves as a guide to designing relevant courses on all the facets of advanced practice nursing. An exciting feature for faculty is the Instructor's Electronic Resource that accompanies the text. This resource includes over 1500 PowerPoint lecture slides that are presented by chapter and include key text, tables, and boxes; an electronic Image Collection containing all images from the text; "Things to Think About" discussion topics and questions for each chapter; teaching strategies for effectively teaching the content of various chapters; and WebLinks to all websites cited in the text. It is available on the Evolve website (*http://evolve.elsevier.com/Hamric/*).

For nursing leaders, educators, and practicing clinicians alike, this book is a clarion call to reach greater consensus regarding our understanding of and preparation for advanced practice nursing and the roles APNs assume so that we speak with increasing authority and consistency to policymakers, to those in other disciplines, and to one another. Clarity regarding advanced practice nursing is a professional imperative—while we are encouraged at the progress being made and the use of our work in this progress, the profession has not yet achieved this clarity at all levels.

APPROACH

We continue to describe advanced practice nursing at its best—as it is being enacted by APNs throughout the country. There is still much work to be done: not all APN students are educated to practice with the competencies described here; too many nurses are in APN roles without the necessary credentials or competencies, and thus true advanced practice nursing is not demonstrated; and there is still too much "alphabet soup" in role titles (for example, CNSs are variously called clinical coordinators, outcomes managers, educators, or consultants).

Roles continue to evolve as nursing matures in its enactment of this level of nursing practice, but advanced practice nursing must be distinct, recognizable, and describable if it is to continue to flourish. It will be clear to the reader that although the diverse roles described in Part III share the core criteria and competencies of advanced practice nursing, they are different and distinct from one another in their role enactment. This should be a cause for celebration as nursing recognizes its strength and range in meeting patient/client needs.

Creating this new edition has once again been a challenging undertaking. We are grateful for the hard work of our contributors, who substantially revised their chapters to portray a cutting-edge understanding of advanced practice nursing. We are privileged to participate with them in shaping this ever-changing area of nursing practice. Advanced practice nursing is a relatively young idea in the profession's evolution. We continue to be impressed by how complex it is to integrate and incorporate the perspectives of all APN specialties. Not all groups have addressed the core concepts of advanced practice nursing or the competencies of APNs in a complete or consistent manner. The literature from the various advanced practice specialty groups remains unfortunately separated, and clinicians and educators tend to read and cite only their own group's literature. One of the major contributions of this book is the effort to solidify our conceptualization of advanced practice nursing and to struggle with the complexities of new and evolving APN roles. Adopting this integrative approach, as challenging as it continues to be, has in our view immeasurably enriched this work.

We encourage readers to examine and apply the ideas put forth in this book, thereby adding to the evidence about the importance and quality of advanced practice nursing. As a growing and critical component of present and future health care delivery systems, APNs are and must continue to be active participants in solving some of the pressing problems in health care delivery. We remain convinced that advanced practice nursing is essential to improving the health and well-being of the citizens of this nation and that increasing numbers of competent, well-prepared APNs will be needed as this century unfolds. As part of our succession planning, we have brought Dr. Mary Fran Tracy into many of the editorial activities that go into an undertaking of this magnitude. We welcome her and look forward to her participation in future editions.

Ann B. Hamric
Judith A. Spross
Charlene M. Hanson

References

American Association of Colleges of Nursing (AACN). (2006). *The essentials of doctoral education for advanced nursing practice.* Washington, DC: Author.

APRN Joint Dialogue Group. (2008). *Consensus model for APRN regulation: Licensure, accreditation, certification, and education.* Draft of April 7, 2008. Chicago, IL: Author.

U.S. Department of Health and Human Services (USDHHS), Division of Nursing. (2006). *The registered nurse population March 2004. Findings from the national sample survey of registered nurses.* Washington, DC: Author.

Contents

Chapter 10
Collaboration, 283

Charlene M. Hanson and Judith A. Spross

Chapter 15
The Blended Role of the Clinical Nurse Specialist and the Nurse Practitioner, 437
Patricia M. Hentz and Ann B. Hamric

Chapter 16
The Certified Nurse-Midwife, 462
Cheryl A. Sarton and Maureen A. Kelley

Chapter 22
Health Policy Issues in Changing Environments, 627
Eileen T. O'Grady and Jean E. Johnson

Chapter 23
Strengthening Advanced Practice Nursing in Organizational Structures: Administrative Considerations, 657
Brenda M. Nevidjon and Cynthia J. Simonson

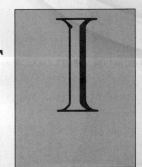

Historical and Developmental Aspects of Advanced Practice Nursing

A Brief History of Advanced Practice Nursing in the United States

Arlene W. Keeling

INTRODUCTION

To understand the challenges facing advanced practice nursing today and determine a path for the future, it is essential to look to the past. This chapter presents some highlights of the history of advanced practice nursing in the United States from the late nineteenth century to the present. It examines four established advanced practice roles—certified registered nurse anesthetists (CRNAs), certified nurse-midwives (CNMs), clinical nurse specialists (CNSs), and nurse practitioners (NPs)—in the context of the social, political, and economic environment of each decade and within the context of the history of medicine, technology, and science. Legal issues and issues related to gender and health care manpower are considered. Although sociopolitical and economic contexts are critical to understanding nursing history, only historical events specifically relevant to the history of advanced practice nursing are included. The reader is encouraged to consult the references of this chapter for further information.

A brief comment on terminology:

The use of the term *specialist* in nursing can be traced to the turn of the twentieth century, when it was used to designate a nurse who had completed a postgraduate course in a clinical specialty area or who had extensive experience and expertise in a particular clinical practice area. With the introduction of the NP role during the 1960s and 1970s, the terms *expanded role* and *extended role* were used, implying a horizontal movement to encompass expertise from medicine and other disciplines. The more contemporary term, *advanced practice,* which began to be seen in the 1980s, reflects a more vertical or hierarchical movement encompassing graduate education within nursing rather than a simple expansion of expertise by development of knowledge and skills used by other disciplines. Since the 1980s, state nursing practice acts have increasingly adopted the term *advanced practice nurses* (APNs) to delineate CRNAs, CNMs, CNSs, and NPs.

LATE NINETEENTH CENTURY: HISTORICAL ROOTS

Nurse Anesthetists. The roots of nurse anesthesia in the United States can be traced to the late nineteenth century. During the 1860s, two key events converged: the widespread use of chloroform anesthesia and the demand for such treatment for wounded soldiers during the American Civil War (1861-1865). This convergence provided Catholic sisters and others with a unique opportunity to assist surgeons.

In 1861, except for Catholic sisters and Lutheran deaconesses, there were few professional nurses in the United States. In fact, only a handful of nurse training schools[1] existed, and for the most part, laywomen cared for families and friends when they were ill. Thus when the first shots were fired on Fort Sumter, thousands of laywomen from both the North and the South volunteered to nurse. For the most part, these women read to patients, served them broths and stimulants such as tea, coffee, and alcohol, and assisted with the preparation of food in diet kitchens. Societal restrictions prohibited them from giving direct patient care.[2] However, this restriction did not hold for the Catholic sisters who nursed, and their work included assisting in surgery, particularly with the administration of chloroform. Because the administration of chloroform was a relatively simple procedure in which the anesthetizer poured the drug over a cloth held over the patient's nose and mouth, the nuns quickly mastered this technique, providing the surgeons with invaluable assistance during the war (Jolly, 1927; Wall, 2005).

In the decade after the Civil War, hospitals throughout the United States opened nurse training schools modeled according to Florence Nightingale's

---

[1]The word *training* was commonly used to describe nursing education in this era.
[2]This is a generalization. Class and race were determining factors in women's nursing duties. Black slaves, for example, provided much direct patient care in the South.

school at St. Thomas Hospital in London. Soon thereafter, most U.S. hospitals used student nurses for staffing rather than employing graduate nurses. One exception to this trend was the increasing use of graduate nurses as nurse anesthetists. Surgeons readily accepted them, valuing the fact that nurse anesthetists concentrated on administering the anesthesia and observing the patient, whereas the medical students who usually assisted the surgeons with anesthesia delivery tended to spend more time watching the surgery than observing the patient.

Dr. William W. Mayo at St. Mary's Hospital in Rochester, Minnesota, was among the first physicians in the country to formally recognize and train nurse anesthetists. In 1889 Mayo hired Edith Granham to be his anesthetist. Subsequently he hired Alice Magaw, whom he later referred to as the "mother of anesthesia" (Keeling, 2007). In 1900 Magaw published the results of her practice in the *St. Paul's Medical Journal*, reporting her "Observations on 1092 Cases of Anesthesia from January 1, 1899 to January 1, 1900":

> In that time, we administered an anesthetic 1,092 times; ether alone 674 times; chloroform 245 times; ether and chloroform combined, 173 times. I can report that out of this number, 1,092 cases, we have not had an accident; we have not had occasion to use artificial respiration once; nor one case of ether pneumonia; neither have we had any serious renal results. Tongue forceps were used but once, the operation was on the jaw and it was quite necessary. (p. 306)

Between 1899 and 1901, the Mayo surgeons added a woman physician anesthesiologist, Dr. Isabelle Herb, and several other nurse anesthetists to their surgical teams—soon becoming world-renowned for their nurse anesthesia training program (Strickland, 1995). By 1913 the Mayo program was 6 months long and included both theoretical training and clinical practice. That year, Sophie Gran Jevene Winton completed her training at Mayo and went on to become a leader in nurse anesthesia. Twenty-one years later, she would be asked to testify about the nature of that education in the Superior Court of California, when the Los Angeles County Medical Association, represented by William Chalmers-Francis, sued nurse anesthetist Dagmar Nelson for the "illegal practice of medicine in violation of the Medical Practice Act" (Keeling, 2007; McGarrel, 1934).

Nurse-Midwives. Like the origins of nurse anesthesia, the origins of nurse-midwifery in America can be traced to the pre-professional work of women. Throughout the eighteenth and nineteenth centuries,

lay midwives, rather than professional nurses or physicians, assisted women in childbirth. Midwives, who were brought to the United States with the slave trade in 1619 and who later came with waves of European immigration, were respected community members. In the late nineteenth and early twentieth centuries, these untrained "old country" midwives would lose respect as "scientific," hospital-based deliveries became the norm. Meanwhile, women in isolated communities throughout the country, particularly in rural settings, continued to employ midwives for deliveries well into the twentieth century.

Psychiatric Specialization in Nursing. The roots of nursing specialization are also embedded in the second half of the nineteenth century. Recognized as the first clinical specialty in nursing, psychiatric nursing had its origins in the Quaker reform movement initiated earlier in the century in England. In the United States, these Quaker reformers challenged the brutal treatment of the insane and advocated "moral treatment," emphasizing gentler methods of social control in a domestic setting (D'Antonio, 1991, p. 411).

The first American training program for psychiatric nurses was founded in 1880 at McLean Hospital in Massachusetts (Critchley, 1985). According to Linda Richards, an 1873 graduate of The New England Hospital School of Nursing, from the outset the McLean Hospital maintained high standards and demonstrated "the value of trained nursing for the many persons afflicted with mental disease" (Richards, 1911, p. 109). Richards served as superintendent of nurses at the Taunton Insane Hospital for 4 years, beginning in 1899. She subsequently organized a nursing school for the preparation of psychiatric nurses at the Worcester Hospital for the Insane and finally went to the Michigan Insane Hospital in Kalamazoo where she remained until 1909 (Richards, 1911). Because of this work, Richards is credited with founding the specialty of psychiatric nursing.

"Primary Care." The idea of using nurses to provide what we now refer to as "primary care" services dates to the late 1800s. During this period of rapid industrialization and social reform, nurses played a major role in providing care for poverty-stricken immigrants in cities throughout the country, particularly in the Northeast. In 1893 Lillian Wald, a young graduate nurse from the New York Training School for Nurses, established the Henry Street Settlement (HSS) House on the Lower East Side of Manhattan. Its purpose was to address the needs of the poor, many of whom lived in overcrowded, rat-infested tenements. For several decades the HSS visiting nurses, like other district nurses, visited thousands of patients with little interference in their work (Wald, 1922). The needs of this disadvantaged community were limitless. According to one HSS nurse (Duffus, 1938):

> There were nursing infants, many of them with the summer bowel complaint that sent infant mortality soaring during the hot months; there were children with measles, not quarantined; there were children with opthalmia [sic], a contagious eye disease; there were children scarred with vermin bites; there were adults with typhoid; there was a case of puerperal septicemia, lying on a vermin-infested bed without sheets or pillow cases; a family consisting of a pregnant mother, a crippled child and two others living on dry bread . . . ; a young girl dying of tuberculosis amid the very conditions that had produced the disease. (p. 43)

In addition to making home visits, the HSS nurses also established a nurses' dispensary in one room of the settlement house, where "simple complaints and emergencies not requiring referral elsewhere were treated" (Buhler-Wilkerson, 2001, p. 107). According to nurse historian Karen Buhler-Wilkerson (2001):

> As the number of ambulatory visits grew, the settlement risked attracting the unwelcome attention of the increasingly disagreeable "uptown docs." The New York Medical Society's recent success in attaching a clause to the Nursing Registration Bill prohibiting nurses from practicing medicine gave the society a new opportunity to disrupt the settlement's neighborly activities. While initially the first aid rooms went unnoticed, by 1904 . . . Lavinia Dock (a colleague of Lillian Wald) wrote to Wald about doctors' concerns that nurses were carrying ointments and even giving pills outside the strict control of physicians. (p. 110)

To resolve this problem, the HSS nurses obtained standing orders for emergency medications and treatments from a group of Lower East Side physicians (Buhler-Wilkerson, 2001). Later, however, conflicts with medicine surfaced again when the HSS nurses expanded their visits to areas of the city outside the Lower East Side. The situation came to a head with the collapse of the stock market in 1929 when uptown physicians, concerned about their own incomes, saw the nurses as an economic threat. That year, the Medical Economic Committee of the Westchester Village Medical Group accused the nurses of practicing medicine. Angered by the accusation, Elizabeth Mackenzie, the Associate Director of Nurses at HSS, defended the HSS nurses in her reply (Mackenzie, 1929):

My dear Dr. Black:

> Your letter . . . addressed to Miss Elizabeth Neary, Supervisor of our Westchester Office, has been referred to me for reply. May I call the attention of your group to the fact that in administering the work in that office, Miss Neary does so as a representative of the HSS Visiting Nurse Service and in accord with definite policies in effect throughout the entire city-wide service. It has been the unvarying policy of the organization over the 35 years of its service to work in close cooperation with the medical profession doing nursing and preventive health work entirely and avoiding any semblance of the "practice of medicine" in competition with the doctors . . . . We will call a meeting . . . to which the members of your group will be invited for a frank discussion of our common problems.

Although the records about this meeting are no longer available, one can assume that the meeting happened and the nurses continued to practice, because HSS remained active until the 1950s. Nonetheless, as is apparent in these two scenarios, from early in the century there is evidence of interprofessional conflicts with medicine as nurses began to expand their scope of practice. There is also evidence of emerging collaboration between the professions as physicians and nurses negotiated solutions to the boundary problems. What is clear, even in these early years, is that nurses were considered "good enough" to care for the poor, whereas physicians would care for those who could pay.

1900-1950s: INNOVATION AND GROWTH

Turn of the Twentieth Century

As immigrants continued to flood into the cities and towns of the Northeast, problems of excessive crowding, tenement house dwelling, and the spread of infectious diseases intensified. Coinciding with the trend toward urbanization and industrialization, medicine was establishing itself as a respectable and economically viable profession, one that was dominated by men. At the same time, the nursing profession made significant progress, particularly in the area of licensure. In 1903, state licensure registration for nurses was initiated in North Carolina, New Jersey, New York, and Virginia. Licensure was a first step in regulating the profession of nursing at the state level. Moreover, it was crucial to the upgrading of nursing education because it determined what requirements a nurse must meet before she would be eligible for licensure. Licensure would set the stage for nursing to move from a trade occupation to a profession.

The Specialties, Circa 1900s

The use of the term *specialist* in nursing can be traced to the turn of the twentieth century when hospitals offered postgraduate courses in a variety of specialty areas including anesthesia, tuberculosis, operating room, laboratory, and dietetics. In the first issue of the *American Journal of Nursing (AJN)*, Katherine Dewitt (1900) described specialty practice and the specialist's need for continuing education in an article titled "Specialties in Nursing" as follows:

> Those who devote themselves to one branch of nursing often do so because of the keen interest they feel in it. The specialist can and should reach greater perfection in her sphere when she gives her entire time to it. Her studies should be continued in that direction, she should try constantly to keep up with the rapid advances in medical science . . . . The nurse who is a specialist can often supplement the doctor's work to a great extent . . . . (p. 16)

Specialists in nursing were important to both patients and physicians. The educational requirements for specialization, the nature of specialty practice, and the definition of a nurse specialist were all issues the profession would later have to address.

1910s: The Impact of the Progressive Era and World War I

In the 1910s the prevalence of infectious diseases in the United States and the persistent problems of high maternal and infant mortality would directly affect the nursing profession. In 1912 the National Organization for Public Health Nursing (NOPHN) was established. That same year, Lillian Wald spearheaded the creation of the Children's Bureau, a federal organization whose early studies of infant and maternal mortality rates led to the government's conclusion that a substantial number of maternal and infant deaths could be prevented by adequate prenatal care. Later in the decade, two significant events coincided: the United States entered the war in Europe, and an influenza epidemic swept the country. Both events would provide new challenges for the nursing profession: (1) the realities of war and the demands for immediate treatment on the battlefield would expand nurses' scope of practice; and (2) the critical shortage of nurses, all too apparent as influenza devastated towns and cities across the country, initiated debates among professional nursing leaders about the use of nurses' aides to meet the health care needs of the nation.

Nurse Anesthetists, Circa 1910s. During the 1910s, nurse anesthetists faced obstacles as well as new opportunities. Early in the decade, the medical profession began to question the right of nurses to administer anesthesia, claiming that these nurses were practicing medicine without a license. In 1911 the New York State Medical Society unsuccessfully declared that the administration of an anesthetic by a nurse violated state law (Thatcher, 1953). A year later, the Ohio State Medical Board passed a resolution specifying that only physicians could administer anesthesia. Despite this resolution, nurse anesthetist Agatha Hodgins established The Lakeside Hospital School of Anesthesia in Cleveland, Ohio, in 1915, culminating in a lawsuit brought against the Lakeside Hospital program by the state medical society. This lawsuit was unsuccessful and resulted in an amendment to the Ohio Medical Practice Act, protecting the practice of nurse anesthesia. However, medical opposition to the practice of nurse anesthesia continued. In a landmark decision, the Kentucky appellate court, in the case of *Frank v. South* (1917), ruled that anesthesia provided by nurse anesthetist Margaret Hatfield did not constitute the practice of medicine if it was given under the orders and supervision of a licensed physician (Dr. Louis Frank). The significance of this decision lay in the fact that the courts declared nurse anesthesia legal but "subordinate" to the medical profession, a decision that would have lasting implications for the specialty and, later, for advanced practice nurses in general (Keeling, 2007).

Later in the decade, opportunities for nurse anesthetists increased when the United States entered the war in Europe (later known as *World War I*) and over a thousand nurses were deployed to Britain and France. The realities of the front were gruesome: shrapnel created devastating wounds, and mustard gas destroyed lungs and caused profound burns (Beeber, 1990). The resulting need for pain relief and anesthesia care for the wounded soldiers created an immediate demand for nurse anesthetists' knowledge and skills. Moreover, the United States' Base Hospital system, established under the leadership of the Mayo doctors and their colleague Dr. George W. Crile of the Lakeside Hospital anesthesia program in Cleveland, supported the employment of nurse anesthetists (Keeling, 2007).

Concurrent with the war effort, scientific investigations into new methods of administering anesthetics were initiated. At the well-established Lakeside Hospital anesthesia program, Crile and nurse anesthetist Agatha Hodgins experimented with combined nitrous oxide–oxygen administration. They also investigated the use of morphine and scopolamine as adjuncts to anesthesia. These scientific advances in clinical anesthesia complicated matters. As the specialty became more complex and increasingly based on new scientific discoveries, increasing numbers of physicians became interested in establishing anesthesia as a medical specialty. As they did so, some medical anesthesia groups again claimed that nurse anesthetists were practicing medicine without a license and once again initiated legal battles. Interprofessional conflict over disciplinary boundary issues seemed inescapable.

Nurse-Midwives, Circa 1910s. It was in the setting of increasing national concern about high maternal-infant mortality rates that heated debates surrounding issues of midwife licensing and control took place. Indeed, lay midwives would soon be blamed for the high maternal and infant mortality rates and the idea of "nurse-midwives" was introduced. In 1914 Dr. Frederick Taussig, speaking at the annual meeting of the NOPHN in St. Louis, proposed that the creation of "nurse-midwives" might solve the "midwife question" and suggested that nurse-midwifery schools be established to train graduate nurses (Taussig, 1914). Later in the decade, the Children's Bureau called for efforts to instruct pregnant women in nutrition and recommended that public health nurses teach principles of hygiene and prenatal care to "granny midwives" (Rooks, 1997). Then in 1918, in response to a study conducted by the New York City health commissioner that indicated the need for comprehensive prenatal care, the Maternity Center Association (MCA) was established. It served as the central organization for a network of community-based maternity centers throughout the city. Overall, the opening decade of the twentieth century was one of continued progress for nurse-midwives.

1920s: The Roaring 20s

In 1920 Congress passed the Nineteenth Amendment to the United States Constitution, granting women the right to vote. That same year, Congress also approved a bill that provided nurses military rank (Dock & Stewart, 1920). Both acts of Congress helped open the decade of the Roaring 20s, a time in which the new-found freedom for women was reflected in their shortened hairstyles, rising hemlines, and use of cigarettes and cosmetics. The decade also saw an increase in acceptance of the scientific basis of medicine and increased use of hospitals, especially for surgery (Howell, 1996). Of particular importance, in 1921 Congress passed the Shepherd-Towner Maternity and Infant Protection Act, providing health care services to mothers and children throughout the nation.

During this decade, the nursing profession undertook a study on nursing education supported by the Rockefeller Foundation. The Goldmark Report, published in 1923, advocated the establishment of collegiate schools of nursing rather than hospital-based diploma programs (Goldmark, 1923). Championed mainly by a group of nursing faculty at Columbia's Teachers College, the report provided a significant opportunity for nursing to become professionalized through collegiate education. Hoping the Goldmark Report would gain for nursing the status the Flexner Report (1910)[3] had gained for medicine, the Columbia nursing faculty group, led by Adelaide Nutting, strongly supported collegiate programs at Yale University and Case Western Reserve University and pressed other colleagues to take advantage of the opportunity. However, hospital administrators and physicians largely ignored the report, arguing that the plan was not practical (Baer, 2001). In the end, although some collegiate programs were established, strong support never materialized for university education for nurses, and the majority of aspiring nurses continued to be trained in diploma schools. In essence, organized nursing's response to the Goldmark Report may be considered a missed opportunity in the profession's history.

Nurse Anesthetists, Circa 1920s. Although the 1920s provided new opportunities for a few nurse anesthetists, it was also a decade in which resistance to their role grew. In 1922 nurse anesthetist Alice M. Hunt responded to a request by Samuel Harvey, a Yale professor of surgery, to "send me a nurse anesthetist" (Thatcher, 1953, p. 101) by accepting the offer herself. The offer included her

---

[3]The Flexner Report ended medical apprenticeship training in the United States, and medical education became university-based after this study (Flexner, 1910).

appointment as an instructor of anesthesia with university rank at the Yale Medical School, a significant and prestigious appointment for a nurse. In contrast to Hunt's experience, however, during the 1920s many nurse anesthetists struggled to find practice opportunities as more physicians began to choose anesthesia as their medical specialty. Medicine was becoming increasingly complex, increasingly scientific, and increasingly controlled by organized medical societies.

Nurse-Midwives, Circa 1920s. During the 1920s the American public's growing acceptance of hospitals and scientific medicine greatly decreased the numbers of women choosing to use lay midwives for deliveries. In fact, many upper and middle class urban white women began to use obstetricians to deliver their babies in hospital delivery rooms (Rinker, 2000). However, nationality and other issues continued to influence women's choices. For example, regardless of class, many urban European immigrants continued to employ midwives to deliver their babies at home. Geographical location, race, poverty, and access to physicians' services also played a part. In rural southern states such as Mississippi, for example, where half the population were black, the majority of women (80% of African-American and 8% of white women) continued to rely on African-American "granny midwives" to deliver their babies (Smith, 1994). The same pattern seen at the turn of the century continued: physician-assisted, hospital births were associated with patients of higher socioeconomic status. Midwives could attend the poor.

The Frontier Nursing Service: A New Model for Nurse-Midwives. In 1925 Mary Breckenridge, a British-trained nurse-midwife, founded the Frontier Nursing Service (FNS) in an economically depressed rural mountain area of Leslie County, Kentucky. British nurse-midwives and American public health nurses whom Breckenridge had sent to England for midwifery training provided midwifery services and nursing care to the isolated Appalachian community through a decentralized network of nurse-run clinics (Breckinridge, 1981; Rooks, 1997). Because there were few roads in the mountainous region, the nurses traveled by horseback to attend births, carrying their supplies in saddlebags. One FNS nurse, Vanda Summers (1938), described how the bags also contained a list

of standing orders, or *Medical Routines*, by which a physician committee supervised their practice:

> The whole of the district work of the FNS in the Kentucky mountains is done with the aid of two pairs of saddle-bags.... The "midwifery" saddle-bags weigh about 42 pounds when packed.... In these bags we have everything needed for a home delivery.... In one of the pockets we carry our *Medical Routines* which tells us what we may— and may not—do. A very treasured possession! (pp. 1183-1184)

The FNS nurses maintained outstanding patient data from the outset. Reflecting on her work in later years, Breckinridge (1981) noted that "trained statisticians were to come later, through a grant from the Carnegie Corporation, but from the start we had records and report sheets and kept them carefully" (p. 166). When findings were analyzed by the Metropolitan Life Insurance Company in 1951, they indicated that 8596 births had been attended, with 6533 occurring in homes, since 1925. More important, the FNS maternal mortality rate of 1.2 per 1000 was significantly lower than the national average of 3.4 per 1000 during the same period (Varney, 1987). Besides caring for patients, the FNS nurses formally organized the Kentucky State Association of Midwives in 1928. Later, this organization would become known as *The American Association of Nurse-Midwives* (AANM) and would play a key role in the progress of this specialty. Meanwhile, the FNS nurses' documentation of the outcomes of their care would serve to advance their cause.

1930s: The Great Depression

By the time President Franklin Roosevelt took the oath of office in March 1933, the United States was mired in an economic depression that involved the entire industrialized world. Over the next 6 years, Roosevelt's social programs under the New Deal would dramatically affect U.S. citizens. Rural rehabilitation programs, including health care programs sponsored by the Farm Security Administration (FSA), would be particularly important for poverty-stricken farmers and their families. In addition, the Depression would change the hospital workforce. During these fiscally stringent times, many private hospitals were forced to close their schools of nursing and hospitals without student labor began to employ graduate nurses to staff their wards. Soon, increasing numbers of unemployed private duty nurses began to turn to hospitals for secure employment, giving up the autonomy of private duty nursing to work in physician-dominated hospital bureaucracies. This change marked a major shift in the nursing workforce during which the majority of nurses became hospital employees rather than independent practitioners. With the shift, nurses also forfeited the freedom to bill for their services. The change would have profound implications for the profession later in the century as nursing services were first considered as part of the room rate and later "bundled" under general hospital services.

Nurse Anesthetists, Circa 1930s. Despite the turmoil of the Depression years, Lakeside Hospital nurse anesthetist Agatha Hodgins established the American Association of Nurse Anesthetists (AANA) in 1931 and served as the organization's first president. At the first meeting of the association, the group voted to affiliate with the American Nurses Association (ANA). However, the AANA was rebuffed, probably because the ANA was afraid to assume legal responsibility for a group that could be charged with practicing medicine without a license (Thatcher, 1953).

The ANA's fears were not unfounded. During the 1930s the devastation of the national economy made jobs scarce and the tension between nurse anesthetists and their physician counterparts continued, with more legal challenges to the practice of nurse anesthesia. In California, the Los Angeles County Medical Association sued nurse anesthetist Dagmar Nelson in 1934 for practicing medicine without a license. Nelson won. According to the judge (McGarrel, 1934):

> The administration of general anesthetics by the defendant Dagmar A. Nelson, pursuant to the directions and supervision of duly licensed physicians and surgeons, as shown by the evidence in this case, does not constitute the practice of medicine or surgery . . . .

In response, William Chalmers-Frances, MD, filed another suit against Nelson in 1936, which again resulted in a judgment for Nelson (*Chalmers-Frances v. Nelson*, 1936). In 1938 the judgment was appealed to the California Supreme Court, which again ruled in favor of Nelson. The case became famous. The courts established legal precedent: the practice of nurse anesthesia was legal and within the scope of nursing practice, *as long as it was done under the guidance of a supervising physician.*

Nurse-Midwives, Circa 1930s. During the decade of the Great Depression, nurse-midwifery also made significant strides. In 1930 a group of MCA board members, including Mary Breckenridge, incorporated as the Association for the Promotion and Standardization of Midwifery and in 1931 opened the Lobenstine Clinic in New York City, the nation's second nurse-midwifery service. Its purpose was not to prepare public health nurses to deliver babies but rather to teach and supervise traditional midwives and nurses with limited obstetrical training. The school set high standards. In fact, most of its first class of six students were college graduates (Rooks, 1997).

In 1939 the entry of Britain into World War II proved to be the catalyst for the establishment of another school for nurse-midwifery in the United States. That year the Kentucky FNS lost many of its British nurse-midwives when they returned to England to work. To deal with this shortage of qualified nurse-midwives, Breckinridge established the Frontier Graduate School of Midwifery, specifically to train American nurses (Buck, 1940).[4] Key to the midwives' success was that they were not posing a threat to private obstetricians: the FNS delivered babies in the backwoods of Kentucky.

"Primary Care," Circa 1930s. In addition to providing midwifery services, the FNS nurses in Leslie County, Kentucky, informally modeled what would become in the 1960s the primary care NP role. In fact, during the 1930s, the FNS continued the work Breckinridge had started in 1928, providing most of the primary health care needed by people living in rural Appalachia. Working out of eight centers that covered about 78 square miles in remote mountainous regions, the FNS nurses had considerable autonomy. They made diagnoses and treated patients, dispensing both herbs and medicines (including morphine). Working from standing orders written by the FNS medical advisory committee, the nurses also dispensed such medicines as aspirin, ipecac, cascara, and castor oil with a wide degree of latitude (Keeling, 2007). That unprecedented autonomy in practice was not always recognized however—even by the FNS nurses themselves. During an interview in 1978, Betty Lester, RN, reflected on her work as assistant field

---

[4]This program was for nurses who already had a degree in nursing (i.e., registered nurses) but was not a *graduate program* in the modern sense of the term.

supervisor in Leslie County in the 1930s, stating (Keeling, 2007):

> See we nurses don't prescribe and we don't diagnose. We can make a tentative diagnosis and we can give that to the doctor, and if there's anything wrong then he'll tell us how to treat it. So they [the doctors] gave us this Routine of things that we could use and the things we could do—and the things we couldn't do. (p. 49)

Indeed, Lester denied the extent of the practice autonomy she had had. Like other registered nurses (RNs) of the era, she had been socialized to defer to physicians' judgment and orders. So, recalling her practice later in her life, Lester acknowledged only that she and her colleagues had made "tentative" diagnoses. In reality, she had practiced on her own because few telephones were in the isolated community and even fewer physicians were available for personal consultation. For all practical purposes, the diagnoses she had made were the only diagnoses and the treatment she had given was the only treatment (Keeling, 2007).

Besides the FNS nurses, other nurses working among the poor in rural areas during the 1930s also practiced with exceptional autonomy. In particular, the FSA nurses "were given unusual latitude in their clinical roles" (Grey, 1999, p. 94) in migrant health programs in the western region of the United States. According to historian Michael Grey (1999), who chronicled the history of rural health programs established by President Franklin D. Roosevelt during the Great Depression:

> With the verbal approval of the camp doctor, they [FSA nurses] could write prescriptions and dispense drugs from the clinic formulary.... They staffed well baby clinics, coordinated immunization programs...decided whether a sick migrant required referral to a physician...and provided emergency care. (p. 94)

Like the FNS nurses, FSA nurses practiced according to standing orders issued by the FSA medical offices and approved by local physicians. As Dr. H. Daniels recalled in a 1984 interview, "Nurses functioned pretty autonomously. They were able to do a lot of what NPs do after a lot of training, but these nurses did it through experience" (Grey, 1999, p. 96). Essential to this practice autonomy for the FNS and FSA nurses, however, was the tacit requirement that the patients be poor and marginalized and have little access to physician-provided medical care.

The same requirements held true for the field nurses working with the Bureau of Indian Affairs (BIA), who often found themselves traveling the reservation alone, making diagnoses and treating patients. In addition to making home visits, the BIA nurses conducted well-baby "nursing conferences," the initial intent of which was health education and disease prevention, not treatment. In actuality, these conferences became what we refer to today as "nurse-run clinics," as Navajo mothers would bring sick infants and children to the "conference" to be seen by the nurse (Keeling, 2007). Reporting on her work at Teec Nos Pas in the Northern Navajo region in May 1931, nurse Dorothy Williams described that reality, referring to the conferences as "clinics" (Williams, 1931):

> Five clinics held this week, three general and two baby clinics. Mothers bathed their babies and were given material to cut out and make gowns for baby. Preschool children were weighed, inspected and mothers advised about diets for underweights [sic] .... Fifty treatments given .... (p. 3)

Indeed, these field nurses, like the FNS and FSA nurses, practiced with relatively little medical supervision.

Clinical Specialization in Psychiatry, Circa 1930s. The 1930s also witnessed growth in the area of psychiatry. In this period, Harry Stack Sullivan's classic writings and the work of Sigmund Freud changed psychiatric nursing dramatically. The emphasis on interpersonal interaction with patients and milieu treatment supported the movement of nurses into a more direct role in the psychiatric care of hospitalized patients. Scientific advances in the field, including the use of insulin and chemotherapies, required nurses to assume an increasingly active role in patient treatment.

1940s: World War II Challenges the Nation and the Profession

During the 1940s, the rise of medical specialization and the increase in technology and scientific knowledge further influenced the trend toward specialization and the expansion of nurses' responsibilities. However, the effect of these factors did not compare with the impact World War II had on the profession. The demands of the battlefront, scientific discoveries made as a result of experiments to protect soldiers from chemical warfare, and the shortage of nurses on the home front would all create opportunities for nurses.

As in other wars, battlefront demands forced nurses to assume responsibilities that went beyond their usual scope of practice. One example of this expansion of the nurse's role and practice autonomy is evidenced in a 1943 *American Journal of Nursing* article on flight nursing, an emerging nursing specialty (White, 1943):

> Once in the air, the nurse is in complete charge of the patients, assisted by a trained staff sergeant . . . . She may have to readjust splints, administer sedatives or stimulants, arrest sudden hemorrhage, treat shock, administer oxygen . . . . She will be responsible for handling any emergency and for doing anything a doctor would have to do, except operate. (p. 344)

It was simple: if a physician was unavailable or too busy with other cases, the nurse's role could expand from "caring" to "curing." In contrast, if a physician was readily available, the nurse was expected to practice within the traditional "caring" boundaries of the profession (Lynaugh & Fairman, 1992; Reverby, 1987).

Scientific discoveries also provided opportunities for the expansion of nursing practice, particularly for what would later become the specialty of oncology nursing. It was during World War II that the United States military's investigations of nitrogen mustard[5] led to the significant scientific discovery that the agent had substantial activity against lymphocytes. This discovery promoted further study of agents that could effectively kill rapidly spreading cancer cells. In fact, the discovery would herald the beginning of the "era of cytotoxic chemotherapy" (Friereich, 1984), a landmark event that would presage major changes in clinical oncology and cancer nursing.

In addition to the demands of the battlefront and the scientific discoveries of the era, the nursing shortages that occurred after the United States entered the war on December 7, 1941, led to federal legislation that would ultimately benefit the profession. Reacting to the nursing shortage, Congress passed the Bolton Act, forming the Cadet Nurse Corps. The bill, sponsored by Congresswoman Frances Payne Bolton and signed into law by President Roosevelt in 1943, subsidized the nursing education of 179,000 students and provided funds to graduate nurses for advanced education to increase the number of nursing instructors

(Spalding, 1943). The Bolton Act not only ensured an adequate supply of nurses for both military and civilian hospitals but also had positive effects on nursing education. Federal funding, paid directly to schools, facilitated the separation of nursing education from nursing service. Moreover, Cadet Nurse Corps funds were also allocated for postgraduate study in certificate programs such as those preparing CRNAs or in programs in administration and education. By the time the program ended, "more than 3 million dollars had been spent for postgraduate study for more than 10,000 registered nurses throughout the country" (U.S. Federal Security Agency, 1950, p. 61).

Nurse Anesthetists, Circa 1940s. Just as World War I benefitted nurse anesthetists, World War II defined anesthesia as a medical specialty (Waisel, 2001). In 1939, just before the United States entered the war, the first written examination for board certification in anesthesiology was given, but the practice of medical anesthesiology still sought legitimacy. By the 1940s, demands for anesthetists, advances in the types of anesthesia available, and continuing education in the field increasingly stimulated physicians' interest in the specialty (Olsen, 1940). The medical journal *Anesthesiology,* established in 1940, further strengthened medicine's claim to anesthesia practice. In particular, the use of the new drug *sodium pentothal* required specialized knowledge of physiology and pharmacology and underscored the emerging view that only physicians could provide anesthesia. In fact, the administration of anesthetics was becoming more complex, and anesthesiologists demonstrated their expertise not only in administering sodium pentothal but also in performing endotracheal intubation and regional blocks (Waisel, 2001). Without a doubt, medicine was increasingly strengthening its hold on the specialty.

Meanwhile, there were shortages of anesthetists on the battlefields. Despite these shortages, the U.S. military would not grant nurse anesthetists a specific designation within the military and experienced nurse anesthetists were required to accept general nurse status. Later, when shortages became severe, the Army Nurse Corps trained staff nurses as anesthetists (*News About Nursing,* 1942). The war years represented a time of growth in the knowledge base for the anesthesia specialty and an expansion in responsibilities for individual CRNAs. Paradoxically, this was also a period in which organized medicine increased its claim over the field of anesthesiology.

---

[5]Although gas warfare was not used in World War II, a stock of mustard gas canisters was held in the Italian port of Bari. An accident involving leakage of one of these canisters rekindled interest begun in World War I about the myelosuppressive effect of nitrogen mustard (Baguley, 2002).

After the war, the specialty of nurse anesthesia continued to take steps to increase its legitimacy. The AANA instituted mandatory certification for CRNAs in 1945. This formal credentialing of CRNAs preceded credentialing of nurses in the other specialties and marked a significant milestone for them as it specified the requirements a nurse had to meet to practice as a nurse anesthetist.

Nurse-Midwives, Circa 1940s. While the United States was at war, nurse-midwives continued their work on the home front. Key to their development in the 1940s was the establishment of a formal organization of practicing nurse-midwives, the AANM, which incorporated in 1941 under the leadership of Mary Breckinridge. By July 1942, the AANM had a "membership of 71 graduate nurses" who had specialty training in midwifery (News Here and There, 1942, p. 832). Three years later, in 1944, the National Organization of Public Health Nurses established a section for nurse-midwives[6] within their organization. This group prepared a roster of all midwives in the country and defined their practice, making it clear that nurse-midwives would continue to practice under physician authority, an idea that was first implemented by Breckinridge in 1928.

In the FNS, the medical advisory board was increasingly concerned over professional boundary issues between medicine and nursing, as evidenced in the introduction to the 1948 version of the Medical Routines which stated (Frontier Nursing Service [FNS], 1948):

> The routines set forth in this book are the orders given by the physicians of the medical advisory committee of the FNS for the use of nurses in the service. They must be followed exactly. No other medications or treatments may be used.... In a grave emergency you may act according to your own judgment, but must report the case in full to the Medical Director. (p. 3)

Changes in leadership on the advisory board, an increase in medical knowledge, the rapid development of new drugs, and a changing economic climate all

played a part in accounting for these stricter controls over FNS nursing practice. Clearly, by mid-century the FNS medical advisory board was trying to reinforce traditional disciplinary boundaries on nursing's scope of practice (Keeling, 2007).

Psychiatric Nursing, Circa 1940s. Because of an increased public awareness of psychiatric problems in returning soldiers, (Critchley, 1985), World War II also affected the specialty of psychiatric nursing. During the 1940s, new treatments were introduced for the care of the mentally ill, including the widespread use of electroshock therapy. The new treatments would require nurses who had specialized knowledge and training to assist with new procedures. According to a 1942 *AJN* article, "Only the nurse skilled in her profession and with additional psychiatric background has a place in mental hospitals today" (Schindler, 1942, p. 861). By 1943 three postgraduate programs in psychiatric nursing had been established. That year, nurse educator Frances Reiter first used the term *nurse clinician* to describe a nurse with advanced "curative" knowledge and clinical competence committed to providing the highest quality of direct patient care (Reiter, 1966). In 1946, after Congress passed the National Mental Health Act designating psychiatric nursing as a core discipline in mental health, federal funding for graduate and undergraduate educational programs and research became available and programs in psychiatric–mental health were included in schools of nursing throughout the United States. Psychiatric nursing knowledge was now widely accepted as essential content in the nursing curriculum. Psychiatric nursing was also becoming established as a graduate level specialty, one that would lead the way for clinical nurse specialization in the next decade.

1950s: The Growth of Hospitals, Scientific Nursing, and the GI Bill

In the period after World War II, optimism about the possibilities of research and scientific knowledge permeated the United States. Without a doubt, specialization and a scientific approach to medical care had captured America's interest. These two factors would set the stage for dramatic changes in health care.

Another important factor was economic as federally funded hospital construction reshaped the settings in which physicians and nurses practiced. In 1946 Congress passed the Hill-Burton Act, which provided large-scale funding to modernize aging

---

[6]Expanded preparation for nurse-midwives also influenced the practice of lay midwives. As the CNMs gained knowledge, they began to share it with the lay midwives. During this decade, minority nurses were also encouraged to become CNMs, albeit in segregated institutions. On March 13, 1942, "the first class of three Negro nurse midwives graduated from the midwifery school operated at the Tuskegee Institute under the auspices of the Macon County Health Department" (Negro Nurse-Midwives, 1942, p. 705).

hospitals and build new ones. These modern hospitals eliminated the large open wards in which nurses could easily observe patients. Instead, the renovated hospitals had long halls with numerous private and semiprivate rooms. The new hospital spaces changed the way in which care was given as the sickest patients were soon grouped together in intensive care units (ICUs) (Fairman & Lynaugh, 1998). This trend contributed to an increase in specialization in nursing while accelerating nursing's invisibility when the costs of nursing care were included with the rate charged for a semiprivate or private room.

In addition to funding new hospitals, the federal government provided funds for nurse education in the post-war years. Nurses returning from World War II were eligible to pursue advanced education under the GI Bill, and many took advantage of the opportunity to return to school. Prompted by the Brown Report of 1948, the National League of Nursing Education (NLNE) established a committee that catalogued all nursing programs, including those leading to a master's degree, in a 1949 issue of *AJN* (Donahue, 1996). Thus federal initiatives during this decade and in the years that followed proved to be critically important to graduate programs in nursing.

Nurse Anesthetists, Circa 1950s. During the 1950s increasing numbers of male physicians were choosing anesthesia as a specialty. However, nurse anesthetists were not to be deterred. In 1952 the AANA established an accreditation program to monitor the quality of nurse anesthetist education. Meanwhile, the United States was once again at war, this time with Korea, and once again, war provided a setting in which opportunities abounded for nurse anesthetists, particularly for men. By the end of the decade, the army had established nurse anesthesia educational programs, including one at Walter Reed General Hospital, which graduated its first class in 1961. This class consisted only of men. Soon after, the Letterman General Hospital School of Anesthesia in San Francisco also graduated an all-male class. This significant movement of men into a nursing specialty was unprecedented.

Nurse-Midwives, Circa 1950s. Numerous factors increased the demand for obstetrical care during the 1950s, not the least of which was the high post-war birth rate. In the 1950s, most urban mothers delivered their babies in hospitals where scientific methods, including the use of scopolamine during labor and general anesthesia during delivery, were the norm. Meanwhile, women in rural areas, especially in the South, continued to rely on "granny midwives" or CNMs to deliver their babies. During this period, nurse-midwives attempted to establish hospital-based practices, and in 1955 Columbia Presbyterian Sloan Hospital opened its doors to nurse-midwives. Concomitantly, Columbia University established a graduate program in maternal nursing, the first to provide midwifery education in an academic medical center. A cooperative program involving Columbia University's Department of Nursing and School of Public Health and Administrative Medicine, the obstetrics and gynecology departments of Presbyterian-Sloan Hospital and Kings County Hospital, and the MCA led to a master of science degree in nursing and a nurse-midwifery certificate (Rooks, 1997). By 1956, three certificate programs and two master's degree programs existed in the United States. Given the conservative mood of the country in this decade and the increasing emphasis on the scientific management for labor and delivery, it is surprising that nurse-midwives fared as well as they did. Overall, they not only held their ground but also made some progress in establishing programs at the graduate level. It is noteworthy that they were among the first specialties to advocate graduate education, a significant move toward advanced practice status.

Psychiatric Clinical Nurse Specialists, Circa 1950s. Psychiatric nursing blossomed as a specialty in the 1950s. In 1954 Hildegarde E. Peplau, professor of psychiatric nursing, established the first master's program in psychiatric nursing in the United States at Rutgers University in New Jersey. Considered the first CNS educational program, this program and the growth of specialty knowledge in psychiatric nursing that ensued provided support for psychiatric nurses to begin exploring new leadership roles in the care of patients with mental illness in both inpatient and outpatient settings. Scholarship in psychiatric nursing also flourished. Among the most significant publications were the writings of Peplau, who proposed the first conceptual framework for psychiatric nursing, *Interpersonal Relations in Nursing, a Conceptual Frame of Reference for Psychodynamic Nursing* (1952), providing theory-based practice for the specialty. Clearly, the link between academia and specialization was becoming stronger and the specialty of psychiatric nursing was leading the way.

American Nurses Association Defines Nursing Practice, Circa 1950s. The seminal work of nurse scholar Virginia Henderson on scientifically based, patient-centered care laid the foundation for changes in nursing that would occur in the second half of the twentieth century. Influenced by both Henderson and Peplau, innovative nurses like France Reiter at New York Medical College initiated a clinical nurse graduate curriculum designed to provide nurses with an intellectual clinical component based on a liberal arts education, in effect supporting a broader role for nurses (Fairman, 2001). However, while academic nursing was making strides toward establishing specialty education and expanding the nurse specialist's scope of practice, the ANA developed a model definition of nursing that would unduly restrict nursing practice for the next several decades. The definition, prepared in 1955 and adopted by many states, read as follows (American Nurses Association [ANA], 1955):

> The practice of professional nursing means the performance for compensation of any act in the observation, care and counsel of the ill . . . or in the maintenance of health or prevention of illness . . . or the administration of medications and treatments as prescribed by a licensed physician . . . . The foregoing shall not be deemed to include acts of diagnosis or prescription of therapeutic or corrective measures. (p. 1474)

Although the ANA may simply have been seeking clarity in defining the discipline's boundaries, its exclusion of the acts of diagnosis and prescription stifled the development of advanced practice nursing. Discussing the impact of the ANA's restrictions on diagnosis and prescription, law professor Barbara Safriet (1992) argued: "Even at the time the ANA's model definition was issued . . . it was unduly restrictive when measured by then current nursing practice" (p. 417). Nurses had been assessing patients for more than 50 years. According to historian Bonnie Bullough (1984), "The fascinating thing about the disclaimer [regarding diagnosis and prescription] is that it was made not by the American Medical Association, but the American Nurses Association . . . . In effect, organized nursing surrendered without any battle over boundaries" (p. 374). The ANA's 1955 definition of nursing would restrict the expansion of nurses' scope of practice for the remainder of the 20th century, as the profession struggled with the dichotomy of "care versus cure" and the legalities of "medical" versus "nursing" diagnosis. In essence, the definition reversed years of hard-won gains in expanding the scope of nursing practice.

1960s: TECHNOLOGY AND ROLE EXPANSION

The federal legislation of the Great Society, the national problems of heart disease and stroke, and the war in Vietnam set the stage for innovation and growth in nursing practice during the 1960s. In 1964 Congress passed the Nurse Training Act, specifically funding nursing education. The Nurse Training Act provided a comprehensive financial package for student grants and loans, as well as for the construction of nursing schools and faculty recruitment and development. A year later, in his 1965 inaugural address, President Lyndon Johnson outlined his plans for the Great Society, proposing a massive legislative agenda that included Medicare and Medicaid programs (under Title XVIII of the Social Security Act), providing millions of Americans with health care benefits. In addition, the agenda included funding for regional medical programs to coordinate state and local efforts to combat cancer, heart disease, and stroke.

Of particular importance to the future of nursing education, the ANA published its "First Position on Education for Nursing" in 1965, calling for nursing education for professional practice to take place in colleges and universities (ANA, 1965). Had that position been enacted formally, it would have united the profession on the issue of nurse preparation for entry into practice. As it was, the position paper incited much debate on the issue but did little else. What became very clear was that although collegiate education in nursing was widely accepted, it would not be the only entry route into the nursing profession. What it did accomplish was the laying of the foundation for master's programs in nursing—only bachelor of science in nursing (BSN)–prepared individuals could go on for advanced education.

Nurse Anesthetists, Circa 1960s. As was the case in wars of other eras, the war in Vietnam provided nurses with opportunities to stretch the boundaries of the discipline as they treated thousands of casualties in evacuation hospitals and aboard hospital ships. Not surprisingly, nurse anesthetists in particular played an active role in the Vietnam War, providing vital services in the prompt surgical treatment of the wounded. According to one account (Jenicek, 1967):

> The nurse anesthetist suddenly became a part of a new concept in the treatment of the severely wounded. The Dust-Off helicopter brings medical aid to severely wounded casualties who formerly would have died before or perhaps during evacuation . . . . Very

often it is a nurse anesthetist who first is available to intubate a casualty, and by so doing may avoid the need for tracheostomy. (p. 348)

Opportunity was not without cost. Of the 10 nurses killed in Vietnam, two were male nurse anesthetists (Bankert, 1989).

Nurse-Midwives, Circa 1960s. During the 1960s nurse-midwives faced both opportunities and obstacles. Some advances were made in defining their role when, in 1962, the American College of Nurse-Midwives (ACNM) established the definitions of the nurse-midwife and nurse-midwifery. These definitions clearly emphasized that the role was an "extension" of nursing practice (American College of Nurse-Midwives [ACNM], 1962). However, the states were slow to grant statutory recognition to CNMs. In fact, as late as 1963, only Kentucky, New Mexico, and New York City had legally sanctioned CNM practice (Rooks, 1997). That same year, only 11% of CNMs who responded to a national survey reported that they were practicing midwifery. This proportion increased to 23% by 1967. However, about one in four of these CNMs was practicing overseas through church and international health organizations. Within the United States, the proportion of CNMs actually practicing midwifery was highest in areas with strong educational programs—particularly in New Mexico, Kentucky, and New York City, where midwives cared primarily for indigent women (ACNM, 1968).

Clinical Nurse Specialists, Circa 1960s. The 1960s are most often noted as the decade in which clinical nurse specialization took its modern form. Nurse educator Hildegarde Peplau (1965) contended that development of areas of specialization is preceded by three social forces: (1) an increase in specialty-related information, (2) new technological advances, and (3) a response to public need and interest. All of these forces clearly helped shape the development of the psychiatric CNS role in the 1960s. The expansion of that role in outpatient mental health was greatly enhanced by the Community Mental Health Centers Act of 1963, as well as the growing interest in child and adolescent mental health care. After the enactment of the 1964 Nurse Training Act, an abundance of CNS master's programs were created. These new clinically focused graduate programs were instrumental in developing and defining the role of the CNS.

With the establishment of the Bethany Hospital Coronary Care Unit (CCU) in Kansas City in 1962, one of the new clinical specialty areas to emerge in the 1960s was coronary care nursing. As CCUs proliferated across the country with the support of federally funded regional medical programs, nurses and physicians acquired specialized clinical knowledge. Together, they discussed clinical questions and negotiated responsibilities (Lynaugh & Fairman, 1992). In doing so, CCU nurses also expanded their scope of practice, developing clinical skills that would be the precursor to a new role—that of nurse practitioner. CCU nurses identified arrhythmias, administered intravenous medications, and defibrillated patients who had lethal ventricular fibrillation, blurring the invisible boundary separating the disciplines of nursing and medicine. In fact, these nurses were diagnosing and treating, "curing," in dramatic life-saving moments. In doing so, they challenged the very definition of nursing that had been published by the ANA only a few years earlier (Keeling, 2004, 2007). What they did not do, however, was differentiate "specialization" from "advanced practice nursing" (a term that would not emerge for decades). That differentiation would come later as master's programs were developed to prepare cardiovascular CNSs and, after that, nurse practitioners.

Although creation of the CCU may have caused confusion about "specialization" and "advanced practice," it unleashed a new era for nurses. The changes that occurred in the clinical setting of the CCU helped establish collegial relationships between nurses and physicians that would be important for APNs in the decades to follow. Collaborative practice became the norm in ICUs and CCUs. "Most importantly, nurses and physicians learned to trust each other . . . ." (Lynaugh & Fairman, 1992, p. 24). In all, the decade was one of unprecedented growth in both the number and variety of ICUs and the latitude and scope of practice for nurses in these areas.

Nurse Practitioners, Circa 1960s. The CCU nurses' work initiated other practice questions for the profession. If specially trained nurses could diagnose and treat life-threatening arrhythmias in CCUs, why couldn't specially trained nurses in pediatrics diagnose and treat a child's sore throat or ear infection? If an ICU nurse could use a stethoscope to listen to a patient's heart and lungs in a highly technological academic medical centers where doctors were readily available, why couldn't a nurse use a stethoscope to examine a patient in a remote, medically underserved area—something that had been done by nurses since the mid-1920s and 1930s? Where were the practice boundaries? Moreover, what education was required?

Although the NP role had been modeled informally in the FNS in the 1930s, it was during the 1960s that the role was first formally described and implemented in outpatient pediatric clinics, originating in part as a response to a shortage of primary care physicians. As the trend toward medical specialization drew increasing numbers of physicians away from primary care, many areas of the country were designated underserved with respect to numbers of primary care physicians. In fact, "report after report issued by the AMA and the Association of American Medical Colleges decried the shortage of physicians in poor rural and urban areas" (Fairman, 2002, p. 163). At the same time, consumers across the nation were demanding accessible, affordable, and sensitive health care, while health care delivery costs were increasing at an annual rate of 10% to 14% (Jonas, 1981).

Pediatric Nurse Practitioners. The landmark event marking the birth of the modern NP role was the establishment of the first pediatric NP (PNP) program by Loretta Ford, RN, and Henry Silver, MD, at the University of Colorado in 1965 (Ford, 1970; Ford & Silver, 1967). This demonstration project, funded by the Commonwealth Foundation, was designed to prepare professional nurses to provide comprehensive well-child care and to manage common childhood health problems. The 4-month program, which certified RNs as PNPs without requiring master's preparation, emphasized health promotion and the inclusion of the family.

A study evaluating the project demonstrated that PNPs were highly competent in assessing and managing 75% of well and ill children in community health settings. In addition, PNPs increased the number of patients served in private pediatric practice by 33% (Ford & Silver, 1967). Like early nurse-midwife and nurse anesthetist data, these positive findings demonstrated support for this new nursing role. Meanwhile, the PNP role was not without significant intraprofessional controversy—particularly with regard to educational preparation. Early on, certificate programs based on the Colorado project rapidly sprang into existence. According to Ford (1991), some of these programs shifted the emphasis of PNP preparation

from a nursing to a medical model. As a result, one of the major areas of controversy in academia was over the fact that NPs made "medical" diagnoses and wrote prescriptions for medications, essentially stepping over the invisible medical boundary into the realm of "curing." Because of this, some nurse educators and other nurse leaders questioned whether the NP role could be conceptualized as being within the discipline of nursing, a profession that had historically been "ordered to care" (Reverby, 1987; Rogers, 1972).

While nursing professors debated the educational preparation of NPs (Keeling, 2007; Rogers, 1972), the NP role attracted considerable attention from professional groups and policymakers. Health policy groups, such as the National Advisory Commission on Health Manpower, issued statements in support of the NP concept (Moxley, 1968). At the grassroots level, physicians accepted the new role and hired nurse practitioners. Indeed, the "horse was out of the barn" in the practice setting.

Physician Assistants. If nurses in academe were upset about NPs, they were even more reactive to the role of the physician assistant (PA) when it was introduced at Duke University in North Carolina in 1965 by Eugene Stead, MD. In fact, organized nursing was opposed to the idea of the PA from the beginning (Ballweg, 1994). According to Christman (1998):

> The idea of having an NP program for medical surgical nursing at Duke, modeled after the PNP program established at Colorado, collapsed because the National League for Nursing (NLN) refused to accredit a program in which physicians would teach much of the curriculum. Moreover, some of the prominent nurses at Duke did not support the idea. (p. 56)

Frustrated by organized nursing's refusal to collaborate to create this new medical-surgical NP, the physicians who conceived of the idea concluded that "nurse leaders were very antagonistic to innovation and change" (Christman, 1998, p. 56). Meanwhile, Duke had recently had experience with training firefighters, ex-corpsmen, and other non–college graduates to resolve personnel shortages in the clinical services of Duke University Hospital. The school proceeded with plans to open a PA program. The 2-year training program defied established concepts of medical education and accepted some applicants who had no prior college education but who had practical experience under battlefield conditions. Moreover, it provided for sharing the knowledge base formerly "owned" by medicine but mandated that the PA would work under the license of a preceptor-physician (Ballweg, 1994). Relationships between PAs and NPs, at least at the academic level, continued to be fraught with tension as more programs developed. At the clinical level, PAs and NPs began to work together.

1970s: BUILDING CREDIBILITY AND DEFINING PRACTICE

The 1970s ushered in a period of rapid growth and development for advanced practice nursing, a decade in which selected roles would become firmly established and the public would begin to recognize an expanded role for nurses with advanced preparation for practice (e.g., see Georgopoulos & Christman, 1970). According to historians Lynaugh and Brush (1996): "What was historically unique . . . was the emerging [public] consensus that nursing, the largest single health care group, should expand its scope of practice to provide direct services to patients, including services previously considered solely in the physician's domain" (p. 38). In fact, in 1971 this new view of nursing was documented in a report to Elliot Richardson, the Secretary of Health, Education, and Welfare, titled "Extending the Scope of Nursing Practice." The report called for nurses in primary, acute, and long-term care to expand their responsibilities to collect medical data and make clinical decisions about patients (Lynaugh & Brush, 1996). Recognizing the need for leadership in the area, the ANA Congress for Nursing Practice published educational standards, described the NP and CNS roles, and attempted to define the expanding scope of nursing practice (ANA Congress for Nursing Practice, 1974). However, considerable conflict developed within the nursing profession as nurses themselves struggled to identify the boundaries of the discipline and the scope of advanced practice nursing. These changes took place within the context of the women's movement, growing public disillusion with government, widespread resistance to continuing the war in Vietnam, and an awareness and concern about environmental issues.

Nurse Anesthetists, Circa 1970s. The 1970s proved to be a difficult decade for nurse anesthetists. In 1972, years after the inception of nurse anesthesia as a specialty role, only four state nurse practice acts specifically mentioned them. Nevertheless, some progress was made in interprofessional relations that year. After years of negotiation, in 1972 the AANA and

the American Society of Anesthesiologists (ASA) issued a "Joint Statement on Anesthesia Practice," promoting the concept of the anesthesia team. However, a few years later, in 1976, the ASA Board of Directors voted to withdraw support from the 1972 statement, endorsing one that explicitly supported physician control and leadership over CRNA practice (Bankert, 1989).

During the mid-1970s, the number of nurse anesthesia educational programs declined significantly, largely because of the closure of many small certificate programs that did not award a master's degree. Physician pressure, inadequate financial support, limited clinical facilities, and lack of accessible universities with which programs could be affiliated contributed to these closures (Faut-Callahan & Kremer, 1996). However, the new requirement that programs offer a graduate degree was not without benefit for CRNAs. In 1973 the University of Hawaii opened the first master's degree program for nurse anesthesia, making it clear that the role was one of advanced practice.

The economic implications of third-party payment also affected nurse anesthetists. Beginning in 1977, the AANA led a long and complex effort to secure third-party reimbursement under Medicare so that CRNAs could bill for their services. The organization would finally succeed in 1989.

Certified Nurse-Midwives, Circa 1970s. The renewed public interest in natural childbirth that stemmed from the women's movement was particularly beneficial to the practice of nurse-midwifery in the 1970s. In fact, the demand for nurse-midwifery services increased dramatically. In addition, sociopolitical developments, including the increased employment of CNMs in federally funded health care projects and the increased birth rate resulting from baby boomers reaching adulthood, converged with inadequate numbers of obstetricians to foster the rapid growth of CNM practice (Varney, 1987). In 1971 only 37% of CNMs who responded to an ACNM survey were employed in clinical midwifery practice. By 1977 this percentage increased to 51%. Not surprisingly, the majority practiced in the rural, underserved areas of the Southwest and Southeast, including Appalachia.

At the national level, physician support for CNM practice became official. In 1971 the ACNM, the American College of Obstetricians and Gynecologists, and the Nurses' Association of the American

College of Obstetricians and Gynecologists issued a joint statement supporting the development and employment of nurse-midwives in obstetrical teams *directed by a physician*. The joint statement, which was critical to the practice of nurse-midwifery, reflected some resolution of the interprofessional tension that had existed through much of the twentieth century. However, it did not provide for autonomy for CNMs. The statement made clear that the medical profession would retain supervisory authority over the practice of nurse-midwifery.

Later in the decade, in 1978, the ACNM revised its definitions of CNM practice and its philosophy, emphasizing the distinct midwifery and nursing origins of the role (ACNM, 1978a, 1978b). This conceptualization of nurse-midwifery as the combination of two disciplines, nursing and midwifery, was unique among the advanced practice nursing specialties. It served to align nurse-midwives with non-nurse midwives, thereby broadening their organizational and political base. Nonetheless, the conceptualization created some distance from other APN specialties that conceptualized the advanced practice role as based solely within the discipline of nursing. This distinction would continue to isolate CNMs from mainstream APNs for the next several decades as they persisted in aligning with non-nurses.

Clinical Nurse Specialists, Circa 1970s. The rapid proliferation of programs and jobs, as well as the emerging role ambiguity and confusion facing them, defined the 1970s for the CNSs (Woodrow & Bell, 1971). During this decade, psychiatric CNSs continued to provide leadership in the educational and clinical arenas and federal funding from the Professional Nurse Traineeship Program provided fiscal support to new programs. In addition, the ANA's Congress for Nursing Practice operationally defined the role of the CNS, and nursing began to conduct evaluative research on the outcomes of CNS care.

Psychiatric CNSs were particularly visible. Early in the decade, a cadre of graduate-prepared psychiatric CNSs assumed roles as individual, group, family, and milieu therapists and obtained direct third-party reimbursement for their services. Soon after, psychiatric nurses identified minimum educational and clinical criteria for CNSs and established national specialty certification through the ANA (Critchley, 1985).

The specialties of critical care and oncology nursing also received attention during the 1970s. The American Association of Critical-Care Nurses, estab-

lished by a small group of concerned nurses at the end of the previous decade, further organized to meet the continuing educational needs of new specialists in the areas of coronary care and intensive care nursing. Only 4 years later, after the first National Cancer Nursing Research Conference sponsored by the ANA and the American Cancer Society (ACS), a group of oncology nurses met to discuss the need for a national organization to support their specialty. Officially incorporated in 1975, the Oncology Nursing Society (ONS) provided a forum for issues related to cancer nursing and supported the growth of advanced practice nursing in this specialty (Oncology Nursing Society, 1994).

By the middle of the decade, the ANA officially recognized the CNS role, defining the CNS as an expert practitioner and a change agent. Of particular significance, the ANA's definition included master's education as a requirement for the CNS (ANA Congress for Nursing Practice, 1974).

As with the other advanced nursing specialties, the development of the CNS role included early evaluation research that served to validate and promote the innovation. Landmark studies by Georgopoulos and colleagues (Georgopoulos & Christman, 1970; Georgopoulos & Jackson, 1970; Georgopoulos & Sana, 1971) evaluated the effect of CNS practice on nursing process and outcomes in inpatient adult health care settings. These and other evaluative studies (Ayers, 1971; Girouard, 1978; Little & Carnevali, 1967) demonstrated the positive effect of the introduction of the CNS in relation to nursing care improvements and functioning.

Overall, the decade of the 70s was one of remarkable progress for the CNS. It was a period in which growth was unprecedented in the health care field in an era of expanding opportunities for women. Moreover, there was an increasing demand from society to cure illness with high-tech solutions and a willingness on the part of hospital administrators to support specialization in nursing and to hire CNSs, particularly in revenue-producing ICUs.

Nurse Practitioners, Circa 1970s. Nurse practitioners also made considerable progress in the 1970s, increasing their visibility within the health care system, negotiating with physicians to expand their scope of practice, and demonstrating their cost-effectiveness in providing quality care. Nevertheless, it was also a period characterized by intraprofessional conflict as some leaders within the nursing community continued to reject the role. In contrast, state legislatures increasingly recognized these expanded roles of RNs, and a group of "pro-NP" nursing faculty, already teaching in NP programs, held their first national meeting in Chapel Hill, North Carolina, in 1974. This meeting would lay the foundation for the formation of the National Organization of Nurse Practitioner Faculties (NONPF).

In the early 1970s, Health, Education, and Welfare Secretary Elliott Richardson established the Committee to Study Extended Roles for Nurses. This group of health care leaders was charged with evaluating the feasibility of expanding nursing practice (Kalisch & Kalisch, 1986). They concluded that extending the scope of the nurse's role was essential to providing equal access to health care for all Americans. According to a 1971 editorial in *AJN*, "The kind of health care Lillian Wald began preaching and practicing in 1893 is the kind the people of this country are still crying for" (Schutt, 1971, p. 53). The committee urged the establishment of innovative curricular designs in health science centers and increased financial support for nursing education. It also advocated standardizing nursing licensure and national certification and developed a model nurse practice law suitable for national application. In addition, the committee called for further research related to cost-benefit analyses and attitudinal surveys to assess the impact of the NP role (U.S. Department of Health, Education, and Welfare [HEW], 1972). This report resulted in increased federal support for training programs for the preparation of several types of NPs including family NPs, adult NPs, and emergency department NPs.

One of the new types of NPs to emerge was the neonatal NP. Originating in the late 1970s in response to a shortage of neonatologists coinciding with restrictions in the total time pediatric residents could devote to neonatal intensive care, the neonatal NP was the forerunner of the acute care NP of the 1990s. These highly skilled, experienced neonatal nurses assumed a wide range of new responsibilities formerly undertaken by pediatric residents, including interhospital transport of critically ill infants and newborn resuscitation (Clancy & Maguire, 1995).

As noted, conflict and discord about the NP role characterized the relationships between NPs and other nurses during this decade. Some members of academia who believed that NPs were not practicing nursing continued to pose resistance to the role

(Ford, 1982). Nurse theorist Martha Rogers, one of the most outspoken opponents of the NP concept, argued that the development of the NP role was a ploy to lure nurses away from nursing to medicine and thereby undermine nursing's unique role in health care (Rogers, 1972). Subsequently, nurse leaders and educators took sides for and against the establishment of educational programs for NPs within mainstream master's programs. Over time, a move toward standardizing NP educational programs at the master's level, initiated by the group of faculty who formed NONPF, would serve to reduce intraprofessional tension.

Despite this resistance within nursing, physicians increasingly accepted NPs in individual health care practices. Working together in local practices, NPs and MDs established collegial relationships, negotiating with each other to construct work boundaries and reach agreement about their collaborative practice. "In the NP-MD dyad, negotiations centered on the NP's right to practice an essential part of traditional medicine: the process or skill set of clinical thinking . . . to perform a physical examination, elicit patient symptoms . . . create a diagnosis, formulate treatment options, prescribe treatment and make decisions about prognosis" (Fairman, 2002, pp. 163-164). The proximity of a supervising physician was thought to be key to effective practice, and "on-site" supervision was the norm. Indeed, grass-roots acceptance of the role depended on tight physician supervision and control of the protocols under which NPs practiced. That supervision was not without benefit to the newly certified, inexperienced NPs. According to Corene Johnson, "Initially, we had to always have a physician on site . . . . I didn't resent that. Actually, I needed the backup" (Fairman, 2002, p. 164).

While physicians and NPs collaborated at the local level, organized medicine began to increase its resistance to the NP role. One of the most contentious areas of interprofessional conflict involved prescriptive authority for nursing. As one author so aptly noted, "Nursing's efforts to obtain the legal authority to prescribe may be seen as the second chapter in the struggle over the use of the word 'diagnosing' in Nurse Practice Acts" (Hadley, 1989, p. 291). Basically, prescriptive authority, regarded as a delegated medical act, depended on NPs' legal right to provide treatment. In 1971 Idaho became the first state to recognize diagnosis and treatment as part of the scope of practice of specialty nurses (Idaho Code 54-1413, 1971). However, "As path-breaking as the statute was, it was still rather restrictive in that any acts of diagnosis and treatment had to be authorized by rules and regulations promulgated by the Idaho State Boards of Medicine and Nursing" (Safriet, 1992, p. 445). Moreover, the Drug Enforcement Act required that practitioners wishing to prescribe controlled substances obtain Drug Enforcement Agency (DEA) registration numbers, and only those practitioners with broad prescriptive authority (e.g., physicians and dentists) could obtain these numbers. In spite of these barriers, by the end of the decade, PNPs obtained legal authority to prescribe drugs for infants and children using standing protocols developed by physicians.[7]

1980s: MATURATION

During the 1980s the ANA provided the leadership needed for APN roles to become institutionalized in the health care system. A critical component of this support was the ANA's 1980 Social Policy Statement, which declared that "specialization in nursing is now clearly established" (ANA, 1980, p. 22)—a statement that also demonstrated the ANA's bias toward the CNS role as opposed to that of the NP. Despite this gain, the lack of consensus about educational preparation for APNs (particularly for NPs) and the titles to identify them continued to plague the profession. According to nurse educator Grace Sills (1983), "The issue of titles was hotly debated in the nursing literature. Nurse clinician, advanced clinical nurse, nurse practitioner—all such titles had different meanings, differing descriptions of the preparation needed and of the performance expected" (p. 566).

On the positive side, however, during the 1980s the concept of advanced nursing practice began to be defined and used in the literature. In 1983 Harriet Kitzman, an associate professor at the University of Rochester, explored the interrelationships between CNSs and NPs (Kitzman, 1983). She used the term *advanced practice* throughout her discussion, applying the term not only to advanced education but also to CNS and NP practice. She noted, "Recognition for advanced practice competence is already established for both NPs and CNSs through the profession's certification programs . . . advanced nursing practice cannot be setting-bound, because nursing needs are not exclusively setting-restricted" (Kitzman, 1983, pp. 284, 288). Building on Kitzman's ideas, Spross and Hamric (1983) proposed the term *advanced*

registered nurse practitioner for a blended CNS/NP model of practice (see Chapter 15). In 1984 an associate professor at the University of Wisconsin–Madison, Joy Calkin, proposed a model for advanced nursing practice, specifically identifying CNSs and NPs with master's degrees as APNs (Calkin, 1984; see Chapter 2 in this textbook). By the end of the decade, the nursing literature increasingly used the term.

The increasing emphasis on cost containment in the 1980s produced legislative and economic changes that affected advanced practice nursing and the health care delivery system as a whole. In particular, the establishment of a prospective payment system in 1983 was a landmark event. This payment system, which used "diagnosis-related groups" (DRGs) to classify billing for hospitalized Medicare recipients, represented an effort to control rising costs and reimbursement to hospitals by shifting reimbursement from "payment for services provided" to "payment by case" (capitation). As a result, hospital administrators put increasing pressure on nurses and physicians to save money by decreasing the length of time patients remained in the hospital. The emphasis on cost containment also heralded budget cuts for hospitals that forced nursing administrators to carefully evaluate the cost-effectiveness of CNSs (then the most commonly employed APNs). The end result was the elimination of some CNS positions by the end of the decade.

The economic climate was not all negative for nursing. In fact, the need to provide cost-effective, quality care to American citizens prompted the Senate Committee on Appropriations to request a report on the contributions of NPs, CNMs, and PAs in meeting the nation's health care needs. The report, released in 1986 and titled "Nurse Practitioners, Physician Assistants and Certified Nurse-Midwives," was based on an analysis of numerous studies that assessed quality of care, patient satisfaction, and physician acceptance. It concluded that "within their areas of competence NPs . . . and CNMs provide care whose quality is equivalent to that of care provided by physicians" (Office of Technology Assessment, 1986, p. 5). However, while the Office of Technology Assessment was conducting this study, the AMA House of Delegates, threatened by the possibility of competition from APNs, passed a resolution to "oppose any attempt at empowering non-physicians to become unsupervised primary care providers and be directly reimbursed" (Safriet, 1992, p. 429).

---

[7]Alaska and North Carolina authorized PNPs to write prescriptions in 1975.

Nurse Anesthetists, Circa 1980s. Despite progress on the educational front, interprofessional conflicts with medicine continued. Although the earlier litigation, *Frank et al. v. South et al.* (1917) and *Chalmers-Frances v. Nelson* (1936) provided the critical legal basis of nurse anesthesia practice, tension between physicians and nurse anesthetists continued, particularly in relation to malpractice policies, antitrust issues, and restraint of trade issues. In 1986 *Oltz v. St. Peter's Community Hospital* established the right of CRNAs to sue for anticompetitive damages when anesthesiologists conspired to restrict practice privileges. A second case, *Bhan v. NME Hospitals, Inc.* (1985), established the right of CRNAs to be awarded damages when exclusive contracts were made between hospitals and physician anesthesiologists. Undeniably, CRNAs were winning the legal battles and overcoming barriers to their practice erected by hospital administrators and physicians.

Like other APNs during the 1980s, nurse anesthetists also had to overcome barriers to reimbursement for their service by third-party payers. The chief problem was that nurse anesthetists could not bill for their services and hospitals had to consider them as a cost center rather than as a revenue-generating service, creating reimbursement disincentives for hospitals to use them (Diers, 1991). Overall, the decade was one of legal success for CRNAs and gradual progress in a difficult economic environment.

Nurse-Midwives, Circa 1980s. By the 1980s the public's acceptance of nurse-midwives had grown and demand for their services had increased among all socioeconomic groups. By the middle of 1982 there were almost 2600 CNMs, the majority located on the East Coast. "Nurse-midwifery had become not only acceptable but also desirable and demanded. Now the problem was that, after years during which nurse-midwives struggled for existence, there was nowhere near the supply to meet the demand" (Varney, 1987, p. 31).

Conflict with the medical profession increased as obstetricians perceived a growing threat to their practices. The denial of hospital privileges, attempts to deny third-party reimbursement, and state legislative battles over statutory recognition of CNMs ensued. In particular, problems concerning "restraint of trade" emerged. In 1980 Congress and the Federal Trade Commission conducted a hearing to determine the extent of the restraint-of-trade issues experienced by CNMs. In two cases, one in Tennessee and one in

Georgia, the Federal Trade Commission obtained restraint orders against hospitals and insurance companies that attempted to limit the practice of CNMs (Diers, 1991)—in essence, assuring CNMs that they could practice. Third-party reimbursement for CNMs was a second issue. In 1980 CNMs working under the Civilian Health and Medical Program of the Uniformed Services (CHAMPUS) for military dependents were the first to receive approval for reimbursement. Third-party payment for CNMs was also included under Medicaid. Statutory recognition by state legislatures was a third problem that would be addressed in the 1980s. By 1984 all states had recognized nurse-midwifery within state laws or regulations (Varney, 1987).

Throughout this decade, nurse-midwifery was immersed in interprofessional struggles over disciplinary boundaries. The support they received in the Office of Technology Assessment study, as well as backing from the Federal Trade Commission and the state legislatures, was critical to their continued survival.

Clinical Nurse Specialists, Circa 1980s. The CNS role continued to be the dominant APN role in the 1980s, with CNSs representing 42% of all APNs (U.S. Department of Health and Human Services [USDHHS], 1996). Of particular significance to the maturation of the CNS role during this decade was the ANA's Social Policy Statement (ANA, 1980), which clearly delineated the criteria required to assume the title of CNS. According to that statement:

> The specialist in nursing practice is a nurse who, through study and supervised clinical practice at the graduate level (masters or doctorate), has become expert in a defined area of knowledge and practice in a selected clinical area of nursing . . . . Upon completion of a graduate program degree in a university graduate program with an emphasis on clinical specialization, the specialist in nursing practice should meet the criteria for specialty certification through nursing's professional society. (p. 23)

In the early 1980s, nurse executives were eager to hire CNSs and the demand for programs increased. In February 1983, the first meeting of the executive committee of the ANA's Council of Clinical Nurse Specialists provided a forum for CNSs and a general repository for documents and information about the role. By 1984 the NLN had accredited 129 programs for preparation of CNSs (National League for Nursing [NLN], 1984). However, about that time, concerns related to the future of the CNS role were surfacing in light of the increasing concern with health care cost containment (Hamric, 1989). Concurrently, some nurse researchers studied the outcomes related to CNS practice. In 1987, for example, McBride and colleagues demonstrated that nursing practice, particularly in relation to documentation, improved as a result of the introduction of a CNS in an inpatient psychiatric setting. By the late 1980s, many CNSs shifted the focus of their practice away from the clinical area and instead focused on the educational and organizational aspects of the CNS role. This shift was supported by the view that CNSs were too valuable to spend their time on direct patient care (Wolff, 1984). Meanwhile, others who asserted that the essence of the CNS role was clinical expertise were publishing articles and books on the topic (Hamric & Spross, 1983, 1989; Sparacino, 1990). In addition, articles describing the practice of CNSs and consensus reports on this APN role began to appear in critical care, oncology, and other nursing specialty journals. These publications helped lay the groundwork for curriculum development in APN specialties.

Also during the 1980s, the ANA Council of Clinical Nurse Specialists (CCNS) and Council of Primary Health Care Nurse Practitioners (CPHCNP) began to explore commonalities of the two roles. In 1988 the councils conducted a survey of all NP and CNS graduate programs and identified considerable overlap in curricula (Forbes, Rafson, Spross, & Koslowski, 1990). Subsequently, between 1988 and 1990, the two councils discussed a proposal to merge, and in 1991 the new Council of Nurses in Advanced Practice was formed. Unfortunately, it was short-lived because of the restructuring of ANA during the early 1990s. Nevertheless, this merger was a landmark event in the organizational coalescence of advanced practice nursing (ANA, 1991).

Nurse Practitioners, Circa 1980s. Significant growth in the numbers of NPs in practice and the fight for prescriptive authority for NPs characterized the 1980s. NP practice increased immeasurably during the 1980s as new types of NPs developed—the most significant of which were the emergency NP, the neonatal NP, and the family NP. By 1984 approximately 20,000 graduates of NP programs were employed, for the most part in settings "that the founders envisioned": outpatient clinics, health maintenance organizations, health departments, community health centers, rural clinics, schools, occupational health clinics, and private offices (Kalisch & Kalisch, 1986,

p. 715). By the late 1980s, however, based on their success in neonatal intensive care units, NPs with specialty preparation were increasingly utilized in tertiary care centers (Silver & McAtee, 1988).

During this period, the multiple roles for NPs created competing interests that would affect NPs' ability to speak with one voice on legislative issues. In an attempt to rectify this situation, the ANA established the CPHCNP in the early 1980s. At about the same time, the Alliance of Nurse Practitioners was established as an umbrella organization for all the various NP associations.

Throughout the 1980s, NPs worked tirelessly to convince state legislatures to pass laws and establish reimbursement policies that would support their practice. Interprofessional conflicts with organized medicine, and to a lesser extent with pharmacists, centered on control issues and the degree of independence the NP was allowed. These conflicts intensified as NPs moved beyond the "physician extender" model to a more autonomous one. In a 1980 landmark case, *Sermchief v. Gonzales* (1983), the Missouri medical board charged two women's health care NPs with practicing medicine without a license (Doyle & Meurer, 1983). The initial ruling was against the NPs, but on appeal, the Missouri Supreme Court overturned the decision, concluding that the scope of practice of APNs may evolve without statutory constraints (Wolff, 1984). In essence, this case provided a model for new state nurse practice acts to address issues related to APN practice with very generalized wording, a change that allowed for expansion in APNs' roles and functions.

The fight for prescriptive authority for NPs also characterized this decade. In 1983 only Oregon and Washington granted NPs statutory independent prescriptive authority. Other states granting prescriptive authority to NPs did so with the provision that the NP be directly supervised by a licensed physician. How prescriptions were handled depended on the availability of the physician, the negotiated boundaries of the individual physician-NP team, and the state in which practice occurred. In some cases that meant that physicians pre-signed a pad of prescriptions for the NP to use at her discretion; in remote area clinics like those in the Frontier Nursing Service, a physician would countersign NP prescriptions once a week; and in other instances the physician would write and sign a prescription on the request of the NP. With the exception of the latter, these practices were of questionable legality (Keeling, 2007).

1990s: RESPONDING TO REGULATORY AND HEALTH CARE CHANGE

The 1990s continued to be a period of growth and change for advanced practice nursing as the profession responded to regulatory and health care change. The 1990s opened with the United States' war with Iraq, a war in which thousands of American military nurses were deployed to the Persian Gulf. The cost of health care was a constant concern, and by 1992, when William Jefferson Clinton was elected President of the United States, the country was in serious need of health care reform. Determined to take a proactive stance in the movement, the ANA wrote its Agenda for Health Care Reform (1992). The plan focused on restructuring the U.S. health care system to reduce costs and improve access to care. Although the Clinton administration's efforts for health care reform failed, radical changes were made by the private sector in which the once dominant "fee-for-service" insurance plans were overtaken by managed care organizations (Safriet, 1998). The changing marketplace created new challenges for APNs as they struggled not only with restrictive, outdated state laws on prescriptive authority but also with "non-governmental, market-based impediments" to their practices (Safriet, 1998, p. 25). In this environment, APNs continued to expand their roles, their educational programs, and their practice settings. In August 1993, representatives of 63 of 66 tri-council organizations attending a national nursing summit agreed to require master's education for advanced practice nursing (Cronenwett, 1995).

Nurse Anesthetists, Circa 1990s. The 1990s saw significant growth in CRNA educational programs, although many of the programs were very small. As the decade opened, there were 17 master's programs in nurse anesthesia; by 1999 there were 82 (Bigbee & Amidi-Nouri, 2000). As of 1998, all accredited programs in nurse anesthesia were required to be at the master's level; however, they were not uniformly located within schools of nursing. Rather, they were housed in a variety of disciplines, including schools of nursing, medicine, allied health, and basic science. As it had been throughout the century, nurse anesthetist programs continued to be regarded by the profession as "on the fringe." By the end of the decade, however, increasing numbers of CRNA programs were offered within graduate nursing programs.

Nurse-Midwives, Circa 1990s. During the 1990s, increasing demand for CNM services resulted in the gradual expansion in the scope of nurse-midwifery practice. CNMs began to provide care to women with relatively high-risk pregnancies in collaboration with obstetricians in some of the nation's academic tertiary care centers (Rooks, 1997). During this decade, two practice models emerged: the CNM service model in which CNMs were responsible for the care of a caseload of women determined to be eligible for midwifery care, and the CNM/MD team model. Nurse-midwives made significant progress in establishing laws and regulations needed to support their practice. In fact, over the course of the decade, every state gave statutory recognition to CNMs. Moreover, CNMs were also granted prescriptive privileges and third-party reimbursement (Rooks, 1997).

By the end of the decade (Dorron & Kelley, 2000), 72% of CNMs had a master's or doctoral degree, and 89% of CNM education programs (39 of 44) were at the master's level. However, the ACNM required only a minimum of a bachelor's degree (rather than a master's degree) to be eligible for ACNM accreditation. This requirement diverged from the trend among other APN specialties to require graduate preparation. At about the same time, economic conditions created new problems for CNMs. The rapid transition to managed care, as well as an increase in the cost of liability insurance, began to threaten nurse-midwifery practice.

Clinical Nurse Specialists, Circa 1990s. The 1990s was also a challenging decade for CNSs, beginning with cutbacks in their employment opportunities because of the financial problems within hospitals and ending with national recognition by the federal government for Medicare reimbursement for their services. In the early 1990s, CNS programs were the most numerous of all the master's nursing programs nationally, serving more than 11,000 students (NLN, 1994). The largest area of specialization was adult health/medical-surgical nursing. However, with the increasing emphasis on primary care in the mid-1990s, the rapid growth of NP programs, the financial challenges faced by hospital administrators, and the introduction of the acute care nurse practitioner (ACNP) role in tertiary care centers, the number of CNS positions in hospitals declined sharply. Consequently, the number of nurses interested in pursuing master's degrees for the CNS role also decreased.

The 1996 Sample Survey of Registered Nurses also revealed that a significant number (7802) of CNSs were also prepared as NPs (see Chapter 3). According to that report, these dual-role–prepared APNs were more likely to be employed as NPs rather than as CNSs. By 1996, of the 61,601 CNSs in the United States, only 23% were practicing in CNS-specific positions (USDHHS, 1996). This low percentage may reflect the fact that CNSs accepted different positions as, for example, administrators or staff educators. It may also reflect the decline in the number of CNS positions available because of budget cutbacks. Certification for CNS practice was particularly complicated. In many specialties, certification examinations were targeted to nurses who were experts by experience, not APNs. APN certification was slow to emerge. For example, it was not until 1995 that the Oncology Nursing Society (ONS) administered the first certification examination for advanced practice in oncology nursing. A further complication was that not all states recognized these examinations for APN regulatory purposes.

Despite these realities, the decade was not without its positive side for CNSs. The creation of the National Association of Clinical Nurse Specialists (NACNS), established in 1995, represented a major step in the organizational development of this specialty. In 1997 CNSs were specifically identified for Medicare reimbursement eligibility in the Balanced Budget Act (Public Law 105-33) (Safriet, 1998). This law, providing Medicare Part B direct payment to NPs and CNSs regardless of their geographical area of practice, allowed both CNSs and NPs to be paid 85% of the fee paid to physicians for the same services. Moreover, the law's inclusion and definition of CNSs corrected a previous omission of this group for reimbursement (Safriet, 1998). The possibility of reimbursement for services was an important step in the continuing development of the CNS role because hospital administrators would continue to focus on the cost of having APNs provide patient care.

Nurse Practitioners, Circa 1990s. During the 1990s, the number of NPs increased dramatically in response to increasing demand, the national emphasis on primary care, and the concomitant decrease in the number of medical residencies in the subspecialties (a factor spurring growth of ACNPs). In 1990 there were 135 master's degree and 40 certificate NP programs. Between 1992 and 1994, the number of institutions offering NP education more than

doubled, from 78 to 158. In 1994 these institutions offered a total of 384 NP tracks in master's programs throughout the United States. By 1998 the number of institutions offering NP education again doubled, representing a total of 769 distinct NP specialty tracks (American Association of Colleges of Nursing [AACN], 1999; National Organization of Nurse Practitioner Faculties [NONPF], 1997). The majority of the programs were at the master's or post-master's level. In fact, by 1998 only 12 post–basic RN certificate programs remained in existence. This rapid expansion created concern about the need for so many programs and the quality of the programs. In the end, most nurse educators supported the master's degree as the educational requirement for NP practice and most used the NONPF guidelines in determining their curricula (NONPF, 1997).

Acute Care Nurse Practitioners. Like the neonatal NP role of the late 1970s, the adult ACNP role grew during this decade in response to residency shortages in ICUs, although this time the shortage was because of decreases in the number of residents available to work in the medical subspecialties. In addition, increasingly complicated tertiary care systems lacked coordination of care. Advanced practice nursing responded quickly to this need, building on the earlier work of Silver and McAtee (1988) to create a role that promoted both quality patient care and nursing's leadership in health care delivery (Daly, 1997). University of Pennsylvania Professors Anne Keane and Theresa Richmond (1993) were among those who documented the emergence of the tertiary NP (TNP), noting:

> The TNP is an advanced practice nurse educated at the master's level with both a theoretical and experiential focus on complex patients with specialized health needs, ... There is precedent for the NP in tertiary care. For example, neonatal nurse practitioners are central to the provision of care in many intensive care nurseries, ... It is our belief that the TNP can provide clinically expert specialized care in a holistic manner in a system that is often typified by fragmentation, lack of communication among medical specialists and a loss of recognition of the patient and patient's needs as central to the care delivered. (p. 282)

From 1992 to 1995, ACNP tracks in master's programs proliferated across the country.[8] Soon, questions abounded about the content of the curriculum. To resolve these, the educators met annually at ACNP consensus conferences, beginning in 1993. The first ACNP certification examination was given in December 1995 by the American Nurses Credentialing Center (ANCC), and by 1997 there were 43 tracks nationwide that prepared ACNPs either at the master's or post-master's level (Kleinpell, 1997). In 2002 ACNPs formally merged with the American Academy of Nurse Practitioners (AANP) with the goal of uniting both primary care and acute care NPs under an umbrella organization. By this time, the ACNP role was beginning to be accepted. ACNPs were employed in multiple specialties including cardiology, cardiovascular surgery, neurosurgery, emergency/trauma, internal medicine, and radiology services (Daly, 2002).

Federal legislation regulating narcotics in the Controlled Substances Act (1991 and 1992) would be of major significance to NP progress in implementing prescriptive authority in this decade. As NPs began to gain prescriptive authority for controlled substances in the different states, they required a parallel authority granted by the federal Drug Enforcement Agency (DEA). In 1991 the DEA first responded to this situation by proposing registration for "affiliated practitioners" (56FR 4181). This proposal called for those NPs who had prescriptive authority pursuant to a practice protocol or collaborative practice agreement to be assigned a registration number for controlled substances tied to the number of the physician with whom they worked. This proposal received much criticism specifically related to the restriction of access to health care and to the legal liability of the prescribers. Because of these criticisms, the proposal was revoked in 1992. Later in the year, in July 1992, the DEA amended its regulations by adding a category of "mid-level providers" (MLPs) who would be issued individual provider DEA numbers as long as they were granted prescriptive authority by the state in which they practiced. The MLP's number would begin with an M for "mid-level provider," rather than an A or B. The MLP provision took effect in 1993, significantly expanding NPs' ability to prescribe.

During this decade, the growth in number of NP programs, the increase in prescriptive authority for NPs, and the autonomy NPs found in their practice

settings converged to make the NP role enticing, and increasing numbers of nurses wanting to be APNs chose the NP role. The problem was that numerous organizations were speaking for the various types of NPs. In the mid-1990s, NPs attempted to unify their organizational voice by establishing the AANP. Membership in this organization included national organizational affiliates, state NP organizations, and individuals. Supposedly, the focus of the organization was to address public policy issues that affected all NPs. However, NPs never unified. Throughout this period, many were angry about the establishment of the AANP. The Alliance of Nurse Practitioners continued to be active, and the American College of Nurse Practitioners was born. In addition, PNPs formed the National Association of Pediatric Nurse Associates and Practitioners (NAPNAP), and nurses interested in women's health formed the Association of Women's Health, Obstetric, & Neonatal Nurses (AWHONN). Multiple certification examinations were developed by these various groups, in addition to the ANCC. In fact, dissension about which group should speak for NPs continued throughout the 1990s and into the twenty-first century.

THE TWENTY-FIRST CENTURY: NEW CHALLENGES

The turn of the twenty-first century brought new challenges to APNs. Computerized charting, the widespread use of the Internet to access information, an emphasis on evidence-based practice, and an increasing awareness of the global community were just a few of the challenges facing the profession. In addition, the September 11, 2001, attacks on the Pentagon and the World Trade Center heightened national awareness of the need to be prepared to respond to terrorism. Also, the threat of emerging infectious diseases (particularly Avian influenza) made the country aware of its lack of preparation for responding to life-threatening pandemics.

Today, America is faced with a health care system at risk of imploding because of spiraling costs. Military conflicts in Afghanistan and Iraq have consumed significant national resources. Along with an increasingly diverse and aging population, increasing percentages of uninsured or underinsured individuals, and a critical nursing shortage, the health care system faces significant problems that must be addressed. Legislative battles continue over the scope of APN prescriptive authority, especially

---

[8]The University of Pittsburgh, Case Western Reserve University, the University of Connecticut, The University of Rochester, Rush Presbyterian University, and the University of Pennsylvania were among the first university schools of nursing to embrace the idea and implement programs, most of which were originally at the post-master's level (Daly, 2002).

for controlled substances. More important, current market forces represent more significant barriers than regulatory ones. As Safriet (1998) noted:

> No longer is governmental prohibition or restriction the only—or even the principal—problem. Now an increase in the competitive chaos of the marketplace has thrown APNs into unfamiliar territory in which private contracting, market-share, and capital requirements may pose potentially serious obstacles. (p. 25)

Full recognition of APNs by insurers and health care organizations is one of the most important challenges. Legislative efforts to secure third-party reimbursement continue to be critical to the economic survival of advanced practice nursing. In addition, with the Institute of Medicine's (2000) report on safety in health care, the nursing and medical professions are undergoing an increased level of analysis by health policy experts. The protection of the public is paramount, as is an attempt to reduce disparities in access to care. Both issues have major implications for advanced practice nursing.

The American Association of Colleges of Nursing and the Doctor of Nursing Practice

A primary example of an attempt to address the current issues in the profession and the nation is the Doctor of Nursing Practice (DNP) developed by the American Association for Colleges of Nursing (AACN) in 2004. This initiative was aimed at ensuring adequate educational preparation for APNs and arose in response to the explosion in needed information for advanced practice nursing, technology and scientific evidence to guide practice, the need to prepare senior level nurses for key leadership positions, and the reality of ever-increasing curricular requirements in master's programs throughout the country. As proposed by the AACN, the DNP would standardize practice entry requirements for all APNs by the year 2015, assuring the public that each APN would have had 1000 supervised clinical hours before entering the practice setting. Moreover, the proposed curriculum for DNPs would include competencies deemed essential for nursing practice in the twenty-first century, including (1) scientific underpinnings for practice, (2) organizational and systems leadership, (3) clinical scholarship and analysis for evidence-based practice, (4) information systems technology, (5) health care policy, (6) interprofessional collaboration, and (7) clinical prevention and population health (AACN, 2006). Although it is too early to evaluate this initiative from an historical

perspective, the national dialogue to move APN education to a practice doctorate offers significant opportunity for the profession to connect scientific evidence and practice. Expanded educational preparation could position APNs to be vital players in the translation of research evidence at the point of care (Magyary, Whitney, & Brown, 2006).

SUMMARY AND CONCLUSIONS: ADVANCED PRACTICE NURSING IN CONTEXT

This brief analysis of the history of advanced practice nursing in the twentieth century reveals several themes:

- Throughout the century, APNs have been permitted by organized medicine and state legislative bodies to provide care to the underserved poor, particularly in rural areas of the nation. However, when that care competes with physicians' reimbursement for their services, significant resistance from organized medicine has occurred and resulted in interprofessional conflict.
- Documentation of the outcomes of practice helped establish the earliest nursing specialties and continues to be of critical importance to the survival of APN practice.
- The efforts of national professional organizations, national certification, and the move toward graduate education as a requirement for advanced practice have been critical to the credibility of advanced practice nursing.
- Intraprofessional and interprofessional resistance to expanding the boundaries of the nursing discipline continue to recur.
- Societal forces including wars, the economic climate, and health care policy have influenced APN history.

Providing care to people in underserved areas has, by default, been assigned to nursing throughout the twentieth and early twenty-first centuries. Moreover, history is clear that the concept of expanding the scope of practice for nurses was inextricably entwined with that assignment. The HSS visiting nurses cared for poor immigrants of the Lower East Side unopposed by physicians until MDs perceived them as a threat. The FNS nurses made diagnoses and treated patients in remote areas of Appalachia with the blessings of the physician committee who supervised them, and the BIA nurses "cured," as best they could, native American Indians in their communities. In other instances, if one considers time as place, "after midnight" nurses expanded their scope of practice by defibrillating patients in CCUs across the nation and army nurses did whatever needed to be done on the battlefront (Keeling, 2004). Only when APNs threatened physicians' practice and income did organized medicine accuse them of practicing medicine without a license. Moreover, organized nursing itself was responsible for resisting the expansion of the scope of practice of nursing. However, it is also clear that when nurses and physicians focused on providing quality care for their patients, they were capable of working collaboratively and interdependently.

Further analysis of the history of advanced practice nursing demonstrates the importance of evaluative research in documenting the contributions of APNs to the health care system and patients' well-being. As evidenced by nurse anesthetist Alice Magaw's 1900 publication on outcomes, the early "APNs" were particularly visionary in their use of data to document their effectiveness. Throughout the century, evaluative research based on measurable outcomes served as a tool for the profession to argue its position to both health care policymakers and the medical profession (Brooten et al., 1986; Hamric, Lindbak, Jaubert, & Worley, 1998; Mitchell-DiCenso et al., 1996; Mundinger et al., 2000; Shah, Brutlomesso, Sullivan, & Lattanzio, 1997). As Beck (1995) stated, "It is inconsistent for a state medical association to maintain a position that quality health care is their objective … [while] … disregarding data demonstrating the positive impact of APNs on health care" (p. 15).

The powerful influence of organizational efforts also emerges as a theme. National organization has been key to progress for advanced practice nursing. Within the development of each of the advanced practice specialties, several common features emerge. Strong national organizational leadership has been clearly demonstrated to be of critical importance in enhancing the growth and protection of the specialty. On the basis of the experience of the two oldest specialties, nurse anesthesia and nurse-midwifery, the process of establishing an effective national organization has taken a minimum of three decades. The history of these specialties reveals that specialty organizations have also played a critical role in the credentialing process for individuals within the specialty. The strength, unity, and depth of the organizational development of the two oldest advanced nursing specialties should serve as a model for the younger developing specialties.

An additional theme to emerge is the importance of professional unity regarding the requisite education of APNs. Early in the twentieth century, specialty education was considered to be postgraduate with a heavy component of on-the-job training; however, that education was commonly post-diploma, not post-baccalaureate, and did not result in a master's degree. These early programs were of variable length and quality. The establishment of credible and stable educational programs has been a crucial step in the evolution of advanced practice nursing. As educational programs moved from informal, institutionally based models with a strong apprenticeship approach to more formalized graduate education programs, the credibility of APN roles increased. State regulations also influenced the evolution of advanced practice as an increasing number of states mandated a master's degree as a prerequisite for APN licensure. This regulatory influence served to unite the advanced practice specialty roles conceptually and legislatively, thereby promoting collaboration and cohesion among APNs.

The powerful influence of interprofessional struggles is apparent in all the advanced specialties, with the possible exception of CNSs. The legal battles between nursing and medicine are longstanding, particularly in relation to nurse anesthesia and nurse-midwifery. Most of these tensions revolve around issues of control, autonomy, and economic competition. However, the outcomes of the legal battles have proven to be positive for nursing for the most part and have helped legitimize APN roles.

Nurse anesthetists, nurse-midwives, and NPs specifically challenged the boundaries between nursing and medical practice. When they did, organized medicine responded, and today, these predictable responses should not be unexpected or underestimated. According to Inglis and Kjervik (1993), "It should be noted that organized medicine, largely through lobbying, has played a central role in creating and perpetuating the states' contradictory and constraining provisions of APN practice" (p. 196).

Controversy within the nursing community was also a strong theme as the specialties developed. CRNAs, and to some extent NPs, developed outside of mainstream nursing, whereas from the start, CNSs developed within the mainstream. Nevertheless, each specialty has had to deal with resistance from other nurses. These intraprofessional struggles can be understood within the context of change: each of the APN specialties represented innovations that challenged the status quo of the nursing establishment and the health care system.

Throughout the century, prescriptive authority for advanced practice nursing, inextricably linked to economic and boundary issues between medicine and nursing, has been a particularly volatile legislative issue. Today, in most states, NPs and CRNAs can prescribe drugs with varying degrees of physician involvement and supervision. Although CNSs can prescribe in many states, they have not received the full recognition that has been granted to the other APN groups. Thus despite a great deal of progress in the role of APNs over the past century and gradual changes in state legislation and third-party reimbursement, APNs have not reached their full potential to fulfill the nation's health care needs. Barriers to enhancement of prescriptive authority for APNs include (1) exclusive reimbursement patterns, (2) anticompetitive practices and resistance of organized medicine, (3) variable state regulation and practice acts, and (4) restrictive DEA registration laws (Beck, 1995; Keeling 2007).

Societal forces have clearly influenced the development of advanced practice nursing. Gender issues have affected all the specialties to some degree because of the unique position of nursing as a female-dominated profession. CRNA and NP roles have been the exceptions, with more men entering these fields. Within nurse-midwifery, the status of women and the status of women's health were powerful forces in the establishment and development of the specialty. Overall, war has served as a catalyst to the development of advanced practice nursing, education, and professional organization, as nurses who expanded their scope of activities in wartime lobbied to continue that expanded practice when back home. Finally, economic changes, particularly in relation to health care financing, have had a powerful effect on the development of advanced practice nursing. The dramatic growth of managed care systems in the 1990s in particular presented new challenges and opportunities for APNs related to reimbursement, scope of practice, and autonomy (Safriet, 1998).

With unremitting changes in nursing and health care, it is apparent that the APN specialties will continue to evolve and diversify (see Chapter 18). As new roles emerge, the history of advanced practice nursing continues to be written. Today, particularly in light of the DNP initiative, the profession is at a critical juncture in which it must decide whether or not it will mandate doctoral level preparation for all advanced practice nursing roles. Agreement on master's preparation for all APNs is relatively new, and disagreements about the need for and requirement of the doctorate (Dracup, Cronenwett, Meleis, & Benner, 2005a; 2005b) may continue to impede progress toward the adoption of standardized educational criteria in the future. Undoubtedly, as law professor Safriet (1998) has argued, consistency in the definition of advanced practice nursing and in the criteria for licensure as an APN is critical to autonomy in practice.

Thus what remains to be seen is whether the profession can unite on issues related to the definition of advanced practice nursing and standardized criteria for educational preparation to ensure that APNs are permitted to practice with the autonomy experienced by other professionals. If that can be done, APNs can make a significant contribution to the transformation of health care in the twenty-first century. As William Shakespeare so aptly noted: "The past is prologue" (2002).

REFERENCES

American Association of Colleges of Nursing (AACN). (1999). *Enrollment and graduations in baccalaureate and graduate programs in nursing.* Washington, DC: Author.

American Association of Colleges of Nursing (AACN). (2006) *Essentials of the DNP.* Retrieved February 8, 2006, from www.aacn.nche.edu.

American College of Nurse-Midwives (ACNM). (1962). *Definition of a certified nurse-midwife.* Washington, DC: Author.

American College of Nurse-Midwives (ACNM). (1968). *Descriptive data, nurse-midwives—U.S.A.* Washington, DC: Author.

American College of Nurse-Midwives (ACNM). (1978a). *Definition of a certified nurse-midwife.* Washington, DC: Author.

American College of Nurse-Midwives (ACNM). (1978b). *Philosophy.* Washington, DC: Author.

American Nurses Association (ANA). (1955). ANA board approves a definition of nursing practice. *American Journal of Nursing, 5,* 1474.

American Nurses Association (ANA). (1965). ANA's first position on education for nursing. *American Journal of Nursing, 65,* 106-111.

American Nurses Association (ANA). (1980). *Nursing: A social policy statement.* Kansas City, MO: Author.

American Nurses Association (ANA). (April 1991). *Report of the Congress for Nursing Practice to ANA Board of Directors on the merger of the Council of Clinical Nurse Specialists and the Council of Primary Health Care Nurse Practitioners into the Council of Nurses.* Washington, DC: Author.

American Nurses Association (ANA). (1992). *Agenda for health care reform.* Washington, DC: Author.

American Nurses Association (ANA) Congress for Nursing Practice. (1974). *Definition: Nurse practitioner, nurse clinician and clinical nurse specialist.* Kansas City, MO: American Nurses Association.

Ayers, R. (1971). Effects and development of the role of the clinical nurse specialist. In R. Ayers (Ed.), *The clinical nurse specialist: An experiment in role effectiveness and role development* (pp. 32-49). Duarte, CA: City of Hope National Medical Center.

Baer, E. (2001). Aspirations unattained: The story of the Illinois Training School's search for university status. In E. Baer, P. D'Antonio, S. Rinker , & J. Lynaugh (Eds.), *Enduring issues in American nursing* (pp. 150-164). New York: Springer.

Baguley, B. (2002). A brief history of cancer chemotherapy. In B. Baguley & D. Kerr (Eds.), *Anticancer drug development* (pp. 1-9). New York: Academic Press.

Ballweg, R. (1994). History of the profession. In R. Ballweg, S. Stolberg, & E.M. Sullivan (Eds.), *Physician assistant* (pp. 1-20). Philadelphia: Saunders.

Bankert, M. (1989). *Watchful care: A history of America's nurse anesthetists.* New York: Continuum.

Beck, M. (1995). Improving America's health care: Authorizing independent prescriptive privileges for advanced practice nurses. *University of San Francisco's Law Review, 29,* 951.

Beeber, L.S. (1990). To be one of the boys: Aftershocks of the WWI nursing experience. *Advances in Nursing Science, 12,* 32-43.

Bhan v. NME Hospitals, Inc. et al., 772 F.2d 1467 (9th Cir. 1985).

Bigbee, J., & Amidi-Nouri, A. (2000). History and evolution of advanced nursing practice. In A.B. Hamric, J.A. Spross, & C.M. Hanson (Eds.), *Advanced nursing practice: An integrative approach* (2nd ed., pp. 3-32). Philadelphia: Saunders.

Breckinridge, M. (1981). *Wide neighborhoods: A story of the Frontier Nursing Service.* Lexington, KY: The University Press of Kentucky.

Brooten, D., Kumar, S., Brown, L.P., Butts, P., Finkler, S.A., Bakewell-Sachs, S. et al. (1986). A randomized clinical trial of early hospital discharge and home follow-up of very-low-birth-weight infants. *New England Journal of Medicine, 315,* 934-939.

Brown, E.L. (1948). *Nursing for the future.* New York: Russell Sage Foundation.

Buck, D.F. (1940). The nurses on horseback ride on. *American Journal of Nursing, 40,* 993-995.

Buhler-Wilkerson, K. (2001). *No place like home: A history of nursing and home care in the United States.* Baltimore: The Johns Hopkins University Press.

Bullough, B. (1984). The current phase of the development of nurse practice acts. *St. Louis Law Journal, 28,* 365-395.

Calkin, J.D. (1984). A model for advanced nursing practice. *Journal of Nursing Administration, 14,* 24-30.

Chalmers-Frances v. Nelson, 6 Cal.2d 402 (1936).

Christman, L. (1998). Advanced practice nursing: Is the physician's assistant an accident of history or a failure to act? *Nursing Outlook, 46,* 56-59.

Clancy, G.T., & Maguire, D. (1995). Advanced practice nursing in the neonatal intensive care unit. *Critical Care Nursing Clinics of North America, 7,* 71-76.

Critchley, D.L. (1985). Evolution of the role. In D.L. Critchley & J.T. Maurin (Eds.), *The clinical specialist in psychiatric mental health nursing* (pp. 5-22). New York: John Wiley & Sons.

Cronenwett, L.R. (1995). Modeling the future of advanced practice nursing. *Nursing Outlook, 43,* 112-118.

Daly, B. (1997). *The acute care nurse practitioner.* New York: Springer.

Daly, B. (2002). ACNP 2002. *Where we've been and where we're going.* Original manuscript, keynote address presented at the April 2002 ACNP Consensus Conference, Charlottesville, VA. The Keeling Collection, Center for Nursing Historical Inquiry, UVA.

D'Antonio, P. (1991). Staff needs and patient care: Seclusion and restraint in a nineteenth-century insane asylum. *Transactions and Studies of the College of Physicians of Philadelphia, 13*(4), 411-423.

Dewitt, K. (1900). Specialties in nursing. *American Journal of Nursing, 1,* 14-17.

Diers, D. (1991). Nurse-midwives and nurse anesthetists: The cutting edge in specialist practice. In L.H. Aiken & C.M. Fagin (Eds.), *Charting nursing's future: Agenda for the 1990s* (pp. 159-180). New York: Lippincott.

Dock, L., & Stewart, I. (1920). *A short history of nursing.* New York: Putnam.

Donahue, P.M. (1996). *Nursing, the finest art: An illustrated history* (2nd ed.). St. Louis: Mosby.

Dorron, M.W., Kelley, M.A. (2000). The certified nurse-midwife. In A.B. Hamric, J.A. Spross, & C.M. Hanson (Eds.), *Advanced nursing practice: An integrative approach* (3rd ed.) (pp. 491-519). Philadelphia: Saunders.

Doyle, E., & Meurer, J. (1983). Missouri legislation and litigation: Practicing medicine without a license. *Nurse Practitioner, 8,* 41-44.

Dracup, K., Cronenwett, L., Meleis, A.I., Benner, P.E. (2005a). Reply to letter to the editor on reflections on the doctorate of nursing practice. *Nursing Outlook, 53*(6), 269.

Dracup, K., Cronenwett, L., Meleis, A.I., Benner, P.E. (2005b). Reflections on the doctorate of nursing practice. *Nursing Outlook, 53*(4): 177-182.

Drug Enforcement Agency (DEA). (1991). *Definition and exemption of affiliated practitioners,* 56 Fed. Reg. 4181.

Duffus, R.L. (1938). *Lillian Wald: Neighbor and crusader.* New York: Macmillan.

Fairman, J. (2001). Delegated by default or negotiated by need?: Physicians, nurse practitioners, and the process of clinical thinking. In E. Baer, P. D'Antonio, S. Rinker, & J. Lynaugh (Eds.), *Enduring issues in American nursing* (pp. 309-333). New York: Springer.

Fairman, J. (2002). The roots of collaborative practice: Nurse practitioner pioneers' stories. *Nursing History Review, 10,* 159-174.

Fairman, J., & Lynaugh, J. (1998). *Critical care nursing: A history.* Philadelphia: University of Pennsylvania.

Faut-Callahan, M., & Kremer, M. (1996). The certified registered nurse anesthetist. In A.B. Hamric, J.A. Spross, & C.M. Hanson (Eds.), *Advanced nursing practice: An integrative approach* (pp. 421-444). Philadelphia: Saunders.

Flexner, A. (1910). *Medical education in the United States and Canada.* New York: Carnegie Foundation.

Ford, L.C. (1970). A nurse for all settings: The nurse practitioner. *Nursing Outlook, 27,* 516-521.

Ford, L.C. (1982). Nurse practitioners: History of a new idea and predictions for the future. In L.H. Aiken (Ed.), *Nursing in the 80s* (pp. 231-248). Philadelphia: Lippincott.

Ford, L.C. (1991). Advanced nursing practice: Future of the nurse practitioner. In L.H. Aiken & C.M. Fagin (Eds.), *Charting nursing's future: Agenda for the 1990s* (pp. 287-299). New York: Lippincott.

Ford, L.C., & Silver, H.K. (1967). The expanded role of the nurse in child care. *Nursing Outlook, 15,* 43-45.

Forbes, K.E., Rafson, J., Spross, J.A., & Kozlowski, D. (1990). The clinical nurse specialist and nurse practitioner: Core curriculum survey results. *Clinical Nurse Specialist, 4*(2), 63-66.

Frank v. South, 175 KY. 416-428 (1917).

Friereich, E. (1984). Landmark perspective: Nitrogen mustard therapy. *Journal of the American Medical Association, 251,* 2262-2263.

Frontier Nursing Service (FNS). (1948). *Medical routines.* Lexington, KY: University of Kentucky, Frontier Nursing Service Collection.

Georgopoulos, B.S., & Christman, L. (1970). The clinical nurse specialist: A role model. *American Journal of Nursing, 70,* 1030-1039.

Georgopoulos, B.S., & Jackson, M.M. (1970). Nursing Kardex behavior in an experimental study of patient units with and without clinical specialists. *Nursing Research, 19,* 196-218.

Georgopoulos, B.S., & Sana, M. (1971). Clinical nursing specialization and intershift report behavior. *American Journal of Nursing, 71,* 538-545.

Girouard, S. (1978). The role of the clinical nurse specialist as change agent: An experiment in preoperative teaching. *International Journal of Nursing Studies, 15,* 57-65.

Goldmark, J. (1923). *Nursing and nursing education in the United States.* (Report of the Committee for the Study of Nursing Education). New York: Garland.

Grey, M. (1999). *New Deal medicine: The rural health programs of the Farm Security Administration.* Baltimore: Johns Hopkins University.

Hadley, E. (1989). Nurses and prescriptive authority: A legal and economic analysis. *American Journal of Law and Medicine, 15*(213), 245-299.

Hamric, A., Lindbak, S., Jaubert, S., & Worley, D. (1998). Outcomes associated with advanced nursing practice prescriptive authority. *Journal of the American Academy of Nurse Practitioners, 10,* 113-118.

Hamric, A.B. (1989). History and overview of the CNS role. In A.B. Hamric & J.A. Spross (Eds.), *The clinical nurse specialist in theory and practice* (2nd ed., pp. 3-18). Philadelphia: Saunders.

Hamric, A.B., & Spross, J. (Eds.). (1983). *The clinical nurse specialist in theory and practice.* New York: Grune & Stratton.

Hamric, A.B., & Spross, J.A. (Eds.). (1989). *The clinical nurse specialist in theory and practice* (2nd ed.). Philadelphia: Saunders.

Howell, J. (1996). *Technology in the hospital.* Baltimore: Johns Hopkins University Press.

Idaho Code 54-1413 (1971).

Inglis, A.D., & Kjervik, D.K. (1993). Empowerment of advanced practice nurses: Regulation reform needed to increase access to care. *Journal of Law, Medicine and Ethics, 21*(2), 193-205.

Institute of Medicine (IOM). (2000). *To err is human: Building a safer health system.* Washington, DC: National Academy of Science Press.

Jenicek, J. (1967). Vietnam—new challenges for the army nurse anesthetist. *Journal of the American Association of Nurse Anesthetists, 67,* 347-352.

Jolly, E. (1927). *Nuns of the battlefield.* Providence, RI: The Providence Visitor Press.

Jonas, S. (1981). *Health care delivery in the United States.* New York: Springer.

Kalisch, P.A., & Kalisch, B.J. (1986). *The advance of American nursing* (2nd ed.). Boston: Little, Brown.

Keane, A,. & Richmond, T. (1993). Tertiary nurse practitioners. *Image: Journal of Nursing Scholarship, 25,* 281-284.

Keeling, A. (2004). Blurring the boundaries between medicine and nursing: Coronary care nursing, circa the 1960s. *Nursing History Review, 12,* 139-164.

Keeling, A. (2007). *Nursing and the privilege of prescription.* Columbus, OH: The Ohio State University Press.

Kitzman, H.J. (1983). The CNS and the nurse practitioner. In A.B. Hamric & J.A. Spross (Eds.), *The clinical nurse specialist in theory and practice* (pp. 275-290). New York: Grune & Stratton.

Kleinpell, R.M. (1997). Acute care nurse practitioners: Roles and practice profiles. *AACN Clinical Issues, 8,* 156-162.

Little, D.E., & Carnevali, D. (1967). Nurse specialist effect on tuberculosis. *Nursing Research, 16,* 321-326.

Lynaugh, J.E., & Brush, B.L. (1996). *American nursing: From hospitals to health systems.* Cambridge, MA: Milbank Memorial Fund and Blackwell Publishers.

Lynaugh, J.E., & Fairman, J. (1992). New nurses, new spaces: A preview of the AACN history study. *American Journal of Critical Nursing, 1*(1), 19-24.

Mackenzie, E. (1929). *Report of the Associate Director, Henry Street Visiting Nurses Service,* December 15, 1928–January 15, 1929, Lillian Wald Collection, Columbia University. Box 46, folder 1.15, 1-3.

Magaw, A. (May 1900). Observations on 1092 cases of anesthesia from January 1, 1899, to January 1, 1900. *St. Paul's Medical Journal,* 306-311.

Magyary, D., Whitney, J, & Brown, M. (2006). Advancing practice inquiry: Research foundations of the practice doctorate in nursing, *Nursing Outlook, 543,* 139-151.

McBride, A.B., Austin, J.K., Chestnut, E.E., Main, C.S., Richards, B.S., & Roy, B.A. (1987). Evaluation of the impact of the clinical nurse specialist in a state psychiatric hospital. *Archives of Psychiatric Nursing, 1,* 55-61.

McGarrel, A. (July 1934. (official reporter) Transcript on appeal, Vol. 1. William Chalmers-Francis and the Anesthesia Section of the *LA County Medical Association v. Dagmar A. Nelson and St. Vincent's Hospital.* Xeroxed copy RG 0811. AANA Executive Office, Historical Files, Chicago, IL.

Mitchell-DiCenso, A., Guyatt, G., Marrin, M., Goeree, R., Willan, A., Southwell, D. et al. (1996). A controlled trial of nurse practitioners in neonatal intensive care. *Pediatrics, 98,* 1143-1148.

Mundinger, M., Kane, R., Lenz, E., Totten, A., Tsai, W.Y., Cleary, P., et al. (2000). Primary care outcomes in patients treated by nurse practitioners or physicians, *JAMA, 283*(1), 59-68.

Moxley, J. (1968). The predicament in health manpower. *American Journal of Nursing, 68,* 1489-1492.

National League for Nursing (NLN). (1984). *Master's education in nursing: Route to opportunities in contemporary nursing, 1984-1985.* New York: Author.

National League for Nursing (NLN). (1994). *Graduate education in nursing: Advanced practice nursing.* New York: Author.

National Organization of Nurse Practitioner Faculties (NONPF). (1997). *Criteria for evaluation of nurse practitioner programs.* Washington, DC: National Task Force on Quality Nurse Practitioner Education.

Negro nurse-midwives. (1942). *American Journal of Nursing, 42,* 705.

News about nursing: Nursing and national defense: Nurse anesthetists in the Army Nurse Corps. (1942). *American Journal of Nursing, 42,* 451.

News here and there: American Association of Nurse-Midwives.(1942). American Journal of Nursing, 42, 832.

Office of Technology Assessment. (1986). *Nurse practitioners, physicians assistants and certified nurse-midwives: A policy analysis.* Washington DC: U.S. Congress, HCS 37. Washington, DC: Author.

Olsen, G.W. (1940). The nurse anesthetists: Past, present and future. *Bulletin of the American Association of Nurse Anesthetists, 8,* 296-299.

Oltz v. St. Peter's Community Hospital, CV 81-271-H-Res (D. Mont. 1986).

Peplau, H.E. (1952). *Interpersonal relations in nursing: A conceptual frame of reference for psychodynamic nursing.* New York: Putnam.

Peplau, H.E. (1965). Specialization in professional nursing. *Nursing Science, 3,* 268-287.

Reiter, F. (1966). The nurse-clinician. *American Journal of Nursing, 66,* 274-280.

Reverby, S.M. (1987). *Ordered to care: The dilemma of American nursing, 1850-1945.* New York: Cambridge University Press.

Richards, L. (1911). *Reminiscences of America's first trained nurse* (reprint). Boston: Whitcomb & Barrows.

Rinker, S. (2000). To cultivate a feeling of confidence: The nursing of obstetric patients, 1890-1940. *Nursing History Review, 8,* 117-142.

Rogers, M.E. (1972). Nursing: To be or not to be. *Nursing Outlook, 20,* 42-46.

Rooks, J. (1997). *Midwifery and childbirth in America.* Philadelphia: Temple University Press.

Safriet, B.J. (1992). Health care dollars and regulatory sense: The role of advance practice nursing. *Yale Journal on Regulation, 9,* 417-488.

Safriet, B.J. (1998). Still spending dollars, still searching for sense: Advanced practice nursing in an era of regulatory and economic turmoil. *Advanced Practice Nursing Quarterly, 4,* 24-33.

Schindler, F. (1942). Nursing in electro-shock therapy. *American Journal of Nursing, 42,* 858-861.

Schutt, B. (1971). A prophet honored. *American Journal of Nursing, 71*(1), 53.

Sermchief v. Gonzales, 660 S.W.2d 683 (1983).

Shah, H., Brutlomesso, K., Sullivan, D., & Lattanzio, J. (1997). An evaluation of the role and practices of the acute care nurse practitioner. *AACN Clinical Issues, 8,* 147-155.

Shakespeare, W. (2002). The Tempest. In S. Orgel & A.R. Braunmuller (Eds.), *William Shakespeare 1564-1616: The complete works* (2.1.245-253). New York: Penguin.

Sills, G.M. (1983). The role, function of the clinical nurse specialist. In N.L. Chaska (Ed.), *The nursing profession: A time to speak* (pp. 563-579). New York: McGraw-Hill.

Silver, H.K., & McAtee, P. (1988). Speaking out: Should nurses substitute for house staff? *American Journal of Nursing, 88,* 1671-1673.

Smith, S. (1994). White nurses, black midwives, and public health in Mississippi, 1920-1950. *Nursing History Review, 2,* 29-49.

Spalding, E. (1943). The Bolton Act provides federal funds for postgraduate programs. *American Journal of Nursing, 43,* 833.

Sparacino, P. (1990). A historical perspective on the development of the CNS role. In P. Sparacino, D.M. Cooper, & P.A. Minarik (Eds.), *The CNS: Implementation and impact* (pp. 3-10), Norwalk, CT: Appleton & Lange.

Spross, J., & Hamric, A.B. (1983). A model for future clinical specialist practice. In A.B. Hamric & J. Spross (Eds.), *The clinical nurse specialist in theory and practice* (pp. 291-306). New York: Grune & Stratton.

Strickland, R. (1995). Isabella Coler Herb MD: An early leader in anesthesiology. *Anesthesia and Analgesia, 80,* 3: 600-605.

Summers, V. (1938). Saddle bag and log cabin technic. *The American Journal of Nursing, 38,* 1183-1189.

Taussig, F.J. (June 1914). The nurse-midwife. *Public Health Quarterly,* 33-39.

Thatcher, V.S. (1953). *A history of anesthesia: With emphasis on the nurse specialist.* Philadelphia: Lippincott.

U.S. Department of Health, Education, & Welfare (HEW) Secretary's Committee to Study Extended Roles for Nurses. (1972). *Extending the scope of nursing practice: A report of the Secretary's Committee* (pp. 3-6). Washington, DC: U.S. Government Printing Office.

U.S. Department of Health and Human Services (HHS). (1996). *The registered nurse population March* 1996. *Findings from the National Sample Survey of Registered Nurses.* Washington, DC: Author.

U.S. Federal Security Agency. (1950). *Cadet Nurse Corps and other federal nurse training programs.* Washington, DC: U.S. Government Printing Office.

Varney, H. (1987). *Nurse-midwifery* (2nd ed.). Boston: Blackwell Scientific.

Waisel, D. (2001). The role of World War II and the European theater of operations in the development of anesthesiology as a physician specialty in the USA. *Anesthesiology, 94,* 907-912.

Wald, L. (1922). *The origin and development of Henry Street Settlement.* Text for Broadcasting, The Westinghouse Electric and Manufacturing Co., Reel #25, Lillian Wald Papers, New York Public Library.

Wall, B.M. (2005). *Unlikely entrepreneurs: Catholic Sisters and the hospital marketplace, 1863-1925.* Columbus: The Ohio State University Press.

White, R. (1943). Army nurses—in the air! *American Journal of Nursing, 43,* 344.

Williams, D. (1931). *Field nurses' narrative report, May 1931.* National Archives and Records Administration, Record Group 75, E779, Box 9.

Wolff, M.A. (1984). Court upholds expanded practice roles for nurses. *Law, Medicine and Health Care, 12,* 26-29.

Woodrow, M., & Bell, J. (1971). Clinical specialization: Conflict between reality and theory. *Journal of Nursing Administration, 1,* 23-27.

CHAPTER 2

Conceptualizations of Advanced Practice Nursing

Judith A. Spross • Marjorie Thomas Lawson*

INTRODUCTION

Fundamental to the sound progress of any practice field is the development of a common language and conceptual framework for communication and for guiding and evaluating practice, education, policy, research, and theory. Although such a foundation is particularly crucial at this stage in the development of advanced practice nursing, a professional consensus on the nature of advanced practice nursing has not yet been reached. In reviewing the literature for this edition, we searched using the term *advanced practice nursing,* the four advanced practice nurse (APN) role phrases, and the authors of models cited in the prior edition. Several types of articles related to model development and advanced practice nursing were identified. These models could be characterized as the following:

- Curriculum models (e.g., Atkins & Ersser, 2000; Curran & Roberts, 2002; Plager, Conger, & Craig, 2003; Thibodeau & Hawkins, 1994; Williams & Kelly, 1998; Williams et al., 1998; Woods, 19)
- Administrative or organizational models (e.g., Gibbins, Green, Scott, & Watson MacDonell, 2000; Valentine, Antai-Otong, Kupecz, Lynn, & Chaffee, 2000; Whitcomb et al., 2002)
- Models that differentiate among advanced practice roles (e.g., Lincoln, 2000; Williams & Valdivieso, 1994)
- Models that differentiate between basic and advanced practice nursing (e.g., Calkin, 1984; Oberle & Allen, 2001)
- Models of the nature of advanced practice nursing (Ball & Cox, 2003; Brown, 1998; Hamric, 1996, 2000, 2005; and see Chapter 3; Mantzoukas & Watkinson, 2007)
- Models of role development of advanced practice nurses (APNs) (e.g., Brown & Olshansky, 1997, and see Chapter 4)
- Models of APN regulation and credentialing (e.g., Raudonis & Anderson, 2002; APRN Joint Dialogue Work Group, 2007a, 2007b; Styles, 1998)

- Models of APN care delivery (Cumbie, Conley, & Burman, 2004; McCabe & Macnee, 2002) and role implementation (Ball & Cox, 2004; Bryant-Lukosius, DiCenso, Browne, & Pinelli, 2004)
- Models that APNs would find useful (e.g., Curley, 1998; Thibodeau & Hawkins, 1994)

In addition to these types of models, professional organizations with interests in defining, educating, and accrediting APNs can be viewed as operating from some conceptualization of advanced practice nursing, whether implicit or explicit. In the previous edition, we identified problems associated with lack of a unified definition of advanced practice and imperatives for undertaking this important work. We concluded, as had Styles and Lewis (2000), that little progress had been made in defining and clarifying advanced nursing practice and made several recommendations. Since that time, a number of organizations have led or participated in important consensus-building initiatives that promise to bring clarity to licensing, accreditation, certification, and educational (LACE) issues in advanced practice nursing. This work is described in detail in Chapter 21. Of particular relevance to this chapter are the Doctor of Nursing Practice (DNP) (American Association of Colleges of Nursing, [AACN], 2006) and the regulatory model of advanced nursing practice that is being developed from a collaboration of national stakeholder organizations (APRN Joint Dialogue Group, 2008).

The purpose of this chapter is to lay the foundation for thinking about the concepts underlying advanced practice nursing and to outline future directions and recommendations that may foster professional consensus on advanced practice nursing. Using published documents from national professional organizations

---

*The authors and editors express their gratitude to Margretta Styles and Carolyn Lewis, authors of this chapter in the first and second editions, for their keen insights and clarity of thinking about advanced practice. We also acknowledge Ann Hamric and Charlene Hanson for their contributions in revising the chapter.

and the literature, the authors focus selectively on the following types of models of APN practice: those promulgated by professional organizations for all APNs and those that address a specific APN role; those that aim to explicate the nature of advanced practice nursing; and conceptualizations that are useful to APNs. The models that relate to identifying and evaluating outcomes of advanced practice nursing have been moved to Chapter 24. This review is not exhaustive. For example, in limiting the scope of this chapter, statements on advanced practice nursing by specialty organizations have not been examined. Although we reviewed articles on conceptualizations of advanced practice nursing proposed by authors writing about advanced practice in foreign countries (e.g., Ball & Cox, 2004; Mantzoukas & Watkinson, 2007), information on the International Council of Nursing (ICN) Advanced Practice Network (International Council of Nursing [ICN], 2006), indicated that advanced practice nursing seemed to be moving in somewhat different directions from advanced practice in the United States. For example, advanced practice nursing may or may not include both clinical nurse specialists (CNSs) and nurse practitioners (NPs). Content from these articles is used to illuminate certain points of specific models or in the discussion of recommendations and future directions. International efforts are underway to examine advanced practice nursing, including issues related to credentialing (Sheer, 2007) (the Evolve website for this chapter contains information and activities relevant to advanced practice nursing internationally). We invite readers to debate and enlarge upon the models, issues, and thinking put forward in this chapter.

THE NATURE, PURPOSES, AND COMPONENTS OF CONCEPTUAL MODELS

What is a conceptual model? What purposes does it serve? What are its components? A number of answers to these questions are in the nursing literature. Fawcett (2000, 2001) identified a conceptual model as "a set of relatively abstract and general concepts that address the phenomena of central interest to a discipline, the propositions that broadly describe these concepts, and the propositions that state relatively abstract and general relations between two or more of the concepts" (2001, p. 380). In describing nurse-midwifery, Carveth (1987) drew heavily from various expert sources to arrive at a clear, comprehensive, and general explanation of a conceptual model, paraphrased as follows.

A conceptual model is that which orders, clarifies, and systematizes selected components of the phenomenon (e.g., nursing) it serves to depict. The components of conceptual models are concepts and relationships (i.e., concepts in meaningful configuration) serving as building blocks that reflect assumptions about the philosophy, values, and practices of a profession. The model then becomes a tool for interrelating concepts in a way in which the concepts can be better understood and explained.

Conceptual models serve many purposes. Models may help APNs articulate professional role identity and function, serving as a framework for organizing their beliefs and knowledge about their professional roles and practice and providing a sound base for further development of knowledge. The Strong Memorial Model, discussed later in this chapter, is such a model. In clinical practice, APNs use conceptual models to understand the bigger picture so that holistic, comprehensive care is provided. Models may also be used to differentiate among levels of nursing practice (e.g., staff nursing and advanced practice nursing as discussed later in Calkin's model). In research and other scholarly activities, investigators use conceptual models to guide the conceptualization of research and theory development. An investigator could decide to focus on the study of one concept or examine relationships among select concepts to elucidate testable theories. For example, research by Fenton (1985) and Brykczynski (1989), described later in this chapter, elucidated new domains of practice for CNSs and NPs, respectively. In education, faculty use conceptual models to plan curricula, identify important concepts and the relationships among them, and make choices about course content and clinical experiences, based on such models. For example, Plager and colleagues (2003) developed a model that helped their faculty differentiate among APN roles and informed the design of the curricula for NPs and CNSs.

Fawcett and colleagues (Fawcett, Newman, & McAllister, 2004; Fawcett & Graham, 2005) raised conceptual questions about advanced practice: What do APNs do that makes their practice "advanced"? To what extent does incorporating activities traditionally done by physicians qualify the practice as "advanced"? Are there nursing activities that are also advanced? Because direct clinical practice is viewed as the central APN competency, what does the word *clinical* mean—does it refer to only hospitals or clinics? Thus a well-thought-out, robust conceptual model helps individuals answer important questions about the phenomenon. Despite the utility and benefits of conceptual models, some difficulties are apparent when the advanced practice nursing literature is examined.

CONCEPTUALIZATIONS OF ADVANCED PRACTICE NURSING: PROBLEMS AND IMPERATIVES

As noted in prior editions of this text, there have been problems with conceptualizations of advanced practice nursing. In addition, when one examines the clinical and professional issues inherent in advanced practice nursing, imperatives for clarifying advanced practice and arriving at a professional consensus on what it is and what it is not are apparent. Four areas of conceptual confusion or uncertainty in the evolution of advanced practice nursing can be identified.

The first issue is that well-defined and consistently applied terms of reference are absent. A core, stable vocabulary, a lingua franca, is needed for definition and model building. The lack of a consistent, stable vocabulary can be seen in the literature. For example, the basic elements or building blocks of conceptual models of advanced practice nursing literature are variously labeled *domains, theories, roles, subroles, hallmarks, competencies, functions, activities, skills,* and *abilities*. The problem in comparing, refining, or developing models is that these terms are used with no universal meaning or frame of reference; occasionally, no definition is offered at all or terms are used inconsistently. In introducing their nurse practitioner (NP) model, Shuler and Davis (1993a) stated, "One of the greatest barriers to using nursing models in practice relates to vocabulary and communication within the models" (p. 11). This instability and inconsistency are evident in the various models cited in this chapter. It is rightly anticipated that conceptual models of the field and its practice change over time. However, the evolution of advanced practice nursing and its comprehension by nurses, policymakers, and others would be enhanced if scholars and practitioners in the field could agree on the use and definition of fundamental terms of reference.

The second issue is that many attempts to articulate models of advanced practice nursing fail to consider extant literature that is directly relevant to such conceptualizing activities. In part, this seems to be because of a lag between the conceptualizing effort and its ultimate publication, as well as the knowledge explosion. For example, some articles reviewed for this chapter with recent publication dates cited work from the 1980s and 1990s; revised publications of these earlier works, though apparently available, were not cited. We note this as a caution to be considered in proposing, evaluating, or refining advanced practice nursing models.

The third issue is a lack of clarity regarding conceptualizations that differentiate between and among levels of clinical practice. There is much to understand about how the practice of APNs differs from the practice of non–master's prepared experts-by-experience and how the practice of an APN certified in a subspecialty such as oncology differs from the practice of a non–master's prepared clinician who is certified at the basic level (not advanced) in the oncology subspecialty (Fawcett et al., 2004; Hanson & Hamric, 2003). For example, many authors who write about advanced practice nursing cite Benner's Model of Expert Practice (1984) without clearly indicating that the model was derived from the study of nurses who were experts-by-experience, not APNs. Certainly, Benner's model is relevant to efforts to conceptualize advanced practice nursing as demonstrated by Fenton's (1985) and Brykczynski's (1989) work. Given that clinical practice is the *raison d'etre* for the profession of nursing and is central to advanced practice nursing, models that help the profession differentiate levels of practice are needed.

The fourth issue is to clarify the differences between advanced practice nursing and medicine (see, for example, the Schuler Model on pp. 56-57). Students struggle with this issue as part of role development (see Chapter 4). This lack of conceptual clarity is apparent in advertisements that invite NPs or physician assistants to apply for the same job. Fawcett, a well-respected nursing leader, asked, "What does it mean to blend nursing and medicine?" (Fawcett et al., 2004; Fawcett & Graham, 2005). In addition, as noted in Chapters 20 and 21, organized medicine expends resources in trying to limit or discredit advanced practice nursing. Hamric, in Chapter 3, asserts that advanced practice nursing is not the junior practice of medicine. The articulation of the seven competencies of advanced nursing practice (Chapters 5 through 11) supports this assertion.

In addition to these problems, imperatives for reaching a conceptual consensus can be identified in three broad, interrelated areas: policymaking, licensing and credentialing, and practice. In the policymaking arena, for example, not all APNs are eligible to be reimbursed by insurers and even those activities that are reimbursable are often billed incident to a physician's care, rendering the work of APNs invisible. Further evidence of the need for consensus is the National Council of State Boards of Nursing (NCSBN) proposal for a uniform licensing compact that would standardize criteria for advanced practice nursing licensure (National Council of State Boards of Nursing [NCSBN], 2002). There has been progress in this area since the previous edition. In the United States, both an NCSBN APRN Committee and an APRN Consensus Work Group has worked to develop a consensus statement on advanced practice nursing (APRN Joint Dialogue Group, 2007a, 2007b, 2008; Stanley & the APRN Consensus Work Group, 2007; see also Chapters 21 and 22 and p. 43 in this chapter). In practice, little is understood about the impact of APN-physician collaboration on practice or strategies for matching the level of nursing knowledge and skill to the needs of patient populations (Brooten & Youngblut, 2006; Calkin, 1984). These illustrations are examples of many professional imperatives for reaching a consensus on the nature and definition of advanced practice nursing. As outlined in Chapters 21 and 22, the profession is at a critical juncture in terms of policymaking: policies created today will have far-reaching effects and will shape every aspect of APN practice—APN education, APN regulation and credentialing, scopes of APN practice, the populations with whom and the environments in which APNs work, compensation for APN activities, and research priorities. To fully appreciate the interrelationships between concepts of advanced practice nursing and their effects on LACE and APN practice, the reader is encouraged to refer back to Chapter 2 when reading Chapters 12 through 18 in Part III and Chapters 21 and 22 in Part IV.

Some conceptual models reviewed in this chapter are more narrowly focused than others. Some advanced practice models are more homogeneous and some are mixed with respect to the phenomenon studied. Some could be seen as micro-models in terms of the unit of analysis, and others could be seen as meta-models, incorporating a number of conceptual frameworks. Some models explain systems; others explain relationships between systems. All these foci are important, depending on the purposes to be served. However, in the development of conceptual models, the phenomenon to be modeled must be carefully defined. For example, is the model intended to encompass the entire field of advanced practice nursing or is it confined to distinctive concepts such as collaborative practice between physicians and

APNs? If a phenomenon and its related concepts are not clearly delimited, it is possible that the model will be so inconsistent as to be confusing or so comprehensive that its impact will be diluted.

Assumptions about the philosophy, values, and practices of the profession are reflected in conceptual models. The present discussion of conceptualizations of advanced practice nursing is guided by two assumptions. The first is that the development and strengthening of the field of advanced practice nursing depends on a professional consensus regarding the nature of advanced practice nursing (a conceptual framework) that can inform APN program accreditation and credentialing and practice. The second is that advanced practice nursing will reach its full potential to the extent that important conceptual components of the framework are delineated. Clarification and consensus on conceptualization of the nature of advanced practice nursing will lead to the following outcomes:

1. Clear differentiation of advanced practice nursing from other levels of clinical nursing practice
2. Clear differentiation between advanced practice nursing and the clinical practice of physicians and other non-nurse providers within a specialty
3. Clear delineation of the similarities and differences among APN roles
4. Regulation and credentialing of APNs that protects the public and ensures equitable treatment of all APNs
5. Clear articulation of federal and state health policies that: (a) recognize and make visible the substantive contributions of APNs to quality, cost effective health care, and patient outcomes; (b) ensure the public's access to APN care; and (c) ensure explicit and appropriate mechanisms to bill and pay for APN care
6. A maximum social contribution by APNs in health care, including improvement in health outcomes and health-related quality of life for the people to whom they provide care
7. The actualization of practitioners of advanced practice nursing—APNs will reach their full potential personally and professionally

CONCEPTUALIZATIONS OF ADVANCED PRACTICE NURSING

Practice with individual clients and patients is the central clinical work of the field. Practice is the reason for which nursing was created. What are the characteristics of advanced practice nursing? How does advanced practice nursing differ from other types of nursing practice, particularly the clinical practice of nurses who are not master's prepared, who are experts-by-experience, and who are often certified in a specialty? What is the scope and purpose of advanced practice nursing? How do APNs' scopes of practice differ from those of other providers offering similar or related services? What knowledge and skills are required? Within what settings does this practice occur? When has a specialty evolved to the point that society needs APNs in a new field? When should health care systems employ APNs, and what types of patients particularly benefit from advanced practice nursing care? For what types of pressing health care problems are APNs a solution in terms of improving outcomes, quality of care, and cost-effectiveness?

These and other questions have encouraged scores of writers to describe advanced practice nursing from a variety of perspectives. The Oncology Nursing Society and the American Association of Critical-Care Nurses have addressed advanced practice nursing in their particular specialties. Specialty and subspecialty models and standards are important to students and APNs but are not addressed in this chapter. As students and readers consider their own APN practices, they may want to review both the history of advanced practice nursing (see Chapter 1) and evolving advanced practice nursing roles (see Chapter 18) to inform their efforts to conceptualize their own practice of advanced nursing.

In the next section, we examine the implicit and explicit conceptualizations of advanced practice nursing promulgated by professional organizations concerned with defining APN practice and with clarifying particular APN roles.

Professional Organizations' Conceptualizations

Although not all of the documents described in this chapter are conceptual models, many include a conceptual framework or reference a conceptual framework. Some of the problems with the absence of a core vocabulary noted previously are apparent as one reads the different approaches taken by organizations, so comparisons are difficult to make because terms of reference and their meanings vary. To help the reader appreciate the challenge of developing a common language to characterize advanced practice, dictionary definitions of terms used in conceptualizations of advanced practice nursing are found in Box 2-1. In spite of differences in terminology, the efforts of the profession to come to grips with a definition of advanced practice nursing are evident in all of these documents. Reflection on and discussion of the various terms used and debate about interpreting them—for example, *roles, domains*, and *competencies*—may contribute to clarification of conceptual models and the emergence of a common language. The descriptions of each model in the following sections are necessarily limited. The reader is encouraged to refer to the original documents and publications to more fully understand advanced practice nursing as described by organizations and individual authors. Website addresses for national APN organizations are found in Chapter 21. The work of the NCSBN, the APRN Consensus Work Group, and the APRN Joint Dialogue Group is discussed at the end of this

Box 2-1   Definition of Terms

Competent Having requisite or adequate ability or qualities; legally qualified or adequate; having the capacity to function or develop in a particular way; (sufficient)

Competence/Competency The quality or state of being competent; the knowledge that enables a person to speak and understand a language

Component A constituent part; ingredient

Domain A sphere of knowledge, influence, or activity

Role A socially expected behavior pattern usually determined by an individual's status in a particular society

Hallmark Distinguishing characteristic, trait, or feature

Sphere An area or range over or within which someone or something acts, exists, or has influence or significance

Scope Space or opportunity for unhampered motion, activity, or thought; extent of treatment, activity, or influence

Standard Something established by authority, custom, or general consent as a model or example; something set up and established by an authority as a rule for the measure of quantity, weight, extent, value, or quality

From Mish, F.C. (Ed.). (2001). *Merriam-Webster's collegiate dictionary* (10th ed.). Springfield, MA: Merriam-Webster, International.

section since it is the result of collaboration of many organizations.

American Nurses Association and the American Board of Nursing Specialties. In addition to standards for basic and advanced nursing practice (American Nurses Association [ANA], 1996, 2004), the ANA has periodically published a social policy statement (ANA, 1980, 1995, 2003). In earlier editions of the statement, specialization, expansion, and advancement were identified as concepts that differentiated advanced practice nursing from basic nursing practice. In addition to explicit recognition of certified nurse-midwives (CNMs), CNSs, certified registered nurse anesthetists (CRNAs), and NPs as APNs, it was noted that APNs use both expanded and specialized knowledge and skills in their practices. According to the 2003 statement, expansion, specialization, and advanced practice were defined as follows (ANA, 2003):

> *Expansion* refers to the acquisition of new practice knowledge and skills, including the knowledge and skills that legitimize role autonomy within areas of practice that may overlap traditional boundaries of medical practice.
>
> *Specialization* is concentrating or delimiting one's focus to part of the whole field of nursing such as ambulatory care, pediatric, maternal-child, psychiatric, palliative care, or oncology nursing.
>
> *Advanced practice* is characterized by the integration of a broad range of theoretical, research-based, and practical knowledge that occurs as part of graduate education. Advanced practice registered nurses are either certified or approved to practice in their expanded, specialized roles. (p. 9)

More recently, the ANA and the American Board of Nursing Specialties (ABNS) staff have been working with other stakeholder organizations, including the National Association of Clinical Nurse Specialists (NACNS), to define CNS competencies, an effort discussed under the APRN Consensus Working and Joint Dialogue Groups.

American Association of Colleges of Nursing. Over the past 5 years, AACN has undertaken two nursing education initiatives that are aimed at transforming nursing education. *The Essentials of Master's Education for Advanced Practice Nursing* (AACN, 1996), which defined curricular elements

and competencies that should be part of master's level education for all APNs, continues to guide master's level APN education. However, AACN has called for all APN preparation to take place at the doctoral level in practice-based programs (Doctor of Nursing Practice [DNP]) by 2015, with master's level education being refocused on preparation of clinical nurse leaders (CNLs). CNLs are not APNs (AACN, 2002) and therefore are not included in our discussion of conceptualizations. Through these initiatives and to the extent that AACN and the Commission on Collegiate Nursing Education (CCNE) influence accreditation, the DNP is likely to become the preferred degree for APNs, though this goal is controversial. Because graduate education for APNs is in transition, a brief overview of both the existing *Essentials* for APN education (AACN, 1996) and the recently approved *Essentials* for DNP education (AACN, 2006) as they relate to advanced nursing practice will be provided. The *Essentials* for master's education (1996) specified three types of core content. The *graduate nursing core* specifies content for all graduate nursing programs whether in advanced practice, administration, or education (e.g., ethics and theory courses). An *advanced practice nursing core* that includes advanced health/physical assessment, advanced physiology and pathophysiology, and advanced pharmacology is specified for APNs. *Specialty core* includes content and clinical practice that help students acquire the knowledge and skills essential to a specific advanced practice role.

The DNP *Essentials* (AACN, 2006) are comprised of eight competencies for DNP graduates (Box 2-2). Graduates are expected to demonstrate the eight Essentials upon graduation. "Essential VIII specifies the foundational practice competencies that cut across specialties and are seen as requisite for DNP practice"(Box 2-3) (AACN, 2006, p. 16). Recognizing that DNP programs will prepare nurses for roles other than APN roles, the authors of the DNP *Essentials* acknowledge that specialty organizations (those related to roles such as the CNSs and NPs) are expected to develop Essential VIII as it relates to the advanced practice role and "to develop competency expectations that build upon and complement DNP *Essentials* I through VIII" (AACN, 2006, p. 17). The advanced practice nursing core described in the 1996 *Essentials* will be required for DNP-APNs (AACN, 2006). Although the DNP remains controversial (Avery & Howe, 2007; American College of Nurse-Midwives [ACNM], 2007b; American Association of

Box 2-2   The Essentials of Doctoral Education for Advanced Nursing Practice

I. Scientific underpinnings for practice	V. Health care policy for advocacy in health care
II. Organizational and systems leadership for quality improvement and systems thinking	VI. Interprofessional collaboration for improving patient and population health outcomes
III. Clinical scholarship and analytical methods for evidence-based practice	VII. Clinical prevention and population health for improving the nation's health
IV. Information systems/technology and patient care technology for the improvement and transformation of health care	VIII. Advanced nursing practice

From American Association of Colleges of Nursing (AACN) (2006). *Essentials of doctoral education for advanced nursing practice.* Retrieved July 24, 2007, from www.aacn.nche. edu/dnp/PDF/essentials.PDF.

Box 2-3   Essential VIII: Advanced Nursing Practice Competencies

I. Conduct a comprehensive and systematic assessment of health and illness parameters in complex situations, incorporating diverse and culturally sensitive approaches.	IV. Demonstrate advanced levels of clinical judgment, systems thinking, and accountability in designing, delivering, and evaluating evidence-based care to improve patient outcomes.
II. Design, implement, and evaluate therapeutic interventions based on nursing science and other sciences.	V. Guide, mentor, and support other nurses to achieve excellence in nursing practice.
III. Develop and sustain therapeutic relationships and partnerships with patients (individual, family, or group) and other professionals to facilitate optimal care and patient outcomes.	VI. Educate and guide individuals and groups through complex health and situational transitions.
	VII. Use conceptual and analytical skills in evaluating the links among practice, organizational, population, fiscal, and policy issues.

From American Association of Colleges of Nursing (AACN) (2006). *Essentials of doctoral education for advanced nursing practice.* Retrieved July 24, 2007, from www.aacn.nche. edu/dnp/PDF/essentials.PDF.

Nurse Anesthetists [AANA], 2006a, 2006b; National Association of Clinical Nurse Specialists [NACNS], 2005; National Organization of Nurse Practitioner Faculties [NONPF], 2006b), the AACN DNP is one of several national initiatives that has contributed to a broader discussion of advanced practice nursing that may lead the profession closer to a clearer definition of advanced practice.

Although not a conceptual model per se, the AACN *Essentials* documents (1996, 2006) include concepts and content that are evident in the educational components of the majority of other documents that address standards of APN practice and education. The response of APN organizations representing the four APN roles to the DNP initiative are briefly discussed on pp. 40-42; readers are encouraged to visit stakeholder organizations' websites for the history and detailed information on organizational responses to AACN's DNP position paper (2004). Initiatives such as AACN's highlight the urgency of conceptualizing advanced practice nursing so that new nursing roles such as the CNL or nurse informaticist can be adequately distinguished from APNs in discussions of advanced practice nursing in agencies, in the boardroom, and in policy arenas.

National Council of State Boards of Nursing. The variation in regulation of advanced practice nurses prompted the leaders of the NCSBN to undertake a number of initiatives to bring more consistency to the licensing of APNs and to the regulation of advanced practice nursing. In 2002 a role delineation study of NPs and CNSs was published (Chornick, 2002). The main conclusion of this study was that there was more overlap in the priority and criticality of activities than differences for these two roles. (Note that such studies comparing NPs and CNSs in specialties suggest that the knowledge base is similar and some activities are similar but there may be important differences in the frequency and types of some activities or interventions (e.g., McMillan, Heusinkveld, Spray, and Murphy, 1999; Becker, Kaplow, Muenzcen, & Hartigan, 2006). Subsequent to Chornick's study and considering the impact of the DNP initiative, the NCSBN APRN Advisory Committee published a *Vision Paper: The Future Regulation of Advanced Practice Nursing* (2006) outlining a proposal for a future regulatory model that contained some controversial recommendations. For example, they recommended that CNSs, unless they would be diagnosing disease and prescribing medications, be regulated based on their basic license, not as APNs. The paper generated a great deal of concern and feedback. Although the *Vision* paper could be considered a conceptualization of APN regulation, NCSBN withdrew the paper for revision. We believe the publication of this draft vision paper generated the momentum along with the AACN's DNP initiative for the national consensus building efforts that are currently underway.

National Organization of Nurse Practitioner Faculties. The mission of the NONPF is to provide leadership in promoting quality NP education. In 1990 NONPF published a set of domains and core competencies for primary care NPs based on Benner's (1984) domains of expert nursing practice and the results of Brykczynski's (1989) study of the use of these domains by primary care NPs (Price et al., 1992; Zimmer, et al., 1990). These domains and core competencies serve as a framework for primary care NP curricula. Subsequent work done to validate the NP domains and competencies resulted in revisions, the most recent of which was published in 2006 (NONPF, 2006a). One purpose of the most recent revision of primary care NP competencies was to eliminate redundancy and facilitate evaluation and measurement of the extent to which competencies are met. Within each domain are a number of specific competencies. For example, for primary care/adult/gerontological NPs, across the seven domains in the following list, students are expected to demonstrate 75 competencies upon graduation (NONPF, 2006a). The domains used in each of the documents are as follows:

1. Management of patient health/illness status
2. The nurse practitioner–patient relationship
3. The teaching-coaching function
4. Professional role (includes leadership)
5. Managing and negotiating health care delivery systems
6. Monitoring and ensuring the quality of health care practice
7. Culturally sensitive care

These domains can be considered an implicit conceptual model, derived from the practice of NPs and empirically validated (NONPF, 2002, 2003). The model is intended to inform curriculum design and regulatory and credentialing mechanisms. These two documents are notable for several reasons: the domains and competencies for NPs were developed collaboratively by stakeholder organizations; a similar collaborative process was used by the group that developed domains and competencies for psychiatric mental health nurse practitioners (PMHNPs); and empirical validation has been used to affirm the domains and competencies for each of the two APN roles.

NONPF's most recent position statement on the practice doctorate (2006b) supports the practice doctorate as "an evolutionary step" in the preparation of NPs and endorses the DNP title for this preparation. NONPF indicated their plan to evaluate the implications of the DNP for modifying the current master's level competencies and increasing the number of clinical hours for DNPs. The NONPF-sponsored National Panel on NP Practice Doctorate Competencies (2006) identified the following nine additional "competency areas" for NP DNP graduates in addition to the NP core competencies:

1. Independent practice
2. Scientific foundation
3. Leadership
4. Quality
5. Practice inquiry
6. Technology and information literacy
7. Policy
8. Health delivery system
9. Ethics

It is interesting to note that these are called *competency areas*, not *competencies* or *domains*. Presumably, in addition to being consistent with the DNP *Essentials*, these areas reflect expanded competencies of some of the 75 NP competencies that are listed under the seven domains.

In addition to the primary care NP competencies, domains and competencies for PMHNPs (NONPF, 2003) and for acute care nurse practitioners (ACNPs) have been published (National Panel on Acute Care NP Competencies, 2004; for further discussion of ACNPs and competencies, see Chapter 14).

National Association of Clinical Nurse Specialists. The NACNS published the "Statement on Clinical Nurse Specialist Practice and Education" in 1998 and revised it in 2004. While acknowledging the early conceptualization of CNS practice as subroles proposed by Hamric and Spross (1983, 1989), the authors of the NACNS statement believed that this conceptualization failed to differentiate CNS practice from that of other APNs and proposed a new statement to resolve the ambiguity about this particular APN role. Three spheres of influence are posited: patient, nurses and nursing practice, and organization/system, each of which requires a unique set of competencies (NACNS, 2004) (Figure 2-1). In addition, the statement outlines expected outcomes of CNS practice for each sphere. For each sphere, competencies that parallel the nursing process are identified. Thus for each sphere, CNSs have sphere-specific competencies of assessment, diagnosis, intervention, and evaluation. Previous descriptions of CNS subroles informed the delineation of CNS competencies.

Several components of conceptual models are incorporated into the NACNS statement: a definition of nursing on which the definition of a CNS is based, assumptions that inform the model, essential characteristics, description of the spheres of influence and associated competencies, and recommendations for graduate education. A key assumption, which has empirical validation, is that CNSs have an impact on patients, nursing practice, and institutional outcomes. In 2005, NACNS published a white paper on the DNP. In the paper, a number of concerns were raised, and the leaders called for extensive dialogue with stakeholders. Since then, NACNS leaders convened a summit of CNS stakeholder organizations (2006) to discuss the DNP. For further information see Chapters 12 and 21.

American Association of Nurse Anesthetists and American College of Nurse-Midwives. Advanced practice nursing models of CRNAs and CNMs are implied in the official statements of the American Association of Nurse Anesthetists (AANA) (2005a, 2005b) and the American College of Nurse-Midwives (ACNM) (2003, 2007a). These statements include scopes of practice, standards, and other documents that describe CRNA and CNM practices. See Chapters 16 and 17 for a thorough discussion of CNM and CRNA practice, respectively.

The CRNA's scope of practice is defined in the most recent revision of the AANA's "Scope and Standards for Nurse Anesthesia Practice" (2005a). The scope is followed by 10 items that we would characterize as clinical competencies or responsibilities (e.g., managing a patient's airway)—the direct clinical practice of CRNAs. CRNAs have seven "additional responsibilities" that are within the CRNA's scope of practice that can be characterized as leadership behaviors, including participation in research. Eleven standards and an interpretation for each are also listed. The purposes of the standards are to (1) provide a guide for evaluating CRNA care, (2) provide a common foundation on which CRNAs can develop a quality practice, (3) help the public understand what they can expect from CRNAs, and (4) support and preserve the basic rights of patients. In an interim position on the DNP, the AANA did not support the DNP for entry into CRNA practice, citing a lack of evidence for "mandatory clinical doctoral degrees" (AANA, 2006a). They remain in dialogue with national stakeholder organizations and have established a task force on doctoral preparation for nurse anesthetists (AANA, 2006b).

The scope of practice for CNMs (and certified midwives [CMs] who are not nurses) is defined in three ACNM documents: The "Core Competencies for Basic Midwifery Practice" (ACNM, 2007a), "Standards for the Practice of Midwifery" (ACNM,

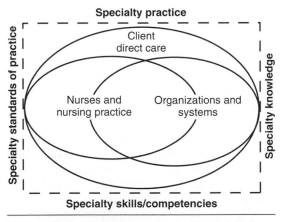

FIGURE **2-1:** National Association of Clinical Nurse Specialists Model. Clinical nurse specialist practice conceptualized as core competencies in three interacting spheres actualized in specialty practice and guided by specialty knowledge and specialty standards. (From National Association of Clinical Nurse Specialists. [2004]. *Statement on clinical nurse specialist practice and education.* Harrisburg, PA: Author.)

2003) and a "Code of Ethics" (ACNM, 2005). The core competencies include 16 hallmarks of the art and science of midwifery and the components of midwifery care, within which are prescribed competencies. Competencies are defined as the "professional responsibilities of CNMs and CMs" (ACNM, 2007a) and detail knowledge, skills, and attitudes expected of a new practitioner. The components of midwifery care are identified as follows:

- Professional responsibilities of CNMs and CMs
- Midwifery management process
- Fundamentals (e.g., knowledge such as anatomy and physiology)
- The primary health care of women
- The childbearing family (includes care of childbearing women and newborns)

These components and associated core competencies are said to make up the foundation on which midwifery curricula practice guidelines are built.

In addition to the competencies, there are eight ACNM standards that midwives are expected to meet (ACNM, 2003) and a Code of Ethics (ACNM, 2005). The standards address such issues as qualifications, safety, patient rights, assessment, documentation, and expansion of midwifery practice. Three ethical mandates related to its mission to promote the health and well-being of women and newborns within their families and communities are identified in the Ethics Code.

In 1998 ACNM issued a statement that was not in support of state-mandated requirements for a master's degree to be licensed as a CNM, a position that conflicted with the standard of graduate education for APNs promoted by most organizations at the time (ACNM, 1998). In 2006 ACNM took the position that by 2010, "completion of a graduate degree will be required for entry into practice"; a particular graduate degree is not specified but the value of preparation in nursing, public health, or other related fields is acknowledged. In addition, persons with a "previously earned graduate degree" will be able to meet the requirements for midwifery practice by completing a certificate. ACNM does not support the DNP as a requirement for entry into nurse-midwifery practice for three reasons. ACNM maintains that midwifery practice is safe based on the rigor of their curriculum standards and outcome data; evidence is insufficient to justify the DNP as a mandatory requirement for CNM; and the costs of attaining such a degree could limit the applicant pool and access to midwifery care (ACNM, 2007b). ACNM reiterated its support of a variety of educational pathways for midwifery preparation, proposes the development of independent schools of midwifery, and supports the DNP as one of many pathways into the profession (ACNM, 2006, 2007b).

The APRN Joint Dialogue Group: A Regulatory Model of Advanced Practice Nursing. Over the past 3 to 4 years, two groups have made significant progress in developing a new regulatory model for APRNs. The APRN Consensus Group was established in 2004 based on a request from AACN and NONPF to the Alliance for APRN Credentialing. The purpose, outlined in the request, was to develop a process for achieving consensus regarding the credentialing of advanced practice nurses (APRN Consensus Work Group, 2007a; APRN Joint Dialogue Group, 2008). Concurrently, the APRN Advisory Committee for NCSBN was charged by the NCSBN Board of Directors with the similar task of creating a future model for APRN regulation (NCSBN, 2006). The Joint Dialogue Group, made up of representatives from the original NCSBN and Consensus groups, has proposed a draft Consensus Model for APRN Regulation (APRN Joint Dialogue Group, 2008).

Organizations represented at the Joint Dialogue Group included ACNM, AANA, NACNS, NCSBN, and NONPF, as well as accrediting bodies. The draft report includes a brief history and consensus development processes; describes the Consensus Model for APRN Regulation (Figure 2-2), including definitions; identifies the titles to be used; defines the term *specialty*; describes the emergence of new roles and population foci; presents strategies for implementation; and proposes a timeline for adoption.

Figure 2-2 depicts the components of the Consensus Model for APRN Regulation: the four recognized APN roles and six population foci. The model also "makes room" for the emergence of new APRN roles. The term *advanced practice registered nurse (APRN)* refers to all four APN roles. An APRN is a nurse who meets the following criteria (APRN Joint Dialogue Group, 2008):

- Completes an accredited graduate-level education program preparing him or her for one of the four recognized APRN roles
- Passes a national certification examination that measures APRN role and population-focused competencies and maintains continued competence as evidenced by recertification in the role and population through the national certification program

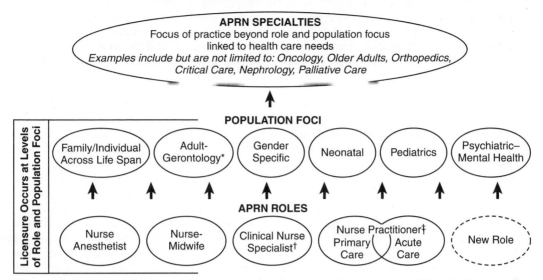

APRN SPECIALTIES
Focus of practice beyond role and population focus
linked to health care needs
*Examples include but are not limited to: Oncology, Older Adults, Orthopedics,
Critical Care, Nephrology, Palliative Care*

POPULATION FOCI

Licensure Occurs at Levels of Role and Population Foci

Family/Individual Across Life Span

Adult-Gerontology*

Gender Specific

Neonatal

Pediatrics

Psychiatric–Mental Health

APRN ROLES

Nurse Anesthetist

Nurse-Midwife

Clinical Nurse Specialist†

Nurse Practitioner‡ Primary Care / Acute Care

New Role

*The population focus *Adult-Gerontology* encompasses the young adult to the older adult, including the frail elderly. APRNs educated and certified in the Adult-Gerontology population are educated and certified across both areas of practice and will be titled Adult-Gerontology CNP or CNS. In addition, all APRNs in any of the four roles providing care to the adult population (e.g. Family or Gender Specific) must be prepared to meet the growing needs of the older adult population. Therefore the education program should include didactic and clinical education experiences necessary to prepare APRNs with these enhanced skills and knowledge.

†The clinical nurse specialist (CNS) is educated and assessed through national certification processes across the continuum from wellness through acute care.

‡The certified nurse practitioner (CNP) is prepared with the acute care CNP competencies and/or the primary care CNP competencies. At this point in time the acute care and primary care CNP delineation applies only to the Pediatrics and Adult-Gerontology CNP population foci. Scope of practice of the primary care or acute care CNP is **not setting-specific** but is based on patient care needs. Programs may prepare individuals across both the primary care and acute care CNP roles. If programs prepare graduates across both roles, the graduate must be prepared with the consensus-based competencies for both roles and must successfully obtain certification in both the acute and the primary care CNP roles.

FIGURE 2-2: **Consensus Model for APRN Regulation.** (From APRN Joint Dialogue Group. [2008]. *Consensus Model for APRN Regulation.* Based on the work of the APRN Consensus Work Group and the NCSBN APRN Advisory Committee. Chicago/Washington, DC: Author.)

- Possesses advanced clinical knowledge and skills preparing him or her to provide direct care to patients; the defining factor for *all* APRNs is that a significant component of the education and practice focuses on direct care of individuals
- Builds on the competencies of registered nurses (RNs) by demonstrating greater depth and breadth of knowledge and greater synthesis of data, by performing more complex skills and interventions, and by possessing greater role autonomy
- Is educationally prepared to assume responsibility and accountability for health promotion and/or maintenance as well as the assessment, diagnosis, and management of patient problems, including the use and prescription of pharmacological and nonpharmacological interventions
- Has sufficient depth and breadth of clinical experience to reflect the intended license
- Obtains a license to practice as an APRN in one of the four APRN roles

In addition to a definition of APRN, an important agreement was that providing direct care to individuals is a defining characteristic of *all* APRN roles. Indeed, the definition of the components of The Consensus Model for APN Regulation begins to address the questions about advanced practice posed on pages 34 and 35.

Broad-based graduate education for the four APRN roles is described: as with the AACN *Essentials* documents (1996, 2006), completion of at least three separate comprehensive graduate courses in advanced physiology/pathophysiology, health assessment, and advanced pharmacology are required. In addition, curricula must address three other areas: the principles of decision making for the particular APN role; preparation in the core competencies identified for the role; and role preparation in one of the six population foci.

It is clear that the Joint Dialogue Group discussed the differences between population foci and specialty. Specialty is a more discrete area of practice than the population focus. The six population foci displayed in Figure 2-2 include adult-gerontology, gender specific, pediatrics, neonatal, psych/mental health and individual/family across the life span. Educational preparation must include a population focus. They note that educational programs preparing APRNs for a specialty must prepare them for one of the six population foci. Thus, for example, students preparing as oncology CNSs would need to acquire the knowledge to sit for the adult health CNS examination; the oncology content would prepare them to sit for the oncology CNS certification examination. Based on this regulatory model, if it is adopted, states would require that APRNs be certified in one of the six population-focused certifications. Certification in the specialty would be optional from a regulatory standpoint; it is conceivable that employers would require both certifications. Subspecialties also exist but, like specialties, would not be subject to licensure.

In elucidation of the model, the APRN Joint Dialogue Group asserted that the four separate processes of licensure, accreditation of educational programs, certification, and education (LACE) "are necessary for adequate regulation of APRNs" (APRN Consensus Work Group, 2007b, p. 10), calling these the "Four Prongs of Regulation" (APRN Consensus Work Group, 2007b). It is expected that a full report will be available in Summer 2008. The comprehensive approach to defining advanced practice nursing and the requirements for LACE has the potential to promote a unified and coherent understanding of advanced practice for the public, the profession, and policymakers.

A related national effort that will inform this evolving conceptualization is the CNS Competency Stakeholder Group convened by ANA and the ABNS. This group is charged with identifying competencies that are common in CNS practice, regardless of specialty. Despite the extensive work done to revise the document and that many programs have used it as the basis for CNS curricula, *The Statement on CNS Practice and Education* [NACNS, 2004] had not, in the

view of some, undergone sufficient validation to be used for accrediting CNS programs.

What is notable, if the APRN Regulatory Model is approved and implemented, is that the diverse stakeholders will have agreed to certain definitions (concepts) that may, at least in the United States, lead to improved clarity about what advanced practice is and is not. (Note that consensus, in this process, did not reflect 100% agreement. A two-thirds majority was defined as consensus. If as many as one third of participating organizations do not agree, such a sizable minority could determine whether or not the "consensus" solves the problem of lack of clarity regarding advanced practice nursing.)

Given the foregoing discussion of conceptualizations inferred from the documents of APN role group organizations, one can appreciate that achieving agreement on the issue of education and certification would be a complex process; achieving consensus on LACE will require ongoing dialogue and collaboration among the stakeholder organizations and policymakers.

Summary/Implications for Advanced Practice Nursing Conceptualizations. From this overview, it is clear that organizations are engaged in a more active dialogue about the nature of advanced practice and have begun a concerted effort to address LACE issues. Although the nature of advanced practice nursing is amplified and clarified by the role-specific documents published by these organizations, the level of conceptualization is more complex than is usually associated with conceptual models. This complexity illustrates the breadth and depth of advanced, specialized practice in the four APN roles and may be one reason why it has been difficult to identify a unified and coherent view of advanced practice nursing.

In conclusion, the organizational models just described enable the reader to understand who engages in advanced practice nursing and in what capacity. Thus these models address primarily professional role identity and function, curriculum planning and accreditation, and clinical practice—some of the purposes identified on p. 34. The descriptive statements about APN roles—CNS, NP, CNM, CRNA—demonstrate that common elements exist across all APN roles. These elements include a central focus on and accountability for patient care; knowledge and skills specific to each APN role; and a concern for patient rights. Table 2-1 was constructed based on the content of official statements of AANA, ACNM, NACNS, and NONPF to illustrate commonalities

Table 2-1 COMPARISON OF AANA, ACNM, NACNS, AND NONPF STATEMENTS ON PRIMARY CRITERIA AND APN COMPETENCIES*

Organization	Primary Criteria					Competencies					
	Graduate Education	Certification (if available)	Practice Focused on Patient/Family	Direct Care	Patient/Family Guidance/ Coaching	Collaboration	Consul- tation	Research	Leader- ship	Ethical Decision Making
AANA	Y	Y	Y	Y	Y	Y (implied)	Y	Y	Y	Y
ACNM	Y	Y	Y	Y	Y	Y	Y	Y	Y	Y
NACNS	Y	Varies†	Y	Y	Y	Y	Y	Y	Y	Y
NONPF	Y	Y	Y	Y	Y	Y	Y	Y	Y	Y

AANA, American Association of Nurse Anesthetists; *ACNM*, American College of Nurse-Midwives; *NACNS*, National Association of Clinical Nurse Specialists; *NONPF*, National Organization of Nurse Practitioner Faculties; *APN*, advanced practice nurse; *CNS*, clinical nurse specialist.

*Each organization's primary statements on the nature of the advanced practice role were used to complete the grid as follows: AANA (1996, 2002, 2005); ACNM (2006); NACNS (2004)†; NONPF (2002, 2006)

†Although NACNS has identified over 40 specialties, CNS certification examinations are not available for all specialties.

across the four roles. Despite the existence of common elements, some organizations have taken stands that may prevent the profession from reaching a consensus on advanced practice nursing. Even so, these models provide templates against which (1) differences among APN roles and practices can be distinguished; (2) educational programs can be developed and evaluated; (3) knowledge and behaviors can be measured for certification purposes; (4) practitioners can understand, examine, and improve their own practice; and (5) job descriptions can be developed.

The proposed APRN Regulatory Model outlines an understandable framework for making decisions regarding advanced practice nursing and LACE issues. It is likely that each role group had to give up something important to them to reach this level of agreement and coherence. Readers should pay attention to both the processes and outcomes of this important collaborative effort as it evolves.

Conceptualizations of the Nature of Advanced Practice Nursing

The APN role-specific models promulgated by professional organizations naturally lead to the following questions: What is common across APN roles? Can an overarching conceptualization of advanced practice nursing be articulated? How can one distinguish among basic, expert, and advanced levels of nursing practice? Some authors have attempted to discern the nature of advanced practice nursing and address these questions. The extent to which they have considered all existing APN roles is not always clear: some authors have considered only the CNS and NP roles.

In this section, the focus is on those frameworks that address the nature of advanced practice nursing. The term *role* is used loosely and variably, sometimes seeming to describe functions, such as management or teaching or research or consultation, and sometimes taking a psychological or sociological perspective on developing social roles or selves in relation to environment. Dictionary definitions add to the confusion by using the terms *role, function, occupation,* and *duties* to define one another. For example, *role* is usually used to refer to titles appearing in legal documents, certification programs, or job descriptions. From this perspective, the CNS, NP, CNM, and CRNA designations represent advanced practice roles. From the present review of a number of frameworks, it can be seen that *domain* and *competency* may be the most commonly used concepts in explaining nursing practice

and advanced practice nursing. However, meanings are not consistent. Because Hamric's model is the only one that is integrative—considers all four APN roles—it is discussed last. Otherwise, the models are discussed in chronological order.

Fenton's and Brykczynski's Expert Practice Domains of the Clinical Nurse Specialist and Nurse Practitioner: Building on Benner's Model of Expert Practice. To appreciate the contributions of Fenton (1985) and Brykczynski (1989) to the understanding of advanced practice, it is important to highlight some of Benner's key findings about nurses who are experts-by-experience. Although many authors have used Benner's (1984) seminal work, *From Novice to Expert,* in their conceptualizations of advanced practice nursing, it is important to note that Benner did not study advanced practice nurses; her research described nurses who were experts-by-experience. In using an interpretive approach to identifying and describing clinical knowledge, Benner defined two key terms as follows (Benner, 1984, pp. 292-293):

- *Competency*: An interpretively defined area of skilled performance identified and described by its intent, function, and meanings
- *Domain*: A cluster of competencies that have similar intents, functions, and meanings

Through the analysis of clinical exemplars discussed in interviews, Benner derived a group of competencies. Clustering the competencies resulted in further identification of seven domains of expert nursing practice. Within her lexicon, these domains are a combination of roles, functions, and competencies, although the three have not been precisely differentiated. The seven domains are as follows (Benner, 1984):

1. The helping role
2. Administering and monitoring therapeutic interventions and regimens
3. Effective management of rapidly changing situations
4. The diagnostic and monitoring function
5. The teaching-coaching function
6. Monitoring and ensuring the quality of health care practices
7. Organizational and work-role competencies

Fenton (1985) and Brykczynski (1989) each independently applied Benner's Model of Expert Practice to APNs, examining the practice of CNSs and NPs, respectively. In a later publication, Fenton and Brykczynski (1993) compared their earlier research findings to identify similarities and differences between CNSs and NPs. They used Benner's understanding of the concepts of domains, competencies, roles, and functions. Fenton and Brykczynski verified that nurses in advanced practice were indeed experts, as defined by Benner, but they demonstrated that APNs possessed something more than experts-by-experience. They identified additional domains and competencies as outlined in Figure 2-3. Across the top of Figure 2-3 are the seven domains identified by Benner and the additional domain found in CNS practice (Fenton, 1985)—that of consultation provided by CNSs to other nurses (the rectangular dotted box, top right). Under this box, there are two new CNS competencies (hexagonal boxes). The third (rounded) box is a new NP competency identified by Brykczynski in 1989. In her study of NPs, Brykczynski also identified an eighth domain—management of health/illness in ambulatory care settings. It would seem that, rather than identify it as a ninth domain, Brykczynski recognized this as a qualitatively different expression of the first two domains identified by Benner—that for NPs the new competencies identified are a result of the integration of the diagnostic/monitoring and administering/monitoring domains. This may reflect differences in both the scope of practice of the NP and the setting characteristics of Brykczynski's subjects compared with Benner's subjects, who were primarily experts-by-experience working in acute care. A close examination of Figure 2-3 also reveals the new competencies identified by Fenton and Brykczynski's work. In the hexagonal boxes, new CNS competencies were identified under the organization and work role domain (e.g., providing support for nursing staff) and the helping role in addition to the consulting domain and competencies. Similarly, in the rectangles with rounded edges, one sees additional NP competencies under seven of the eight domains (e.g., detecting acute or chronic disease while attending to illness under the diagnostic/administering domains). Their findings offer possible answers to questions posed at the beginning of the chapter. By examining the extent to which APNs demonstrate the seven domains found in experts-by-experience and uncovering differences, the findings offer a possible explanation of the differences between expert and advanced practice. In addition, they also described ways in which two advanced practice nursing roles, CNSs and NPs, may be different with regard to practice domains and competencies.

In considering the applications of the Benner Model and the refinements to CNS practice made by Fenton's (1985) and Benner's (1985) own reflections on expertise in oncology CNSs, Spross and Baggerly (1989) made recommendations for further development. With some modification, their recommendations for further research apply to contemporary advanced practice nursing: (1) studies to confirm Fenton and Brykczynski's findings in CNS and NP roles and to determine whether new domains and competencies have emerged in contemporary advanced practice across all four APN roles; (2) studies to elucidate the teaching/coaching domain as it relates to educating nurses and other staff; (3) studies to understand the ways in which APN competencies develop in direct-entry graduate students and RN graduate students; and (4) studies to compare the non-master's-prepared clinician's competencies with the APN's competencies to further distinguish components of expert versus advanced practice nursing,

Calkin's Model of Advanced Nursing Practice. Calkin's model (1984) was the first to explicitly distinguish the practice of experts-by-experience from advanced practice nursing as practiced by CNSs and NPs. Calkin developed the model to help nurse administrators determine how to differentiate advanced practice nursing from other levels of clinical practice in personnel policies. She proposed that this could be accomplished by matching (1) patient responses to health problems (as nursing was defined in the ANA 1980 social policy statement) with (2) the skill level and (3) the knowledge level of nursing personnel. In Calkin's model, three curves were overlaid on a normal distribution chart. Calkin depicted the skills and knowledge of novices, experts-by-experience, and APNs in relation to knowledge required in caring for patients whose responses to health care problems (i.e., health care needs) ranged from simple and common to complex and complicated (Figure 2-4). A closer look at Figure 2-4, *A*, shows, as one would expect, that there are many more human responses (the highest and widest curve) than a beginning nurse would have the knowledge and skill to manage. The impact of experience is illustrated in Figure 2-4, *B*. The highest and widest curve is effectively the same, but because of experience, expert nurses have more knowledge and skill (the curves are higher and somewhat wider, but their additional skill and knowledge do not yet match the range of responses they may encounter in the patients for whom they care). In Figure 2-4, *C*, APNs, by virtue of education and experience, have knowledge and skill that enable them to respond to a

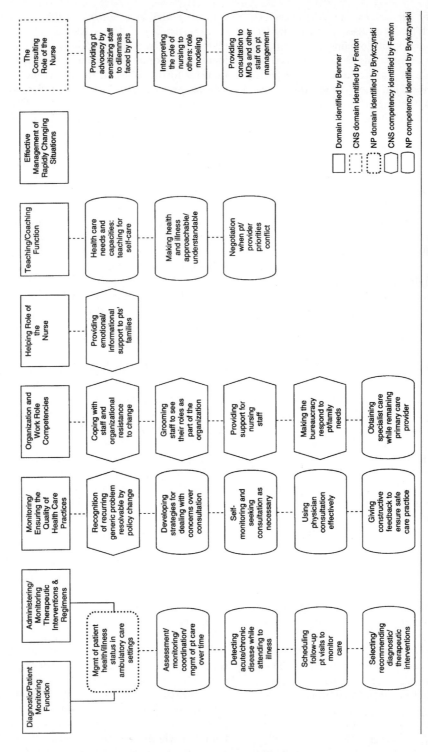

FIGURE 2-3: Fenton's and Brykczynski's **Expert Practice Domains of the Clinical Nurse Specialist (CNS) and Nurse Practitioner (NP).** (From Fenton, M.V., & Brykczynski, K.A. [1993]. Qualitative distinctions and similarities in the practice of clinical nurse specialists and nurse practitioners. *Journal of Professional Nursing, 9,* 313-326.)

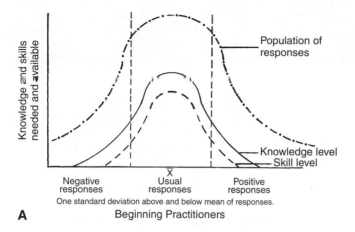

A   Beginning Practitioners

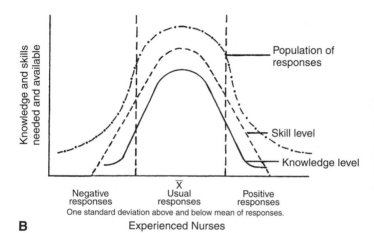

B   Experienced Nurses

FIGURE **2-4:** Calkin's **Model of Advanced Nursing Practice.** Patient responses correlated with the knowledge and skill of beginning practitioners **(A),** experienced nurses **(B),** and advanced practice nurses **(C).** (From Calkin, J.D. [1984]. A model for advanced nursing practice. *Journal of Nursing Administration, 14,* 24-30.)

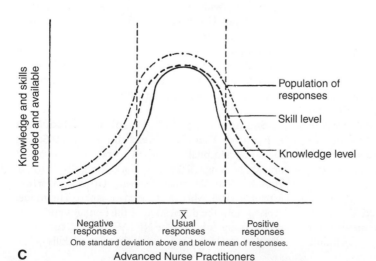

C   Advanced Nurse Practitioners

wider range of human problems. The three curves in Figure 2-4, *C,* parallel each other; this suggests that even as less-common human responses arise in clinical practice, APNs, in theory, can respond to these unusual problems.

Calkin used the framework to explain how APNs perform under different sets of circumstances: when there is a high degree of unpredictability; when there are new conditions or a new patient population or new sets of problems; and when there are a wide variety of health problems requiring the services of "specialist generalists," as she called them. She defined what APNs do in terms of functions. For example, when patients' health problems elicit a wide range of human responses with continuing and substantial unpredictable elements, the APN should do the following (Calkin, 1984, p. 28):

- Identify and develop interventions for the unusual by providing direct care
- Transmit this knowledge to nurses and, in some settings, to students
- Identify and communicate the need for research or to carry out research related to human responses to these health problems
- Anticipate factors that may lead to unfamiliar human responses
- Provide anticipatory guidance to nurse administrators when the changes in the diagnosis and treatment of these responses may require altered levels or types of resources

A principal advantage to Calkin's model is that the skills, education, and knowledge of the nurses needed are considered based on patient needs. It provides a framework for scholars to use in studying the function of APNs in a variety of work situations, and it should be a useful conceptualization for administrators who must maximize a multilevel nursing workforce and thus need to rationalize the use of APNs. However, the model has been left for others to test. Brooten's recent work on the concept of "nurse dose," based on years of empirical research, offers a similar understanding of the differences among beginners, experts-by-experience, and APNs. They propose, as did Calkin, that one needs to understand patients' needs/responses and the expertise, experience, and education of nurses in order to match nursing care to the needs of patients but did not cite Calkin's work (Brooten & Youngblut, 2006).

Brown's Framework for Advanced Practice Nursing. Brown (1998) developed a framework for the entire field of advanced practice nursing, including

the environments that surround and impact upon practice (Figure 2-5). She synthesized existing literature to propose a conceptual framework that included 4 main and 17 specific concepts (the specific concepts are in parentheses): environments (society, health care economy, local conditions, nursing, advanced practice community); role legitimacy (graduate education, certification, licensure); advanced practice nursing (scope, clinical care, competencies, managing health care environments, professional involvement in health care discourse); and outcomes (patient, health care system, the nursing profession, individual APN outcomes).

The central concept, conceptually and visually, is advanced practice nursing. Brown (1998) proposed a definition of advanced practice nursing: "professional health care activities that (1) focus on clinical services rendered at the nurse-client interface, (2) use a nursing orientation, (3) have a defined but dynamic and evolving scope, and (4) are based on competencies that are acquired through graduate nursing education" (p. 161).

This comprehensive model is one of the few that explicates the relevant components of a conceptual framework as described in the beginning of this chapter. Brown defines the concepts or "building blocks" of the model, articulates assumptions, and proposes linkages among concepts that could be tested. The model is comprehensive in that it addresses both the nature of the practice and the context in which the practice occurs. She notes the importance of a nursing orientation, particularly when APNs perform activities traditionally done by physicians. Brown notes that scope is "defined but dynamic and evolving" (p. 161), an observation that reflects the rapidity with which knowledge accrues and practice changes. The model is sufficiently explicated that it could be used for all of the purposes conceptual models can serve: differentiating practice, designing curricula, and evaluating advanced practice. Like the NONPF model, Brown uses domains and competencies to describe the work of APNs.

Strong Memorial Hospital's Model of Advanced Practice Nursing. APNs at Strong Memorial Hospital developed a model of advanced practice nursing (Ackerman, Clark, Reed, Van Horn, & Francati, 2000; Ackerman, Norsen, Martin, Wiedrich, & Kitzman, 1996; Mick & Ackerman, 2000). The model evolved from the delineation of the domains and competencies of the acute care NP (ACNP) role, conceptualized as a role that "combines the clinical skills of the

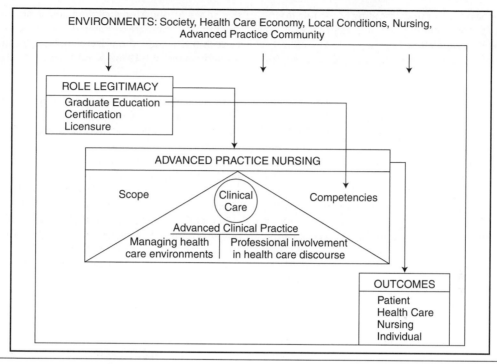

FIGURE **2-5:** Brown's **Framework for Advanced Practice Nursing.** (From Brown, S.J. [1998]. A framework for advanced practice nursing. *Journal of Professional Nursing, 14,* 157-164.)

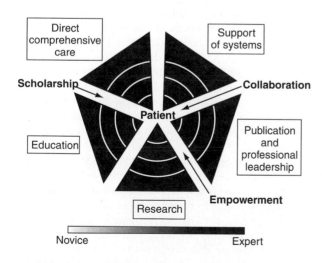

FIGURE **2-6:** The Strong Memorial Hospital's **Model of Advanced Practice Nursing.** (From Ackerman, M.H., Norsen, L., Martin, B., Wiedrich, J., & Kitzman H.J. [1996]. Development of a model of advanced practice. *American Journal of Critical Care, 5,* 68-73.)

NP with the systems acumen, educational commitment, and leadership ability of the CNS" (Ackerman et al., 1996, p. 69). The five domains are direct comprehensive patient care, support of systems, education, research, and publication and professional leadership. All domains have direct and indirect activities associated

with them. In addition, necessary, unifying threads influence each domain, which are illustrated as circular and continuous threads in Figure 2-6: collaboration, scholarship, and empowerment (Ackerman et al., 1996). These threads are operationalized in each practice domain. Ackerman and colleagues (2000) noted that the model is based on an understanding of the role development of APNs—the concept of novice (APN) to expert (APN) is foundational to the Strong Model.

Direct comprehensive care includes a range of assessments and interventions performed by APNs including history taking; physical assessment; requesting and/or performing diagnostic studies; performing invasive procedures; interpreting clinical and laboratory data; prescribing medications and other therapies; and case management of complex, critically ill patients. The support of systems domain includes indirect patient care activities that support the clinical enterprise and serve to improve the quality of care. These activities include consultation; participating or leading strategic planning; quality improvement initiatives; establishing and evaluating standards of practice; precepting students; and promoting APN practice. The education domain includes a variety of activities such as evaluating educational programs, providing formal and informal education to staff, educating patients and families, and identifying and disseminating educational resources. The research domain addresses both the use and conduct of research. The publication and professional leadership domain includes those APN functions involved with disseminating knowledge about the ACNP role, participating in professional organizations as a member or leader, influencing health and public policy, and publishing. APNs are expected to exert influence within and outside their institution.

The unifying threads of collaboration, scholarship, and empowerment are attributes of advanced practice that exert influence across all five domains and characterize the professional model of nursing practice. Collaboration ensures that the contributions of all caregivers are valued. APNs are expected to create and sustain a culture that supports scholarly inquiry whether it is questioning a common nursing practice or developing and disseminating an innovation. APNs support the empowerment of staff, ensuring that nurses have authority over nursing practice and opportunities to improve practice.

The Strong Model is a parsimonious model that has many similarities with other advanced practice conceptualizations. For example, its domains are consistent with the competencies delineated in the Hamric Model. Unlike the Hamric Model, which posits direct care as the central competency that informs all other advanced nursing practice competencies, in the Strong Model all domains of practice, including direct care, are considered "mutually exclusive of each other and exhaustive of practice behaviors" (Ackerman et al., 1996, p. 69). Like the Synergy Model, discussed later, role development is incorporated within the model (novice to expert). As described in the original article, the Strong Model emerged from consideration of the ACNP as a combined CNS/NP role—we consider this a blended role (see Chapter 15) which is not the same as the ACNP role described in this textbook (see Chapter 14)—highlighting our point that work remains to be done on a unifying conceptualization of advanced nursing practice. Even so, we agree with the authors' conclusion that the model may be useful to other APNs and administrators (Ackerman et al., 1996). It is notable that this model was the result of a collaborative effort between practicing APNs and APN faculty members. One could infer that such a model would be useful for guiding clinical practice and planning curricula, two of the purposes of conceptual models outlined earlier in the chapter.

Oberle and Allen: The Nature of Advanced Practice Nursing. For Oberle and Allen (2001), current conceptualizations of advanced practice nursing were limited: particular gaps were the lack of clear distinctions between the expert practice of experienced nurses and the expert practice of APNs, as well as the lack of nursing theories to address such levels of practice. The authors note that although the literature on expert nursing is mostly focused on expertise as it unfolds in the context of relationships, the literature on advanced practice nursing seems to focus more on expertise as "skills acquisition and critical thinking abilities" (p. 148).

According to Oberle and Allen (2001), any conceptualization of advanced practice nursing should be embedded in a conceptual understanding of nursing. To elucidate their model of advanced practice nursing, the authors first proposed a conceptualization of nursing practice. They refer to practice as *praxis*, a term that captures the values-oriented, reflective, and creative nature of the work of nurses. They conceive of nursing as a dialectical (back-and-forth) process between the nurse's knowledge and his or her experiences and relationships with patients. In this process, the nurse considers general and particular knowledge, synthesizes this knowledge, and generates options for care that he or she can offer to the patient. By this they mean that experiences with patients (and, presumably, reflection on these experiences) extend nurses' knowledge; this new knowledge informs their practice with subsequent patients; experiences with applying the new knowledge gained from experience and reflection again inform and extend their thinking—a dialectical process that occurs over and over. As nurses accumulate experience, this dialectical process that occurs in relationships with patients contributes to developing expertise.

The conceptualization of advanced practice nursing proposed by Oberle and Allen (2001) is illustrated in Figure 2-7. Each of the elements in the model is described in Box 2-4. Oberle and Allen (2001) differentiate between experts-by-experience and APNs as follows: "The inherent difference between expert and advanced practice is that the expert nurse's knowledge base is largely experientially acquired, whereas the APN has a greater store of theoretical knowledge acquired through graduate study" (p. 151).

Although Figure 2-7 is meant to illustrate advanced practice nursing, the elements in the model are the same as those used for the authors' textual description of experts-by-experience; there are not separate illustrations of the two levels of practice. Differences between experts-by-experience and APNs are described in the text. Oberle and Allen (2001) proposed that graduate education is a process in which students (presumably experts-by-experience) have experiences that lead to transformations in self and in practice, a dialectical process that results in "transformative practice" (p. 152). Although the notion of transformative practice is provocative and likely to resonate with students and faculty, neither the model nor the text helps the reader understand what this transformative practice is and how it is different from the practice of experts-by-experience.

Oberle and Allen acknowledged that they do not consider the specifics of advanced practice. Neither did they address the environment or contexts of practice in their model, which we consider a limitation of the model. Environment is a significant theoretical concept for nursing in general and for advanced

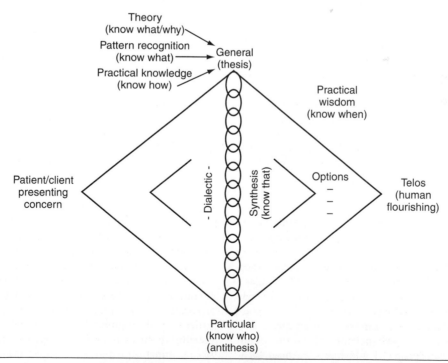

FIGURE **2-7:** Oberle and Allen's **Conceptualization of Advanced Practice.** (From Oberle, K., & Allen, M. [2001]. The nature of advanced practice nursing. *Nursing Outlook, 49,* 148-153.)

Box 2-4 ELEMENTS OF OBERLE AND ALLEN'S CONCEPTUALIZATION OF ADVANCED PRACTICE NURSING

Patient/client presenting concern—Problem or potential problem for which an individual needs nursing care.

General and particular knowledge—Nurses move back and forth between global knowledge (e.g., the features of an illness or the nursing care that usually works for a particular problem) and specific knowledge (specifics about the individual patient or situation).

GENERAL KNOWLEDGE
• Theory—Know what and know why.
• Pattern recognition—Know what.
• Practical knowledge—Know how.

PARTICULAR KNOWLEDGE
• Client's meanings, desired outcomes, and acceptable actions—Know who.

• *Dialectic*—The process by which nurses consider general and particular knowledge and synthesize this information to generate options and propose actions to the patient to move the patient toward his or her goals.
• *Synthesis*—Know that [a particular action is called for in a specific situation].
• *Practical wisdom*—Know when [a particular action ought to be taken]. The dialectical process and experience with synthesis, informed by praxis, lead to the development of "practical wisdom."
• *Telos*—Human flourishing (the object of nursing care, of which health is a part—health is a resource for human flourishing; Oberle & Allen, p. 150)
• *Options*—possibilities for actions identified by nurse

From Oberle, K., & Allen, M. (2001). The nature of advanced practice nursing. *Nursing Outlook, 49,* 148-153.

practice nursing in particular—a concept that is addressed, for example, in Brown's and Hamric's models. Another limitation of Oberle and Allen's model is the emphasis on practical experience in nursing. With more and more career changers entering nursing through direct-entry programs that prepare APNs, future conceptualizations of advanced practice nursing will need to take into account how non-nursing experience helps graduate nursing students experience the dialectical process that is at the heart of praxis and helps them develop the practical wisdom that is essential to effective nursing practice. Graduate APN students who do not have nursing experience are encouraged to reflect on and expand on this model, considering how their life and professional experiences account for their experience of transformation and their mastery of advanced practice nursing.

Shuler's Model of Nurse Practitioner Practice: A Theoretical Framework. Shuler's efforts to integrate both nursing and medical knowledge skills into the NP role led her to develop a conceptual model that would make apparent the unique contribution NPs made to patient care and outcomes. Thus Shuler purposefully addressed the need for a model that reflects the acquisition of expertise by the NP in two health care disciplines: nursing and

medicine. Shuler's Nurse Practitioner Practice Model (Figure 2-8 on pp. 56-57) is a complex systems model that is holistic and wellness oriented. It is both definitive and detailed in terms of how the NP-patient interaction, patient assessment, intervention, and evaluation should occur (Shuler & Davis, 1993a). Its complexity is likely to overwhelm beginning NP students, and its value for understanding NP practice may not become clear until they have experience as practicing NPs. To simplify the presentation of the model, Table 2-2 outlines key model constructs and related theories, many of which should be familiar to students. Knowing that these familiar concepts are embedded in this very complex model may help readers as they read about and examine Figure 2-8. To fully understand the model, the reader should go back to the original publication; the following discussion highlights selected elements.

Within NP practice, Shuler conceptualizes patient visits as fitting into one of three categories: episodic (Figure 2-8, patient/NP throughput A); comprehensive examination with an existing acute (Figure 2-8, patient/NP throughput B1) or chronic (Figure 2-8, patient/NP throughput B2) problem; or comprehensive examination without an existing health problem (Figure 2-8, patient/NP throughput C). Input categories are similar regardless of the type of visit. Students

Table 2-2 Model Constructs and Underlying Theoretical Concepts Included in Shuler's Model of Nurse Practitioner Practice

Model Constructs	Wholistic [sic] Patient Needs	NP-Patient Interaction	Self-Care	Health Prevention	Health Promotion	Wellness
Underlying Theoretical Concepts	Basic needs Wellness activities Health/illness Psychological health Family Culture Social support Environmental health Spirituality	Contracting Role modeling Self-care activities Teaching/learning Contracting Culture Family Social support Environmental health	Wellness activities Preventative health activities Health promotion activities Compliance Problem solving Teaching/learning Contracting Culture Family Social support Environmental health	Primary prevention Secondary prevention Tertiary prevention Preventative health behavior Family Culture Environmental health	Health promotion behavior Wellness Family Culture Environmental health Social support	Self-care activities Wellness activities Disease prevention activities Health promotion activities Family Culture Social support Environmental health Spirituality Contracting Teaching/learning

From Shuler, P.A., & Davis, J.E. (1993a). The Shuler nurse practitioner practice model: A theoretical framework for nurse practitioner clinicians, educators, and researchers, Part 1. *Journal of the American Academy of Nurse Practitioners, 5,* 11-18.

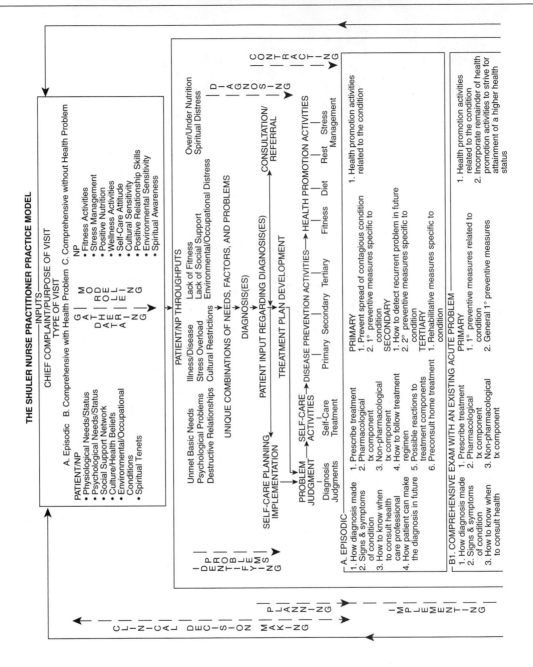

THE SHULER NURSE PRACTITIONER PRACTICE MODEL

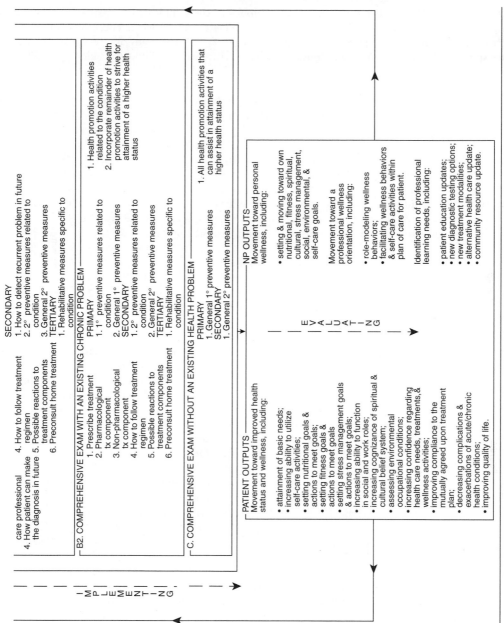

FIGURE 2–8: **The Shuler Nurse Practitioner Practice Model.** (From Shuler, P.A., & Davis, J.E. [1993a]. The Shuler Nurse Practitioner Practice Model: A theoretical framework for nurse practitioner clinicians, educators, and researchers, Part 1. *Journal of the American Academy of Nurse Practitioners, 5,* 11-18.)

can see the integration of nursing and medicine in the Inputs box; in addition to information that one would assess in the usual history and physical, the NP incorporates spiritual elements, traditionally considered part of nursing assessment. NP characteristics are also viewed as inputs in that NPs' own wellness orientations may exert influence on NP-patient interactions and patient outcomes through role modeling. Throughputs vary somewhat according to the type of visit. A close look at the throughputs indicates that both patient data from the history, physical, and other assessments and NP interventions are identified. The Outputs box could be viewed as outcomes—patient outputs such as reduced complications and adherence to treatment and NP outputs such as adoption of healthy behaviors and identification of professional learning needs.

In addition to integrating nursing and medicine, the model incorporates concepts from a number of disciplines (e.g., psychology). From the figure alone, the reader will appreciate that it is most ambitious; it incorporates multiple theoretical constructs within a systems framework that integrates internal and external environments and input-throughput-output processes. From our review we discerned that the systems model incorporates the following: (1) the four concepts of nursing's metaparadigm (person, health, nursing, and environment); (2) the nursing process; (3) humanistically based assumptions about patients and nurse practitioners; and (4) theoretical concepts underlying practice model constructs. Indeed, the model could be characterized as a network or system of frameworks.

Shuler's model is intended "to impact the NP domain at four levels: theoretical, clinical, educational, and research" (Shuler & Davis, 1993a, p. 17). Clinical application of the Shuler Model is intended to ensure demonstration of the NP's combined (i.e., nursing and medicine) role with the proposed benefits for both the practitioner and the patient and to provide a framework by which NP services can be evaluated (Shuler & Davis, 1993b). For example, if NPs purposefully include patients in the assessment, planning, intervention, and evaluation processes, an improvement in patient adherence to a mutually agreed upon treatment/wellness plan would be anticipated.

Shuler and Davis (1993b) published a template for conducting a visit with guidelines on what types of information should be solicited during a comprehensive examination when there is an existing health problem—the template is 17 pages long! The scope and intent of the model are enormous. Although it is difficult to imagine ready implementation into the busy NP practices of today, Shuler and colleagues have proposed examples of applying the model, which included (1) providing care to patients with an existing health problem seen for a comprehensive examination (Shuler & Davis, 1993b), (2) delivering primary care through school-based health centers (Shuler, 2000), and (3) providing holistic health care to older adults (Shuler, Huebscher, & Hallock, 2001). These examples illustrate the model's comprehensiveness and vastness. The ability to use the entire framework in the context of individual patient encounters may prove overwhelming, especially for NP students. Faculty may be able to use the complete model to help NP students see how nursing and medical knowledge and skills come together in this advanced practice role or to demonstrate the complexity of NP practice—the view from the mountaintop, if you will. However, the model may be best utilized when a student or reader isolates and tries to grasp one or two constructs and then visualizes these constructs within the larger whole. For practicing NPs, the model's benefit may lie in providing NPs with a guide on how to promote and retain the nursing focus on care in the context of a combined role that integrates medical knowledge and skills into nursing.

Ball and Cox's Restoring Patients to Health—Outcome and Indicators of Advanced Nursing Practice in Critical Care: A Theory of Legitimate Influence. One of the few empirical studies of advanced practice nursing is an international, grounded theory study of NPs, CNSs, and *clinical nurse consultants*—a term used in Australia for those in CNS-like positions) (Ball & Cox, 2003, 2004). Subjects (n = 36) from the United States, Canada, the United Kingdom, and Australia participated; they were required to be master's prepared or graduate students preparing for an advanced practice role. The investigators conducted interviews and made observations of the participants over a 3-year period. The theory that emerged from this study was a "Theory of Legitimate Influence" (Figure 2-9). The figure illustrates the range of activities in which APNs engage to "enhance patient stay" and "improve patient outcomes." This study provides empirical support for many of the competencies described in the conceptualizations reviewed in this chapter (Table 2-3). The work of these authors suggests that the activities of

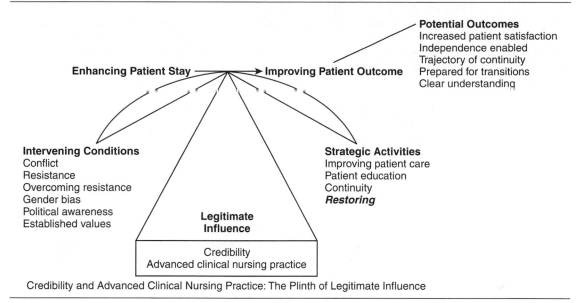

FIGURE **2-9:** Ball & Cox's **Theory of Legitimate Influence.** (From Ball, C., & Cox, C.L. [2003]. Restoring patients to health: Outcomes and indicators of advanced nursing practice in adult critical care, Part 1. *International Journal of Nursing Practice, 9,* 356-367.)

Table 2-3   COMPARISON OF CONCEPTS IN BALL AND COX'S THEORY OF LEGITIMATE INFLUENCE AND HAMRIC'S SEVEN APN COMPETENCIES

Hamric Competency	Ball and Cox Concept
Direct care	Credibility Advanced clinical practice Restoring
Expert coaching and guidance	Patient education Continuity
Consultation	Legitimate influence Credibility
Research	Improving patient care
Collaboration	Conflict
Leadership	Improving patient care (Addressing/overcoming) resistance (Recognizing/addressing) gender bias Political awareness Legitimate influence
Ethical decision making	Established values

APNs, in this case NPs and CNSs, are strategic and focused and that some activities involve direct service to patients, whereas others are aimed at communication and system issues.

Hamric's Integrative Model of Advanced Practice Nursing. One of the earliest efforts to synthesize a model of advanced practice that would apply to all APN roles was developed by Hamric

(1996). Hamric, whose early conceptual work was done on the CNS role (Hamric & Spross, 1983, 1989), proposed an integrative understanding of the core of advanced practice nursing, based on literature from all APN specialties (Hamric, 1996, 2000, 2005). She proposed a conceptual definition of advanced practice nursing and defining characteristics that included primary criteria (graduate education, certification in the specialty, and a focus on clinical practice with patients) and a set of core competencies (direct clinical practice, collaboration, coaching and guidance, research, ethical decision making, consultation, and leadership). This early model was further refined together with Hanson and Spross in 2000 and in 2005 was based on dialogue among the editors of this text (the editors determined that no change from 2004 was necessary for this edition; see Chapter 3). Key components of the model (Figure 2-10) are the primary criteria for advanced nursing practice, seven advanced practice competencies with direct care as the core competency on which the other competencies depend, and environmental and contextual factors that must be managed for advanced practice nursing to flourish.

The revisions to the Hamric Model since 1996 highlight the dynamic nature of a conceptual model; at the same time, the fact that essential features remain the same demonstrates the inherent stability and robustness of Hamric's model, particularly when many potentially transformative advanced practice nursing initiatives are afoot. Models are refined over time according to changes in practice, research, and theoretical understanding. This model forms the understanding of advanced practice nursing used throughout this text and has provided the structure for each edition of the book.

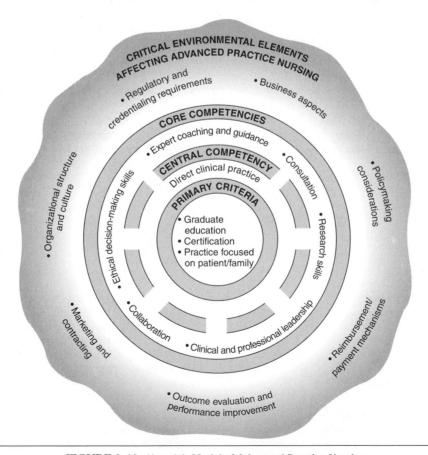

FIGURE **2-10:** Hamric's **Model of Advanced Practice Nursing**.

Using Hamric's model, some contributors to this text further elaborate the specific competencies she proposed (see Chapter 3) by describing and graphically depicting concepts relevant to the specific competency. These competencies include coaching (Spross, Clarke, & Beauregard, 2000; Spross, 2005; see Chapter 6), consultation (Barron & White, 2000, 2005; see Chapter 7), and ethical decision making (Reigle & Boyle, 2000; Hamric & Reigle, 2005; see Chapter 11).

A recent review of the literature provides support for Hamric's integrative conceptualization of advanced practice nursing (Mantzoukas & Watkinson, 2007). The purpose of the review was to identify "generic features" of advanced nursing practice. They identified seven generic features: (1) use of knowledge in practice; (2) critical thinking and analytical skills; (3) clinical judgment and decision making; (4) professional leadership and clinical inquiry; (5) coaching and mentoring; (6) research skills; and (7) changing practice. The first three generic features are consistent with the direct care competency in Hamric's model; that three of the seven characteristics seem directly related to clinical practice supports the notion that direct care is a central competency. The remaining four features are consistent with the three competencies of leadership, expert guidance and coaching, and the research competency in Hamric's model.

Hamric's conceptualization of advanced practice nursing informed the development of the DNP *Essentials* (AACN, 2006). For example, the research competency of APNs (DePalma & McGuire, 2005; see Chapter 8) informed the development of Essential III, "Clinical Scholarship and Analytical Methods for Evidence-Based Practice." Given the emphasis of this competency on evaluation of practice, drawing on an existing conceptualization of this competency made sense. DNP-prepared clinical administrators who employ APNs will have a sound understanding of and ability to perform or oversee this particular competency. More important, development of Essential VIII, "Advanced Nursing Practice" drew on two key competencies—expert coaching and guidance (Spross, 2005; see Chapter 6) and direct clinical practice (Brown, 2005; see Chapter 5)—to inform the content on DNP-prepared APNs.

Summary/Implications for Advanced Practice Nursing Conceptualizations. When one considers conceptualizations of advanced practice nursing described by professional organizations and individual authors, similarities and differences emerge. Many conceptual models address competencies that APNs must possess. All are in agreement that the direct care of patients is central to APN practice. Some models (e.g., Calkin Model and Strong Model) address the issue of skill mix as it relates to APNs, an issue of concern to administrators who hire APNs. On the other hand, consultation and collaboration competencies are infrequently addressed. There is a fairly consistent emphasis on outcomes—how APN practice influences patient and institutional outcomes. However, different models may emphasize different competencies. Some models address concepts such as research, scholarly inquiry, and ethics more explicitly than others. A notable difference across models is the extent to which the concept of environment as it relates to APN practice is addressed. In the next section we review models that have not necessarily emerged from an APN perspective, but they are ones that APNs may find useful as they develop and evaluate their own practices.

Based on this review, can one begin to answer the questions about advanced practice raised on p. 34. The answer is a qualified "yes." For example, the authors of the Schuler Model and the Dunphy-Winland Model acknowledge the challenge of integrating or blending medicine and nursing as it relates to nurse practitioner practice. The Calkin Model provides some information on why the profession might distinguish among novice, expert, and advanced levels of practice. As education and credentialing of APNs have evolved, with a requirement for a second license for APNs, there is now regulatory "justification" for the term *advanced*. There have been many forays into conceptualizing advanced practice nursing with little research to test the models and little "crosstalk" among stakeholders (until recently). It remains to be seen whether the promising work of the NCSBN (2006), APRN Consensus Work Group (2007) and the APRN Joint Dialogue Group (2007a, 2007b, 2008) will clarify advanced nursing practice for the profession and the public.

MODELS THAT ADVANCED PRACTICE NURSES WILL FIND USEFUL IN THEIR PRACTICE

Other models exist that can contribute to conceptualizing and studying advanced practice nursing. In addition to the ones described in the following sections, conceptual models of APN role development that help students, faculty, and APNs understand how an individual APN's knowledge and practice evolve over time are fully explored in Chapter 4.

Models Useful for Differentiating Levels of Nursing Practice

The American Association of Critical-Care Nurses Synergy Model. The American Association of Critical Care Nurses created the Synergy Model (Figure 2-11) in an effort to link nursing practice with patient outcomes (Curley, 1998). Components of the model are patients' characteristics; nurses' competencies; and patient, nurse, and system level outcomes. Patients' capacity for health and their vulnerability to illness are influenced by biological, genetic, psychological, and socioecological determinants. The Synergy Model posits a unique cluster of personal characteristics that arise from these determinants and exist

along a continuum that parallels health and illness states: stability, complexity, predictability, resiliency, vulnerability, participation in decision making and care, and resource availability (Box 2-5). An important function of the nurse is to ensure the patient's "safe passage" through the health care situation.

Nursing competencies are derived from the needs of patients and also exist along continua. The eight nursing competency continua are clinical judgment, advocacy and moral agency, caring practices, facilitation of learning, collaboration, systems thinking, diversity of responsiveness, and clinical inquiry (Box 2-6). The continua for these competencies range from "competent" (level 1) to "expert" (level 5). A discussion of the interpretation of these levels is beyond the scope of this chapter. The reader is referred to the American Association of Critical-Care Nurses website *(www.aacn.org)* and

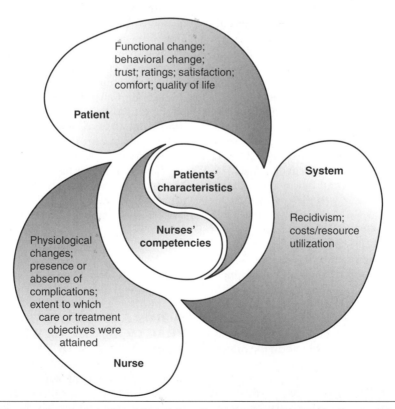

FIGURE **2-11:** The American Association of Critical-Care Nurses' **Synergy Model**. The Synergy Model delineates three levels of outcomes: those derived from the patient, those derived from the nurse, and those derived from the health care system. (From Curley, M.A.Q. [1998]. Patient-nurse synergy: Optimizing patient's outcomes. *American Journal of Critical Care, 7,* **64**-72.)

Box 2-5 THE SYNERGY MODEL: THE SEVEN CONTINUA OF PATIENT CHARACTERISTICS

1	2	3	4	5
Minimally resilient				Highly resilient
Highly vulnerable				Minimally vulnerable
Minimally stable				Highly stable
Minimally complex				Highly complex
Not predictable				Highly predictable
Few resources available				Many resources available
No participation in decision making and care				Full participation in decision making and care

Adapted from American Association of Critical-Care Nurses. (2003). *The AACN Synergy Model for patient care.* Retrieved December 7, 2003, from www.aacn.org/certcorp/certcorp.nsf/vwdoc/SynModel?opendocument.

publications (American Association of Critical-Care Nurses, 2003; Curley, 1998).

Outcomes are conceptualized as being derived from patient, nurse, and/or system. For example, trust of the caregiver and patient satisfaction are patient outcomes that arise or are derived from the patient. Physiological outcomes are derived from the nurse (i.e., the nurse's interventions). System level outcomes are derived from the hospital or insurer (e.g., readmission to the hospital for a preventable complication).

The model is interesting for several reasons. Certification examinations are based on the conceptualization of levels of competency and represent an effort to ensure conceptual coherence between the nature of the practice and how one's knowledge of the practice is tested. Because certification examinations are based on the model, it seems likely that programs preparing APNs in critical care would use the model to structure curricula. APNs have used the model to understand complex cases (e.g., Collopy, 1999; Moloney-Harmon, 1999). Finally, the model is beginning to be used to understand differences among critical care APN roles (Becker, Kaplow, Muenzen, & Hartigan, 2006). In addition, like the NACNS, Hamric, and DNP conceptualizations, the Synergy Model addresses patient, nurse, and system.

Models Useful for Studying Outcomes of Advanced Practice Nursing

Brooten's Model of Transitional Care. Brooten used a conceptual framework proposed by Doessel and Marshall (1985). Doessel and Marshall

Box 2-6 THE SYNERGY MODEL: THE EIGHT CONTINUA OF NURSE CHARACTERISTICS/ NURSING COMPETENCIES

	1	2	3	4	5
Clinical judgment	Competent				Expert
Advocacy/Moral agency	Competent				Expert
Caring practices	Competent				Expert
Collaboration	Competent				Expert
Systems thinking	Competent				Expert
Response to diversity	Competent				Expert
Clinical inquiry or Innovator/Evaluator	Competent				Expert
Facilitator of patient and family learning	Competent				Expert

Adapted from American Association of Critical-Care Nurses. (2003). *The AACN Synergy Model for patient care.* Retrieved December 7, 2003, from www.aacn.org/certcorp/certcorp.nsf/vwdoc/SynModel?opendocument.

synthesized medical and economic concepts to propose a definition of quality of health care whose key concepts were outcomes, patient satisfaction, and cost. Brooten and colleagues (Brooten et al., 1988) integrated these three concepts into their evaluation of outcomes of APN transitional care with different populations such as very-low-birth-weight infants, hospitalized older patients, and women who had undergone cesarean deliveries. APN transitional care was defined as "comprehensive discharge planning designed for each patient group plus APN home follow-up through a period of normally expected recovery or stabilization" (Brooten et al., 2002, p. 370). Brooten's model was intended to address outlier patient populations (e.g., those patients who were complex, who were at high risk for complications, who represented a significant proportion of those whose care was expensive). Across all studies, care was provided by NPs and/or CNSs whose clinical expertise was matched to the needs of the patient population. APN care was associated with improved patient outcomes and reduced costs (see Chapter 24).

Research conducted by Brooten and others who have used this model provided empirical support for several elements important to a conceptualization of advanced practice nursing. In a summary of the studies conducted to date, the investigators identified several factors that contribute to APNs' effectiveness: content expertise, interpersonal skills, knowledge of systems, the ability to implement change, and the ability to access resources (Brooten, Youngblut, Deatrick, Naylor, & York, 2003). This finding provides empirical support for the importance of the APN competencies of direct care, collaboration, coaching, and systems leadership. Two other important findings were the existence of patterns of morbidity within patient populations and an apparent "dose effect" (i.e., outcomes seemed to be related to how much time, how many interactions patients had with APNs, and numbers and types of APN interventions) (Brooten et al., 2003). Subsequently, based on this program of research, Brooten and Youngblut (2006) proposed a conceptual explanation of "nurse dose." Their proposed explanation suggests that nurse dose depends on patient and nurse characteristics. For the nurse, differences in education and experience can influence the dose of nursing needed. Their conceptualization of nurse dose—which has empiric support—may enable the profession to better define differences among novice, expert, and advanced levels of nursing practice.

Taken together, findings from this program of research suggest that characteristics of patients and characteristics and dose of APN interventions are likely to be important to any conceptualization of advanced practice nursing. Finally, the fact that this program of research has used both NPs and CNSs to intervene with patients provides support for elucidating a conceptual model that encompasses characteristics, competencies, and other concepts that are common across advanced practice nursing roles.

A similar model, the care transitions model, builds on this work (Coleman, Parry, Chalmers, & Min, 2006). Exemplar 2-1 shows how graduate CNS students used the content in this chapter to synthesize Hamric's conceptualization of APN practice with NACNS's spheres of influence to explain the advanced practice activities they used in implementing a project to improve transitional care of hospitalized older adults at high risk of readmission.

Models Useful for Conceptualizing Interdisciplinary Practice

Dunphy and Winland-Brown's Circle of Caring: A Transformative Model. A central premise of Dunphy and Winland-Brown's model (1998) is that the health care needs of individuals, families, and communities are not being met in a health care system that is dominated by medicine and one in which medical language (i.e., the International Classification of Disease Codes [ICD-10-CM]) is the basis for reimbursement. They proposed the *Circle of Caring: A Transformative Model* to foster a more active and visible nursing presence in the health care system and to explain and promote medical-nursing collaboration. Dunphy and Winland-Brown's transformative model (Figure 2-12 on p. 67) is a synthesized problem-solving approach to advanced practice nursing that builds on both nursing and medical models (Dunphy & Winland-Brown, 1998).

The authors argued that a model such as theirs is needed because nursing and medicine have two very different traditions, with the medical model being viewed as primarily reductionistic and nursing being regarded as primarily humanistic. Neither a nursing nor a medical model of practice, in isolation or in combination, provides a structure that allows APNs to be recognized for their day-to-day practice and the positive patient health outcomes that can be attributed to APNs' care. The model's authors viewed the development of nursing diagnoses as an attempt to differentiate nursing care from medical care. Though this

An assignment for clinical nurse specialist (CNS) students in the first author's class required them to submit an abstract for presentation at the annual university-sponsored research symposium, Thinking Matters (Unnold, Erickson, Spross, & Warrick, 2007). Two students were working on implementation of the evidence-based Care Transition Intervention (CTI) (Coleman et al., 2006). The CTI is aimed at helping patients assume more responsibility for their health. The CTI consists of four pillars: medication reconciliation, the Personal Health Record (PHR) maintained by the patient (to facilitate communication between patient and providers and information transfer), timely postdischarge appointments with primary care or specialty provider, and a list of red flags with instructions for managing worsening health problems. A care transition coach conducts a medication reconciliation (compares discharge medications with medications taken at home before hospitalization) and teaches patients about the four pillars: how to take medications, how to maintain the PHR, strategies for communicating with providers, and self-management behaviors and skills

for "red flags" (worsening symptoms).

Two students functioned as CTI coaches. The purpose of their project was to reduce rehospitalization in older adults at high risk for readmission. In planning their poster presentations, one student decided to explain how she operationalized the Care Transition Intervention Coach role using Hamric's seven advanced practice nurse (APN) competencies (Hamric, 2005; see Chapter 3) with NACNS' three spheres of influence (NACNS, 2004). During seminar discussions, the students and faculty synthesized these two conceptualizations—creating the figure first, then using the figure to guide the analysis and categorization of their CTI activities. Part of the student's poster is reproduced in the figure below and in the table on p. 66. The figure is a graphic representation of our synthesized conceptualization of relationships between and among the spheres of influence and competencies. The table operationalizes the conceptualization by describing specific advanced practice actions that students performed to implement the Care Transition Intervention.

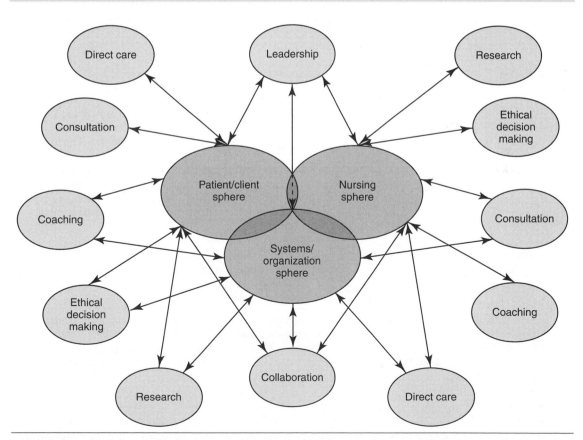

Clinical Nurse Specialist (CNS) competencies and spheres of influence. (Adapted from Unnold, R., Erickson, V., Spross, J., & Warrick, C. [2007]. Helping patients through health transitions: The role of the clinical nurse specialist in system change. Unpublished Poster Presentation University of Southern Maine. Adapted from Hamric, 2005 and NACNS, 2004.)

ADVANCED PRACTICE COMPETENCIES WITHIN THE THREE SPHERES OF CNS INFLUENCE

	Patient/Client Sphere	Nursing Sphere	Systems/Organization Sphere
Direct Care	Medication reconciliation Advanced health assessment	Recognizing and reporting urgent clinical findings	CTI protocol Developing clinical and data forms for project Participating in and leading project team meetings
Leadership	Adapting priorities to meet patient needs (e.g., facilitating discharge to home [the patient's goal] not to long-term care facility [doctor's recommendation])	CNS role model for staff Meeting facilitation Enlisting stakeholder buy-in Dealing with staff time constraints and priorities	Project management IRB applications Anticipating potential conflicts and addressing them early and effectively Maintaining a flexible schedule to be available to enroll patients and consult with team
Research	Preparation of two IRB applications (two agencies)	Education on CTI protocol CNS student role	Implementing CTI protocol Submission of protocol revision to IRBS
Coaching	Chronic disease management Personal Health Record (PHR) Utilization	Staff meeting Clinical rounds	Disseminating CTI information to staff on participating units
Consultation	Consulted with: Gerontology CNS and physician Home care staff	Consulted with: CNS/CNL Home care staff Geriatric CNS Care coordinator	Consulted with: PHO staff MMC and USM IRB Dr. Coleman and UCSC team Course faculty and students
Collaboration	With patients and families	Attended staff meetings Participated in interdisciplinary clinical rounds CNS student to student Faculty/student CNS/CNL	Clinical seminar and preceptor discussions on role implementation, challenges and successes
Ethical Decision Making	Eliciting informed consent from subjects	Seminar discussion of double agency (conflict between clinician and student researcher role)	Complied with standards Informed consent Explained project to clinical and administrative staff

CNS, Clinical nurse specialist; *CTI,* Care Transitions Intervention; *IRB,* Institutional Review Board; CDSM, chronic disease self-management; *CNL,* clinical nurse leader; *PHO,* Physician Hospital Organization; *MMC,* Maine Medical Center; *USM,* University of Southern Maine; *UCHSC,* University of Colorado Health Sciences Center.

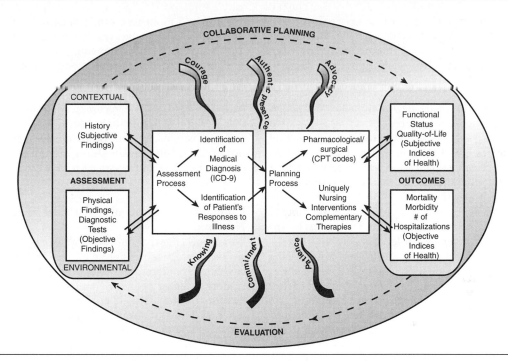

FIGURE 2-12: Dunphy and Winland-Brown's Circle of Caring Model. (From Dunphy, L.M., & Winland-Brown, J.E. [1998]. The circle of caring: A transformative model of advanced practice nursing. *Clinical Excellence for Nurse Practitioners, 2,* 241-247.)

initiative gave nurses a taxonomy for naming problems that are within the nursing domain to treat, nursing diagnoses are not recognized by current reimbursement systems, even though APNs may use them in the context of their practices. Dunphy and Winland-Brown further noted the challenge facing APNs to identify and cost out the unique characteristics of advanced practice nursing that are associated with improved patient outcomes.

The Circle of Caring Model was proposed to incorporate the strengths of medicine and nursing in a transforming way. The conceptual elements are the processes of assessment, planning, intervention, and evaluation with a feedback loop. Each of these processes is greatly enriched by a multiparadigmatic perspective. Integrating a nursing model with a traditional medical model permits the following to occur:

- The assessment and evaluation are contextualized, incorporating subjective and environmental elements into traditional history taking and physical examination.

- The approach to therapeutics is broadened to include holistic approaches to healing and makes nursing care more visible.

- Measured outcomes include patients' perceptions of health and care, not just physiological outcomes and resource utilization.

The assessment-planning-intervention-evaluation processes in linear configuration are encircled by caring. Caring is actualized through interpersonal interactions with patients and caregivers to which NPs bring patience, courage, advocacy, authentic presence, commitment, and knowing (Dunphy & Winland-Brown, 1998). Conceptual definitions of these terms would add to the understanding of how these processes interact with and affect the caregiving of APNs. The authors suggested that the model promotes the incorporation of the lived experience of the patient into the provider-patient interaction and that the process of caring is prerequisite to APNs providing effective and meaningful care to patients.

The Circle of Caring is seen as an integrated model of caregiving that incorporates the discrete strengths of both nursing and medicine. This is an important concern for many graduate students. They struggle with integrating their nursing expertise and philosophy with new knowledge and skills that were traditionally viewed as medicine. Though the authors view the concept of caring as a way to bridge the gap between advanced practice nursing and medicine and raise awareness, the model provides no clear guidance on how faculty can help students or how students themselves can use the model to bridge the gap.

Several issues remain to be considered. Dunphy and Winland-Brown intended that the model be applied on both the micro-level of one-to-one relationships in acute care and the macro-level of caring for communities and populations, although the feasibility, desirability, and implementation of the latter are not specifically addressed. For example, if one goal of proposing the model is to resolve differences about the diagnostic language used by medicine and nursing to obtain reimbursement, the model offers no specific mechanism for APNs to resolve this issue using the model. Indeed, the model does not seem sufficiently described to guide policymaking. The conceptual significance of encircling the four practice processes with the six caring processes is unclear. Practically, one would expect the caring processes, which appear to be attitudes and values, to be integrated throughout each practice step in a value-added collaborative model. Since the model was first proposed, we did not find literature that indicated it has been tested empirically. Such testing would help determine whether the model (1) is applicable to all advanced practice nursing roles; (2) has the potential to be used to distinguish expert-by-experience practice from advanced practice; (3) is viewed by other disciplines as having an interdisciplinary focus that would promote collaboration; and (4) would result in more visibility for NPs and other APNs within the health care system.

RECOMMENDATIONS AND FUTURE DIRECTIONS

It is understandable that students may feel overwhelmed at the variety of conceptualizations and inconsistency in terminology. The challenge for students is to find a model that works for them—that enables them to understand and evaluate their practices and to attend to the profession's efforts to create a coherent, stable, and robust conceptualization of advanced practice nursing.

Based on this review of models of advanced practice nursing and recognizing the advances made in this area since the previous edition, we have formulated some recommendations for further work on conceptualizing advanced practice in three areas: conceptualizations of advanced practice nursing, consensus building around advanced practice nursing, and research on APN practice and outcomes.

Conceptualizations of Advanced Practice Nursing

We acknowledge that our review of extant models of advanced practice nursing is rather cursory, is focused on U.S. literature, and may be incomplete—it is more a survey or overview than a review of the literature. Although there is some agreement on selected elements of advanced practice, by and large, there has been no comprehensive synthesis of existing work and limited evidence that new conceptualizations build on earlier work. To promote a unified conceptualization of advanced practice nursing, we suggest the following be undertaken:

1. A rigorous content analysis of the statements published by national and international professional organizations that describe the advanced practice nursing of recognized APNs (CNMs, CNSs, CRNAs, NPs) (this would be a natural evolution of the work done by the NCSBN, APRN Consensus Work Group, and APRN Joint Dialogue Groups to inform future work)
2. A similar content analysis of statements that address advanced practice nursing promulgated by specialty organizations
3. A review of recent role delineation studies of the four APN roles
4. A comprehensive integrative review of the advanced practice literature (building on the work of Mantzoukas and Watkinson, [2007])
5. Based on recommendations 1 through 3, a synthesis of results should be generated that can be used to propose a definition of the phenomenon—advanced practice nursing—and related concepts
6. Use the results of 1 through 5 to inform revisions of the DNP *Essentials*, standards,

and other documents that address APN education, credentialing, and licensing for existing and new APN roles

Consensus Building Around Advanced Practice Nursing

We believe a collaboratively developed conceptualization of advanced practice nursing is a prerequisite for building consensus among APNs, stakeholder organizations, and policymakers—this is a priority for the profession. This work is critical to ensuring that patients will continue to benefit from advanced practice nursing. The work of the APRN Joint Dialogue and Consensus Work Groups represents substantial progress in this area, as does the international work that is underway (Sheer, 2007). We recommend that a consensus on advanced practice nursing address the following:

1. A common language regarding advanced practice nursing:
   - For titling and criteria that must be met for credentialing and regulation. The proposed Consensus Model for APRN Regulation language (NCSBN, APRN Consensus Work Group, APRN Joint Dialogue Group) represents an important step in the development of a common language for educating and credentialing APNs as well as a process for creating and credentialing new APN roles.
   - For competencies and responsibilities of APNs. It is evident from this review that there is still a need for common language to describe advanced practice nursing—there is no clear articulation of the differences among Essentials, domains, competencies, and hallmarks and how these may be different from standards of care.
2. Disagreement on the nature and credentialing of advanced practice nursing should be resolved by continued efforts to foster true consensus by:
   - Addressing the legitimate concerns of these organizations (e.g., impact on access to care, grandfathering existing APNs)
   - Establishing priorities for negotiation and resolution by stakeholder groups and initiating a process for resolving them if disagreements remain.

NCSBN's vision paper and AACN's DNP initiative may have directly and indirectly pushed the profession to tackle the issue of conceptualization of advanced practice nursing. The work of the APRN Consensus Work Group, NCSBN APRN Advisory Committee, and Joint Dialogue Group is a substantive effort in this direction. The responses of NACNS, NONPF, ACNM, and AANA to the DNP initiative and the extent to which they will support and endorse the APRN Joint Dialogue Group report are likely to influence the evolution of advanced practice nursing in the next decade—including the extent to which we reach agreement within the profession, the extent to which we influence policy related to advanced practice, and whether the public recognizes and requests the services of APNs.

These consensus-building efforts are needed if our profession is to remain attractive to new nurses and new APNs and make room for evolving APN roles. Such consensus is critical if the profession is to make the expertise of APNs prepared 20 years ago available to the public and is particularly important considering the shortage of nurses.

Research on Advanced Practice Nurses and Outcomes

Theory-based research on APNs' contributions to improved patient outcomes and cost-effectiveness is needed to inform and validate the conceptualizations of advanced practice nursing. Increased knowledge about advanced practice nursing is critical (see Chapter 24): the worth of any service depends on the extent to which practice meets the needs and priorities of health care systems, the public policy arena, and society in general. In addition to research that links advanced practice nursing with outcomes, we recommend the following:

1. That promising conceptual models of advanced practice nursing be refined based on research that validates key concepts and tests theoretical propositions associated with such models.
2. That research on APNs examines the interpersonal processes they use in the course of coaching patients and collaborating with colleagues within and across disciplines—across many of the models reviewed in this chapter the APN's skill in communication and collaboration is considered important. We hypothesize that advanced communication skills contribute to APNs' effectiveness. APNs can contribute descriptive data on the interpersonal strategies they use in practice to

enable researchers to examine links between these less tangible aspects of APN care and patient outcomes.

3. That studies be undertaken to examine advanced practice nursing across APN roles and between physician and APN practice. Such studies can determine whether the assumption that a core set of competencies is used by all APNs is valid regardless of APN role. In addition, the activities that differentiate one APN role from another and those that distinguish APNs from physicians can be identified.

When there is a better empirical understanding of the similarities and differences across APN roles and between physicians and APNs, this knowledge must be packaged and presented to colleagues in other disciplines, to policymakers, and to the public. Such information is important to educating physicians, consumers, and policymakers about the meaning and relevance of advanced practice nursing to the health of our society.

For further discussion of research directions relevant to advanced practice nursing, see Chapter 24.

SUMMARY

Conceptual models serve many purposes for the fields they seek to describe. If the nursing profession can achieve consensus on a conceptual model of advanced practice nursing, then considerable progress will have been made. The future of advanced practice nursing will depend on the extent to which practice meets the needs and priorities of the society, health care systems, and the public policy arena. A stable, robust model of advanced practice nursing will serve to guide the evolution of advanced practice nursing and ensure that patients will have access to APN care.

We have identified problems and imperatives related to conceptualizing advanced practice nursing, reviewed a number of models, and made some recommendations for future work on conceptualizing advanced practice nursing that address the problems and imperatives. The nursing profession, nationally and internationally, is at a critical juncture with regard to advanced practice nursing. The need to move forward with one voice on this issue is urgent if APNs and the nursing profession as a whole are to fulfill their social contract with the individuals, the institutions, and the communities we serve. A unified conceptualization of advanced practice nursing will focus the efforts of the profession

on preparing APNs, promulgating policies, and fostering research that can enable the realization of the outcomes put forward at the beginning of this chapter (p. 36), including maximizing the social contribution of APNs to the health needs of society and promoting the actualization of APNs.

REFERENCES

Ackerman, M., Clark J., Reed, T., Van Horn, L., & Francati, M. (2000). A nurse practitioner managed cardiovascular intensive care unit. In J. Hickey, R. Ouimette, & S. Venegoni (Eds.), *Advanced practice nursing: Changing roles and clinical applications* (pp. 470-480). Philadelphia: Lippincott.

Ackerman, M.H., Norsen, L., Martin, B., Wiedrich, J., & Kitzman, H.J. (1996). Development of a model of advanced practice. *American Journal of Critical Care, 5,* 68-73.

American Association of Colleges of Nursing (AACN). (1996). *Essentials of master's education for advanced practice nursing.* Washington, DC: Author.

American Association of Colleges of Nursing (AACN). (2002). *The clinical nurse leader, developing a new nurse.* Retrieved July 22, 2007, from www.aacn.nche.edu/CNL/pdf/CNLFactSheet.pdf.

American Association of Colleges of Nursing (AACN). (October 2004). *AACN position statement on the practice doctorate in nursing.* Washington, DC. AACN. Retrieved July 27, 2007, from www.aacn.nche.edu/DNP/pdf/DNP.pdf.

American Association of Colleges of Nursing (AACN). (2006). Essentials of doctorate education for advanced nursing practice. Retrieved July 24, 2007, from www.aacn.nche.edu/DNP/pdf/Essentials.pdf.

American Association of Critical-Care Nurses. (2003). *The AACN Synergy Model for patient care.* Retrieved December 7, 2003, from www.aacn.org/certcorp/certcorp.nsf/vwdoc/SynModel?opendocument.

American Association of Nurse Anesthetists (AANA). (2005a). *Scope and standards for nurse anesthesia practice.* Park Ridge, IL: Author. Retrieved July 13, 2007, from www.aana.com/uploadedFiles/Resources/Practice_Documents/scope_stds_nap07_2007.pdf.

American Association of Nurse Anesthetists (AANA). (2005b). *Qualifications and capabilities of certified registered nurse anesthetists.* Retrieved July 14, 2007, from www.aana.com/becomingcrna.aspx?ucNavMenu_TSMenuTargetID=102&ucNavMenu_TSMenuTargetType=4&ucNavMenu_TSMenuID=6&id=112.

American Association of Nurse Anesthetists (AANA). (2006a). *Interim position statement on the DNP as entry into advanced practice for nurse anesthesia.* Retrieved July 13, 2007, from www.aana.com/professionaldevelopment.aspx?ucNavMenu_TSMenuTargetID=131&u cNavMenu_TSMenuTargetType=4&ucNavMenu_TSMenuID=6&id=1742&terms=DNP&se archtype=1&fragment=True.

American Association of Nurse Anesthetists (AANA). (2006b). *The doctorate in nursing practice (DNP): Background, current status, and future activities.* Retrieved July 12, 2007, from www.aana.com/professionaldevelopment. aspx?ucNavMenu_TSMenuTargetID=131&u cNavMenu_ TSMenuTargetType=4&ucNavMenu_TSMenuID=6&id 1742&terms=DNP&se archtype=1&fragment=True.

American College of Nurse-Midwives (ACNM). (1998). *State mandated master's degrees: A tip sheet for ACNM legislative contacts Number 18.* Retrieved July 22, 2007, from www. acnm.org/display.cfm?id=517.

American College of Nurse-Midwives (ACNM). (2003). *Standards for the practice of midwifery.* Retrieved July 12, 2007, from www.acnm.org/display.cfm?id=485.

American College of Nurse-Midwives (ACNM). (2005). *Code of ethics with explanatory statements.* Retrieved July 14, 2007, from www.midwife.org/siteFiles/education/Code-OfEthicswithExplanatoryStatements2005.pdf.

American College of Nurse-Midwives (ACNM). (2006). Mandatory degree requirements for entry into midwifery practice. Retrieved July 14, 2007, from www.midwife.org/ siteFiles/position/Mandatory_Degree_Requirements_ 3.06.pdf.

American College of Nurse-Midwives (AACN). (2007a). *Core competencies for basic midwifery practice.* Washington, DC: Author. Retrieved July 12, 2007, from www.acnm.org/site-Files/education/Core_Competencies_for_Basic_ Midwifery_Practice_6_07.pdf.

American College of Nurse-Midwives (AACM). (2007b). *Midwifery education and the doctor of nursing practice.* Retrieved July 14, 2007, from www.midwife.org/siteFiles/ position/Midwifery_Ed_and_DNP_6_07.pdf.

American Nurses Association (ANA). (1980). *Nursing: A social policy statement.* Kansas City, MO: Author.

American Nurses Association (ANA). (1995). *Nursing's social policy statement.* Washington, DC: Author.

American Nurses Association (ANA). (1996). *Scope and standards of advanced practice registered nursing.* Washington, DC: Author.

American Nurses Association (ANA). (2003). *Nursing's social policy statement* (2nd ed.). Washington, DC: Author.

American Nurses Association (ANA). (2004). *Scope and standards of advanced practice registered nursing.* Washington, DC: Author.

APRN Consensus Work Group. (2007a). *APRN Consensus Work Group Report* (draft), May 21, 2007. Chicago: Author

APRN Consensus Work Group. (2007b). *Consensus statement on advanced practice registered nursing report of APRN consensus work group* (Draft). Washington, DC: Author.

APRN Joint Dialogue Group. (2007a). *Meeting Notes for March 8-9, 2007.*

APRN Joint Dialogue Group. (2007b). *Report of the APRN Joint Dialogue Group.* Based on the work of the NCSBN APRN Committee and the Alliance for APRN Credentialing/APRN Consensus Group. Chicago and Washington DC: Author.

APRN Joint Dialogue Group. (2008). *Consensus Model for APRN Regulation.* Based on the work of the APRN Consensus Work Group and the NCSBN APRN Advisory Committee. Chicago/Washington, DC: Author.

Atkins, S., & Ersser, S. (2000). Education for advanced nursing practice: An evolving framework. *International Journal of Nursing Studies, 37,* 523-533.

Avery, M., & Howe, C. (2007). The DNP and entry into midwifery practice: An analysis. *Journal of Midwifery and Women's Health, 52*(1), 14-22.

Ball, C., & Cox, C. (2003). Restoring patients to health— Outcomes and indicators of advanced nursing practice in adult critical care, Part 1. *International Journal of Nursing Practice, 9,* 356-367.

Ball, C., & Cox, C. (2004). The core components of legitimate influence and the conditions that constrain or facilitate advanced nursing practice in adult critical care, Part 2. *International Journal of Nursing Practice, 10,* 10-20.

Barron, A., & White, P.A. (2000). Consultation. In A.B. Hamric, J.A. Spross, & C.M. Hanson (Eds.), *Advanced nursing practice: An integrative approach* (2nd ed., pp. 217-246). Philadelphia: Saunders.

Barron, A., & White, P.A. (2005). Consultation. In A.B. Hamric, J.A. Spross, & C.M. Hanson (Eds.), *Advanced nursing practice: An integrative approach* (3rd ed., pp. 225-255). Philadelphia: Saunders.

Becker, D., Kaplow, R., Muenzen, P., & Hartigan, C. (2006). Activities performed by acute and critical care advanced practice nurses: American Association of Critical-Care Nurses study of practice. *American Journal of Critical Care, 2,* 130-148.

Benner, P. (1984). *From novice to expert.* Menlo Park, CA: Addison-Wesley.

Benner, P. (1985). The oncology clinical nurse specialist as expert coach. *Oncology Nursing Forum, 12,* 40-44.

Brooten, D., Brown, L., Munro, B., York, R., Cohen, S., Roncoli, M., et al. (1988). Early discharge and specialist transitional care. *Image: Journal of Nursing Scholarship, 20,* 64-68.

Brooten, D., Naylor, M., York, R., Brown, L., Munro, B., Hollingsworth, A., et al. (2002). Lessons learned from testing the quality cost model of advanced practice nursing (APN) transitional care. *Journal of Nursing Scholarship, 34,* 359-375.

Brooten, D., & Youngblut, J. (2006). Nurse dose as a concept. *Journal of Nursing Scholarship, 38*(1), 94-99.

Brooten, D., Youngblut, J., Deatrick, J., Naylor, M., & York, R. (2003). Patient problems, advanced practice nurse (APN) interventions, time and contacts among five patient groups. *Journal of Nursing Scholarship, 35*(1), 73-79.

Brown, M.A., & Olshansky, E.F. (1997). From limbo to legitimacy: A theoretical model of the transition to the primary care nurse practitioner role. *Nursing Research, 46,* 46-51.

Brown, S.J. (1998). A framework for advanced practice nursing. *Journal of Professional Nursing, 14,* 157-164.

Brown, S. (2005). Direct clinical practice. In A. Hamric, J. Spross, & C. Hanson (Eds.), *Advanced nursing practice: An integrative approach* (3rd ed., pp. 143-185). Philadelphia: Saunders.

Bryant-Lukosius, D., DiCenso, A., Browne, G., & Pinelli, J. (2004). Advanced practice nursing roles: Development, implementation and evaluation. *Journal of Advanced Nursing, 48*(5), 519-529.

Brykczynski, K.A. (1989). An interpretive study describing the clinical judgment of nurse practitioners. *Scholarly Inquiry for Nursing Practice, 3,* 75-104.

Calkin, J.D. (1984). A model for advanced nursing practice. *Journal of Nursing Administration, 14,* 24-30.

Carveth, J.A. (1987). Conceptual models in nurse-midwifery. *Journal of Nurse-Midwifery, 32,* 20-25.

Chornick, N. (2002). *Role delineation study of nurse practitioners (NPs) and clinical nurse specialist (CNSs).* Retrieved July 19, 2007, from www.ncsbn.org/ICN_Poster(5_CNS).pdf.

Coleman, E., Parry, C., Chalmers, S., & Min, S.J. (2006). The Care Transitions Intervention: Results of a randomized controlled trial. *Archives of Internal Medicine, 166,* 1822-1828.

Collopy, K. (1999). The Synergy Model in practice: Advanced practice nurses guiding families through system. *Critical Care Nurse, 19*(5), 80-85.

Cumbie, S., Conley, V., & Burman, M. (2004). Advanced practice nursing: Model for comprehensive care with chronic illness. *Advances in Nursing Science, 27,* 70-80.

Curley, M.A.Q. (1998). Patient-nurse synergy: Optimizing patients' outcomes. *American Journal of Critical Care, 7,* 64-72.

Curran, C., & Roberts, W. (2002). Columbia University's competency and evidence-based acute care nurse practitioner program. *Nursing Outlook, 50,* 232-237.

DePalma, J., & McGuire, D. (2005). Research. In A. Hamric, J. Spross & C. Hanson (Eds.), *Advanced nursing practice: An integrative approach* (3rd ed., pp. 257-305). Philadelphia: Saunders.

Doessel, D., & Marshall, J. (1985). A rehabilitation of health outcomes in quality assessment. *Social Science and Medicine, 21*(12), 1319-1328.

Dunphy, L.M., & Winland-Brown, J.E. (1998). The circle of caring: A transformative model of advanced practice nursing. *Clinical Excellence for Nurse Practitioners, 2,* 241-247.

Fawcett, J. (2000). *Analysis and evaluation of contemporary nursing knowledge: Nursing models and theories.* Philadelphia: Davis.

Fawcett, J. (2001). Integrating conceptual models, theories, research, and practice. In D. Robinson & C. Kish (Eds.), *Core concepts in advanced practice nursing* (pp. 380-391). St. Louis: Mosby.

Fawcett, J., & Graham, I. (2005). Advanced practice nursing: Continuation of the dialogue. *Nursing Science Quarterly, 18,* 37-41.

Fawcett, J., Newman, D., & McAllister, M. (2004). Advanced practice nursing and conceptual models of nursing. *Nursing Science Quarterly, 17*(2), 135-138.

Fenton, M.V. (1985). Identifying competencies of clinical nurse specialists. *Journal of Nursing Administration, 15,* 31-37.

Fenton, M.V., & Brykczynski, K.A. (1993). Qualitative distinctions and similarities in the practice of clinical nurse specialists and nurse practitioners. *Journal of Professional Nursing, 9,* 313-326.

Gibbins, S., Green, P., Scott, P., & Watson MacDonell, J. (2000). The role of the clinical nurse specialist/neonatal nurse practitioner in a breastfeeding clinic: A model of advanced practice. *Clinical Nurse Specialist, 14*(2), 56-59.

Hamric, A.B. (1996). A definition of advanced practice nursing. In A.B. Hamric, J.A. Spross, & C.M. Hanson (Eds.), *Advanced nursing practice: An integrative approach* (pp. 25-41). Philadelphia: Saunders.

Hamric, A.B. (2005). A definition of advanced practice nursing. In A.B. Hamric, J.A. Spross, & C.M. Hanson (Eds.), *Advanced nursing practice: An integrative approach* (3rd ed., pp. 85-108). Philadelphia: Saunders.

Hamric, A.B. (2000). A definition of advanced practice nursing. In A.B. Hamric, J.A. Spross, & C.M. Hanson (Eds.), *Advanced nursing practice: An integrative approach* (2nd ed., pp. 53-74). Philadelphia: Saunders.

Hamric, A.B., & Reigle, J. (2005). Ethical decision making. In A.B. Hamric, J.A. Spross, & C.M. Hanson (Eds.), Advanced nursing practice: An integrative approach (3rd ed., pp. 379-412). Philadelphia: Saunders.

Hamric, A.B., & Spross, J.A. (1983). A model for future clinical specialist practice. In A.B. Hamric & J.A. Spross (Eds.), *The clinical nurse specialist in theory and practice* (pp. 291-306). New York: Grune & Stratton.

Hamric, A.B., & Spross, J.A. (1989). *The clinical nurse specialist in theory and practice* (2nd ed) Philadelphia: Saunders

Hanson, C.M., & Hamric, A.B. (2003). Reflections on the continuing evolution of advanced practice nursing. *Nursing Outlook, 51*(5), 203-210.

International Council of Nurses (ICN). (2006). *Definitions and characteristics of the (APN) role.* Retrieved July 12, 2007, from www.aanp.org/inp%20apn%20network/practice%20issue/role%20definitions.asp.

Lincoln, P. (2000). Comparing CNS and NP role activities: A replication. *Clinical Nurse Specialist, 14*(6), 269-277.

Mantzoukas, S., & Watkinson, S. (2007). Review of advanced nursing practice: The international literature and developing the generic features. *Journal of Clinical Nursing, 16,* 28-37.

McCabe, S., & Macnee, C. (2002). Weaving a new safety net of mental health care in rural America: A model of integrated practice. *Issues in Mental Health Nursing, 23,* 263-278.

McMillan, S.C., Heusinkveld, K.B., Spray, J.A.& Murphy, C.M. (1999). Revising the blueprint for the AOCN Examination using a role delineation study for advanced practice oncology nursing. *Oncology Nursing Forum, 26*:529-537.

Mick, D., & Ackerman, M. (2000). Advanced practice nursing role delineation in acute and critical care: Application of the Strong Model of advanced practice. *Heart & Lung, 29*(3), 210-221.

Moloney-Harmon, P. (1999). The Synergy Model: Contemporary practice of the clinical nurse specialist. *Critical Care Nurse, 19*(2), 101-104.

National Association of Clinical Nurse Specialists (NACNS). (1998). *Statement on clinical nurse specialist practice and education.* Glenview, IL: Author.

National Association of Clinical Nurse Specialists (NACNS). (2004). *Statement on clinical nurse specialist practice and education.* Harrisburg, PA: Author.

National Association of Clinical Nurse Specialists (NACNS). (2005). *White paper on the nursing practice doctorate.* Retrieved July 28, 2007, from www.nacns.org/nacns_dnpwhitepaper2.pdf.

National Association of Clinical Nurse Specialists' (NACNS) Board. (2006). Executive Summary: 2006 CNS Summit July 21-22, Indianapolis, Ind. *Clinical Nurse Specialist, 21*: 50-51.

National Council of State Boards of Nursing (NCSBN). (2002). *Nurse licensure compact.* Retrieved March 11, 2004, from www.ncsbn.org/nlc/aprncompact.asp.

National Council of State Boards of Nursing (NCSBN). (2006). *The future regulation of advanced practice nurses.* Retrieved July 19, 2007, from www.ncsbn.org/Draft_APRN_Vision_Paper.pdf.

National Organization of Nurse Practitioner Faculties (NONPF). (2002). *Nurse practitioner primary care competencies in specialty areas: Adult, family gerontological, pediatric, and women's health.* Retrieved March 6, 2004, from www.nonpf.com/finalaug2002.pdf.

National Organization of Nurse Practitioner Faculties (NONPF). (2003). *Psychiatric–mental health nurse practitioner competencies.* Retrieved March 6, 2004, from www.nonpf.com/finalcomps03.pdf.

National Organization of Nurse Practitioner Faculties (NONPF). (2006a). *Domains and core competencies of nurse practitioner practice.* Retrieved July 13, 2007, from www.nonpf.com/NONPF.

National Organization of Nurse Practitioner Faculties. (2006b). *Statement on the practice doctorate in nursing: Response to recommendations on clinical hours and degree title.* Retrieved July 13, 2007, from www.nonpf.com/NONPF2005/PracticeDoctorateResourceCenter/PDstatement1006.htm.

National Panel on Acute Care Nurse Practitioner Competencies. (2004). *Acute care nurse practitioner competencies.* Washington, DC: National Organization of Nurse Practitioner Faculties (NONPF).

National Panel for NP Practice Doctorate Competencies. (2006). *Practice doctorate nurse practitioner entry level competencies.* Washington, DC: National Organization of Nurse Practitioner Faculties.

Oberle, K., & Allen, M. (2001). The nature of advanced practice nursing. *Nursing Outlook, 49,* 148-153.

Plager, K., Conger, M., & Craig, C. (2003). Education for differentiated role development for NP and CNS practice: One nursing program's approach. *Journal of Nursing Education, 42*(9), 406-416.

Price, M.J., Martin, A.C., Newberry, Y.G., Zimmer, P.A., Brykczynski, K.A., & Warren, B. (1992). Developing national guidelines for nurse practitioner education: An overview of the product and the process. *Journal of Nursing Education, 31,* 10-15.

Raudonis, B., & Anderson, C. (2002). A theoretical framework for specialty certification in nursing practice. *Nursing Outlook, 30,* 247-252.

Reigle, J., & Boyle, R.J. (2000). Ethical decision-making skills. In A.B. Hamric, J.A. Spross, & C.M. Hanson (Eds.), *Advanced nursing practice: An integrative approach* (2nd ed., pp. 273-295). Philadelphia: Saunders.

Sheer, B. (2007). ICN Advanced Practice Nursing Network meets in Japan. *Nurse Practitioner World News, 12*(8), 10-11.

Shuler, P.A. (2000). Evaluating student services provided by school-based health centers: Applying the Shuler Nurse Practitioner Practice Model. *Journal of School Health, 70,* 348-352.

Shuler, P.A., & Davis, J.E. (1993a). The Shuler Nurse Practitioner Practice Model: A theoretical framework for nurse practitioner clinicians, educators, and researchers, Part 1. *Journal of the American Academy of Nurse Practitioners, 5,* 11-18.

Shuler, P.A., & Davis, J.E. (1993b). The Shuler Nurse Practitioner Practice Model: Clinical application, Part 2. *Journal of the American Academy of Nurse Practitioners, 5,* 73-88.

Shuler, P.A., Huebscher, R., & Hallock, J. (2001). Providing wholistic health care for the elderly: Utilization of the Shuler Nurse Practitioner Practice Model. *Journal of the American Academy of Nurse Practitioners, 13,* 297-303.

Spross, J.A. (2005). Expert coaching and guidance. In A.B. Hamric, J.A. Spross, & C.M. Hanson (Eds.), *Advanced nursing practice: An integrative approach* (3rd ed., pp. 187-224). Philadelphia: Saunders.

Spross, J.A., & Baggerly, J. (1989). Models of advanced nursing practice. In A.B. Hamric & J.A. Spross (Eds.), *The clinical nurse specialist in theory and practice* (2nd ed., pp. 19-40). Philadelphia: Saunders.

Spross, J.A., Clarke, E.B., & Beauregard, J. (2000). Expert coaching and guidance. In A.B. Hamric, J.A. Spross, & C.M. Hanson (Eds.), *Advanced nursing practice: An integrative approach* (2nd ed., pp. 183-216). Philadelphia: Saunders.

Stanley, J., & APRN Consensus Work Group. (2007). *Consensus statement on advanced practice registered nursing report of APRN consensus work group* (Draft). Washington, DC: Author.

Styles, M. (1998). An international perspective: APN credentialing. *Advanced Practice Nursing Quarterly, 4*(3), 1-5.

Styles, M.M., & Lewis, C. (2000). Conceptualizations of advanced nursing practice. In A.B. Hamric, J.A. Spross, & C.M. Hanson (Eds.), *Advanced nursing practice: An integrative approach* (2nd ed., pp. 25-41). Philadelphia: Saunders.

Thibodeau, J.A., & Hawkins, J.W. (1994). Moving toward a nursing model in advanced practice. *Western Journal of Nursing Research, 16,* 205-218.

Unnold, R., Erickson, V., Spross, J., & Warrick, C. (2007). Helping patients through health transitions: The role of the clinical nurse specialist in system change. Unpublished poster presentation, University of Southern Maine.

Valentine, N. Antai-Otong, D., Kupecz, D., Lynn, M., & Chaffee, M. (2000). Advanced practice nursing in the Department of Veterans Affairs: A model for the future. In J. Hickey, R. Ouimette, & S. Venegoni (Eds.), *Advanced practice nursing: Changing roles and clinical applications* (pp. 378-389). Philadelphia: Lippincott.

Whitcomb, R., Wilson, S., Chang-Dawkins, S., Durand, J., Pitcher, D., Lauzon, C., et al. (2002). Advanced practice nursing: Acute care model in progress. *Journal of Nursing Administration, 32*(3), 123-125.

Williams, C.A., & Valdivieso, G.C. (1994). Advanced practice models. A clinical comparison of clinical nurse specialist and nurse practitioner activities. *Clinical Nurse Specialist, 8,* 311-318.

Williams, C., Pesut, D., Boyd, M., Russell, S., Morrow, J., & Head, K. (1998). Toward an integration of competencies for advanced practice mental health nursing. *Journal of the American Psychiatric Nurses Association, 4*(2), 48-56.

Williams, D., & Kelley, M. (1998). Core competency-based education, certification, and practice: The nurse-midwifery model. *Advanced Practice Nursing Quarterly, 4*(3), 63-71.

Woods, L.P. (1997). Conceptualizing advanced nursing practice: Curriculum issues to consider in the educational preparation of advanced practice nurses in the UK. *Journal of Advanced Nursing, 25,* 820-828.

Zimmer, P., Brykczynski, K., Martin, A., Newberry, Y., Price, M., & Warren, B. (1990). *National guidelines for nurse practitioner education.* Seattle, WA: National Organization of Nurse Practitioner Faculties.

A Definition of Advanced Practice Nursing

Ann B. Hamric

INTRODUCTION

The advanced practice of nursing builds on the foundation and core values of the nursing discipline. According to the American Nurses Association (ANA) (American Nurses Association [ANA], 2003), contemporary nursing practice has six essential features: (1) inclusion of the full range of human experiences and responses to health and illness without restriction to a problem-focused orientation; (2) practice based on the integration of objective and subjective experience; (3) the ability to apply scientific knowledge to diagnostic and treatment processes; (4) the ability to provide a caring relationship that facilitates health and healing; (5) advancement of nursing's knowledge base through scholarly inquiry; and (6) the promotion of social justice through influencing public policy. These characteristics are equally essential for advanced practice nursing. Core values that guide nurses in practice include advocating for patients; respecting patient and family values and informed choices; viewing individuals holistically within their environments, communities, and cultural traditions; and maintaining a focus on disease prevention, health restoration, and health promotion (ANA, 2001; Creasia & Parker, 2006; Hood, 2006). These core professional values also inform the central perspective of advanced practice nursing.

Advanced practice nursing is a dynamic and evolving entity. Although differing interpretations are still evident at this stage of its development, the definition proffered here has been relatively stable throughout the four editions of this book. Consensus is growing within the profession regarding the primary criteria and core competency requirements for any advanced practice nurse (APN) role (in the regulatory arena, the alternative term *advanced practice registered nurse* or *APRN* is most commonly used) (APRN Joint Dialogue Group, 2008). Ongoing efforts to standardize the definition of advanced practice nursing (American Association of Colleges of Nursing [AACN], 1995; ANA, 1996, 2003; Hamric, 1996, 2000, 2005; National Council of State Boards of Nursing [NCSBN], 1993; 2002), however,

have not yet resulted in full clarity within or outside the profession. Different interpretations of advanced practice (AACN, 2006; ANA, 2005), debates about who is and is not an APN, and discrepancies in educational preparation for APNs remain. For advanced practice nursing to achieve its full potential and for new APN roles to evolve, the profession must agree on the key issues of definition, education, and credentialing.

In this chapter, advanced practice nursing is defined and the scope of practice of APNs is discussed. Various APN roles are differentiated, and key factors in advanced practice nursing environments are identified. The importance of a common and unified understanding of the distinguishing characteristics of advanced practice nursing is emphasized in this chapter and throughout the book.

DISTINGUISHING BETWEEN SPECIALIZATION AND ADVANCED PRACTICE NURSING

Before the definition of advanced practice nursing can be explored, it is important to distinguish between specialization in nursing and advanced practice nursing. Specialization involves concentration in a selected clinical area within the field of nursing. All nurses with extensive experience in a particular area of practice (e.g., pediatric nursing, trauma nursing) are specialized in this sense. As the profession has advanced and responded to changes in health care, specialization and the need for specialty knowledge have increased. Thus few nurses are generalists in the true sense of the word (Kitzman, 1989). Although family nurse practitioners (NPs) traditionally represented themselves as generalists, they are specialists in the sense discussed here because they have specialized in one of the many facets of health care, namely primary care. As Keeling notes in Chapter 1, early specialization involved primarily on-the-job training or hospital-based training courses, and many nurses continue to develop specialty skills through practice experiences and continuing education. Examples of currently evolving specialties include genetics nursing, forensic nursing, and clinical research nurse coordination. As specialties mature, they may develop graduate-level clinical preparation and incorporate the competencies of advanced practice nursing as the concept is defined in this chapter (Hanson & Hamric, 2003; see also Chapter 18). This progression is clearly seen in such APN roles as those of the certified registered nurse anesthetist (CRNA) and the NP.

The nursing profession has responded in a variety of ways to the increasing need for specialization in both clinical and clinical support arenas. The creation of specialty organizations, such as the American Association of Critical-Care Nurses and the Oncology Nursing Society, has been one response. The creation of APN roles—the CRNA and certified nurse-midwife (CNM) roles early in nursing's evolution and the clinical nurse specialist (CNS) and NP roles more recently—has been another response. A third response has been the development of specialized faculty, nursing researchers, and nursing administrators. Nurses in all of these roles can be considered specialists in an area of nursing (e.g., education, research and administration); some of these roles may involve advanced education in a clinical specialty as well. However, they are not necessarily advanced practice nursing roles. Advanced practice nursing includes specialization but also involves expansion and educational advancement (ANA, 1995; Cronenwett, 1995). In addition to specialization, *Nursing's Social Policy Statement* (ANA, 2003) defined these elements as follows:

> Expansion refers to the acquisition of new practice knowledge and skills, including the knowledge and skills that authorize role autonomy within areas of practice that overlap traditional boundaries of medical practice . . . . Advanced practice is characterized by the integration and application of a broad range of theoretical and evidence-based knowledge that occurs as a part of graduate nursing. (p. 9)

As compared with basic nursing practice, APN practice is further characterized by (1) significant role autonomy, (2) responsibility for health promotion in addition to diagnosis and management of patient problems including prescribing pharmacological and nonpharmacological interventions, and (3) the greater complexity of clinical decision making and leadership in organizations and environments (ANA, 1996; APRN Joint Dialogue Group, 2008).

DISTINGUISHING BETWEEN ADVANCED NURSING PRACTICE AND ADVANCED PRACTICE NURSING

In 2004 the American Association of Colleges of Nursing (AACN) adopted a "Position Statement on the Practice Doctorate in Nursing," which recommended doctoral-level educational preparation for individuals at the most advanced level of nursing practice. This Doctor of Nursing Practice (DNP) degree was further recommended to be the required level of education for APNs by 2015. The DNP position statement (AACN, 2004) advanced a broad definition of advanced nursing practice as

> . . .any form of nursing intervention that influences health care outcomes for individuals or populations, including the direct care of individual patients, management of care for individuals and populations, administration of nursing and health care organizations, and the development and implementation of health policy. (p. 3)

A definition this broad goes beyond advanced practice nursing to include other advanced nursing specialties not involved in providing direct clinical care to patients, such as administration, policy, informatics, and public health. One reason for such a broad definition was the desire to have the DNP degree be available to nurses practicing at the highest level in many varied *specialties*, not only those in APN roles. A decision was reached by the original DNP Task Force (AACN, 2004) that the DNP degree was not to be a "clinical" doctorate, as was advocated in early discussions (Mundinger et al., 2000) but, rather, a "practice" doctorate in an expansive understanding of the term *practice*. The AACN's *The Essentials of Doctoral Education for Advanced Nursing Practice* (2006) distinguishes between roles with an aggregate/systems/organizational focus ("advanced specialties") and roles with a direct clinical practice focus (APN roles of CNS, NP, CRNA, and CNM), while recognizing that these two groups share some essential competencies.

Advanced practice nursing is a concept that applies to roles that include direct patient care to individual patients and families (see the following section). These roles involve expanded clinical skills and abilities and require a different level of regulation than do non-APN roles. Consequently, a distinction between the terms *advanced nursing practice* and *advanced practice nursing* is necessary. This book focuses on advanced practice nursing and the varied roles of APNs. DNP programs that prepare students for APN roles will have different curricula from those preparing students for administration, informatics or other specialties that do not have a direct practice component (AACN, 2006).

DEFINING ADVANCED PRACTICE NURSING

In 1996 O'Malley and colleagues wrote, "In most settings, the role of APNs has not been fully understood …. APNs are still not identified by the public as primary care providers, partially due to misunderstanding of their roles" (O'Malley, Cummings, & King, 1996, p. 63). Since that time, APNs have made significant progress in the public and policy arenas. However, the concept of advanced practice nursing continues to be defined in various ways in the nursing literature. The *Cumulative Index to Nursing and Allied Health Literature* defines advanced practice broadly as anything beyond the staff nurse role: "The performance of additional acts by registered nurses who have gained added knowledge and skills through post-basic education and clinical experience" (Advanced Nursing Practice, 2007). As just noted with the DNP definition, a definition this broad incorporates many specialized nursing roles, not all of which should be considered advanced practice nursing.

Advanced practice nursing is often defined as a constellation of four roles: the NP, CNS, CNM, and CRNA (APRN Joint Dialogue Group, 2008; Donley, 1995; NCSBN, 2002; Stanley, 2005). In the past, some authors discussed advanced practice nursing only in terms of selected roles such as NP and CNS (Lindeke, Canedy, & Kay, 1997; Rasch & Frauman, 1996) or the NP role exclusively (Hickey, Ouimette, & Venegoni, 2000; Mundinger, 1994; Thibodeau & Hawkins, 1994). Defining advanced practice nursing in terms of particular roles limits the concept and denies the reality that some nurses in these four roles are not using the core competencies of advanced practice nursing in their practices. These definitions are also limiting because they do not incorporate evolving APN roles, such as the blended CNS/NP (see Chapter 15). Thus it seems preferable to define advanced practice nursing as a concept without reference to particular roles (Davies & Hughes, 1995).

A definition should also clarify the critical point that advanced practice nursing involves advanced *nursing* knowledge and skills; it is not a *medical* practice, although APNs perform expanded medical therapeutics in many roles. Throughout nursing's history,

nurses have assumed "medical" roles. For example, common nursing tasks such as blood pressure measurement and administration of chemotherapeutic agents were once performed exclusively by physicians. When APNs begin to transfer new skills or interventions into their repertoire, they become nursing skills, informed by the clinical practice values of the profession.

In addition, advanced practice nursing needs to be understood in a conceptually clear fashion that recognizes the core competencies that all APNs share. Conceptual clarity can guide educational curricula to ensure that all APNs learn the core competencies so essential to successful practice.

CORE DEFINITION OF ADVANCED PRACTICE NURSING

As can be seen from this brief review, advanced practice nursing has been defined in different and sometimes contradictory ways. The definition proposed in this chapter builds on and extends the understanding of advanced practice nursing proposed in the first three editions of this book. Important assertions of this discussion are as follows:

- Advanced practice nursing is a function of educational and practice preparation and a constellation of primary criteria and core competencies.
- Direct clinical practice is the central competency of any APN role and informs all the other competencies.
- All APNs share the same core criteria and competencies, though the actual clinical skill set varies depending on the needs of the APN's specialty patient population.

Actual practices differ significantly based on the particular role adopted and the organizational framework within which the role is performed. Because particular APN roles have different expectations and include additional competencies specific to them, it is both necessary and preferable to retain varied job titles that reflect these actual practices, rather than reduce all APNs to one title.

In spite of the need to keep job descriptions and job titles distinct in practice settings, it is critical that the public's acceptance of advanced practice nursing be enhanced and confusion decreased. As Safriet (1993, 1998) noted, nursing's future depends on reaching consensus on titles and consistent preparation for title holders. The burden is clearly on the nursing profession and its APNs to be clear, concrete, and consistent about APN titles and their functions in discussions with nursing's larger constituencies: consumers, other health care professionals, health care administrators, and health care policymakers.

Conceptual Definition

The ANA's *Scope and Standards of Advanced Practice Registered Nursing* (1996) summarized conceptual elements of APN practice as follows:

> Advanced practice registered nurses manifest a high level of expertise in the assessment, diagnosis, and treatment of the complex responses of individuals, families, or communities to actual or potential health problems, prevention of illness and injury, maintenance of wellness, and provision of comfort. The advanced practice registered nurse has a master's or doctoral education concentrating in a specific area of advanced nursing practice, had supervised practice during graduate education, and has ongoing clinical experiences. Advanced practice registered nurses continue to perform many of the same interventions used in basic nursing practice. The difference in this practice relates to a greater depth and breadth of knowledge, a greater degree of synthesis of data, and complexity of skills and interventions. (p. 2)

Integrating this earlier understanding leads to the following conceptual definition:

> **Advanced practice nursing is the application of an expanded range of practical, theoretical, and research-based competencies to phenomena experienced by patients within a specialized clinical area of the larger discipline of nursing.**[1]

The term *competencies* refers to any area of skillful performance; seven core competencies combine to distinguish nursing practice at this level. Competencies include activities undertaken as part of delivering advanced nursing care directly to patients, including assessment, diagnosis, planning, intervention/treatment, and evaluation. Some competencies are processes that APNs use in all dimensions of their practice, such as collaboration and leadership. Through graduate education and practice experiences, APNs expand their capability to provide and direct care. Although certain activities may also be performed by physicians and other health care professionals, the experiential, theoretical, and philosophical perspectives of nursing make these activities advanced nursing practice when they are carried out by an APN. In addition, advanced practice nursing involves highly developed nursing skills, as well

as performance of selected medical therapies, as the defining characteristics will clarify. The nursing profession needs to be clear on this point, for *the advanced practice of nursing is not the junior practice of medicine.*

This definition recognizes that not all nursing competencies are research based at this point in nursing's evolution. Expanded theoretical knowledge is a key element of advanced practice. In addition, a strong experiential component is necessary to develop the competencies and clinical practice expertise that characterize advanced practice nursing. Although graduate education in nursing provides a critical foundation for the expanded knowledge and theory base necessary to support advanced practice nursing, in-depth clinical experiences are equally critical. Graduate education and clinical practice experience work together to develop the APN. The definition also emphasizes the patient-focused and specialized nature of advanced practice nursing. Finally, the critical importance of ensuring that any type of advanced practice is grounded within the larger discipline of nursing is made explicit.

Advanced practice nursing is further defined by three primary criteria and seven core competencies, one of them central to the others. This discussion and the chapters in Part II isolate each of these core competencies to clarify them. The reader should recognize that this is only a heuristic device for clarifying the conceptualization of advanced practice nursing used in this book. In reality, these elements are integrated into an APN's practice; they are not separate and distinct features. The concentric circles in Figures 3-1 through 3-3 represent the seamless nature of this interweaving of elements. In addition, an APN's skills function synergistically to produce a whole that is greater than the sum of its parts. The essence of advanced practice nursing is found not only in the primary criteria and competencies demonstrated but also in the synthesis of these elements, along with individual nurse characteristics, into a unified composite practice (Davies & Hughes, 1995) that conforms to the conceptual definition presented earlier.

Many nurses who are not in APN roles have developed some of these competencies; this is particularly true of experts-by-experience, who are often seen as exemplary nurses (see Chapter 2). What sets APN practice apart, however, is the *expectation* that every APN encompasses all of these competencies and seamlessly blends them in everyday practice. It is also important to understand that each of the competencies that are described in Part II of this book have specific definitions in the context of advanced

---

[1]The term *patient* is intended to be used interchangeably with *individual* and *client.*

practice nursing. For example, clinical, professional, and systems leadership has a definition for the APN that differs from that for a nursing administrator or a staff nurse.

Primary Criteria

Certain criteria (or qualifications) must be met before a nurse can be considered an APN. Although these baseline criteria are not *sufficient* in and of themselves, they are *necessary* core elements of advanced practice nursing. The three primary criteria for advanced practice nursing are shown in Figure 3-1 and include an earned graduate degree with a concentration in an advanced practice nursing role and specialty, national certification of practice at an advanced level within a given specialty, and a practice that is focused on patients and their families. These criteria are most often the ones used by states to regulate APN practice (APRN Joint Dialogue Group, 2008) because they are objective and easily measured (see Chapter 21).

Graduate Education. First, the APN must possess an *earned graduate (master's or DNP) degree with a concentration in an APN role.* Advanced practice students acquire specialized knowledge and skills through study and supervised practice at either the master's or the doctoral level. Curricular content includes theories and research findings relevant to the core of a particular advanced nursing specialty. Because APNs assess, manage, and evaluate patients at the most independent level of clinical nursing practice, all APN curricula contain specific courses in advanced health/physical assessment, advanced pathophysiology, and advanced

pharmacology (AACN, 1995; 2006). This expansion of practice skills is acquired through clinical experience in addition to faculty-supervised practice, with most master's programs requiring a minimum of 500 clinical hours and DNP programs requiring 1000 hours. As noted previously in the ANA's definition, there is consensus that a master's education in nursing is a baseline requirement for advanced practice nursing (nurse-midwifery is the latest APN specialty to agree to this requirement; a graduate degree will be required for CNM practice by 2010) (American College of Nurse-Midwives [ACNM], 2006; see also Chapter 16).

Why is graduate educational preparation necessary for advanced practice nursing? Graduate education is a more efficient and standardized way to inculcate the complex competencies of APN-level practice than nursing's traditional on-the-job or apprentice training programs (see Chapter 18). As the knowledge base within specialties has grown, so too has the need for formal education at the graduate level. In particular, the research skills necessary for evidence-based practice (EBP) and the theory base required for advanced practice nursing mandate education at the graduate level.

Some of the differences between basic and advanced practice in nursing are apparent in the range and depth of APNs' clinical knowledge; in APNs' ability to anticipate patient responses to health, illness, and nursing interventions; in their ability to analyze clinical situations and explain why a phenomenon has occurred or why a particular intervention has been chosen; in the reflective nature of their practice; in their skill in assessing and addressing nonclinical variables that influence patient care; and in their attention to the consequences of care and improving patient outcomes. Because of the interaction and integration of graduate education in nursing and extensive clinical experience, APNs are able to exercise a level of discrimination in clinical judgment that is unavailable to other experienced clinicians (Spross & Baggerly, 1989).

Professionally, requiring graduate preparation is important to create parity among all APN roles so that all can move forward together in addressing policymaking and regulatory issues. This parity advances the profession's standards and ensures more uniform credentialing mechanisms. Creating a normative educational expectation also enhances nursing's image and credibility with other disciplines. Indeed, decisions by other health care providers, such

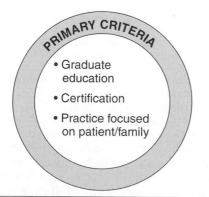

PRIMARY CRITERIA

- Graduate education
- Certification
- Practice focused on patient/family

FIGURE **3-1:** Primary criteria of advanced practice nursing.

as pharmacists, physical therapists, and occupational therapists, to require doctoral preparation for entry into their professions provided compelling support for nursing to establish the practice doctorate for APNs to achieve parity with these disciplines (AACN, 2006). Nursing has a particular need to achieve greater credibility with medicine. Organized medicine has historically been eager to point to nursing's internal differences in APN education as evidence that APNs are inferior providers.

The new clinical nurse leader (CNL) role represents a new understanding of the master's credential. Historically, master's education in nursing was by definition specialized education (see Chapter 1). However, the master's-prepared CNL is described as a "generalist," a staff nurse with expanded leadership skills at the point of care (AACN, 2003). Even though these nurses have expanded leadership skills and graduate-level education, they are clearly not APNs. APN graduate education is highly specialized and involves preparation for an expanded scope of practice, neither of which characterizes CNL education.

Certification. The second primary criterion is *professional certification for practice at an advanced level within a clinical specialty*. The continuing growth of specialization has dramatically increased the amount of knowledge and experience required to practice safely in modern health care settings. National certification examinations have been developed by specialty organizations and are used to determine whether nurses meet beginning standards for practice in a particular clinical specialty. Historically, these examinations tested the specialty knowledge of experienced nurses and not knowledge at the advanced level of practice. Two notable exceptions are the CNM and CRNA certifying examinations (see Chapter 1). As regulatory groups, particularly state boards of nursing, have increasingly used the certification credential to recognize APN providers, the picture has changed and more APN-specific certifications have been developed (see Chapter 21). NPs now have a number of certification options for both primary care and acute care practices.

Although the American Nurses Credentialing Center has sponsored CNS certification examinations in adult health (formerly *medical-surgical*) and psychiatric areas for years, advanced practice certification examinations in particular specialties have been slow to develop. However, the number of ex-amination options for CNSs is increasing. For example, the Oncology Nursing Society began administering an advanced practice certification examination in 1995, and advanced practice certifications for CNSs exist in such specialties as acute and critical care nursing (see Chapter 18 for additional examples).

The latest regulatory proposal from a joint consensus group that includes the National Council of State Boards of Nursing (NCSBN) and multiple APN stakeholder groups is that APNs will be required to pass certification examinations at the level of role (CNS, NP, CRNA, and CNM) population focus (areas such as adult-gerontology, individual/family, neonatal, and family [APRN Joint Dialogue Group, 2008]). Regulation will focus on these broad role and population foci rather than on particular specialties. Even though APN regulation is becoming more standardized, a need exists for the continued development of specialty examinations at the advanced practice nursing level. This is most pressing and challenging for CNSs, many of whose specialty areas have no advanced examination.

Why is it important that national certification at an advanced practice level be a primary criterion for advanced practice nursing? As early as 1980, in the seminal document *Nursing: A Social Policy Statement*, the ANA definitively stated (ANA, 1980):

> [T]he public needs clear evidence that a nurse who claims to be a specialist does indeed have expertise of a particular kind. The profession of nursing has a social obligation to the public to satisfy that need, which it does by means of certification of specialists and by accreditation of the graduate programs that educate specialists in nursing practice. These two methods by which the public is protected against false claims are in accord with the prerogative of self-regulation (within the profession) that society has accorded as a trust to its professions. It is in the absence of such within-profession credentialing that the public turns to the law for its protection. Through credentialing of those nurses who claim competence at an expert level, the nursing profession assures the public that these claims of a higher standard of nursing competence are not false. (p. 24)

Continuing variability in graduate curricula make sole reliance on the criterion of graduate education insufficient to protect the public. For example, a survey of CNS programs in the United States (Walker et al., 2003) revealed tremendous variability in both program length (varying from 27 to 60 credit hours required) and clinical practice experiences (ranging from 3 to 42 credit hours required). Given this example of program variability, it is difficult to argue that graduate education alone can provide sufficient evidence of competence for regulatory purposes. National certifying examinations provide a consistent standard that each APN must meet to demonstrate beginning competency for an advanced level of practice in his or her specialty. Finally, certification enhances title recognition in the regulatory arena, which promotes the visibility of advanced practice nursing and enhances the public's access to APN services.

Table 3-1 on p. 86 lists numbers of APNs and numbers certified in the United States from 1996 through 2004. Certification percentages have increased for all APN specialty groups, with CRNAs and CNMs having the consistently highest percentage of certified practitioners. Although CNSs continue to lag behind other specialties in percentage certified, they have made steady gains in this area since the early 1990s.

It is critically important that certifying organizations work to clarify the certification credential as appropriate only for *currently practicing* APNs. Given the centrality of the direct clinical practice component to the definition of advanced practice nursing, certification examinations must establish a significant number of hours of clinical practice as a requirement for maintaining APN certification. Some faculty and nursing leaders who do not maintain a direct clinical practice component in their positions have been allowed to sit for certification examinations and represent themselves as APNs. Statements such as "Once a CNS, always a CNS," which are heard with NPs and CNMs as well, perpetuate the mistaken notion that an APN title is a professional attribute rather than a practice role. Such a misunderstanding is confusing both inside and outside of nursing; by definition, these individuals are no longer APNs (see the next section).

Practice Focused on Patient/Family The third primary criterion is *a practice focused on patients and their families.* As noted in describing DNP graduates, the AACN DNP Task Force differentiated APNs from other roles using this primary criterion. They noted two general role categories (AACN, 2006): "roles which specialize as an advanced practice nurse (APN) with a focus on care of individuals; and roles that specialize in practice at an aggregate, systems, or organizational level. This distinction is important as APNs face different licensure, regulatory, credentialing, liability, and reimbursement issues than those who practice at an aggregate, sys-

tems, or organizational level" (p. 17). This criterion does not imply that direct practice is the only activity that APNs undertake, however. APNs also educate others, participate in and conduct research, and serve as consultants (Brown, 1998); they understand and are involved in practice contexts to identify and effect needed system changes, and they work to improve the health of their specialty populations (AACN, 2006). With that said, to be considered an APN role, the patient/family direct practice focus must be primary.

Historically, APN roles have been associated with direct clinical care; as the ANA (1996) noted, "The term advanced practice is used to refer exclusively to advanced clinical practice" (p. 16). Recent work is solidifying this understanding. The APRN Joint Dialogue Group (2008) makes clear that the provision of direct care to individuals as a significant component of their practice is *the* defining factor for all APRNs. The centrality of direct clinical practice is further reflected in the core competencies presented in the next section.

As noted earlier, there are other important specialized roles in the profession—notably, educators, administrators, and researchers. Master's level programs have been developed for staff development and clinical educators. All of these roles are valuable and vital to the profession's continued development. They are "critical to the preparation of nurses for practice, the provision of environments that are conducive to nursing practice, and the continued development of the knowledge base that nurses use in practice" (ANA, 1995, p. 15). Some of the nurses in these roles possess advanced practice knowledge and skills as well and may be certified in their specialty. However, their differing focus on staff nurses, students, or systems, rather than on patients and families, means that they are not considered APNs by this definition.

This requirement for a patient-focused practice puts some community health nurses in a gray area between advanced practice nursing and specialized practices of program development or consultation. Some APNs in community-based practices take a community view of their practice and consider the community to be their patient or client. Certainly, the broad perspective of the APN encompasses the community and society in which care is provided (AACN, 2006; Davies & Hughes, 1995); effecting positive outcomes for populations of patients is an important expectation for APNs in general. The National Organization of Nurse Practitioner

Faculties (NONPF) has integrated community health concepts into NP education and considers them to be a core competency of NP practice (National Organization of Nurse Practitioner Faculties [NONPF], 2000).

However, advanced practice nursing is focused on and realized at the level of clinical practice with patients and families. As long as APNs in community health practices maintain a direct clinical practice focused on patients and their families in addition to programmatic or consultative responsibilities, they are APNs by this definition. Community/public health specialists who do not have a patient-focused practice but, rather, focus on community assessment, monitoring community health status, and developing policies and program plans are more appropriately considered advanced specialty nurses rather than APNs (AACN, 2006; Hanson & Hamric, 2003). Community/public health nursing leaders have differentiated their specialty from this understanding of advanced practice nursing in two reports (ANA, 2005; Association of Community Health Nursing Educators Task Force on Community/Public Health Master's Level Preparation, 2000). The competencies they list for the community/public health specialty differ from the core APN competencies outlined here, particularly with regard to direct clinical practice.

Why limit the definition of advanced practice nursing to roles that focus on clinical practice to patients and families? There are many reasons. Nursing is a practice profession. The nurse-patient interface is at the core of nursing practice; in the final analysis, the reason the profession exists is to render nursing services to individuals in need of them. Clinical practice expertise in a given specialty develops from these nurse-patient encounters and lies at the heart of advanced practice nursing. In addition, ongoing direct clinical practice is necessary to maintain and develop an APN's expertise. Without regular immersion in practice, the cutting-edge clinical acumen and expertise found in APN practices cannot be sustained. In addition, the knowledge base needed for APN roles also differs from that for non-APN roles.

If every specialized role in nursing were considered advanced practice nursing, the term would become so broad as to lack meaning and explanatory value. (For further discussion, see Cronenwett [1995].) Distinguishing between APN roles and other specialized roles in nursing can help clarify the concept of advanced practice nursing to consumers, to other health care providers, and even to other nurses. In addition, the monitoring and regulation of advanced practice nursing are increasingly important issues as APNs work toward more authority for their practices (see Chapter 21). If the definition of advanced practice nursing included nonclinical roles, development of sound regulatory mechanisms would be impossible.

It is critical to understand that this definition of advanced practice nursing is not a value statement but, rather, a differentiation of one group of nurses from other groups for the sake of clarity within and outside the profession. Some nurses with specialized skills in administration, research, and community health have viewed the direct practice requirement as a devaluing of their contributions. Some faculty who teach clinical nursing but do not themselves maintain an advanced clinical practice have also felt disenfranchised because they are not considered APNs by virtue of this primary criterion. Perhaps this problem has been exacerbated with use of the term *advanced*, because this term can inadvertently imply that nurses who do not fit into the APN definition are not "advanced" (i.e., are not as well prepared or highly skilled as APNs).

The contention advanced in this book is that no value difference exists between specialized nurses and APNs—both groups are equally important to the overall growth and strengthening of the profession. The profession must be able to differentiate its various roles without such differentiation being viewed as a disparagement of any one group. Thus it is critical to understand that this definition of advanced practice nursing is not a value statement but, rather, a differentiation of one group of nurses from other groups for the sake of clarity within and outside the profession. As the ANA (1995) noted, all nurses—whether their focus is clinical practice, educating students, conducting research, planning community programs, or leading nursing service organizations—are valuable and necessary to the integrity and growth of the larger profession. However, all nurses—particularly those with advanced degrees—are *not the same,* nor are they necessarily APNs. Historically, the profession has had difficulty differentiating itself and has struggled with the prevailing lay notion that "a nurse is a nurse is a nurse." This antiquated view does not match the reality of the health care arena, nor does it celebrate the diverse contributions of all the various nursing roles and specialties.

SEVEN CORE COMPETENCIES OF ADVANCED PRACTICE NURSING

Direct Clinical Practice: The Central Competency

As noted earlier, the primary criteria are necessary but insufficient elements of the definition of advanced practice nursing. Advanced practice is further defined by a set of seven core competencies that are enacted in each APN role. The first core competency of direct clinical practice is central to and informs all of the others (Figure 3-2). In one sense, it is "first among equals" of the seven core competencies that define advanced practice nursing. Although APNs do many things, excellence in direct clinical practice provides the foundation necessary for APNs to execute the other competencies, such as consultation, patient and staff teaching, and leadership within organizations.

However, clinical expertise alone should not be equated with advanced practice nursing. The work of Patricia Benner and her colleagues (Benner, 1984; Benner, Hooper-Kyriakidis, & Stannard, 1999; Benner, Tanner, & Chesla, 1996) is a major contribution to an understanding of clinically expert nursing practice. These researchers extensively studied expert nurses in acute care clinical settings and described the engaged clinical reasoning and domains of practice seen in clinically expert nurses. Although some of the participants in this research were APNs (in the most recent report [Benner et al., 1999], 16% of the nurse participants were APNs), the majority were nurses with extensive clinical experience who did not have APN preparation. Calkin (1984) characterized these latter nurses as "experts by experience." (See Chapter 2 for a discussion of Calkin's conceptual differentiation between levels of nursing practice.) Benner and colleagues have not discussed differences in the practices of APNs as compared with other nurses they have studied. In fact, they stated, "'Expert' is not used to refer to a specific role such as an advanced practice nurse. Expertise is found in the practice of experienced clinicians and advanced practice nurses" (Benner et al., 1999, p. 9).

Although clinical expertise is a central ingredient of an APN's practice, the direct care practice of APNs is distinguished by six characteristics: (1) use of a holistic perspective, (2) formation of therapeutic partnerships with patients, (3) use of expert clinical thinking and skillful performance, (4) use of reflective practice, (5) reliance on research evidence as a guide to practice, and (6) use of diverse health and illness management approaches (see Chapter 5). These characteristics help distinguish the practice of the expert by experience from that of the APN. Of importance, APN clinical practice is also informed by a population focus (AACN, 2006) as APNs work to improve the care for their specialty patient population even as they care for individuals within the population. As previously noted, experiential knowledge and graduate education combine to develop these characteristics in an APN's clinical practice.

The specific content of the direct practice competency differs significantly by specialty. For example, the clinical practice of a CNS dealing with critically ill children differs from the expertise of an NP managing the health maintenance needs of older adults or a CRNA administering anesthesia in an outpatient surgical clinic. In addition, the amount of time spent in direct practice differs by APN specialty. CNSs in particular may spend the majority of their time in activities other than direct clinical practice (see Chapter 12). So it is important to understand this competency as a central defining characteristic of advanced practice nursing rather than an expectation that APNs only engage in direct clinical practice.

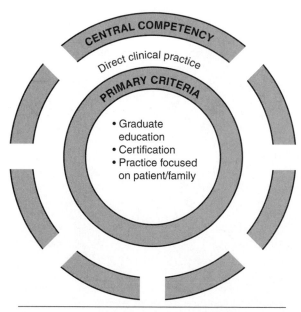

FIGURE **3-2:** Central competency of advanced practice nursing.

Additional Advanced Practice Nurse Core Competencies

In addition to the central competency of direct clinical practice, six additional competencies further define advanced practice nursing regardless of role function or setting. These competencies have repeatedly been identified as essential features of advanced practice nursing (AACN, 1995; ANA, 1995, 2003; Davies & Hughes, 1995; Hamric & Spross, 1989; National Association of Clinical Nurse Specialists [NACNS], 2004; NCSBN, 1993; NONPF, 2006). As shown in Figure 3-3, these additional core competencies are as follows:

- Expert coaching and guidance of patients, families, and other care providers
- Consultation
- Research
- Clinical, professional, and systems leadership
- Collaboration
- Ethical decision making

These competencies are not unique to advanced practice nursing, although they are defined in some specific ways with respect to APN practice (e.g., see the description of ethical decision making in Chapter 11). Experienced staff nurses may master several of these competencies over time, and such nurses are seen as exemplary performers. In fact, these nurses are often encouraged to enter graduate school to become APNs. What distinguishes APN practice is the *expectation* that these competencies are visible in the practice; that is, they are basic elements of the practice of every APN. Similarly, many competencies taught in graduate programs are important components of other specialized nursing roles. For example, collaboration, consultation, and leadership are important competencies for nursing administrators. The uniqueness of advanced practice nursing is seen in the synergistic interaction between direct clinical practice and this constellation of competencies. In Figure 3-3, the openings between the central practice competency and these additional competencies represent the fact that the APN's direct practice skill interacts with and informs all the other competencies. For example, APNs consult with other providers who seek their practice expertise to plan care for specialty patients. They are able to provide expert guidance and coaching for patients going through health and illness transitions because of their direct practice experience and insight.

These complex competencies develop over time. No APN emerges from a graduate program fully prepared to enact all of them. However, it is critical that graduate

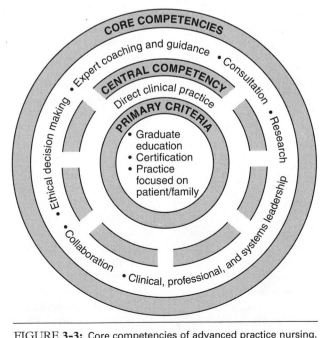

FIGURE **3-3:** Core competencies of advanced practice nursing.

programs provide exposure to each competency in the form of didactic content, as well as practical experiences so that new graduates can be tested for initial credentialing and be given a base on which to build their practices. These key competencies are described in detail in subsequent chapters and so are not further elaborated here.

Scope of Practice

The term *scope of practice* refers to the legal authority granted to a professional to provide and be reimbursed for health care services. This authority for practice emanates from many sources, such as state and federal laws and regulations, the profession's code of ethics, and professional practice standards. For all health care professionals, scope of practice is most closely tied to state statutes; for nursing, these statutes are the nurse practice acts of the various states. As previously discussed, APN scope of practice is characterized by specialization; expansion of services provided, including diagnosing and prescribing; and autonomy to practice (ANA, 2003; APRN Joint Dialogue Group, 2008). The scopes of practice differ among the various APN roles; various specialty organizations have provided detailed and specific descriptions for their specialties. Carving out an adequate scope of APN practice authority has been an historic struggle for most of the advanced practice specialties (see Chapter 1), and this continues to be a hotly debated issue among and within the health professions. Significant variability in state practice acts continues such that APNs can perform certain activities, notably prescribing certain medications and practicing without physician supervision, in some states but may be constrained from performing these same activities in another state (Lugo, O'Grady, Hodnicki, & Hanson, 2007).

The Pew Commission's Taskforce on Health Care Workforce Regulation (Finocchio, Dower, Blick, Gragnola, & the Taskforce on Health Care Workforce Regulation, 1998) noted that the tension and turf battles between professions and the increased legislative activities in this area "clog legislative agendas across the country" (p. ii). These battles are costly and time consuming, and lawmakers' decisions related to scope of practice are too often distorted by campaign contributions, lobbying efforts, and political power struggles rather than being based on empirical evidence. The Pew Commission Taskforce report contains a number of recommendations that directly address scope-of-practice concerns, including the need for a national policy advisory body to research, develop, and publish national scopes of practice and continuing competency standards (see Chapter 21 for further discussion). Encouraging progress is being made on these issues, particularly interdisciplinary scopes of practice (NCSBN, Association of Social Work Boards, Federation of State Boards of Physical Therapy, Federation of State Medical Boards, National Association of Boards of Pharmacy, & National Board for Certification in Occupational Therapy, 2006) and APN scope of practice (APRN Joint Dialogue Group, 2008), though much remains to be done.

DIFFERENTIATING ADVANCED PRACTICE ROLES: OPERATIONAL DEFINITIONS OF ADVANCED PRACTICE NURSING

As noted earlier, it is critical to the public's understanding of advanced practice nursing that APN roles and resulting job titles reflect actual practices. Because actual practices differ, job titles should differ. This is particularly evident when considering CRNA practice as compared with that of a family NP. The following corollary is also true: If the actual practices do not differ, the job titles should not differ. For example, some institutions have retitled their CNSs as *clinical coordinators* or *clinical educators,* even though these APNs are continuing to enact a CNS practice. This change in job title renders the CNS practice less clearly visible in the clinical setting and thereby obscures CNS role clarity. As noted earlier, differences among roles must be clarified in ways that promote understanding of advanced practice nursing rather than divide the profession. This spirit of promoting understanding and clarity informs the ensuing discussion. A key assumption is that all of these APN roles are valuable in meeting the needs of patients in current and evolving health care settings.

Table 3-1 provides national sample survey data on RNs prepared to practice as APNs, from 1996 to 2004. As of 2004, an estimated 240,460 RNs, or 8.3% of the RN population, were prepared in at least one APN role (U.S. Department of Health & Human Services [USHHS], 2006). Only 8% of these individuals were from racial or ethnic minority backgrounds as compared with 10.7% of the overall RN population. The overall number of RNs prepared as APNs represents a 22.5% increase as compared with 2000 data. An estimated 82.8% of all APNs are either CNSs or NPs. When changes in each specialty are compared

Table 3-1 NUMBER OF ADVANCED PRACTICE NURSES IN THE UNITED STATES

APN Category	1996*			2000†			2004‡		
	Total No.	% Currently in Nursing	% Nationally Certified	Total No.	% Currently in Nursing	% Nationally Certified	Total No.	% Currently in Nursing	% Nationally Certified
CRNAs	30,386	86.7	84.4	29,844	85.7	84.4	32,523	89.6	95.3
CNMs	6,534	81.7	87.9	9,232	85.7	88.4	13,684	89.3	93.7
CNSs	53,799	90.5	23.6	54,374	87	36.5	57,832	85.1	44.7
NPs	63,191	88.2	63.5	88,186	89	74	126,520	87.7	77.6
Blended CNS/NP Preparation (not included in CNS or NP numbers)	7,802	100	70.9	14,643	95.7	73.4	14,689	93.4	Not reported

*From U.S. Department of Health & Human Services (USHHS), Division of Nursing. (1996). *The registered nurse population March 1996: Findings from the national sample survey of registered nurses.* Washington, DC: Author.
†From U.S. Department of Health & Human Services (USHHS), Division of Nursing. (2002). *The registered nurse population March 2000: Findings from the seventh national sample survey of registered nurses.* Washington, DC: Author.
APN, Advanced practice nurse; *CRNAs,* Certified registered nurse anesthetists; *CNMs,* certified nurse-midwives; *CNSs,* clinical nurse specialists; *NPs,* nurse practitioners.
‡From U.S. Department of Health & Human Services (USHHS), Division of Nursing. (2006). *The registered nurse population: Findings from the March 2004 national sample survey of registered nurses.* Washington, DC: Author.

over time, different patterns are evident in the different APN specialties. CRNA numbers show a 9% increase from 2000 to 2004. CNMs experienced the greatest percentage growth (48.2%), though this is based on a small sample and only 62.3% of CNMs reported graduate preparation. CNSs have increased by 6.4% since 2000.

The APN role that has shown the most significant growth is the NP. The number of RNs educated as NPs increased by 43.5% between 2000 and 2004 (excluding blended CNS/NPs) and more than doubled from 1996 to 2004. The number of RNs with dual preparation as a CNS and an NP remained relatively stable in those same 4 years, with only a 0.3% increase as compared with an 88% increase between 1996 and 2000. For the first time, the 2004 National Sample Survey notes that there are APNs with other blended role preparation, notably combining NP and CNM credentials; these APNs represent 21% of nurse-midwives. The breakdown of various APN roles is shown in Figure 3-4.

In addition to each role's unique competencies, differentiation among APNs occurs in a number of dimensions. The nature of the patient population receiving APN care, organizational expectations, emphasis given to specific competencies, and practice characteristics unique to each role also serve to distinguish the practice of one APN group from others. These differences between APN roles are not rigid demarcations but, rather, are fluid and involve overlapping areas. Nursing's scope of practice is dynamic and continually evolving, and this is especially true at the boundaries of the discipline,

where advanced practice occurs (ANA, 1995). The intent of this discussion is not to create stereotypical divisions or to deny the dynamic and evolving nature of advanced practice nursing but, rather, to describe key differences that are evident in actual practices at this stage in APN evolution (see Chapter 18 for further discussion of evolving APN roles).

Advanced practice nursing is applied in the four established and in emerging roles. These APN roles can be considered to be the operational definitions of the concept of advanced practice nursing. Figure 3-5 shows the differing "shapes" of APN roles. The shapes used in the figure do not have any particular significance; rather, they are meant to illustrate that roles differ along varying dimensions, as noted earlier. Figure 3-5 also shows that although each APN role has the common definition, criteria, and competencies of advanced practice nursing at its center, it has its own distinct form. For example, the American College of Nurse-Midwives [ACNM] (2007), the NONPF (2006), the NACNS (2004), and the American Association of Nurse Anesthetists (2002) have identified additional core competencies for the CNM, NP, CNS, and CRNA roles, respectively. Some of these distinctive features of the various roles are listed here. Differences and similarities among roles are further explored in Part III.

The CNS role was originally distinguished by four traditional subroles: clinical expert, consultant, educator, and researcher (Hamric & Spross, 1989; see also Chapter 12). More recently, the NACNS (2004) has

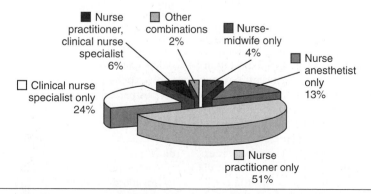

FIGURE **3-4:** Registered nurses prepared for advanced practice, March, 2004. (From U.S. Department of Health & Human Services [USHHS], Division of Nursing. [2006]. *The registered nurse population March 2004: Findings from the national sample survey of registered nurses.* Washington, DC: Author.)

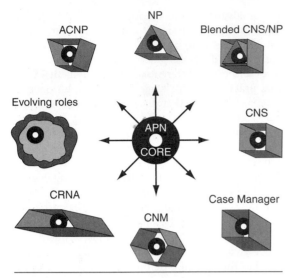

FIGURE **3-5:** Different advanced practice roles. *ACNP,* Acute care nurse practitioner; *NP,* nurse practitioner; *CNS,* clinical nurse specialist; *CNM,* certified nurse-midwife; *CRNA,* certified registered nurse anesthetist.

distinguished CNS practice by characterizing "spheres of influence" in which the CNS operates. These include the patient/client sphere, the nursing personnel sphere, and the organization/network sphere. CNSs are first and foremost clinical experts who provide direct care to patients with complex health problems. CNSs not only learn consultation processes, as do other APNs, but also function as formal consultants to nursing staff and other care providers within their organizations. Developing, supporting, and educating nursing staff to improve the quality of patient care is a core part of the nursing personnel sphere. Managing system change in complex organizations to build teams and improve nursing practices and "massaging the system" (Fenton, 1985) to advocate for patients are additional role expectations of the CNS. Expectations regarding research activities have been central to this role since its inception.

NPs, whether in primary care or acute care, possess advanced health assessment, diagnostic, and clinical management skills that include pharmacology management (see Chapters 13 and 14). Their focus is expert direct care, managing the health needs of individuals and their families. Incumbents in the classic NP role provide primary health care focused on wellness and prevention; NP practice also includes caring for patients with minor, common acute conditions

and stable chronic conditions. The newer acute care NP (ACNP) brings practitioner skills to a specialized patient population within the acute care setting. The ACNP's focus is the diagnosis and clinical management of acutely or critically ill patient populations in a particular specialized setting. Acquisition of additional medical diagnostic and management skills, such as interpreting computed tomography (CT) and magnetic resonance imaging (MRI) scans, inserting chest tubes, and performing lumbar punctures, also characterizes this role.

The blended CNS/NP role (see Chapter 15) combines the CNS's in-depth specialized knowledge of a particular patient population with the NP's primary health care expertise. It is important to clarify that CNSs who acquire NP skills are not necessarily functioning in a blended role. Many work as NPs in either primary care NP or ACNP roles as described earlier. The blended CNS/NP provides primary and specialty care, including clinical management, to a complex patient population, such as children with diabetes. A unique feature of this role is the provision of primary and specialized care such that the blended CNS/NP crosses setting boundaries to provide continuity of care. An additional characteristic that distinguishes this role from that of the ACNP is the expectation of CNS competencies in the three spheres of influence noted earlier. For example, this role combines individual patient management with expectations to develop nursing staff and effect change in complex organizational practices. In addition to acquisition of the advanced practice core competencies, education for this role must include functional role preparation for both the CNS and the NP roles. Blended role APNs must ensure that their roles are carefully structured to allow time and emphasis in the three spheres of influence.

The CNM (see Chapter 16) has advanced health assessment and intervention skills focused on women's health and childbearing. CNM practice involves independent management of women's health care. CNMs focus particularly on pregnancy, childbirth, the postpartum period, and care of the newborn, but their practices also include family planning, gynecological care, and primary health care for women (ACNM, 2007). The CNM's focus is on providing direct care to a select patient population.

CRNA practice (see Chapter 17) is distinguished by advanced procedural and pharmacological management of patients undergoing anesthesia. CRNAs practice independently, in collaboration with physicians, or as employees of a health care institution. Like

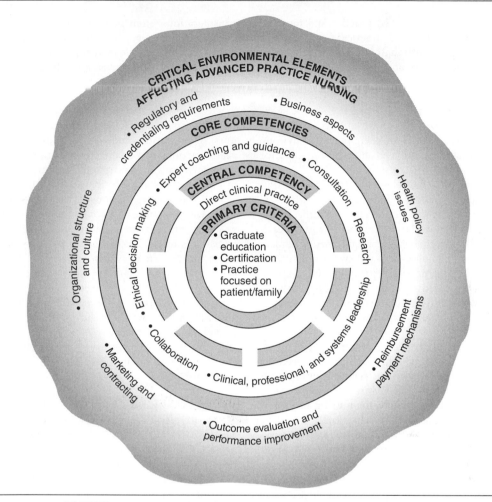

FIGURE **3-6:** Critical elements in advanced nursing practice environments.

CNMs, their primary focus is providing direct care to a select patient population. Both CNM and CRNA practices are also distinguished by well-established national standards, national examinations, and certification for practice at the advanced specialty level.

These differing roles and their similarities and distinctions are explored in detail in subsequent chapters. In addition, newly evolving opportunities for advanced practice nursing are discussed in Chapter 18. This brief discussion underscores the rich and varied nature of advanced practice nursing and the necessity for retaining and supporting different APN roles and titles in the health care marketplace. At the same time, a consistent definition of advanced practice nursing undergirds each of these roles.

CRITICAL ELEMENTS IN MANAGING ADVANCED PRACTICE NURSING ENVIRONMENTS

The health care arena is increasingly fluid and changeable—some would even say it is chaotic. Advanced practice nursing does not exist in a vacuum or a singular environment. Rather, this level of practice occurs in an increasing variety of health care delivery environments. These diverse environments are complex admixtures of interdependent elements. The term *environment* refers to any milieu in which an APN practices, ranging from a community-based rural health care practice for a primary care NP to a complex tertiary health care organization for an ACNP. Certain core features of these environments dramatically shape advanced practice and must be managed by APNs for their practices to survive and thrive (Figure 3-6). Although not technically part of the core definition of advanced practice nursing, these environmental features are included here to frame the understanding that APNs must be aware of these key elements in any practice setting. Furthermore, APNs must be prepared to contend with and shape these aspects of their practice environment to be able to fully enact advanced practice nursing.

The environmental elements that affect APN practice include managing reimbursement and business aspects of the practice; dealing with marketing and contracting considerations; understanding legal, regulatory and credentialing requirements; understanding and shaping health policy considerations; strengthening organizational structures and cultures to support advanced practice nursing; and enabling outcome evaluation and performance improvement. Part IV of this book explores these elements in depth.

Common to all of these environmental elements is the increasing use of technology and the need for APNs to master a variety of new technologies to improve patient care and health care systems. The ability to use information systems/technology and patient care technology is an essential element of DNP curricula (AACN, 2006). Electronic technology is changing health care practice in documentation formats, coding schemas, communications, Internet use, and provision of care across state lines through telehealth practices. These changes in turn are reshaping all seven APN core competencies. Proficiency in the use of new technologies is increasingly necessary to support clinical practice, to implement quality improvement initiatives, and to provide leadership to evaluate outcomes of care and care systems (AACN, 2006).

Managing the business and legal aspects of practice is increasingly critical to APN survival in the competitive health care marketplace. All APNs must understand the reimbursement issues and legal constraints within their organizations, regardless of setting. Given the increasing competition among physicians, APNs, and nonphysician providers, APNs must be prepared to assertively and knowledgeably market their services. Marketing oneself as a new NP in a small community may look different from marketing oneself as a CNS in a large health system, but the principles are the same. Marketing

considerations often include the need to advocate for and actively create positions that do not currently exist. Contract considerations are much more complex at the APN level, and all APNs, whether newly graduated or experienced, must be prepared to enter into contract negotiations.

Health policy at state and federal levels is an increasingly potent force shaping advanced practice nursing; regulations and policies that flow from legislative actions can enable or constrain APN practices. Variations in the strength and number of APNs in various states attest to the power of this environmental factor. Organizational structures and cultures, whether those of a community-based practice or a hospital unit, are also important facilitators of or barriers to advanced practice nursing; APN students must learn to assess and intervene to build organizations and cultures that strengthen APN practice. Finally, APNs are accountable for the use of evidence-based practice to ensure positive patient and system outcomes. Measuring the favorable impact of advanced practice nursing on these outcomes and effecting performance improvements are essential activities that all APNs must be prepared to undertake.

IMPLICATIONS OF THE DEFINITION OF ADVANCED PRACTICE NURSING

Many of the implications of this definition have been noted throughout the chapter, such as the need for an individual nurse to meet the primary criteria and core competencies of advanced practice nursing to be considered an APN. In addition, other implications for education, regulation and credentialing, practice, and research flow from this understanding of advanced practice nursing. The current work of the APRN Joint Dialogue Group (2008) makes the important point that effective communication between legal/regulatory groups, accreditors, certifying organizations, and educators (LACE) is necessary to advance the goals of advanced practice nursing. Decisions made by each of these groups affect and are affected by all the others. Historically, advanced practice nursing has been hampered by the lack of consensus in APN definition, terminology, educational and certification requirements, and regulatory approaches. The Joint Dialogue Group, by combining stakeholders from each of the LACE areas, may help achieve needed consensus on APN practice, education, certification, and regulation.

Implications for Advanced Practice Nursing Education

Graduate programs should provide anticipatory socialization experiences to prepare students for their chosen APN role. Graduate experiences should include practice in all the competencies of advanced practice nursing, not just direct clinical practice. For example, students who have no theoretical base or guided practice experiences in consultative skills or clinical, professional, and systems leadership will be ill-equipped to demonstrate these competencies on assuming a new APN role. In addition, APN students need to understand the critical elements in health care environments, such as the business aspects of practice and health care policy, that must be managed if their practices are to survive and grow. However, even with the best graduate education, no APN new to practice can be expected to perform all the role components and competencies with equal skill.

All APN roles require at least a specialty master's education; it is anticipated that master's programs will continue even as the new DNP degree is being developed for advanced practice nursing. The profession has embraced a wide variety of graduate educational models for preparing APNs, including direct-entry programs for non-nurse college graduates and RN-to-MSN programs. Whether doctoral preparation for advanced practice nursing will supplant these various master's programs by 2015, as proposed by the AACN, remains to be seen. Debate on the issue of the DNP continues (Dracup, Cronenwett, Meleis, & Benner, 2005; Fulton & Lyon, 2005; Marion et al., 2003; Mundinger et al., 2000) (see also Part III for views of leaders in each APN role). Various educational models differ in clinical experience hours, program length, and academic requirements (Marion, O'Sullivan, Crabtree, Price, & Fontana, 2005; O'Sullivan, Carter, Marion, Pohl, & Werner, 2005). Ensuring quality and standardization of APN education in the various specialties is a professional imperative and, indeed, is a goal of DNP-level preparation. As previously noted, the variability in some master's programs in terms of both content and clinical hours constrains the profession's ability to guarantee a highly skilled, uniformly educated APN to the public.

Implications for Regulation and Credentialing

Federal and state regulations have limited the potential of APN roles by not recognizing advanced practice nursing or by placing APNs in dependent positions with respect to their physician colleagues. Although encouraging progress has been made in states with restrictive practice acts, APNs and their advocates must continue to work actively for removal of these barriers if advanced practice nursing is to flourish.

Clarifying regulatory requirements for advanced practice nursing helps clarify the concept to nursing's external stakeholders, such as legislators, insurers, and other disciplines. This clarification depends on an integrated understanding of the concept of advanced practice nursing. Significant progress in unifying education and certifying requirements among all the various APN specialties can be seen over the past 10 years. It is gratifying to see the progress being made toward an integrative view of APN regulation based on this definition of advanced practice nursing. In particular, the primary criteria of graduate education, advanced specialty certification, and focus on direct clinical practice for all APN roles have been affirmed as the key elements in regulating and credentialing advanced practice nurses (APRN Joint Dialogue Group, 2008). Such internal cohesion can go a long way toward removing barriers to the public's access to APN care.

One implication for credentialing flows from the increasingly diverse specialty and role base of advanced practice nursing. Just as no APN can be characterized as a "generalist," no one APN program can prepare students for the full depth and breadth of advanced practice nursing. As a consequence, APNs must practice and be certified in the specific specialty and role for which they have been educated. APNs who wish to change specialties or roles need to return to school for education targeted to that area. The days are past when a primary care NP could take a job in a specialized acute care practice without further education to prepare for that specialty. This issue of aligning APN job expectations with education and certification is not always well understood by practice environments, by educators, or even by APNs themselves. However, the need to ensure congruence between particular APN specialties and roles and education, certification, and subsequent practice has been identified by regulators, and more stringent regulations regarding this issue are being promulgated (APRN Joint Dialogue Group, 2008).

Implications for Research

As noted in Chapter 8, APNs may be involved in research at different levels. A baseline expectation is the use of evidence-based practice and the ability to assist others to incorporate research evidence into their practices. Being actively involved in research related to patient care (at whatever level the APN is comfortable) is a crucial ingredient of advanced practice nursing. The practice doctorate initiative identified the increased need for leadership in evidence-based practice and application of knowledge to solve practice problems and improve health outcomes as reasons for moving to the DNP degree for APN practice (AACN, 2006). If research is to be relevant to care delivery and to nursing practice at all levels, APNs must be involved. APNs need to recognize the importance of advancing both the profession's and the health care system's knowledge about effective patient care practices and to realize that they are a vital link in building this knowledge. Further, APNs are in a key position to uncover the knowledge embedded in expert clinical practice (Benner, 1984).

Related to this research involvement is the necessity for more research differentiating basic and advanced practice nursing and identifying the patient populations that benefit most from APN intervention. For example, there is compelling empirical evidence that APNs can effectively manage chronic disease—preventing or mitigating complications, reducing rehospitalizations, and increasing patients' quality of life. This evidence is presented in each of the chapters of Part III and in Chapter 24. Linking advanced practice nursing to specific patient outcomes remains a major research imperative for this century.

Likewise, research is needed on the outcomes of the different APN educational pathways in terms of APN graduate experiences and patient outcomes. Such data would be invaluable in continuing to refine advanced practice education. Outcomes achieved by graduates from DNP programs need similar study in comparison to master's-level APN graduates; in critiquing the need for the DNP degree, Fulton & Lyon (2005) noted the absence of research data on whether there are weaknesses in current master's-level graduates.

Implications for Practice Environments

Because of the centrality of direct clinical practice, APNs must hold onto and make explicit their direct patient care activities. They must also articulate the importance of this level of care for patients. In addition, it is important to identify those patients who most need APN services and ensure that they receive this care.

APN roles require considerable autonomy and authority to be fully enacted. Practice settings have not always structured APN roles to allow sufficient autonomy or accountability for achievement of the patient

and system outcomes that are expected of advanced practitioners. It is equally important to emphasize that APNs have expanded responsibilities. Expanded authority for practice requires expanded responsibility for practice. APNs must demonstrate a higher level of responsibility and accountability if they are to be seen as legitimate providers of care and full partners on provider teams responsible for patient populations. This willingness to be accountable for practice will also promote consumers' and policymakers' perceptions of APNs as credible providers in line with physicians.

The APN leadership competency mandates that APNs serve as visible role models and mentors for other nurses (Cronenwett, 1995; see Chapter 9). Leadership is not optional in APN practice—it is a requirement. APNs must be a visible part of the solution to the health care system's problems. For this goal to be realized, each APN must practice leadership in his or her daily activities. In practice environments, APNs need structured time and opportunities for this leadership, including mentoring activities with new nurses.

The fact that new APNs require a considerable period of role development before they can master all of the components and competencies of their chosen role has important implications for employers of new APNs. Employers should provide experienced preceptors, some structure for the new APN, and ongoing support for role development (see Chapter 4 for further recommendations).

Finally, APN roles must be structured in practice environments to allow APNs to enact advanced nursing skills rather than simply substitute for physicians. It is certainly the case that APNs gain additional skills in medical diagnosis and therapeutic interventions, including the knowledge needed for prescriptive authority. However, *advanced practice nursing is a value-added complement to medical practice, not a substitution for it.* This is particularly an issue for CRNA, NP, and ACNP roles, which involve the addition of substantial medical therapeutics in practice. As the number of physicians increases, particularly the number of physicians prepared in family practice and the new "hospitalist" practices, this distinction must be clear in the minds of employers, insurers, and APNs themselves. As advanced practice nursing evolves, it is becoming clear that APNs represent a choice and alternative for patients seeking care. Consequently, the understanding of what APNs bring to health care must be articulated to multiple stakeholders to enable informed patient choice.

CONCLUSION

Since the first edition of this text in 1996, substantial progress has been made toward clarifying the definition of advanced practice nursing. This progress is enabling APNs, educators, administrators, and other nursing leaders to be clear and consistent about the definition of advanced practice nursing so that the profession speaks with one voice.

This is a critical juncture in the evolution of advanced practice nursing as new educational programs and proliferating specialties emerge in an increasingly chaotic health care system. APNs must continue to clarify that the advanced practice of nursing is not the junior practice of medicine but, instead, represents an important alternative practice that is complementary to, rather than competing with, medical practice. In some situations, patients need advanced nursing and not medicine; identifying these situations and matching APN resources to patient need are important priorities for transforming the current health care system. APNs must be able to clearly and forcefully articulate their defining characteristics so that their practices will survive and thrive amidst the continued cost cutting in the health care sector.

For a profession to succeed, it must have internal cohesion and external legitimacy and have them at the same time (Safriet, 1993). Clarity about the core definition of advanced practice nursing and recognition of the primary criteria and competencies necessary for all APNs enhance nursing's external legitimacy. At the same time, recognizing the differences among APNs and the legitimacy of different advanced practice nursing roles enhances nursing's internal cohesion.

REFERENCES

Advanced Nursing Practice. (2007). *Cumulative index to nursing and allied health literature.* Retrieved from the index on July 8, 2007.

American Association of Colleges of Nursing (AACN). (1995). *The essentials of master's education for advanced practice nursing.* Washington, DC: Author.

American Association of Colleges of Nursing (AACN). (2003). *White paper on the role of the clinical nurse leader.* Washington, DC: Author.

American Association of Colleges of Nursing (AACN). (2004). *Position statement on the practice doctorate in nursing.* Washington, DC: Author.

American Association of Colleges of Nursing (AACN). (2006). *The essentials of doctoral education for advanced nursing practice.* Washington, DC: Author.

American Association of Nurse Anesthetists. (2002). *Scope and standards for nurse anesthesia practice.* Park Ridge, IL: Author.

American College of Nurse-Midwives (ACNM). (2006). *Position statement: Mandatory degree requirements for entry into midwifery practice.* Washington, DC: Author.

American College of Nurse-Midwives (ACNM). (2007). *Core competencies for basic midwifery practice.* Washington, DC: Author.

American Nurses Association (ANA). (1980). *Nursing: A social policy statement.* Kansas City, MO: Author.

American Nurses Association (ANA). (1995). *Nursing's social policy statement.* Washington, DC: Author.

American Nurses Association (ANA). (1996). *Scope and standards of advanced practice registered nursing.* Washington, DC: Author.

American Nurses Association (ANA). (2001). *Code of ethics for nurses with interpretive statements.* Washington, DC: Author.

American Nurses Association (ANA). (2003). *Nursing's social policy statement* (2nd ed.). Washington, DC: Author.

American Nurses Association (ANA). (2005). *Public health nursing: Scope and standards of practice.* Washington, DC: Author.

APRN Joint Dialogue Group. (2008). *Consensus Model for APRN Regulation.* Based on the work of the APRN Consensus Work Group and the NCSBN APRN Advisory Committee. Chicago/Washington, DC: Author

Association of Community Health Nursing Educators Task Force on Community/Public Health Master's Level Preparation. (November 2000). *Graduate education for advanced community/public health nursing practice.* Louisville, KY: Author.

Benner, P. (1984). *From novice to expert.* Menlo Park, CA: Addison-Wesley.

Benner, P., Hooper-Kyriakidis, P., & Stannard, D. (1999). *Clinical wisdom and interventions in critical care.* Philadelphia: Saunders.

Benner, P., Tanner, C.A., & Chesla, C.A. (1996). *Expertise in nursing practice: Caring, clinical judgment, and ethics.* New York: Springer.

Brown, S.J. (1998). A framework for advanced practice nursing. *Journal of Professional Nursing, 14,* 157-164.

Calkin, J.D. (1984). A model for advanced nursing practice. *Journal of Nursing Administration, 14,* 24-30.

Creasia, J.L., & Parker, B. (Eds.). (2006). *Conceptual foundations: The bridge to professional nursing practice* (4 ed.). St. Louis: Mosby.

Cronenwett, L.R. (1995). Molding the future of advanced practice nursing. *Nursing Outlook, 43,* 112-118.

Davies, B., & Hughes, A.M. (1995). Clarification of advanced nursing practice: Characteristics and competencies. *Clinical Nurse Specialist, 9,* 156-160.

Donley, S.R. (1995). Advanced practice nursing after health care reform. *Nursing Economics, 13,* 84-88.

Dracup, K., Cronenwett, L., Meleis, A.I., & Benner, P.E. (2005). Reflections on the doctorate of nursing practice. *Nursing Outlook, 53,* 177-182.

Fenton, M.V. (1985). Identifying competencies of clinical nurse specialists. *Journal of Nursing Administration, 15,* 31-37.

Finocchio, L.J., Dower, C.M., Blick, N.T., Gragnola, C.M., & the Taskforce on Health Care Workforce Regulation. (1998).

Strengthening consumer protection: Priorities for health care workforce regulation. San Francisco: Pew Health Professions Commission.

Fulton, J.S., & Lyon, B.L. (2005). The need for some sense making: Doctor of Nursing Practice. *Online Journal of Issues in Nursing, 10*(3), Manuscript 3. Retrieved July, 20, 2005, from www.nursingworld.org/ojin/topic28/tpc28_3.htm.

Hamric, A.B. (1996). A definition of advanced nursing practice. In A.B. Hamric, J.A. Spross, & C.M. Hanson (Eds.), *Advanced nursing practice: An integrative approach* (pp. 42-56). Philadelphia: Saunders.

Hamric, A.B. (2000). A definition of advanced nursing practice. In A.B. Hamric, J.A. Spross, & C.M. Hanson (Eds.), *Advanced nursing practice: An integrative approach* (2nd ed., pp. 53-73). Philadelphia: Saunders.

Hamric, A.B. (2005). A definition of advanced nursing practice. In A.B. Hamric, J.A. Spross, & C.M. Hanson (Eds.), *Advanced nursing practice: An integrative approach* (3rd ed., pp. 85-108). Philadelphia: Saunders.

Hamric, A.B., & Spross, J.A. (Eds.). (1989). *The clinical nurse specialist in theory and practice* (2nd ed.). Philadelphia: Saunders.

Hanson, C.M., & Hamric, A.B. (2003). Reflections on the continuing evolution of advanced practice nursing. *Nursing Outlook, 51,* 203-211.

Hickey, J.V., Ouimette, R.V., & Venegoni, S.L. (2000). *Advance practice nursing: Changing roles and clinical applications* (2nd ed.). Philadelphia: Lippincott.

Hood, L.J. (2006). *Leddy and Pepper's conceptual bases of professional nursing* (6 ed.). Philadelphia: Lippincott Williams & Wilkins.

Kitzman, H. (1989). The CNS and the nurse practitioner. In A.B. Hamric & J.A. Spross (Eds.), *The clinical nurse specialist in theory and practice* (2nd ed., pp. 379-394). Philadelphia: Saunders.

Lindeke, L.L., Canedy, B.H., & Kay, M.M. (1997). A comparison of practice domains of clinical nurse specialists and nurse practitioners. *Journal of Professional Nursing, 13,* 281-287.

Lugo, N.R., O'Grady, E.T., Hodnicki, D.R., & Hanson, C.M. (2007). Ranking state nurse practitioner regulation: Practice environment and consumer healthcare choice. *American Journal of Nurse Practitioners, 11*(4), 8-24.

Marion, L., Viens, D., O'Sullivan, A., Crabtree, K., Fontana, S., & Price, M. The practice doctorate in nursing: Future or fringe? *Topics in Advanced Practice Nursing eJournal, 3*(2). Retrieved May 21, 2003, from www.medscape.com/ viewarticle/453247.

Marion, L.N., O'Sullivan, A.L., Crabtree, M.K., Price, M., & Fontana, S.A. (2005). Curriculum models for the practice doctorate in nursing. *Topics in Advanced Practice Nursing eJournal, 5*(1). Retrieved March 16, 2005, from www.medscape.com/viewarticle/500742.

Mundinger, M.O. (1994). Advanced practice nursing: Good medicine for physicians? *New England Journal of Medicine, 330,* 211-214.

Mundinger, M., Cook, S., Lenz, E., Piacentini, K., Auerhahn, C., & Smith J. (2000). Assuring quality and access in advanced practice nursing: A challenge to nurse educators. *Journal of Professional Nursing, 16,* 322-329.

National Association of Clinical Nurse Specialists (NACNS). (2004). *Statement on clinical nurse specialist practice and education* (2nd ed.). Glenview, IL: Author.

National Council of State Boards of Nursing (NCSBN). (1993). *Position paper on the regulation of advanced nursing practice.* Chicago: Author.

National Council of State Boards of Nursing (NCSBN). (2002). *Position paper on the regulation of advanced practice nursing.* Chicago: Author.

National Council of State Boards of Nursing (NCSBN), Association of Social Work Boards, Federation of State Boards of Physical Therapy, Federation of State Medical Boards, National Association of Boards of Pharmacy, & National Board for Certification in Occupational Therapy. (2006). *Changes in healthcare professions' scope of practice: Legislative considerations.* (Brochure). Chicago: Authors.

National Organization of Nurse Practitioner Faculties (NONPF). (2000). *Challenges and opportunities for integrating community health in nurse practitioner programs.* Washington DC: Author.

National Organization of Nurse Practitioner Faculties (NONPF). (March, 2006). *Domains and core competencies of nurse practitioner practice.* Washington, DC: Author.

O'Malley, J., Cummings, S., & King, C.S. (1996). The politics of advanced practice. *Nursing Administration Quarterly, 20,* 62-72.

O'Sullivan, A., Carter, M., Marion, L., Pohl, J., & Werner, K. (2005). Moving forward together: The practice doctorate in nursing. *Online Journal of Issues in Nursing, 10*(3), Manuscript 4. Retrieved August 21, 2006 from www.nursinworld.org/ojjn/topic28/tpc28_4.htm.

Rasch, R.F.R., & Frauman, A.C. (1996). Advanced practice in nursing: Conceptual issues. *Journal of Professional Nursing, 12,* 141-146.

Safriet, B.J. (February 1993). *Keynote address: One strong voice.* Paper presented at the National Nurse Practitioner Leadership Summit, Washington, DC.

Safriet, B.J. (1998). Still spending dollars, still searching for sense: Advanced practice nursing in an era of regulatory and economic turmoil. *Advanced Practice Nursing Quarterly, 4,* 24-33.

Spross, J.A., & Baggerly, J. (1989). Models of advanced practice. In A.B. Hamric & J.A. Spross (Eds.), *The clinical nurse specialist in theory and practice* (2nd ed., pp. 19-40). Philadelphia: Saunders.

Stanley, J.M. (Ed.). (2005). *Advanced practice nursing: Emphasizing common roles* (2nd ed.). Philadelphia: F.A. Davis.

Thibodeau, J.A., & Hawkins, J.W. (1994). Moving toward a nursing model in advanced practice. *Western Journal of Nursing Research, 16,* 205-218.

U.S. Department of Health and Human Services (USHHS), Division of Nursing. (2006). *The registered nurse population March 2004. Findings from the national sample survey of registered nurses.* Washington, DC: Author.

Walker, J., Gerard, P.S., Bayley, E.W., Coeling, H., Clark, A.P., Dayhoff, N., et al. (2003). A description of clinical nurse specialist programs in the United States. *Clinical Nurse Specialist, 17,* 50-57.

Role Development of the Advanced Practice Nurse

Karen A. Brykczynski

INTRODUCTION

What is it like to become an advanced practice nurse (APN)? Role development in advanced practice nursing is described here as a process that evolves over time. The scope of nursing practice has expanded and contracted in response to societal needs, political forces, and economic realities (Levy, 1968; Safriet, 1992). Historical evidence suggests that the expanded role of the 1970s was common nursing practice during the early 1900s (DeMaio, 1979). Yet, the core of nursing is not defined by the tasks nurses perform. This task-oriented perspective is inadequate and disregards the complex nature of nursing. Nursing practice is distinguished by an orientation to holistic care; a philosophy of collaboration with patients, their families, and other health professionals; a tradition of care and concern; a disciplinary matrix; a rich and varied history; and an ever-growing body of knowledge. Recognition of the knowledge that develops as nurses expand their scope of practice and incorporate new knowledge and skill into their repertoire is required for advancing understanding of clinical nursing practice (Benner, 1985).

In the current cost-constrained environment, the pressure to be cost-effective and to make an impact on outcomes is greater than ever. Yet literature indicates that the initial year of practice is one of transition (Brown & Olshansky, 1998; Brykczynski, 1996; Kelly & Mathews, 2001) and an APN's maximum potential may not be realized until approximately 5 or more years in practice (Cooper & Sparacino, 1990). This chapter explores the complex processes of APN role development with the objectives of providing (1) understanding of related concepts and research; (2) anticipatory guidance for APN students; (3) role facilitation strategies for new APNs, APN preceptors, faculty, administrators, and interested colleagues; and (4) guidelines for continued role evolution. Specific concepts and strategies for faculty teaching APNs are included in the Evolve website.

This chapter consolidates literature from all of the APN specialties—including clinical nurse specialists

(CNSs), nurse practitioners (NPs), certified nurse-midwives (CNMs), and certified registered nurse anesthetists (CRNAs)—to present a generic process relevant to all APN roles. Some of this literature is foundational to understanding issues of role development for all APN roles and, although dated, remains relevant. The discussion is separated into the educational component of APN role acquisition and the occupational or work component of role implementation. This division in the process of role development is intended to clarify and distinguish the changes occurring during role transitions experienced during the educational period (role acquisition) and the changes occurring during the actual performance of the role after program completion (role implementation). Strategies for enhancing APN role development are described. The chapter concludes with summary comments and suggestions regarding facilitation of future APN role development and evolution.

PERSPECTIVES ON ADVANCED PRACTICE NURSE ROLE DEVELOPMENT

Professional role development is a dynamic, ongoing process that, once begun, spans a lifetime. The concept of graduation as commencement, whereby one's career begins on completion of a degree, is central to understanding the evolving nature of professional roles in response to personal, professional, and societal demands (Gunn, 1998). Professional role development literature in nursing is abundant and complex, involving multiple component processes. These include (1) aspects of adult development, (2) development of clinical expertise, (3) modification of self-identity through initial socialization in school, (4) development and integration of professional role components, and (5) subsequent resocialization in the work setting. Like socialization for other professional roles, such as those of attorney, physician, teacher, and social worker, the process of becoming an APN involves aspects of adult development, as well as professional socialization. The professional socialization process in advanced practice nursing involves identification with and acquisition of the behaviors and attitudes of the "aspired to" advanced practice group (Waugaman & Lu, 1999, p. 239). This includes learning the specialized language, skills, and knowledge of the particular APN group; internalizing its values and norms; and incorporating these into one's professional nursing identity and other life roles (Cohen, 1981).

NOVICE-TO-EXPERT SKILL ACQUISITION MODEL

Acquisition of knowledge and skill occurs in a progressive movement through stages of performance from novice to expert as described by Dreyfus and Dreyfus (1986, 1996), who studied diverse groups, including pilots, chess players, and adult learners of second languages. The skill acquisition model has broad applicability and can be used to better understand many different skills, which range from playing a musical instrument to writing a research grant. The most widely known application of this model is Benner's (1984) observational and interview study of clinical nursing practice situations from the perspective of new nurses and their preceptors in hospital nursing services. Although this study included several APNs, it did not specify a particular education level as a criterion for expertise. As noted in Chapter 3, there has been some confusion about this criterion. The skill acquisition model is a situation-based model, not a trait model; therefore the level of expertise is not an individual characteristic of a particular nurse. Rather, it is a function of the nurse's familiarity with a particular situation in combination with his or her educational background. This model could be used to study the level of expertise required for other aspects of advanced practice including coaching and guidance, consultation, collaboration, research, ethical decision making, and clinical, professional and systems leadership.

According to the Dreyfus model, there is a generic process of skill acquisition through which humans proceed in stages from novice to expert as they acquire new psychomotor, perceptual, and judgment skills (Dreyfus & Dreyfus, 1996). The progression from novice to expert is incremental but not necessarily stepwise or linear. Instead, as with growth and development or healing processes, plateaus, setbacks, and even stagnation can occur, as well as occasional leaps forward. The competent level is a critical juncture in the development of expertise. Some individuals do not advance to expertise because they do not become sufficiently engaged in their practice. A change from "acting like," sometimes referred to as the *imposter phenomenon* (Arena & Page, 1992; Brown & Olshansky, 1997, 1998; Huffstutler & Varnell, 2006), to individualized embodiment of the new role occurs as the individual moves up to the proficient level. In other words, it takes time and practice for new skills to become fully owned or embodied. Embodiment of a skill occurs after repeated experiences of performing the skill "as if" one actually could do it skillfully. It is a kind of "going through the motions" until, over time, the skill is transformed from the halting, stepwise performance of the novice to the holistic, fluid performance of the expert.

The proficient level represents a discontinuous, qualitative leap from the competent level whereby intuition, defined as "holistic situation recognition" (Dreyfus & Dreyfus, 1986, p. 28), replaces analytically reasoned responses. According to this model, expertise develops over time through direct personal encounters, which alter preconceptions and prior understanding. The deep situational understanding associated with expertise involves holistic pattern recognition, described as "the intuitive ability to use patterns without decomposing them into component features" (Dreyfus & Dreyfus, 1986, p. 28). Decomposition of situations into abstract attributes is associated with earlier skill levels.

Deliberative rationality, a fine-tuning of intuition, takes place at the expert level, replacing the calculative rationality characteristic of other levels (Dreyfus & Dreyfus, 1986). Deliberative rationality is a detached, meditative reflection on goals and possible ways to achieve the goals, whereas calculative rationality is the inferential reasoning exhibited by less-than-expert performers when they apply and modify theoretical principles and rules. Deliberative rationality is involved in distinguishing a novel situation or a situation in which the initial grasp may be incorrect from a situation in which experience can be trusted. Such personal expert knowledge is not totally idiosyncratic; it can be shared in ways such as the identification of maxims, common meanings, and exemplars that convey the contextual understanding of clinical situations (Benner, 1984; Benner, Hooper-Kyriakidis, & Stannard, 1999; Benner, Tanner, & Chesla, 1996; Brykczynski, 1991, 1999; Horvath et al., 1994).

Figure 4-1 shows a typical APN role development pattern in terms of this skill acquisition model. A major implication of the novice-to-expert model for advanced practice nursing is the claim that even experts can be expected to perform at lower skill levels when they enter new situations or positions. Hamric and Taylor's (1989) report that experienced

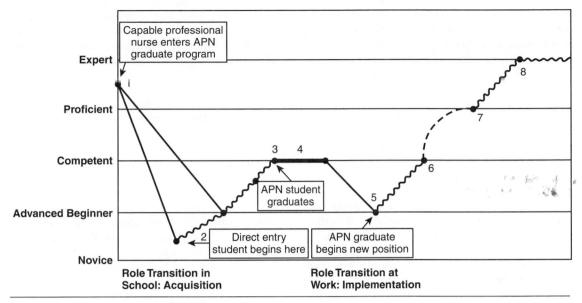

FIGURE **4-1:** Typical advanced practice nurse (APN) role development pattern:

1. APNs may begin graduate school as proficient or expert nurses. Some enter as competent RNs with limited prac- tice experience. Depending on previous background, the new APN student will revert to novice level or advanced- beginner level upon assuming the student role.
2. A direct-entry APN student or non-nurse college graduate (NNCG) student with no nursing experience would begin the role transition process at the novice level.
3. The graduate from an APN program is competent as an APN student but has no experience as a practicing APN.
4. A limbo period is experienced while the APN graduate searches for a position and becomes certified.
5. The newly employed APN reverts to advanced-beginner level in the new APN position as role trajectory begins again. The imposter phenomenon may be experienced here (Arena & Page, 1992; Brown & Olshansky, 1998).
6. Some individuals remain at the competent level. There is a discontinuous leap from the competent to the proficient level.
7. Proficiency develops only if there is sufficient commitment and involvement in practice along with embodiment of skills and knowledge.
8. Expertise is intuitive and situation-specific, meaning that not all situations will be managed expertly. Refer to text discussion for details.

NOTE: Refer to Dreyfus Skill Acquisition Model for further details (Benner, 1984; Benner, Tanner, & Chesla, 1996; Dreyfus & Dreyfus, 1986; 1996). For the purpose of illustration, this figure is more linear than the individualized role development trajectories that actually occur.

CNSs starting a new position experience the same role development phases as new graduates, only over a shorter period, supports this claim.

Figure 4-1 shows the overall trajectory expected during APN role development; however, each APN ex- periences a unique pattern of role transitions and life transitions concurrently. For example, a professional nurse who functions as a mentor for new graduates may decide to pursue an advanced degree as an APN. As an APN graduate student, this nurse will experience the challenges of acquiring a new role, the anxiety as- sociated with learning new skills and practices, and the dependency of being a novice. At the same time, if this nurse continues to work as a registered nurse, his or her functioning in this work role will be at the competent,

proficient, or expert level (depending on experience and the situation). On graduation, the new APN may experience a limbo period, during which the nurse is no longer a student and not yet an APN, while search- ing for a position and meeting certification require- ments (see later discussion). Once in a new APN posi- tion, this nurse may experience a return to the advanced-beginner stage as he or she proceeds through the phases of role implementation. Even after making the transition to an APN role, progression in role im- plementation is not a linear process. As Figure 4-1 indi- cates, there are discontinuities, with movement back and forth as the trajectory begins again. Years later, the APN may decide to pursue yet another APN role. The processes of role acquisition, role implementation, and novice-to-expert skill development will again be experienced (although altered and informed by previous experiences) as the postgraduate student acquires additional skills and knowledge. Role development involves multiple, dynamic, and situational processes, with each new undertaking being characterized by passage through earlier transitional phases with some movement back and forth, horizontally or vertically, as different career options are pursued.

Direct-entry students who are non-nurse college graduates (NNCGs) and APN students with little or no experience as nurses before entry into an APN graduate program would be expected to begin their APN role development at the novice level as shown in Figure 4-1. Some evidence indicates that while these inexperienced-nurse students may lack the intuitive sense that comes with clinical experience, they avoid the role confusion associated with "letting go" of the traditional RN role commonly reported with experienced-nurse students (Heitz, Steiner, & Burman, 2004). This finding has implications for APN education as the profession moves toward the Doctor of Nursing Practice (DNP) as the preferred educational pathway for APN preparation (American Association of Colleges of Nursing [AACN], 2006).

Another significant implication of the Dreyfus model (Dreyfus & Dreyfus, 1986, 1996) for APNs is the observation that the quality of performance may deteriorate when performers are subjected to intense scrutiny, whether their own or that of someone else (Roberts, Tabloski, & Bova, 1997). The increased anxiety experienced by APN students during faculty on-site clinical evaluation visits or during videotaped testing of clinical performance in simulated situations is an example of responding to such intense scrutiny. A third implication of this skill acquisition model for APNs is the need to accrue experience in actual situations over time, so that both practical and theoretical knowledge are refined, clarified, personalized, and embodied, forming an individualized repertoire of experience that guides advanced practice performance. As the profession encourages new nurses to move more rapidly into APN education, students, faculty, and educational programs must search for creative ways to incorporate both the practical and theoretical knowledge necessary for advanced practice nursing.

ROLE CONCEPTS AND ROLE DEVELOPMENT ISSUES

This discussion of professional role issues incorporates role concepts described by Hardy and Hardy (1988) along with the concept that different APN roles repre-sent different subcultural groups within the broader nursing culture (Leininger, 1994). APNs can be described as tricultural and trilingual (Johnson, 1993). They share background knowledge, practices, and skills of three cultures: (1) biomedicine, (2) mainstream nursing, and (3) everyday life. They are fluent in the languages of biomedical science, nursing knowledge and skill, and everyday parlance. Some APNs, CNMs for example, are socialized into a fourth culture as well, that of midwifery. Others are also fluent in more than one everyday language. Just as APN roles can be conceptualized as encompassing skills and knowledge from more than one culture, they can also be seen as encompassing aspects of both male and female occupational gender roles. Because APNs are multicultural, multilingual, and androgynous, they are able to work effectively with many different people in an increasingly diverse world.

The concepts of role stress and strain discussed by Hardy and Hardy (1988) are useful for understanding the dynamics of role transitions (Table 4-1). Hardy and Hardy described *role stress* as a social structural condition in which role obligations are ambiguous, conflicting, incongruous, excessive, or unpredictable. *Role strain* is defined as the subjective feeling of frustration, tension, or anxiety experienced in response to role stress. The highly stressful nature of the nursing profession needs to be recognized as the background within which individuals seek advanced education to become APNs (Aiken, Clarke, Sloan, Sochalski, & Silber, 2002; Dionne-Proulx & Pepin, 1993). Role strain can be minimized by the identification of potential role stressors, development of strategies to cope with them, and rehearsal of situations designed for application of those strategies; however, the difficulties experienced by neophytes in new positions cannot be eliminated. As noted previously, expertise is holistic, involving bodily perceptual skills and shared background knowledge, as well as cognitive ability. A school-work, theory-practice, ideal-real gap will remain because of the nature of human skill acquisition.

Judith Spross (personal communication, July 25, 2003) pointed out that Bandura's (1977) social-cognitive theory of self-efficacy may be of interest to APNs in terms of understanding what motivates individuals to acquire skills and what builds confidence as skills are developed. Self-efficacy theory has been used widely to further understanding of skill acquisition with patients (Burglehaus, 1997; Clark & Dodge, 1999; Dalton & Blau, 1996). Self-efficacy theory has also been applied to mentoring APN students (Hayes, 2001) and to training health care professionals in skill acquisition (Parle, Maguire, & Heaven, 1997).

Table 4-1   SELECTED ROLE CONCEPTS

Concept	Definition	Examples
Role stress*	A situation of increased role performance demand	Returning to school while maintaining work/family responsibilities
Role strain*	Subjective feeling of frustration, tension, or anxiety in response to role stress	Feeling of decreased self-esteem when performance is below expectations of self or significant others
Role stressors*	Factors that produce role stress	Financial, personal, or academic demands and role expectations that are ambiguous, conflicting, excessive, or unpredictable
Role ambiguity*	Unclear expectations, diffuse responsibilities, uncertainty about subroles	All professional positions have some degree of ambiguity because of the evolving nature of roles and expansion of skills and knowledge
Role incongruity*	A role with incompatibility between skills and abilities and role obligations or incompatibility between personal values, self-concept, and role obligations	An adult NP in a role requiring pediatric skills and knowledge
Role conflict*	Occurs when role expectations are perceived to be mutually exclusive or contradictory	Intraprofessional role conflict between APNs and other nurses
		Interprofessional role conflict between APNs and physicians
Role transition*†	A dynamic process of change over time as new roles are acquired	Changing from a staff nurse role to an APN role
Role insufficiency†	Feeling inadequate to meet role demands	New APN graduate experiencing the *imposter* phenomenon (Arena & Page, 1992; Brown & Olshansky, 1998)
Role supplementation†	Anticipatory socialization	Role-specific educational components in graduate program

*Adapted from Hardy, M.E., & Hardy, W.L. (1988). Role stress and role strain. In M.E. Hardy & M.E. Conway (Eds.), *Role theory: Perspectives for health professionals* (2nd ed., pp. 159-239). Norwalk, CT: Appleton & Lange.
†Adapted from Schumacher, K.L., & Meleis, A.I. (1994). Transitions: A central concept in nursing. *Image: The Journal of Nursing Scholarship, 26,* 119-127.
NP, Nurse practitioner; *APN,* advance practice nurse.

Role Ambiguity

Role ambiguity (see Table 4-1) develops when there is a lack of clarity about expectations, a blurring of responsibilities, uncertainty regarding role implementation, and the inherent uncertainty of existent knowledge. According to Hardy and Hardy (1988), role ambiguity characterizes all professional positions. They point out that role ambiguity might be positive in that it offers opportunities for creative possibilities. It can be expected to be more prominent in professions undergoing change, such as those in the health care field. Role ambiguity has been widely discussed in relation to the CNS role (Chase, Johnson, Laffoon, Jacobs, & Johnson, 1996; Hamric, 2003; Payne & Baumgartner, 1996; Redekopp, 1997; see also Chapter 12), but it is a relevant issue for other APN roles as well (Kelly & Mathews, 2001), particularly as APN roles evolve (Stahl & Myers, 2002).

Role Incongruity

Role incongruity is intrarole conflict, which Hardy and Hardy (1988) described as developing from two sources. Incompatibility between skills and abilities and role obligations is one source of role incongruity. An example of this is an adult APN hired to work in an emergency department with a large percentage of pediatric patients. Such an APN will find it necessary to enroll in a family NP or pediatric NP program to gain the necessary knowledge to eliminate this role incongruity. This is a growing issue as NP roles become more specialized. Another source of role incongruity is incompatibility among personal values, self-concept, and expected role behaviors. An APN interested primarily in clinical practice may experience this incongruity if the position he or she obtains requires performing administrative functions. An example comes from Banda's (1985) study of psychiatric liaison CNSs in acute care hospitals and community health agencies. She reported that they viewed consultation and teaching as their major functions, whereas research and administrative activities were associated with role strain.

Role Conflict

Role conflict develops when role expectations are perceived to be contradictory or mutually exclusive. APNs may experience conflict with varying demands of their role, as well as both intraprofessional and interprofessional role conflict.

Intraprofessional Role Conflict. APNs experience *intraprofessional* role conflict for a variety of reasons. The historical development of APN roles has been fraught with conflict and controversy in nursing education and nursing organizations, particularly for CNMs (Varney, 1987), NPs (Ford, 1982), and CRNAs (Gunn, 1991; see also Chapter 1). Relationships among these APN groups and nursing as a discipline have improved markedly in recent years, yet difficulties remain (Fawcett, Newman, & McAllister, 2004; Roberts, 1996; Watson, 1995).

Communication difficulties that underlie intraprofessional role conflict occur in four major areas: (1) at an organizational level, (2) in educational programs, (3) in the literature, and (4) in direct clinical practice. Kimbro (1978) initially described these communication difficulties in reference to CNMs, but they are relevant for all APN roles. The fact that CNSs, NPs, CNMs, and CRNAs each have specific organizations with different certification requirements, competencies, and curricula creates boundaries and sets up the need for formal lines of communication. Communication gaps occur when courses and textbooks are not shared among APN programs in which more than one specialty is offered in the same school. Specialty-specific journals are another formal communication barrier, because APNs may read primarily within their own specialty and not keep abreast of larger APN issues. In clinical settings, some APNs may be more concerned with providing direct clinical care to individual patients whereas staff nurses and other APNs may be more concerned with 24-hour coverage and smooth functioning of the unit or the institution. These differences may set the stage for intraprofessional role conflict.

During the 1980s and 1990s when there was more confusion about delineation of roles and responsibilities between RNs and NPs, RNs would sometimes demonstrate resistance to NPs by refusing to take vital signs, obtain blood samples, or perform other support functions for patients of NPs (Brykczynski, 1985; Hupcey, 1993; Lurie, 1981) and they were not admonished by their supervisors for these negative behaviors. These behaviors are suggestive of horizontal violence (a form of hostility), which may be more common during nursing shortages (Thomas, 2003). Roberts (1983) first described horizontal violence among nurses as oppressed-group behavior wherein nurses who were doubly oppressed as women and as nurses demonstrated hostility toward their own less-powerful group instead of toward the more powerful oppressors. Recognizing that intraprofessional conflict among nurses is similar to oppressed-group behavior can be useful in the development of strategies to overcome these difficulties (Bartholomew, 2006; Brykczynski, 1997; Farrell, 2001; Freshwater, 2000; McKenna, Smith, Poole, & Coverdale, 2003; Roberts, 1996; Rounds, 1997; see also Chapter 9). According to Rounds (1997), horizontal violence is less common among NPs as a group than among RNs generally. Over the years as the NP role has become more accepted by nurses, there appear to be fewer instances of these hostile passive-aggressive behaviors toward NPs. However, they are still reported in APN transition literature (Heitz et al., 2004; Kelly & Mathews, 2001).

One way to address these issues would be to include APN position descriptions in staff nurse orientation programs. Curry's (1994) claim that thorough orientation of staff nurses to the APN role (including clear guidelines and policies regarding responsibility issues) is an important component of successful integration of NP practice in an emergency department setting is also applicable to other roles and settings. Another significant strategy for minimizing intraprofessional role conflict is for the new APN, as well as APN students, to spend time getting to know the nursing staff to establish rapport and learn as much as possible about the new setting from those who really know what is going on—the nurses. This action affirms the value and significance of nurses and nursing and sets up a positive atmosphere for collegiality and intraprofessional role cooperation and collaboration. In Kelly and Mathews' (2001) study of new NP graduates, such a strategy was exactly what new NPs regretted not having incorporated into their first positions.

Interprofessional Role Conflict. Conflicts between physicians and APNs constitute the most common situations of *interprofessional* conflict. Major sources of conflict for physicians and APNs are the perceived economic threat of competition, limited resources in clinical training sites, lack of experience working together, and the historical hierarchy. The relationship between anesthesiologists and CRNAs is an ongoing exemplar for examination of the issues of interprofessional role conflict between physicians and APNs (Exemplar 4-1).

The complementary nature of advanced practice nursing to medical care is a foreign concept for some physicians who view all health care as an extension of medical care and see APNs simply as physician extenders. This misunderstanding of advanced practice nursing underlies physicians' opposition to independent roles for nurses because they believe APNs want to practice medicine without a license (see Chapters 1 and 3). The fact that nursing has its own knowledge and skill base is a novel idea for physicians who see nursing as a subset of medicine. When APNs are viewed as direct competitors, it is understandable that some physicians would be reluctant to be involved in assisting with APN education (National Commission on Nurse Anesthesia Education, 1990). In addition, some nurse educators have held the belief that physicians should not be involved in teaching or acting as preceptors for APNs. Improved relationships between APNs and physicians will require redefinition of the situation by both groups.

The Pew Commission's (O'Neil & the Pew Health Profession Commission, 1998) advocacy for an interdisciplinary vision for all health professionals and the Institute of Medicine's (IOM) (Institute of Medicine [IOM], 2003) recommendation that the health professional workforce be prepared to work in interdisciplinary teams underscore the imperative of interdisciplinary collaboration (Fagin, 1992; see also Chapter 10). Competency in interdisciplinary collaboration is critical for APNs because it is central to APN practice. This content is incorporated into the leadership and interprofessional partnership components of *The Essentials of Doctoral Education for Advanced Nursing Practice* (AACN, 2006).

Nurse-midwives have been in the forefront of developing collaborative relationships with physicians for many years (American College of Nurse-Midwives [ACNM], 2006; Long & Sharp, 1982; Rooks, 1983, 1999; Rooks & Haas, 1986). All APN groups would benefit from attention to the progress that CNMs have made in collaboration with physicians. The joint practice statement of the American College of Nurse-Midwives (ACNM) and the American College of Obstetricians and Gynecologists can be used as a model for other APN groups (Roberts, 2001; see also the ACNM's website *[www.acnm.org]*). Problems with

---

 EXEMPLAR 4-1   **Interprofessional Role Conflict: The Case of CRNAs and Anesthesiologists**

For many years, nurse anesthetists have provided high-quality anesthesia care in a variety of settings, and they are the sole anesthesia providers in more than 65% of rural hospitals (Blumenreich, 2000). According to the American Association of Nurse Anesthetists (AANA) (AANA, 2007), over 30,000 certified registered nurse anesthetists (CRNAs) provide quality anesthesia care to more than 65% of all patients undergoing surgical or other medical interventions that necessitate the services of an anesthetist. The fact that nurse anesthetists predated the first physician anesthesiologists by many years (see Chapter 1) may explain in part why the relationship between anesthesiologists and CRNAs has historically been interpreted by anesthesiologists as one of direct competition, thus creating an adversarial stance. Over the years, this relationship might be characterized as a cold war with overt offensives mounted periodically by anesthesiologists.

In 1970 CRNAs outnumbered anesthesiologists by 1.5 to 1. By 2000 anesthesiologists outnumbered CRNAs (Blumenreich, 2000). This is one of the

factors underlying recent conflicts over CRNA autonomy (see the AANA website *[www.aana.com]* for updates on this issue). Another factor is the decision made by the Centers for Medicare and Medicaid Services, after study of the available evidence in 1997, to reimburse nurse anesthetists directly under Medicare (Kleinpell, 2001). In response, anesthesiologists and the American Medical Association (AMA) launched a major campaign against CRNA autonomy in the operating room, claiming that supervision of CRNAs by physicians is essential for public safety (Federwisch, 1999; Kleinpell, 2001; Stein, 2000; see also Chapter 17). This struggle with physicians over limiting the scope of practice of CRNAs is ongoing and reflects the experiences of other advanced practice nurse (APN) groups as well. An example of this continuing struggle is the Scope of Practice Partnership (SOPP), a coalition recently formed by the AMA with other physician organizations, to mount initiatives to limit the scope of practice of non-physician clinicians (Waters, 2007).

previous joint practice statements were that they included varying interpretations of physician supervision. "The problematic sentence that referred to a maternity care team 'directed by a qualified obstetrician gynecologist' now states that the team 'must include an obstetrician gynecologist with hospital privileges or other physicians with hospital privileges to provide complete obstetric care'" (Roberts, 2001, p. 269). The revised joint practice statement "places responsibility for the outcomes of care with the provider who is directly managing the care" (Roberts, 2001, p. 269). The ACNM (2006) opposes requirements for signed collaborative agreements as a condition for licensure, reimbursement, clinical privileging and hospital credentialing, or prescriptive authority for CNMs or certified midwives (CMs).

Collaboration between nurses and physicians can be beneficial for both groups, as well as for the public (see Chapter 10). One way to promote positive interprofessional relationships is to provide education and practice experiences that include APN students, medical students, and both physician and APN faculty to enhance mutual understanding of both professional roles (Kelly & Mathews, 2001). Developing such interdisciplinary experiences is difficult because of different academic calendars and clinical schedules. However, such obstacles can be overcome if these interdisciplinary activities are considered essential for improved health care delivery and if they have administrative support.

ROLE TRANSITIONS

Role transitions are defined here as dynamic processes of change that occur over time as new roles are acquired (see Table 4-1). Five essential factors influence role transitions (Schumacher & Meleis, 1994): (1) personal meaning of the transition, which relates to the degree of identity crisis experienced; (2) degree of planning, which involves the time and energy devoted to anticipating the change; (3) environmental barriers and supports, which refer to family, peer, school, and other components; (4) level of knowledge and skill, which relates to prior experience and school experiences; and (5) expectations, which are related to role models, literature, media, and the like. The role strain experienced by individuals in response to role insufficiency (see Table 4-1 for definitions) that accompanies the transition to APN roles can be minimized, although certainly not completely prevented, by (1) individualized assessment of these five essential factors, (2) development of strategies to cope with them, and (3) rehearsal of situations designed for application of these strategies. Entering

graduate school may be associated with a ripple effect of concurrent role transitions in family, work, and other social arenas (Klaich, 1990).

Advanced Practice Nurse Role Acquisition (in Graduate School)

The personal meaning of role transitions is a major focus of literature in nursing role development. In a review of APN role development literature from certificate and graduate NP programs, alterations in self-identity and self-concept emerged as a consistent theme, with role acquisition experiences commonly described as identity crises (see Brykczynski, 1996, for a detailed discussion of this earlier work).

In their study of NP students, Roberts and colleagues (1997) reported findings very similar to those observed decades earlier by Anderson, Leonard, and Yates (1974). Anderson and colleagues described the process of role development observed in three NP programs (a graduate program, a post-baccalaureate certificate program, and a continuing education program), whereas Roberts and colleagues described a current graduate NP program. Anderson and colleagues' (1974) description of NP students' progression from dependence to interdependence being accompanied by regression, anxiety, and conflict was found to be similar to observations made by Roberts and colleagues (1997) in graduate NP students over a period of 6 years (Table 4-2). For many years, my NP faculty colleagues and I have observed similar role transition processes in teaching role and clinical courses for graduate NP students. In a more recent discussion of role transition experiences for neonatal NPs, Cusson and Viggiano (2002) made the important point that even positive transitions are stressful.

Roberts and colleagues (1997) observed 100 NP graduate students and reviewed their student clinical journals. They identified three major areas of transition as students progressed from dependence to interdependence: (1) development of professional competence, (2) change in role identity, and (3) evolving relationships with preceptors and faculty. The lowest level of competence coincided with the highest level of role confusion. This occurred at the end of the first semester and the beginning of the second semester in the three-semester program examined (Roberts et al., 1997). It seems that the most intense transition period comes at the end of the students' first clinical immersion experience. Faculty can help students by identifying such periods of high stress in their particular program so that support can be built in during those periods.

Table 4-2 Role Acquisition Process in School

Stage	Descriptive Characteristics
I: Complete dependence	Immersion in learning medical components of care Role transition associated with role confusion and anxiety Decreased appreciation for psychosocial components of health and illness concerns Loss of confidence in clinical skills; feelings of incompetence
II: Developing competence	Ongoing clinical preceptorship experiences Didactic classes that incorporate medical diagnostic and both nursing and medical therapeutic components along with personal experience of illness components Renewed sense of appreciation for the value of nursing knowledge and skills More realistic self-expectations of clinical performance, although still uncomfortable about accountability Increased confidence in ability to succeed in learning and making a valid contribution to care Initial formation of own philosophy and standards of practice
III: Independence	Comfortable with ability to conduct holistic assessments (both physical and psychosocial) Concentration on intervention and management options Conflicts with preceptors occur as student and preceptor challenge one another Conflicts with faculty relate to management options, clinical evaluations, examination questions, concern over not being taught all there is to know
IV: Interdependence	Renewed appreciation for the interdependence of nursing and medicine Development of individualized version of the advanced practice role

Adapted from Anderson, E.M., Leonard, B.J., & Yates, J.A. (1974). Epigenesis of the nurse practitioner role. *American Journal of Nursing 10*, 12-16; Roberts, S.J., Tabloski, P., & Bova, C. (1997). Epigenesis of the nurse practitioner role revisited. *Journal of Nursing Education, 36*, 67-73.

Roberts and colleagues (1997) have described the first transition as involving an initial feeling of loss of confidence and competence accompanied by anxiety (see Table 4-2, stage I). Initial clinical experiences were associated with the desire to observe rather than to provide care, the inability to recall simple facts, the omission of essential data from history taking, feelings of awkwardness with patients, and difficulty prioritizing data. The students' focus at this time was almost exclusively on acquiring and refining assessment skills and continued development of physical examination techniques. By the end of the first semester, students reported returning feelings of confidence and the regaining of their former competence in interpersonal skills. Although they were still tentative about diagnostic and treatment decisions, students reported feeling more comfortable with patients as some of their basic nursing abilities began to return (see Table 4-2, stage II).

Transitions in nursing role identity occurring during the first two stages were associated with feelings of role confusion. Students were dismayed at how slow and inefficient they were clinically and reported feelings of self-doubt and lack of confidence in their abilities to ever function in the "real world" of health care. They sought shortcuts in attempts to increase their efficiency. They reported profound feelings of responsibility regarding diagnostic and treatment decisions and at the same time increasingly realized the limitations of clinical practice when they were confronted with the real-life situations of their patients. They recalled finding it easy to second-guess physicians' decisions in their previous nursing roles, but now they found those decisions more problematic when they were responsible for making them. They joked about feeling like adolescents. This is the point that Cusson and Viggiano (2002) are making when they comment, in reference to neonatal NPs, that the infant really does look different when viewed from the head of the bed rather than the side of the bed. They explain that "rather than taking orders, as they did as staff nurses, NNPs must synthesize incredibly complex information and decide on a plan of action. Experienced neonatal nurses often guide house staff regarding care decisions and writing orders to match the care that is being given. However, the shift in responsibility to actually writing the orders can be very intimidating" (p. 24).

Roberts and colleagues (1997) observed that a blending of the APN student and the former nurse developed during stage II as students renewed their appreciation for their previous interpersonal skills as teachers, supporters, and collaborators and again perceived their patients as unique individuals in the context of their life situations. Students developed increased awareness of the uncertainty involved in the process of making definitive diagnostic and treatment decisions. Although these insights served to demystify the clinical diagnostic process, the students' anxiety about providing care increased. In spite of current attempts to reduce diagnostic and treatment uncertainty through evidence-based practice, a basic degree of uncertainty is inherent in clinical practice. Learning about strategies to cope with clinical decision making in situations of uncertainty, such as ruling out the worst-case scenario, seeking consultation, and monitoring patients closely with phone calls and follow-up visits, can decrease anxiety and promote increased confidence (Brykczynski, 1991).

The transition in the relationships between students and preceptors and students and faculty in the study by Roberts and colleagues (1997) involved students feeling anxious that they were not learning enough and would never know enough to practice competently. Students felt frustrated and perceived that faculty and preceptors were not providing them with all the information that they needed. Then during the third stage (see Table 4-2), as they felt more confident and competent, students began to question the clinical judgments of their preceptors and faculty. This process is thought to help students advance from independence to interdependence—the last stage of the transition process. Much of the conflict at this juncture appeared to derive from students' feelings of "ambivalence about giving up dependence on external authorities" (Roberts et al., 1997, p. 71) such as preceptors and faculty and assuming responsibility for making independent judgments based on their own assessments from their clinical and educational experiences and the literature. The relevance of these role acquisition processes for other APN roles has not been reported. This is another area in which research would be helpful.

Until recently, the literature on APN role acquisition in school has focused exclusively on individuals who were already nurses. A commonly held assumption among nurses is "the more clinical experience, the better" for acquiring the necessary knowledge and skill to take on complex APN roles. It is usual for at least 1 year of nursing practice to be required for admission to APN programs. The process of role acquisition for students in direct-entry APN master's programs that admit NNCGs may differ because these individuals were not functioning as nurses before they entered the program. Rich and Rodriguez (2002) point out "anecdotally, strong biases against NNCGs exist. It is not uncommon for nurse practitioners or physicians to refuse to precept NNCG NP students" (p. 31).

They conducted a qualitative study of nurses' perceptions of NNCG NPs and purposely sought out those with biases against NNCGs in recruiting nurse participants for this study by inviting clinicians to participate who had refused to precept NNCG students. Forty-two questionnaires were mailed, but only the first 14 were analyzed for their report because saturation (a qualitative research term indicating that data were repetitive) was reached at that point. Six of the 14 female nurse participants were NPs. They ranged in age from 31 to 71 years, and their educational background varied from baccalaureate to doctorate with 10 having master's degrees. They reported that "those taking the time to complete and return the questionnaire clearly had opinions about non-nurse college graduates" (Rich & Rodriguez, 2002, p. 33). The findings included three themes supporting the benefit of acquiring nursing experience before learning an APN role. A fourth theme highlighting the positive aspects of NNCGs such as being strong academically, highly motivated, and confident was also identified.

In their qualitative study of family nurse practitioner (FNP) role transition, Heitz and colleagues (2004) found differences in role acquisition experiences between FNP students who were inexperienced nurses and FNP students who were experienced nurses. Feelings of insecurity, inadequacy, vulnerability, and being overwhelmed were typical, but role confusion was reported primarily by the more experienced RN students as they went through the "letting go" of the RN role and "taking on" of the FNP role. Further investigation is indicated to explore the similarities and differences in the role development experiences of students in all types of programs.

Strategies to Facilitate Role Acquisition

The anticipatory socialization to APN roles that occurs in graduate education is analogous to a process that Kramer (1974) described for undergraduate RNs that she called "immunization." The overall objective is to expose role incumbents to as many real-life experiences as possible during the educational program to minimize reality shock and role insufficiency on graduation and initial role implementation. Role content can be incorporated into APN curricula in a variety of ways such as (1) in the overall framework for designing an APN curriculum, (2) in a specific role course, (3) as part of specific assignments, or (4) in role seminars that span an entire curriculum. Hamric and Hanson (2003) asserted that it is an ethical mandate for all APN educators, regardless of specialty, to provide graduates with up-to-date knowledge of professional role and regulatory issues, in addition to concentration on clinical competence. The importance of explicit role preparation for the complex and challenging roles of graduates of DNP programs is recognized in the curriculum proposed by the American Association of Colleges of Nursing (AACN) (AACN, 2006). If there is not a separate role course, careful attention must be paid to this curriculum component so that it does not become integrated out of existence.

Specific strategies for facilitating role acquisition can be categorized according to three major purposes: (1) role rehearsal; (2) development of clinical knowledge and skills, including strategies for dealing with uncertainty; and (3) creation of a supportive network. These are presented on the Evolve website. For adequate role rehearsal, APN students should experience all aspects of the core competencies (see Chapter 3) directly, while faculty and fellow students are available to help them process or debrief these experiences (Hamric & Taylor, 1989; Hupcey, 1990). APN students should be cautioned that other nurses, physicians, other providers, and administrators in the work setting may value only clinical expertise and not the other core competencies. Strategies for enhancing understanding of how the core competencies are embedded in each APN role include preparation of short-term and long-term goals to use as guides in development of professional portfolios, analysis of existing position descriptions, and development of the ideal position description. These are also helpful for guiding students in their search for an initial APN position.

The development of clinical knowledge and skills for APN role acquisition can be promoted by planning for realistic clinical experiences with the support of faculty and preceptors nearby. Emphasis on realism and a holistic situational perspective are important in clinical experiences for helping students understand that the complex clinical judgments involved in APN assessment and management of patient situations over time are not simply technical medical knowledge but, rather, a hybrid of nursing and medical knowledge and experience. Studies of APN practice demonstrate that advanced practice roles incorporate a holistic approach that blends elements of nursing and medicine (Brown, 1992; Brykczynski,

1999; Grando, 1998; Johnson, 1993; see also Chapter 5). Teaching and learning experiences for all of the APN role components should integrate elements of research and theory and be incorporated into specialty APN courses to build on the knowledge gained in the traditional graduate core and clinical support courses in the curriculum. New APN graduates can benefit from familiarity with role transition processes by not expecting to be able to fully and expertly demonstrate all APN role components immediately on graduation.

Clinical mentoring by preceptors is an important component of ensuring realistic clinical learning experiences (Hayes, 2001; Kelly & Mathews, 2001; Kleinpell-Nowell, 2001). A survey of 258 graduating NP students at 10 institutions indicated that students who selected their own preceptor scored higher on mentoring and self-efficacy than those whose preceptors were assigned by faculty (Hayes, 1998). In addition, students with non-nurse preceptors scored lower than those with nurse preceptors. These findings need to be considered in planning preceptor arrangements. A mix of APN and non-nurse preceptors during the program can be quite valuable. Hayes (2001) observed that requiring students to locate their own preceptors can be problematic for some students who may not have the necessary professional connections to identify a qualified preceptor.

Careful planning for the first APN position after program completion is important. Reports of the transition experiences of new NP graduates during their first year after graduation suggested that the first position can be critical in terms of solidifying the NP's career (Brown & Olshansky, 1997; Heitz et al., 2004; Kelly & Mathews, 2001). Preparation of students for fulfillment of APN roles on graduation should be a collaborative effort of students, faculty, and preceptors. The need for position descriptions that clearly outline roles and responsibilities has been emphasized as essential for smooth role transition (Cooper & Sparacino, 1990; Hamric & Taylor, 1989; McMyler & Miller, 1997). The transition to the first position is a process—not an event that needs to be a focus of role content in APN programs (Hamric & Hanson, 2003; Hunter, Bormann, & Lops, 1996). Several NP faculty believe that the role disillusionment of some new APNs may be reflected in frequent position changes or staying in the same registered nurse job after graduation from an APN program (C. Hanson, personal communication, August 30, 2003). Substantive role courses are critical to smooth the path to full APN role implementation (Hamric & Hanson, 2003; Hunter et al., 1996).

Finally and perhaps most important, an overall strategy for enhancing APN clinical knowledge and skill is for faculty to maintain competency in clinical practice. Clinical competency enhances the faculty's ability to evaluate students clinically, to discuss clinically relevant examples in classes, to serve as preceptors for students, and to evaluate the care provided in preceptorship sites. The clinical competence of faculty is important to prevent a wide gap between education and practice, to enhance faculty credibility, and to foster realistic expectations for new APN graduates.

Establishing a peer support system, planning social functions with faculty and preceptors, and creating a virtual community can facilitate the development of a support network. Computer literacy is critical for networking and access to the high-quality materials available on websites (Table 4-3), in literature searches, and on personal digital assistants. The importance of forming a support network was emphasized by study findings (Kelly & Mathews, 2001; Kleinpell-Nowell, 2001). The establishment of a system for self-directed learning activities during the

first few years after program completion forms the basis for maintaining competence throughout one's career (Gunn, 1998). The establishment of a process for lifelong learning should be initiated during the APN educational program as students create a computer-based self-monitoring system that includes clinical and role transition experiences over time to serve as a reality check or timetable. On graduation, continuing education program attendance could be incorporated into this monitoring system to facilitate compilation of necessary documentation for certification along with ongoing self-evaluation and role development.

Advanced Practice Nursing Role Implementation (at Work)

After successfully emerging from the APN educational process, new APN graduates face yet another transition from the student role to the professional APN role (see Figure 4-1). APN graduates can be expected to experience attitudinal, behavioral, and value conflicts as they move from the academic world, in which holistic care is highly valued, to the work world, in which organizational efficiency is paramount. Anticipatory

Table 4-3　Useful Internet Sites for Creating a Support Network

Website	Organization	Selected Highlights
www.aahcdc.org/	Association of Academic Health Centers	Interdisciplinary education and practice in prevention Resources for building a practice
www.nonpf.com	National Organization of Nurse Practitioner Faculties	NP competencies, publications, resource centers
www.aanp.org	American Academy of Nurse Practitioners	Certification, legislative news, links to international sites
www.nacns.org	National Association of Clinical Nurse Specialists	Position statement on CNS practice and education
www.acnpweb.org	American College of Nurse Practitioners	Headlines, NP legislation ACNP outcome studies page
http://nursingworld.org	American Nurses Association	Credentialing center, patient safety/advocacy
www.napnap.org	National Association of Pediatric Nurse Practitioners	Scope of practice for PNPs, healthy eating initiative
www.aana.com	American Association of Nurse Anesthetists	Scope and standards; click on "Resources" for professional practice documents
www.acnm.org	American College of Nurse-Midwives	Position statements; click on "Continuing Education & Practice Resources"
www.ncsbn.org	National Council of State Boards of Nursing	APRN vision paper—programs and services News releases—media room

ACNP, Acute care nurse practitioner; *APRN,* advanced practice registered nurse; *CNS,* clinical nurse specialist; *NP,* nurse practitioner; *PNPs,* pediatric nurse practitioners.

guidance is needed for role transition yet again. The process of APN role implementation is an example of a situational transition (Schumacher & Meleis, 1994), which has been described in the literature as a progressive movement through phases (Baker, 1979; Hamric & Taylor, 1989; Oda, 1977; Page & Arena, 1991). There is general agreement that significant overlap and fluidity exist among the phases. However, for purposes of discussion, the phases will be considered sequentially.

Hamric and Taylor's (1989) study of CNS role development and Brown and Olshansky's (1997) study of NP role transition are two major investigations in which APN role implementation processes are described. Additional studies that contribute to understanding of the transitional processes as APNs implement their roles include the longitudinal survey of acute care NP practice (Kleinpell-Nowell, 1999, 2001), in which the first six cohorts to take the adult acute care national certification examination were followed annually for 5 years; Kelly and Mathews' (2001) qualitative focus group study of 21 recent NP graduates; and Heitz and colleagues' (2004) qualitative study of nine FNPs' role transition experiences. Findings from these studies will be incorporated into this discussion of APN role implementation.

Hamric and Taylor (1989) described seven phases of CNS role development along with associated characteristics and developmental tasks derived from analysis of questionnaires returned by 100 CNSs (see Table 4-4). All but 2 of the 42 CNSs in their first positions for 3 years or less experienced progression through the first three phases (identical to those phases identified by Baker [1979]). Most of the CNS respondents went through these three phases within 2 years. Phase 1, Orientation (Table 4-4), is characterized by enthusiasm, optimism, and attention to mastery of clinical skills. The second phase, Frustration, is associated with feelings of conflict, inadequacy, frustration, and anxiety. Arena and Page (1992) identified the imposter phenomenon as a feature of CNS practice that could interfere with effective role implementation. In retrospect, it appears that the imposter phenomenon is one of the distressing features of the frustration phase. The next phase, Implementation, is described as one of role modification in response to interactions with others. This phase is associated with a renewed or returning perspective.

CNSs with more than 3 years of experience described their role development experiences in terms very different from Baker's (1979) phases. Content analysis of these data led to a description of four additional phases (see Table 4-4). Experienced CNSs identified the Integration phase, which was characterized by "self-confidence and assurance in the role, high job satisfaction, an advanced level of practice, and signs of recognition and respect for expertise within and outside the work setting" (Hamric & Taylor, 1989, p. 56). Only 10% of the CNSs with less than 5 years of experience in the role met the criteria for this phase, whereas 50% of those with more than 6 years of experience could be categorized as being in this phase. The Integration phase was typically reached after 3 to 5 years in the CNS role. This fourth phase of Integration (thought to be reached only after successful transition through the earlier phases) is characterized by refinement of clinical expertise and integration of role components appropriate for the particular situation.

Hamric and Taylor (1989) also described three negative phases not evident in previous literature. The Frozen phase is described as being associated with frustration, anger, and lack of career satisfaction. Restructuring of role responsibilities and changing organizational expectations characterize the Reorganization phase. The Complacent phase is characterized by comfort, stability, and maintenance of the status quo. Unlike the Integration phase, these additional phases share a negative, nonproductive character. One might speculate that APNs experiencing these negative phases would be more vulnerable to position changes in today's cost-constrained health care system.

The complexity of APN role development processes is further demonstrated by findings from Brown and Olshansky's (1997) longitudinal grounded theory study of the role transition experiences of 35 novice NPs conducted at 1 month, 6 months, and 12 months for two different cohorts of graduates during their first year of practice. They described a four-stage process of moving from "limbo to legitimacy" during the first year of practice, which is outlined in Table 4-5. Related developmental tasks and strategies included in Table 4-5 were specifically developed for this chapter. The first stage, "Laying the Foundation," was not described in previous literature. During this stage, new graduates take certification examinations, obtain necessary recognition or licensure from state boards of nursing, and look for positions. This stage has been shortened because of the availability of certification examinations by computer.

Table 4-4   PHASES OF APN ROLE DEVELOPMENT

Phase	Characteristics	Developmental Tasks	Facilitation Strategies
Orientation	Enthusiasm, optimism, eager to prove self to setting Anxious about ability to meet self- and institutional expectations Expects to make change	Learn formal and informal organizations Learn key players; begin establishing relationship and power base Explore expectations to see whether compatible with own Identify and clarify role to self and others	Structure an orientation plan Establish mutually agreed upon role expectations Circulate literature on APN role Meetings with key individuals Peer networking Identify with a role model/mentor Set reasonable 3- to 6-month goals Concentrate on clinical mastery Postpone recommendations for major changes Join key committees
Frustration*	Discouragement and questioning as a result of unrealistic expectations (either self- or employer); difficult and slow-paced change; resistance encountered Feelings of inadequacy in response to the overwhelming problems encountered, pressure to prove worth	Develop more realistic expectations Work on time management and setting priorities Develop short-term goals or projects to obtain tangible results/feedback Develop support system within and/or outside work setting	Schedule debriefing sessions Practice time management Review initial logs/Update professional portfolio Continue seeking peer and mentor support Maintain communication with administrators Consult with experts Organize resources for easy accessibility
Implementation	Returning optimism and enthusiasm as positive feedback received and expectations realigned Organization and reorganization of role tasks, modified in response to feedback Implementing and balancing new subroles Regaining sense of perspective *May* focus on specific project(s)	Enhance visibility and power base within informal and formal organizations; build coalitions and networks Identify tangible accomplishments Complete transition to advanced practice level if necessary Continue to reassess and refocus direction	Reassess demands, priorities, goals Plan for performance and outcome evaluation Sustain communication with peers, administrators, and others

Adapted by Brykczynski, K.A. from Hamric, A.B., & Taylor, J.W. (1989). Role development of the CNS. In A.B. Hamric & J.A. Spross (Eds.), *The clinical nurse specialist in theory and practice* (2nd ed., p. 48). Philadelphia: Saunders.
*The *imposter* phenomenon (Arena & Page, 1992) may be experienced during the Frustration phase.
APN, Advanced practice nurse; CNS, clinical nurse specialist.

Table 4-4   PHASES OF APN ROLE DEVELOPMENT—cont'd

Phase	Characteristics	Developmental Tasks	Facilitation Strategies
Integration	Self-confident and assured in role Rates self at advanced level of practice Activities reflect wide recognition, influence in area of specialty Continuously feels challenged; takes on new projects; expands practice Either moderately or very satisfied with present position Congruence between personal and organizational goals and expectations	Continued role evolution and skill development to strengthen all role components and competencies Share expertise and experience with others through publications, research, professional activities Maintain flexible approach Be alert for signs of complacency or boredom	Continue debriefing sessions Plan for role expansion and refinement Schedule performance and outcome evaluations Develop broader professional interests Formulate short- and long-term goals for further development
Frozen	Self-confident, assured in role; rates self at intermediate or advanced practice level Experiencing anger/frustration reflecting experience Conflict between self-goals and those of organization/supervisor Reports sense of being unable to move forward because of forces outside of self	Obtain feedback from supervisor and peers Reevaluate self-goals in relation to CNS role and organization Objective assessment of organization: Is there potential for compatibility? Attempt to redesign or renegotiate the role Consider career move/change If unsuccessful, consider change in position/career direction	
Reorganization	Reports earlier experiences that represent integration Organization experiencing major changes Pressure to change role in ways that are incongruent with own concept of CNS role and/or personal goals	Open discussion with change agents Attempt compromise to preserve integrity of role and still meet needs of organization If unsuccessful, change position/title or negotiate job change	
Complacent	Experiences self in role as settled and comfortable Variable job satisfaction Questionable impact on organization	Need to reenergize Reconfigure role to allow growth by identifying changing needs of patient population or institution	

Table 4-5   TRANSITION STAGES IN FIRST YEAR OF PRIMARY CARE PRACTICE

Stage*	Characteristics*	Developmental Tasks	Facilitation Strategies
Laying the foundation	Period of role identity confusion immediately after graduation Not yet an NP, but no longer a student Feelings of worry, confusion, and insecurity about ability to practice successfully as an NP	Recuperate from school Initiate a job search and secure a position Obtain certification	Take time out to recuperate from the pressures of school Plan rewards for self Maintain peer support network Refine professional portfolio and use it to analyze available positions in terms of future goals
Launching	Discomfort of advanced-beginner level of knowledge and skills Feelings of unreality, insecurity—"the imposter phenomenon" Pervasive performance anxiety Daily stress Time pressure	Develop realistic expectations Incorporate feeling of legitimacy into NP role identity Cope with anxiety Mobilize problem-solving skills Work on time management and setting priorities† Develop support system†	Plan for longer appointments initially Anticipate need for time to feel comfortable in new role Realize that the transition process is time limited Schedule debriefing sessions with experienced MD or APN Seek peer and mentor support regularly Learn time-saving tips Clarify appropriate patient problems to work with initially Monitor internal self-talk—be positive
Meeting the challenge	Decreased anxiety Increased feeling of legitimacy Increased confidence develops along with increased competence Increased acceptance and comfort with the uncertainty inherent in primary care	Expand recognition of practice concerns to include the work environment Gain situational knowledge and skill in managing clinical problems Identify tangible accomplishments† Develop individualized style of approaching patients and organizing care	Schedule a 6-month evaluation Maintain communication with peers, administrators, and others† Modify expectations to be more realistic Learn from repetitive practice Structure work situation so that resources are readily available Practice strategies to manage uncertainty Gain ability to handle uncertainty

*Data from Brown, M.A., & Olshansky, E. (1997). From limbo to legitimacy: A theoretical model of the transition to the primary care nurse practitioner role. *Nursing Research 46*, 46-51; Brown, M.A., & Olshansky, E. (1998). Becoming a primary nurse practitioner: Challenges of the initial year of practice. *The Nurse Practitioner, 23*, 46, 52, 58, 61-66.
†Adapted by Brykczynski, K.A. from Hamric, A.B., & Taylor, J.W. (1989). Role development of the CNS. In A.B. Hamric & J.A. Spross (Eds.), *The clinical nurse specialist in theory and practice* (2nd ed., p. 48). Philadelphia: Saunders.
APN, Advanced practice nurse; *NP*, nurse practitioner; *MD*, doctor of medicine.

Table 4-5   Transition Stages in First Year of Primary Care Practice—cont'd

Stage*	Characteristics*	Developmental Tasks	Facilitation Strategies
Broadening the perspective	Feeling of enhanced self-esteem Solid feeling of legitimacy and competence Realistic and positive feelings about future practice	Acknowledge strengths and identify ways to incorporate additional challenges Identify larger system problems and seek solutions (All the developmental tasks from the Integration phase of Table 4-4 would be appropriate here also†)	Schedule a 12-month evaluation to reflect on progress and accomplishments Continue to seek verification and feedback from colleagues Make changes in work situation to increase support and effectiveness Inform staff and colleagues about NP role Affirm self-worth (Facilitation strategies from the Integration phase of Table 4-4 would be useful here also†)

The second stage, Launching, was defined as beginning with the first NP position and lasting at least 3 months. During this stage, the new graduate NP experiences the anxiety associated with the crisis of confidence and competence that accompanies taking on a new position and the return to the advanced-beginner skill level (Benner et al., 1996; Dreyfus & Dreyfus, 1986, 1996). As the advanced beginner becomes increasingly aware of the number of elements relevant to actual performance in the role, he or she may become overwhelmed with the complexity of the skills required for the role and exhausted by the effort required for mastery. New NPs in Kelly and Mathews' (2001) study described similar experiences of exhaustion and frustration with lack of control over time. This is the at-work version of the crisis of confidence and competence experienced during stage I of the in-school role acquisition process (see Table 4-2).

The feeling of being "an imposter" or "a fake," described by Brown and Olshansky (1997), Arena and Page (1992), and Huffstutler and Varnell (2006), was first reported in the psychological literature in reference to high-achieving women (Clance & Imes, 1978). Clinical symptoms associated with this phenomenon (generalized anxiety, lack of self confidence, depression, frustration) are commonly reported by APNs experiencing the frustration or launching phase. It is related to feeling unable to meet one's own expectations and those of others (Clance & Imes, 1978) and feelings of inadequacy and constantly being tested (Arena & Page, 1992). Harvey and Katz (1985) clarified that this phenomenon is typically a temporary experience associated with taking on a new role or beginning a new job. There is no evidence relating to whether or not new male APNs experience this phenomenon. Heitz and colleagues' (2004) study related similar role transition experiences of self-doubt, disillusionment, and turbulence and also reported that engaging in positive self-talk was helpful. They suggested that issues of gender and age may underlie differing perceptions of personal commitments and sacrifices as obstacles to surmount in role transition.

Although Brown and Olshansky (1997, 1998) did not relate their findings about NP role transition to Hamric and Taylor's (1989) findings about CNS role development, there appear to be many similarities in the results of the two studies. The characteristics of the Launching stage are very similar to those described by Hamric and Taylor (1989) for the Frustration phase. Brown and Olshansky's (1997, 1998) third stage, Meeting the challenge, is associated with feelings of regaining confidence and increasing competence. This stage has much in common with Hamric and Taylor's (1989) Implementation phase, which is noted for returning optimism and enthusiasm as expectations are realigned. The last stage, Broadening the perspective, is characterized by feelings of legitimacy and competency as NPs. This last stage is quite similar to Hamric and Taylor's (1989) fourth stage of Integration, during which the role is expanded and refined.

Rich (2005) investigated the relationship between duration of experience as an RN and NP clinical skills in practice among NPs who graduated within 4 years from three universities in the Northeast. One hundred and fifty NPs completed the self-report instrument assessments of their clinical skills (a response rate of 21%), and 60% of the collaborating physicians completed assessments of their NP clinical skills. Findings from the NP self-report data indicated that duration of practice experience as an RN was not correlated with level of competency in NP practice skills. "An unexpected finding was that there was a significant negative correlation between years of experience as an RN and NP clinical practice skills as assessed by the collaborating physicians" (Rich, 2005, p. 55). Data describing which role development phase the NP participants were experiencing would have been helpful for enhancing understanding of the findings. The finding that collaborating physicians rated the NPs as more clinically competent than the NPs rated themselves (Rich, 2005) would be expected for NPs in the Frustration or Launching phases (see Tables 4-4 and 4-5). Inclusion of assessments of both role development and clinical competency in APN follow-up studies would be helpful for building on the existing knowledge base.

Strategies to Facilitate Role Implementation

The four major developmental phases (Orientation, Frustration, Implementation, and Integration) identified by Hamric and Taylor (1989) to describe CNS role development are combined with strategies for facilitating APN role implementation (see Table 4-4). Table 4-5 lists the four stages of NP role implementation and their characteristics as identified by Brown and Olshansky (1997) and includes developmental tasks and strategies for facilitating NP role development in an attempt to link this study with those findings from the Hamric and Taylor (1989) study. The reader is encouraged to compare and contrast Tables 4-4 and 4-5 to glean relevant content for their particular APN role.

The four major phases described by Hamric and Taylor (1989) are used here to structure discussion of strategies to facilitate role implementation. The importance of being patient and recognizing that it takes time to fully develop in a new APN role was stressed by NPs in Kleinpell-Nowell's surveys (1999, 2001). A strategy to facilitate role implementation for all APNs during the Orientation phase is development of a structured orientation plan. Brown and Olshansky (1997, 1998) noted the importance of clarification of values, needs, and expectations and of recognition that transitional experiences are time limited. They also point out the importance of anticipatory guidance and realizing that these transition experiences follow a common pattern in new graduates. An APN in a new position (whether experienced in the role or not) needs to be aware of the importance of being informed about the organizational structure, philosophy, goals, policies, and procedures of the agency.

Networking was emphasized by NPs in Kleinpell-Nowell's surveys (1999, 2001). Peer support both within and outside the work setting is important, as noted by Hamric and Taylor (1989). New NPs stressed the importance of getting to know other nurses in the work setting, gaining their respect, and forming key alliances with them to enhance optimal functioning in their new positions (Kelly & Mathews, 2001). Designating a more experienced APN in the work setting as a mentor would be helpful and provide support for all APNs new to a position. APNs who serve as preceptors for students might be particularly effective mentors for new graduates (Hayes, 2005). The importance of careful selection of a mentor was reported by NPs in the study by Kelly and Mathews (2001). Additional strategies suggested for networking within the system include developing peer support groups, being accessible to colleagues by beeper or cell phone, and getting involved in interdisciplinary committees (Page & Arena, 1991). APNs should be encouraged to join local APN groups for peer support, legislative and political updates, and networking opportunities. Numerous Internet sites are also available for networking as noted earlier.

Page and Arena (1991) recommended that CNSs schedule and devote the major portion of their time during the Orientation phase to direct patient care to substantiate the clinical expert role. They also suggested making appointments with nursing leaders, physicians, and other health care professionals during this phase to garner administrative support. They recommended distributing business cards and making the job description available for discussion. They also counseled new CNSs to withhold suggestions for change until they have had the opportunity to more fully assess the system. When a new APN joins the staff of an organization, the administrator should send a letter describing the APN's background experiences and new position to key people in the organization.

Hamric and Taylor (1989) observed that the Frustration phase might come and go and may overlap other phases. They noted that painful affective responses are typical of this very difficult phase. They suggested that monthly sessions for sharing concerns with a group of peers and an administrator might facilitate movement through this phase. Strategies identified as helpful for energizing movement from the Frustration phase to the Implementation phase include obtaining assistance with time management (Allen, 2001); participating in support groups to ameliorate feelings of inadequacy; engaging in discussions for conflict resolution and role clarification; reassessing priorities and setting realistic expectations; and focusing on short-term, visible goals.

Page and Arena (1991) suggested keeping a work portfolio to document activities so APN progress is more readily visible. This can be an expansion of the portfolio and self-monitoring system begun during the APN program. Brown and Olshansky (1997) pointed out that organized sources of support such as phone calls, seminars, planned meetings with mentors, and scheduled time for consultation can significantly decrease feelings of anxiety. They note that recognition of the discomfort arising from moving from "expert back to novice" and realization that previous expertise can be valuable in the new role may help reduce feelings of inadequacy. They suggest that new APNs request reasonable time frames for initial patient visits, because novices take longer than experienced practitioners, and this may be key to successful adjustment to a new position.

During the Implementation phase, it is important for the APN to reassess demands to prevent feeling overwhelmed. Priorities may need to be readjusted, and short-term goals may need to be reformulated. Brown and Olshansky (1997, 1998) observed that competence and confidence are fostered through repetition. They also recommend scheduling a formal evaluation after approximately 6 months in which feedback about areas of strength and needs for improvement can be ascertained. Strategies mentioned

as important during this time include seeking administrative support through involvement in meetings, maintaining visibility in clinical areas, and developing in-service programs with input from staff (Page & Arena, 1991). After some time in the Implementation phase, APNs may plan and execute small-scale projects to demonstrate their effectiveness in their new roles.

Hamric and Taylor's (1989) survey data indicated that CNSs maximize their role potential during the Integration phase. Satisfactory completion of the earlier phases appears to be essential for passage into the Integration phase. One strategy for enhancing and maintaining optimal role implementation during this phase is having a trusted colleague who can act as a safe sounding board for "feedback, constructive criticism, and advice" (Hamric & Taylor, 1989, p. 79). During this phase, it is important to have a plan to guide continued role expansion and refinement, such as the portfolio mentioned earlier. Seeking appointment to key committees is important to increase recognition of APNs in the organization. Administrative support and constructive feedback from a trusted mentor continue to be important. Development of a promotional system that offers professional advancement in the APN practice role remains a challenge for practitioners and administrators. Page and Arena (1991) observed that less time is required for establishing relationships and assessing the system during this phase; therefore more time can be devoted to areas of scholarly interest. Brown and Olshansky (1997, 1998) pointed out the importance of formulating short-term goals to further development.

Whether the Frozen, Reorganization, and Complacent phases are distinct developmental phases or variations of the Implementation and Integration phases, they are clearly negative resolutions for APNs and their organizations. Table 4-4 includes strategies described by Hamric and Taylor (1989) for enhancing role development in these phases (see the earlier editions of this chapter for further discussion of these phases). APNs should engage in periodic self-assessment so that they recognize beginning signs associated with these phases, such as feelings of anger or dissatisfaction, conflict between self-goals and those of the organization or supervisor, feeling pressure to change one's APN role in ways that are incongruent with one's concept of the role, and feelings of complacency. Early recognition of problems and taking proactive steps to deal with organizational changes can help prevent or ameliorate the negative feelings associated with these phases.

Further analysis of the relationships between the stages described by Brown and Olshansky (1997, 1998) for NPs and the phases described by Hamric and Taylor (1989) for CNSs is needed. The relevance of these frameworks for transition processes experienced by other APNs also needs study. Further refinement of these findings could promote their incorporation into APN teaching, research, and practice. Questions of interest are (1) Is the Laying the Foundation stage common to other APN groups? (2) Do the negative phases Frozen, Reorganization, and Complacent appear after 3 years of practice in APN groups other than CNSs? and (3) How do role acquisition and role implementation experiences of APN graduates of DNP programs compare with those reported here for master's-prepared APNs?

Facilitators and Barriers in the Work Setting

Aspects of the work setting exert a major influence on APN role definitions and expectations, thereby affecting role ambiguity, role incongruity, and role conflict. Findings from a survey by McFadden and Miller (1994) of CNSs identify access to support services, such as computers, statistical consultation, and secretarial and library services, as a facilitator of role development. Factors found to promote NP role development include being recognized as a primary care provider; having one's own examination room; and being supported by co-workers, administrators, and patients (Andrews, Hanson, Maule, & Snelling, 1999; Hupcey, 1993; Kelly & Mathews, 2001; Lurie, 1981). Practical strategies identified by Bonnel, Belt, Hill, Wiggins, and Ohm (2000) for initiating NP practice in nursing facilities included proactive communication, developing a consistent system for visits, setting up the physical environment, and building a team approach to care. Factors found to impede NP role development include pressure to manage care for large numbers of patients, resistance from staff nurses, and lack of understanding of the NP role (Andrews et al., 1999; Hupcey, 1993; Kelly & Mathews, 2001, Lurie, 1981). More recent constraints operating in today's health care settings that affect not only APNs but also other providers and office staff include new billing and coding guidelines, Health Insurance Portability and Accountability Act (HIPAA) regulations, monitoring for fraud and abuse, sexual harassment, and demands to integrate technology into practice.

The ability to incorporate teaching and counseling into the patient encounter may be a function of skill development gained with experience in the APN role. This observation may be used as a rationale for structuring more time for visits and fewer total patients for new APNs, with gradual increases in caseloads as experience is accrued. Research indicates that NPs incorporate counseling and teaching into the flow of patient visits—capturing the teachable moment (Brykczynski, 1985; Johnson, 1993; Lurie, 1981; see also Chapter 13 for examples). Future plans to redesign primary care payment systems to blend monthly patient panel fees with fee-for-service charges and include incentives for patient-centered care performance are promising for APNs because such payment systems highlight and support the additional dimensions of care that APNs can provide (Davis, Schoenbaun, & Audet, 2005).

Administrative factors that should be considered include whether APNs are placed in line or staff positions; whether they are unit based, population based, or in some other arrangement; who evaluates them; and whether they report to administrative or clinical supervisors. Baird and Prouty (1989) maintained that the organizational design should have enough flexibility to change as the situation changes. The placements of various APN positions may differ even within one setting, depending on size, complexity, and distribution of the patient population (Andrews et al., 1999; Baird & Prouty, 1989; see also Chapter 23).

Issues of professional versus administrative authority underlie the importance of the structural placement of the APN within the organization. Effectiveness of the APN role is enhanced when there is a mutual fit between the goals and expectations of the individual and the organization (Cooper & Sparacino, 1990; see also Chapter 23). Clarification of goals and expectations before employment and periodic reassessments can minimize conflict and enhance role development and effectiveness.

Continued Advanced Practice Nurse Role Evolution

CNMs, CRNAs, NPs, and CNSs have attained positive recognition and support for role confirmation in clinical positions in many settings in the United States (Andrews et al., 1999). However, in spite of the increasing familiarity and popularity of these APN roles, some health care settings have employed few if any APNs and some staff members have had minimal experience working with APNs. In some areas of the

United States, physicians or physician assistants are preferred over APNs. Even experienced APNs can expect to encounter resistance to full implementation of their roles if they seek positions in institutions with no history of employing APNs. Andrews and colleagues (1999) described their experiences introducing the NP role into a large academic teaching hospital. They delineate helpful strategies for marketing the new NP role to staff, patients, and the surrounding community, as well as ways to set up the necessary infrastructure to support the new role in the institution. They refer to this process as "evolutionary."

The meaning of evolution of established APN roles varies according to the type of APN role. For example, for CNMs, role evolution refers to broadening the scope of practice to include primary health care (Kinsley, 2005). For over a decade, midwifery has encompassed primary care management of women in their *Core Competencies for Basic Midwifery Practice* (ACNM, 2007; see also the ACNM's website *[www.acnm.org]*). Integrating these competencies into midwifery practice without increasing program length constitutes a threefold challenge for CNMs to (1) incorporate didactic and clinical content into educational programs, (2) address the educational gap between new graduates and practicing CNMs, and (3) define and clarify the appropriate scope of primary health care practice for CNMs (Stuart & Oshio, 2002; see also Chapter 16).

The emphasis on cost containment in the health care delivery system has led to the trend of having acute care NPs staff intensive care units to compensate for the shortage of house staff physicians (Rosenfeld, 2001; Sechrist & Berlin, 1998; see also Chapters 14 and 18).

In addition, evolution of APN roles is also reflected in expansion of practice to multiple areas or sites, often in blended role CNS/NP practices (see Chapter 15). Although responsibility for multiple areas in the same facility has been typical of many CNS roles for years, it is an evolutionary process for most other APN roles. Multi-site roles might signify practice responsibilities at different sites or multiple areas of responsibility in the same site, and they may combine both inpatient and outpatient responsibilities (Stahl & Myers, 2002). Stahl and Myers' clinical practices are exemplars of APN practice evolving to multiple sites, which constitute a strategy for extending APN resources and trying to use them more efficiently. Stahl is a CNS whose practice has evolved from the full range of CNS

practice for four medical cardiac units at a tertiary care center to also include support primarily in education, consultation, and program development at two additional hospitals. Myers is an adult NP who directs a hepatitis C program for a specialty physician group with 11 physicians at nine practice locations, and she also provides direct care for patients at four of the sites.

The complexity of multi-site roles can be overwhelming if the APN does not develop a certain degree of comfort with ambiguity. Stahl and Myers relied on Quinn's (1996) wisdom for developing the leader within by expecting to "build the bridge as you walk on it" (p. 83) and learning "how to get lost with confidence" (p. 86). Their commitment to being continuous learners is a useful model for APNs to follow as they experience the situational transitions that are inevitable as clinical practices evolve. Stahl and Myers (2002) used the National Association of Clinical Nurse Specialists' (NACNS, 1998) position statement (an updated version is now available on the NACNS website [see Table 4-3]) describing three spheres of CNS influence to stimulate creativity and guide their APN practices as they evolve into new and multiple practice settings.

Current plans for the evolution of APN programs from the master's to the doctoral level follow the pattern of the historical development of many APN programs. Whether programs will move to the doctoral level is no longer a question; instead, the issue now is how to facilitate the transition (O'Sullivan, Carter, Marion, Pohl, & Werner, 2005). In the case of NPs, Mundinger (2005) asserted that DNP preparation is necessary so that NPs will be prepared for comprehensive care inclusive of both inpatient and outpatient management. This objective is congruent with Ford's (1979) perspective of the NP as the nurse for all settings. The issue of how non-clinician graduates of DNP programs will be distinguished from APN clinician graduates will be of interest as these programs develop over time.

As individual APNs mature into their respective roles and become comfortable and confident in the more technical components of their roles, greater concentration on the unique nature of APN practice can be expected. In their study of CNSs, Hamric and Taylor (1989) found that freedom to develop their unique APN role, availability of feedback from a mentor, support to broaden their influence and take on new projects, and recognition of their contributions enabled experienced CNSs to stay energized in their clinical practice roles. As Peplau (1997) advocated, nurse leaders must emphasize what nurses do for patients. The claim that nurses provide patient-centered care and that APN practice incorporates patient education, family assessment, involvement, and support, and community awareness and connections (Neale, 1999) needs to be documented. For example, Kelly and Mathews (2001) found that graduates with from 1 to 7 years of experience as NPs found it difficult to adhere to ideals of holistic care and health promotion given the pressures of the clinical situation. Continued research that demonstrates positive outcomes of APN care is essential for APN practice to make an impact on health care policy (Brooten et al., 2002; Murphy-Ende, 2002; Russell, VorderBruegge, & Burns, 2002; Ryden et al., 2000; see also Chapter 24). Rashotte (2005) advocates for dialogical forms of research to evoke the more holistic and humanistic aspects of what it means to be an APN to complement the predominant instrumental and economic perspectives underlying the majority of APN research. Greater research activity and increasing involvement in the larger arena of health policy may also represent continuing role evolution for APNs.

Evaluation of Role Development

Evaluation is fundamental to enhancing role implementation (see Chapter 25). Development of a professional portfolio to document APN accomplishments can be useful for both performance and impact (process and outcome) evaluation. Performance evaluation for APNs should include self-evaluation, peer review, and administrative evaluation (Cooper & Sparacino, 1990; Hamric & Taylor, 1989). Use of a competency profile can be helpful for organizing evaluation in a dynamic way that allows for changes in role implementation over time as expertise, situations, and priorities change (Callahan & Bruton-Maree, 1994). The competency profile can be used to assess performance in each of the core APN competencies. APN programs need to include content and skill development regarding self-evaluation and peer evaluation of role implementation so that individuals can learn to monitor their practice and identify difficulties early to avoid moving into negative developmental phases (Hamric & Hanson, 2003).

Outcome evaluation is important to demonstrate the effectiveness of each APN role. Ongoing development of appropriate outcome evaluation measures, such as patient outcomes and patient satisfaction, is

important (Ingersoll, McIntosh, & Williams, 2000; see also Chapters 24 and 25). The existence of a reward system to provide for career advancement through a clinical ladder program and accrual of additional benefits is particularly important for retaining APNs in clinical roles. In less structured situations, APNs can negotiate for periodic reassessments and salary increases through options such as profit sharing.

The evaluation process broadens to incorporate interdisciplinary review when APN practice includes hospital privileges, prescriptive privileges, and third-party reimbursement. This expansion of the evaluation process has both positive and negative aspects. Advantages to the review process associated with securing and maintaining hospital privileges include the multiple aspects that are considered in the evaluation, the variety of perspectives, and the visibility afforded APNs. APNs should seek key positions on hospital review committees to promote APN roles within organizations. A major difficulty in implementing interdisciplinary peer review is lack of interaction between and among the incumbents of the various health professional groups during their formative educational programs (Brykczynski, 1999). The resurgence of interest in developing and implementing interdisciplinary educational experiences between nursing students and medical students is encouraging (AACN, 2006; Hamric & Hanson, 2003; IOM, 2003; O'Neil, 1998, see also Table 4-3, Association of Academic Health Centers website highlights).

CONCLUSION

Role development experiences for APNs are described as a two-phase process that consists of role acquisition in school and role implementation after graduation. The limits of the educational process in preparing graduates for the realities of the work world are acknowledged. Students, faculty, preceptors, and administrators need to be informed about the human skill acquisition process and its stages, the processes of adult and professional socialization, identity transformation, role acquisition, role implementation, and overall career development. Knowing (theoretical knowledge) and actually experiencing (practical knowledge) are very different phenomena, but at least students and new graduates can be forewarned about the transition experiences in school and the turbulence that can be expected during the first year of practice. Anticipatory guidance can be provided through role rehearsal experiences, such as clinical preceptorships and role seminars. Students need to be encouraged to begin networking with practicing APNs through local, state, and national APN groups. This networking is especially important for APNs who will not be practicing in proximity to other APNs. Experienced APNs and new APN graduates can form mutually beneficial relationships.

Although anticipatory socialization experiences in school can facilitate role acquisition, they cannot prevent the transition that occurs with movement into a new position and actual role implementation. APN programs should have a firm foundation in the real world. However, a certain degree of incongruence or conflict between academic ideals and work-world realities will continue to exist (Ormond & Kish, 2001). APNs must take a leadership role in guiding and directing planned change and guard against mere maintenance of the status quo. Establishing mentor programs for new APNs in the work setting is one way to develop and maintain support for the developmental phases of role implementation described here.

APN role development has been described as dynamic, complex, and situational. It is influenced by many factors, such as experience, level of expertise, personal and professional values, setting, specialty, relationships with co-workers, aspects of role transition, and life transitions. Frameworks for understanding APN role development processes have been discussed along with strategies for facilitating role acquisition and role implementation. Ongoing evolution of APN roles in response to organizational and health care system changes and demands will continue. Future research studies to assess the applicability of this information for all APN specialty groups and for APN graduates of DNP programs are needed to further the understanding of APN role development.

REFERENCES

Aiken, L.H., Clarke, S.P., Sloan, D.M., Sochalski, J., & Silber, J.H. (2002). Hospital nurse staffing and patient mortality, nurse burnout, and job dissatisfaction. *JAMA: The Journal of the American Medical Association, 288*, 1987-1995.

Allen, D. (2001). *Getting things done: The art of stress-free productivity.* New York: Penguin Books.

American Association of Colleges of Nursing (AACN). (2006). *The essentials of doctoral education for advanced nursing practice.* Retrieved October 28, 2007, from www.aacn.nche.edu/DNP/pdf/Essentials.pdf.

American Association of Nurse Anesthetists (AANA). (2007). *Qualifications and capabilities of the certified registered nurse anesthetist.* Author. Retrieved June 4, 2007, from www.aana.com.

American College of Nurse-Midwives (ACNM). (2006). *Requirements for signed collaborative agreements between physicians and certified nurse-midwives (CNMs) or certified midwives (CMs).* Retrieved June 1, 2007, from www.acnm.org.

American College of Nurse-Midwives (ACNM). (2007). *Core competencies for basic midwifery practice.* Washington, DC: Author. Retrieved October 28, 2007, from www.acnm.org/siteFiles/descriptive/Core_Competencies_6_07_3.pdf.

Anderson, E.M., Leonard, B.J., & Yates, J.A. (1974). Epigenesis of the nurse practitioner role. *American Journal of Nursing, 74*, 1812-1816.

Andrews, J., Hanson, C., Maule, S., & Snelling, M. (1999). Attaining role confirmation in nurse practitioner practice. *Clinical Excellence for Nurse Practitioners, 3*, 302-310.

Arena, D.M., & Page, N.E. (1992). The imposter phenomenon in the clinical nurse specialist role. *Image: The Journal of Nursing Scholarship, 24*, 121-125.

Baird, S.B., & Prouty, M.P. (1989). Administratively enhancing CNS contributions. In A.B. Hamric & J.A. Spross (Eds.), *The clinical nurse specialist in theory and practice* (2nd ed., pp. 261-283). Philadelphia: Saunders.

Baker, V. (1979). Retrospective explorations in role development. In G.V. Padilla (Ed.), *The clinical nurse specialist and improvement of nursing practice* (pp. 56-63). Wakefield, MA: Nursing Resources.

Banda, E.E. (1985). *Role problems, role strain: Perception and experience of clinical nurse specialist.* Unpublished master's thesis, Boston University School of Nursing, Boston, MA.

Bandura, A. (1977). Self-efficacy: Toward a unifying theory of behavioral change. *Psychological Review, 84*, 191-215.

Bartholomew, K. (2006). *Ending nurse to nurse hostility: Why nurses eat their young and each other.* Mission, KS: Opus Communications.

Benner, P. (1984). *From novice to expert: Excellence and power in clinical nursing practice.* Menlo Park, CA: Addison-Wesley.

Benner, P. (March/April 1985). The oncology clinical nurse specialist: An expert coach. *Oncology Nursing Forum, 12*(2), 40-44.

Benner, P., Hooper-Kyriakidis, P., & Stannard, D. (1999). *Clinical wisdom and interventions in critical care: A thinking-in-action approach.* Philadelphia: Saunders.

Benner, P., Tanner, C.A., & Chesla, C.A. (1996). *Expertise in nursing practice: Caring, clinical judgment and ethics.* New York: Springer-Verlag.

Blumenreich, G.A. (2000). Legal briefs: Supervision. *AANA Journal, 68*, 404-409.

Bonnel, W., Belt, J., Hill, D., Wiggins, S., & Ohm, R. (2000). Challenges and strategies for initiating a nursing facility practice. *Journal of American Academy of Nurse Practitioners, 12*(9), 353-359.

Brooten, D., Naylor, M.D., York, R., Brown, L.P., Munro, B.H., Hollingsworth, A.O., et al. (2002). Lessons learned from testing the quality cost model of advanced practice nursing (APN) transitional care. *Journal of Nursing Scholarship, 34*, 369-375.

Brown, M.A., & Olshansky, E.F. (1997). From limbo to legitimacy: A theoretical model of the transition to the primary care nurse practitioner role. *Nursing Research, 46,* 46-51.

Brown, M.A., & Olshansky, E.F. (1998). Becoming a primary care nurse practitioner: Challenges of the initial year of practice. *The Nurse Practitioner, 23*(7), 46, 52-66.

Brown, S.J. (1992). Tailoring nursing care to the individual client: Empirical challenge of a theoretical concept. *Research in Nursing and Health, 15,* 39-46.

Brykczynski, K.A. (1985). Exploring the clinical practice of nurse practitioners. *Dissertation Abstracts International, 46,* 3789B. (University Microfilms No. DA8600592)

Brykczynski, K.A. (1991). Judgment strategies for coping with ambiguous clinical situations encountered in family primary care. *Journal of the Academy of Nurse Practitioners, 3,* 79-84.

Brykczynski, K.A. (1996). Role development of the advanced practice nurse. In A.B. Hamric, J.A. Spross, & C.M. Hanson (Eds.), *Advanced nursing practice: An integrative approach* (pp. 89-95). Philadelphia: Saunders.

Brykczynski, K.A. (1997). Holism: A foundation for healing wounds of divisiveness among nurses. In P.B. Kritek (Ed.), *Reflections on healing. A central nursing construct* (pp. 234-241). New York: National League for Nursing.

Brykczynski, K.A. (1999). An interpretive study describing the clinical judgment of nurse practitioners. *Scholarly Inquiry for Nursing Practice: An International Journal, 13,* 141-166.

Burglehaus, M. (1997). Physicians and breastfeeding: Beliefs, knowledge, self-efficacy and counseling practices. *Canadian Journal of Public Health, 88,* 383-387.

Callahan, L., & Bruton-Maree, N. (1994). Establishing measures of competence. In S.D. Foster & L.M. Jordan (Eds.), *Professional aspects of nurse anesthesia practice* (pp. 275-290). Philadelphia: FA Davis.

Chase, L.K., Johnson, S.K., Laffoon, T.A., Jacobs, R.S., & Johnson, M.E. (1996). CNS role: An experience in retitling and role clarification. *Clinical Nurse Specialist, 10,* 41-45.

Clance, P., & Imes, S. (1978). The imposter phenomenon in high achieving women: Dynamics and therapeutic intervention. *Psychotherapy: Theory, Research and Practice, 15,* 241-247.

Clark, N., & Dodge, J. (1999). Exploring self-efficacy as a predictor of disease management. *Health Education & Behavior, 26,* 72-89.

Cohen, H.A. (1981). *The nurse's quest for a professional identity.* Menlo Park, CA: Addison-Wesley.

Cooper, D.M., & Sparacino, P.S.A. (1990). Acquiring, implementing, and evaluating the clinical nurse specialist role. In P.S.A. Sparacino, D.M. Cooper, & P.A. Minarik (Eds.), *The clinical nurse specialist: Implementation and impact* (pp. 41-75). Norwalk, CT: Appleton & Lange.

Curry, J.L. (1994). Nurse practitioners in the emergency department: Current issues. *Journal of Emergency Nursing, 20,* 207-215.

Cusson, R.M., & Viggiano, N.M. (2002). Transition to the neonatal nurse practitioner role: Making the change from the side to the head of the bed. *Neonatal Network: NN, 21,* 21-28.

Dalton, J., & Blau, W. (1996). Changing the practice of pain management: An examination of the theoretical basis of change. *Pain Forum, 5,* 266-272.

Davis, K., Schoenbaum, S.C., & Audet, A. (2005). A 2020 vision of patient-centered primary care. *Journal of General Internal Medicine, 20,* 953-957.

DeMaio, D. (1979). The born-again nurse. *Nursing Outlook, 27*(4), 272-273.

Dionne-Proulz, J., & Pepin, R. (1993). Stress management in the nursing profession. *Journal of Nursing Management, 1,* 75-81.

Dreyfus, H.L., & Dreyfus, S.E. (1986). *Mind over machine: The power of human intuition and expertise in the era of the computer.* New York: Free Press.

Dreyfus, H.L., & Dreyfus, S.E. (1996). The relationship of theory and practice in the acquisition of skill. In P. Benner, C.A. Tanner, & C.A. Chesla, *Expertise in nursing practice: Caring, clinical judgment and ethics* (pp. 29-47). New York: Springer-Verlag.

Fagin, C.M. (1992). Collaboration between nurses and physicians no longer a choice. *Nursing & Health Care, 13,* 354-363.

Farrell, G.A. (2001). From tall poppies to squashed weeds: Why don't nurses pull together more? *Journal of Advanced Nursing, 35,* 26-33.

Fawcett, J., Newman, D.M.L., & McAllister, M. (2004). Advanced practice nursing and conceptual models of nursing. *Nursing Science Quarterly, 17*(2), 135-138.

Federwisch, A. (1999). CRNA autonomy: Nurse anesthetists fight latest skirmish. *Nursing & Allied Health Week (Greater Dallas/Fort Worth edition), 4,* 16.

Ford, L.C. (1979). A nurse for all settings: The nurse practitioner. *Nursing Outlook, 27,* 516-521.

Ford, L.C. (1982). Nurse practitioners: History of a new idea and predictions for the future. In L.H. Aiken (Ed.), *Nursing in the 1980s: Crises, opportunities, challenges* (pp. 231-247). Philadelphia: Lippincott.

Freshwater, D. (2000). Crosscurrents: Against cultural narration in nursing. *Journal of Advanced Nursing, 32,* 481-484.

Grando, V.T. (1998). Articulating nursing for advanced practice nursing. In T.J. Sullivan (Ed.). *Collaboration: A health care imperative* (pp. 499-514). New York: McGraw-Hill.

Gunn, I.P. (1991). The history of nurse anesthesia education: Highlights and influences. Report of the National Commission on Nurse Anesthesia Education. *Journal of the American Association of Nurse Anesthetists, 59,* 53-61.

Gunn, I.P. (1998). Setting the record straight on nurse anesthesia and medical anesthesiology education. *CRNA: The Clinical Forum for Nurse Anesthetists, 9,* 163-171.

Hamric, A.B. (2003). Defining our practice: A personal perspective (Letter to the editor). *Clinical Nurse Specialist, 17*(2), 75-76.

Hamric, A.B., & Hanson, C.M. (2003). Educating advanced practice nurses for practice reality. *Journal of Professional Nursing, 19,* 262-268.

Hamric, A.B., & Taylor, J.W. (1989). Role development of the CNS. In A.B. Hamric & J. Spross (Eds.), *The clinical nurse specialist in theory and practice* (2nd ed., pp. 41-82). Philadelphia: Saunders.

Hardy, M.E., & Hardy, W.L. (1988). Role stress and role strain. In M.E. Hardy & M.E. Conway (Eds.), *Role theory: Perspectives for health professionals* (2nd ed., pp. 159-239). Norwalk, CT: Appleton & Lange

Harvey, J., & Katz, C. (1985). *If I'm so successful, why do I feel like a fake? The imposter phenomenon.* New York: St Martin's Press.

Hayes, E. (1998). Mentoring and nurse practitioner student self-efficacy. *Western Journal of Nursing Research, 20,* 521-525.

Hayes, E. (2005). Mentoring research in the NP preceptor/student relationship. In L. Rauckhorst (Ed.), *Mentoring: Ensuring the future of NP practice and education.* Washington, DC: National Organization of Nurse Practitioner Faculties.

Hayes, E.F. (2001). Factors that facilitate or hinder mentoring in the nurse practitioner preceptor/student relationship. *Clinical Excellence for Nurse Practitioners, 5,* 111-118.

Heitz, L.J., Steiner, S.H., & Burman, M.E. (2004). RN to FNP: A qualitative study of role transition. *Journal of Nursing Education, 43*(9), 416-420.

Horvath, K.J., Secatore, J.A., Alpert, H.B., Costa, M.J., Powers, E.M., Stengrevics, S.S., et al. (1994). Uncovering the knowledge embedded in clinical nurse manager practice. *Journal of Nursing Administration, 24,* 39-44.

Huffstutler, S.Y., & Varnell, G. (2006). The imposter phenomenon in new nurse practitioner graduates. *Topics in Advanced Practice Nursing eJournal, 6*(2).

Hunter, L.P., Bormann, J.E., & Lops, V.R. (1996). Student to nurse-midwife role transition process: Smoothing the way. *Journal of Nurse-Midwifery, 41,* 328-333.

Hupcey, J.E. (1990). The socialization process of master's level nurse practitioner students. *Journal of Nursing Education, 29,* 196-201.

Hupcey, J.E. (1993). Factors and work settings that may influence nurse practitioner practice. *Nursing Outlook, 41,* 181-185.

Ingersoll, G.L., McIntosh, E., & Williams, M. (2000). Nurse-sensitive outcomes of advanced practice. *Journal of Advanced Practice, 32,* 1272-1281.

Institute of Medicine (IOM). (2003). *Health professions education: A bridge to quality.* Washington, DC: National Academies Press.

Johnson, R. (1993). Nurse practitioner-patient discourse: Uncovering the voice of nursing in primary care practice. *Scholarly Inquiry for Nursing Practice: An International Journal, 7,* 143-157.

Kelly, N.R., & Mathews, M. (2001). The transition to first position as nurse practitioner. *Journal of Nursing Education, 40,* 156-162.

Kimbro, C.D. (1978). The relationship between nurses and nurse-midwives. *Journal of Nurse-Midwifery, 22,* 28-31.

Kinsley, M. (2005). You've come a long way! *Nursing Spectrum (New York/New Jersey), 17*(20), 4-5.

Klaich, K. (1990). Transitions in professional identity of nurses enrolled in graduate educational programs. *Holistic Nursing Practice, 4,* 17-24.

Kleinpell, R. (2001). Nurse anesthetists hold fast under physicians' blast of supervision ruling. *The Nursing Spectrum, 11,* 26-27.

Kleinpell-Nowell, R. (1999). Longitudinal survey of acute care nurse practitioner practice: Year 1. *AACN Clinical Issues, 10,* 515-520.

Kleinpell-Nowell, R. (2001). Longitudinal survey of acute care nurse practitioner practice: Year 2. *AACN Clinical Issues, 12,* 447-452.

Kramer, M. (1974). *Reality shock.* St. Louis: Mosby.

Leininger, M.M. (1994). The tribes of nursing in the United States. *Journal of Transcultural Nursing, 6,* 18-22.

Levy, J. (1968). The maternal and infant mortality in midwifery practice in Newark, NJ. *American Journal of Obstetrics and Gynecology, 77,* 42.

Long, W.N., & Sharp, E.S. (1982). Relationships between professions: From the viewpoint of the physician and nurse-midwife in a tertiary center. *Journal of Nurse Midwifery, 27,* 14-24.

Lurie, E.E. (1981). Nurse practitioners: Issues in professional socialization. *Journal of Health and Social Behavior, 22,* 31-48.

McFadden, E.A., & Miller, M.A. (1994). Clinical nurse specialist practice: Facilitators and barriers. *Clinical Nurse Specialist, 8,* 27-33.

McKenna, B.G., Smith, N.A., Poole, S.J., & Coverdale, J.H. (2003). Horizontal violence: Experiences of registered nurses in their first year of practice. *Journal of Advanced Nursing, 42,* 90-96.

McMyler, E.T., & Miller, D.J. (1997). Two graduating master's students struggle to find meaning. *Clinical Nurse Specialist, 11,* 169-173.

Mundinger, M.O. (2005). Who's who in nursing: Bringing clarity to the Doctor of Nursing Practice. *Nursing Outlook, 53,* 173-176.

Murphy-Ende, K. (2002). Advanced practice nursing: Reflections on the past, issues for the future. *Oncology Nursing Forum, 29,* 106-112.

National Association of Clinical Nurse Specialists (NACNS). (1998). *Statement on clinical nurse specialists practice and education.* Harrisburg, PA: Author.

National Commission on Nurse Anesthesia Education. (1990). Summary of Commission findings: Issues and review of supporting documents. *Journal of the American Association of Nurse Anesthetists, 58,* 394-398.

Neale, J. (1999). Nurse practitioners and physicians: A collaborative practice. *Clinical Nurse Specialist, 13,* 252-258.

Oda, D. (1977). Specialized role development: A three-phase process. *Nursing Outlook, 25,* 374-377.

O'Neil, E.H., & the Pew Health Profession Commission. (December 1998). *Re-creating health professional practice for a new century: The fourth Report of the Pew Health Professions Commission.* San Francisco, CA: Pew Health Professions Commission.

Ormond, C., & Kish, C.P. (2001). Role acquisition. In D. Robinson & C.P. Kish (Eds.), *Core concepts in advanced practice nursing* (pp. 269-285). St. Louis: Mosby.

O'Sullivan, A.L., Carter, M., Marion, L., Pohl, J.M., & Werner, K.E. (2005). Moving forward together: The practice doctorate in nursing. *Online Journal of Issues in Nursing, 10*(3), Manuscript 4. Retrieved October 28, 2007, from www.medscape.com/viewarticle/514546_1.

Page, N.E., & Arena, D.M. (1991). Practical strategies for CNS role implementation. *Clinical Nurse Specialist, 5,* 43-48.

Parle, M., Maguire, P., & Heaven, C. (1997). The development of a training model to improve health professionals skills, self-efficacy, and outcome expectancies when communicating with cancer patients. *Social Science & Medicine, 44,* 231-240.

Payne, J.L., & Baumgartner, R.G. (1996). CNS role evolution. *Clinical Nurse Specialist, 10,* 46-48.

Peplau, H. (June 1997). *Keynote address.* Presented at International Congress of Nurses, Vancouver, British Columbia, Canada.

Quinn, R.E. (1996). *Deep change: Discovering the leader within.* San Francisco: Jossey-Bass.

Rashotte, J. (2005). Knowing the nurse practitioner: Dominant discourses shaping our horizons. *Nursing Philosophy, 6,* 51-62.

Redekopp, M.A. (1997). Clinical nurse specialist role confusion: The need for identity. *Clinical Nurse Specialist, 11,* 87-91.

Rich, E.R. (2005). Does RN experience relate to NP clinical skills? *The Nurse Practitioner, 30*(12), 53-56.

Rich, E.R., & Rodriquez, L. (2002). A qualitative study of perceptions regarding the non-nurse college graduate nurse practitioner. *The Journal of the New York State Nurses' Association, 33*(2), 31-35.

Roberts, J. (2001). Revised "Joint Statement" clarifies relationships between midwives and physician collaborators. *Journal of Midwifery & Women's Health, 46,* 269-271.

Roberts, S.J. (1983). Oppressed group behavior: Implications for nursing. *Advances in Nursing Science, 5,* 21-30.

Roberts, S.J. (1996). Breaking the cycle of oppression: Lessons for nurse practitioners? *Journal of the Academy of Nurse Practitioners, 8*(5), 209-214.

Roberts, S.J., Tabloski, P., & Bova, C. (1997). Epigenesis of the nurse practitioner role revisited. *Journal of Nursing Education, 36,* 67-73.

Rooks, J.P. (1983). The context of nurse midwifery in the 1980s: Our relationships with medicine, nursing, lay-midwives, consumers and health care economists. *Journal of Nurse-Midwifery, 26,* 3-8.

Rooks, J.P. (1999). The midwifery model of care. *Journal of Nurse Midwifery, 44,* 370-374.

Rooks, J.P., & Haas, J.E. (Eds.). (1986). *Nurse midwifery in America.* Washington, DC: American College of Nurse-Midwives Foundation.

Rosenfeld, P. (2001). Acute care nurse practitioners: Standard in ambulatory care, they're also useful in hospitals. *American Journal of Nursing, 101*(5), 61-62.

Rounds, L.R. (1997). The nurse practitioner: A healing role for the nurse. In P.B. Kritek (Ed.), *Reflections on healing: A central nursing construct* (pp. 209-223). New York: National League for Nursing.

Russell, D., VorderBruegge, M., & Burns, S.M. (2002). Effect of an outcomes-managed approach to care of neuroscience patients by acute care nurse practitioners. *American Journal of Critical Care, 11,* 353-364.

Ryden, M.B., Snyder, M., Gross, C.R., Savik, K., Pearson, V., Krichbaum, K., et al. (2000). Value-added outcomes: The use of advanced practice nurses in long-term care facilities. *The Gerontologist, 40,* 654-662.

Safriet, B.J. (1992). Health care dollars and regulatory sense: The role of advanced practice nursing. *Yale Journal on Regulation, 9,* 417-488.

Schumacher, K.L., & Meleis, A.I. (1994). Transitions: A central concept in nursing. *Image: The Journal of Nursing Scholarship, 26,* 119-127.

Sechrist, K.R., & Berlin, L.E. (1998). Role of the clinical nurse specialist: An integrative review of the literature. *AACN Clinical Issues, 9,* 306-324.

Stahl, M.A., & Myers, J. (2002). The advanced practice nursing role with multisite responsibilities. *Critical Care Nursing Clinics of North America, 14,* 299-305.

Stein, T. (2000). Struggling for autonomy: Dispute between CRNAs and anesthesiologists continues. *Nurseweek (California Statewide Edition), 13,* 31.

Stuart, D., & Oshio, S. (2002). Primary care in nurse-midwifery practice: A national survey. *Journal of Midwifery & Women's Health, 47,* 104-109.

Thomas, S.P. (2003). "Horizontal Hostility," Nurses against themselves: How to resolve this threat to retention. *American Journal of Nursing, 103*(10), 87-91.

Varney, H. (1987). *Nurse-midwifery* (2nd ed.). Boston: Blackwell Scientific.

Waters, R. (March 2007). Scope of practice legislative fights expected to return in 2007. *JNP The Journal for Nurse Practitioners, 3*(3), 195.

Watson, J. (1995). Advanced nursing practice . . . and what might be. *N & HC Perspectives on Community, 16,* 78-83.

Waugaman, W.R., & Lu, J. (1999). From nurse to nurse anesthetist: The relationship of culture, race, and ethnicity to professional socialization and career commitment of advanced practice nurses. *Journal of Transcultural Nursing, 10,* 237-247.

PART II

Competencies of Advanced Practice Nursing

Direct Clinical Practice

Mary Fran Tracy

INTRODUCTION

Direct care is the central competency of advanced practice nursing. This competency informs and shapes the execution of the other six competencies. Direct care is essential for a number of reasons. To consult, collaborate, and lead clinical staff and programs effectively, an APN must have clinical credibility. With the deep clinical and systems understanding that APNs possess, they facilitate the care processes that ensure achievement of outcomes for individuals and groups of patients. Advanced practice occurs within a health care system that is constantly changing— changing delivery models, reimbursement structures, regulatory requirements, population-based management, and even proposed changes in the basic educational requirements for advanced practice nurses through the Doctor of Nursing Practice (DNP) degree. The challenge many APNs face is how to maintain the characteristics of care that have helped patients achieve positive health outcomes and afforded APN care a unique niche in the health care marketplace. Characteristics such as use of a holistic perspective and the formation of therapeutic partnerships with patients to co-produce individualized health care are challenged by management approaches and cost-containment strategies that emphasize standardization of care to achieve population-based outcome targets. Conversely, characteristics of APN care such as health promotion, fostering self-care, and patient education are valued by these managed care programs because they result in appropriate use of health care system resources and sustain quality.

This chapter describes the direct clinical practice of APNs and helps readers understand how it differs from the practice of experts-by-experience, describes strategies for balancing direct care with other competencies, and describes strategies for retaining a direct care focus. The six characteristics of APN practice are identified. In addition, implications of the DNP as it relates to this core competency are discussed.

DIRECT CARE ACTIVITIES

Direct Care and Indirect Care

Direct care is the central APN competency (see Chapter 3). The APN is using advanced clinical judgment, systems thinking, and accountability in providing evidence-based care at a more advanced level than the care provided by the expert registered nurse. The APN is prepared to facilitate individuals through complex health care situations by use of education, counseling, and coordination of care (American Association of Colleges of Nursing [AACN], 2006). Although an expert registered nurse may, at times, demonstrate components of care that are at an advanced level, it is care that is gained through experience and is exemplary (not expected) at that level. Essentials I and II of practice doctorate education for APNs delineates that APN-level care is demonstrated through advanced, refined assessment skills and implementing and evaluating practice interventions based on integrated knowledge from multiple sciences such as biophysical, psychosocial, behavioral, cultural, economic, and nursing science (AACN, 2006). Graduate-level APN education provides a foundation for the evolution of practice over time as necessitated by health care and patients. This advanced level of practice is an expected competency of all APNs, not an exemplary skill that is intermittently or inconsistently displayed by staff or expert nurses.

For the purposes of this chapter, the terms *direct care* and *direct clinical practice* refer to the activities and functions APNs perform within the patient-nurse interface (Brown, 2005). Depending on the focus of an APN's practice, the patient may, and often does, include family members/significant others. The activities that occur in this interface or as direct follow-up to what occurred there are unique because they are interpersonally and physically co-enacted with a particular patient for the purpose of promoting that patient's health or well-being. Many

Box 5-1   EXAMPLES OF ADVANCED PRACTICE NURSE INDIRECT CARE ACTIVITIES

- Consultation with other health care providers (physicians, nurses, pharmacists)
- Writing prescriptions and orders
- Discharge planning
- Care coordination
- Communication with managed care and insurance organizations
- Guidance of bedside nurses
- Unit rounds
- Researching care guidelines

important processes transpire at this point of care including the following:

- The patient-provider therapeutic partnership is established.
- Health problems become mutually understood through information gathering and effective communication.
- Health, recovery, or palliative goals are expressed by the patient.
- Management and treatment options are explored.
- Physical acts of diagnosis, monitoring, treatment, and therapy are performed.
- Education, support, coaching, counseling, and comfort are provided.
- Decisions regarding future actions to be taken by each party are made.
- Future contact is planned.

Advanced practice nursing activities occurring before and adjacent to the patient-nurse interface have a great influence on the direct care that occurs in the interface; however, either they are not performed with an individual patient or their main purpose is tangential to the direct care of the patient. Activities such as collaboration, consultation, and mentoring of staff may all be occurring in relation to the direct care interface. It is often difficult to separate out these indirect care interventions that are equally necessary for adequate fulfillment of the APN role and care of the patient (Box 5-1). For instance, when an APN consults with another provider regarding the nature of a patient's condition or the care that should be recommended to a patient, the APN is engaging in advanced clinical practice but it is not direct care. Even though there may be direct contact with the patient during the consultation and the APN is accountable for the consultation, the primary purpose of that contact is to acquire information and understanding to use in formulating recommendations for the patient's direct care provider (see Chapter 7). Thus according to the definition of direct care used in this chapter, the APN is engaged in

clinical practice but he or she is not providing direct care to the patient. The direct care role of the clinical nurse specialist (CNS) may not be as apparent to observers as it is for nurse practitioners (NPs), certified registered nurse anesthetists (CRNAs), and certified nurse-midwives (CNMs) because the CNS frequently shifts from direct to indirect activities depending on the situation and the providers involved (Exemplar 5-1). For CNSs, these shifts may occur within one patient encounter and certainly across a day. Most APNs will have a role in ensuring that others are providing quality and safe care through indirect practice.

APN roles tend to diverge when comparing the amount of time spent in each of the direct care activities (Lincoln, 2000; Scott, 1999; Verger, Marcoux, Madden, Bojko, & Barnsteiner 2005). For example, more than 72% of CNSs reported performing patient and family education, counseling, and psychosocial assessments daily, with 24% to 37% performing physical care and physical examinations and ordering laboratory tests and medications daily. By contrast, more than 84% of NP respondents reported performing these activities on a daily basis (Lincoln, 2000). Other studies support the fact that NPs and CNMs are spending the majority of their time in direct care with patients (Holland & Holland, 2007; McCloskey, Grey, Deshefy-Longhi, & Grey, 2003; Rosenfeld, McEvoy, & Glassman 2003; Swartz et al., 2003).

This delineation of direct and indirect practice is not intended to denigrate clinical activities that occur outside the patient-nurse interface—quite the contrary. These clinical activities and functions should be recognized as influencing what happens in the interface and as having a significant impact on patient outcomes. Because these other clinical activities so significantly affect patient outcomes, they should be valued by the nursing community and by health care systems. In the current environment of cost containment and technological development, all activities that enhance patients' health, recovery, and adjustment are critical components of care delivered by APNs. Ball

EXEMPLAR 5-1   **Examples of Direct Care and Indirect Care Provided by Advanced Practice Nurses**

DIRECT CARE EXAMPLE

The medical intensive care unit (MICU) acute care nurse practitioner (ACNP) was called into a patient's room by a novice staff nurse. On quick visual assessment of the patient and room and a verbal update by the nurse, the ACNP ascertained that this was a 65-year-old male with acute respiratory distress syndrome who was intubated and on a ventilator with FiO_2 at 60%. Current SaO_2 reading was 84%, blood pressure was 88/60 and dropping, and heart rate was 110 beats per minute. The patient was sedated, and his skin was pale. The alarm on the ventilator was sounding with high peak inspiratory pressures. The staff nurse appeared anxious and stated she had been unable to determine why the alarm was sounding. When the nurse noticed that that the patient's status was deteriorating, she called for the ACNP to help.

Recognizing that it was not an appropriate time to talk the staff nurse through troubleshooting the ventilator, the ACNP assumed responsibility for the nursing interventions by increasing the FiO_2 on the ventilator and hyperventilating the patient. However, she explained each action she was taking to the staff nurse. The ACNP suctioned the patient and removed a large mucus plug. The patient's color slowly returned to pink, the blood pressure started to increase, the heart rate started to decrease, and the SaO_2 rose to 92%.

After ensuring the patient was stable and the ventilator was functioning and returning the ventilator to the original settings, the ACNP reviewed the situation with the staff nurse. She reviewed each step, describing indicators and appropriate actions to take, and answered the staff nurse's questions. In this case, the ACNP assumed direct care activities for the patient to address an urgent situation.

INDIRECT CARE EXAMPLE

The MICU clinical nurse specialist (CNS) was approached by an experienced staff nurse who was struggling to develop an interpersonal relationship with the family of a complex critically ill patient. The family was very anxious and was having difficulty synthesizing the information the staff nurse was trying to provide them.

Rather than intervene directly with the family, the CNS recognized that this would be a good opportunity for the staff nurse to develop and expand her skills at interpersonal relationship building. The CNS explored with the nurse the interventions she had already attempted and reviewed with her the literature regarding family stressors in critical care, family needs, and the goal of assessing and addressing what the family perceives as their educational and care needs. Armed with the information, the nurse felt comfortable in working with family to assess their priority educational and psychosocial needs to obtain the resources and information they needed.

The CNS could have intervened by establishing a direct relationship with the family, which would have been providing direct care. In this instance, however, she determined it was more important to assist the staff nurse in development of the relationship as a growth opportunity and to form an ongoing partnership with family with whom she would be interacting on a continuing basis.

and Cox (2003), based on a study of CNSs and NPs (see Chapters 2 and 6), found that APNs engaged in a range of "strategic activities," an excellent characterization of the direct and indirect but "adjacent" actions that make up the clinical practice of APNs.

Researchers are beginning to understand the specific activities that constitute the direct care component of various advanced practice nursing roles. However, it is difficult to make generalizations about these activities because the APNs studied had different roles and worked in different settings with different populations. Different classification schemas were used to categorize APN actions. For instance, in some studies, investigators used the term *activities* to classify APN

actions; in others, the term *interventions* was used. The variability in terminology and definitions makes it difficult to compare results across APN roles, settings, and populations. Nevertheless, a review of these studies yields some insights into the extent and nature of direct care activities in APN roles.

Many direct care activities performed are similar across APN roles and include physical examinations and assessments, patient and family education and counseling, ordering laboratory tests and medications, and performing procedures (Lincoln, 2000; Scott, 1999; Verger et al., 2005). Verger and colleagues (2005) surveyed pediatric critical care NPs regarding their direct care activities, which included physical assessments, patient and family teaching, and performing such procedures as venipuncture, IV insertions, lumbar punctures, feeding tube placements, endotracheal intubations, and central line placements. CNMs reported expansion of their direct care procedures to include first-assisting during cesarean sections and performing endometrial biopsies (Holland & Holland, 2007).

Regardless of population being cared for, surveillance was a key direct care activity of APNs identified in two studies (Brooten, Youngblut, Deatrick, Naylor, & York, 2003; Hughes et al., 2002). Surveillance was described in the areas of watching for physical and emotional signs and symptoms and monitoring dressing and wound care, laboratory results, medications, nutrition, and caretaking/parenting. Thus surveillance refers to an APN's vigilant assessment of patient status, the rapid identification and diagnosis of subtle or emergent conditions; and quick intervention to prevent or reverse a potentially negative outcome. APNs in these studies also used extensive teaching, guidance, and counseling in many of the same areas in which they were using surveillance. The extent of surveillance and teaching may fluctuate depending on the phase of care and the particular population being cared for.

In summary, direct care activities make up a large part of what most APNs do, although there is considerable variation in what activities are performed and how much time is devoted to the direct care function across roles, settings, and patient populations.

SIX CHARACTERISTICS OF DIRECT CLINICAL CARE PROVIDED BY ADVANCED PRACTICE NURSES

APNs function in many roles and settings and with different populations. Despite such variability in role implementation, there is a similarity in the components of direct care provided. Characteristics of advanced practice nursing care extend across advanced practice roles, health care settings, and populations of patients. These characteristics include the following:

- Use of a holistic perspective
- Formation of therapeutic partnerships with patients
- Expert clinical thinking and skillful performance
- Use of reflective practice
- Use of evidence as a guide to practice
- Use of diverse approaches to health and illness management

These characteristics are evident in the literature cited earlier. Moreover, there is accumulating research evidence supporting these features of APN practice as having positive influences on patient outcomes. Throughout this chapter, the empirical evidence cited regarding claims about APN practice is illustrative and not based on a systematic review of research. The research regarding outcomes of APN practice is addressed comprehensively in Chapter 24.

The six characteristics of advanced direct care practice have their roots in the traditional values of the nursing profession. These values are defined within nursing's social contract with society as outlined by the American Nurses Association (ANA) (American Nurses Association [ANA], 2003):

- Nurses view humans holistically, considering a patient's mind, body, and spirit
- Health and illness are experiences that are not mutually exclusive and have cultural and contextual aspects.
- The patient-nurse relationship involves mutual participation, which takes into account the values of both.
- Health care systems and policies impact both society and nursing.

Nurses in advanced practice roles often have a deep commitment to the values on which these characteristics rest and are able to persuasively advocate and incorporate these values in daily practice. The expanded scope of practice of APN roles often enables APNs to fully enact these characteristics in their daily interactions with patients. An overview of strategies for enacting these characteristics is provided in Box 5-2.

USE OF A HOLISTIC PERSPECTIVE

Holism Described

Holism has a variety of meanings. A broad view is that holism involves a deep understanding of each patient as a complex and unique person who is embedded in a temporally unfolding life. The holistic perspective recognizes the multiple dimensions of each person—biological, psychological, social, and spiritual—and that the relationships among these dimensions result in a whole that is greater than the sum of the parts. The broad perspective also recognizes that the individual is "a unitary whole in mutual process with the environment"(American Holistic Nurses Association, 2007). This comprehensive and integrated view of human life and health is enacted in the health care encounter as attention to the full

Box 5-2   CHARACTERISTICS OF ADVANCED DIRECT CARE PRACTICE AND STRATEGIES
             FOR ENACTING THEM

USE OF A HOLISTIC PERSPECTIVE
Take into account the complexity of human life.
Recognize and address how social, organizational,
   and physical environments affect people.
Consider the profound effects of illness, aging,
   hospitalization, and stress.
Consider how symptoms, illness, and treatment
   affect quality of life.
Focus on functional abilities and requirements.

**FORMATION OF THERAPEUTIC PARTNERSHIPS
WITH PATIENTS**
Use a conversational style to conduct health care
   encounters.
Encourage the patient to actively participate in
   decision making.
Look for potential cultural influences on health
   care discourse.
Listen to the indirect voices of patients who are
   noncommunicative.
Advocate the patient's perspective and concerns
   to others.

**EXPERT CLINICAL REASONING AND SKILLFUL
PERFORMANCE**
Acquire specialized knowledge and know-how.
Seek out supervision when performing a new skill.
Invest in deeply understanding the patient situations
   in which you are involved.
Generate and test alternative lines of reasoning.
Trust your hunches—check them out.
Be aware of when you are time pressured and
   likely to make thinking errors.
Consider multiple aspects of the patient's situation
   when you are deciding how to treat.
Make sure you know how to use technical
   equipment safely.
Make sure you know how to interpret data
   produced by monitoring devices.
Pay attention to how you move and touch patients
   during care.
Anticipate ethical conflicts.
Acquire computer-related skills for accessing and
   managing patient data and practice information.

USE OF REFLECTIVE PRACTICE
Explore your personal values, belief systems, and
   behaviors.
Identify your basic assumptions about health care,
   the APN role, and the rights and responsibilities
   of patients.
Consider how your assumptions impact your
   judgments.
Talk to colleagues and your teachers about your
   clinical experiences.
Consider use of a journal to document
   experiences.
Assess your current skill and comfort in reflection.

USE OF EVIDENCE AS A GUIDE TO PRACTICE
Learn how to search health care databases for
   studies related to specific clinical topics.
Read research reports related to your field of
   practice.
Seek out systematic revision of research and
   research-based clinical guidelines.
Acquire skills in appraising the various forms
   of evidence.
Work with colleagues to consider research-based
   improvements in care.

**DIVERSE APPROACHES TO HEALTH AND ILLNESS
MANAGEMENT**
Use interpersonal interventions to influence pa-
   tients.
Acquire proficiency in new ways of treating and
   helping patients.
Help patients maintain health and capitalize on
   their strengths and resources.
Provide preventive services appropriate to your
   field of practice.
Know what is allowed under managed care con-
   tracts.
Negotiate with managed care case managers for
   noncovered services when necessary.
Coordinate services among care sites and multiple
   providers.
Acquire knowledge about complementary and alternative therapies.

range of factors influencing patients' experiences (Box 5-3). Incorporation of holism into care results in new pathways of the patient's story, movement into the healing domain, and optimal use of holistic nursing that promotes healing across the entire life span (Dossey, 2001).

Another view is that holism incorporates several perspectives including the following (Newman, 1997; Waite, Harker, & Messerman, 1994):
- Viewing the patient as an integral part of larger social, physical, and energy environments

Box 5-3   Factors to Consider When Helping the Patient Holistically

- The patient's view of his or her health or illness
- Patterns of physical symptoms and amount of distress they cause
- The effect of physical symptoms on the patient's daily functioning and quality of life
- Symptom management approaches that are acceptable to the patient
- Life changes that could affect the patient's physical or psychological well-being (e.g., relationship breakup, job change, intrafamily conflict, retirement, death of a beloved person)
- The context of the patient's life, including the nuclear family unit, social support, job responsibilities, financial situation, health insurance coverage, responsibilities for the care of others (e.g., children, chronically ill spouse or partner, older parents)
- Spiritual and life values (e.g., independence, religion, beliefs about life, acceptance of fate)

- Assuming that the mind, body, and spirit are closely related, so that one dimension should not be considered in isolation from the others
- Focusing on the meanings patients assign to health, illness experiences, and health care choices
- Viewing patients' current behaviors and responses as consistent with their life span patterns of response and choice

Clearly, high-tech care environments with many health care providers, each focused on a particular aspect of a patient's condition and treatment, require designated coordinators who have a comprehensive and integrated appreciation of the patient and his or her experience of care as a whole. APNs' capacity to "keep the pieces together" and promote continuity of care in a way that focuses care on the unique individual is undoubtedly why many clinical programs have an APN member or coordinator (see "Management of Complex Situations" on p. 147). In an ethnographic study of one high-tech environment, neonatal intensive care units, APNs were found to emphasize holism, caring, and health (Beal, 2000). The Shuler Nurse Practitioner Practice Model is based on a holistic understanding of human health and illness in older adults that integrates medical and nursing perspectives (Shuler, Huebscher, & Hallock, 2001; see also pp. 54-58 in Chapter 2).

Holism and Health Assessment

When working with a relatively healthy person, the APN seeks to understand the person's life goals, functional interests, and health risks to preserve quality of life in the future. In contrast, when working with an ill patient, the APN is interested in what the person views as problems, how he or she is responding to problems, and what the problems and responses mean to the individual in terms of daily living and life goals. In a study of 199 primary care clinical situations (Burman, Stepans, Jansa, & Steiner, 2002), NPs were found to engage in holistic assessment and to ground their decision making within the context of the patient's life.

The ability to function in daily activities and relationships is an important consideration for patients when they evaluate their health, so it is an appropriate and essential focus for holistic, person-centered assessment. Most functional assessment formats focus on (1) how patients view their health or quality of life; (2) how they accomplish self-care and household or job responsibilities; (3) the social, physical, financial, environmental, and spiritual factors that augment or tax their functioning; and (4) the strategies they and their families use to cope with the stresses and problems in their lives.

In pediatrics, measures of functional status for children with asthma (American Academy of Pediatrics, 2007) and for children with chronic physical disorders (Stein & Jessop, 1990) have been developed. In adults, APNs may choose to use a *disease-* or *problem-focused* tool such as one that measures functional status in heart failure patients (Rector, Anand, & Cohn, 2006) or a widely used *general* measure such as the Short Form-36 Health Status Profile (SF-36), which measures overall health, functional status, and well-being in adults and is available in several languages (Ware & Sherbourne, 1992).

Nursing Model or Medical Model

As APNs take on responsibilities that formerly were in the purview of physicians, some have expressed concern that APNs are being asked to function within a medical model of practice rather than within a holistic nursing model. This concern is particularly

Box 5-4   NURSING-FOCUSED PRACTICE INTERVENTIONS

- Engagement of patients in their own care
- Patient education
- Care planning
- Physical and occupational therapy referrals
- Use of communication skills

- Promotion of continuity of care
- Teaching of nursing staff
- Advance directive discussions
- Wellness/health promotion model

raised when APNs substitute for physicians. However, evidence exists that a nursing orientation is an enduring component of APN practice, even when medical management is part of the role (Blasdell, Klunick, & Purseglove, 2002; Hoffman, Tasota, Scharfenberg, Zullo, & Donahoe, 2003; Hoffman, Happ, Scharfenberg, diVirgilio-Thomas, & Tasota, 2004; Lambing, Adams, Fox, & Divine, 2004; Sidani, et al., 2006) (Box 5-4). Activities described in these studies clearly reflect a nursing-focused practice.

Statements from professional organizations indicate that APNs value their nursing orientation and their medical functions. For instance, the description of APNs in the ANA's nursing social policy statement includes strong endorsement of both specialized and expanded knowledge and skills within the context of holistic values (ANA, 2003). On the theoretical front, several models of advanced practice blend nursing and medical orientations (see the Shuler Nurse Practitioner Practice Model, pp. 54-58, and the Dunphy-Winland models, p. 67, in Chapter 2).

FORMATION OF THERAPEUTIC PARTNERSHIPS WITH PATIENTS

The Institute of Medicine has recommended patient-centered care as the foundation of safe, effective, and efficient health care (Institute of Medicine [IOM], 2001). The person-centered, holistic perspective of APNs serves as the foundation for the types of relationships they co-create with patients. It is well known that APNs develop therapeutic partnerships by engaging in social story exchanges, expressing positive regard for patients, asking about patients' home lives, and helping patients plan how they can follow health and illness management recommendations (Brown, 1999; Courtney & Rice, 1997; Flesner & Clawson, 1998; Grando, 1998). APNs are well prepared to develop therapeutic relationships as the cornerstone of patient-centered care (see Chapter 6).

Development and maintenance of therapeutic relationships with patients and families is one of the key criteria in *The Essentials of Doctoral Education for*

Advanced Nursing Practice that is specific and foundational to advanced practice nursing (AACN, 2006). Research reveals that APNs form collaborative relationships with patients. Dontje, Corser, Kreulen, and Teitelman (2004) described the primary care environment as particularly conducive to developing sustained partnerships with patients. In a synthesis of the literature, a review of qualitative data, and reflection on their own clinical experiences, the authors identified the following as goals of therapeutic partnerships in primary care: self-management of care, promotion of shared decision making, and a holistic approach to care that promotes continuity. The authors posited that these characteristics of APN partnerships may contribute to high-quality care—through adoption of preventive care practices, improved patient satisfaction, appropriate utilization of resources, and overall better patient outcomes—although more research is needed in this area.

Shared Decision Making

In addition to eliciting information that increases understanding of the patient's illness experience, APNs, in the studies cited previously, encouraged patients to participate in decisions regarding how their diseases and illnesses should be managed. There is a continuum of patient involvement in making decisions for their own health care. At one end of the continuum are patients who want to be fully engaged in a partnership with providers in making decisions, whereas at the other end of the continuum are patients who want to rely on family members or care providers to make all treatment decisions. This may include patients who are older, who are sicker, and who have cultural beliefs that lead them to defer decisions to others. Regardless of where the patient falls on this continuum, it is still incumbent on the provider to establish a collaborative partnership to ensure that regardless of whom the patient wants to make decisions, it is done in congruence with the patient's beliefs and values.

APNs should individually determine each patient's preference for participation in decision making and be sensitive to the fact that patients' preferences may change over time as they get to know the provider better and as different kinds of health problems arise. Once the patient's preference has been elicited, the provider should tailor his or her communication and decision-making style to the patient's preference. Many patients have not had prior health care experiences in which shared decision making was even a possibility, but when offered the opportunity, many choose it— tentatively in some cases, enthusiastically in others. "Trying on" a more active role may require some help from the provider, such as explaining how it would work and which responsibilities are the patient's and which are the provider's. Providers can encourage patients to bring up issues by asking open-ended questions such as "So, how have you been?" and focused-but-open questions such as "So, how are things going at home?" Patients can be encouraged to participate in decision making by offering them explicit opportunities in the form of questions such as "Does one of those approaches sound better to you than the other?" Gradually, patients approached in this way will learn that health care encounters will be organized around their concerns, not around a series of questions asked by the provider, and that they should feel safe to express their concerns and preferences.

Open and honest communication is foundational to a shared decision-making philosophy. APNs have reported more advanced communication skills than those reported by basic RNs (Sivesind et al., 2003). The ability to adapt communication styles is a needed skill of APNs (Lawson, 2002; McCourt, 2006) and can result in patients who report that they have more knowledge and control of their own care.

APNs must be cognizant of their own personal beliefs and value systems in a partnership in which they are coaching patients in decision making. While they are uniquely prepared to facilitate the holistic management of the physical, psychosocial, and spiritual aspects of care in these particular situations, APNs may be involved in interactions in which it is difficult for them to help patients make decisions. If the APN is unconscious of or has unresolved issues of his or her own, he or she may risk exercising undue or unintentional influence on patients' decisions in emotionally charged situations (Bialk, 2004). Bringing one's own beliefs and values to consciousness prior to a discussion focused on patient decision making, reflecting on one's own cognitive and affective responses to such discussions, and debriefing with a colleague can help APNs maintain a therapeutic approach (or

determine when it is appropriate for another clinician to become involved).

Cultural Influences on Partnerships

Another important factor affecting whether and how persons want to participate in health care decision making is their cultural background. It is easy to forget that not all cultures value individual autonomy as much as North Americans of Anglo-Saxon ancestry do. Increasingly, recognizing and respecting the cultural identification of patients is being viewed as essential to building meaningful partnerships. Cultural groups form along lines of racial, national origin, religious, professional, organizational, sexual orientation, or age-group identification. Some cultural groups are easier to identify than others. Physical differences in appearance often tip off the provider to the fact that he or she is dealing with a person of a different cultural orientation. Other cultural identifications are less obvious—for example, people with religious beliefs about fate, God as healer, or treatment taboos. However, it is important to avoid making assumptions about cultural beliefs simply based on physical appearance or dress. In today's increasingly diverse society, many families have blended traditional beliefs and practices from multiple cultures.

The DNP *Essentials* identifies the need for APNs to synthesize and incorporate principles of cultural diversity into preventive and therapeutic interventions for individuals and populations (AACN, 2006). The preparation of APNs in the area of cultural competence and culturally appropriate care is key, since the demographics of nurses and APNs do not match the overall demographics of the United States population (McNeal & Walker, 2006; Ndiwane et al., 2004). Interactions that are complicated by cultural misunderstandings can result in incomplete or inaccurate assessments and even misdiagnosis and suboptimal outcomes (Barakzai, Gregory, & Fraser, 2007; Sobralske & Katz, 2005). The APN needs to individualize care based on an assessment of the cultural influences on both the perception of illness and reporting of symptoms. Otherwise, differences in perceptions can cause confusion, misunderstandings, and even conflicts that disrupt the patient-provider relationship and discourse. Moreover, they often complicate attempts to resolve misunderstandings because different cultural groups approach conflict negotiation differently. In every encounter, the provider should expect that the patient may have values that are different in some ways from his or her own and must make a special effort to ensure that the care being given meets the patient's needs and is acceptable to him or her.

Therapeutic Partnerships with Noncommunicative Patients

Some patients are not able to enter fully into partnership with APNs because they are too young, have compromised cognitive capacity, or are unconscious. Clinical populations who may be unable to participate fully in shared decision making are listed in Box 5-5. Unfortunately, staff nurses working with noncommunicative patients can become so focused in providing care that they forget about having meaningful interactions with the patient (Alasad & Ahmad, 2005). APNs can role model alternative forms of communication so noncommunicative patients can receive optimal care.

Although these patients may have limited ability to speak for themselves, they are not entirely without opinion or voice. Situations in which patients will experience temporary alterations in cognition or verbal ability can often be anticipated (e.g., during general anesthesia and during intubation), and the APN can discuss patients' preferences for handling possible events beforehand and elicit their wishes.

In the absence of this kind of prior dialogue, experts who work with patients who cannot verbalize their concerns and preferences learn to pay close attention to how patients are responding to what happens to them; facial expressions, body movement, and physiological parameters are used to ascertain what causes the patient discomfort and what helps alleviate it. In a study of persons who had experienced and recovered from unconsciousness (Lawrence, 1995), 27% of the patients reported being able to hear, understand, and respond emotionally while they were unconscious. These findings suggest that nurses should communicate with unconscious patients by providing them with interventions such as reassurance, bodily care, pain relief, explanations, and comforting touch. APNs should view these interactions as not merely one-way imparting of information but also providing key emotional support (Alasad & Ahmad, 2005; Geraghty, 2005).

There are tools that can be used for patients who are conscious but unable to communicate. Unfortunately, many nurses are not adequately educated in using alternative methods of communication and, if they are, may not be familiar or comfortable with the particular method required for an individual patient (Hemsley et al., 2001). Other barriers include having access to communication devices and time pressures that may not allow providers to adequately engage in a process that can take more time.

Alternative sources of information about patients who are unable to respond physically or to communicate should also be identified. For example, siblings visiting an adolescent male with a major head injury would be able to tell you what kind of music he likes to listen to and would probably even bring you a tape or CD to play for the patient. His mother would know what has caused him to have skin reactions in the past. Responding to his father's offhand comment that he cannot stand to be without his glasses when he is not wearing his contact lenses would most likely help both father and son. All of these are ways of building partnership with an unconscious teenager in an intensive care unit (ICU). In adults and adolescents, advance directives, heath care proxy documents, and organ donation cards are other sources of information regarding patients' wishes. Thus noncommunicative patients are not without voices, but hearing their voices does require presence, attentiveness, and relationship. Box 5-6 summarizes options for the APN in engaging with noncommunicative patients.

Box 5-5   PATIENT POPULATIONS UNABLE TO PARTICIPATE FULLY IN PARTNERSHIP

- Infants and preverbal children
- Anesthetized patients
- Unconscious/comatose patients
- People in severe pain
- Patients receiving medications that impair cognition
- People with dementia
- People with psychiatric conditions that seriously impair rational thought
- People with conditions that render them incapable of speech and conversation
- People with congenital or acquired cognitive limitations
- People whose primary language is different from the provider's

Box 5-6   Techniques for Communicating with Noncommunicative Patients

- Maintain verbal interactions with patient throughout care.
- Explain procedures and cares.
- Monitor tone of voice so you are not inadvertently relaying emotional subcontext to the actual words used.
- Use appropriate touch for reassurance.
- Use other communication devices such as alphabet and word boards, writing, computers, electronic communication devices.

- Consider use of interpreters for foreign languages and sign language.
- Use other sources of information for patient's likes and dislikes—family, primary care providers, friends.
- Use physiological cues as appropriate to evaluate patient responses to care and treatments—grimacing, frowning, turning away from touch, relaxing facial muscles, blood pressure and heart rate responses.

EXPERT CLINICAL THINKING AND SKILLFUL PERFORMANCE

Few studies clearly differentiate between the expert skills of the APN and the practice of the basic RN. An expert's clinical judgment is characterized by the ability to make fine distinctions among features of a particular condition that were not possible during beginning practice. Benner's studies of expert clinical judgment, though not with APN participants, inform this discussion of APNs' clinical expertise (1984). Tanner reviewed the literature regarding clinical judgment and found that it requires three main categories of knowledge (Tanner, 2006). The first is scientific and theoretical knowledge that is widely applicable. The second is knowledge based on experience that fills in gaps and assists in prompt identification of clinical issues. The final category is knowledge that is very individualized based on the interpersonal connection with the patient.

Knowledge

APNs' specialized knowledge accrues from a variety of sources including graduate and continuing education, clinical experience, professional reading, reflection, mentoring, and exchange of information and ideas with colleagues within and outside nursing. The integration of knowledge from these sources provides a foundation for the expert clinical thinking that is associated with advanced direct care practice. Once an APN has been in practice for a while, formalized knowledge and experiential knowledge become so mixed together that they may not be distinguishable to the outside observer. Illness trajectories and presentations of prior patients make an impression and come to mind when a patient with a similar problem is seen later (Benner, 1984). The expert also remembers what interventions worked and did not work in certain situations. Timetables of progress that most patients attain in certain situations (e.g., the time after surgery when patients' energy levels return) create expectations for patients who fit into that population (Benner, Tanner, & Chesla, 1996). Eventually, the expert's clinical knowledge consists of a complex network of memorable cases, prototypic images, research findings, thinking strategies, moral values, maxims, probabilities, behavioral responses, associations, illness trajectories and timetables, therapeutic information, and domain-relevant concepts. Thus experts have extensive, varied, and complex knowledge networks that can be activated to help them understand clinical situations and events. These networks comprise both internal resources and external resources. The APN may mentally review internal resources such as educational knowledge, typical cases, and previously experienced cases when confronted with a complex or challenging case. But the APN is also cognizant of when internal resources are no longer adequate and knows when to refer to external resources for consultation, more data, or guidance.

Clinical Thinking

Clinical reasoning brings together the clinical knowledge of the provider with specific observations, perceptions, events, and facts from the situation at hand to produce an understanding of what is occurring (O'Neill, 1995). Sometimes the understanding is arrived at by using cognitive processes to logically consider evidence and alternative explanations. At other times the insight or understanding "arrives" intuitively, that is, through direct apprehension without recourse to deliberate reasoning (Benner et al., 1996; Tanner, 2006). In these situations, APNs can use reflective practice to "sort" through the intuition to better understand the components and identify new insights. With experience, they are then able to repackage these insights and incorporate them into their experiential learning to prospectively and deliberately use the information in the next relevant case.

APN experts have the ability to rapidly scan a situation (e.g., past records, patient's appearance, and the patient's unexpressed concern or discomfort) and identify salient and relevant information. The APN is able to purposely suspend judgment about personal strongly held beliefs that may be proposed by others, such as "he's a difficult patient" or "she's just drug seeking." The ability to do this ensures as much objectivity as possible in caring for patients. For example, research has shown that expert CNSs are able to transcend the labeling of a "difficult patient" to problem resolution through use of patient respect, communication skills, and increased self-efficacy (Wolf & Robinson-Smith, 2007). Relying heavily on their perceptions, observations, and assessment skills, APNs quickly activate one or several lines of reasoning regarding what might be going on. They then conduct a more focused assessment to determine which one best explains the situation at hand. These lines of reasoning can be informal, personal theories about the specific patient situation; their formulation draws from personal knowledge of the particular patient, from personal knowledge acquired from previous experiences, and from formalized domain-specific knowledge (Tanner, 2006). In implementing the solutions, these lines of reasoning can be tested by performing a clinical intervention and noting how the patient responds. Throughout this process, the APN may be teaching and role modeling with staff to assist in staff nurse self-awareness and reflection. A novice APN may need to work through the situation in a very formal, logical way and be more deliberate about the use of formal educational knowledge, enriching it over time with experiential knowledge (Tanner, 2006).

It has been shown that the values and underlying knowledge a nurse brings to a situation also has a profound influence on his or her assessment of the patient. Results of one study demonstrated that a nurse's philosophy regarding aging could influence his or her assessment of acute confusion in older adults (McCarthy, 2003). Whether a nurse's attitude toward confusion comes from a perspective of decline, vulnerability, or healthfulness will greatly influence how the nurse intervenes on behalf of that patient (McCarthy, 2003). A nurse's moral opinion of drug addiction and interpretation of behavior as drug seeking may have more influence on the treatment of a patient's pain rather than the actual assessment of the pain.

Most patient accounts unfold in a fairly predictable way, and the APN arrives at a diagnosis and/or intervention with considerable confidence in his or her clinical inferences. At other times, however, there is uncertainty and lack of understanding regarding the situation. The uncertainty may pertain to information the patient provides, to the diagnosis, to the best approach to management, or to how the patient is responding (Brykczynski, 1991). When there is ambiguity, experts often break into conscious problem solving or "detective-like thinking and questioning" (Benner et al., 1996; Benner, Hooper-Kyriakidis, & Stannard, 1999) to try to figure out what is going on.

Knowing the patient may be critical to perceptive and accurate clinical reasoning. Knowing the patient as an individual with certain patterns of responses enables experienced nurses to detect subtle changes in a patient's condition over time (Tanner, 2006; Tanner, Benner, Chesla, & Gordon, 1993). The extent to which any nurse knows a patient may be associated with that nurse's ability to do the following:

- Recognize that risk factors are present
- Detect early indicators of a problem (i.e., a slight change in pattern)
- Take timely preventive action
- Recognize nonfitting and atypical data

Nonfitting data suggest to experts that they need to generate new or additional hypotheses because the current observations and parameters do not fully explain the clinical picture as it has been or as it should be. For example, when faced with a nonfitting sign or symptom, the nurse may generate alternative hypotheses pertaining to the onset of a complication or to the worsening of the disease process (Burman et al., 2002).

Thinking Errors

The clinical acumen of APNs and the inferences, hypotheses, and lines of reasoning they generate are highly dependable. However, as practice becomes repetitive, APNs may develop routine responses, and they then run the risk of making certain types of thinking errors (Schön, 1992). Errors of expectancy occur when the correct diagnosis is not generated as a hypothesis because a set of circumstances, in either the clinician's experience or the patient's circumstances, predisposes the clinician to disregard it. For example, the NP who over several years has seen an older woman for problems associated with chronic pulmonary disease may fail to consider that the most recent onset of shortness of breath and fatigue could be related to worsening aortic stenosis; the NP has come to expect pulmonary disease, not cardiac disease.

Erroneous conclusions are also more likely when the situation is ambiguous, that is, when the meaning or reliability of the data is unclear, the interpretation of the data is not clear-cut, the best approach to treatment is debatable, or one cannot say for sure whether the patient is responding well to treatment (Brykczynski, 1991). To avoid errors in these kinds of situations, experts often revert to the use of maxims to guide their thinking (Brykczynski, 1989). One of the maxims that NPs use to deal with uncertain diagnoses is "When you hear hoofbeats in Kansas, think horses, not zebras." This reminds clinicians who are about to make a diagnosis that occurs infrequently to consider the incidence of the condition in the population. Thus an older adult with respiratory problems seen in a suburban office is unlikely to have tuberculosis; pneumonia is a more likely diagnosis. Because tuberculosis is rare in the population of which the older adult is a member, the clinical data for tuberculosis should be quite convincing if that diagnosis is proposed.

Poor judgment can also result from tunnel vision; overgeneralization; influence by a recent, dramatic experience; premature closure (Croskerry, 2003); and fixation on certain problems to the exclusion of others (Benner et al., 1999). Faulty thinking is not the only source of error in clinical decision making. Other sources include inaccurate observations, misinterpretation of the meaning of data, a sketchy knowledge of the particular situation, and a faulty or outdated model of the disease, condition, or response.

It is important that APNs recognize the potential for and avoid leaping to conclusions and making snap judgments. It can become easy to allow biases to lead us to premature diagnoses without fully listening to or assessing patients (Paul & Heaslip, 1995). The expert APN has learned to constantly scan data and look for deviations. The ability to effectively differentiate between significant and insignificant data is needed to have safe practice (Paul & Heaslip, 1995). See Box 5-7 for actions that APNs can do to prevent thinking errors.

Time Pressures

Regardless of setting, practitioners worry about the effect time pressures have on the accuracy and completeness of their clinical thinking and decision making. The IOM's galvanizing report on errors and patient safety cited studies in which between 3% and 46% of hospitalized patients in the United States are harmed by error or negligence (IOM, 2000); the committee called for transformation and redesign of the health care system. The wide variation is the result of varying definitions of what constitutes adverse events and various methods of detecting their occurrence. A heavy workload is associated with feelings of pressure, being rushed, cognitive overload, and fatigue adding to already burdened clinicians; these feelings clearly contribute to unsafe acts and omissions in care (IOM, 2000). Evidence in support of this inference comes from studies of nurse staffing in hospitals in which fewer hours of nursing care per patient per day and less care provided by registered nurses were associated with poorer patient outcomes (Aiken, Clarke, Sloane, Sochalski, & Silber, 2002; Kovner, Jones, Zhan, Gergen, & Basu, 2002; Needleman, Buerhaus, Mattke, Steward, & Zelevinsky, 2002). Effectively addressing the issues of time pressures and insufficient hours of nursing care requires culture change, process redesign, and appropriate use of technology. The patient safety movement has led to a variety of efforts aimed at preventing errors: root cause analysis of sentinel

---

Box 5-7   ACTIONS TO USE TO AVOID THINKING ERRORS

- Listen fully to patients' concerns and descriptions of their problems.
- Listen to input from other providers as to their assessments and perspectives.
- Pay attention to intuition that points to an incongruence in data.
- Avoid reliance on knowledge derived solely from rote memorization or repetition, but

critically think through the source of knowing and how it relates to the individual patient.
- Remain constantly open to re-evaluation of working diagnoses and treatments.
- Be aware of personal biases and assumptions.
- Continually evaluate what is "critical" data in each patient case.

events, improved work processes, redesign of delivery systems, use of technological aids, communication training, human factors analysis, and team building. All of these factors can have significant direct and indirect effects on workload, fatigue, and time available for direct patient care.

The effects of a heavy workload on patient outcomes in nonhospital settings are less understood; thus actions to address this issue have received less attention. However, as lengths of visits or contact times are decreased or the number of patients practitioners are expected to see in a day is increased, it is logical to assume that the number of errors in clinical thinking will increase. Each contact requires the practitioner to "reset" his or her clinical reasoning process by closing out one thinking project and starting on an entirely new one. This resetting, which is done back-to-back many times during a day, is cognitively and physically demanding. How these performance expectations affect clinical reasoning accuracy is unknown.

Moreover, time pressures often get compounded by hassles. Hassles come in the form of interruptions, noise in the environment, missing supplies, and system glitches that make clinical data or even whole charts unavailable to providers. These hassles likely interfere with providers' ability to concentrate on what the patient is saying and disrupt their efforts to make clinical sense of patients' accounts. In many settings, providers are required to multitask. They start a task but must attend to another task before completing the original one. This clearly increases the risks of failure to obtain needed information, broken lines of thought, technological missteps, omissions in care, and failure to respond to patients' requests for service (Ebright, Patterson, Chalko, & Render, 2003).

In a descriptive study of emergency department physicians, the number of times physicians were interrupted or required to change to another task while in the process of performing a task was counted (Chisholm, Collison, Nelson, & Cordell, 2001). On average, in a 3-hour period the physicians saw 12 patients and performed 68 tasks. In the 3-hour period, they were interrupted an average of 31 times and required to change tasks 21 times. The investigators concluded that emergency physicians are "interrupt-driven." Admittedly, the emergency department may be an extreme example of a multitasking environment, but other settings also impose interruptions at a very high rate. An experienced APN may be more skilled at focusing on and prioritizing tasks and quickly dismissing interruptions and extraneous information. The novice APN, conversely, may take longer to perform tasks (allowing for more interruptions) and need more assistance with consultations or accessing resources (Phillips, 2005). As time pressures for clinicians increase, organizational efforts to monitor for errors and potential errors and seek correction when there are system weaknesses are actions APNs owe patients—and themselves as providers functioning in busy environments.

Many patients are sensitive to the pace with which staff and providers greet them, talk with them, and do things, particularly those activities that involve verbal interaction and physical contact. Some patients respond to the fast-paced talk and hurried movements of providers by not bringing up some of the questions they had intended to ask. Others may just get flustered and forget to mention important information; still others may become hostile and withhold information. Thus error in the form of information omission by the patient enters the clinical reasoning and decision-making process.

In summary, clinical thinking is a complex task. It involves drawing on knowledge in memory and attending to multiple sources of situational input, some of which are difficult to interpret. Often, multiple clinical issues must be addressed during a patient encounter, and there are several ways of thinking about each issue. These complexities make clinical thinking a challenging task, even under the best of circumstances. Situational awareness—perceptions of the current environment in which the APN is functioning—can make the APN more cognizant of the potential for error and improve diligence to thought process at critical junctures such as when writing orders, when performing procedures, or during handoffs (Phillips, 2005).

Direct Care and Information Management

Health care is an information-rich environment. It has been said that health care encounters occur essentially for the exchange of information—between the patient and the care provider and among care providers themselves (IOM, 2001). With the adoption of information technology, health care information management has become increasingly complex. Inadequate resources and difficulty in accessing information at the time it is needed further complicate the situation. (IOM, 2001). The IOM report recommended that government, health care leaders, and vendors work collaboratively to quickly build an information infrastructure to eliminate handwritten clinical data by the end of 2010. It is believed that appropriate use of these systems will decrease errors in prescribing and dosing, increase appropriate use of best practice guidelines, reduce redundancy, improve access to information for both patients and providers, and improve quality of care. The direct care practice of APNs is directly influenced by these changes.

The DNP *Essentials* task force recognized the increasing importance of information systems for APN practice and education. Essential IV of the DNP *Essentials* requires that APNs be prepared to participate in design, selection, and evaluation of systems that are utilized for outcomes and quality improvement, exhibit leadership in the area of legal and ethical issues related to information systems, and be knowledgeable about how to evaluate consumer sources of information available through technology (AACN, 2006). With rapid changes in technology, it will be an ongoing challenge throughout an APN's career to remain current in this area.

Even basic competence in the use of computers can be a challenge for some APNs. Wilbright and colleagues (2006) surveyed 454 nursing staff at all role levels in their self-reported skill in 11 key areas of computer use. Although the APNs did report excellent to good skills at entering orders and accessing laboratory results, they rated their skills as fair or poor in 5 of 11 areas that were deemed essential to their role. The skills included bookmarking websites, copying and pasting files, entering data into spreadsheets, searching MEDLINE or CINAHL, and setting patients up for return clinic appointments. If APNs struggle with these basic skills, it will be difficult for them to use tools and their time optimally to care for their patients.

Well-functioning information systems can ease the workload of the APN by optimizing the management of extensive data. However, information technology needs much more development to overcome challenges that APNs may face on a daily basis in their use, such as workflow disruptions, lack of interfaces between systems, and inappropriate use of order entry warning alerts (DePhillips, 2007; Feldstein et al., 2004; Staggers, Thompson, & Snyder-Halpern, 2001). Computer technology may actually require increased staff time when it is used for complex order entry and clinical documentation.

Health care institutions and private practices are rapidly implementing information systems across the country, so it is likely that APNs will work in an environment in which a system is being implemented or upgraded. In a survey of primary care pediatric practices, it was reported that the larger the size of the practice, the more likely it was that they had an information system. Smaller practices reported difficulty in implementing them, chiefly because of system expense. Even with systems in place, only one third of practices had decision support components available such as prompts for immunizations or alerts for abnormal laboratory values (Kemper, Uren, & Clark, 2006). APNs can have an impact on how these systems function to make them user-friendly and efficient at the direct care interface. Although APNs may feel they have neither the time, inclination, nor expertise to participate in these implementations, user input is imperative and ultimately affects direct care.

As information systems are implemented, APNs need to be cognizant of the potential for at least a temporary increase in errors, reduced charge capture, incomplete or difficult-to-access information, and increased time for routine tasks. Implementation of these systems is a major undertaking because it takes time to re-equilibrate workflow and organization skills regardless of APN experience. When information systems are well-implemented and utilized, the APN will be able to use and view data in new ways to improve patient care.

To obtain the information they need to take care of patients, APNs need to be able to use personal digital assistants (PDAs) and desktop computers to access essential information. PDAs improve care at the point of care by decreasing time to access information, decreasing potential for error through access to current information, and increasing opportunities for care planning (Krauskopf & Wyatt, 2006). APNs can feel overwhelmed with these devices if they are not familiar with them because of fear of loss of data, multiple options in devices, cost, and intimidation related to use. There are numerous resources such as free software, web-based purchasing advice, and resources for learning about PDAs and increasing one's expertise in using PDAs clinically (Krauskopf & Wyatt, 2006).

Although information systems and electronic resources can be great tools in the APN's repertoire, the APN must be constantly aware that these technologies bring with them their own pitfalls and unique potential for errors. APNs can play important roles in evaluating proposed technology and information management systems and the impact they have on APN practice and patient care.

Ethical Reasoning

Clinical reasoning is inextricably linked to ethical reasoning. Clinical reasoning generates possibilities of what could be done in a situation, whereas ethical reasoning adds the dimension of what should be done in the situation (see Chapter 11). Advances in health care and medical technology have increasingly resulted in gaps between care that is medically possible and care that is actually in the best interest of the patient. These gaps may be most notable when dealing with decisions regarding withdrawing or withholding nutrition, hydration, or a treatment; when dealing with reproductive technology or human genetics; and when cost must figure into clinical treatment decisions. These situations are at high risk for becoming ethically problematic.

The literature regarding how to resolve ethical issues is extensive. One approach, incorporating preventive or prospective ethical considerations into clinical thinking and decision making, makes a great deal of sense (Forrow, Arnold, & Parker, 1993). This approach places an emphasis on preventing ethical conflicts from developing rather than waiting until a conflict arises; it does so by shaping the process of clinical care so that potential value conflicts are anticipated and discussed before outright conflict occurs. In addition to emphasizing early communication among the patient, significant others, and the provider(s) about values, preventive ethics requires explicit, critical reflection on the institutional factors that lead to conflict (Forrow, Arnold, & Parker, 1993). A third aspect of preventive ethics is an effort to create and preserve trust and understanding among providers, as well as between providers and patients (and their families). Thus the use of preventive ethics can be considered proactive in that it requires providers to consider how the routine processes of care either foster or prevent conflicts from occurring or, at the very least, ensure that such issues are identified at an early stage.

Many questions about preventive ethics remain (Dowdy, Robertson, & Bander, 1998). When in a patient's illness should the values issues be discussed? How can they be raised without frightening patients and families? What information should be discussed? Is it better to discuss specific but hypothetical future clinical scenarios or to discuss a patient's more general goals and values? Even when these questions are unanswered, the preventive approach has the potential to avoid conflicts because clinicians integrate ethical reasoning into clinical reasoning at an earlier point in time than when a traditional conflict-based ethics approach is used. APNs can use this approach with routine encounters with patients. For example, during an encounter with a healthy patient, an APN may be able to say, "I'd like to discuss an important issue with you while you're well so I will know how to best help you." Such issues could include pain management, advance directives, or organ donation.

The concept of moral distress is being recognized increasingly as an issue for all nurses, including APNs. *Moral distress* is defined as knowing what the ethically appropriate action should be but encountering barriers that discourage the provider from carrying out the action (American Association of Critical-Care Nurses, 2004; Rushton, 2006). This results in internal conflict that is not resolved. The extent of moral distress has been reported as ranging from 30% to 70% in health care providers (Corley, 1995; Redman & Fry, 2000). Barriers to acting upon ethical positions include lack of resources and support, conflicts of interest, and rigid rules (Rushton, 2006).

Laabs (2005) found that among primary care NPs, distress was most frequently caused by patient refusal of appropriate treatment. This created a conflict for the NPs between promoting patient autonomy and beneficence on the part of the NP, resulting in feelings of frustration and powerlessness. Some NPs changed jobs, and others considered leaving advanced practice altogether.

The American Association of Critical-Care Nurses has developed a model to address this moral distress—*the 4 A's Model to Rise Above Moral Distress* (2004). APNs can use this model to understand and work toward resolution of distressing situations. The 4 A's include the following (American Association of Critical-Care Nurses, 2004; Rushton, 2006):

- Ask—explore and understand where the distress is coming from
- Affirm—confirm the distress and consider one's professional obligations
- Assess—utilize self-awareness, reflection, and evaluation to assess barriers, opportunities, and potential consequences in preparation for action
- Action—put into place actions that will initiate resolving the distress, anticipating setbacks and ways to cope with them

Encountering these situations can feel overwhelming but can also be opportunities for an APN to reassess current beliefs and values. The APN can use concurrent and retrospective reflection on these situations as a growth and development experience that can be used in positive, proactive interventions with future patient encounters (Rushton, 2006). APNs can role model addressing moral distress by leading forums that promote open, honest communication; establishing positive interdisciplinary collaboration; and offering to debrief and review cases as opportunities for learning.

Skillful Performance

Although the health care professions place high value on knowledge and expert clinical reasoning, it is important to keep in mind that the public values skillful performance in physical examinations, delivery of treatments, diagnostic procedures, and comfort care. Most graduate schools require students to perform a specific set of procedural skills recommended by a national specialty organization before they complete their program. However, little is known about how APNs acquire competency in new or expanded procedural skills once they are in practice. Presumably, competency of APNs to perform specific procedures and treatments is initially ensured through the processes agencies use to credential and grant privileges to APNs. After that, the responsibility for acquiring new competencies lies with the individual APN and the employing agency. When an APN or an agency recognizes that patients would receive better care if the APN would perform a new procedure, an agreement should be reached regarding exactly what new procedure the APN will perform, the conditions under which the procedure will be done, how the APN will acquire the necessary skill, and how supervision will be provided during the learning period. The APN must also be aware that refinement of the technical component is only a piece of the procedure. He or she must also understand indications, contraindications, complications, and consequences of performing the procedures (Hravnak, Tuite, & Baldisseri, 2005).

The types of skills nurses have performed have evolved over time. For example, it used to be within the physician's scope of practice (and outside the nurse's) to measure blood pressure and to administer chemotherapy. With the advent of the APN role, APNs have acquired new performance skills when it made sense within their role and for the comfort, convenience, and satisfaction of patients. It is key for APNs to be cognizant of the scope of their role, regulatory requirements of the states, and the reasonableness of acquiring the skill.

Advanced Physical Assessment

Discussion continues about what actually constitutes advanced physical assessment in the differentiation between the basic RN and APN practice. In one survey, 99 APNs, physician assistants (PAs), and their corresponding preceptor physicians were asked to rank the importance of 87 competencies as an advanced skill (Davidson, Bennett, Hamera, & Raines, 2004). All skills were ranked fairly high as being necessary for advanced practice care. Those skills ranked highest as advanced skills were cardiac assessments, such as rhythm interpretation, and women's health skills, such as gynecological and breast examinations. Competencies such as head, neck, and throat and skin assessment skills were rated lower on the advanced skill priority scale. The authors reported that higher-rated skills appeared to need more use of clinical judgment to interpret or differentially diagnose when compared with lower-rated skills that tended to be more demonstration or technical skills.

Another component to advanced assessment is the use of evidence in assessment and formatting a diagnosis (Munro, 2004). APNs should be skilled at understanding and utilizing the concepts of sensitivity, specificity, and the kappa statistic to differentiate the likelihood of presence or absence of disease based on physical signs and the reliability of that finding. The increased use of technology does not preclude the importance of the physical assessment in accurate diagnosis (Munro, 2004).

Adverse Events and Performance Errors

Since the publication of the IOM's report "To Err is Human," medical errors have been prominent in the public eye as well as a focus of reform for health care institutions (IOM, 2000). Ideally, institutions and care providers should focus on improving reliability of complicated systems to prevent failures or quickly identify, redesign, and rectify failures that do occur. Improving reliability ensures that care is consistently and appropriately provided (Nolan, Resar, Haraden, & Griffin, 2004). Traditionally, institutions and providers have been reluctant to be forthcoming with patients when errors or "near misses" have occurred. That stance is slowly changing with the movement toward increasing transparency in care and a focus on addressing system dysfunction to improve patient safety. This change is relevant to APNs as it relates to their direct care role and the potential to be involved in near-miss or medical error situations. It would be to the APN's advantage to be cognizant of the institution's or practice group's policies related to appropriate actions when errors occur. APNs may find themselves involved in these situations as a result of the many issues already presented such as thinking errors and time pressures.

APNs involved as caregivers in these types of events should anticipate the need to readily inform the patient and family of the event. Honest, open communication and sensitivity will help preserve trust and support ongoing care and may reduce emotional trauma (Gallagher, Waterman, Ebers, Fraser, & Levinson, 2003; Vincent, 2003). Medical research shows that patients expect to be told of medical errors and were more likely to consider legal recourse if the physician withheld information about the error (Witman, Park, & Hardin, 1996).

A consensus group of Harvard hospitals (Massachusetts Coalition for the Prevention of Medical Errors, 2006) recommends four steps in communicating about adverse events:

1. Tell the patient what happened immediately, but leave details of how and why for later when a thorough review has occurred.
2. Take responsibility for the incident.
3. Apologize and communicate remorse.
4. Inform the patient and family what will be done to prevent similar events.

APNs involved in incidents should anticipate the need for their own emotional support during this time. APNs should take advantage of training and educational opportunities on how to communicate bad news and ways to promote safety.

USE OF REFLECTIVE PRACTICE

To continually grow and develop, APNs must be reflective practitioners. APNs may be familiar with multiple methods of learning—didactic, small group projects, clinical experiences with preceptors—but may be less familiar with this method of learning that will be useful to them throughout their careers. Reflective practice is a way to take the experiences a practitioner has (positive or negative) and explore them for the purpose of clarifying meaning, critically analyzing, and synthesizing and using learning to improve practice (Atkins & Murphy, 1995; Schön, 1992). The goal is to turn experience into personal knowledge by seeking insights that are not available with superficial recall (Atkins & Murphy, 1995; Rolfe, 1997; Schön, 1992). Research findings have been reported that show reflective practice by nurses is a valuable learning method, may increase self-

confidence as a practitioner, and may promote accountability (Astor, Jefferson, & Humphrys, 1998; Davies, 1995; Wong et al., 1997).

Forms of clinical supervision are frequently employed in behavioral nursing. Barron and White describe clinical supervision in this realm as a relationship between a more experienced and a more novice nurse in which the expected outcome is to assist the less-experienced nurse in professional development of knowledge, skills, and autonomy (see Chapter 7, p. 195). In these cases, clinical supervision may be used as a debriefing with a trusted and more experienced colleague of a situation that has been complex, intense, or characterized by uncertainty.

Reflection is not just a retrospective activity—it may occur prospectively or concurrently (Atkins & Murphy, 1995) while providing care. Retrospective reflection occurs when an APN takes the opportunity to consider how a situation could have been handled differently. Prospective reflection may occur when an APN prepares to enter a difficult or uncertain clinical situation; one draws on experience and scientific knowledge to plan an approach and anticipates possible reactions or outcomes. Reflection can also occur concurrently. Concurrent reflection is termed *reflection-in-action* and can promote flexibility and adaptation of interventions to suit the situation. Reflection-in-action may be the goal of a more expert practitioner who has honed the skill of reflection (Benner et al., 1999). Although Benner's work was done with bedside staff nurses, it may be applicable to APNs as well, as research by Bryzcznski and Fenton suggested (see Chapter 2). Several models have been proposed to gain expertise in reflective practice (Atkins & Murphy, 1995; Johns, 2000; Kim, 1999) although they utilize similar processes to guide the practitioner through the reflective process. The model Spross proposed (see Chapter 6) explains expert coaching as a process that relies on self-reflection to fully integrate technical competencies, clinical competencies, and interpersonal competencies; it may equally apply to the direct care competency. Deliberate self-reflection allows the APN to anticipate alternative possibilities, remain flexible in challenging and changing situations, and strategically integrate the results of self-reflection with best practices to match interventions to patient and family needs.

Strengthening skills in self-reflection can be done in a number of ways for the APN—through solitary self-evaluation, with a supervisor or teacher, or in small groups of supportive colleagues. With experience, the

APN may be asked to be the mentor in guiding others through a self-reflective process. Regardless of which model is used for reflection, the following tips can be considered:

- If reflection occurs in a small group, participants must feel safe to express thoughts, emotions, and thinking processes without fear of judgment.
- Practitioners need to gain awareness of personal values, beliefs, and behaviors.
- Practitioners need to develop the skills to articulate a situation with both objective and subjective details.
- Critical debriefing and analysis are used to identify practitioner goals in the situation, extent of knowledge that was present or missing, feelings on the part of the practitioner and patient, consequences of actions, and what alternative options existed.
- Knowledge gained through this process can be integrated with current knowledge to change interventions in a current situation or improve approaches in future situations.
- Evaluation of this reflective process supports masterful practice and creates lasting improvements in practice.

Several barriers exist to using reflection in daily practice. Lack of time may result in care and interventions becoming very routine. Utilization of a reflective practice process will require dedicated time. If not thoughtfully arranged, it may seem to be extraneous and a "nice thing to do" rather than a necessary component to the APN role. Acknowledging that we do not always know the right answer can be difficult for an APN who is trying to establish a practice and role. In addition, reflection may elicit emotions that may be painful or difficult to deal with. It takes experience and skill to use reflection, which is particularly important when an APN is very involved in a situation. Novice APNs may need guidance in performing reflection to assist in ascertaining meaning and making connections that otherwise might be missed (Johns, 2000). Finally, some may see reflective practice discussions as official surveillance or a confessional when supervisors are involved and depending on the context (Clouder & Sellars, 2004). However, when reflective thinking is developed and incorporated into one's practice, it can be a means to demonstrate professional accountability for practice and a source of life-long learning (Clouder & Sellars, 2004). Knowledge from reflection informs future clinical decision making, especially in those situations for which no benchmarks or best practice guidelines exist.

USE OF EVIDENCE AS A GUIDE TO PRACTICE

An important form of knowledge that must be brought to bear on clinical decision making, for individuals and for populations, is the ever-increasing volume of research findings. For the nursing profession, the use of research findings as a basis for practice is more than the latest trend. The profession has been exploring and considering the issues of research utilization intensively since the early 1970s. Historically, CNSs led efforts in many agencies to move toward research-based practice (DePalma, 2004; Hanson & Ashley, 1994; Hickey, 1990; Mackay, 1998; Stetler, Batista, Vernale-Hannon, & Foster, 1995). They have brought research findings to the attention of the nursing staff and interdisciplinary teams and worked to develop the research appraisal skills of nursing staffs. The profession, agencies, and APNs themselves view evidence-based practice skills as central to APNs' research competency and as a more appropriate expectation of APNs than the conduct of research itself (see Chapter 8). This is particularly delineated in Essentials III and VII of the DNP *Essentials,* in which the criteria focus on the ability of the APN to synthesize, analyze, and apply pertinent data to care for populations and individuals (AACN, 2006).

Identifying and locating research findings is much easier than it was just 5 years ago. However, clinicians often do not have sufficient experience in the use of various search engines available to retrieve information from databases. Research has shown that clinicians are not skilled in either writing a researchable question that is clearly articulated or in searching for evidence (Meats, Brassey, Heneghan, & Glasziou, 2007). APNs could benefit from education on simple tools that could greatly increase the efficiency of their searches. APNs in all settings engaging in an evidence-based practice project would be well served by developing a relationship with a health care librarian who can assist with searches (Pond, 1999), save time, and prevent the omission of relevant evidence.

Research evidence can be used in a variety of ways. Differentiating between research-sensitive practice, research-based practice, and evidence-based practice provides a useful way of thinking about how APNs can incorporate evidence into their practices.

Research-Sensitive Practice

Research-sensitive practice is practice in which the individual clinician brings research findings to bear on practice in an unstructured way. To do this, an APN would (1) read primary research reports and summaries of research findings on a regular basis, (2) informally evaluate the soundness of the methods, and (3) adjust or fine-tune his or her own practice on the basis of credible findings. This is the form of research utilization in which every professional nurse should engage. It is part of staying abreast of new knowledge in one's area of clinical practice.

Research-sensitive practice could take the form of setting time aside to systematically scan clinical journals for reports relevant to one's clinical specialty. Alternatively, an APN could join or form a multidisciplinary group that meets monthly to discuss several research reports on topics of mutual interest. Some APNs keep a small notebook in which to jot down clinical issues and questions about which they have uncertainty. Then once a month, they use the 2 hours of library time that is built into their schedules to find studies about these issues. The recorded questions help them use the limited library time in the most efficient manner.

Research-Based Practice

Research-based practice is a more systematic, rigorous, and precise way of translating research findings into practice. The research-based practice process is used within an organization to design a standard of care for a population of patients. The research-based practice process is more formal because research-based care will be widely used as a guide to care and therefore the scientific conclusions on which it is based must be as free of bias and error as possible. In general terms, the process involves three steps: (1) locating, evaluating, and summarizing the science; (2) translating the science into clinical recommendations; and (3) strategically implementing the recommendations. The recommendations may take the form of a clinical practice guideline, a decision algorithm, a clinical protocol, the components of a clinical program, or change in policies or procedures.

Evidence-Based Practice

It would be ideal to have all of practice based on research. However, in reality, research frequently does not exist on which to base decisions. Sackett (1998) defined evidence-based practice as the explicit and judicious integration of best evidence with clinical expertise and patient values. Using only external evidence to make practice decisions is as unacceptable as using only individual clinical expertise.

Usually when APNs are involved in designing care for a population of patients, all forms of objective evidence should be used; this would include quality improvement data, data from internal databases, expert opinion panels, consensus statements, data from benchmarking partners, and data from state and national databases (e.g., the Centers for Disease Control and Prevention [CDC]). Agency-specific information, collected to pinpoint the nature of a problem, is particularly useful evidence that should be combined with the more general knowledge gained from research evidence (Brown, 2001).

Theory-Based Practice

The preceding discussion of research-based practice recognizes how research evidence informs practice but ignores the role of theory. APNs are becoming comfortable with the idea of research evidence as a guide to practice, yet the idea of theory-based practice is less familiar. It should not be, because contrary to common perception, theory can be a very practical tool. Theory often brings together research findings in a way that helps practice be more purposeful, systematic, and comprehensive.

In the past, most discussions of theory-based practice addressed the use of conceptual models of nursing to guide care (Bonamy, Schultz, Graham, & Hampton, 1995; Hawkins, Thibodeau, Utley-Smith, Igou, & Johnson, 1993; Laschinger & Duff, 1991; Sappington & Kelley, 1996). However, more recently, emphasis has shifted to middle-range theories, which guide practice more specifically. Middle-range theories typically address a particular patient experience (e.g., living with rheumatoid arthritis) or problem (e.g., managing chronic pain); thus their range of applicability is relatively narrow. However, this narrow range of applicability allows them to be developed to address specific issues encountered in clinical practice. Schwartz-Barcott, Patterson, Lusardi, and Farmer (2002) make a strong case for developing theories by using fieldwork so that the theories will be more closely aligned to the realities practicing nurses encounter. Another approach to developing theories that are more specific to clinical situations is to generate a middle-range theory from one of the broader conceptual models. For instance, Whittemore and Roy (2002) developed a middle-range theory describing adaptation to diabetes mellitus based on the concepts and theoretical statements of the broader Roy Adaptation Model.

A 1999 analysis of the nursing literature identified 22 middle-range theories that met certain criteria (Liehr & Smith, 1999). The list of theories generated by that analysis is provided in Box 5-8. The list provides a sampling of the middle-range theories currently available to practicing nurses. In looking at this list, the reader can see that the topics of the theories are substantively specific, although some are more specific than others. "Balance between analgesia and side effects" is more specific and less abstract than "Resilience." An APN in a particular field may find that only one or two of these theories are applicable to his or her area of practice. However, as middle-range theories are developed for other topics, APNs will be able to use several of these types of theories to guide different aspects of practice (Smith & Liehr, 2003).

DIVERSE APPROACHES TO HEALTH AND ILLNESS MANAGEMENT

APNs' holistic approach to care and their commitment to using research evidence as a basis for care contribute to how they help patients. Generally, APNs use a variety of interventions to effect change in the health status or quality of life of an individual or family and tailor their recommendations, approaches, and treatment to individual patients (Hughes et al., 2002). Interpersonal interventions that are psychosocial in nature are frequently referred to as *support interventions.* Support interventions are somewhat distinct from educational interventions, which are informational in nature. Coaching uses a combination of support and education strategies (see Chapter 6). Then, of course, there are discrete physical actions, which are frequently categorized as nonpharmacological and pharmacological interventions. These distinctions are arbitrary because good clinicians probably craft interventions that are a combination of various types as they seek to alleviate, prevent, or manage specific physical symptoms, conditions, or problems.

Interpersonal Interventions

Support is not a discrete intervention; it is a composite of interpersonal interventions based on the patient's unique psychological and informational needs. Supportive interpersonal interventions include providing reassurance, giving information, coaching, affirming,

Box 5-8   Middle-Range Theories

TOPIC	AUTHOR(S)
Uncertainly in illness	Mishel
Nurse-midwifery care	Thompson et al.
Facilitating growth and development	Kinney
Self-transcendence	Reed
Hazardous secrets and reluctantly taking charge	Burke et al.
Women's anger	Thomas
Caring	Swanson
Negotiating partnership	Powell-Cope
Unpleasant symptoms	Lenz et al.
Cultural brokering	Jezewski
Homelessness-hopelessness	Tollett & Thomas
Balance between analgesia and side effects	Good, Moore, & Good
Chronotherapeutic intervention for postsurgical pain	Auvil-Novak
Nurse-expressed empathy and patient distress	Olso & Hanchett
Interpersonal perceptual awareness	Brooks & Thomas
Resilience	Polk
Individualized music intervention for agitation	Gerdner
Affiliated individuation as a mediator for stress	Acton
Chronic sorrow	Eakes, Burke, & Hainsworth
Acute pain management	Huth & Moore
Psychological adaptation	Levesque et al.
Peaceful end of life	Ruland & Moore

From Liehr, P., & Smith, M.J. (1999). Middle range theory: Spinning research and practice to create knowledge for the new millennium. *Advances in Nursing Science, 14,* 81-91.

providing anticipatory guidance, guiding decision making, listening actively, expressing understanding, and being available. Each of these interventions can be described in terms of the circumstances for which it is indicated. For example, reassurance is indicated when a patient is experiencing uncertainty, distress, or lack of confidence; active listening is indicated when a patient has a strong need to tell his or her story. The actions that constitute these interventions are not mutually exclusive. For instance, giving factual information can be reassuring, instructional, guiding, or all of these things at the same time.

In practice, these interpersonal interventions are blended, and APNs may not be consciously aware of when they are doing one and when they are doing another. This is as it should be. APNs have no need to think "Now I'm doing active listening; now I'm going to do anticipatory guidance." Instead, APNs interact with patients in ways that intermingle the conceptually separate interventions. This crafting of support evolves as the APN talks with patients; infers their worries, fears, and concerns; and, without a great deal of conscious thought, acts to alleviate their distress. A patient may experience the interaction as just a good talk with the APN or as a feeling of being understood. However, support is a complex nursing intervention that is strategically crafted and purposefully administered and often makes a difference in how the patient feels and acts.

Telehealth, Information Technology, and Direct Care

Telehealth (sometimes known as *telemedicine*) has traditionally been utilized by physicians. Now with expanding technology, telehealth is offering expanding service and roles for APNs (Reed, 2005). Telehealth can offer opportunities both for APNs who practice in rural settings and who need timely access to specialized services for consultation and for specialty APNs who can now reach patients in isolated areas to provide them access to needed care. Telehealth is not a substitute for routine care but, rather, is complementary to the health care patients already receive (Jenkins & White, 2001). Telehealth uses a variety of equipment including computers, video cameras, faxes, and telephones and can involve a variety of services.

There are multiple examples of the impact telehealth can have on improving patient care. The area of genetics in general has been rapidly expanding and with it the opportunity to provide APN genetic counseling through telemedicine (Lea, 2006). Providing genetic counseling

through this format offers care individualized to patients and families while allowing them to remain in their home communities. In this project in the northeastern United States, APNs provide genetic evaluations, test interpretations, and counseling. APNs are able to partner with maternal-child and primary care providers to improve access to care.

Rural areas have taken advantage of telehealth to provide primary care where there are shortages of providers or specialists. Telehealth in these projects has facilitated consultations and communication with specialists. Outcomes of these initiatives have been improved patient outcomes, effective care, and increased satisfaction for patients and providers (Armer, 2003; Henderson, 2006). Though barriers were identified, it would be anticipated that with time and improved technological resources, some of these barriers could be removed.

Another emerging example is the initiation of electronic ICUs (e-ICUs)—locations onsite or offsite that house a complement of nurses and intensivists who provide additional monitoring of patients who are in a traditional ICU. Video cameras and electronic interfaces with hemodynamic monitoring and diagnostic equipment transmit data that allow these "remote" providers to be an "extra set of eyes," at the bedside for APNs or physicians, who may need an immediate intensivist consult. These e-ICUs can be helpful in a multitude of settings from rural to urban.

DISCRETE MANAGEMENT AND TREATMENT INTERVENTIONS

Preventive Services in Primary Care

Health promotion and disease prevention interventions are tools that APNs in primary care regularly use to help people achieve and maintain a high quality of life. The preventive services include the following:

- Counseling regarding personal health practices that can protect a person from disease or promote screening for the presence of disease
- Immunization to prevent specific diseases
- Chemoprevention (e.g., use of aspirin for prevention of cardiovascular events)

Discernment is needed in the use of these interventions because time and effort can be wasted if their use is not based on current scientific knowledge and tailored to the individual person or community. In addition, the public is confused regarding many of the preventive recommendations because new research evidence has been unseating long-established recommendations, such as the value of breast self-examination. The U.S. Preventive Services Task Force's "Guide to Clinical Preventive Services" (2003) and the Canadian Task Force on Preventive Health Care (2007) provide specific preventive guidelines for many health conditions. These guidelines include valuable summaries of the state of the science for each recommendation, and the U.S. guidelines provide cost-effectiveness analyses, which summarize the benefits, harms, and costs of alternative strategies.

An important point made in an earlier version of the "Guide to Clinical Preventive Services" (U.S. Preventive Services Task Force, 1996) is that primary prevention in the form of counseling aimed at changing health-related behavior may be more effective than diagnostic screening and testing. Many healthy people, as well as people who have had a recent health scare, are quite receptive to, even eager for, information and guidance about how to stay healthy and avoid age-related disabilities. However, other people who engage in one or several unhealthy behaviors can be quite defensive and resistant to talking about their risks and how behavior changes could reduce risks. Introducing behavior change issues with unreceptive people requires a high level of interpersonal skill and a good sense of timing. An APN must consider that it is possible that no health care provider has previously attempted to discuss the problem (e.g., smoking, lack of exercise, alcohol abuse) with the person, even though signs of a problem have existed for quite a while (Stafford & Blumenthal, 1998).

Talking about the risks of the current behavior and the benefits of the behavior change is not enough. To be effective, counseling regarding these issues should also include a discussion of how the person perceives the burden of changing a personal behavior; that is, what would be lost and what would be required to make the change? The provider must elicit how much effort will be required, what would give the individual the confidence to change, and what forms of self-help assistance are acceptable to the individual. Then, and only then, can a specific recommendation about a strategy or program be made. Theoretical models that can be useful in planning a behavior change program or protocol include the Transtheoretical Model *(www. uri.edu/research/cprc/transtheoretical.htm)* and the Health Belief Model *(www.etr.org/recapp/theories/hbm /index.htm#majorconcepts)*. Both models include provider strategies for building the person's self-efficacy (i.e., confidence in one's ability to take action).

Clinicians also have at their disposal a wide array of screening tools, some of which are better with certain populations or age-groups than others. For example, the U.S. Preventive Services Task Force (2003) recommends against routinely screening women older than age 65 for cervical cancer if they have had adequate recent screening with normal Papanicolaou test results and are not otherwise at risk; they also recommend against performing routine Papanicolaou tests for women who have had a total hysterectomy as treatment for benign disease. Staying current with the latest screening recommendations in one's area of practice ensures that care is provided in a way that is both scientific and cost-effective.

Preventive Services in Hospitals and Home Care

The preventive services provided in inpatient and home care settings are somewhat different from those provided in primary care. Many of the actions and assessments performed on behalf of acutely ill patients are aimed at early detection and prevention of problems related to treatment, disease progression, self-care deficits, or the hospital environment itself. Complications typically result from a complex set of factors, such as inadequate delivery systems or failure to assess patients for risk of complications common to their condition. Nurses assist patients by preventing adverse events and complications, including adverse medication reactions, unexpected physiological decline, poor communication, pressure ulcers, and death. This function is also referred to as *surveillance* or *rescuing* (as in rescuing from a bad course of events or death) (Aiken, Sochalski, & Lake, 1997). As mentioned earlier, in five studies of APN interventions with diverse patient groups, surveillance was the predominant APN function (Brooten et al., 2003).

In the home setting, APNs serve as advisors and partners. In addition to assessment and surveillance, coaching and guidance is particularly important. The patient may be new to the role of partner in this setting (Holman & Lorig, 2004). APNs work with patients to prioritize measures that might prevent rehospitalizations. Interventions may include teaching about reportable signs and symptoms, guidance on how to communicate with their providers, and assistance in making connections between behaviors and situations in the home that directly impact health status.

Therapeutic Interventions

The decision about whether to treat can be difficult, because the practitioner is faced with several probabilities that do not all lead to the same decision.

Moreover, there is often pressure from patients to "do something." When deciding whether and how to treat patients, clinicians consider the following five types of information:

- The degree of certainty about the diagnosis, condition, or symptom
- What is known about the effectiveness of the various treatment alternatives
- What is known about the risks of the treatment alternatives
- The clinician's comfort with a particular treatment or intervention
- The patient's preference for a certain kind of treatment or management

The most clear-cut situation is when the condition is definitely present, a particular treatment is known to be highly effective, the treatment can be expected to be low in risk for the particular patient, and both the clinician and the patient are comfortable with the treatment. Unfortunately, many (probably most) therapeutic decisions are not so clear-cut. Instead, the weight of factors in support of a particular treatment and the weight of those against treatment or in support of another treatment are close to equivalent.

The treatment and management interventions that APNs perform include a wide variety of self-care modalities and low-tech, nonpharmacological modalities (Day & Horton-Deutsch, 2004; Fowler, 2006; Hiltunen et al., 2005; Riegel et al., 2006). However, even when technological and pharmacological modalities are used, they are selected based on the consideration of many factors. In a study of 10 collaborative pairs of physicians and NPs, NPs and physicians were identical in their final recommendations related to medication management, although the processes used to reach decisions were different (Flesner & Clawson, 1998). The NPs elicited more information about the context of the patients' lives and available resources and collaborated with patients more frequently to work out the details of implementing the management plans.

When prescribing or recommending medications, APNs consider the patient's financial status, the patient's previous experience with similar medications, the ease of taking the medication, how many other medications the person is taking, how often the medications must be taken, the side effect profiles of the drugs being considered, and potential drug and disease interactions (Brown & Grimes, 1993). A descriptive study of the safety and effectiveness of APN prescriptive authority revealed that the 33 NPs in the project prescribed medications for 90% of 1708 patients; 42% had one drug prescribed per visit, and 31% had two drugs prescribed per visit (Hamric, Worley, Lindebak, & Jaubert, 1998). This would seem to be a low number of prescribed medications, but further study of the extent to which APNs recommend prescription drugs as compared with the extent to which other providers who care for similar patients do is needed before it can be established that a lower use of prescription drugs is characteristic of APNs.

As previously discussed, considerable evidence indicates that APNs use a broad range of interventions, with substantial reliance on self-care and low-tech interventions. Surveillance, teaching, guidance, counseling, and case management are interventions that are used much more often than procedural interventions (Brooten et al., 2003). The frequency with which the various categories of interventions were used varied moderately with patient populations.

The nursing interventions classification project (Bulechek & McCloskey, 1999), the Omaha classification system, and the home health care classification are well along the road to capturing the full range of treatments and interventions nurses use (Henry, Holzemer, Randell, Hsieh, & Miller, 1997). In addition, they have the potential to ensure that, in the future, nursing interventions currently not recognized by the Current Procedural Terminology (CPT) system as contributing to patients' outcomes will be integrated into diagnostic, intervention, billing, and other taxonomies. In February of 2003, the U.S. Department of Health and Human Services authorized the test of a proposed modification to the billing codes used for Medicare and Medicaid. The new codes are called the *advanced billing concept (ABC) codes* and include intervention codes from the intervention classification systems developed and used by nurses. Although this is only a testing phase, it does hold promise for a billing system that will enable APNs to bill for services they provide that are not billable under the current CPT system.

The repertoire of interventions used by individual APNs clearly depends on the problems experienced by the population of patients with whom they work. Acute care nurse practitioners (ACNPs), CNMs, CRNAs, and CNSs use repertoires of therapeutic interventions different from those used by APNs who provide primary care. The methods of practice an individual APN uses also depend on the methods of practice used by colleagues in their settings and on what is allowed by their reimbursement systems. Nevertheless, APNs must make an effort to constantly extend and refine their repertoire beyond the interventions learned during graduate education.

Complementary and Alternative Therapies

The extent of public use of complementary and alternative therapies (CAT) was well documented in the early 1990s and mid-1990s by Eisenberg and colleagues when they reported that approximately 33% of Americans were using at least one unconventional therapy and this was supported in further studies (Eisenberg et al., 1993; Eisenberg et al., 1998; Ni, Simile, & Hardy, 2002). This use has resulted in recognition by the government and establishment of the National Center for Complementary and Alternative Therapies. The use among certain ethnic groups is often higher than the national average. Many patients use alternative therapies in conjunction with conventional medical services; hence these therapies are also referred to as *integrative therapies.*

The effectiveness and safety of alternative and complementary therapies vary widely. Some have been scientifically studied (e.g., relaxation, guided imagery, glucosamine and chondroitin for osteoarthritis), whereas others have not been studied at all. Of concern is that some may interact with other medications the patient is receiving (Norred, 2002; Scott & Elmer, 2002). Another issue particular to dietary supplements and herb therapy is the lack of control over ingredients (Barnes, 2003; Tesch, 2002). Providers are caught between the desire of patients to use alternative therapies and reservations about their safety, often in the face of insufficient scientific evidence.

APNs are incorporating complementary and alternative treatments into their practices in a variety of ways, albeit with some caution (Allaire, Moos, & Wells, 2000; Hayes & Alexander, 2000; Sohn & Loveland Cook, 2002; Thomas, 2003). APNs have expressed interest in being able to provide CAT for patients even if it means expanding their scope of practice (Patterson, Kaczorowski, Arthur, Smith, & Mills, 2003). They are increasing their engagement in these therapies, are more willing to ask patients about CAT practices, and are counseling patients on appropriate use. Many APNs report a need to increase their own knowledge about CAT to fully incorporate it into care. An interim solution to this situation may be for an APN to consider developing a collaborative relationship with expert CAT providers. In summary, because patients are using CAT, APNs seem to believe that it is better that they do so with provider guidance and awareness.

Individualized Interventions

One goal of treatment decision making is to choose from among several possible interventions and to use the one that will have the highest probability of achieving the outcomes the patient most desires. Usually that probability is increased by "particularizing" the treatment or action to the individual patient (Benner et al., 1996, p. 24). Particularizing requires that the recommendation or action take the following into account:

- The acceptability of the treatment to the patient
- What has worked for the patient in the past
- The patient's motivation and ability to use or follow the treatment (self-care)
- The likelihood that the patient will continue to use the treatment even if side effects are experienced
- The financial burden of the treatment
- The health literacy of the patient

Nursing has always believed that individualizing nursing care, that is, tailoring care to the unique characteristics of the person and his or her situation, produces the best patient outcomes. In contrast, standardization of care and control of wide variation are important to quality control and cost containment. Clearly, a blending of the two perspectives is required to produce care that is effective for an individual and congruent with available resources. This can be accomplished by adopting evidence-based standards and guidelines to provide a framework for care while acknowledging that at the point of care (i.e., in the patient-provider interface) interventions and management may need to be tailored to reflect the patient's unique situation and needs (Brown, 2001).

Unfortunately, research support for the effectiveness of individualized interventions in general is not as strong as most APNs would like. The extent to which the equivocal nature of the evidence is a function of methodological difficulties in studying individualized interventions is unknown. Part of the difficulty stems from the various ways in which health messages may be customized: personalized, targeted, tailored, and individualized (Ryan & Lauver, 2002). An integrative research review of 20 studies in which interventions with varying degrees of customization to the individual were delivered revealed that in only half of the studies were better patient outcomes achieved with tailored interventions as compared with standard interventions (Ryan & Lauver, 2002). The authors of the review proposed that another reason for the modest support for the efficacy of customized interventions is that patients with certain characteristics are more affected by these interventions than others; such uneven effects across subgroups would offset each other and present an appearance of little or no benefit. Even when a tailored intervention does not result in changed behavior or produce better patient outcomes, it may have other benefits. An example of this collateral gain was found in a study of 43 women with gynecological cancer (Ward, Donovan, Owen, Grosen, & Serlin, 2000). The individualized sensory and coping message for pain management intervention did not have a demonstrable effect on analgesic use, pain intensity scores, or pain interference with life, but the women who received the individualized intervention reported that it contained useful information that helped them to feel more comfortable taking pain medication and to discuss pain more openly with a doctor or nurse.

Many patients are using computers to access information and educate themselves about their health and diseases. Patients may actually come to appointments knowing more about their disease than the APN does (McMullan, 2006). Although this can be disconcerting, it is important to recognize this as information-seeking behavior and capitalize on the opportunity to work with the patients to help them gain the information they need (Cutilli, 2006). Patients vary widely in terms of how much information they want and how they want information presented. Allowing them to make choices about how and what they learn should help prevent content overload and enhance relevancy of information given, thus producing better retention and application. Along similar lines, computer-based programs have been developed to counsel patients who are faced with major treatment decisions (Cherkin et al., 2002; Frosch, Kaplan, & Felitti, 2001; Morgan et al., 2000). Programs can be designed to allow the patients to acquire information that is most important to them and to help them sort out their values, priorities, and preference in the specific situations they face. Undoubtedly, computer-based learning and decision-making tools will be more acceptable to some groups of patients than others.

Essential IV of the DNP *Essentials* states that APNs should have expertise in evaluating consumer resources and help patients use reputable websites. It will be important for APNs to help consumers discern between websites that are reputable and offer valid information and those that may not have accurate evidence. The Internet is being used for patients with similar or rare diseases to connect with each other as support in a way that may never have been possible for them before the advent and ease of use of the Internet. APNs can also direct patients to state health department websites as excellent sites for accessing helpful information such as immunization schedules, tobacco cessation tools, and information on diabetes care, sexually transmitted diseases, tuberculosis, and newborn screening (Alpi, 2005).

MANAGEMENT OF COMPLEX SITUATIONS

APNs' direct care often involves management and coordination of complex situations; many illustrations of this advanced practice nursing characteristic may be found in the chapters on specific advanced practice nursing roles (see Chapters 12 through 17). In some settings, APNs have been designated as the providers responsible for coordination of complex follow-up care (Dellasega & Zerbe, 2002) or for education of patients at high risk for complications (Brooten et al., 2003; Naylor et al., 1999). APNs manage diverse patient conditions and care requirements, which include the following:

- Confusion in older hospitalized patients and acute care of the elderly (ACE) units
- Risk for complications in older adults admitted to the emergency department (Mion et al., 2003)
- Pain in patients who are chronically or terminally ill
- Acute pain (Musclow, Sawhney, & Watt-Watson, 2002)
- Transitional care needs of frail rural older adults (Dellasega & Zerbe, 2002)
- Long-term mechanical ventilation (Burns & Earven, 2002)
- Heart failure patients (Riegel et al., 2006; Brooten et al., 2003)
- Neurosurgical patients (Yeager, Shaw, Casavant, & Burns, 2006)
- Organ failure and care needs of patients awaiting transplantation (McNatt & Easom, 2000)
- Critically ill neonates

Many CNSs have been called in on a consultation and found a need for skilled communication, advocacy, or coordination of the various providers' plans—or some combination thereof (Exemplar 5-2). The patient's condition may not be improving because wound care, pain management, and physical

EXEMPLAR 5-2   Management of Complex Patient Situations

C.M. is a diabetes clinical nurse specialist with 20 years of experience. She works in an 800-bed academic medical center where she is accountable for overall outcomes of glycemic control in the inpatient setting; she is also responsible for evaluating, treating, and educating patients with complex diabetes needs.

C.M. has been asked to consult on and write treatment recommendations for a 30-year-old Somali woman. Before seeing the patient, C.M. reviewed the chart to ascertain patient history and information. The patient was diagnosed with type II diabetes mellitus (DM) 11 years ago and had been on oral hypoglycemic agents, though not well controlled. She has been managed by multiple providers over the years. The patient was not married and had two sons—13 and 17 years of age—both have been diagnosed with type I DM.

Documentation in the chart indicated that the patient had been admitted to the hospital in ketoacidosis caused by presumed nonadherence to her regimen. The health care team had initiated an insulin infusion but had not initiated the diabetic ketoacidosis (DKA) protocol and had been having difficulty getting the patient's glucoses in the target range.

When C.M. entered the patient's room, she saw an African woman with truncal obesity, a puffy face, acne, and facial hair. The patient did not make eye contact and appeared standoffish. The patient was reluctant to answer questions. C.M. recognized the need to proceed thoughtfully in developing a relationship with the patient and establish trust. C.M. also realized that multiple visits would be required to fully ascertain the extent of needs for this complex patient. From C.M.'s experience and knowledge base, she knew that the symptomatology of DM in the African population is different from the typical Caucasian presentation of DM. Type I symptoms in the African population may not be as severe on initial presentation and not reflect ketosis; therefore this population can be misdiagnosed with type II DM and started on oral agents when they actually have type I DM and should be treated with insulin. C.M. suspected this may be the case with this patient. In addition, on first glance, C.M. immediately suspected that the patient may have had other endocrine issues (e.g., adrenal dysfunction or polycystic ovary syndrome [PCOS]) because of the presence of puffy face, acne, and facial hair.

C.M. decided the priority for this initial visit was to focus on the physical care aspects while clarifying the diagnosis and prescribing appropriate treatment to control the patient's glucose. She performed a physical examination and ordered the following diagnostics:
- C-peptide and antibodies (to differentiate between type I and type II DM)
- Fasting cortisol
- ACTH stimulation test
- Estradiol/androgen panel
- 24-hour urine
- Endocrinologist consult
- Initiation of the standardized DKA protocol

C.M. returned the following day with the intent to explore knowledge and psychosocial areas with the patient. Again the patient was wary in her interaction but started to have better eye contact. C.M. started by asking about the patient's psychosocial situation and determined that, the patient was making ends meet financially. However, there were income issues, and the C.M. determined that a social work referral was in order. The patient described having a good relationship with her sons and acknowledged an extensive family support system in the community. She identified herself as a Christian, not Muslim as most people assumed. C.M. then started to ask about the physical signs she had noticed on the previous visit by asking how long the patient had had acne and facial hair. At that point, the patient started to cry and stated that C.M. was the first person to have ever asked her about it. They were clearly distressing symptoms for the patient, and she relayed that she had tried multiple over-the-counter products to try to resolve the acne without success. C.M. shared with the patient what she suspected may be happening with other endocrine issues and reassured her that if that were the case, prescription dermatology creams and hormone therapies would help resolve the symptoms. It was at this point that the patient realized that C.M. was committed to helping her and a therapeutic relationship began to develop. The patient was now more receptive to allowing a full knowledge assessment.

C.M. discovered that the patient understood DM well and knew how to count carbohydrates and how to use that knowledge in planning meals. Although the patient spoke English well, C.M. discovered that the patient could not read English and had some visual disturbances. What had been labeled as nonadherence was really an inability to read and see health care instructions. When C.M. reviewed the diagnostic test results, it was

EXEMPLAR 5-2   Management of Complex Patient Situations—cont'd

determined that the patient had Cushing syndrome, PCOS, and type I DM rather than type II. Over the following days, in educational sessions with C.M., the patient quickly gained knowledge about insulin and how to administer it and became proficient at using a magnifier to read the insulin syringe. C.M. developed instructional tools that did not require the ability to read complicated English. Whenever the patient's sons were present, they were included in the teaching.

The patient was eventually discharged to home with new knowledge of insulin and type I management, as well as knowledge of her new diagnoses and medications, ongoing support from external social services, and a referral to a physician group that could manage the health needs of the entire family and provide continuity of care over time.

HIGHLIGHTS OF ADVANCED PRACTICE NURSING CARE OF A COMPLEX PATIENT
This case exemplifies the role an APN can play in making accurate diagnoses and optimizing care for a complex patient. C.M. exhibited the following:
- Use of evidence and knowledge of unique population-based data that were applied to an individual patient, which resulted in prompt correction of a diabetes misdiagnosis
- Expert clinical assessment and intervention skills that identified new endocrine diagnoses and assisted in rapid correction of glycemic control
- Holistic approach to care, incorporating cultural assessment, psychosocial needs, barriers to knowledge
- Individualized interventions to meet patient needs
- An interpersonal approach that allowed for rapid development of a trusting, therapeutic relationship with a patient who was traditionally wary of health care providers who had consistently misidentified her as noncompliant

---

therapy have not been well thought out and coordinated. Family members may be angry because plans keep changing and they are receiving conflicting information from various providers. Typically, the CNS talks with the patient and family to become familiar with their concerns and objectives and then brokers a new plan of care that reflects the patient's and family's needs and preferences, as well as the clinical objectives of the involved providers. The agreed-upon plan must also be consistent with the care authorized by the third-party payers for the patient, or a special agreement must be negotiated. This brokering requires broad clinical knowledge regarding the objectives of various providers, interpersonal skill in dealing with the results of misunderstandings, diplomacy to encourage stakeholders to see each other's points of view, and a commitment to keeping the patient's needs at the center of what is being done.

Helping Patients Manage Chronic Illnesses
Another type of complex situation that APNs manage effectively is chronic illness. Chronic diseases such as multiple sclerosis, cognitive degeneration, psoriasis, heart failure, chronic lung disease, cancer, acquired immunodeficiency syndrome, and organ failure with subsequent transplantation affect individuals and families in profound ways. Most chronic illnesses are characterized by a great deal of uncertainty—uncertainty about the future life course, the effectiveness of treatment, the chances of leading a happy life, bodily functions, medical bills, and intimate relationships (Mast, 1995). Spouses and significant others of people with chronic illness often bear considerable emotional and caregiving burdens. For a variety of reasons related to the characteristics of advanced practice nursing, APNs are successful in providing care to persons with chronic conditions and their families.

Among the reasons that APNs are successful in providing care to persons with chronic illness is their advocacy of patient self-care. It has been proposed that the key to self-care by patients with chronic illness is to provide self-management education in conjunction with traditional patient education (Bodenheimer, Lorig, Holman, & Grumbach, 2002). Self-management education is aimed at promoting confidence to carry out new behaviors, teaching the identification and solving of problems, and setting patient-directed short-term goals (Bodenheimer et al., 2002; Lorig, Ritter, & Gonzalez, 2003).

Partnership in management of chronic illness requires a change in roles for patients and providers. Patients develop daily management skills, changes in behaviors, and accurate reporting of symptoms. While providers continue as advisers and partners, they now also become teachers, a role that many are not adequately prepared to enact (Holman & Lorig, 2004). In this new partnership, patients develop more knowledge and experience over time and they know the most about the real consequences of chronic disease and their behaviors.

The benefits of emphasizing self-care are supported by research showing that when patients are given information about illnesses and helped to manage their illnesses such as heart failure, asthma, and arthritis, their courses of illness and quality of life are improved (Bodenheimer et al., 2002; Lorig, 2003; Riegel et al., 2006). Moreover, the evidence suggests that health education for self-management works in part by building patients' self-confidence about controlling their lives in spite of the presence of disease (Bodenheimer et al., 2002). Hence many self-management, educational interventions for persons with chronic conditions are being designed to bolster patients' sense of self-efficacy related to coping with the associated disabilities and gaining control over the impact of the disease on their lives. In addition, APNs can help patients make good decisions that are specific to the context of their disease and their home situation (Riegel et al., 2006).

There are barriers to using a self-management education program in today's health care environment. Some of these include lack of trained personnel in this intervention, a patient dependence on the medical model that has been facilitated by health care providers, and a lack of reimbursement for these services (Bodenheimer & Grumbach, 2007). Regardless, results of this model are compelling and need to be promoted because the aging of the U.S. population will only result in increasing numbers of patients living with chronic illness.

APNs who see chronically ill patients, either in a primary care setting or in a specialty setting, improve care by coordinating the services patients receive from multiple providers. Chronic illnesses often affect several body systems or have numerous sequelae. Thus persons who are chronically ill often receive care from a primary care provider and several other clinicians including physicians and APN specialists, social workers, physical therapists, and dietitians. Without coordination, families coping with chronic illness can find themselves in an "agency maze" (Burton, 1995, p. 457). This vivid phrase captures the confusing experiences that ensue when the agencies and providers rendering care to a family do not communicate with one another. Families do not know where to go for help, and as a result, many resort to a trial-and-error approach to getting what they need. They often suffer the negative effects of misinformation, repetitive intake interviews, denial of service, conflicting approaches, and unsolved problems. A resource-savvy APN can often assess such situations and intervene to reduce stress, improve communications, and benefit patients and families. By contacting other providers to develop a coordinated management plan and by linking patients with suitable agencies, the APN can do much to relieve the burdens of chronic illness on a family.

Through the use of diverse approaches and individualized, interpersonal, and therapeutic interventions, APNs have the skills and resources to partner in managing populations throughout the care continuum from preventive care to the most complex care required by patients with chronic conditions. This is important in light of the increasing complexity of patients in today's society.

CONDITIONS CONDUCIVE TO PROVISION OF HIGH-QUALITY DIRECT CARE BY ADVANCED PRACTICE NURSES

Although APNs are committed to providing quality care, the conditions under which they work can impact their ability to provide that care. A discussion of some of these conditions follows.

Healthy Work Environments

It is becoming increasingly recognized that healthy work environments are necessary to achieve excellent nursing practice and safe, quality patient care and outcomes (American Association of Critical-Care Nurses, 2005; Registered Nurses' Association of Ontario, 2006). Standards such as true collaboration, skilled communication, developing authentic leaders, and professionalism in nursing are key to establishing healthy work environments. Many forms of system analysis, organizational redesign, planning, and coordination are needed to develop and sustain the processes of direct care that help patients attain good health outcomes at reasonable cost. APNs working in unhealthy environments can commit increased numbers of errors and can experience moral distress, burnout, frustration, and low morale. APNs have long recognized the need for development of organizational systems that support patient care processes, and they have actively participated in and often led such efforts.

Consultation, Collaboration, and Referral

Consultation, collaboration, and referral are crucial to high-quality direct care (Kleinpell et al., 2002). No single clinician can be knowledgeable about all the problems and issues that arise in daily practice, even in a specialized practice. Wise clinicians are aware of the limits of their knowledge and experience. Consulting with other providers who have special expertise, managing complex care as part of a team, and referring patients who have conditions or problems outside their scope of practice—or even outside their comfort zone—are actions that clinicians owe patients. Examples of strong collaborative teams are evident in perinatal care that demonstrate improved infant outcomes, cost savings, fewer operative deliveries, and fewer medical resources (Brooten et al., 2003; Jackson et al., 2003). These matters are addressed extensively in Chapters 7 and 10.

Clinical Guidelines

Evidence-based clinical practice guidelines can be useful decision-making and planning aids for clinicians. Many guidelines have been developed in close association with providers, are based on systematic and thorough reviews of research evidence, and have attained a balance between optimal care and economic reality. However, contractors also use clinical guidelines to ensure quality, limit variation, and control resource use. Guidelines should be based on research evidence that is evaluated and summarized by a credible panel, either inside or outside the system, to ensure that the guidelines serve to both incorporate science into practice and contain costs. Providers involved in the care of patients with the condition the guideline addresses should have the opportunity to adapt guidelines produced by others. Ideally, contractors and clinicians should review proposed guidelines and negotiate problematic recommendations in advance to avoid situations in which the care of the individual becomes the focus of negotiation. In addition, con-

tractors and clinicians should acknowledge that although the guidelines may serve most patients well, some patients will require treatment and interventions not recommended in the guidelines. An explicit method for advocating for individual needs should be available to clinicians.

Population-Based Data to Inform Practice

The hallmark of the APN role that differentiates it from other advanced nursing roles is the direct care that the APN provides in the patient interface. Although this is a key component of the role, it is expected that APNs also utilize a clinical prevention and population health focus (AACN, 2006). Clinical prevention refers to the health promotion and risk reduction components of individual health care that are learned as a result of aggregate population data. APNs are considered to be nursing leaders in achieving national health goals for individuals and populations. Interventions outlined in the *Healthy People 2010* campaign (U.S. Department of Health and Human Services, 2007) can frequently be instituted or recommended by APNs regardless of their roles or settings. Monitoring for current vaccinations, advocating for tobacco cessation with patients, assisting in healthy diets, and identifying opportunities for increasing physical activity are all population-identified behaviors that can be implemented at the individual level. These interventions are key to addressing the ever-rising disease rates of diabetes, obesity, lung cancer, and asthma. The *Healthy People 2010* website (*www.healthypeople.gov*) is a great resource for APNs and patients to identify basic health care information. In addition, APNs should be cognizant of the ever-changing information related to infectious diseases and emergency preparedness based on today's world climate.

APNs can use population trends to inform direct care and improve the assessments and interventions used at the direct care interface. Population data are frequently based on the diseases and conditions that are prevalent in the geographical setting in which the APN practices. Examples of this include the following:

- Monitoring for metabolic syndrome in the southeast United States
- Assessing for asthma in Virginia
- Surveillance for neurological disorders in Minnesota
- Cognizance of altitude-based disorders in mountain states

• High suspicion for tuberculosis in homeless patients with pulmonary symptoms living in densely populated urban settings

Aggregated, individual clinical outcomes are also useful in evaluation of program and practice effectiveness. By requiring that care administered and individual outcomes be documented in standardized ways, the health care system can conduct programmatic evaluations of clinical outcomes. Population-based evaluations can also be used by APNs to evaluate and improve the care they provide. Such evaluations can help answer questions such as "Is the specific care I/we provide patients the best way of managing their health or illness?" and "Are my/our patients doing as well as similar patients who are cared for by other providers?" Conducting such an evaluation involves (1) identifying groups of patients (i.e., populations) who have high costs of care, less than optimal outcomes, or both; (2) monitoring and analyzing variances in outcomes and costs; (3) examining processes of care to determine how management of the condition could be improved; and (4) incorporating management methods found to be effective in research or best practice networks.

To serve patients well, clinical recommendations must take into account the financial structure of the patient's health care plan. Thus APNs may need to familiarize themselves with how several financing systems work, as well as the specifics of several contractual agreements. Evaluation of the degree to which desirable outcomes are attained enables health care systems to compare their effectiveness with that of a comparable system or to evaluate the relative effectiveness of a new program or process of care. These kinds of evaluations and comparisons can lead to the identification of best practice methods at the health care system level. Use of services, readmission rates, complication rates, and average total cost per case are examples of population outcomes used in these kinds of evaluations and comparisons.

Contracts

The contractual arrangements APNs' practice groups enter into with various health care systems have become more complex in recent years. Although the specific nature of these contracts is beyond the scope of this chapter (see Chapter 20 for a more detailed discussion), APNs' direct care delivery is most definitely affected by the terms of these contracts. Providers are encouraged to practice preventive health care and constrain their use of costly services such as specialty referrals, hospitalization, and expensive technology. Financial incentives to avoid use of resources create a conflict of interest for providers, which may result in withholding of tests, treatments, and services from patients who really should have them. Thus the contractual arrangements that integrated health care delivery systems make between care provider groups along the continuum from acute to long-term care influence what, where, and how illness is managed.

An APN should know who negotiates and manages contracts for advanced practice nursing services in his or her organization. From the contracting manager the APN can learn who the top payers for advanced practice nursing services are, what managed care agreements have the most effect on the APN's service line, and how the rate of reimbursement relates to the cost of providing the service (e.g., which services/programs are operating within their reimbursement rate and which are not). The APN should ask to be informed when new contracts are being negotiated and when changes in existing contracts are under discussion so that solutions to problems can be sought and new opportunities can be explored.

CONCLUSION

The central competency of advanced practice nursing is direct care regardless of the specific role of CNS, NP, CRNA, or CNM. APNs are currently providing direct health care services that positively affect patients' health care outcomes and that are qualitatively different from those provided by other health care professionals. Of importance, these services are valued by the public and are cost-effective. APNs are able to offer this essential care through use of the six characteristics that make up APN direct care: use of a holistic perspective, formation of therapeutic partnerships with patients, expert clinical thinking and skillful performance, use of reflective practice, use of evidence as a guide to practice, and use of diverse approaches to health and illness management. Together, these characteristics form a solid foundation for providing scientifically based, person-centered, and outcome-validated health care. Research evidence supports each of these claims and hence substantiates the nursing profession's and the public's confidence in the care provided by APNs. As APNs continue to expand the scope and settings of their practice, it will be imperative that these six characteristics continue to be substantiated by solid research in each of the roles. In addition, research will be important in documenting the optimal "nurse dose" of APN intervention as we will continue to face challenges in caring for culturally diverse, aging, chronically ill populations.

REFERENCES

Aiken, L., Sochalski, J., & Lake, E. (1997). Studying outcomes of organizational change in health services. *Medical Care, 35*(Suppl.), NS6-NS18.

Aiken, L.H., Clarke, S.P., Sloane, D.M., Sochalski, J., & Silber J.H. (2002). Hospital nurse staffing and patient mortality, nurse burnout, and job satisfaction. *JAMA, 288*(16), 1987-1993.

Alasad, J., & Ahmad, M. (2005). Communication with critically ill patients. *Journal of Advanced Nursing, 50,* 356-362.

Allaire, A.D., Moos, M.K., & Wells, S.R. (2000). Complementary and alternative medicine in pregnancy: A survey of North Carolina certified nurse-midwives. *Obstetrics and Gynecology, 95,* 19-23.

Alpi, K.M. (2005). State health department websites: Rich resources for consumer health information. *Journal of Consumer Health on the Internet, 9,* 33-44.

American Academy of Pediatrics. (2007). *Children's health survey for asthma.* Elk Grove Village, IL: Author. Retrieved November 2, 2007, from www.aap.org/ research/chsa.htm.

American Association of Colleges of Nursing (AACN). (2006). *The essentials of doctoral education for advanced nursing practice.* Retrieved November 2, 2007, from www.aacn.nche.edu/DNP/pdf/Essentials.pdf.

American Association of Critical-Care Nurses. (2004). *Moral distress position statement.* Aliso Viejo, CA: Author.

American Association of Critical-Care Nurses. (2005). *AACN standards for establishing and sustaining healthy work environments.* Aliso Viejo, CA: Author.

American Holistic Nurses Association. (2007). *What is holistic nursing?* Retrieved November 2, 2007, from www.ahna.org/about/whatis.html.

American Nurses Association (ANA). (2003). *Nursing's social policy statement* (2nd ed.). Washington, DC: Author.

Armer, J.M. (2003). A case study of the use of telemedicine by advanced practice nurses in Missouri. *Journal of Continuing Education in Nursing, 34,* 226-233.

Astor, R., Jefferson, H., & Humphrys, K. (1998). Incorporating the service accomplishments into pre-registration curriculum to enhance reflective practice. *Nurse Education Today, 18,* 567-575.

Atkins, S., & Murphy, K. (1995). Reflective practice. *Nursing Standard, 9,* 31-37.

Ball, C., & Cox, C.L. (2003). Restoring patients to health: Outcomes and indicators of advanced nursing practice in adult critical care. Part 1. *International Journal of Nursing Practice, 9,* 356-367.

Barakzai, M.D., Gregory, J., & Fraser, D. (2007). The effect of culture on symptom reporting: Hispanics and irritable bowel syndrome. *Journal of the American Academy of Nurse Practitioners, 19,* 261-267.

Barnes, J. (2003). Quality, efficacy, and safety of complementary medicines: Fashions, facts and the future. Part I. Regulation and quality. *British Journal of Clinical Pharmacology, 55,* 226-233.

Beal, J.A. (2000). A nurse practitioner model of practice in the neonatal intensive care unit. *MCN The American Journal of Maternal Child Nursing, 25,* 18-24.

Benner, P.A. (1984). *From novice to expert: Excellence and power in clinical practice.* Menlo Park, CA: Addison-Wesley.

Benner, P.A., Hooper-Kyriakidis, P., & Stannard, D. (1999). *Clinical wisdom and interventions in critical care: A thinking-in-action approach.* Philadelphia: Saunders.

Benner, P.A., Tanner, C.A., & Chesla, C.A. (1996). *Expertise in nursing practice: Caring, clinical judgment, and ethics.* New York: Springer-Verlag.

Bialk, J.L. (2004). Ethical guidelines for assisting patients with end-of-life decision making. *MedSurg Nursing, 13,* 87-90.

Blasdell, A.L., Klunick, V., & Purseglove, T. (2002). The use of nursing and medical models in advanced practice: Does education affect the nurse practitioner's practice model? *Journal of Nursing Education, 41,* 231-233.

Bodenheimer, T., & Grumbach, K. (2007). *Improving primary care.* New York: McGraw-Hill/Lange.

Bodenheimer, T., Lorig, K., Holman, H., & Grumbach, K. (2002). Patient self-management of chronic disease in primary care. *JAMA, 288,* 2469-2475.

Bonamy, C., Schultz, P., Graham, K., & Hampton, M. (1995). The use of theory-based practice in the Department of Veterans' Affairs Medical Centers. *Journal of Nursing Staff Development, 11,* 27-30.

Brooten, D., Youngblut, J.M., Deatrick, J., Naylor, M., & York, R. (2003). Patient problems, advanced practice nurse (APN) interventions, time and contacts among five patient groups. *Journal of Nursing Scholarship, 35,* 73-79.

Brown, S.A., & Grimes, D.E. (1993). *Nurse practitioners and certified nurse-midwives: A meta-analysis of studies on nurses in primary care roles.* Washington, DC: American Nurses Publishing.

Brown, S.J. (1999). Patient-centered communication. *Annual Review of Nursing Research, 17,* 85-104.

Brown, S.J. (2001). Managing the complexity of best practice health care. *Journal of Nursing Care Quality, 15,* 1-8.

Brown, S.J. (2005). Direct clinical practice. In Hamric, A.B., Spross, J.A., & Hanson, C.M. (Eds.). *Advanced practice nursing: An integrative approach* (3rd ed.). Philadelphia: Saunders.

Brykczynski, K.A. (1989). An interpretive study describing the clinical judgment of nurse practitioners. *Scholarly Inquiry for Nursing Practice 3,* 75-104.

Brykczynski, K.A. (1991). Judgment strategies for coping with ambiguous clinical situations encountered in primary family care. *Journal of the American Academy of Nurse Practitioners, 3,* 79-84.

Bulechek, G.M., & McCloskey, J.C. (Eds.). (1999). *Nursing interventions classification: Effective nursing treatments* (3rd ed.). Philadelphia: Saunders.

Burman, M.E., Stepans, M.B., Jansa, N., & Steiner, S. (2002). How do NPs make clinical decisions? *The Nurse Practitioner, 27,* 57-64.

Burns, S.M., & Earven, S. (2002). Improving outcomes for mechanically ventilated medical intensive care unit patients using advanced practice nurses: A 6-year experience. *Critical Care Nursing Clinics of North America, 14,* 231-243.

Burton, D. (1995). Agency maze. In I.M. Lubkin (Ed.), *Chronic illness: Impact and interventions* (3rd ed., pp. 457-480). Boston: Jones & Bartlett.

Canadian Task Force on Preventive Health Care. (2007). *Evidence-based clinical prevention.* Retrieved November 2, 2007, from www.ctfphc.org/index.html.

Cherkin, D.C., Deyo, R.A., Sherman, K.J., Hart, L.G., Street, J.H., Hrbek, A., et al. (2002). Characteristics of visits to licensed acupuncturists, chiropractors, massage therapists, and naturopathic physicians. *Journal of the American Board of Family Practice, 16,* 463-472.

Chisholm, C.D., Collison, E.K., Nelson, D.R., & Cordell, W.H. (2001). Emergency department workplace interruptions: Are emergency physicians "interrupt-driven" and "multitasking"? *Academic Emergency Medicine, 7,* 1239-1243.

Clouder, L., & Sellars, J. (2004). Reflective practice and clinical supervision: An interprofessional perspective. *Journal of Advanced Nursing, 46,* 262-269.

Corley, M.C. (1995). Moral distress of critical care nurses. *American Journal of Critical Care, 4,* 280-285.

Courtney, R., & Rice, C. (1997). Investigation of nurse practitioner–patient interactions: Using the Nurse Practitioner Rating Form. *Nurse Practitioner, 22,* 46-48, 54-57, 60 (passim).

Croskerry, P. (2003). Cognitive forcing strategies in clinical decision-making. *Annals of Emergency Medicine, 41,* 110-121.

Cutilli, C.C. (2006). Accessing and evaluating the Internet for patient and family education. *Orthopaedic Nursing, 25,* 333-338.

Davidson, L.J., Bennett, S.E., Hamera, E.K., & Raines, B.K. (2004). What constitutes advanced assessment? *Journal of Nursing Education, 43,* 421-425.

Davies, E. (1995). Reflective practice: A focus for caring. *Journal of Nursing Education, 34,* 167-174.

Day, P.O., & Horton-Deutsch, S. (2004). Using mindfulness-based therapeutic interventions in psychiatric nursing practice. Part 1. Description and empirical support for mindfulness-based interventions. *Archives of Psychiatric Nursing, 18,* 164-169.

Dellasega, C., & Zerbe, T.M. (2002). Caregivers of frail rural older adults: Effects of an advanced practice nursing intervention. *Journal of Gerontological Nursing, 28,* 40-49.

DePalma, J.A. (2004). Advanced practice nurses' research competencies: Competency I—Using evidence in practice. *Home Health Care Management and Practice, 16,* 124-126.

DePhillips, H.A. III. (2007). Initiatives and barriers to adopting health information technology. *Disease Management and Health Outcomes, 15,* 1-6.

Dontje, K., Corser, W., Kreulen, G., & Teitelman, A. (2004). A unique set of interactions: The MSU sustained partnership model of nurse practitioner primary care. *Journal of the American Academy of Nurse Practitioners, 16,* 63-69.

Dossey, B.M. (2001). Holistic nursing: Taking your practice to the next level. *Nursing Clinics of North America, 36,* 1-22.

Dowdy, M.D., Robertson, C., & Bander, J.A. (1998). A study of proactive ethics consultation for critically and terminally ill patients with extended lengths of stay. *Critical Care Medicine, 26,* 252-259.

Ebright, P.R., Patterson, E.S., Chalko, B.A., & Render, M.L. (2003). Understanding the complexity of registered nurse work in acute care settings. *Journal of Nursing Administration, 33*(12), 630-638.

Eisenberg, D., Kessler, R., Foster, C., Norlock, F., Calkings, D., & Delbanco, T. (1993). Unconventional medicine in the United States. *New England Journal of Medicine, 328,* 246-252.

Eisenberg, D.M., Davis, R.B., Ettner, S.L., Appel, S., Von Rampay, M., & Kessler, R.C. (1998). Trends in alternative medicine in the United States, 1990-1997: Results of a follow-up national survey. *JAMA, 280,* 1569-1575.

Feldstein, A., Simon, S.R., Schneider, J., Krall, M., Laferriere, D., Smith, D.H., et al. (2004). How to design computerized alerts to ensure safe prescribing practices. *Joint Commission Journal on Quality and Safety, 30,* 602-613.

Flesner, M., & Clawson, J. (1998). Clinical management by family nurse practitioners and physicians in collaborative practice: A comparative analysis. In T.J. Sullivan (Ed.), *Collaboration: A health care imperative.* New York: McGraw-Hill.

Forrow, L., Arnold, R.M., & Parker, L.A. (1993). Preventive ethics: Expanding the horizons of clinical ethics. *The Journal of Clinical Ethics, 4,* 287-294.

Fowler, T.L. (2006). Alcohol dependence and depression: Advanced practice nurse interventions. *Journal of the American Academy of Nurse Practitioners, 18,* 303-308.

Frosch, D.L., Kaplan, R.M., & Felitti, V. (2001). The evaluation of two methods to facilitate shared decision making for men considering the prostate-specific antigen test. *Journal of General Internal Medicine, 16,* 391-398.

Gallagher, T.H., Waterman, A.D., Ebers, A.G., Fraser, V.J., & Levinson, W. (2003). Patients' and physicians' attitudes regarding the disclosure of medical errors. *JAMA, 289,* 1001-1007.

Geraghty, M. (2005). Nursing the unconscious patient. *Nursing Standard, 20,* 54-64.

Grando, V.T. (1998). Articulating nursing for advanced practice nursing. In T.J. Sullivan (Ed.), *Collaboration: A health care imperative.* New York: McGraw-Hill.

Hamric, A.B., Worley, D., Lindebak, S., & Jaubert, S. (1998). Outcomes associated with advanced nursing practice prescriptive authority. *Journal of the American Academy of Nurse Practitioners, 10,* 113-118.

Hanson, J.L., & Ashley, B. (1994). Advanced practice nurses' application of the Stetler Model for research utilization: Improving bereavement care. *Oncology Nursing Forum, 21,* 720-724.

Hawkins, J.W., Thibodeau, J.A., Utley-Smith, Q.E., Igou, J.F., & Johnson, E.E. (1993). Using a conceptual model for practice in a nursing wellness centre for seniors. *Perspectives, 17,* 11-16.

Hayes, K.M., & Alexander, I.M. (2000). Alternative therapies and nurse practitioners: Knowledge, professional experience, and personal use. *Holistic Nursing Practice, 14,* 49-58.

Hemsley, B., Sigafoos, J., Balandin, S., Forbes, R., Taylor, C., Green, V.A., et al. (2001). Nursing the patient with severe communication impairment. *Journal of Advanced Nursing, 35,* 827-835.

Henderson, K. (2006). TelEmergency: Distance emergency care in rural emergency departments using nurse practitioners. *Journal of Emergency Nursing, 32,* 388-393.

Henry, S.B., Holzemer, W.L., Randell, C., Hsieh, S.F., & Miller, T.J. (1997). Comparison of nursing interventions classification and current procedural terminology codes for categorizing nursing activities. *Image: The Journal of Nursing Scholarship, 29,* 133-138.

Hickey, M. (1990). The role of the clinical nurse specialist in the research utilization process. *Clinical Nurse Specialist, 4,* 93-96.

Hiltunen, E.F., Winder, P.A., Rait, M.A., Buselli, E.F., Carroll, D.L., & Rankin, S.H. (2005). Implementation of efficacy enhancement nursing interventions with cardiac elders. *Rehabilitation Nursing, 30,* 221-229.

Hoffman, L.A., Happ, M.B., Scharfenberg, C., diVirgilio-Thomas, D., & Tasota, F.J. (2004). Perceptions of physicians, nurses, and respiratory therapists about the role of acute care nurse practitioners. *American Journal of Critical Care, 13,* 480-488.

Hoffman, L.A., Tasota, F.J., Scharfenberg, C., Zullo, T.G., & Donahoe, M.P. (2003). Management of patients in the intensive care unit: Comparison via work sampling analysis of an acute care nurse practitioner and physicians in training. *American Journal of Critical Care, 12,* 436-443.

Holland, M.L., & Holland, E.S. (2007). Survey of Connecticut nurse-midwives. *Journal of Midwifery & Women's Health, 52,* 106-115.

Holman, H., & Lorig, K. (2004). Patient self-management: A key to effectiveness and efficiency in care of chronic disease. *Public Health Reports, 119,* 239-243.

Hravnak, M., Tuite, P., & Baldisseri, M. (2005). Expanding acute care nurse practitioner and clinical nurse specialist education: Invasive procedure training and human simulation in critical care. *AACN Clinical Issues, 16,* 89-104.

Hughes, L.C., Robinson, L., Cooley, M.E., Nuamah, I., Grobe, S.J., & McCorkle, R. (2002). Describing an episode of home nursing care for elderly postsurgical cancer patients. *Nursing Research, 51*(2), 110-118.

Institute of Medicine (IOM). (2000). Kohn, L.T., Corrigan, J.M., & Donaldson, M.S. (Eds.). *To err is human: Building a safer health system.* Washington, DC: National Academy Press.

Institute of Medicine (IOM). (2001). Committee on Quality of Health Care in America, W.C. Richardson (Chair) (Eds.). *Crossing the quality chasm: A new health system for the 21st century.* Washington, DC: National Academy Press.

Jackson, D.J., Lang, J.M., Swartz, W.H., Ganiats, T.G., Fullerton, J., Ecker, J., et al. (2003). Outcomes, safety, and resource utilization in a collaborative care birth center program compared with traditional physician-based perinatal care. *American Journal of Public Health, 93,* 999-106.

Jenkins, R.L., & White, P. (2001). Telehealth advanced nursing practice. *Nursing Outlook, 49,* 100-105.

Johns, C. (2000). *Becoming a reflective practitioner.* London: Blackwell Science.

Kemper, A.R., Uren, R.L., & Clark, S.J. (2006). Adoption of electronic health records in primary care pediatric practices. *Pediatrics, 118,* e20-e24.

Kim, H.S. (1999). Critical reflective inquiry for knowledge development in nursing practice. *Journal of Advanced Nursing, 29,* 1205-1212.

Kleinpell, R.M., Faut-Callahan, M., Lauer, K., Kremer, M.J., Murphy, M., & Sperhac, A. (2002). Collaborative practice in advanced practice nursing in acute care. *Critical Care Nursing Clinics of North America, 14,* 307-313.

Kovner, C., Jones, C., Zhan, C., Gergen, P.J., & Basu, J. (2002). Nurse staffing and postsurgical adverse events: An analysis of administrative data from a sample of U.S. hospitals, 1990-1996. *Health Services Research, 37,* 611-629.

Krauskopf, P.B., & Wyatt, T.H. (2006). Even techno-phobic NPs can use PDAs. *The Nurse Practitioner, 31,* 48-52.

Laabs, C.A. (2005). Moral problems and distress among nurse practitioners in primary care. *Journal of the American Academy of Nurse Practitioners, 17,* 76-83.

Lambing, A.Y., Adams, D.L.C., Fox, D.H., & Divine, G. (2004). Nurse practitioners' and physicians' care activities and clinical outcomes with an inpatient geriatric population. *Journal of the American Academy of Nurse Practitioners, 16,* 343-352.

Laschinger, H.K., & Duff, V. (1991). Attitudes of practicing nurses towards theory-based nursing practice. *Canadian Journal of Nursing Administration, 4,* 6-10.

Lawrence, M. (1995). The unconscious experience. *American Journal of Critical Care, 4,* 227-232.

Lawson, M.T. (2002). Nurse practitioner and physician communication styles. *Applied Nursing Research, 15,* 60-66.

Lea, D.H. (2006). Expanding nurses' roles in telemedicine and genetic services. *MCN The American Journal of Maternal Child Nursing, 31,* 185-189.

Liehr, P., & Smith, M.J. (1999). Middle range theory: Spinning research and practice to create knowledge for the new millennium. *Advances in Nursing Science, 14,* 81-91.

Lincoln, P.E. (2000). Comparing CNS and NP role activities: A replication. *Clinical Nurse Specialist, 14,* 269-277.

Lorig, K. (2003). Self-management education: More than a nice extra. *Medical Care, 41,* 699-701.

Lorig, K., Ritter, P.L., & Gonzalez, V. (2003). Hispanic chronic disease self-management: A randomized community-based outcome trial. *Nursing Research, 52,* 361-369.

Mackay, M.H. (1998). Research utilization and the CNS: Confronting the issues. *Clinical Nurse Specialist, 12,* 232-237.

Massachusetts Coalition for the Prevention of Medical Errors. (2006). *When things go wrong: Responding to adverse events.* Retrieved November 2, 2007, from www.macoalition.org.

Mast, M.E. (1995). Adult uncertainty in illness: A critical review of research. *Scholarly Inquiry for Nursing Practice, 9,* 3-24.

McCarthy, M.C. (2003). Situated clinical reasoning: Distinguishing acute confusion from dementia in hospitalized older adults. *Research in Nursing and Health, 26,* 90-101.

McCloskey, B., Grey, M., Deshefy-Longhi, T., & Grey, L.J. (2003). APRN practice patterns in primary care. *Nurse Practitioner, 28*(4), 39-44.

McCourt, C. (2006). Supporting choice and control? Communication and interaction between midwives and women at the antenatal booking visit. *Social Science and Medicine, 62,* 1307-1318.

McMullan, M. (2006). Patients using the Internet to obtain health information: How this affects the patient-health professional relationship. *Patient Education and Counseling, 63,* 24-28.

McNatt, G.E., & Easom, A. (2000). The role of the advanced practice nurse in the care of organ transplant recipients. *Advances in Renal Replacement Therapy, 7,* 172-176.

McNeal, G.J., & Walker, D. (2006). Enhancing success in advanced practice nursing: A grant-funded project. *Journal of Cultural Diversity, 13,* 10-19.

Meats, E., Brassey, J., Heneghan, C., & Glasziou, P. (2007). Using the Turning Research into Practice (TRIP) database: How do clinicians really search? *Journal of the Medical Library Association, 95,* 156-163.

Mion, L.C., Palmer, R.M., Meldon, S.W., Bass, D.M., Singer, M.E., Payne, S.M., et al. (2003). Case finding and referral model for emergency department elders: A randomized clinical trial. *Annals of Emergency Medicine, 41,* 69-71.

Morgan, M.W., Deber, R.B., Llewellyn-Thomas, H.A., Gladstone, P., Cusimano, R.J., O'Rourke, K., et al. (2000). Randomized, controlled trial of an interactive videodisc decision aid for patients with ischemic heart disease. *Journal of General Internal Medicine, 15,* 685-693.

Munro, N. (2004). Evidence-based assessment: No more pride or prejudice. *AACN Clinical Issues, 15,* 501-505.

Musclow, S.L., Sawhney, M., & Watt-Watson, J. (2002). The emerging role of advanced nursing practice in acute pain management throughout Canada. *Clinical Nurse Specialist, 16,* 63-66.

Naylor, M.D., Brooten, D., Campbell, R., Jacobsen, B.S., Mezey, M.D., Pauly, M.V., et al. (1999). Comprehensive discharge planning and home follow-up of hospitalized elders: A randomized clinical trial. *JAMA, 281,* 613-620.

Ndiwane, A., Miller, K.H., Bonner, A., Imperio, K., Matzo, M., McNeal, G., et al. (2004). Enhancing cultural competencies of advanced practice nurses: Health care challenges in the twenty-first century. *Journal of Cultural Diversity, 11,* 118-121.

Needleman, J., Buerhaus, P., Mattke, S., Steward, M., & Zelevinsky, K. (2002). Nurse-staffing levels and the quality of care in hospitals. *New England Journal of Medicine, 346,* 1715-1722.

Newman, M. (1997). Experiencing the whole. *Advances in Nursing Science, 20,* 34-39.

Ni, H., Simile, C., & Hardy, A.M. (2002). Utilization of complementary and alternative medicine by United States adults: Results from the 1999 National Health Interview Survey. *Medical Care, 40,* 353-358.

Nolan, T., Resar, R., Haraden, C., & Griffin, F.A. (2004). *Improving the reliability of health care.* IHI Innovation Series white paper. Cambridge, MA: Institute for Healthcare Improvement.

Norred, C.L. (2002). Complementary and alternative medicine use by surgical patients. *Journal of American Operating Room Nurses, 76,* 1013-1021.

O'Neill, E.S. (1995). Heuristics reasoning in diagnostic judgment. *Journal of Professional Nursing, 11,* 239-245.

Patterson, C., Kaczorowski, J., Arthur, H., Smith, K., & Mills, D.A. (2003). Complementary therapy practice: Defining the role of advanced nurse practitioners. *Journal of Clinical Nursing, 12,* 816-823.

Paul, R.W., & Heaslip, P. (1995). Critical thinking and intuitive nursing practice. *Journal of Advanced Nursing, 22,* 40-47.

Phillips, J. (2005). Neuroscience critical care: The role of the advanced practice nurse in patient safety. *AACN Clinical Issues, 16,* 581-592.

Pond, F. (1999). Searching for studies. In S.J. Brown (Ed.), *Knowledge for health care practice: A guide to using research evidence* (pp. 41-58). Philadelphia: Saunders.

Rector, T.S., Anand, I.S., & Cohn, J.N. (2006). Relationships between clinical assessments and patients' perceptions of the effects of heart failure on their quality of life. *Journal of Cardiac Failure, 12,* 87-92.

Redman, B.K., & Fry, S.T. (2000). Nurses' ethical conflicts: What is really known about them? *Nursing Ethics, 7,* 360-366.

Reed, K. (2005). Telemedicine: Benefits to advanced nursing practice and the communities they serve. *Journal of the American Academy of Nurse Practitioners, 17,* 176-180.

Registered Nurses' Association of Ontario. (2006). *Collaborative practice among nursing teams.* Toronto, Canada: Author.

Riegel, B., Dickson, V.V., Hoke, L., McMahon, J.P., Reis, B.F., & Sayers, S. (2006). A motivational counseling approach to improving heart failure self-care: Mechanisms of effectiveness. *Journal of Cardiovascular Nursing, 21, 232-241.*

Rolfe, G. (1997). Beyond expertise: Theory, practice, and the reflexive practitioner. *Journal of Clinical Nursing, 6,* 93-97.

Rosenfeld, P., McEvoy, M.D., & Glassman, K. (2003). Measuring practice patterns among acute care nurse practitioners. *Journal of Nursing Administration, 33*(3), 159-165.

Rushton, C.H. (2006). Defining and addressing moral distress: Tools for critical care nursing leaders. *AACN Advanced Critical Care, 17,* 161-168.

Ryan, P., & Lauver, D.R. (2002). The efficacy of tailored interventions. *Journal of Nursing Scholarship, 34,* 331-337.

Sackett, D.L. (1998). Evidence-based medicine. *Spine, 23,* 1085-1086.

Sappington, J., & Kelley, J.H. (1996). Modeling and role-modeling theory: A case of holistic care. *Journal of Holistic Nursing, 14,* 130-141.

Schön, D.A. (1992). *The reflective practitioner: How professionals think in action* (2nd ed.). San Francisco: Jossey-Bass.

Schwartz-Barcott, D., Patterson, B.J., Lusardi, P., & Farmer, B.C. (2002). From practice to theory: Tightening the link via three fieldwork strategies. *Journal of Advanced Nursing, 39,* 281-289.

Scott, G. N., & Elmer, G.W. (2002). Update on natural product–drug interactions. *American Journal of Health-System Pharmacy, 59,* 339-347.

Scott, R.A. (1999). A description of the roles, activities, and skills of clinical nurse specialists in the United States. *Clinical Nurse Specialist, 13,* 183-190.

Shuler, P.A., Huebscher, R., & Hallock, J. (2001). Providing wholistic health care for the elderly: Utilization of the Shuler Nurse Practitioner Practice Model. *Journal of the American Academy of Nurse Practitioners, 13,* 297-303.

Sidani, S., Doran, D., Porter, H., LeFort, S., O'Brien-Pallas, L.L., Zahn, C., et al. (2006). Processes of care: Comparison between nurse practitioners and physician residents in acute care. *Canadian Journal of Nursing Leadership, 19*(1), 69-85.

Sivesind, D., Parker, P.A., Cohen, L., Demoor, C., Bumbaugh, M., Throckmorton, T., et al. (2003). Communicating with patients in cancer care. *Journal of Cancer Education, 18,* 202-209.

Smith, M.J., & Liehr, P.R. (2003). *Middle range theory for nursing.* New York: Springer.

Sobralske, M., & Katz. J. (2005). Culturally competent care of patients with acute chest pain. *Journal of the American Academy of Nurse Practitioners, 17,* 342-349.

Sohn, P.M., & Loveland Cook, C.A. (2002). Nurse practitioner knowledge of complementary alternative health care: Foundation for practice. *Journal of Advanced Nursing, 39,* 9-16.

Stafford, R.S., & Blumenthal, D. (1998). Specialty differences in cardiovascular disease prevention practices. *Journal of the American College of Cardiology, 32,* 1238-1243.

Staggers, N., Thompson, C.B., & Snyder-Halpern, R. (2001). History and trends in clinical information systems in the United States. *Journal of Nursing Scholarship, 33,* 75-81.

Stein, R.E., & Jessop, D.J. (1990). Functional status II (R): A measure of child health status. *Medical Care, 28,* 1041-1055.

Stetler, C.B., Bautista, C., Vernale-Hannon, C., & Foster, J. (1995). Enhancing research utilization by clinical nurse specialists. *Nursing Clinics of North America, 30,* 457-473.

Swartz, M.K., Grey, M., Allan, J.D., Ridenour, N., Kovern, C., Walker, P.H., et al. (2003). A day in the lives of APNs in the U.S. *The Nurse Practitioner, 28,* 32-39.

Tanner, C.A. (2006). Thinking like a nurse: A research-based model of clinical judgment in nursing. *Journal of Nursing Education, 45*(6), 204-211.

Tanner, C.A., Benner, P., Chesla, C., & Gordon, D.R. (1993). The phenomenology of knowing a patient. *Image: The Journal of Nursing Scholarship, 25,* 273-280.

Tesch, B.J. (2002). Herbs commonly used by women: An evidence-based review. *Disease-A-Month: DM, 48,* 671-696.

Thomas, L.A. (2003). Clinical management of stressors perceived by patients on mechanical ventilation. *AACN Clinical Issues, 14,* 73-81.

U.S. Department of Health and Human Services. (2007). *Healthy People 2010.* Retrieved November 2, 2007, from www.healthypeople.gov.

U.S. Preventive Services Task Force. (1996). *Guide to clinical preventive services: Report of the U.S. Preventive Services Task Force* (2nd ed.). Baltimore: Williams & Wilkins.

U.S. Preventive Services Task Force. (2003). *Guide to clinical preventive services: Report of the U.S. Preventive Services Task Force* (3rd ed.). Baltimore: Williams & Wilkins.

Verger, J.T., Marcoux, K.K., Madden, M.A., Bojko, T., & Barnsteiner, J.H. (2005). Nurse practitioners in pediatric critical care: Results of a national survey. *AACN Clinical Issues, 16,* 396-408.

Vincent, C. (2003). Understanding and responding to adverse events. *New England Journal of Medicine, 348,* 1051-1056.

Waite, M.S., Harker, J.O., & Messerman, L.I. (1994). Interdisciplinary team training and diversity: Problems, concepts and strategies. In D. Wieland, D. Benton, B.J. Kramer, & G.D. Dawson (Eds.), *Cultural diversity and geriatric health care: Challenges to the health care professions* (pp. 68-82). New York: Haworth Press.

Ward, S., Donovan, H.S., Owen, B., Grosen, E., & Serlin, R. (2000). An individualized intervention to overcome patient-related barriers to pain management in women with gynecologic cancers. *Research in Nursing and Health, 23,* 393-405.

Ware, J.E., & Sherbourne, C.D. (1992). The MOS 36-item short form health survey (SF-36): I. Conceptual framework and item selection. *Medical Care, 30,* 473-483.

Whittemore, R., & Roy, C. (2002). Adapting to diabetes mellitus: A theory synthesis. *Nursing Science Quarterly, 15,* 311-317.

Wilbright, W.A., Haun, D.E., Romano, T., Krutzfeldt, T., Fontenot, C.E., & Nolan, T.E. (2006). Computer use in an urban university hospital: Technology ahead of literacy. *Computers, Informatics, Nursing: CIN, 24,* 37-43.

Witman, A.B., Park, D.M., & Hardin, S.B. (1996). How do patients want physicians to handle mistakes? A survey of internal medicine patients in an academic setting. *Archives of Internal Medicine, 156,* 2565-2569.

Wolf, Z.R., & Robinson-Smith, G. (2007). Strategies used by clinical nurse specialists in "difficult" clinician-patient situations. *Clinical Nurse Specialist, 21,* 74-84.

Wong, F.K.Y., Loke, A.Y., Wong, M., Tse, H., Kan, E., & Kember, D. (1997). An action research study into the development of nurses as reflective practitioners. *Journal of Nursing Education, 36,* 476-481.

Yeager, S., Shaw, K.D., Casavant, J., & Burns, S.M. (2006). An acute care nurse practitioner model of care for neurosurgical patients. *Critical Care Nurse, 26,* 57-64.

CHAPTER 6

Expert Coaching and Guidance

Judith A. Spross

INTRODUCTION

Patient education is a central and well-documented function of all nurses in any setting, and evidence of its effectiveness is well established (Lindemann, 1988; Redman, 2004; Theis & Johnson, 1995). Patient education provided by advanced practice nurses (APNs) is best conceptualized as interpersonal processes of expert coaching and guidance through life transitions such as illness, childbearing, and bereavement. National initiatives aimed at improving quality and safety emphasize patient empowerment or activation and patient-centered care (Institute of Medicine [IOM], 2001; Milbank Memorial Fund and the Center for the Advancement of Health [Milbank report],[1] 1999; Nolan, Resar, Haraden, & Griffin, 2004; Robert Wood Johnson Foundation [RWJ report],[2] 2000), which are key elements of coaching.

To provide patient-centered care, health professionals are supposed to demonstrate that they can do the following (Greiner & Knebel, 2003):

> Identify, respect and care about patients' differences, values, preferences and expressed needs; relieve pain and suffering; coordinate continuous care; listen to, clearly inform, communicate and educate patients; share decision making and management and continuously advocate disease prevention, wellness and promotion of health lifestyles, including a focus on population health. (p. 4)

These competencies are consistent with expectations of health professionals (HealthSciences Institute, 2005; 2007) and of APNs' direct care and coaching competencies (American Association of Colleges of Nursing [AACN], 2006). In addition, programs to help patients manage chronic illnesses suggest that APNs play a role in activating or motivating patients to make changes in their lifestyles (Brooten et al., 2002; Brooten, Youngblut, Deatrick, Naylor, & York, 2003; Brooten & Youngblut, 2006; Litaker et al., 2003;

Parry, Kramer, & Coleman, 2006). APNs' skill in expert coaching and guidance will be central to efforts to redesign and transform health care systems to become more patient-centered.

Teaching and coaching are recognized as core competencies of APNs (AACN, 2006; National Association of Clinical Nurse Specialists [NACNS], 2004; National Organization of Nurse Practitioner Faculties [NONPF], 2006; National Panel on Acute Care Nurse Practitioner Competencies, 2004; National Panel for Psychiatric Mental Health NP Competencies, 2003). Spross and colleagues synthesized their own practice and teaching experiences with interdisciplinary theoretical, research, and clinical literature to develop a model of coaching: Coaching through transitions is the complex, interpersonal process APNs use to enlist patients' active and effective participation in their care (Clarke & Spross, 1996; Spross, 2005; Spross, Clarke, & Beauregard, 2000). In this chapter, the use of the terms *coach* and *coaching*, rather than *education*, is deliberate because these terms imply the existence of a relationship that is fundamental to effective teaching. Coaching people through transitions is a relatively invisible, intangible, but complex process that must be made more explicit if APNs are to be seen by consumers and policymakers as a solution to health policy concerns such as access to and continuity of care and if they are to secure reimbursement for the care they provide.

Numerous resources exist to help APNs develop and implement educational programs for individuals and groups and therefore are not included here. This chapter focuses on the APN competency of expert coaching and guidance. Strategies for acquiring and implementing the skills needed to coach effectively are presented. Selected issues in guidance and coaching are discussed. Although the primary focus of the chapter is on coaching of patients and families, applications of the coaching model to student and staff education are also discussed.

---

[1]Hereafter called the *Milbank report*.
[2]Hereafter called the *RWJ report*.

EXPERT COACHING AND GUIDANCE BY ADVANCED PRACTICE NURSES

Many studies document the nature, focus, content, and amount of time APNs spend in teaching and counseling, as well as the outcomes of these interventions (see Chapter 24). Teaching and counseling are significant clinical activities in nurse-midwifery (Holland & Holland, 2007; Scupholme, Paine, Lang, Kumar, & DeJoseph, 1994) and clinical nurse specialist (CNS) (Parry et al., 2006; Scott, 1999) practice. Studies of nurse practitioners (NPs) indicate that they spend a significant proportion of their direct care time in teaching and counseling (Brown, 1995; Brown & Waybrant, 1988; Lincoln, 2000; Mezey, Dougherty, Wade, & Mersmann, 1994). A study of NP students revealed that many of their interventions were also directed toward education. Of 3733 patient visits, Knowledge Deficit was one of the top four nursing diagnoses made by NP students (O'Connor, Hameister, and Kershaw, 2000). Using the Nursing Intervention Classification (NIC) system, O'Connor and colleagues (2000) also found that patient education was one of the top four intervention classifications used by NP students. A study of an APN telephone intervention to enhance recovery of patients post–cardiac surgery showed no effect on the outcomes measured (health-related quality of life, symptom distress, satisfaction with care, and unexpected health care contacts) (Tranmer & Parry, 2004). This may have been because the same APNs delivered some of the "usual care" (preparing for discharge) in addition to providing the intervention of telephone follow-up, so the intervention may not have been different enough from usual care.

Quantitative studies, qualitative studies, and anecdotal reports suggest that coaching patients and staff through transitions is embedded in the practices of nurses, including APNs (Barnsteiner, Gillis-Donovan, Knox-Fischer, & McKlindon, 1994; Benner, Hooper-Kyriakidis, & Stannard, 1999; Dick & Frazier, 2006) and that APN-led patient education and monitoring programs for specific clinical populations indicate that patient education and coaching are central to their effectiveness (Brooten et al., 2002; Crowther, 2003; George et al., 1999; Larson, Neverett, & Larsen, 2001; Parry et al., 2006).

The Quality-Cost Model of Early Discharge and Nurse Specialist/Advanced Practice Nurse Transitional Care

Readers should become familiar with the program of research conducted by Brooten, Naylor, and others to examine the impact of APN care on various clinical populations (Brooten et al., 1986, 1988, 1994, 2002, 2003). These studies provide substantive evidence of the range and focus of teaching activities undertaken by CNSs and NPs who provided interventions to patients across several studies. Controlled trials of APN care that involved teaching and coaching activities have demonstrated statistically significant differences in patient outcomes and resource use (Brooten et al., 1986, 1994; Naylor et al., 1999). Interventions in these studies occurred in hospitals and during the post-discharge period. APNs in these studies used a holistic focus that requires clinical expertise (including sufficient patient contact), interpersonal competence, and systems leadership skills to improve outcomes (Brooten et al., 2003). Early work in this program of research documented that APNs provided teaching and counseling during face-to-face contacts in the home and through regular telephone contact, services that were regarded by researchers as critical (Brooten et al., 1986). Analysis of CNSs' interventions revealed that 68% could be categorized as teaching (Brooten et al., 1988, 1991). Other types of interventions were liaison, consultation, and referral; encouragement of self-care and infant care; and reassurance and reinforcement of the patient's actions (Brooten et al., 1988, 1991). Secondary analysis of data identified the interventions APNs delivered to five clinical populations in the studies of transitional care: older adults, women with high-risk pregnancies or those who have had cesarean deliveries, women who have had hysterectomies, and very-low-birth-weight infants (Brooten et al., 2003; Naylor, Bowles, & Brooten, 2000). Using the Omaha classification system, the investigators classified 9488 APN interventions. They identified four categories of problems: the environment, psychosocial, physiological, and human-related behavior. They also identified four categories of interventions: health teaching, guidance, and/or counseling; treatments and procedures; case management; and surveillance (Brooten et al., 2003). Across groups, the most frequent intervention was surveillance; health teaching was the second or third most frequent intervention, depending on the patient population. The focus of teaching was usually related to the issues for which the APN was providing surveillance.

The Care Transitions Intervention Model

Coleman (a physician) and colleagues described a model of transitional care for patients with chronic illness that used fewer resources such as APN time and is, therefore, less expensive (Coleman & Berenson,

2004; Coleman et al., 2004; Coleman, Parry, Chalmers, & Min, 2006; Parry et al., 2006). This model builds on the work of Brooten, Naylor, and others cited earlier. Transitional care has been defined as "a set of actions designed to ensure the coordination and continuity of health care as patients transfer between different locations or different levels of care within the same location" (American Geriatrics Society, 2002). The Care Transitions Model is based on four concepts or pillars: medication self-management; use of a dynamic patient-centered record (called the *personal health record* or *PHR*); follow-up with providers; and knowledge/self-management of one or more conditions. This model has two key components—structured interactions with a transition coach (an APN or RN "trained in education and advocacy with older adults" [Parry et al., 2006]) and a PHR. The structured interactions consisted of weekly visits to the patient in the hospital or rehabilitation setting; a home visit that occurred within 48 to 72 hours of discharge; three follow-up phone calls at 2, 7, and 14 days post-discharge; and 24-hour access to the transition coach. Coaches did not function as health care providers—rather, they were facilitators and educators who taught and encouraged patients to become more active and informed participants in their care. Patients were taught to pay attention to factors that made them vulnerable during transitions, ways to manage their chronic condition (including "red flags"—what signs and symptoms they could self-manage and which of these to report), and how to communicate with providers. Similar to the studies by Brooten, Naylor, and others, outcomes for the 976 patients in this study improved (e.g., reduced rehospitalizations).

More research on the process of patient coaching used by APNs and how it promotes adherence to therapies and self-care is needed. The observations that education and coaching generally improve outcomes and that telephone follow-up has been one of the important APN activities in studies of APN care and patient outcomes (Brooten et al., 2003; George et al., 1999; Naylor et al., 1999) suggest several directions for research. Evidence that APNs make a difference in outcomes for older adults has led to a call for health policy changes that would require employment of more APNs in long-term care to provide direct care as well as educate and coach staff and families in meeting the health care needs of this vulnerable population (Wells, 2002).

Studies that identify the process and the "dose" of APN-delivered interventions (Brooten & Youngblut,

2006)—as well as the differential effects and costs of APN coaching, registered nurse coaching, and coaching by other clinicians—are needed. The effects of Internet-based information and education and the role of APNs in helping patients use this information effectively should be studied. Finally, effective strategies for teaching patients who are illiterate must be identified.

The foregoing selective review supports the premise that expert guidance and coaching are key foci of the APN's direct care role. Expert coaching and guidance are broad competencies of which patient education about disease, symptom management, preparation for procedures, and other issues is a part. APNs must understand the basic principles of patient education and the specific educational needs of their clinical populations. To be effective coaches, APNs must be aware of the research in their specialties and be responsible for knowing the theoretical and scientific bases for patient teaching and coaching in their specialties and practice settings. Examples of APNs' integration of specialty knowledge with principles of patient education to operationalize the coaching competency are incorporated in the chapters on the different APN roles in Part III.

COACHING THROUGH TRANSITIONS: A SYNTHESIS OF THEORETICAL PERSPECTIVES

Coaching: An Interdisciplinary Perspective

The word *coach* is derived from the Middle English word *coche,* meaning "wagon or carriage, a means of conveyance from one destination to another." Modern use of *coach* to mean a *teacher* is apt: a coach facilitates the safe passage of a person in transition from one situation to another. Coaching is complex interpersonal work that helps people who are facing personal transitions or journeys. These meanings of coaching can be applied to nurse-patient, faculty-student, preceptor-student, and mentor-protégé relationships.

Coaching has been used in several disciplines to describe interactions between experts and learners that focus on developing the learner's knowledge and skill in an area that is within the coach's expertise (Frisch, Elliott, Atsaides, Salva, & Denney, 1982; Hops, 1983; Pelligrini & Urbain, 1985; Spross, 1994; Wells-Federman, Stuart-Shor, & Webster, 2001). A review of interdisciplinary literature supports the use of *coach* and *coaching* as terms that describe the teaching functions of APNs and inform the elucidation of the

Model of APN Expert Coaching and Guidance described on p. 167. The fact that *coach* and *coaching* are common terms may also make it easier for APNs to communicate with consumers and policymakers about what they do. Because the nature of coaching by nurses and APNs and the "mechanism of action" by which APN coaching works to facilitate or activate patient behavior change are not well understood, selected observations made about coaching in other disciplines are discussed.

In sports, coaches create and present complex challenges that develop athletes' physical and psychological capacities while providing support and motivation (Lombardo, 1987; Sullivan & Wilson, 1991) and use their interpersonal and leadership skills to strengthen athletes' performance and self-concept (Lombardo, 1987). Coaches can do this, in part, because they themselves are competent, secure in their self-concepts, and self-accepting (Lombardo, 1987). A recent integrative review of sports coaching resulted in a coaching schematic that included roles, goals, typical actions, required knowledge, and factors influencing coach development (Abraham, Collins, & Martindale, 2006).

Situations that require expert coaching are those in which the problems are complex: a technical solution is unavailable and would be inadequate anyway, and the problem demands adaptive work (Heifetz, 1994). Coaching can be viewed as identifying the adaptive task and helping people uncover opportunities for personal growth by helping them clarify their goals, decide what matters most to them, acknowledge trade-offs and losses, and develop coping strategies. Becoming a parent, losing a job, adjusting to and living with a chronic illness, coping with national disasters and traumatic losses, and facing impending death are examples of transitions requiring complex, adaptive work that can be facilitated by APNs.

In a qualitative study of nurses' clinical experiences, Benner (1984) identified the teaching-coaching role as one of seven domains of nursing practice. Subsequent studies, based on Benner's work, have confirmed that APNs demonstrate this role as part of their practice (Benner et al., 1999; Dick & Frazier, 2006; Fenton, 1984; Fenton & Brykczynski, 1993; Steele & Fenton, 1988). Benner (1985) elaborated on the teaching-coaching role of APNs who work with patients with chronic illness: "Coaches learn what the illness means to the individual, what the adaptive demands, tasks, and resources are for the patient at different stages in the illness" (p. 43). APNs use their knowledge of a patient and knowledge from previous experiences with similar patients to craft patient-specific coaching interventions.

Other nurses have used the term *coaching* to characterize the nature of nurses' relational, therapeutic interventions with patients. Table 6-1 summarizes selected nursing conceptualizations of coaching. These descriptions of coaching by nurses are consistent with the concepts of coaching from other disciplines discussed previously. In describing coaching as the interpersonal process nurses use to help those who suffer, Spross (1996) summarized the elements of the nurse-patient relationship connoted by the term *coaching*:

> Coaching captures the essence of the relationships nurses create with patients on which their effectiveness depends.... It is a term that permits the experience of intense emotions on both sides; it captures the temporal nature of the relationship (which may be brief or extended); it suggests both the one-sided aspect (the coach has information and expertise needed by the patient) and the mutuality (opportunities for personal growth) in the relationship; and it conveys the contractual or voluntary nature of the relationship (if the relationship is not working despite the best efforts of both, another coach may need to be found). (pp. 197-198)

This brief overview speaks to the complexity of the process of coaching and the importance of tailoring coaching and guidance to the particular needs of patients. The interdisciplinary perspective can help APNs deepen their understanding of coaching and articulate coaching processes. It is clear that the coaching competency is inextricably linked with the direct clinical care competency. Coaching can be viewed as a relational, multidimensional process that involves all aspects of being human—cognitive, affective, behavioral, physical, social, and spiritual. In the process of delivering care, APNs are coaching patients, their families, staff, colleagues, and even themselves.

Transitions

Transitions—physiological, developmental, situational, and organizational—make up the natural course of human lives. Transitions are paradigms for life and living. Like life, they may be predictable or unpredictable, joyous or painful, obvious or barely perceptible, chosen and welcomed or unexpected and feared. Bridges (1980), in a classic text on change and transition, described three phases of transition: an ending or leaving; a period of chaos, confusion,

Table 6-1 NURSING CONCEPTUALIZATIONS OF COACHING

	Benner (1985)	Spross (1994)	Wilkie et al. (1995)	Carrieri-Kohlman et al. (1996)	Lewis & Zahlis (1997)	Benner et al. (1999)
Purpose/focus of coaching	To teach and coach patients	To ameliorate suffering	To teach patients with lung cancer to report pain perception and changes in pain perceptions to clinicians	To increase patients' self-efficacy in performing exercises and decrease anxiety to decrease dyspnea	To help clients (patients and significant others) process thoughts and feelings related to breast cancer experience; to enhance cognitive-behavioral management and self-care skills	An embodied clinical leadership skill in which relational skills are used to help others in their understanding, their judgment, their skilled know-how, and their openness to seeing new possibilities
Characteristics or elements of the coaching interaction or protocol	Capturing readiness to learn. Assisting patients to integrate implications of illness and recovery. Eliciting patients' understanding of situation. Providing interpretation of each patient's condition and giving a rationale for procedures. Making culturally avoided aspects of an illness approachable and understandable	Permits the experience of intense emotions on both sides. Temporal aspects of the relationship (brief or extended). Relationship is both one-sided (nurse has knowledge and skills needed by patient) and mutual (relationship is an opportunity for personal growth for nurse and patient). Relationship is, at least theoretically, voluntary and contractual	Encourages patients to mark a self-assessment tool to record pain intensity. Encourages patients to report pain characteristics to clinicians. Emphasizes and reinforces that pain characteristics reported by patients are important for clinicians' pain treatment decisions	Nurse coach teaches coping skills. Nurse coach collaborates with patient to set goals for exercise session based on prior performance and clinical factors. Nurse coach teaches relaxation and breathing exercises. Nurse coach reinforces information given and encourages patients	Attending to the story. Encircling the experience. Inviting the work. Exploring solutions. Anchoring the skill through feedback, self-monitoring, and homework. Setting up success	Envisions realistic possibilities. Makes excellent judgment. Is able to balance patient's need for safety with team members' need to learn. Is able to help others learn to interpret, forecast, and respond to patient transitions
Type of article/book	Qualitative research	Theoretical synthesis	Quantitative research (pilot study)	Quantitative research (experimental design)	Qualitative research	Qualitative research

and distress; and a new beginning. Bridges indicated that, for some people, "transitionality" might be a semipermanent state. Schumacher and Meleis (1994) asserted that transition is a central concept in nursing, and Chick and Meleis (1986) offered a clinically useful definition of it:

> Transition is a passage from one life phase, condition, or status to another.... Transition refers to both the process and outcome of complex person-environment interactions. It may involve more than one person and is embedded in the context and the situation. (pp. 239-240)

Chick and Meleis (1986) also characterized the process of transition as having phases during which individuals experience (1) a disconnectedness from their usual social supports, (2) a loss of familiar reference points, (3) old needs that remain unmet, (4) new needs, and (5) old expectations that are no longer congruent with the changing situation. Becoming a parent, giving up cigarettes, learning how to cope with chronic illness, and dying in comfort and dignity are just a few examples of transitions. Transitions can also be characterized according to type, conditions, and universal properties. Schumacher and Meleis (1994) have identified nursing therapeutics that support or facilitate transitions, and education is one of them. Other models and concepts inform the author's conceptualization of APN coaching through transition (Table 6-2).

A Typology of Transitions. Schumacher and Meleis (1994) proposed that nurses are involved in four categories of transitions: developmental, health/illness, situational, and organizational. *Developmental transitions* are those that reflect life-cycle transitions, such as adolescence, parenthood, and aging. For the purposes of discussing coaching by APNs, developmental transitions are considered to include any transition with an intrapersonal focus, including changes in life cycle, self-perception, motivation, expectations, or meanings.

Health/illness transitions were described by Schumacher and Meleis (1994) primarily as illness-related and range from adapting to a chronic illness to returning home after a stay in the hospital. Such transitions can include modifying risk factors, adapting to the physiological and psychological demands of pregnancy, and numerous other clinical phenomena. Some health/illness changes are self-limiting (e.g., the physiological changes of pregnancy), whereas others are long-term and may be reversible or irreversible. Although Schumacher and Meleis excluded acute self-limiting illnesses (e.g., a cold) from the notion of transition, other variables are likely to influence whether a transition occurs as a result of a self-limiting illness (e.g., if a cold prevents a person from attending an important event). Because health/illness transitions are often the primary incentive for seeking health care, these are discussed in more detail.

In this chapter, health/illness transitions are defined as transitions that are driven by an individual's experience of the body in a holistic sense. Prior "embodied" experiences may play a role in the expression or the trajectory of a patient's health/illness experience. Alonzo (2000), based on the results of studies of patients with acute myocardial infarctions, has proposed a model of the impact of cumulative adversity on the course of chronic illness and individuals' abilities to cope. For example, the memory of the stress of repeated, invasive procedures experienced during one hospitalization for treatment of an acute myocardial infarction (AMI) may prevent a patient from seeking timely health care for a subsequent AMI. Some health care experiences may elicit or reactivate posttraumatic stress disorder or other significant emotional responses in vulnerable individuals (Alonzo, 2000; Capasso, 1998).

In the adverse childhood experiences (ACE) study (Felitti, 2002; Felitti et al., 1998), the impact of adverse experiences in childhood, such as abuse and trauma, on adults' health was examined. Health concerns such as smoking and obesity appear to have strong relationships with adverse childhood experiences. In a clinical case study analyzed in light of the ACE study findings, Felitti (2002) proposed a reordering of the patient's health problems. Although diabetes and hypertension were the "presenting concerns" in a 70-year-old woman, Felitti suggested that the childhood sexual abuse (uncovered during history taking) be the treatment priority. Effective treatment of the other illnesses would depend on acknowledging this history and guiding the patient to appropriate therapy.

These studies suggest that APNs' assessment of health/illness transition experiences may be even more complicated than our existing understanding of chronic illness and trauma. Felitti (2002) acknowledged that this understanding of illness, especially chronic conditions, is daunting for providers, especially those in primary care. Nevertheless, theories regarding adverse experiences in childhood and in health care and the potential for cumulative trauma and complex

Table 6-2 Models and Concepts That Informed Conceptualization of Coaching Through Transition

Model or Concept	Author(s)	Comments
Chronic illness trajectory framework	Corbin & Strauss (1992)	Describes principles of framework; Chronic illness has a course that varies over time; Nurses collaborate with patients to shape the trajectory
Cumulative adversity and posttraumatic stress disorders	Alonzo (2000)	Describes potential adverse impact of multiple health care experiences in patients who have had myocardial infarctions; Proposes model for understanding cumulative adversity
Adverse childhood experiences	Felliti (2002); Felliti et al. (1998)	Provides evidence of impact of childhood trauma on adult health
Self-help model	Braden (1990, 1993)	Describes five stages of response to chronic illness; Notes that nursing interventions can facilitate the acquisition of self-help behaviors
Transtheoretical model of change	Prochaska et al. (1994)	Describes phases of behavioral change
Self-care in chronic illness model	Connelly (1993)	Is an extension of health belief model
Transitional care	Brooten et al. (1988); Brooten et al. (2003); Coleman et al., 2004, Lamm et al. (1991); Naylor et al. (1999)	Describes discharge from hospital to home as a transition that can be shaped by nursing interventions
Self-efficacy	Bandura (1977); Carrieri-Kohlman et al. (1996); Clark & Dodge (1999); Lev (1997); McDougall (1999)	Addresses interaction among factors that influence behavior change; Accounts for changes in motivation, self-confidence, and behavior that result from interventions
Patient-centered communication (PCC)	Brown (1999); Squier (1990)	Describes empirical support for components of PCC (see Box 6-1)
Motivational interviewing	Borelli (2006); Lorig et al. (1999)	Interactions aimed at eliciting reasons for ambivalence regarding behavior change and for increased motivation for adopting new behaviors
Comforting-interaction relationship model	Morse et al. (1997)	Addresses patient and nurse factors; Notes that comforting relationship is negotiated by means of nurse-patient interactions
Therapeutic relationships	Peplau (1952); Travelbee (1971)	Addresses existential and spiritual aspects of relationship
Transition experiences	Benner et al. (1999), Chick & Meleis (1986); Coleman et al. (2004); Schumacher & Meleis (1994)	Delineates types and process of transitions

emotional and physical responses may help us better understand the nature and outcomes of coaching.

The other types of transitions described by Schumacher and Meleis (1994) are *situational transitions* and *organizational transitions*. Situational transitions include changes in educational, professional, and family roles and transitions that occur as a result of changes in intangible or tangible structures or resources (e.g., role changes and financial reversals) that are specific to individuals and their relationships. *Organizational transitions* are those that occur in the environment—within agencies, between agencies, or in society—and reflect changes in structures and resources at a system level. *Health/illness, developmental,* and *situational* transitions are the ones most likely to lead to clinical encounters between APNs and patients in which expert coaching is required. However, APNs must also be skilled in dealing with organizational transitions, which tend to affect structural and contextual aspects of providing care. Wise APNs pay attention to all four types of transitions in their personal and professional lives, because transitions can affect the development and effectiveness of APNs' expert coaching.

In practice, the APN is aware of the possibility of multiple transitions occurring as a result of one salient transition. While eliciting information on the primary transition that led the patient to seek care, the APN is attending to verbal, nonverbal, and intuitive cues to identify other transitions and meanings associated with the primary one. Attending to the possibility of multiple transitions enables the APN to tailor coaching to the individual's particular needs and concerns. Table 6-3 lists some situations, based on this typology, that require APN coaching.

Characteristics, Conditions, and Outcomes of Transitions. Transitions can be characterized along the dimensions of time, the nature of the process that occurs, and the type of change that occurs (Schumacher & Meleis, 1994). All transitions seem to unfold over time, as opposed to being one-time events. A single event may precipitate the transition, but the transition is experienced over some period of time. The process that occurs is directional, entailing movement from one state to another, and is often described as occurring in stages. The type of change tends to be substantive and internal, rather than incidental or superficial; transitions affect personal identities, roles, relationships, functional status, and behaviors (Schumacher & Meleis, 1994). The experience of transition can vary considerably for both individuals and groups and from one day to the next as a result of conditions that affect the transition (Corbin & Strauss, 1992; Schumacher & Meleis, 1994).

Outcomes of transitions proposed by Schumacher and Meleis (1994) include subjective well-being, role mastery, and well-being of relationships. Quality-of-care outcomes can also be used as indicators of successful transitions. Increasingly, this notion of transition is informing the way we think about health care as patients move across providers and settings (American Geriatrics Society, 2002; Coleman & Berenson, 2004). When one considers the direct, individual effects of coaching by APNs, the most relevant outcomes are those that are patient-related. Examples include morbidity; mortality; medical complications; comfort; functional, physiological, or mental status; stress level; coping strategies; quality of

Table **6-3**   Transition Situations That Require Coaching

Health/Illness	Developmental	Situational	Organizational
Pregnancy/labor	Parenting	Job loss or change	Mergers
Hospitalization	Adverse childhood	Divorce	Policy changes
Risk reduction	experiences	Natural disasters/national	Change in leadership
Lifestyle changes	Puberty	disasters	Change in organizational
Chronic condition	Suffering	Quality of life	structure
Disability	Loss of significant	Change in social supports	
Weight loss or	others	Social isolation	
gain	Caregiving for older	Financial reversals or	
Symptoms	relatives	windfalls	
Violence	Changes in sexual	Change in living situations	
	function or activity	Community trauma	

NOTE: The situations are categorized according to the initiating change. Many of these transitions have reciprocal impacts across categories.

life; adherence to treatment; patient satisfaction; and caregiver burden (Kolcaba, 1992; Lang & Marek, 1992; Naylor, Munro, & Brooten, 1991; Peplau, 1994). Organizational or cost outcomes that might be affected by coaching processes include lengths of stay, cost of care, proportion of services that receive reimbursement, and use of health care services (Lang & Marek, 1992; Naylor et al., 1991). This description of transitions as a focus for APN coaching underscores the need for and the importance of a holistic orientation when APNs help individuals with their health and illness concerns.

THE FOUNDATIONS OF ADVANCED PRACTICE NURSE COACHING THROUGH TRANSITIONS

A Model of Advanced Practice Nurses' Expert Coaching and Guidance

This author has defined coaching by APNs "as a complex, dynamic, collaborative, and holistic interpersonal process that is mediated by the APN-patient relationship and the APN's self-reflective skills" (Spross, 2005; Spross & Clarke, 1996; Spross et al., 2000). APNs integrate self-reflection and the techni-

cal, clinical, and interpersonal competencies they have acquired through graduate education and experience with patients' understandings, experiences, and goals to shape transitional experiences and accomplish therapeutic and educational goals. Expert coaching by APNs depends on the interaction of four factors: clinical competence, technical competence, interpersonal competence, and self-reflection (Figure 6-1), which are further influenced by individual APN and patient factors as well as contextual ones. The interaction of self-reflection with these three areas of competence drives the ongoing expansion and refinement of expertise in advanced practice nursing.

Several assumptions that underlie this model of the APN's coaching and guiding must be made explicit:

- It is assumed that APNs involve the patient's significant other or the patient's proxy as appropriate.
- Although technical competence and clinical competence may be sufficient for teaching a task, they are insufficient for coaching patients through transitions. For example, patients with diabetes may be taught how to monitor their blood sugar levels and administer insulin

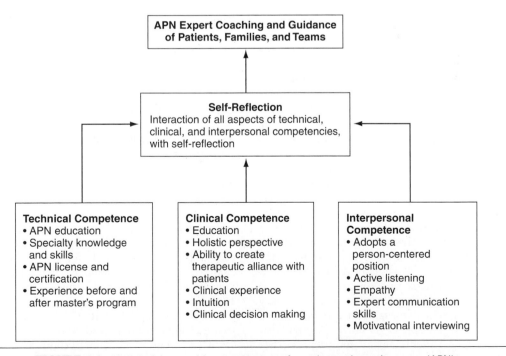

FIGURE **6-1:** Model of the coaching competency of an advanced practice nurse (APN).

with technical accuracy, but if the lifestyle impacts of the transition from health to chronic illness are not evaluated, then coaching and guidance cannot occur. Failure to assess the need for coaching may influence clinical outcomes.

- The clinical and didactic content of graduate education extends the APN's repertoire of assessment skills, technical skills, interpersonal behaviors, and self-reflection abilities, enabling the APN to coach in situations that are broader in scope or more complex in nature.
- The APN is able to be explicit about the processes and outcomes of coaching.
- The coaching competency develops over time during and after graduate education.
- APNs can articulate the nuances of coaching to preceptees, protégés, and staff.
- APNs attend to the patterns of encounters and strategies they have used to coach and can apply or adapt these experiences readily to coach patients in future situations.

The basis for expert APN coaching is the interaction of interpersonal, technical, and clinical competence with self-reflection and consideration of individual and contextual factors. Expert coaching requires that APNs be self-aware and self-reflective as an interpersonal transaction is unfolding so that they can shape communications and behaviors to maximize the therapeutic and educational goals of the clinical encounter. The ability to self-reflect and focus on the process of coaching as it is occurring implies that APNs are capable of the simultaneous execution of other skills. While interacting with a patient, APNs integrate physical, cognitive, and intuitive skills such as physical examination, interviewing, attending to their own noncognitive reactions and those of the patient, and interpreting these multiple sources of information. One might compare the process to simultaneous translation of a speech into several languages as it is being given. The difference is that the simultaneous translations are being carried out by one APN, not several translators. De la Cuesta (1994) characterized this as the "'product' [or outcome] taking shape...in the very process of the interaction" (p. 457). Throughout the process one is aware of the individual and contextual factors that may affect the coaching encounter. Recently, Hanley and Fenton (2007) have suggested that nurses, and therefore APNs, are able to "improvise" in ways that are therapeutic and meaningful for patients. They defined improvisation as "comprising the nurse's

knowledge, ability to relate and be sensitive to the needs of patients, capacity for creating change and practical use of resources" (p. 129). Improvisation is usually spontaneous but thoroughly grounded in the nurse's masterful practice.

Given that the goals of health care are preventing future illness, decreasing chronicity, limiting relapses or exacerbations of illnesses, alleviating suffering, and responding to crises, Squier (1990) wondered why the study of the quality of provider-patient relationships is not given more priority—at least as much as is given to technological treatments. To address this question, Squier analyzed existing literature, including studies of physicians and APNs, and has proposed a model linking a clinician's empathic understanding with a patient's adherence to therapeutic regimens. He hypothesized that empathic understanding has two components: cognitive and affective. Clinicians' cognitive ability to accurately take the perspective of the patient enables them to communicate effectively and reflect this understanding back to the patient. Patients are then more likely to elaborate the concerns that brought them to the clinician. Clinicians' emotional sensitivity to patients' emotions and underlying concerns helps reduce the anxiety and stress that often affect the health problems for which patients are consulting clinicians. Squier also described phases of the clinician-patient consultation and the patient outcomes associated with each phase—the ultimate outcomes being improved adherence to preventive and therapeutic strategies (self-care) and better health. These early findings suggest that APNs are "naturals" at motivational interviewing, a key coaching strategy in helping patients adjust to illness.

Technical Competence and Clinical Competence

Technical and clinical competences are well-defined aspects of established advanced practice nursing roles, and their importance to coaching cannot be overestimated. However, these two factors are not addressed in detail in this chapter. As specialties in advanced practice nursing evolved, specialty organizations published standards for the technical and clinical knowledge and skills required for advanced practice with particular populations. Chapters 1 and 18 document the evolution of these aspects of various APN roles, and Part III illustrates the specific technical and clinical skills APNs need.

An important part of clinical competence is clinical experience with the populations that are the

APN's focus. Pre-graduate school experiences, experiences within graduate clinical practica, and post-master's clinical experiences provide the grist for analyzing, developing, and making visible the coaching competency of APNs. Ongoing development of APNs' coaching competency depends on applying self-reflection to clinical experiences to acquire new coaching knowledge and skills that cannot be found in any textbook. Over the course of caring for patients, nurses learn the many ways people experience and manage health, birth, illness, pain, suffering, and death (Benner, 1985, 1991; Benner et al., 1999). These clinical experiences enable APNs to identify coaching alternatives that help other patients understand, learn, change, modulate, and control experiences of transition.

Interpersonal Competence

Interpersonal competence encompasses a set of advanced communication and relationship skills that enable APNs to communicate effectively and to establish therapeutic, caring relationships. These two components are briefly described, and theoretical and research support for interpersonal competence as an integral part of coaching is provided.

Advanced Communication Skills. During patient encounters, APNs adopt an open, flexible, non-hierarchical stance and communicate this in words

and actions (Brown, 1995; Kasch & Knutson, 1985). They convey an attitude of openness, elicit and respond to feelings, express concern, confirm the patient's experience, and provide positive reinforcement (Quirk & Casey, 1995). They attend to nonverbal cues exhibited by the patient, significant others, other team members, and the APNs' own reactions. APNs use these cues to ask additional questions, to probe the meanings hidden in patient reports, to reshape the interaction as it is unfolding, and to identify issues that may need to be further assessed when the encounter has ended. APNs summarize, recap, and interpret as they coach. Verbal and nonverbal skills that characterize a person-centered approach to interviewing are listed in Box 6-1.

In recent studies of APN coaching and group education (Lorig et al., 1999; Parry et al., 2006), coaches use motivational interviewing—a type of interviewing aimed at understanding and resolving a patient's ambivalence about change and building a desire on the part of the patient (motivation) to adopt new behaviors (Borrelli, 2006; Lorig et al., 1999). This type of interviewing is consistent with a person-centered style of interaction since it gives the patient an opportunity to air his or her concerns about the impact of changing or not changing. Patients are not given specific suggestions until they have decided to change. In this style of interviewing, the APN engages in active and careful listening and poses strategic

---

Box 6-1   SKILLS ASSOCIATED WITH A PERSON-CENTERED STYLE OF COMMUNICATION

- Allowing patients to tell their stories using their own language and chronology
- Using a conversational style of interviewing
- Using motivational interviewing
- Eliciting patients' thoughts, perspectives, expectations, values, and goals
- Asking about the contexts of patients' lives and the impact of health/illness concerns
- Encouraging self-disclosure
- Responding to patients' indirect and nonverbal clues regarding emotions and problems
- Providing patients with self-care information and enabling patients' participation in health care decision making
- Creating shared understandings with patients

- Developing health care plans collaboratively with patients
- Expressing concern for patients' well-being
- Responding empathically
- Creating social connectedness with patients by means of humor, touch, and appropriate self-disclosure
- Using open-ended questions and paraphrasing to elicit information and validate patients' communications
- Using a tone of voice and pace of speech appropriate to the topic being discussed
- Making eye contact and using a forward-leaning posture

Data from Borrelli, B. (2006). Using motivational interviewing to promote patient behavior change and enhance health (electronic version). *Medscape*, 1-16. Retrieved August 11, 2007, from www.medscape.com/viewprogram/5757_pnt; Brown, S.J. (1999). Patient-centered communication. *Annual Review of Nursing Research, 17*, 85-104; Montgomery, C.L. (1993). *Healing through communication*. Newbury Park, CA: Sage; Quirk, M., & Casey, L. (1995). Primary care for women: The art of interviewing. *Journal of Nurse-Midwifery, 40*, 97-103.

questions. Questions are asked in ways that engage the patients in self-reflection—What keeps you from changing? What would help you take action? Can an intermediate goal be identified?

APNs must also demonstrate cultural competence in their communications with patients and create a climate of cultural safety (Betancourt, Green, & Carrillo, 2002; Polaschak, 1998), using verbal and nonverbal skills. Polaschak (1998) noted that cultural safety is not so much about the cultural differences between the clinician and patient but, rather, demonstrating an awareness of how persons of a particular group are perceived. APNs understand not only how the ways in which patients are different will affect patient care but also how clinicians' perceptions of a particular patient or patient population will affect the team's approach to assessment and care (Exemplar 6-1). Patients may avoid seeking care because they are deeply aware, usually based on experience, of how they are perceived—they may not feel safe and seek health care services only when a problem is far advanced.

The content of APNs' communications, whether verbal or written, is equally important. The literature on health communication indicates that effective health communication has the following attributes: accuracy, accessibility, balance (e.g., risks and benefits are clearly outlined), consistency, culturally competent, evidence-based, a broad reach (gets to the largest possible number of people affected by the condition), credible and reliable, repeated over time, timely, and understandable (Department of Health and Human Services [DHHS], 2000; IOM, 2004; Stableford & Mettger, 2007). The APN strives to ensure that communications with patients—whether verbal or written—meet these criteria.

Several features allow these communication skills to be characterized as advanced. A primary feature is that the interactions are strategic even when they are spontaneous (Ball & Cox, 2003; Hanley & Fenton, 2007). For example, APNs prepare themselves, however briefly, for an encounter. This may entail a thorough look at the chart, a quick scan of results and notes since the last visit, or simply setting an intention to be present to a patient in the middle of a harried, time-packed day. Another feature is the collaborative negotiation of goals. Once engaged in the encounter, APNs will collaborate with the patient to set goals and intentions—at the beginning, clarifying the reason for the encounter and, at the end, establishing goals to be worked on before the next encounter. APNs attend to a broad range of verbal and nonverbal cues, quickly determine those that are priorities, and tailor the interaction to address the important issues that are embedded in the patient's language—issues that may be more or less relevant to the clinical problem at hand but are central to the patient. A third characteristic is the APN's deliberate, focused, and listening *presence*. Particular encounters are rarely constrained by individual or contextual factors because the APN remains undistracted and fully present in interactions. If the APN is hurried or harried and knows it is affecting "presence," he or she acknowledges this and may renegotiate what can be accomplished in a particular visit. APNs' communications are informed by evidence, their experiences, and the patient's preferences and goals. Novice APNs may experience more difficulty demonstrating such presence because of concern about their technical competence, awareness of what the next, more demanding task or encounter is, time pressures, and other sources of anxiety that can interfere with "being present."

 EXEMPLAR 6-1   **Advanced Practice Nurse Coaching and Cultural Competence**

A graduate CNS student reflecting on her experience with a homeless patient, noted that when she heard in report that her patient had a challenging wound care regimen and was homeless, she made a number of (negative) judgments about what this meant. Before entering his room, she made the decision to set these judgments aside and set the intention to be open and respectful and learn from this man. She was first surprised by his neat appearance. She learned that the man had been so disabled by his chronic illness (the work he used to perform required him to be on his feet all day,

making him vulnerable to wounds and infections) that he lost his job and, ultimately, his home. Her patient had negotiated his life creatively—determined to "look like" he was working while looking for work. He knew in which public places he could find a place to wash up and, sometimes, shower and have his clothes cleaned. He spent his days at the library when he was not interviewing for a job. This experience forever changed the student—a lesson in suspending judgment to understand and care effectively.

Therapeutic Relationships. Establishing a caring, therapeutic relationship with a patient demands that the APN be emotionally responsive, not distant. APNs who rely only on scientific and technical competencies in their relationships with patients are unlikely to appreciate patients' holistic responses or enable patients to express themselves holistically (Gadow, 1980). The nurse and patient enter the relationship as whole persons, complete with talents, goals, needs, and wishes. However, the focus of the interpersonal process is on addressing the patient's potentials and goals (Martocchio, 1987; Montgomery, 1993). Nurses reveal themselves through their eyes, tone of voice, affect, body language, and silences. The APN "who withholds parts of herself (or himself) is unlikely to allow the patient to emerge as a whole, or to comprehend that wholeness if it does emerge" (Gadow, 1980, p. 87). Montgomery (1993) found that clinicians had predispositional qualities consistent with caring: a person orientation rather than role orientation, concern for the human element in care, person-centered intention, transcendence of judgment, hopeful orientation, lack of ego involvement, and expanded personal boundaries. She also described the properties of caring behaviors (Box 6-2).

Studies of nurses in basic and advanced practice suggest that a caring, person-centered relationship underlies successful coaching interventions (Benner, 1984; Brown, 1999; Fenton, 1984; Lamb & Stempel, 1994; Morgan, 1994; Parry et al., 2006; Steele & Fenton, 1988). Selected findings that support the importance of interpersonal competence to APN coaching are summarized here.

Parry and colleagues (2006), in a qualitative study of 32 of the 976 patients who had participated in the care transitions intervention, identified three overlapping categories that described the patients' experience of the coaching intervention. The first category was "continuity throughout the care transition." The intervention was viewed as having provided continuity and direction at each stage of the transition from one health care setting to the other: patients felt "supported, comforted, and safe" (p. 46). The second category was "self-management knowledge and skills." Patients identified two key components in this category. Patients reported that the home visit during which they were coached in medication management and knowledge of "red flags," including signs of disease complications and adverse drug reactions, was crucial. Many subjects mentioned that the coach supported their ability to communicate effectively with other providers by helping them generate questions and engaging in role playing. The third category was "the coaching relationship: the importance of the caring relationship." Most patients noted the importance of meeting the coach before discharge—in addition to feeling cared about, the coach's knowledge, experience, interest, and organizational skills were relevant to patients and their willingness to become more involved in their care. The investigators observed that the patients' perception of feeling cared about may have been related to the coach's accessibility and frequent follow-up activities.

A caring, person-centered approach demands an involved, current, individualized, contextual understanding of the patient (Tanner, Benner, Chesla, & Gordon, 1993). This understanding serves to bridge the differences between APNs and their patients and enables patients to share power and collaborate with APNs to develop a realistic plan of care. If a patient is to be coached effectively in making transitions that are genuinely his or her own, both the nurse and the patient must enter the relationship as whole persons. Some people may regard this caring, person-centered approach as an unreachable ideal, given the complexity of care and time pressures. However, in most situations, the skilled APN can establish rapport immediately and determine the priorities for assessment and

---

Box 6-2   PROPERTIES OF CARING EXPRESSED AS BEHAVIORS

- Empowerment through mobilization of resources
- Accessibility
- Advocacy
- Authenticity
- Nonjudgmental stance

- Responsiveness
- Commitment
- Being present
- Creating positive meaning and hope
- Competence

Data from Martocchio, B. (1987). Authenticity, belonging, emotional closeness, and self representation. *Oncology Nursing Forum, 14,* 23-27; Montgomery, C.L. (1993). *Healing through communication.* Newbury Park, CA: Sage; Parry, C., Kramer, H.M., & Coleman, E.A. (2006). A qualitative exploration of a patient-centered coaching intervention to improve care transitions in chronically ill older adults. *Home Health Care Services Quarterly, 25*(3/4), 39-53.

intervention while sustaining this person-centered approach. For example, critical care CNSs are skilled in coaching families facing the loss of a loved one due to a traumatic brain injury: they facilitate "bad news" conversations, interpret the intricacies of brain death, and provide comfort to the grief-stricken survivors in rapidly evolving situations. They perform such coaching with skill and compassion while attending to competing needs, demands, and schedules of other patients and colleagues. APNs must develop strategies for staying personally centered and patient-centered in a variety of circumstances, including those with time constraints.

Self-Reflection

The fourth component of the APN expert coaching model is self-reflection—the deliberate, internal examination of experience in order to learn from it. The APN uses self-reflection during interactions with patients, as well as retrospectively. Schön (1983) described these as "reflection-in-action" and "reflection-on-action." Reflection-in-action is the ability to pay attention to phenomena as they are occurring, giving free rein to one's intuitive understanding of the situation as it is unfolding. The APN is not restricted to using only familiar patterns of thought. APN coaching is analogous to the flexible and inventive playing of a jazz musician; APNs can attend to what is happening in the moment and respond with a varied repertoire of exploratory and transforming actions. In the APN-patient relationship, reflective practice is simultaneously doing and learning and coming to know. Reflection-in-action can be compared to the Zen concept of mindfulness (Tremmel, 1993). Mindfulness means paying attention to "right here, right now" and investing the present moment with full concentration. Reflection-in-action, or mindfulness, involves awareness of the world and awareness of multiple aspects of consciousness—thoughts, feelings, behaviors.

Reflection or looking within involves attending to one's own thinking processes (Bartels, 1998; Pugach & Johnson, 1990). As an extension of the work done by Jackson (1986) on expert teaching, APN coaches might be characterized as those who "see more" than nonexperts do. "Seeing more" refers to the practice of "paying attention" (Jackson, 1986). APNs are sensitive to possibilities—within patients, within the processes of the clinical encounter, and within themselves. They anticipate what might happen during the encounter or after the patient leaves. They are sensitive to incipient difficulty: APNs' sensibilities, processes (including reflection), and skills interact to shape their encounters with patients, to support patients, and to enable patients to navigate transitions to achieve mutually determined goals. The capacity to reflect mindfully in action and on action is not readily mastered and requires continual practice (Tremmel, 1993). However, certain qualities and characteristics can be developed to facilitate self-reflection. These include motivation, commitment, open-mindedness, self-awareness, the ability to describe phenomena or situations, critical analysis, and the ability to synthesize and evaluate (Atkins & Murphy, 1994). APNs should pay attention to both positive and negative experiences. What made this effective? Why didn't this work? APNs may be more likely to reflect on negative experiences because the feeling of failure is more uncomfortable than the feeling of satisfaction or success. However, reflecting on satisfying, successful experiences can provide clues to interventions that will be effective in future interactions. One of the key aspects of self-reflection is paying attention to feelings. Experienced nurses and APNs are more likely than inexperienced ones to pay attention to feelings or intuition. However, novice APNs need to be taught to recognize that their affective responses to situations are clues to their developing expertise as clinicians and coaches.

Other Factors

A variety of other factors can influence the coaching process; many of these are well described in Chapter 5 in relation to clinical decision making (e.g., time pressures, thinking errors). Individual factors such as demographic characteristics, health status, cultural differences, mood, years of experience, and competing priorities may affect the APN's attention and ability to coach in any particular encounter. Similarly, individual patient and family factors (some are discussed in the section that follows) can affect their ability to interact with the APN and respond to coaching interventions. Contextual factors—everything from whether or not an activity will be reimbursed, staffing, relationships with others on the caregiving team—can also affect coaching.

ADVANCED PRACTICE NURSE COACHING: ASSESSMENT, PROCESSES, AND OUTCOMES

Assessment

Patient assessment is the basis for determining which coaching interventions will be used. APNs use whatever physical and psychological assessment procedures, skills, or tools they need to evaluate the patient's concerns. They understand that assessments have multiple purposes: (1) to gain an understanding of the patient and establish a therapeutic relationship, (2) to identify patients' health-related concerns and goals, and (3) to collect data. They make conscious efforts to build a partnership that will work by conveying concern, being honest and dependable, and displaying professional knowledge and self-confidence. The person-centered approach adopted by nurses has been described by several researchers as "knowing the patient" (Jenny & Logan, 1992; Radwin, 1996; Tanner et al., 1993). This entails getting to know the patient as a person and learning the patient's pattern of responses, including experiences, habits, practices, preferences, usual demeanor, and self-presentation (Jenny & Logan, 1992). APNs use their observations of themselves, the patients, and the interactive process to decode patients' behaviors and the content of their communications for significance (Kasch & Dine, 1988). They need to grasp the patient's perspective, including salient aspects of the patient's self-definition (Olesen, Schatzman, Droes, Hatton, & Chico, 1990). This expert assessment is critical to the selection of coaching interventions to help people remain healthy, make lifestyle changes, reduce risk, or manage chronic illness.

Assessment must extend beyond the individual to include consideration of the patient's relationships, communities, and social milieu, because social and contextual variables often influence the APN's ability to provide effective care. Both the APN's and the patient's cultural and political values influence their understanding of health, illness, language, identity, social roles, and historical issues. For example, domestic violence, child abuse, malnutrition, substance abuse, and stress-induced illnesses are responses to political, economic, social, and personal problems. APNs may find that coaching their patients requires that they expose social and political inequities that affect people's health so that they can be addressed (Hagedorn, 1995; Kendall, 1992). Otherwise, the core issues in many patients' transitions will be invisible and unidentified and the coaching strategies used will be superficial, unfocused, and ineffective.

Subjective phenomena like meaning and expectations influence the anticipation and experience of transition and its unfolding (Corbin & Strauss, 1992; Neimeyer, 2001; Schumacher & Meleis, 1994) and should be assessed. Meanings and expectations about

a transition are often colored by memories and prior experiences. Meanings may be positive, negative, or neutral. Transitions may require the reconstruction of meaning. Regardless of whether the meaning of the transition is positive or negative, patients may experience uncertainty, grief, guilt, stress, or other emotional responses. Expectations may be accurate and realistic, or they may be unrealistic and even fantastic. Cognitive variables such as knowledge, self-care skills, motivation, coping style, habitual stressors, and personal preferences for control affect people's experience of and ability to accept, adjust to, or adapt to transitional experiences (Alonzo, 2000; Brooten et al., 1991; Corbin & Strauss, 1992; Jenny & Logan, 1992; Kasch & Dine, 1988; Neimeyer, 2001; Schumacher & Meleis, 1994). The environment—including resources, relationships, social support, setting of care, and contextual variables—can mediate transitions (Brooten et al., 1991; Corbin & Strauss, 1992; Schumacher & Meleis, 1994). Family and work responsibilities that may interfere with therapeutic self-care must be identified. Planning, including problem and need identification, organization of phase-related interventions, and communication, influences the success of the transition. Physical and emotional well-being also determine how the transition process is experienced (Schumacher & Meleis, 1994). The nature of the health concern; the severity of symptoms, perceived vulnerability, and seriousness; and the degree of predictability or certainty about one's experience of the body can make for smooth or chaotic transitions.

APNs identify missing information that they might need for coaching and variables that might enhance or hinder coaching. Throughout the interaction, they try to clarify the adaptive task, regulate distress (Heifetz, 1994), respond to patients' needs for information, and create a physically and interpersonally comforting environment (Kasch & Lisnek, 1984). For example, an APN might observe that a patient is becoming fatigued during an examination. In addition to providing for rest and changing the pace of the examination, the APN may explore the causes, duration, and significance of the fatigue.

Several points can be made about the assessment aspects of coaching through transitions. First, not every encounter will involve a transition. Even in routine situations, the APN's coaching competence can result in efficient care delivery, improved patient satisfaction, and return business—all valued outcomes in today's health care environments. Second, not every individual immersed in a transitional situation is interested in moving or adjusting; a person can become stuck or immobilized by the demands of the transition, the underlying nature of the illness (e.g., borderline personality disorder), or personal factors such as limited social support or cognitive ability. Even so, APNs can often help patients who are immobilized. These are often the patients for whom physicians, staff nurses, or novice APNs seek the help of an experienced APN. By working effectively with difficult cases, APNs expand their repertoire of coaching interventions (Exemplar 6-2). Some patients who are stuck simply need a new coach—someone with a different approach or personality. A smaller population may be help rejecters; in this case, coaching is unlikely to be effective and such patients can only be "maintained." Third, although some conscious patients may reject help, noncommunicative patients can often be coached effectively. For example, the APN who is providing palliative care may talk to the dying person about letting go, review aspects of the patient's life, and provide comforting touch interventions. The APN observes responses that indicate relaxation and peace (e.g., less restlessness and moaning).

Processes and Outcomes

Coaching processes used by APNs foster involvement, choice, and autonomy—motivating or activating patients to participate in their own care. The concept of intervention mapping (Bartholomew, Parcel, & Kok,

1998) may also be used to plan care for individuals; an individualized assessment often leads APNs to tailor a standard treatment to improve adherence and the likelihood of reaching a desired outcome.

In coaching a patient, APNs have four main tasks: interpreting unfamiliar diagnostic and treatment demands, coaching the patient through alienated stances (e.g., anger, hopelessness), identifying changing relevance as demands or symptoms of the illness change, and ensuring that cure is enhanced by care (Benner, 1985). These tasks can be accomplished through coaching processes. Coaching processes and outcomes can be categorized by focus: bodily or physical, affective/interpersonal/spiritual, cognitive/behavioral, and social (Spross, 1996). Table 6-4 can be used by students and graduates to facilitate self-reflection (What processes do I typically use? Which work best?), to design coaching protocols (Which strategies are likely to work for this population, based on the evidence?), and to develop outcome evaluation plans for coaching interventions (see Chapter 25).

APNs attend to issues of timing and sequencing in teaching and counseling patients. Thus they may need to coach a patient to become motivated before beginning to teach him or her a particular task. APNs integrate coaching into processes of consultation, collaboration, and referral. They use their knowledge of the patient to mobilize resources and interpret the patient's needs to team members, consultants, and

 EXEMPLAR 6-2   **Advanced Practice Nurse Coaching and Posttraumatic Stress**

Ms. A. was a 35-year-old African-American woman who came to the anesthesia pain unit for an outpatient procedure—a stellate ganglion block for treatment of chronic pain. Assessment revealed that she understood the procedure, including the purposes and the risks. She knew that an intravenous (IV) line would be placed. As the anesthesiology fellow was inserting the IV line, Ms. A. began to cry, shake, and sweat and said she felt afraid. The clinical nurse specialist (CNS) asked the fellow to stop the procedure and give the CNS an opportunity to further assess the patient. The patient indicated that she had not expected such a reaction and had had IV lines placed before. However, after further questioning by the CNS, the patient indicated that the last time she had had an IV line placed was while she was in the emergency department, 10 years before, after she had been raped and beaten. The experience of having the IV

started reproduced the distress and fear she felt then. Ms. A. was offered the option of rescheduling the procedure, but she did not want to do that because she was counting on having the procedure to ameliorate her pain. Ms. A. chose to receive additional antianxiety medication. She was also coached in the standard relaxation exercise that was part of the stellate ganglion block protocol and was reassured that the CNS would remain with her throughout the procedure. Post-procedure discharge planning included referral to a counselor she had seen in the past who had been helpful. In addition, a debriefing session was held with Ms. A. She was advised that future invasive procedures could reproduce the reaction of the prior trauma and that she should include both the original traumatic event and the reaction to the block procedure when relaying her health history.

family caregivers. Knowing the patient enables APNs to take risks, adopt stances that are unusual or unpopular, and make the system work to shape patients' transitional experiences, a quality of the APN direct care competency that has been described as "fearlessness" (Koetters, 1989). Therefore coaching is a holistic process, and although there is a primary focus or target, coaching behaviors often have effects across all dimensions of the patient's experience.

The case in Exemplar 6-3 illustrates the following aspects of coaching: recognizing the need for coaching early in a patient encounter and the risks of not coaching (poor pain management, poor rehabilitation outcome, alienation between staff and patient); identifying the multiple levels of coaching needed (patient, staff, post-discharge caregivers); and using relationships with patients and colleagues to shape a positive outcome in a complex situation.

Table 6-4 ADVANCED PRACTICE NURSES' COACHING PROCESSES AND POSSIBLE OUTCOMES

Dominant Focus	Coaching Processes	Possible Outcomes*
Physical	Demonstrating self-care or self-monitoring skills Describing the likely physical trajectory of the health or illness concern, including physical and psychological demands, tasks, and resources Describing the possibilities inherent in the physical transitions experienced Identifying risk factors Implementing pain and symptom management Interpreting the person's experiences of the body Offering alternative (e.g., more hopeful) interpretations of bodily sensations/functions Offering strategies to modify risk factors Providing assistance with hygiene and toileting and conducting invasive procedures and other physical interventions while preserving dignity Using comforting touch	Effective self-care (e.g., fewer symptoms) Improved functional status Improved mental status (e.g., as a result of decreased pain or normalized blood sugar levels) Increased physical comfort
Affective, interpersonal, spiritual	Accepting the person as he or she is Acknowledging the person's courage, strength, or other personal qualities Acknowledging both expressed and possible fears and concerns Attuning oneself to patient's needs and goals Being available/present Being honest Bonding, establishing a therapeutic alliance Comforting through touch, behavior, and interactions Counseling Eliciting expectations, fears, meanings, and values Enabling Encouraging, praising Ensuring safe passage Expressing confidence in patients and their abilities Inspiring/inspiriting Listening Keeping a vigil Making a commitment to help Offering hope Reassuring Supporting Validating	Acceptance of help from others Decreased anxiety, stress, or uncertainty Decreased spiritual distress Finding meaning Hope Improved quality of life Increased motivation Increased ability to initiate self-care Increased comfort, decreased suffering Revised future agendas Self-acceptance Self-report of satisfaction with decision making Self-transcendence

Continued

Table 6-4   ADVANCED PRACTICE NURSES' COACHING PROCESSES AND POSSIBLE OUTCOMES—cont'd

Dominant Focus	Coaching Processes	Possible Outcomes*
Cognitive, behavioral	Challenging Coaching in communication and technical skills Communicating strategically Confronting and identifying contradictions Dealing with conflict Demonstrating and role modeling Establishing goals Explaining Guiding, offering a map Identifying adaptive tasks Identifying the goals of interventions Improving problem-solving skills Intervention mapping Mediating Monitoring Motivating Negotiating Offering options Presenting challenges Providing cognitive strategies to alter negative thought patterns Providing feedback Reframing expectations, goals, and meanings Setting tasks Using a variety of teaching strategies Using humor Using cognitive coping strategies	Behavior/lifestyle change Change in beliefs or attitudes Decreased stress Effective self-care and problem solving related to clinical issues Improved functional status Improved quality of life Increased self-efficacy
Social	Advocating Bonding Collaborating with the patient and with other providers Facilitating important relationships Interpreting patients' behaviors, needs, and goals to members of the health care team and patients' families Keeping tradition Mobilizing community, financial, and social resources Strengthening social supports through teaching, consultation, and referral	Affection Alienation and stigmatization averted or minimized Comfort Decreased caregiver burden Decreased costs of care Improved satisfaction with care Improved self-care Satisfaction with social support

Adapted from Spross, J.A. (1996). Coaching and suffering: The role of the nurse in helping people face illness. In B.R. Ferrell (Ed.), *The human dimensions of suffering* (Table 8.3, pp. 198-199). Boston: Jones & Bartlett. (The reader is encouraged to refer to this publication for additional references from which the coaching processes were derived.)

*Although most outcomes are patient and family related, some systems outcomes are included to help the reader connect the individual coaching by advanced practice nurses with organization-level outcomes.

DEVELOPMENT OF ADVANCED PRACTICE NURSES' COACHING COMPETENCE

Becoming an expert coach requires a combination of education, experience, interpersonal competence, and self-reflection on one's practice. Although scientific and technical knowledge are essential for effective coaching, it is in the coaching of patients that the art of advanced practice nursing is fully expressed. APNs need a highly nuanced range of interpersonal skills to coach people through multifaceted transitions. The strategies used to develop coaching expertise are designed to prepare

EXEMPLAR 6-3 Advanced Practice Nurse Coaching and Complex Pain Management

A clinical nurse specialist (CNS) collaborated with a psychologist in the care of a patient named Jack who had complex care needs. Jack had been admitted to a rehabilitation hospital after a left hip arthroplasty and left tibial traction pin. His immediate postoperative course had been complicated by a staphylococcal infection at the surgical site, for which he was still receiving intravenous antibiotics. Jack had a history of substance abuse and had been in a methadone maintenance program. Jack was well known to the staff because he had been in the rehabilitation hospital one year earlier after a Girdlestone surgical procedure was performed on his right hip. During both admissions, pain management was a significant problem. He became easily frustrated and impatient and expressed his anger verbally. These characteristics were exacerbated when he was in moderate to severe pain. For example, requests for pain medications were made in demanding and insistent tones. Jack currently reports pain in his left hip and left lower leg, as well as some right shoulder and paralumbar pain. According to the nursing assessment, his pain intensity data are as follows: worst pain is 10/10, least pain is 9/10, and average pain is 9/10. He receives Percocet, 2 tablets every 6 hours prn, and his pain is never below 9/10. Jack did not complete high school and is disabled. His parents are divorced. He has nieces and nephews he adores and has been motivated to stay clean because he is not permitted to see them if he is abusing drugs.

The CNS performed an initial thorough assessment of Jack's pain. During this assessment, she initiated coaching by reviewing with him what they had learned during the prior admission about how to manage his pain by using a combination of scheduled opioids and nondrug interventions. Jack expressed frustration that he was not as independent as he had been during the prior admission. The CNS explained that during the prior admission, he had had the use of his "good" leg to compensate for what the treated leg could not do. Although he had made a good recovery, the leg treated last year was not functional enough to support his weight and compensate for the temporary loss of function in the leg being treated during this admission. He acknowledged that this made sense. The CNS knew from having reviewed the admission orders that she would need to talk to the physicians to get the analgesics changed to a more frequent, around-the-clock schedule so Jack could participate effectively in therapies.

The CNS and the psychologist conferred and agreed to share responsibility for coaching, with the CNS having a primary focus on the patient and the psychologist having a primary focus on the staff. The CNS had been working with the staff for more than a year to improve pain management practices on the unit. However, the staff would need coaching because they were being challenged to apply what they learned about pain management to a patient whose history they believed made use of opioids for pain risky. The psychologist would help the staff understand this patient and the reasons for treating pain with opioids in an addict who had had surgery, and, if needed, help staff see when their attitudes and misconceptions might be interfering with Jack's care. Jack needed coaching regarding appropriate ways to communicate his pain and his responses to pain management interventions to avoid alienating staff and to maximize participation in therapy. In addition, the CNS would work with the nurses and physicians on titrating analgesics to effect. Given Jack's history, he was likely to need more analgesic, not less.

The psychologist noticed during the course of working with Jack that staff often assumed that Jack was "drug seeking" if he requested medications for pain. Staff had other concerns that needed attention: fear of giving too much pain medication, weaning Jack from analgesics as soon as possible (regardless of pain intensity level or impact of unrelieved pain on progress in rehabilitation), and concern that Jack would relapse with regard to substance abuse. The psychologist listened to and acknowledged the staff's issues. He offered them new information to encourage them to modify their thinking about how pain in addicts should be managed. Both the psychologist and the CNS were able to show staff the effectiveness of their interventions: when Jack's pain was well managed, his participation in therapy was better. If someone had withheld or forgotten Jack's medication, it showed in a decreased level of activity during physical and occupational therapy.

The CNS coached Jack in effective ways to communicate his frustration and explained why angry and blaming communications might make it harder for some staff to help him. Both the psychologist and the CNS used cognitive restructuring strategies to help Jack think differently about his problems and learn ways to increase his threshold for frustration. For example, when Jack reported that nothing was going right or that he could not

Continued

EXEMPLAR 6-3 Advanced Practice Nurse Coaching and Complex Pain Management—cont'd

do anything, events of the day were reviewed for evidence of some progress. The links between his thinking and behavior were identified. When Jack became an outpatient, the psychologist and the CNS praised his self-care and adherence to treatment plans. Jack had been discharged 4 weeks after admission with an effective analgesic regimen so he could continue to make progress at home. Before his discharge, the psychologist and the CNS collaborated with the social worker to find

and then coach a primary care physician in the most effective strategies to help Jack because Jack was at high risk of being lost to follow-up. The staff also gained a better understanding of how to manage pain in a patient with a history of substance abuse. The staff's success with managing Jack's pain enabled them to better manage the pain of the occasional future patient who happened to have a co-morbid addiction.

APNs for reflective practice and a person-oriented interactive style, which are foundational abilities that APNs must develop to become skilled coaches.

In this author's opinion, at least two types of experiences, during and after graduate education, in the APN's direct care role, refine and extend one's coaching abilities. Continuous contact with patients over time provides students and APNs with experiences that let them observe how health and illness issues evolve over time. For example, acute care APNs learn the common features of weaning trajectories for patients on ventilators. This knowledge informs their coaching of families—"when we first begin weaning we will do this and you can expect this to happen." In primary care, an NP who has coached many patients in increasing their exercise by using a pedometer knows what goals might be achievable and what factors will impede or facilitate adopting the new behavior and uses this information to coach patients. However, one-time, episodic encounters also contribute to one's coaching expertise. For example, APNs in the organ donation field may see a family only once or twice, but over multiple encounters with many families they learn the different directions "bad news" conversations can take and recognize cues that lead them to use the most appropriate communications and actions for the particular situation. Another example of one-time experiences that develop the coaching competency is an unusual diagnosis such as Ludwig's angina or acute intermittent porphyria; the lessons from one experience with unusual illnesses will be available if and when APNs encounter them again. Thus continuous contact experiences with patients enable APNs to recognize within-patient patterns that help them coach subsequent patients with similar diagnoses and illness trajectories. Episodic or one-time encounters help APNs recognize across-patient patterns—lessons that can be applied in the next similar encounter. In either case, coaching is embedded in a deep knowledge of practice and sound empirical knowledge of the specialty.

Graduate Nursing Education: The Influence of Faculty and Preceptors

Graduate faculty and clinical preceptors are highly influential role models for APN students seeking to develop coaching skills. Faculty can assist APN students to develop as coaches by being reflective themselves. In particular, faculty need to name and evaluate the processes and pedagogies to which they were exposed, distinguishing between effective, respectful experiences of being taught or coached and ineffective, disrespectful ones. Students who have been effectively coached by teachers and preceptors will know experientially what respectful coaching "feels like." They will be more likely to reproduce these behaviors with patients. Schön (1987) called this the "hall of mirrors" effect. The teacher, in the very process of supervising and coaching the student, exemplifies the coaching repertoire that the student is attempting to acquire. If disrespectful, ineffective teaching is recognized for what it is—a position-centered style—then students also learn how not to coach.

Clinical preceptors play a particularly salient role with APN students. In effect, there is a "double exposure" to coaching: the student experiences being coached, and the student observes how patients are coached by the preceptor. Similarly, preceptors need to be able to coach students while coaching patients. A person-centered style of interaction on the part of the preceptor is just as important to developing APN students' coaching skills as it is to helping patients accomplish their health goals. It is possible to have preceptors who use a person-centered style of interaction with patients yet, because of their own student experiences, adopt a position-centered style of interacting with students. Very experienced APNs can be novice preceptors (Meng & Morris, 1995), so that preceptors themselves may need coaching by faculty and feedback from students to develop in their preceptor roles. Just as APNs tailor their coaching to meet individual patient needs, so APN preceptors need to tailor their coaching of students to the level of the student and the situation (Davis, Sawin, & Dunn, 1993).

Faculty and APN preceptors need to make students aware of the range of coaching strategies used in the classroom and the clinical area. This is one way students learn how to coach. What was ineffable and undervalued in the process of coaching becomes defined, contextualized, reproducible, and valued (McKinnon & Erickson, 1988). Developing coaching competence requires attention to all ways of knowing, including personal knowing (Diemert Moch, 1990). Therefore faculty and APN preceptors need to facilitate student reflection on their experiences and intuitions. APN students should reflect on their previous student experiences, identifying and evaluating effective and ineffective coaching. Bringing these educational moments to full consciousness and naming them are key first steps to envisioning coaching processes that students will want to emulate or identifying approaches that should be discarded.

Strategies for Developing and Applying the Coaching Competency

Coaching activities can be conceptualized along two dimensions: the degree of structure and the focus. Activities may be very structured (e.g., a lecture) or unstructured (e.g., storytelling). The focus of the APN's coaching may be individuals or groups.

Less traditional strategies must be used if the APN's interpersonal repertoire and self-reflective abilities are to be enlarged. Expressive writing (Fulwiler, 1987; Sorrell, 1994; Van Manen, 1989) enables students and graduates to recapture important experiences in nursing and reflect on them to arrive at new insights and interpretations. Keeping a journal, storytelling, and writing poetry are other examples.

Journal writing helps students and APNs reflect on the experience of being new or uncertain of their skills and can lead to discussions of developmental tasks such as embracing novicehood or learning to trust one's hands, heart, gut, and observations. Storytelling is another expressive strategy in which stories, the products of reflection, are relayed orally (Mattingly,

1998). Storytelling can build community and mutual respect among nurses (Lindesmith & McWeeny, 1994). Sharing stories from practice enables APN students to establish a shared history and provides a means of offering and receiving support. The process promotes critical thinking, strengthens collegiality, and builds self-esteem and rapport (Lindesmith & McWeeny, 1994). Through journals and storytelling, cues and strategies for coaching used by different APN students and preceptors became available to a larger group of learners. APNs can encourage storytelling among patients and families. In fact, APNs in palliative care often ask family members, whose loved one is not able to communicate, to tell them about the loved one (e.g., memories, personality, interests).

Written exemplars of coaching and group debriefing of coaching experiences facilitate self-reflection on coaching and expand one's coaching repertoire. Monturo (2003) noted that in a study of APNs providing transitional care to cancer patients, the APN interveners met regularly to discuss their experiences and support each other. In some cases, the discussion gave Monturo and her colleagues specific ideas that they could use in subsequent encounters.

Aesthetic approaches to developing interpersonal competence can also enhance APNs' coaching skills. Some of the most profound experiences in which nurses are involved can never be known through scientific and transactional writing because of the limitations of these styles of writing. Poetry, literature, and film can be potent triggers for developing reflective practice. They can help students and novice APNs understand what an experience of illness might be for a patient. For example, movies with plots involving illness or disability, such as *Heartsounds, Passion Fish, Marvin's Room,* and *Regarding Henry,* can help students assess needs for coaching, evaluate clinicians' effective and ineffective interpersonal styles, and articulate the gaps in care that might require advanced practice nursing intervention.

Students can develop coaching competence by developing and implementing patient education. For example, a student could negotiate with a preceptor to co-lead a self-management group for patients with a chronic condition, using motivational interviewing and other chronic disease management strategies (Lorig et al., 1999, 2001a; Lorig, Sobel, Ritter, Laurent, & Hobbs, 2001b). Other activities could include developing limited literacy tools or evaluating existing patient education materials with regard to the appropriateness of content and health literacy level (Foltz & Sullivan,

1999; Quirk, 2000); assessing the cost-effectiveness of a patient education initiative (Welch, Fisher, & Dayhoff, 2002); or evaluating the reliability and appropriateness of health information on the Internet (Clark & Gomez, 2001; Health Summit Working Group, 1999). The Internet is a resource used by many health care consumers. Students should know the health information resources likely to be used by their patient populations and be able to advise patients on those that are reliable and regularly updated.

EXPERT COACHING AND GUIDANCE: SELECTED ISSUES

In today's health care environment, particular issues seem to demand the expert coaching skills of APNs. The following topics represent opportunities or initiatives that are worthy of APNs' attention as the American health care system engages in efforts to transform itself from a fragmented, inequitable, and cumbersome system into one that is patient-centered, effective, efficient, and responsive.

Helping Patients Manage Chronic Illness

As the incidence of chronic conditions such as asthma and diabetes has increased, national organizations have undertaken efforts to prevent illness- or medication-related complications and to improve health-related quality of life for consumers. Consumer involvement in preventing errors is one strategy that is being used and, if successful, will support use of APNs to coach populations of patients who need their advanced skills. For example, through collaboration between the National Council on Patient Information and Education (2003) and the Agency for Healthcare Research and Quality, a brochure titled, "Your Medicine: Play it Safe" was distributed *(www.ahrq.gov/news/press/pr2003/safemedpr. htm)*. Patients are advised to discuss both prescription and over-the-counter medications with their health care providers. More recently, NCPIE (2007) has developed a national action plan to promote adherence to medication, part of its "Educate Before you Medicate" campaign.

In addition to national policy efforts to improve chronic disease management, numerous efforts to help patients manage their chronic illnesses such as the Care Transitions Intervention Model described on pp. 160-161 in this chapter rely on coaching interventions to motivate and empower patients and families to make lifestyle changes, adhere to recommended therapies, and communicate effectively and assertively with providers.

APNs involved in helping patients manage chronic illness, particularly APNs involved in programs to promote self-care, are encouraged to become familiar with the following reports: Milbank report, 1999; RWJ report, 2000; Department of Health, United Kingdom, 2001; IOM, 2001). Authors of these reports provide suggestions on training health professionals how to establish self-care management programs to ensure that programs are covered by insurance. Although these reports were published a number of years ago and some change has occurred, much work remains to ensure adoption of the recommendations. APNs can use the reports to assess the extent to which the recommendations that support patient coaching have been adopted by their employing agencies and the payers who reimburse them for their services.

Based on the research cited earlier and the model of coaching proposed in this chapter, APNs possess several skills that make them well suited to manage chronic illness as direct care providers and to lead and evaluate disease management programs. APNs think and practice in patient-centered ways. The breadth and depth of their clinical experience and their knowledge of their specialty's science and best practices together with patient assessment data allow APNs to anticipate the likely trajectory of a patient's illness course. They can identify barriers to adherence or participation in follow-up, and recognize discrepancies between the patient's personal health goals and clinicians' therapeutic goals. APNs coach patients and clinicians to prepare for the expected events associated with an illness trajectory, provide ways to handle the unexpected, overcome barriers, close the gaps between patient and clinician understandings of the health/illness issue, promote continuity of care, and bring the clinician's preventive or therapeutic goals and patient goals into alignment with the patient's preferences, capabilities, and resources. APNs are skilled at managing the boundaries where evidence-based practice standards and clinical benchmarks meet the particulars of a patient encounter.

APNs who participate in the design and execution of chronic illness management studies should ensure that the characteristics of the clinicians delivering the interventions are included in descriptions of intervention protocols and, when appropriate, the analyses account for clinician characteristics when the interventions are evaluated. Such analyses are important for determining the most efficacious and cost-effective approaches to education and coaching and determining the "nurse-dose" needed.

If coaching is effective and if efficient patient education and coaching are a means of reducing the costs of health care, better understanding of the teaching/coaching processes used by APNs and how they promote adherence to therapies and self-care is needed

Health Disparities and Patient Navigator Programs

In 2005, President Bush signed into law the Patient Navigator, Outreach, and Chronic Disease Prevention Act (National Patient Advocate Foundation [NPAF], 2005). Navigation services include identifying financial resources for treatment, arranging for transportation or childcare during appointments for diagnostic and treatment appointments, ensuring that culturally sensitive caregivers and translators are available throughout the diagnostic and treatment course, coordinating care, and ensuring that the appropriate medical records are available for every patient appointment. The use of "patient navigators" is aimed at reducing disparities in health care access and providing treatment for vulnerable populations. Populations who are vulnerable and less likely to receive timely preventive and therapeutic health care include racial and ethnic minorities, members of lower socioeconomic groups, residents of rural areas, and other underserved populations (National Cancer Institute, 2004). Thus far, most published descriptions of patient navigator programs are in oncology (Bruce, 2007; Houlahan, 2006; Seek & Hogle, 2007; Wilson, Holder, & Torres, 2006). Some nurse navigators are nurses who have been patients and have been through the experience; others are experienced staff nurses in the specialty (Bruce, 2007) or APNs (Bruce, 2007; Seek & Hogle, 2007). In some reports, an APN was involved in planning and overseeing the program (Wilson, Holder, & Torres, 2006). In reports of nurse navigator programs, rationales for initiating such programs were not always based on addressing health disparities—loss of market share for a population also served as an incentive (Seek & Hogle, 2007). Published reports suggest that such programs result in improved patient knowledge and satisfaction, improved adherence to appointments and treatment plans, increased volume, and reduced cancer treatment delays (from diagnosis to start of therapy). However, dialogue about navigator programs suggests that, within oncology nursing, questions about the use of yet another title, *navigator,* are being raised (Griffin-Sobel, 2006; Rochon & Cawthorne, 2006). It remains to be seen how this role as it relates to health professionals will evolve.

Some navigator programs are led by lay people, usually people who have experienced a similar illness journey. The program *Patient Navigator LLC* (www. patientnavigator.com) is designed to "empower patients with the information they need to understand their diagnosis and treatment options, communicate with doctors, ask the right questions, and find the answers they need" (Patient Navigator LLC, 2007). Fees are charged for this service, and the website includes a disclaimer that medical advice is not provided.

Empirical support for the concept of navigating the health care system was identified in an assessment of the concerns and needs of children with epilepsy and their parents (McNelis, Buelow, Myers, & Johnson, 2007). "Navigating the healthcare system" was a specific theme under the category "Difficulties, struggles, problems" that emerged from focus groups conducted with 11 children and 15 parents. The kinds of problems parents identified were directly related to coaching as conceptualized here: insufficient information concerning medications, questions to ask, and how to find answers to pressing questions.

APNs should regularly determine patients' needs for "navigator (coaching) services" within their specialty and determine best ways to address common coaching needs—ensuring that the persons providing the navigator services possess the appropriate knowledge and skills. Whether the navigator is an APN, a staff nurse, or an expert patient should be based on a deliberate assessment of the patient population's needs, the complexity and duration of the processes and services involved, and available resources. APNs also need to be aware of proposed or existing patient navigator programs and participate in developing, evaluating, and improving such programs, whether they are funded by grants or by the employing institution. They can help other stakeholders determine what background is appropriate for the navigator; this may depend on the nature and complexity of the illness, the purpose of the program (is it just coordination or is coaching patients throughout an illness the primary goal?), and other clinical and institutional factors. More navigator programs are likely to emerge, given the nursing shortage as well as the high priority placed on overcoming barriers to health care access, preventive services, and treatments.

Evidence-Based Practice and Patient-Centered Care

Chapter 5 addresses the role of APNs in applying middle-range theories to practice, highlighting theories APNs are likely to use. Middle-range theories that have informed health education and counseling interventions for many clinical populations include self-efficacy (Bandura, 1977; Clark & Dodge, 1999; Lev, 1997), the Transtheoretical Model of Behavior Change (Prochaska, Norcross, & DiClemente, 1994), and the Health Belief Model (Becker, 1974). Given the importance of behavior change to improving health and coping with illness, applying these theories to better understand the expert coaching and guidance competency could yield important insights from both a nursing perspective and an interdisciplinary perspective.

Some commentators have noted the inherent tension between the requirements for evidence-based practice and the high value nurses place on individualizing care (Brown, 2001; Kitson, 2002). The challenge for APNs is to hold onto these two values. They must apply evidence-based standards to ensure reliability of care; at the same time, they must recognize and articulate when and why the standard will not serve the patient. Such variations should be grounded in accurate assessments and an understanding of the patient's health status, quality of life, goals, preferences, and resources. Such understanding typically arises from the APN's coaching interactions.

Health Literacy

The Institute of Medicine (IOM, 2004) estimated that over 90 million Americans have difficulty understanding and acting on information about their health concerns. *Health literacy* is the degree to which individuals have the capacity to obtain, process, and understand basic health information and services needed to make appropriate health decisions (DHHS, 2000). Addressing health literacy is but one aspect of effective health communication (DHHS, 2000). An important consideration in implementing the APN coaching and guidance competency is the extent of health illiteracy in the United States. Health illiteracy is believed to be associated with nonadherence to treatment and disease complications, more frequent use of health resources including hospitalization, and difficulty accessing health care (IOM, 2004; Rudd, 2005; Stableford & Mettger, 2007), all of which contribute to escalating health care costs (Pawlak, 2005). An integrative review of literature on health literacy in older adults concluded that older adults may be at higher risk for marginal or inadequate health literacy, not only because of factors generally associated with health illiteracy such as less education and lower socioeconomic status but also because of declining sensory abilities,

multiple co-morbidities, and the demands of coping with multiple illnesses and providers (Cutilli, 2007). APNs must integrate health literacy assessment into their practices and take literacy concerns into account throughout efforts to help patients manage their health concerns, whether coaching individual patients or preparing educational materials to be used by patients. Health literacy is more complex than being able to read and follow medication and treatment regimens—it may involve managing everyday activities such as grocery shopping and meal preparation. For example, patients with diabetes, hypertension, and heart failure are advised to read and interpret nutritional labels to control these diseases. In addition, efforts to help patients manage such illnesses require an interdisciplinary approach (Johnson Lloyd, Ammary, Epstein, Johnson, & Rhee, 2006).

Assessment of functional health literacy must be done sensitively. Years of education completed may not be an adequate indicator of reading and computational literacy (Davis, Michielutte, Askov, Williams, & Weiss, 1998). In addition, people with higher levels of education who experience a new diagnosis or other stresses may be unable to process complex information and consequently may benefit from use of limited literacy materials (Foltz & Sullivan, 1999; Stableford & Mettger, 2007). A variety of tools are available to assist clinicians in assessing patient literacy (Pawlak, 2005; Quirk, 2000; Root & Stableford, 1999). APNs involved in developing programmatic approaches to patient education must ascertain that materials are appropriate to the literacy level of participants in educational programs. Educational materials should use "plain language," that is, text that exemplifies clear communication (National Institutes of Health, 2007; Stableford & Mettger, 2007). The term *plain language* is also used to describe the approach to developing such materials: "evidence-based standards are used in structuring, writing and designing [materials] to create reading ease" (Stableford & Mettger, 2007, p. 75). Plain language text is accessible, engaging, and reader-friendly. Stableford and Mettger noted that reading levels alone are insufficient to determine whether text was prepared using plain-language principles. They also assert that addressing health literacy effectively will mitigate many of the problems that are the focus of national initiatives including reducing health disparities and improving quality and safety. Readers are encouraged to read the Stableford and Mettger article (2007) to gain an understanding of the clinical and policy issues associated with health illiteracy and to learn more about barriers to and strategies for improving the quality and utility of patient educational materials.

Numerous resources exist to help APNs improve their abilities to assess health literacy and to prepare useful, readable instructional materials (Box 6-3). The Harvard School of Public Health (2007) site is particularly useful; it includes slides documenting the problem of health literacy and its effects on health, as well as links to numerous resources. As APNs work to improve the quality of educational materials for patients with limited literacy, they may encounter resistance to simplifying language and educational tools (Stableford & Mettger, 2007); therefore slides and other resources that document the extent and impact of health illiteracy may be useful.

Telehealth and Coaching

It is clear that use of health information technology (HIT) is growing as clinicians and researchers discover new ways to deliver health services to those who might not otherwise have access, and this will affect APN practice (Reed, 2005). In Chapter 25, Mahn DiNicola describes the types of HIT knowledge and skills that APNs will need as use of telehealth becomes commonplace. How will this affect coaching? Examples from the literature will help the reader anticipate the future of "telecoaching." Boodley, a family nurse practitioner, described her practice, providing primary care using telehealth technology for employees at a site 250 miles away

from her (2006). Boodley described the technology requirements for offering this service. To link the patient and provider sites, a broadband computer network is needed. The patient site has a cart that contains camera equipment, an electronic stethoscope, and the clinical tools one would need to do an assessment. The patient has a "presenter" in attendance, usually an RN, who can manipulate the clinical equipment and cameras as directed by the APN. The camera transmits images; thus not only can the patient and the APN see each other but also, as the assessment progresses, with the aid of the presenter, the APN performs a history and physical. The APN can view the patient's ears and listen to heart, breath, and bowel sounds by means of the technology that relays images and sound via computer. Prescriptions can be entered electronically at the provider site and downloaded at the patient site. Boodley described both the benefits and the limits of physical assessment via HIT. Laboratory tests can be conducted at the patient site and the results transmitted to the APN. Boodley noted the possibilities for educating patients with chronic illness using this technology and is exploring expansion of her telehealth practice.

In another report, Tsai (2006) explored the impact of computer technology on immigrants' adaptation to stress created by resettlement. In this qualitative study of 13 parents and 16 children, the author found that computer technology was used by families to overcome four specific barriers: language, economic survival, loss of social networks, and social disconnection. This study

---

Box 6-3   Selected Health Literacy Resources

Institute of Medicine. (2004). Health literacy: A prescription to end confusion (Executive Summary). Website: http://books.nap.edu/execsumm_pdf/10883.pdf

Harvard School of Public Health, Department of Society, Human Development and Health. Website: www.hsph.harvard.edu/healthliteracy/index.html (This site has a bibliography, hints on preparing materials, and a slide show that provides an overview of the health literacy problem.)

Department of Health and Human Services, *Healthy People 2010: Section 11, Health Communication.* (Website: www.healthypeople.gov/document/html/volume1/11healthcom.htm (This site provides background on health literacy and criteria for effective communication.)

National Institutes of Health. *Clear communication: An NIH health literacy initiative.* Website: www.nih.gov/icd/od/ocpl/resources/improving-healthliteracy.htm (This site provides selected evidence that effectively addresses health literacy, improves outcomes, and lists resources for where one can learn more about health literacy.)

Health Resources and Services Administration:
- Self-sufficiency matrix—Assessment tool (developed to assess homeless patients but may be useful for other underserved/vulnerable populations). Website: www.hrsa.gov/homeless/main_pages/lcw/materials/data/01ssm.pdf
- Health literacy resources including ideas for building a health literacy curriculum. Website: http://ruralhealth.hrsa.gov/RHC/RHCHLR.htm

is particularly interesting because Stableford and Mettger (2007) noted that web resources are less useful to vulnerable populations, including those who are not health literate. Tsai found that parents who were not computer literate were aware of the value of Internet resources and had their children retrieve information. As APNs work with patients, particularly vulnerable populations, assessing their direct and indirect use of technology may help APNs make decisions about use of web-based resources to address patients' coaching needs.

Coaching "Difficult" Patients

Descriptions of APN encounters and exemplars in this text reflect the fact that APNs frequently care for patients whom other clinicians regard as "difficult"—patients or patient situations that others might characterize as difficult. APNs often see these patients and situations as demanding or challenging. APNs recognize that when clinicians describe patients as "difficult," patients can experience stigmatization, marginalization, discrediting, and disconfirmation (Robinson Wolf & Robinson Smith, 2007)—dehumanizing experiences that are not consistent with nursing's values. Thus APNs frequently bring a "let me roll up my sleeves and try to understand what is going on" perspective to this work; they are tenacious, staying with a patient, a family, or a situation until some resolution or accommodation has been achieved. This is an area about which little has been written, and yet APNs frequently find themselves assuming clinical leadership in such situations. In their review of the literature, Robinson Wolf and Robinson Smith (2007) identified a range of patients and situations that were characterized as difficult: physical aspects of an illness; patient attitudes (e.g., never satisfied) and knowledge (knowing "too much" about medications); and social factors. They surveyed a random sample of CNSs to determine what strategies they used. CNSs reported three strategies of 83 that were both priority strategies and were the ones most frequently used: respect the patient's dignity; approach the patient and family with respect, openness, and dignity; and show the patient and family they are respected.

Liaschenko interviewed nurses about strategies they used when working with patients they "did not like" (1994). "Not liking" was defined as "difficulty in establishing and maintaining a relationship in the face of patients who evoke strong negative emotions from nurses for serious reasons" (p. 83). Unlike the situations described by Robinson Wolf and Robinson Smith (2007), the serious reasons included "those who rejected and sabotaged the nurse's care, who endangered others, who made threats to nurses, and who were guilty of morally reprehensible acts, especially those where others were harmed such as in child abuse" (Liaschenko, 1994, p. 83). She noted that nurses experienced these situations as ethical dilemmas. One reason for the dilemma was that rather than speaking of a therapeutic partnership, nurses spoke of "creating a connection" to patients so that they could provide nursing care. The second reason for ethical concern was the nurses' perception that the situation reflected on the nurse's moral character. Nurses did not speak of duty—their central concern was "the kind of person the nurse is and how they preserve moral ideals and actions under adverse circumstances" (Liaschenko, 1994, p. 84). Liaschenko characterized the work of establishing a positive connection—the central moral task—as creating a bridge between self and other. This is morally and cognitively demanding work; Liaschenko suggested that even under these circumstances, nurses did not assume a routine and disengaged persona. Indeed, in one exemplar, a nurse demonstrated her recognition that this stance was beginning to happen in a situation in which she had been physically threatened. Her horror at this realization and her ability to transcend it and create a bridge so that she could care for the patient are instructive. Although this was not a study of APNs, Liaschenko highlights a type of experience APNs may experience. The self-reflective APN may recognize his or her inability to establish a therapeutic relationship only when the repertoire of coaching skills he or she has developed in caring for difficult patients has not worked. APNs who are able to create moral bridges in such situations can provide important clinical and moral leadership when they and their colleagues are challenged to provide safe, reliable, and quality care under adverse circumstances.

CONCLUSION

APNs coach patients through transitions. In the APN, graduate education and technical, clinical, and interpersonal competence interact with self-reflection to produce a diverse set of coaching skills and the ability to invent new coaching processes during novel clinical encounters. Coaching is an extremely complex skill that depends on APNs' personal and professional qualities. Although coaching processes occur simultaneously, they are not automatic. APNs can usually describe the intent of coaching interventions and explain their selection of one approach over another. What may seem automatic is actually very deliberate: the APN has learned what has worked in similar encounters and uses it over and over. In using a person-centered style with a patient, the APN remains open to cues that the approach may not work in this particular encounter, thereby remaining flexible and aware of alternatives. An observer seeing the APN in action may think these processes are automatic because of how natural they seem. That such interactions appear to occur naturally arises from the APN's mindfulness of the encounter and the patient's and the APN's own responses.

In many arts and sports, coaches no longer perform the skill they coach and yet are still able to coach effectively. The nature of the health care environment and the delivery of clinical services are dynamic and complex. A nurse's coaching expertise can still develop when the nurse's primary responsibility shifts from direct care to another area within nursing, such as teaching or administration. However, the coaching processes that are developed will be related to the learners—students or staff. The ability to coach patients depends on direct care experiences in which new human responses, possibilities for growth, and new coaching strategies are revealed through APNs' encounters with patients and families as they experience health and illness and new technologies and therapies. There is evidence that APN coaching has salutary effects on patient outcomes. The challenge for APNs is to determine the most efficient and effective means of adopting these best practices related to expert coaching and guidance that will enable patients and their families to cope with transitions and improve health and health-related quality of life.

Numerous factors in contemporary health care have increased the focus on patient education, expert coaching, and guidance as a means of improving patient-centeredness, treatment adherence, effectiveness, and efficiency and achieving cost and quality outcomes. The contemporary emphasis on meeting benchmarks associated with pay for performance (see Chapter 25), the increasing incidence of chronic diseases, and the emphasis on chronic disease management and self-care to prevent complications, among other mandates and quality and safety initiatives, will serve to make the APN coaching competency more apparent to the public, colleagues, and policymakers.

REFERENCES

Abraham, A., Collins, D., & Martindale, R. (2006). The coaching schematic: Validation through expert coach consensus. *Journal of Sports Sciences, 24,* 549-564.

Alonzo, A. (2000). The experience of chronic illness and posttraumatic stress disorder: The consequences of cumulative adversity. *Social Science & Medicine, 50,* 1475-1484.

American Association of Colleges of Nursing (AACN). (2006). *The essentials of doctoral education for advanced nursing practice.* Washington, DC. Author.

American Geriatrics Society. (2002). *American Geriatrics Society position statement : Improving the quality of transitional care for persons with complex care needs.* Retrieved July 29, 2007, from www.americangeriatrics.org/products/positionpapers/complex_care.shtml.

Atkins, S., & Murphy, K. (1994). Reflective practice. *Nursing Standard, 8,* 49-54.

Ball, C., & Cox, C.I. (2003). Restoring patients to health: Outcomes and indicators of advanced nursing practice in adult critical care, Part 1. *International Journal of Nursing Practice, 9,* 356-367.

Bandura, A. (1977). Self-efficacy: Toward a unifying theory of behavioral change. *Psychological Review, 84,* 191-215.

Barnsteiner, J.H., Gillis-Donovan, J., Knox-Fischer, C., & McKlindon, D.D. (1994). Defining and implementing a standard for therapeutic relationships. *Journal of Holistic Nursing, 12,* 35-49.

Bartels, J.E. (1998). Developing reflective learners: Student self-assessment as learning. *Journal of Professional Nursing, 14,* 135.

Bartholomew, L.K., Parcel, G.S., & Kok, G. (1998). Intervention mapping: A process for developing theory- and evidence-based health education programs. *Health Education & Behavior: The Official Publication of the Society for Public Health Education, 25,* 545-563.

Becker, M. (1974). *The health belief model and personal health behavior.* Thorofare, NJ: Charles B. Slack.

Benner, P. (1984). *From novice to expert: Excellence and power in clinical nursing practice.* Menlo Park, CA: Addison-Wesley.

Benner, P. (1985). The oncology clinical nurse specialist as expert coach. *Oncology Nursing Forum, 12,* 40-44.

Benner, P. (1991). The role of experience, narrative, and community in skilled ethical comportment. *Advances in Nursing Science, 14,* 1-21.

Benner, P., Hooper-Kyriakidis, P., & Stannard, D. (1999). *Clinical wisdom and interventions in critical care: A thinking-in-action approach.* Philadelphia: Saunders.

Betancourt, J., Green, A., & Carrillo, J. (2002). *Cultural competence in health care: Emerging frameworks and practical approaches.* Retrieved August 9, 2007, from www.cmwf.org/usr_doc/betancourt_culturalcompetence_576.pdf.

Boodley, C.A. (2006). Primary care telehealth practice. *Journal of the American Academy of Nurse Practitioners, 18,* 343-345.

Borrelli, B. (2006). Using motivational interviewing to promote patient behavior change and enhance health (electronic version). *Medscape*, 1-16. Retrieved August 11, 2007, from www.medscape.com/viewprogram/5757_pnt.

Braden, C. (1990). Learned self-help response to chronic illness experience: A test of three alternative learning theories. *Scholarly Inquiry for Nursing Practice, 4,* 23-41.

Braden, C. (1993). Research program on learned response to chronic illness experience: Self-help model. *Holistic Nursing Practice, 8,* 38-44.

Bridges, W. (1980). *Transitions: Making sense of life's changes.* Reading, MA: Addison-Wesley.

Brooten, D., Brown, L., Hazard Munro, B., York, R., Cohen, S., Roncoli, M., et al. (1988). Early discharge and specialist transitional care. *Image: The Journal of Nursing Scholarship, 20,* 64-68.

Brooten, D., Gennaro, S., Knapp, H., Jovene, N., Brown, L., & York, R. (1991). Functions of the CNS in early discharge and home follow-up of very low birthweight infants. *Clinical Nurse Specialist, 5,* 196-201.

Brooten, D., Kumar, S., Brown, L., Butts, P., Finkler, S., Bakewell-Sachs, S., et al. (1986). A randomized clinical trial of early hospital discharge and home follow-up of very low birthweight infants. *New England Journal of Medicine, 315,* 934-939.

Brooten, D., Naylor, M., York, R., Brown, L., Hazard Munro, B., Hollingsworth, A., et al. (2002). Lessons learned from testing the quality cost model of advanced practice nursing (APN) transitional care. *Journal of Nursing Scholarship, 34,* 369-375.

Brooten, D., Roncoli, M., Finkler, S., Arnold, L., Cohen, A., & Mennutti, M. (1994). A randomized clinical trial of hospital discharge and nurse specialist home follow-up of women with unplanned cesarean birth. *Obstetrics and Gynecology, 84,* 832-838.

Brooten, D., & Youngblut, J. (2006). Nurse dose as a concept. *Journal of Nursing Scholarship, 38*(1), 94-99.

Brooten, D., Youngblut, J., Deatrick, J., Naylor, M., & York, R. (2003). Patient problems, advanced practice nurse (APN) interventions, time and contacts among five patient groups. *Journal of Nursing Scholarship, 35,* 73-79.

Brown, M., & Waybrant, K. (1988). Health promotion, education, counseling, and coordination in primary health care nursing. *Public Health Nursing, 5,* 16-23.

Brown, S. (2001). Managing the complexity of best practice health care. *Journal of Nursing Care Quality, 15*(2), 1-8.

Brown, S.J. (1995). An interviewing style for nursing assessment. *Journal of Advanced Nursing, 21,* 340-343.

Brown, S.J. (1999). Patient-centered communication. *Annual Review of Nursing Research, 17,* 85-104.

Bruce, S. (March 2007). Oncology nurses help patients navigate the cancer journey: Taking the wheel. *ONS Connect.*

Capasso, V. (1998). The theory is the practice: An exemplar. *Clinical Nurse Specialist, 12,* 226-229.

Carrieri-Kohlman, V., Gormley, J.M., Douglas, M.K., Paul, S.M., & Stulbarg, M.S. (1996). Exercise training decreases dyspnea and the distress and anxiety associated with it: Monitoring alone may be as effective as coaching. *Chest, 110,* 1526-1535.

Chick, N., & Meleis, A. (1986). Transitions: A nursing concern. In P. Chinn (Ed.), *Nursing research methodology: Issues and implementation* (pp. 237-258). Rockville, MD: Aspen.

Clark, N.M., & Dodge, J.A. (1999). Exploring self-efficacy as a predictor of disease management. *Health Education & Behavior: The Official Publication of the Society for Public Health Education, 26,* 72-89.

Clark, P., & Gomez, E. (2001). Details on demand: Consumers, cancer information, and the Internet. *Clinical Journal of Oncology Nursing, 5,* 19-24.

Clarke, E.B., & Spross, J.A. (1996). Expert coaching and guidance. In A.B. Hamric, J.A. Spross, & C.M. Hanson (Eds.), *Advanced practice nursing: An integrative approach* (pp. 139-164). Philadelphia: Saunders.

Coleman, E., Smith, J., Frank, J., Min, S.-J., Parry, C., & Kramer, A. (2004). Preparing patients and caregivers to participate in care delivered across settings: The care transitions intervention. *Journal of the American Geriatric Society, 52,* 1-9.

Coleman, E.A., & Berenson, R.A. (2004). Lost in transition: Challenges and opportunities for improving the quality of transitional care. *Annals of Internal Medicine, 140,* 533-536.

Coleman, E.A., Parry, C., Chalmers, S., & Min, S.J. (2006). The care transitions intervention: Results of a randomized control trial. *Archives of Internal Medicine, 166,* 1822-1828.

Connelly, C. (1993). An empirical model of self-care in chronic illness. *Clinical Nurse Specialist, 7,* 247-253.

Corbin, J., & Strauss, A. (1992). A nursing model for chronic illness management based upon the trajectory framework. In P. Woog (Ed.), *The chronic illness trajectory framework: The Corbin and Strauss Model* (pp. 9-28). New York: Springer-Verlag.

Crowther, M. (2003). Optimal management of outpatients with heart failure using advanced practice nurses in a hospital-based heart failure center. *Journal of the American Academy of Nurse Practitioners, 15,* 260-265.

Cutilli, C.C. (2007). Health literacy in geriatric patients: An integrative review of the literature. *Orthopaedic Nursing, 26,* 43-48.

Davis, M., Sawin, K., & Dunn, M. (1993). Teaching strategies used by expert nurse practitioner preceptors: A qualitative study. *Journal of the American Academy of Nurse Practitioners, 5,* 27-33.

Davis, T.C., Michielutte, R., Askov, E.N., Williams, M.V., & Weiss, B.D. (1998). Practical assessment of adult literacy in health care. *Health Education & Behavior: The Official Publication of the Society for Public Health Education, 25,* 613-624.

de la Cuesta, C. (1994). Relationships in health visiting: Enabling and mediating. *International Journal of Nursing Studies, 31,* 451-459.

Department of Health and Human Services (DHHS). (2000). Healthy People 2010 (Section 11: Health Communication).

Retrieved August 10, 2007, from www.healthypeople.gov/document/html/volume1/11healthcom.htm#_Toc490471359.

Department of Health, United Kingdom. (2001). *The expert patient: A new approach to chronic disease management for the 21st century.* Retrieved November 1, 2003, from United Kingdom, National Health Service, Department of Health website: www.doh.gov.uk/healthinequalities/ ep_report.pdf.

Dick, K., & Frazier, S.C. (2006). An exploration of nurse practitioner care to homebound frail elders. *Journal of the American Academy of Nurse Practitioners, 18,* 325-334.

Diemert Moch, S. (1990). Personal knowing: Evolving research and practice. *Scholarly Inquiry for Nursing Practice, 4,* 155-170.

Felitti, V. (2002). The relationship between adverse childhood experiences and adult health: Turning gold into lead. *The Permanente Journal, 6,* 1-7.

Felitti, V., Anda, R., Nordenberg, D., Williamson, D., Spitz, A., Edwards, V., et al. (1998). Relationship of childhood abuse and household dysfunction to many of the leading causes of death in adults: The Adverse Childhood Experiences (ACE) study. *American Journal of Preventive Medicine, 14,* 245-258.

Fenton, M. (1984). Identification of the skilled performance of master's prepared nurses as a method of curriculum planning and evaluation. In P. Benner (Ed.), *From novice to expert* (pp. 262-274). Menlo Park, CA: Addison-Wesley.

Fenton, M., & Brykczynski, K. (1993). Qualitative distinctions and similarities in the practice of clinical nurse specialists and nurse practitioners. *Journal of Professional Nursing, 9,* 313-326.

Foltz, A., & Sullivan, J. (1999). Limited literacy revisited. *Cancer Practice, 7,* 145-150.

Frisch, M., Elliott, C., Atsaides, J., Salva, D., & Denney, D. (1982). Social skills and stress management training to enhance patients' interpersonal competencies. *Psychotherapy Theory, Research and Practice, 19,* 349-358.

Fulwiler, T. (1987). *Teaching with writing.* Upper Montclair, NJ: Boynton/Cook.

Gadow, S. (1980). Existential advocacy: Philosophical foundations of nursing. In S. Spicker & S. Gadow (Eds.), *Nursing: Images and ideas* (pp. 79-101). New York: Springer-Verlag.

George, M.R., O'Dowd, L.C., Martin, I., Lindell, K.O., Whitney, F., Jones, M., et al. (1999). A comprehensive educational program improves clinical outcome measures in inner-city patients with asthma. *Archives of Internal Medicine, 159,* 1710-1716.

Greiner, A., & Knebel, E. (2003). *Health professions education: A bridge to quality.* Washington, DC: Institute of Medicine.

Griffin-Sobel, J. (2006). The Editor Responds (letter in response to Rochon, Cawthorne letter). *Clinical Journal of Oncology Nursing, 10,* 450.

Hagedorn, S. (1995). The politics of caring: The role of activism in primary care. *Advances in Nursing Science, 17,* 1-11.

Hanley, M., & Fenton, M. (2007). Exploring improvisation in nursing. *Journal of Holistic Nursing, 25,* 126-135.

Harvard School of Public Health, Department of Society, Human Development, and Health, *Health Literacy Studies,* home page. Accessed August 10, 2007, from www.hsph.harvard.edu/healthliteracy/index.html

Health Summit Working Group. (1999). *Criteria for assessing the quality of health information on the Internet: Policy paper, Mitretek Systems.* Retrieved November 2, 2003, from http://hiti web.mitretek.org/docs/policy.html.

HealthSciences Institute. (2005). *Chronic care competency model.* HealthSciences Institute, Chicago, IL. Retrieved July 25, 2007, from www.chroniccare.org/documents/FullCCP-CompetencyModel.pdf.

HealthSciences Institute. (2007). *Chronic care professional certification program.* HealthSciences Institute, Chicago, IL. Retrieved July 25, 2007, from www.chroniccare.org/profdev_CCcert.html.

Heifetz, R. (1994). *Leadership without easy answers.* Cambridge, MA: Belknap Press.

Holland, M.L., & Holland, E.S. (2007). Survey of Connecticut nurse-midwives. *Journal of Midwifery & Women's Health, 52,* 106-115.

Hops, H. (1983). Children's social competence and skill: Current research, practices, and future directions. *Behavioral Therapy, 14,* 3-18.

Houlahan, M.J. (2006). Implementing a foundation grant for a nurse navigator to improve the experience of the newly diagnosed breast cancer patient. *Oncology Nursing Forum, 33*(2), 398-398.

Institute of Medicine (IOM), Committee on Quality Health Care in America. (2001). *Crossing the quality chasm: A new health system for the 21st century.* Washington, DC: National Academies Press.

Institute of Medicine (IOM). (2004). *Health literacy: A prescription to end confusion.* Washington, DC: Author.

Jackson, P. (1986). *The practice of teaching.* New York: Teacher's College Press.

Jenny, J., & Logan, J. (1992). Knowing the patient: One aspect of clinical knowledge. *Image: The Journal of Nursing Scholarship, 24,* 254-258.

Johnson Lloyd, L.L., Ammary, N.J., Epstein, L.G., Johnson, R., & Rhee, K. (2006). A transdisciplinary approach to improve health literacy and reduce disparities. *Health Promotion Practice, 7*: 331-335.

Kasch, C., & Dine, J. (1988). Person-centered communication and social perspective taking. *Western Journal of Nursing Research, 10,* 317-326.

Kasch, C., & Knutson, K. (1985). Patient compliance and interpersonal style: Implications for practice and research. *Nurse Practitioner, 10,* 52-64.

Kasch, C., & Lisnek, P. (1984). Role of strategic communication in nursing theory and research. *Advances in Nursing Science, 6,* 56-71.

Kendall, J. (1992). Fighting back: Promoting emancipatory nursing actions. *Advances in Nursing Science, 15,* 1-15.

Kitson, A. (2002). Recognising relationships: Reflections on evidence-based practice. *Nursing Inquiry, 9*(3), 179-186.

Koetters, T.L. (1989). Clinical practice and direct patient care. In A.B. Hamric & J.A. Spross (Eds.), *The clinical nurse specialist in theory and practice* (2nd ed., pp. 107-124). Philadelphia: Saunders.

Kolcaba, K. (1992). Holistic comfort: Operationalizing the construct as a nurse-sensitive outcome. *Advances in Nursing Science, 15*, 1-10.

Lamb, G., & Stempel, J. (1994). Nurse case management from the client's view: Growing as insider-expert. *Nursing Outlook, 42*, 7-13.

Lamm, B., Dungan, J., & Hiromoto, B. (1991). Long-term lifestyle management. *Clinical Nurse Specialist, 5*, 182-188.

Lang, N., & Marek, K. (1992). Outcomes that reflect clinical practice. In *Patient outcomes research: Examining the effectiveness of nursing practice* (NIH Publication No. 93-3411, pp. 27-38). Washington, DC: Department of Health and Human Services.

Larson, L., Neverett, S., & Larsen, R. (2001). Clinical nurse specialist as facilitator of interdisciplinary collaborative program for adult sickle cell population. *Clinical Nurse Specialist, 15*, 15-22.

Lev, E. (1997). Bandura's theory of self-efficacy: Applications to oncology. *Scholarly Inquiry for Nursing Practice, 11*, 21-37.

Lewis, F.M., & Zahlis, E. (1997). The nurse as coach: A conceptual framework for clinical practice. *Oncology Nursing Forum, 24*, 1695-1702.

Liaschenko, J. (1994). Making a bridge: The moral work with patients we do not like. *Journal of Palliative Care, 10*(3), 83-89.

Lincoln, P.E. (2000). Comparing CNS and NP role activities: A replication. *Clinical Nurse Specialist, 14*, 269-277.

Lindemann, C. (1988). Nursing research in patient education. *Annual Review of Nursing Research, 6*, 29-60.

Lindesmith, K., & McWeeny, M. (1994). The power of storytelling. *Journal of Continuing Education in Nursing, 25*, 186-187.

Litaker, D., Mion, L.C., Plavasky, L., Kippes, C., Mehta, N., & Frolkis, J. (2003). Physician-nurse practitioner teams in chronic disease management: The impact on costs, clinical effectiveness, and patients' perception of care. *Journal of Interprofessional Care, 17*(3), 223-237.

Lombardo, B. (1987). *The humanistic coach: From theory to practice.* Springfield, IL: Charles C Thomas.

Lorig, K.R., Ritter, P., Stewart, A.L., Sobel, D.S., Brown, B.W., Bandura, A., et al. (2001a). Chronic disease self-management program: 2-year health status and health care utilization outcomes. *Medical Care, 39*, 1217-1223.

Lorig, K.R., Sobel, D.S., Ritter, P.L., Laurent, D., & Hobbs, M. (2001b). Effect of a self-management program on patients with chronic disease. *Effective Clinical Practice, 4*, 256-262.

Lorig, K.R., Sobel, D.S., Stewart, A.L., Brown B.W. Jr, Ritter, P.L., González, V.M., et al. (1999). Evidence suggesting that a chronic disease self-management program can improve health status while reducing utilization and costs: A randomized trial. *Medical Care, 37*, 5-14.

Martocchio, B. (1987). Authenticity, belonging, emotional closeness, and self representation. *Oncology Nursing Forum, 14*, 23-27.

Mattingly, C. (1998). *Healing dramas and clinical plots: The narrative structure of experience.* Cambridge, United Kingdom: Cambridge University Press.

McDougall, G.J. Jr. (1999). Cognitive interventions among older adults. *Annual Review of Nursing Research, 17*, 219-240.

McKinnon, A., & Erickson, G. (1988). Taking Schön's ideas to a science teaching practicum. In P. Grimmett & G. Erickson (Eds.), *Reflection in teacher education* (pp. 113-137). New York: Teacher's College Press.

McNelis, A.M., Buelow, J., Myers, J., & Johnson, E.A. (2007). Concerns and needs of children with epilepsy and their parents. *Clinical Nurse Specialist, 21*, 195-202.

Meng, A., & Morris, D. (1995). Continuing education for advanced nurse practitioners: Preparing nurse-midwives as clinical preceptors. *Journal of Continuing Education in Nursing, 26*, 180-184.

Mezey, M., Dougherty, M., Wade, P., & Mersmann, C. (1994). Nurse practitioners, certified nurse-midwives, and nurse anesthetists: Changing care in acute care hospitals in New York City. *Journal of the New York State Nurses' Association, 25*, 13-17.

Milbank Memorial Fund and Center for the Advancement of Health (Milbank report). (1999). *Patients as effective collaborators in managing chronic conditions.* Retrieved November 1, 2003, from The Milbank Memorial Fund website: www.milbank.org/ 990811chronic.html.

Montgomery, C.L. (1993). *Healing through communication.* Newbury Park, CA: Sage.

Monturo, C.A. (2003). The advanced practice nurse in research: From hospital discharge to home. *Oncology Nursing Forum, 30*, 27-28.

Morgan, A. (1994). Client education experiences in professional nursing practice: A phenomenological perspective. *Journal of Advanced Nursing, 19*, 792-801.

Morse, J.M., Havens, G.D., & Wilson, S. (1997). The comforting interaction: Developing a model of nurse-patient relationship. *Scholarly Inquiry for Nursing Practice, 11*, 321-343.

National Association of Clinical Nurse Specialists (NACNS). (2004). *Statement on clinical nurse specialist practice and education* (2nd ed.). Harrisburg, PA: Author.

National Cancer Institute. (2004). *Patient navigator research program* (RFA-CA-05-019). Retrieved July 29, 2007, from http://grants.nig.gov/grants/guide/rfa-files/RFA-CA-05-019.html.

National Council on Patient Information and Education (NCPIE). (2003). *Your medicine: Play it safe.* Retrieved November 2, 2003, from www. talkaboutrx.org/playitsafe_bro.pdf.

National Council on Patient Information and Education (NCPIE) (Ed.). (2007). *Educate before you medicate: Enhancing prescription adherence: A national action plan.* Bethesda, MD: Author. Retrieved August 10, 2007, from www.talkaboutrx.org/documents/enhancing_prescription_medicine_adherence.pdf.

National Institutes of Health. (August 2007). *Clear communication: An NIH literacy initiative.* Retrieved August 10, 2007, from www.nih.gov/icd/od/ocpl/resources/improvinghealthliteracy.htm.

National Organization of Nurse Practitioner Faculties (NONPF). (2006). *Domains and core competencies of nurse practitioner practice.* Retrieved July 13, 2007, from www.nonpf.com.

National Panel on Acute Care Nurse Practitioner Competencies. (2004). *Acute care nurse practitioner competencies.* Washington, DC: National Organization of Nurse Practitioner Faculties (NONPF).

National Panel for Psychiatric Mental Health NP Competencies. (2003). *Psychiatric-mental health nurse practitioner competencies.* Retrieved, July 13, 2007, from www.nonpf.com/finalcomps03.pdf.

National Patient Advocate Foundation (NPAF). (July 1, 2005). *Patient Navigator, Outreach, and Chronic Disease Prevention Act of 2005 bill summary.* Retrieved July 29, 2007, from www.npaf.org/index.php?p=318.

Naylor, M., Bowles, K., & Brooten, D. (2000). Patient problems and advanced practice nurse interventions during transitional care. *Public Health Nursing, 17,* 94-102.

Naylor, M., Munro, B., & Brooten, D. (1991). Measuring the effectiveness of nursing practice. *Clinical Nurse Specialist, 5,* 210-215.

Naylor, M.D., Brooten, D., Campbell, R., Jacobsen, B.S., Mezey, M.D., Pauly, M.V., et al. (1999). Comprehensive discharge planning and home follow-up of hospitalized elders. *JAMA: The Journal of the American Medical Association, 281,* 613-620.

Neimeyer, R. (2001). *Traumatic loss and the reconstruction of meaning: Innovations in end-of-life care, 3.* Retrieved April 16, 2004, from www2.edc.org/lastacts/archives/archives Nov01/editorial.asp.

Nolan, T., Resar, R., Haraden, C., & Griffin, F.A. (2004). *Improving the reliability of health care.* Cambridge, MA: Institute for healthcare improvement. Retrieved August 24, 2007, from www.ihi.org/IHI/Results/WhitePapers/ImprovingtheReliabilityofHealthCare.htm.

O'Connor, N.A., Hameister, A.D., & Kershaw. T. (2000). Developing a database to describe the practice patterns of adult nurse practitioner students. *Journal of Nursing Scholarship, 32,* 57-63.

Olesen, V., Schatzman, L., Droes, N., Hatton, D., & Chico, N. (1990). The mundane ailment and the physical self: Analysis of the social psychology of health and illness. *Social Science and Medicine, 30,* 449-455.

Parry, C., Kramer, H.M., & Coleman, E.A. (2006). A qualitative exploration of a patient-centered coaching intervention to improve care transitions in chronically ill older adults. *Home Health Care Services Quarterly, 25*(3/4), 39-53.

Patient Navigator LLC. (2007). *Information.* Retrieved July 29, 2007, from www.patientnavigator.com/content/view/11/33/.

Pawlak, R. (2005). Economic considerations of health literacy. *Nursing Economic$, 23,* 173-180.

Pelligrini, D., & Urbain, E. (1985). An evaluation of interpersonal cognitive problem solving training with children. *Journal of Psychology and Psychiatry, 26,* 17-41.

Peplau, H. (1952). *Interpersonal relations in nursing: A conceptual frame of reference.* New York: G.P. Putnam.

Peplau, H. (1994). Quality of life: An interpersonal perspective. *Nursing Science Quarterly, 7,* 10-15.

Polaschak, N.R. (1998). Cultural safety: A new concept in nursing people of different ethnicities. *Journal of Advanced Nursing, 27,* 452-457.

Prochaska, J.O., Norcross, J.C., & DiClemente, C.C. (1994). *Changing for good.* New York: William Morrow.

Pugach, M., & Johnson, L. (1990). Developing reflective practice through structured dialogue. In R. Clift, W. Houston, & M. Pugach (Eds.), *Encouraging reflective practice in teacher education* (pp. 186-207). New York: Teacher's College Press.

Quirk, M., & Casey, L. (1995). Primary care for women: The art of interviewing. *Journal of Nurse-Midwifery, 40,* 97-103.

Quirk, P. (2000). Screening for literacy and readability: Implications for the advanced practice nurse. *Clinical Nurse Specialist, 14,* 26-32.

Radwin, L.E. (1996). "Knowing the patient": A review of research on an emerging concept. *Journal of Advanced Nursing, 23,* 1142-1146.

Redman, B.K. (2004). *Advances in patient education.* New York: Springer Publishing.

Reed, K. (2005). Telemedicine: Benefits to advanced practice nursing and the communities they serve. *Journal of the American Academy of Nurse Practitioners, 17,* 176-180.

Robert Wood Johnson Foundation (RWJ report). (2000). *Patient education and consumer activation in chronic disease: Report of the planning meeting on patient education and consumer activation in chronic conditions,* Princeton, NJ. Retrieved November 1, 2003, from http://www.rwjf.org/files/publications/other/PatientEducation.pdf.

Robinson Wolf, Z., & Robinson Smith, B. (2007). Strategies used by clinical nurse specialists in "difficult" clinician-patient situations. *Clinical Nurse Specialist, 21,* 74-84.

Rochon, E., & Cawthorne, L. (2006). Reader suggests navigator role (letter). *Clinical Journal of Oncology Nursing, 10,* 450.

Root, J., & Stableford, S. (1999). Easy-to-read consumer communications: A missing link in Medicaid managed care. *Journal of Health Politics, Policy and Law, 24,* 1-26.

Rudd, R.E. (2005). *Literacy and health literacy.* Retrieved July 29, 2007, from the Harvard School of Public Health, Health Literacy website www.hsph.harvard.edu/healthliteracy/hlslides.pdf; www.hsph.harvard.edu/healthliteracy/overview.html.

Schön, D. (1983). *The reflective practitioner: How professionals think in action.* New York: Basic Books.

Schön, D. (1987). *Educating the reflective practitioner: Toward a new design for teaching and learning in the professions.* San Francisco: Jossey-Bass.

Schumacher, K., & Meleis, A. (1994). Transitions: A central concept in nursing. *Image: The Journal of Nursing Scholarship, 26,* 119-127.

Scott, R.A. (1999). A description of the roles, activities, and skills of clinical nurse specialists in the United States. *Clinical Nurse Specialist, 13,* 183-190.

Scupholme, A., Paine, L., Lang, J., Kumar, S., & DeJoseph, J. (1994). Time associated with components of clinical services rendered by nurse-midwives: Sample data from phase II of nurse-midwifery care to vulnerable populations in the United States. *Journal of Nurse-Midwifery, 39,* 5-12.

Seek, A.J., & Hogle, W.P. (2007). Modeling a better way: Navigating the healthcare system for patients with lung cancer. *Clinical Journal of Oncology Nursing, 11,* 81-85.

Sorrell, J. (1994). Remembrance of things past through writing: Esthetic patterns of knowing in nursing. *Advances in Nursing Science, 17,* 60-70.

Spross, J.A. (1994). *Coaching: An interdisciplinary perspective.* Unpublished manuscript, Doctoral Program in Nursing, Boston College.

Spross, J.A. (1996). Coaching and suffering: The role of the nurse in helping people face illness. In B. Ferrell (Ed.), *Suffering* (pp. 173-208). Boston: Jones & Bartlett.

Spross, J.A., & Clark, E.B. (1996). Expert coaching and guidance. In A.B. Hamric, J.A. Spross, & C.M. Hanson (Eds.), *Advanced nursing practice: An integrative approach.* Philadelphia: Saunders.

Spross, J.A., Clarke, E.B, & Beauregard, J. (2000). Expert coaching and guidance. In A.B. Hamric, J.A. Spross, & C.M. Hanson (Eds.), *Advanced nursing practice: An integrative approach* (pp.183-215). Philadelphia: Saunders.

Spross, J.A. (2005). Expert coaching and guidance. In A.B. Hamric, J.A. Spross, & C.M. Hanson (Eds.), *Advanced practice nursing: An integrative approach* (3rd ed.). Philadelphia: Saunders.

Squier, R. (1990). A model of empathic understanding and adherence to treatment regimens in practitioner-patient relationships. *Social Science and Medicine, 30,* 325-339.

Stableford, S., & Mettger, W. (2007). Plain language: A strategic response to the health literacy challenge. *Journal of Public Health Policy, 28,* 71-93.

Steele, S., & Fenton, M. (1988). Expert practice of clinical nurse specialists. *Clinical Nurse Specialist, 2,* 45-52.

Sullivan, P., & Wilson, D. (1991). The coach's role. In G. Cohen (Ed.), *Women in sport: Issues and controversies* (pp. 230-237). Newbury Park, CA: Sage.

Tanner, C., Benner, P., Chesla, C., & Gordon, D. (1993). The phenomenology of knowing the patient. *Image: The Journal of Nursing Scholarship, 25,* 273-280.

Theis, S., & Johnson, J. (1995). Strategies for teaching patients: A meta-analysis. *Clinical Nurse Specialist, 9,* 100-105, 120.

Tranmer, J.E., & Parry, M.J.E. (2004). Enhancing postoperative recovery of cardiac surgery patients: A randomized clinical trial of an advanced practice nursing intervention. *Western Journal of Nursing Research, 26,* 515-532.

Travelbee, J. (1971). *Interpersonal aspects of nursing.* Philadelphia: F.A. Davis.

Tremmel, R. (1993). Zen and the art of reflective practice in teacher education. *Harvard Educational Review, 63,* 434-458.

Tsai, J.H.C. (2006). Use of computer technology to enhance immigrant families' adaptation. *Journal of Nursing Scholarship, 38,* 87-93.

Van Manen, M. (1989). By the light of anecdote. *Phenomenological Pedagogy, 7,* 232-253.

Welch, J., Fisher, M., & Dayhoff, N. (2002). A cost-effectiveness worksheet for patient education programs. *Clinical Nurse Specialist, 16,* 187-192.

Wells, T.J. (2002). When a dose of advanced practice nursing is the treatment. *Journal of the American Geriatrics Society, 50,* 2092-2093.

Wells-Federman, C., Stuart-Shor, E., & Webster, A. (2001). Cognitive therapy: Applications for health promotion, disease prevention, and disease management. *Nursing Clinics of North America, 36,* 93-113.

Wilkie, D.J., Williams, A.R., Grevstad, P., & Mekwa, J. (1995). Coaching persons with lung cancer to report sensory pain: Literature review and pilot study findings. *Cancer Nursing, 18,* 7-15.

Wilson, B., Holder, R., & Torres, M. (2006). Nurse navigator: Clinical leader in patient-centric stat lung cancer clinic [abstract]. *Oncology Nursing Forum, 33,* 398.

INTRODUCTION

Consultation is an important aspect of advanced practice nursing. Historically, the nursing literature on consultation focused on the clinical nurse specialist (CNS) role. As advanced practice nursing has evolved, the consultation competency has received more attention and is explicitly addressed as a role expectation. The American Association of Colleges of Nursing (AACN) (AACN, 2006) has highlighted consultation as an essential aspect for the Doctor of Nursing Practice (DNP). In elaborating the Essentials of DNP education, the AACN emphasizes the need for exquisite skills in the areas of collaboration and consultation for DNP-prepared advanced practice nurses (APNs). Collaboration is considered in depth in Chapter 10. The complexities of today's health care settings require that all APNs offer and receive consultation and understand the distinctions, practically and legally, between consultation and collaboration.

We (the authors of this chapter) are a psychiatric CNS with a background in psychiatric liaison nursing who is currently working as a part-time psychiatric CNS in an oncology and bone marrow transplant inpatient unit and a primary care nurse practitioner (NP) with a gerontology and adult health emphasis. We are nursing faculty members. The synergy that developed from our collaboration and the sharing of experiences and perspectives was enriching and energizing and perhaps underscores the most fundamental points of this book—that there is much common ground across roles, that APNs have much to offer one another, and that together they can effect important changes in patient care.

This chapter has several goals. First, *consultation* is distinguished from *supervision, collaboration, referral,* and *co-management.* We are concerned that these terms continue to be used interchangeably in practice without clear distinctions. Each term suggests very distinct relationships and responsibilities. For example, consultation is a role function used by APNs to offer their own clinical expertise to other colleagues or to seek additional information to enhance their own practice. Because consultation is often confused with co-management, supervision, and referral in practice settings, these terms are defined to distinguish them from consultation. We then describe our model of consultation in advanced practice and discuss the purposes and processes of consultation. Current realities of practice are considered, and issues are explored. Our goal is to provide more clarity regarding the nature of consultation because it has the potential to increase access to APNs' expert nursing care. APNs can also develop their own consultative skills and use their expertise to enhance their colleagues' nursing practice.

Although all APNs seek and provide consultation, the literature on consultation in specific APN roles varies. Certified nurse-midwives (CNMs), for example, specifically address consultation as an expectation, and consultation has long been a specific expectation for those in CNS positions. Consultation as a competency is less frequently mentioned in the certified registered nurse anesthetist (CRNA) and NP literature, even though they are likely to consult and be consulted in practice. We highlight the importance and value of incorporating consultation as a core competency of all APN roles. All APNs have much to offer one another, as well as other colleagues, as consultants. We draw on the more extensive literature on CNS consultation to discuss APN consultation in general and use our experiences as a CNS and an NP, respectively, to illustrate the consultation competency in practice. Provision of care to patients with complex needs requires continual development of this competency. The sharing of expertise through a consultative relationship is an important way to enhance clinical understanding and promote professional development.

The enduring works of Caplan (1970), Caplan and Caplan (1993), and Lipowski (1974, 1981, 1983) continue to inform our thinking, writing, and practice. A number of the sources used to prepare this chapter are considered classics or have ongoing relevance despite their early publication dates. We reviewed the literature using the following search terms in combination with the term *consultation: documentation guidelines; Medicare; reimbursement; professional practice; quality standards; information control; legal issues; benefit-cost analysis; psychiatry; billable services and nursing; telemedicine;* and *technology.*

CONSULTATION AND ADVANCED PRACTICE NURSING

Whereas APNs across roles and specialties are offering consultation in practice, the literature related to consultation continues to be found in the CNS literature (Ingersoll & Jones, 1992; Norwood, 1998; Scott & Beare, 1993), with the notable exceptions of the work of Monicken (1995) and Manley (1998). Barron and White (2005) emphasized the importance of consultation across advanced practice nursing roles. The significance of consultation as an essential aspect of DNP education (AACN, 2006) highlights the importance of consultation as a focus for education, practice, and scholarship for all APNs.

Sabatier (2002) described a creative partnership between a university nursing school and a medical center. An institute was developed to enhance shared activities between clinicians and academicians. Nursing consultation was viewed as the primary means of offering access to expertise within the medical center, university, and larger community of nurses. The institute brokered the sharing of nursing expertise and coordinated the consultation activities locally, regionally, and even internationally. Forsyth, Rhudy, and Johnson (2002) described the consultation role of the nurse educator in staff development and outlined how the principles of consultation described by Barron and White (1996) and Caplan (1970) can be adapted for educational consultation. Stichler (2002) described the role of the nurse as independent consultant. She focused on practical issues to be considered by nurses who want to share their expertise and leadership skills through consultation. She did not address APNs directly, although she acknowledged that the consultants to whom she posed her questions emphasized the importance of a graduate level degree in an area related to the consultation need.

Although consultation is part of every APN's practice (Barron and White, 1996, 2000, 2005), the CNS and CNM role expectations seem to address the competency most specifically (American College of Nurse-Midwives [ACNM], 1992, 1997; Barron, 1983,

1989; Barron & White, 1996, 2000, 2005; National Association of Clinical Nurse Specialists, 2004; see also Chapters 12 and 16). Faut-Callahan and Kremer (2000, 2005) (see also Chapter 17) discuss consultation in the CRNA role. Skalla and Hamric (2000) and Skalla, Hamric, and Caron (2005) discussed the importance of consultation for the blended role of the CNS and NP (see also Chapter 15). Similarly, Mahn-DiNicola and Zazworsky (2005) described the consultation competency of the APN case manager role. For other advanced practice nursing roles, consultation seems to have been less formally described. In CNS roles, consultation is often directed toward staff nurses as a way of directly or indirectly influencing patient care. Although CNSs might serve as consultants to physicians and other clinicians, staff nurses and their patients are their primary clients.

APNs should be aware that state laws and regulations may mandate a "consulting" or "collaborating" physician for advanced practice and prescriptive privileges. The wording of such mandates often directly states or implies a hierarchical relationship between APN and physician, which is contrary to the description of consultation being put forth here. Minarik and Price (1999) described the critical importance of conceptual clarity for legislative and regulatory reform. At the state and federal levels, medical societies have attempted to limit advanced practice nursing, so the terminology included in the legislation describing the relationship between physicians and APNs is of enormous significance. Minarik and Price (1999) made the compelling argument that the practical effect of the language of legislation related to financing of health care can be devastating to advanced practice nursing, even though state boards of nursing are clear in their regulations about the appropriateness of the expanded scope of practice for APNs. APNs must be sophisticated readers of legislative proposals that include mandated relationships between physicians and APNs. Because legislation is drafted regarding both scope of practice and direct reimbursement for practice, APNs need to be clear and articulate about the implications of such terms as *collaboration, supervision, direction,* and *consultation.* Medical societies may propose such terminology with a clear intent to mandate hierarchical relationships with physicians to limit advanced practice nursing. Because mandated relationships between APNs and physicians may constrain advanced practice nursing consultation, APNs should be aware of the statutes and norms that regulate their practices.

The goals and outcomes of consultation are relevant to ongoing efforts to reform health care. APNs can help bring about the national goal of high-quality, cost-effective health care for every American. Through consultation, APNs create networks with other APNs, physicians, and other colleagues, offering and receiving advice and information that can improve patient care and their own clinical knowledge and skills. Interacting with colleagues in other disciplines can enhance interdisciplinary collaboration (see Chapter 10). Consultation can also help shape and develop the practices of consultees and protégés, thereby indirectly but significantly improving the quality, depth, and comprehensiveness of care available to populations of patients and families. Consultation offers APNs the opportunity to positively influence health care outcomes beyond the direct patient care encounter.

Given the importance of consultation for all APNs, it is surprising that so little emphasis is reflected in other advanced practice nursing literature. With the exception of CNS practice, consultation within advanced practice nursing may be less visible, less common, or just not a major publication emphasis; but consultation activities may be an important variable in explaining the effectiveness of APNs. It is surprising that a recent review of the NP literature by the authors revealed no research related to consultation in primary care settings. Given the complexity of care needs addressed in these settings, the wide-ranging needs of an aging population, and significant time constraints in practice, developing and studying consultation as a core competency in NP practice is imperative. We urge all APNs to recognize the significance of consultation within their practices and to communicate the issues, concerns, and successes of this aspect of practice. Advanced practice nursing researchers must also study the role that timely consultations play in the high-quality, cost-effective care delivered by APNs. Consultation is a variable that should be considered in health care outcomes research. Looking specifically at advanced practice nursing consultation and its impact on patient and institutional outcomes may illuminate the role APNs play in improving care delivery processes.

DEFINING CONSULTATION

The term *consultation* is used in many ways. It is sometimes used to describe direct care: the practitioner is in consultation with the patient. It is also used interchangeably with the terms *referral* and *collaboration.*

For example, a staff nurse might request consultation with the oncology CNS so that the CNS would assume management of the patient's pain, which really is a referral. The term *consultation* is also used when there is a hierarchical or supervisory relationship and the person without decision-making authority presents an issue to the person with such authority for a decision. For example, a psychiatric CNS might consult with the psychiatrist regarding admission of a person to the hospital for inpatient treatment or the primary care NP might consult with an NP specializing in acquired immunodeficiency syndrome (AIDS) care about a patient. Some consultants always see the patient being considered, and some consultants never see the patient being considered. Thus how the term is being used in a given situation may be unclear, and it may be difficult to determine exactly what is being requested and what is expected. The more precisely the word *consultation* is defined, the more likely consultation will be used for its intended purposes. Because consultation is a core competency of advanced practice nursing, such precision is needed for communication within and outside the profession regarding advanced practice nursing roles and patient care. Consultations can enhance patient care and promote positive professional relationships; however, it is important to understand the differences between consultation and other types of professional interactions. Table 7-1 summarizes these differences, which are further described in the remainder of this section.

Distinguishing Consultation from Co-management, Referral, and Collaboration[1]

Providing direct care involves a variety of interactions with colleagues. The terms *consultation, collaboration, co-management,* and *referral* are, at times, used interchangeably but should not be. Lack of clarity about the specific process being used for clinical problem solving leads to confusion about roles and clinical accountability. The primary characteristic that distinguishes consultation from co-management, referral, and supervision is the degree to which one assumes responsibility for the direct clinical management of a

---

[1]In this chapter, we use the term *collaboration* to refer to a specific advanced practice nursing competency (Chapter 10) and the term *co-management* to refer to a specific type of collaborative interaction (Table 7-1). Thus we consider co-management one of many collaborative processes used by APNs. In the American College of Nurse-Midwives (ACNM) documents, the terms *co-management* and *collaboration* are used synonymously (ACNM, 1992, 1997).

Table 7-1   Clarifying Definitions of Clinical Consultation, Co-Management, Referral, and Supervision

Type of Interaction	Goals	Focus	Responsibility for Clinical Outcomes
Clinical consultation	To enhance patient care and/or improve skills and confidence of consultee	Consultant may or may not see patient directly Degree of focus on consultee's skill is negotiated with consultee	Remains with consultee, who is free to accept or reject the advice of consultant
Co-management	To enhance patient care through availability of expertise of two (or more) professionals working together to optimize outcomes	Both professionals see patient directly and coordinate their care with one another (e.g., physician may monitor complex medication regimen while APN focuses on adaptation and human responses)	Shared
Referral	To enhance patient care by relinquishing care (or aspects of care) to another professional whose expertise is perceived to be more essential to care than that of the professional making the referral	Establish connection between patient and professional who is accepting referral Negotiate responsibilities for outcomes	Negotiated, but responsibility is often assumed (at least for aspects of care) by professional accepting referral
Supervision	To enhance patient care by overseeing the work of a less senior professional	Develop skill of the supervisee	Supervisor and supervisee

problem that falls within one's area of expertise. Consultation is an interaction between two professionals in which the consultant is recognized as having specialized expertise (Caplan, 1970; Caplan & Caplan, 1993). The consultee requests the assistance of that expert in handling a problem that he or she recognizes as falling within the expertise of the consultant. Co-management is the process whereby one professional manages some aspects of a patient's care while another professional manages other aspects of the same patient's care. Often, co-management takes place between professionals who consider themselves part of the same interdisciplinary team. Effective co-management requires excellent communication, coordination, and collaborative skills.

The ACNM (2003) distinguished consultation, collaboration, and referral in the care of the high-risk patient in its position statement on collaborative management. *Consultation* occurs when the CNM

requests the advice of a physician or other health care team member and the CNM maintains primary responsibility for the patient's care. The ACNM uses the term *collaboration* to describe the process whereby the CNM and physician jointly manage the care of the woman or newborn. *Referral,* another frequently encountered term, describes a situation in which the clinician making the referral relinquishes responsibility for care (or aspects of care), either temporarily or permanently.

Caplan and Caplan (1993), Spross (1989), Hanson and Spross (1996), and Hanson, Spross, and Carr (2000) discussed collaboration in some depth (see Chapter 10). Collaboration is raised as an issue for consideration in relation to consultation because it has been our experience that APNs are confused about the differences between collaboration and consultation. In Chapter 10, Hanson and Spross offer a thoughtful definition of collaboration, which is slightly modified from the one they proposed in 1996:

> Collaboration is a dynamic, interpersonal process in which two or more individuals make a commitment to each other to interact authentically and constructively to solve problems and to learn from each other in order to accomplish identified goals, purposes, or outcomes. The individuals recognize and articulate the shared values that make this commitment possible.

This definition suggests that collaboration is a process that underlies the professional interactions involved in consultation, co-management, referral, and supervision. Therefore in the discussion of consultation, collaboration is assumed to be essential to the process.

Distinguishing Consultation from Clinical and Administrative Supervision

Caplan and Caplan (1993), Critchley (1985), and Lewis and Levy (1982) described clinical supervision in mental health practice. The term *clinical supervision,* as used in mental health, describes an ongoing supportive and educational process between a more senior, expert clinician and a less senior, novice clinician. The goals of clinical supervision are to develop the knowledge, skills, self-esteem, and autonomy of the supervisee (Caplan & Caplan, 1993). Unlike the consultant, the supervisor is generally responsible for safeguarding the care of the supervisee's patients and is accountable in that respect for the work of the supervisee (Caplan & Caplan, 1993). Thus the process of supervision can be helpful for enhancing the practice of clinicians, especially novice clinicians, regardless of specialty area. In this sense of the term, APNs can be competent supervisors. Some characteristics of clinical supervision distinguish it from consultation, and it is important that the supervisor and supervisee understand that supervision is different from consultation. Also, unlike the consultant, who is often an outsider to the organization or unit in which the consultation occurs, the supervisor and supervisee are commonly employed by the same organization and work together in the same clinical area. The clinical supervisor and supervisee are generally in hierarchical positions, with the supervisor being in a higher position (Caplan & Caplan, 1993). Although the ultimate goal of clinical supervision and consultation is the same (namely, assisting another professional to enhance knowledge, skills, and abilities as he or she cares for patients and families), the processes, relationships, and responsibilities are different.

Administrative supervision (e.g., vice president for nursing for APN employees) has much in common with clinical supervision (e.g., hierarchical relationship, responsibility for professional development of APNs). However, in administrative supervision, interactions are likely to focus on operations and the APN's ability to meet job responsibilities rather than on the day-to-day clinical management of patients.

BACKGROUND

Consultation in Mental Health Practice

Gerald Caplan, the father of mental health consultation theory (Simmons, 1985), recognized that many more needs were to be addressed in the Israeli community in which he worked than could possibly be met by available mental health professionals (Caplan & Caplan, 1993). In the late 1940s, Caplan and a small team of psychologists and social workers were expected to meet the mental health needs of 16,000 new immigrant children in Jerusalem. He developed his consultation model in response to these pressing needs. By consulting with other professionals, such as teachers and counselors, he found that the recipients of consultation could effectively meet many of the mental health needs of the children. Both the need that gave rise to this model and the model itself are relevant to APNs, who must consider strategies that enable patients and families, beyond their direct practice reach, to benefit from advanced practice nursing knowledge and skills.

Lipowski (1981) also developed a model of mental health consultation for use in the general hospital setting. He stressed that it is essential for consultants to understand the context of the consultation situation. He recommended that consultation include an evaluation of the patient, the patient's interactions with the staff, and the specific needs of the consultee (the staff member). The family and social supports are considered as well. The consultant carefully communicates with the staff and provides regular follow-up of the patient for the course of the hospitalization. Although Caplan's and Lipowski's models were developed for application in mental health, they have informed our evolving model of advanced practice nursing consultation.

Types of Consultation

According to Caplan (1970), there are four different types of consultation. *Client-centered case consultation* is the most common type of consultation. The primary goal of this type of consultation is assisting the consultee to develop an effective plan of care for a patient who has a particularly difficult or complex problem. In client-centered case consultation, the consultant often sees the patient directly to complete an assessment of the patient and to make recommendations to the consultee for the consultee's management of the case. This is often a one-time evaluation. Follow-up by the consultant is sometimes needed. The primary goal is to assist the consultee in helping the patient. A positive experience with handling that specific case will enhance the consultee's ability so that future patients with similar problems can be treated more effectively.

In *consultee-centered case consultation,* improving patient care is important but the emphasis is focused directly on the consultee's difficulty in handling the situation. Thus the primary goals are to assess the consultee's needs and address the problem effectively. In consultee-centered case consultation, the task for the consultant is to understand and remedy the problems of the consultee in managing a particular case. A usual problem is lack of knowledge, skill, confidence, or objectivity. Thus the consultant may educate the consultee further on the issues presented by the patient or may suggest alternative strategies for dealing with the problem. This is probably the most common type of consultation sought by APNs. The consultant may seek to bolster the confidence of the consultee in handling the problem if, in the opinion of the consultant, the consultee has the ability and potential to do so. If the problem presented by the consultee is a lack of professional objectivity, the consultant can help the consultee identify the factors interfering with the consultee's ability to see the patient realistically. The consultee may hold a stereotyped view of the patient, or perhaps the patient's difficulties in some way mirror or symbolize the consultee's personal difficulties and cloud the consultee's ability to see the reality of the situation. Effective consultation can foster orderly reflection and extend the frames of reference used by the consultee to solve clinical problems (Caplan & Caplan, 1993). Both client-centered and consultee-centered case consultations have been important activities in traditional CNS practice.

Program-centered administrative consultation focuses on the planning and administration of clinical services. *Consultee-centered administrative consultation* focuses on the consultee's (or group of consultees') difficulties as they interfere with the organization's objectives. APNs may be involved in all four types of consultation at various times. This chapter specifically considers client-centered case consultation and consultee-centered case consultation because the focus of this chapter is the process of interacting with other professionals regarding the care of individual patients. These are the most common types of consultation in which APNs will engage.

A MODEL OF ADVANCED PRACTICE NURSING CONSULTATION

Principles of Consultation
The model of advanced practice nursing consultation that we propose is based on the following principles of consultation derived from the field of mental health (Caplan, 1970; Caplan & Caplan, 1993; Lipowski, 1981):

- The consultation is usually initiated by the consultee.
- The relationship between the consultant and consultee is nonhierarchical and collaborative.
- The consultant always considers contextual factors when responding to the request for consultation.
- The consultant has no direct authority for managing patient care.
- The consultant does not prescribe but makes recommendations.
- The consultee is free to accept or reject the recommendations of the consultant.
- The consultation should be documented.

Description of the Model
Barron (1989) proposed a model of consultation for CNSs that was based on the nursing process and incorporated principles from the work of Caplan (1970) and Lipowski (1974, 1981, 1983). This model, expanded by Barron and White (1996), has evolved into the model of advanced practice nurse consultation shown in Figure 7-1. APNs tend to have a holistic orientation and an understanding of systems theory that will enable them to apply this consultation model in practice. At the center of Barron and White's proposed model are the purposes and outcomes of consultation that are essentially the same. Surrounding the center is the ecological field of the consultation. Consultations are embedded in the context of the specific circumstances surrounding the consultation request, so the ecological field in which the consultation takes place must be understood to provide effective consultation (Caplan & Caplan, 1993). This involves an appreciation of the

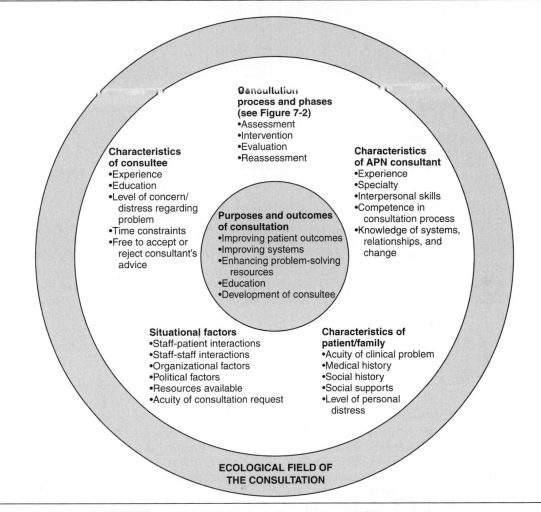

Consultation
process and phases
(see Figure 7-2)
•Assessment
•Intervention
•Evaluation
•Reassessment

**Characteristics
of consultee**
•Experience
•Education
•Level of concern/
  distress regarding
  problem
•Time constraints
•Free to accept or
  reject consultant's
  advice

**Characteristics
of APN consultant**
•Experience
•Specialty
•Interpersonal skills
•Competence in
  consultation process
•Knowledge of systems,
  relationships, and
  change

**Purposes and outcomes
of consultation**
•Improving patient outcomes
•Improving systems
•Enhancing problem-solving
  resources
•Education
•Development of consultee

Situational factors
•Staff-patient interactions
•Staff-staff interactions
•Organizational factors
•Political factors
•Resources available
•Acuity of consultation request

**Characteristics of
patient/family**
•Acuity of clinical problem
•Medical history
•Social history
•Social supports
•Level of personal
  distress

**ECOLOGICAL FIELD OF
THE CONSULTATION**

FIGURE **7-1:** A model of advanced practice nurse (APN) consultation.

interconnection and interrelatedness of the systems and contexts influencing the consultation problem and process. Thus the consultation process is an integral part of the ecological field. The process—in which the consultant evaluates the request, performs an assessment, determines the skills required to address the problem, intervenes, and evaluates the outcome—is expanded in Figure 7-2. Other elements of the ecological field include the characteristics of the consultant, characteristics of the consultee, characteristics of the patient and family, and situational factors. We assume that there are reciprocal influences among the purposes, process, and contextual factors that can affect consultation processes

and outcomes. Each component of the model is elaborated in the following sections.

Purposes and Outcomes

The purpose of a consultation may be to improve care delivery processes and patient outcomes, enhance health care delivery systems, extend the knowledge available to solve clinical problems, foster the ongoing professional development of the consultee, or a combination of these goals. Consultants should be aware that the purposes for which they have been consulted may contract or expand during the process of consulting. Often, APN consultants accomplish several purposes at once. If additional purposes

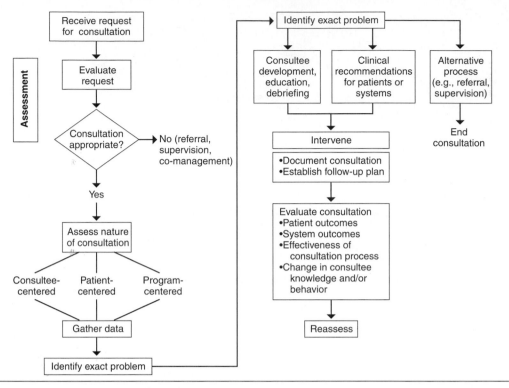

FIGURE **7-2:** Algorithm for consultation process.

and possible outcomes are uncovered during consultation, these should be made clear to the consultee. The consultee may want the consultant's assistance with a patient but does not have the time or interest to focus on his or her own development. Patients may also reveal information that requires a shift in the consultation's focus, purpose, and outcome. Over the course of the consultation, being explicit about the goal or outcome of the consultation is essential if APNs are to evaluate the impact of consultation on practice.

The Consultation Process for Formal Consultation

Figure 7-2 presents an algorithm of the consultation process. With experience and expertise, the process may occur fairly rapidly so that the expert consultant may not be aware of using these steps consciously. In addition, in some situations the problem for which help is sought is clear-cut and the consultation is brief. These types of consultations are discussed later in the chapter.

Once a request for consultation is received, assessment of the consultation problem begins with evaluation of the request itself. An important component of assessment is confirming with the consultee that consultation is, in fact, the appropriate strategy for addressing the problem (rather than a referral, for example). At this stage, the consultant and consultee may decide that an alternative process is needed (e.g., a shift to co-management or referral). The consultant confirms that the problem has been accurately identified and falls within the realm of the consultant's expertise and clarifies the nonhierarchical nature of the relationship between the consultant and consultee. The consultant also confirms that the consultee will remain clinically responsible for the patient who is the focus of the consultation. The consultant must remember that the consultee is ultimately free to accept or reject his or her recommendations. Once the request itself has been considered, the consultant gathers information from the consultee about the specific nature of the problem. The consultant tries to determine whether the patient has unusually difficult and complex problems (patient-centered consultation) and whether the problem results from the consultee's lack of knowledge, skill, confidence, or objectivity (consultee-centered consultation). Once the request, the nature of the relationship, and appropriateness of consultation have been established, the consultant focuses on gathering data related to the consultation problem. This may include direct assessment of the patient. The consultant considers the ecological field of the consultation, which includes the systems and contexts that may influence the patient and family, the consultee and staff, and the setting in which the consultation takes place. Some requests for consultation are quite focused and require that the consultant identify aspects of the ecological field that are priorities for assessment and attention. Others require more comprehensive assessment.

The consultant uses available resources such as patient records, direct assessment of the patient, and interviews with staff and family to identify the exact problem or problems that are to be the focus of consultation. This may or may not be the problem for which help has been sought. Some consultation problems are simple and do not require extensive data collection. Others are complex and may require extensive chart review for a long-standing problem or calls to referring clinicians when incomplete data have been provided. The consultant shares the identified problem with the consultee and validates this with the consultee. If part of the problem is the consultee's lack of expertise, the consultant will want to use tact as the problem is identified and discussed. Interpersonal qualities of the consultant are crucial and are discussed later in this chapter.

Once the specific problem or problems have been identified, the consultant and consultee consider interventions that will address the problem(s). The consultant may intervene directly with the consultee by using such approaches as education, assistance with reinterpretation of the problem, or identification of appropriate resources if the problem is the consultee's lack of experience. If the problem results from a particularly difficult patient situation, the consultant may assist with the process of clinical decision making by providing alternative perspectives on the problem and recommending specific interventions. More data may be needed to further analyze the situation, and a decision may need to be made about whether the consultee or consultant will gather more data. If the consultee accepts the recommendations of the consultant, together they negotiate how

the interventions will be carried out and by whom. If the consultant is to intervene directly with the patient, the consultee must understand his or her ongoing responsibility for the patient and agree to the consultant's interventions. Together they identify additional resources and determine the time frame for the consultation (one time or ongoing).

After the intervention, the consultant and consultee engage in evaluation. Evaluation of the success or lack of success of the intervention and the overall consultation is essential to the consultation process. If the problem is resolved, evaluation offers an opportunity for review, confirmation of the enhanced effectiveness of the consultee in managing the problem (underscoring the new skills and abilities or understanding of the situation by the consultee), and closure. If problems remain, reassessment offers the consultant and consultee another opportunity for problem solving.

Formal and Informal Consultation

The process of consultation described previously is comprehensive and formal. The consultant brings clinical expertise, as well as an understanding and appreciation of the process of consultation, to the problem presented. According to the model, the consultant considers all elements of the nursing process in relation to the consultation problem. However, what about the quick questions to the consultant, when what is needed is a piece of information and a quick description of how to apply the information? Are these brief interactions, sometimes called "corridor consultations," related to a circumscribed problem true consultations? Absolutely, but the consultant needs to make a conscious decision about responding in a brief and simple way to the request and needs to consider with the consultee whether the quick response addresses the problem. Sometimes the problem presented oversimplifies a complex concern requiring a more comprehensive approach. If the consultant and consultee consider the problem together, they can determine whether the quick response is adequate or whether consultation is needed. Conversely, sometimes what is truly needed is a short answer to a clinical question or validation that the approach to the problem is appropriate.

Staff nurses sometimes equate this brief type of consultation with consultation in general because they have experienced only this type of consultation with physicians, who quickly impart information and are then off to the next patient. The idea of the roving clinical expert dropping by with tidbits of expert advice is indeed the notion non-APNs can have of a consultant. That is another reason that it is important to make a conscious decision about responding in a brief way to the consultation request. In the informal situation, the consultee may not realize that a more comprehensive and thorough investigation of the problem and solutions with the consultant is possible. Also, some clinical situations require a more formal approach to the consultation problem. We suggest that APNs consider the kinds of problems in practice that require a formal approach and develop a system for integrating nurse-nurse and interdisciplinary consultations that make advanced practice nursing skills more visible and extend their knowledge and skills.

Ecological Field of the Consultation Process

Characteristics of the Advanced Practice Nurse Consultant. In addition to theoretical understanding, self-awareness and interpersonal skills are essential for the consultant (Barron, 1989; Barron & White, 1996, 2000, 2005). For a model of consultative practice to be implemented, it is critical that APNs first value themselves and the specialized expertise they have developed. One must appreciate one's skills and knowledge before the possibilities for consultation can be envisioned (see Chapters 3 and 5). APNs have developed specialized expertise in the direct care of underserved populations, such as the homeless; frail older adults; persons who are chronically mentally ill, home-bound, or institutionalized; and patients with human immunodeficiency virus (HIV) infection. The knowledge and skills acquired by APNs could serve to inform and expand the practices of staff nurses, other APNs, and health care professionals of various disciplines involved in the care of these populations of patients. However, APNs must first appreciate that they have valuable understanding and knowledge to share.

Ideally, consultants know themselves well: they are aware of their own personal issues, strengths, weaknesses, and motives. A good consultant must be able to suspend judgment and avoid stereotyping. When consultation is sought, often a fresh perspective is needed. Self-understanding allows the consultant to see consultation issues realistically and without prejudice. It is not uncommon for a consultant to step into a highly emotionally charged situation. Self-awareness, understanding, and being able to remain centered and self-possessed are key to remaining ob-

jective and clear. It can be meaningful and helpful for the consultant to have a trusted colleague or supervisor with whom to share and review consultation situations. Such discussions can offer support and enhance the consultant's understanding of personal and interpersonal responses to the consultation material.

The consultant should also be able to establish warm, respectful, and accepting relationships with consultees. The initiation of a consultation request is often associated with a sense of vulnerability on the part of the consultee, who recognizes that assistance is required to help manage the situation at hand. The consultant must communicate (and sincerely believe) that the problem and the consultee are important and worthy of consideration. The consultant must also communicate confidence in the consultee's ability to overcome the difficulties resulting in the consultation request. When the consultant creates a climate of trust and acceptance, the consultee can then be willing to risk vulnerability and genuineness with the consultant. When a respectful, trusting connection is made between the consultant and consultee, a deep examination of the problem, implications, and solutions is possible.

An APN is sometimes the consultee, and often the APN requests consultation from a physician. As a consultee, the APN should be able to identify and articulate the nature of the problem for which help is being sought. It may be necessary to clarify the collegial, nonhierarchical nature of the consultation relationship. When consulting with an APN colleague or physician, an APN has often already tried alternative plans or is thinking about possible directions to take based on knowledge of the patient or clinical situation. Consultants find such information useful in planning their approaches to the consultation. Dialogue with APN colleagues and physicians can improve the effectiveness and efficiency of the consultation and can strengthen collaboration among colleagues. In addition to their intrapersonal knowledge and interpersonal skills, APNs must be competent in the consultative process.

To be an effective consultant, an APN must be knowledgeable about systems, relationships, and change (see Chapter 9). Although skill in consultation develops over time, the attributes of the consultant and the consultation process described here can help novice APNs who are open to learning approach consultation with confidence (see the "Developing Consultation Skills in Advance Practice Nurse Students" section on pp. 207-208).

Characteristics of the Consultee. The consultee identifies a problem that exists in a clinical situation because of uncertainty, complexity, or a lack of knowledge on his or her part and believes that increased knowledge and assistance with clinical decision making would enhance practice. Characteristics of the consultee may need to be considered. Education, experience, the consultee's level of distress regarding the clinical problem for which help is sought, organizational skills, and availability to problem-solve with the consultant are factors that can influence the consultation.

Patient and Family Factors. Among factors to consider are the acuity and complexity of the clinical problem; the patient's medical history, social history, and social supports; and other resources. Depending on the nature of the problem, it may be important to consider concurrent stresses being experienced by the patient and family. An acute problem may demand the consultant's immediate assistance, requiring a shift in the consultant's priorities. A complex or unusual problem may take more time to solve.

Situational Factors. In this model, *situational factors* refer to those inherent within the organization and staff caring for the patient. Numerous situational factors can affect the consultation process. The quality of relationships and interactions between staff and patients or among staff members themselves may be important issues. For example, a patient perceived as being nonadherent to some therapy may be responding to conflicts among team members that the patient has inferred from clinicians' behaviors. A clinician may seek validation from a consultant as a way of getting support for an unpopular but potentially productive approach to a clinical problem. Time pressures and lack of adequate resources can affect consultation. Organizational factors include legal factors, regulatory considerations, and credentialing mechanisms for specialty practice. Organizational politics, power imbalances, and rapid or frequent system changes also are to be considered. All of these factors can affect the consultee's view of the importance of the request. For APNs, the status of advanced practice nursing and APNs in a particular agency or state may influence consultation. For example, organizational policies and procedures regarding consultation, statutes regarding APN-physician "consulting" relationships, protocol agreements, reimbursement policies, and degree of prescriptive authority may affect the consultation process.

COMMON ADVANCED PRACTICE NURSE CONSULTATION SITUATIONS

Depending on one's particular advanced practice nursing role, certain consultation situations may be more common than others. APNs are most likely to receive requests for patient- and consultee-centered case consultations. These types of consultations are described in this section. Experienced APNs may extend their consultative skills into other types of consultations, such as program-centered consultations. The exemplars included here vary in the complexity of consultations and the extent to which aspects of the consultation model are made explicit. The reader is encouraged to examine the ways in which the proposed model of advanced practice nursing consultation is applied and consider ways in which it can be applied in his or her own practice.

Advance Practice Nurse–Advance Practice Nurse Consultation

Within their specialty or setting, APNs may take for granted the available APN consulting resources. They may not think of their interactions regarding patient care as consultation because they occur in the hallway or over coffee. Consultation among APNs may be more or less formal, depending on the culture of the unit or clinic, the relationships among the APNs, and the specialty populations seen in the facility. Consultations are likely to involve specific patient issues; for example: "Could you look at this rash? I've never seen one quite like this before"; or "I've done everything I can think of to try to make sure this pregnant teen comes to her prenatal visits, and she still misses them. Here's what I've done . . . . Can you think of anything else before I get the city department of social services involved?"

Norwood (1998) discussed the importance of and practicalities related to APNs seeking consultation from other APNs. She noted that APNs readily think of themselves as consultants but may overlook opportunities for seeking consultation. She outlined the following factors as relevant when APNs consider the use of a consultant: cost savings, objectivity, politics, when not to seek consultation, and issues to consider in choosing a consultant.

In many settings, APNs may have some clinical and supervisory responsibilities. For example, a senior APN may supervise other APNs and staff and also

EXEMPLAR 7-1   CNS-to-CNS Consultation on a Severely Burned Patient

The medical-surgical clinical nurse specialist (CNS) consulted the psychiatric liaison CNS regarding the care of a young man with severe burn injuries who had been transferred to the surgical service from the intensive care unit (ICU). An initial problem to be addressed was the frequent and painful dressing changes. The patient disliked the lingering effects of narcotic analgesia for the dressing changes but clearly needed assistance with pain relief during the dressing changes. The medical-surgical CNS asked whether the psychiatric liaison nurse could teach the patient relaxation and imagery strategies for use during the dressing changes (and if the strategies proved to be helpful for the patient, could also teach the staff to coach the patient with these tools). The medical-surgical CNS also recognized that the patient would have to confront many complex and difficult psychosocial issues as he recovered. His hands and face were significantly burned. He would likely be permanently disfigured and disabled. She requested that the liaison nurse

provide additional supportive care to the patient and be available to the staff as they planned for the psychosocial dimension of his care.

The patient and staff found relaxation and imagery techniques to be quite helpful for the dressing changes. The liaison CNS and staff planned the patient's care together with the clear intention of providing a climate of trust, acceptance, and openness with the hope that the patient would experience himself as whole and respected and worthwhile in his relationships with them. In spite of his severe and disfiguring burns, the nurses could experience the beauty of the patient's humanity as they established intentional relationships with him. They helped him experience the depths of himself, which transcended the limits established by the burns. They helped him plan his first visit with his young child, preparing the patient for potential reactions and helping the patient prepare his child for his first visit. Follow-up mental health care was arranged at the time of discharge.

have a patient caseload. The supervisory relationship may constrain the consultation process as it is described here. An APN seeking consultation from a supervisor may worry that such a request reflects poorly on his or her clinical competency. The nature of the relationship (i.e., whether it is with a colleague or a supervisor) can affect the consultation process. Given our belief that a nonhierarchical relationship is essential for true consultation, it may be more accurate to refer to interactions with a supervisor *as problem solving*. Regardless of what the interaction is called, these types of interactions are important for professional development and optimal patient care. As APNs integrate consultation more explicitly into their practices and reflect on the process and outcomes of consultation, future discussions might illuminate this consultation dilemma.

Exemplar 7-1 describes a formal CNS-to-CNS consultation that is both client-centered and consultee-centered. Exemplar 7-2 describes an informal consultee-centered consultation between a primary care NP and a psychiatric/mental health NP. Exemplar 7-3 illustrates a formal consultee-centered consultation that is between a primary care NP and a CNS/NP specializing in HIV/AIDS; this consultation also led to a plan to co-manage the patient. Exemplar 7-4 illustrates an informal consultation that led to a referral.

The exchange between a primary care NP and psychiatric NP in Exemplar 7-2 depicts consultee-centered consultation. The expert provided important knowledge and suggestions aimed at enhancing the NP's practice yet was not responsible for how the NP used this information. The consultant provided important perspectives and new information that indirectly affected the patient's care yet was not responsible for the consultee's decision making or outcomes of care. If a psychiatric consultation was necessary and had been initiated by the primary care NP and was accepted by the patient, this would be an example of how this informal, consultee-centered consultation led to a request for a formal, client-centered case consultation.

Exemplar 7-3 highlights both formal consultation and co-management of a client whose needs are chronic and complex and require the resources of many professionals. The CNS/NP specialist in HIV/AIDS provided consultee-centered consultation enhancing the knowledge base of the primary care NP and providing insight into the expected course of adjustment of patients with AIDS as well as suggestions for community-based support. The primary care NP continued providing primary care and monitoring the patient's response to treatment and

EXEMPLAR 7-2 NP-to-NP Consultation on Adolescent Health Care

A primary care nurse practitioner (NP) caring for an adolescent patient was concerned about the high-risk sexual practices her patient reported. Despite the rapport and long-standing nature of the relationship with her patient, the NP felt the need for additional expertise to facilitate caring for this patient. The NP sought the consultation of a psychiatric NP colleague with clinical and research expertise in the area of adolescent health care. The consultant provided some of the latest research on adolescents and high-risk sexual activities and advised the primary care NP to consider other factors that could be influencing the adolescent's behavior. The consultant advised the primary care NP of findings that would warrant further evaluation by a psychiatrist or psychiatric NP to determine the adolescent's need for more specialized care. The primary care NP scheduled a visit with the adolescent and incorporated the consultant's suggestions into her assessment. Specifically, she elicited new information about factors that might be motivating the teenager to engage in high-risk sexual activities, and the primary care NP modified her communications with the teen to focus more on nurturing her and promoting self-care.

 EXEMPLAR 7-3 NP-to-CNS/NP Consultation on Infectious Disease

Ms. L. is a 29-year-old female who has been followed regularly for primary care through her young adulthood in the family practice. She presented 2 years ago with symptoms initially thought consistent with bronchitis. Her symptoms worsened, and she was eventually hospitalized and diagnosed with pneumocystis pneumonia. A diagnosis of acquired immunodeficiency syndrome (AIDS) was then made. Ms. L. was subsequently referred to the infectious disease specialists in a tertiary setting for ongoing management of AIDS; she continued to have her general primary care needs met at the family practice. The primary care nurse practitioner (NP) was pleased that her patient wanted to continue to be cared for in the family practice but was challenged by the increasing complexities in management of her new illness and the patient's struggles in coping with this disease. The primary care NP scheduled a telephone consultation with the advanced practice nurse (APN) in the infectious disease clinic where Ms. L. received her care for AIDS. The APN was a blended-role CNS/NP who had extensive knowledge and experience in the care of clients with human immunodeficiency virus (HIV) and AIDS. She was able to provide the primary care NP with specific knowledge regarding expected and unusual side effects of the medication regimen and commonly encountered drug-drug interactions. While the CNS/NP would continue to prescribe and oversee the medication regimen, they discussed what they would do to co-manage Ms. L.'s care. The NP agreed that she felt comfortable with managing common side effects and would collaborate to monitor Ms. L. for any problems with adherence to the treatment regimen between visits to the specialty clinic. When discussing how the patient was coping, the CNS/NP reassured the NP that her patient's response was appropriate for her stage of illness and suggested communication strategies that might further assist the patient in dealing with the reactions of family, co-workers, and friends. In addition, they acknowledged that the NP was likely to have more opportunities to help Ms. L. with coping with the disease, so the CNS/NP agreed to send the NP some recent, relevant literature on the unique challenges of integrating the experience of living with AIDS into one's life. The CNS/NP provided information on a support group and other resources that the patient might find helpful.

adjustment to the illness, co-managing Ms. L.'s illness with the HIV/AIDS CNS/NP and her colleagues at the specialty clinic.

Exemplar 7-4 demonstrates that an informal consultation may lead to a change in care. In this case, the APN expert's recommendation of a referral illustrates how a consultation may lead to a referral to a third party for assessment, treatment, and co-management when it may be more beneficial for the patient. Although the consultant's role was an important first step, additional care was determined to be the best course of action because neither the consultant nor the primary care APN could provide the range of services deemed necessary for the patient.

EXEMPLAR 7-4 NP-to-CNS Consultation for a Disabled Man Living in the Community

Mr. S. is a 56-year-old man residing in a group home. He has a diagnosis of mental retardation with an intelligence quotient (IQ) consistent with a mild range of mental retardation. In addition, he has a seizure disorder requiring daily medications and laboratory monitoring of the medication. He attends a sheltered workshop 5 days a week and is able to manage his activities of daily living; however, he requires supervision for cooking, shopping, and managing money. The staff at the group home provide the needed support but have noticed over the past few months that he has become agitated and less cooperative around the house. The patient and his caseworker presented to the family practice where he receives his ongoing care. After a careful workup ruled out a physical cause of the behavior change, it was determined that he would need additional monitoring and support, as well as a behavior modification intervention. The primary care NP sought the consultation of a CNS expert in the care of the older mentally retarded population. The consultant shared clinical experiences in caring for this population and cited the lack of research in the area of behavioral change in the mentally retarded population. She also recommended a physician colleague whose subspecialty is assessing and treating these issues in the mentally retarded population.

Advanced Practice Nurse–Physician Consultation

When consulting with other APNs or physicians, an APN is likely to be fairly far along in the problem-solving process. The need for consultation is often related to the consultee's level of diagnostic uncertainty (Calman, 1992). Experienced APNs often have a clear definition of the problem and a preliminary plan to address it that they wish to validate or reformulate, depending on the consultant's advice.

The need for statutory language that clearly describes the autonomous nature of advanced practice nursing has been addressed (Birkholz & Walker, 1994; Safriet, 1992) and continues to inform regulation of practice. The ACNM (1992, 2003) was deliberate in describing the various kinds of interactions CNMs have, primarily with physicians. Unfortunately, as noted earlier, APN-physician consultative relationships have often been structured by laws and regulations that mandate or imply a supervisory relationship, which can reinforce stereotypical nurse-physician relationships. Many organizational cultures reinforce traditional nurse-physician relationships and the behavioral norms associated with them. One of the major challenges facing advanced practice nursing educators is to explicitly address students' prior socialization to nurse-physician relationships that may undermine full expression of autonomous advanced practice nursing. When a hierarchical relationship exists between an APN and a physician, the APN who consults with a physician may defer to the physician's decisions, downplaying or ignoring firsthand knowledge of the patient. However, numerous descriptions of successful collaborative practices between physicians and APNs exist

(Barron & White, 1996). Such practices embrace the collaborative relationships we believe are key to effective consultations (see Chapter 10).

In some APN-physician exchanges, true consultation occurs; however, much of the language that defines relationships between APNs and physicians involve the terms *co-management, referral,* and *supervision.* Truly collaborative relationships between physicians and APNs ensure consultation that is bidirectional. Physicians in primary care often consult APNs regarding such issues as assisting patients in making lifestyle changes or in coping with the effects of chronic illness. Many APNs in primary care have special expertise in women's health care and are sought out by physicians for consultation on such issues. Physicians might then choose to co-manage patients with APNs so that patients benefit from the expertise of both professionals. APNs in turn might consult a physician regarding a patient in a medically unstable condition, which evolves into co-management by the physician and APN, with each assuming responsibility for the outcomes of decision making. Consultation between APNs and physicians can highlight the strengths of each, that is, the APN's deep appreciation for the human responses related to health and illness and the physician's deep understanding of disease and treatment. When both areas of expertise are available to patients and their families, truly holistic, comprehensive, and individualized care is offered.

As APN knowledge evolves and deepens, an emerging issue in relation to APN-physician consultation is the crossing of traditional nurse-physician boundaries. As APNs become more and more specialized, the knowledge embedded in practice may be more closely related to what is generally thought of as medical practice. For example, an oncology CNS may have very highly developed skills in the area of pain management. As a physician consults with the CNS regarding an individual patient, the CNS may make recommendations for specific medications. Regardless of whether the APN has prescriptive authority, an appreciation for the inherent shifts in the usual "professional territories" of nurses and physicians and the need for flexibility is helpful. Tact and understanding of the long-standing boundaries that are being crossed can bring the consultation relationship to a new level.

Advanced Practice Nurse–Staff Nurse Consultation

As CNSs implemented their consultative roles, it became apparent that the culture of nursing had not adopted consultation as an important strategy in providing patient care (Barron, 1983). Staff nurses were expected to take care of the patients themselves. A novice might consult a head nurse or more senior nurse, but staff members were expected to know how to solve problems and use the policy-and-procedure manual. Part of implementing consultation meant teaching staff members how and when to consult. In the early days, CNSs often engaged in active case finding to identify the patients who needed the knowledge and skills they had, because CNSs were not "assigned" to patients and staff nurses. By building this kind of clinical caseload, they demonstrated to staff how consultation might be helpful. Of note, CNSs tended to do direct consultation with patients, as well as to consult with other professionals to assist the staff with problem solving and enhancing patient care. For example, staff nurses might call the medical-surgical CNS regarding a patient with Guillain-Barré syndrome because they had had no experience caring for patients with this disorder. The CNS may have had little or no experience as well but would mobilize the resources needed, such as arranging in-services by the neuroscience or rehabilitation CNS, providing articles, being available to staff on all shifts as they implement unfamiliar assessments, and assisting with care plan development. The CNS would initiate processes (including additional consultation) and provide knowledge directly.

Once relationships are established and staff perceive that the APN consultant is approachable, respectful, and helpful, then staff will initiate contact with the consultant when complex clinical

issues arise. In Exemplar 7-5, intensive care unit nurses requested a psychiatric liaison nursing consultation. The staff and consultant had a well-established relationship.

MECHANISMS TO FACILITATE CONSULTATION

Mechanisms to facilitate consultation need to be considered by all APNs, regardless of setting. Consultation is an explicit role expectation for CNSs and often a daily activity for these APNs. Payment for consultation services is improving in some APN roles, but APNs need a clear understanding of the requirements for payment. As health care becomes more community focused and as APNs provide care to increasingly diverse and vulnerable populations, the breadth and depth of skills required for these newer roles will be considerable. APN-APN consultation is an important means of developing such skills.

In some situations, an APN may seek a patient-centered consultation with another APN and the APN who is consulted may be reimbursed. For example, if the primary care NP in Exemplar 7-2 referred the teen to a psychiatric CNS or if a geriatric NP referred an older female patient to another NP who specializes in urinary incontinence management, these consultants would probably be reimbursed. However, current mechanisms do not provide for reimbursement of indirect patient care activities, even though those activities may improve outcomes for patient care (Sebus, 1994), such as the initial, informal consultation with the psychiatric CNS described in Exemplar 7-2. To the extent that APNs and other disciplines can demonstrate the benefits of consultation, this shortcoming of the current payment system for health care services should be addressed as part of reform efforts. Historically, the focus on reimbursement has been for direct care activities and capitation-based reimbursement. To the extent that research begins to identify the impact of indirect care activities (e.g., some types of consultation) on patient and institutional outcomes, reimbursement for consultation may become available. In the meantime, creative strategies for funding consultation need to be developed. For example, incorporating APN consultation into critical pathways for selected populations may be one strategy for ensuring the cost-effectiveness of capitation-based reimbursement and of building in bottom-line consideration of consultation services. We were unable to find any current payers who

EXEMPLAR 7-5   CNS-to–ICU Staff Consultation on a Young Man Who Overdosed on Acetaminophen

A young man had been admitted to the intensive care unit several hours before consultation was sought, after he had taken an overdose of acetaminophen. Unfortunately, a large quantity of acetaminophen had been ingested the night before, and many hours had passed before he and his family sought medical assistance. His medical condition was grave. The psychiatric service and liaison clinical nurse specialist (CNS) had been consulted to assess the suicidal risk and make recommendations for the treatment of the patient. The nurses were very concerned about the young man and his family. The patient was expressing regret about the overdose, saying he was no longer suicidal. He was terrified by the potential for slipping into liver failure and dying. His mother was beside herself with guilt. The night before admission, the patient had come home intoxicated, telling his mother that he had taken the acetaminophen. She did not believe him; she thought he was looking for sympathy to avoid getting into trouble for drinking. She also reasoned that if he had taken the acetaminophen, it was no big deal; after all, it was a relatively mild and safe drug. When he woke up in the morning very ill, she brought him to the local emergency department for care. He was treated initially and sent by ambulance to the medical center.

The gastroenterologist was not at all confident that liver failure could be prevented. The psychiatrists assessed the patient to no longer be at risk of suicide. Everyone involved was deeply moved and distressed by the tragedy they were witnessing. The nurses requested that the liaison CNS be available for additional supportive care for the patient, support and referral for the family, and assistance in planning nursing care for the patient.

After about a day and a half, the patient slipped into a coma. It became clear that he was dying. His mother had accepted referral to her local mental health center, which was arranged by the psychiatric consult service and liaison nurse. For the first 2 days, the mother was in the unit most of the time. She spoke openly with staff and the liaison CNS about her guilt, regret, and pain.

After her son became comatose, she did not spend much time in the unit. She said it was just too painful for her to see him deteriorate. Other family members and friends spent a great deal of time in the unit. The liaison CNS stopped by the unit frequently, talking with staff and with family members. Everyone (including the liaison nurse) had a great need to talk through the sorrow and sense of impotence in the situation. Everything that could be done was being done, but that was not enough to change the outcome.

The patient had lived for 5 days, but on Friday evening, when the liaison CNS was leaving for the weekend, it was clear that death was not far away. She invited the staff to call her if they needed her over the weekend. The nurses called her and asked her to come very late on Friday evening. They sensed that the patient would die within a matter of minutes or hours, and they were concerned about how to respond to his mother when he actually died.

The CNS came in and was present with the family and friends to support the patient in the process of dying. His mother did not return to the hospital. Hands were held, songs chanted, and tears shed as the patient peacefully died. Unit nurses were in and out of the room also, being present as time allowed. After the emotionally tumultuous week with the young patient, there was some sense of satisfaction in knowing that if his death could not be prevented, a peaceful death could be facilitated. The family and friends expressed their deep gratitude for that facilitation.

The client-centered consultation focused primarily on the needs of the patient and family. The consultant and staff regularly shared their own feelings of impotence and despair with one another as they discussed the care of the patient. That sharing and planning helped shape the nursing perspective in the situation and clarify the goal of promoting a peaceful and comfortable death, once cure was no longer a viable goal. The consultation contributed to an active and compassionate nursing presence in the midst of tragedy and pain.

provide reimbursement for any advanced practice nursing consultation activities related to indirect care. Although Medicare provides some reimbursement for case management activities of primary care providers, consultation activities currently are not included.

Boyd and colleagues (1991) described CNS revenue-generating activities at their hospital in Columbia, South Carolina. They described relevant strategies for APNs as they creatively considered sources of funding for consultation services. They obtained third-party reimbursement for patient education and direct patient care. Other revenue was generated by selling instructional and informational tapes and books written and produced by CNSs. Notably, they also received substantial funding from grants. APNs also need to look to professional organizations for assistance in developing mechanisms to market and facilitate nursing consultation. In particular, specialty organizations and their journals may have practice-specific ideas for establishing and funding consultative activities. Until the issues of financing and reimbursement in the health care delivery system are resolved and include mechanisms to reimburse more consultative activities, creative strategies for this activity will be the responsibility of the profession.

In addition to funding considerations, it is important to consider new settings and potential sources and beneficiaries of advanced practice nursing consultation. APNs from varying specialties can form networks within organizations or geographical locations and identify specific expertise to be shared through consultation among members of the network. APNs within an agency can develop and initiate an explicit process for consultation so that staff within the agency are clear as to how to request an APN consultation and what to reasonably expect from the consultant. When the APN is involved in collaborative relationships, clarification of the possibilities for consultation could be discussed and negotiated. The consultant's services could be made available to interdisciplinary teams—even teams in which the APN is a member. Interdisciplinary teams exist in many settings. In addition to working collaboratively on such teams, APNs can offer valuable consultative services. Staff nurses in these settings may be without the benefit of abundant resources to enhance practice and professional development. APNs could offer such opportunities through consultation.

When APNs are the primary providers of care, such as in nursing homes and community health centers, opportunities for consultation may be missed or minimized because the most common interactions are collaborative or co-managerial or because of time constraints. Yet in these settings, the outcome of consultation is often improved patient care. APNs should consider documenting the consultations they are able to offer in those settings in somewhat standard and easily retrievable forms, such as computerized databases. If information about such consultations were easy to access, patterns and outcomes of consultation activities would be more apparent and the effectiveness of consultation could be more easily studied.

As APNs move into innovative practices, they should determine which consultative services they will market and what types of APNs and other consultants are available and will be needed. Consultation between APNs offers the additional benefit of collegial networking. CRNAs are establishing private independent practices (see Chapter 17). As independent practitioners, they are offering their services in home health (particularly to assist in the respiratory care of patients who require ventilators), in pain clinics, and in obstetrical care settings. Consultation with other APNs in those settings, in addition to the direct care they offer, has the potential to enhance the knowledge and practice of APNs and creates co-management and collaborative possibilities for all of the APNs involved.

ISSUES IN ADVANCED PRACTICE NURSE CONSULTATION

Developing Consultation Skills in Advanced Practice Nurse Students

For APNs to learn the theoretical and practical issues involved in the development of consultative abilities, relevant content must be included in graduate education curricula. In highlighting consultation as an essential aspect of DNP education, the AACN (2006) recognized consultation as a central competency for all APN practice. In addition to faculty-initiated experiences with consultation, APN students have much to offer one another as they move through DNP programs. Consulting with peers on challenging clinical issues can offer students experiences with the consultation process and help them begin to think of themselves as consultants as APN role identity is being formed.

Graduate educators and APN students could collaborate on much-needed research to evaluate the effects of consultative activities on patient outcomes. Research related to consultation could serve as an ideal focus for capstone scholarly projects in DNP programs. Learning how to evaluate and consider the implications related to the outcomes of care is considerably valuable for students. Focusing on the impact of APN consultation would raise many important issues for DNP student consideration. Documentation of the value and cost-effectiveness of consultation could help inform curricular decisions. Findings could also be presented by APN educators and students to insurers and policymakers who determine policy and payment for health care services.

Reflecting on practice is an important skill and attitude to cultivate in DNP students. Reflecting on consultation activities can help students begin to understand the depth and breadth of APN consultation over time. Gurka (1991) suggested that research questions could emerge from analysis of one's own consultations. In an analysis of her own practice, there were three major outcomes of CNS consultation. The first was prevention of complications. The CNS was able to identify high-risk situations and intervene to prevent complications. The second was the maintenance of standards of care and the development of new standards. The CNS's consultation activities ensured that high-quality standards of care were consistently maintained. The third outcome she identified was improvement in staff nurses' clinical judgment skills. Encouraging the process of reflection on practice, with a focus on outcomes of care, can help build important practice "habits" with benefits to the students beyond acquisition of consultation skills.

Developing comfort and skill with seeking, providing, and evaluating consultation is an important goal for DNP education. APNs are expected to influence patients, other providers, and the systems in which they work. Therefore, when APNs graduate, they should be equipped with knowledge, skill, and confidence in the consultation process. Effective consultation, whether it is sought or provided, enables APNs to establish credibility, build collaborative relationships with other members of the health care team, and influence the processes and outcome of care.

Using Technology to Provide Consultation

The use of new technologies to enhance care delivery has affected every aspect of the health care delivery system. APNs should review how consultation activities delivered through these new modalities can enhance the capacity to affect care. Equally important is thoughtful consideration of the potential concerns that might arise in embracing these mechanisms to enhance patient care through consultation. Clarity about the definition of telehealth activities and understanding current legal and ethical issues related to access, privacy, confidentiality, security, jurisdiction, and licensure standards are essential for APNs.

"Telehealth is defined as the use of electronic communication networks to transmit data or information that focuses on health promotion, disease prevention, diagnosis, consultation, education, and/or therapy" (Thede, 2001). Mahn-DiNicola and Zazworsky (2005) described technologies used to increase access to health care by removing the barriers of time and distance as encompassing the use of telephones, teleconferencing, videoconferencing, computers, interactive video transmission of data, and links to health care instruments. Undoubtedly, these technologies will be used with increasing frequency and creativity in the years to come with benefits in terms of increasing access to the health care professionals, improving rapid diagnosis of emergent conditions, and enhancing more frequent monitoring of chronic conditions.

Telehealth technologies are innovative and evolving. Unnold (2006), describing the possibilities of new technologies to assist APNs with home care complexities, proposed ways that the use of telehealth could enhance the management of wounds, as one example of a health problem that causes much suffering and great expense. With the use of high-resolution video equipment, APNs with expertise in wound care could offer their consultation services to a large group of patients and nurses. It is easy to recognize the health benefits of such creative uses of technology, yet neither the answers to the questions being raised about such technology nor the research about the effectiveness of technology strategies to deliver health care is keeping pace with the speed of the proliferation of the technological possibilities in health care. APN consultants should be aware of the questions yet to be answered. A concern of major significance to APNs is the issue of jurisdiction. As described by Hanson in Chapter 21, the complexities regarding telehealth and telepractice are ongoing. The National Council of State Boards of Nursing (NCSBN) has developed a mutual recognition model whereby state boards of nursing can participate in a nurse licensure compact (NLC) granting practice privileges to nurses who meet uniform requirements in the states participating in the NLC. The NLC is similar to the U.S. drivers compact in which drivers may drive across state lines but must adhere to the driving laws of the state in which they are driving. The NCSBN held a summit in December of 2006 (National Council of State Boards of Nursing [NCSBN], 2006) to promote the increased portability of nursing licenses to reduce barriers affecting telehealth and interstate nursing practice. As of June, 2007, twenty-one states have implemented a mutual recognition model for registered nurses and two states have NLC implementation pending *(www. NCSBN.org)*. Because of the lack of uniformity in relation to APN practice, however, mutual recognition for APNs is lagging far behind (Hanson, 2005; Hardin & Langford. 2001). The website for the NCSBN, *www. NCSBN.org*, posts current information regarding NLC and mutual recognition issues.

Reimbursement for telehealth is limited. Hutcherson (2001) described Medicare payment for teleconsultation as being limited to two-way interactive video encounters in which the patient is part of the session. Solomons (2006) discussed the need for the teleconsultation to be part of the physician's prescribed plan of care in order for Medicare to reimburse for services. Medicaid reimbursement, though funded through federal grants, allows for more discretion at the state level in relation to payment for services. Solomons (2006) noted that 26 states have initiatives related to payment for telehealth services. However, covered services and rates of payment vary greatly from state to state.

Privacy, security, and access to telehealth are additional ongoing concerns. Thede (2001) stressed that telehealth poses special requirements for security and privacy that go beyond the patient, caregivers, and third-party payers; the need for security related to the online sharing of private medical information deserves special attention. Ohler and Daine (2001) considered risks related to security of health-related e-mail communication. Confidentiality and the potential for miscommunication pose significant concerns. Providing information through e-mail and telecommunication across state lines raised concerns about liability and about differences in nurse practice acts regarding scope of practice, as just noted. They suggested that documentation guidelines and protocols be established for the application of any telecommunication and recommended further research on confidentiality and security issues in telehealth practice. Maddox (2003) raised the paradox that telehealth, while intending to increase access to health care, particularly for the disadvantaged, requires that recipients of such services be literate and have the technology available to them—assumptions that may be problematic for the very populations intended to benefit from these new approaches.

Research related to the processes and outcomes of telehealth strategies is needed. In a 2001 review of literature, Roine, Ohinmaa, and Hailey critiqued more than 1000 studies and found little evidence to support positive outcomes or cost-effectiveness related to consultation activities using technology. No studies that reported outcomes occurring over time were found; however, examples of successful programs were reported anecdotally. Most of the studies documented the use and application of telemedicine but did not link use to outcome or cost savings. The most-studied telemedicine technologies were the submission of recent diagnostic studies in advance of a patient transfer to another facility, videoconferencing, electronic referrals with subsequent e-mail communication, and telepsychiatry with psychiatrists providing phone consultation.

Use of telemedicine in the treatment of patients with injuries related to trauma in rural areas was reported to be lifesaving in a recent study by Ricci and colleagues (2003). The authors analyzed 41 teletrauma consults in a rural emergency department, and results of the study suggest that at least three lives were saved and overall enhancement of clinical care was considered improved. The number of deaths of patients involved in trauma in rural areas is reported to be twice the number of those in urban areas, justifying the continued study of such consultation activities in emergency settings.

Telenurse practice has been described in the literature, and some initial research has linked telephone follow-up to quality of care and patient outcomes. Larson-Dahn (2001) reported an analysis of quality indicators of telephone contact with patients and identified many of the complexities of providing telephone-based care. She identified such indicators as critical thinking, use of established protocols, and issues of continuity of care in her pilot study involving analysis of 10 telephone encounters for each of the five nurses recruited for her study. Patient outcomes were not measured but were recommended as a critical measure to be studied in the future. In addition, entrepreneurs in health care are designing business models around telephonic coaching of patients by nurses, although being an APN is not a requirement. See Chapter 6 for a discussion of telecoaching.

The application of technology in delivering health-related information has not been well studied in terms of process and outcomes. APNs should consider the potential opportunities that exist to enhance consultation activities with these modalities, but they should exercise caution regarding their implementation until legislative and policy initiatives related to access, security, and mutual recognition of APN practice across state lines are more fully developed and future research elucidates specific processes, outcomes, and concerns related to innovative telehealth strategies and practices.

Documentation and Legal Considerations

Although it has been stressed that the consultee remains clinically responsible for the patient who is the focus of the consultation, it is critical to appreciate that APN consultants are accountable for their practices relative to the consultation problem. For each edition of this text, the authors consulted with nurse-attorneys regarding current legal trends as they apply to consideration of APN consultative services.[2] Kim Larkin, RN, JD, (personal communications, June 18, 2003; April 2, 2007) stressed the importance of APNs adhering to all standards of care for their specialties as they offer consultation. She emphasized also the importance of APNs understanding that a duty of care is assumed by the APN when the APN-patient relationship is established as the result of a contract, either expressed or implied (Larkin, personal communication, April 2, 2007). Generally, the relationship is established when the APN sees the patient directly. Clarity regarding the assumption of the duty of care and the inherent legal responsibilities that are assumed with that duty is paramount (see Chapter 21).

The consultee requesting the consultation has an established duty of care for the patient, as well. Although the consultee is responsible for accepting of rejecting the consultant's recommendations, ultimately, the consultant's recommendations must reflect proper professional skill and adherence to specialty standards. The identification of an urgent or emergent situation that would fall within the consultant's area of expertise may necessitate stepping out of the consultation role (described on p. 211) to ensure that the urgent clinical issues are addressed.

Larkin emphasized the importance of APN consultants understanding professional standards of practice, state regulations, nurse practice acts, and institutional policies as they relate to consultation. This is because these would be used in a court of law to determine the elements of a malpractice claim (duty of care, standards, breach of standards, and damages) if the nurse consultant were to be sued (Larkin, personal communication, June 18, 2003). APNs also need to know when a consultation with a physician, rather than with another APN, would be considered as the standard of care.

Careful documentation of the consultation by the APN consultant in the patient record is appropriate and important when the APN consultant has seen the patient directly. The consultant's assessment of the problem and recommendations for clinical problem solving should be clearly described in the consultation documentation. There are times when the consultant should document recommendations even when the patient is not seen directly. When the consultant offers specialized expertise that impacts the processes and outcomes of care (e.g., the cardiovascular CNS offering interpretations of electrocardiograms; the oncology CNS making recommendations regarding monitoring for side effects of chemotherapy), consultation assessments and recommendations should be recorded in the medical record even in the absence of direct patient contact by the consultant.

Informal consultation obligations are not as clearly defined as formal consultation obligations. Whereas a duty of care may be assumed by the APN consultant when direct contact with the patient occurs, it is less clear-cut in relation to informal consultations. Larkin (personal communication, June 18, 2003) stressed the importance of clarifying with the consultee the nature of the consultation relationship. Consultants need to be explicit that when they do not see the patient directly, they are not actually caring for the patient. In informal consultations, the APN generally does not know the patient, the patient is not aware of the consultation, and there is no reimbursement for the consultation. Larkin noted in 2007 that, in the past, such informal consultations would not have established a duty of care but the legal trends are shifting somewhat for informal medical consultations. Although she could not find evidence for a malpractice suit involving an APN consultant, courts increasingly are allowing medical malpractice suits to proceed against physician specialists or consultants, consulted informally by the primary physician. Courts are seeking to address the following questions in relation to informal consultation: Did a physician/patient relationship exist with the consultant? If so, was there a breach in the duty of care by the consultant? Did the consultant go beyond giving general advice and participate in the patient's care? Given the consultant's expertise, should it have been "foreseeable" to the consultant that the treating physician would subordinate his or her medical judgment in reliance on the consultant's opinion? While this trend to consider informal medical consultants in malpractice suits is new, it is limited. There is

---

[2]The authors would like to acknowledge the contributions of Marie Snyder, RN, MS, JD, and Kathleen Moore, RN, JD, for their important contributions to earlier editions of this chapter. Their legal wisdom has informed the authors' understanding of the complex considerations related to APN consultation.

recognition from a public policy perspective that identifying the existence of a physician-patient relationship with the informal consultant would have a chilling effect on the free flow of information between professionals and could undermine the treating physician's control over the patient's care. It could also have a negative impact on care and medical education by limiting the comparison of problem-solving approaches among practitioners (Larkin, personal communication, April 2, 2007).

For informal consultations, opinions differ about whether or not the APN should record the consultation in the patient's medical record. On the one hand, as administrative specialist and colleague Dr. Amanda Coakley (personal communication, July 3, 2007) stressed, the APN consultant's recommendations should always be reflected in the record, even if the consultation is informal, so that the recommendations can be integrated into the ongoing plan of care for the patient. On the other, the informality of the consultation may imply either a casual encounter, without a full discussion of the patient circumstance, or an encounter focused on the needs of the consultee for additional information, education, or opportunity for reflection—issues generally not reflected in medical records.

APNs should document all informal consultations—if not in the medical record, then in their own files—including their assessments and recommendations in relation to the informal consultation problem. Such records provide documentation if legal concerns arise in relation to the informal consultation. APNs need to make well-considered judgments about where and what to document about informal consultations.

While informal consultation by APNs is a very important aspect of the APN consultant role, Larkin emphasized that APNs should consider a number of issues to limit liability as informal consultants (personal communication, April 2, 2007). When APNs are "on call" as employees of health maintenance organizations (HMOs) or party to managed care or other insurance contracts, they need to know the on-call agreements and contracts with hospitals and organizations that would be applicable to their on-call work. They may be responsible for seeing all who seek care in such circumstances. When on-call APNs are involved in a specific clinical situation, they should be clear about (1) whether or not they are entering into a relationship with the patient through their activities as a consultant and (2) when it would be reasonably

foreseeable that the treating consultee would rely on them as consultants. Larkin had the following suggestions for informal APN consultations:

- Include a disclaimer to emphasize that the consultation is not a formal consultation.
- Keep conversations short.
- Frame responses in general terms.
- Suggest several possible answers, and note that all depend on the specifics of the case.
- Be cautious of evaluating any test results and rendering a specific diagnosis.
- Keep communications about a particular patient to a minimum.
- Document informal consultations for the consultant's records with the inquiring person's name, the date, the nature of the inquiry, and the advice given; if a conflict arises, then the consultant has a record.

Larkin cautioned that the boundary between informal and formal consultation is not always clear; APNs should not hesitate to suggest a formal consultation and comprehensive evaluation when they feel that a comprehensive consideration of the problem is warranted.

The increased responsibilities inherent in all aspects of advanced practice nursing expose APNs to increased liability (Poteet, 1989; Scott & Beare, 1993; Survillo & Levine, 1993). Unresolved issues remain in relation to legal considerations of APN consultation practice. With the evolving use of telehealth technology and the shifting legal climate, the consultation role for APNs will likely become increasingly complex. Therefore when they offer consultation, as in all areas of practice, APNs should be knowledgeable about current legal and practice trends and make carefully considered judgments based on specialty standards and the best available data.

Stepping Out of the Consultation Process

The APN must recognize that unusual circumstances could necessitate abandoning the consultation process and assuming the stance of clinically responsible expert (Barron, 1983, 1989). If the APN became aware that the patient being considered during the consultation was in a dangerous situation and the consultee was unable or unwilling to intervene on behalf of the patient, the consultant would then assume direct responsibility for ensuring that safety needs were addressed. It is unusual that consultees, once aware of safety concerns, are unable or unwilling to address them, but it does happen. Barron described such a circumstance (1989). She was consulted by the coronary care unit (CCU) nursing staff because of a patient's unwillingness to adhere to the safety guidelines of his care protocol. The patient had had a myocardial infarction 2 days earlier. It became apparent during the consultant's psychosocial assessment of the patient that he was delirious. Recognizing the potentially dangerous implications of the delirium, the consultant went directly to the intern (having discussed her plan with the consultee, who fully supported her direct action) to share her concern and to recommend that the cause of the delirium be evaluated. The intern and then the resident minimized the delirium and attributed the patient's symptoms to psychological distress. The consultant then initiated a psychiatric consultation by discussing her concerns with one of the psychiatrists on the consultation and liaison service and asked that he contact the attending CCU physician and offer psychiatric consultation. The psychiatrist consultant agreed with the liaison nurse consultant, and an investigation into the causes of the delirium revealed that the patient's digitalis level exceeded the therapeutic range. A potentially dangerous and correctable problem was identified.

Developing the Practice of Other Nurses

An outcome of nursing consultation, especially consultation over time, is to enhance the professional development and practice of nurse consultees. Consultation can clearly enhance the clinical knowledge and practice of nurses requesting consultation. One of the most satisfying aspects of the consultative process is to watch consultees master new skills and become more clinically expert.

A goal for consultation is to enable the consultee to manage future similar situations effectively. When the consultant and consultee evaluate the effectiveness of the consultation, they can recognize and reinforce helpful problem-solving strategies, which can then be applied in the future. As APNs engage in self-reflection and include staff in that reflection, they model a critical aspect of practice.

Evaluation of the consultation itself with the consultee is enormously important. It can enhance the learning and skill of both the consultee and the consultant. APNs can contribute to the development of other APNs in a meaningful way through the consultation process. APNs can also enhance their own professional development and practices by receiving nursing consultation.

Consultation Practice Over Time

For APNs whose work includes substantial consultation, observations can be made about its evolution. Initially, consultants must market their services to potential consultees. Setting, niche identification, workload, and experience are all issues that contribute to the time and focus an APN may have for consultation efforts. For novice APNs, marketing may consist of demonstrating expertise and offering consultation services. Over time, staff and colleagues will recognize the APN's skill and the APN may need to develop strategies to deal with large numbers of requests. Setting priorities and identifying alternative resources when the consultant's caseload is full are important activities as the consultation practice becomes more and more recognized and valued. Identifying other APNs who can consult on similar issues may be a useful strategy for balancing requests with availability.

Clarifying availability and the timing of responses to requests is essential if consultees are to continue to consider consultation as a helpful, timely option for assistance with complex clinical situations. Negotiating directly with the consultee at the time of the request (or shortly thereafter) allows the consultant to express to the consultee the importance and worth of the request, even if the consultant cannot meet the need directly. It also provides the opportunity to consider appropriate alternative resources to assist the consultee in addressing the clinical problem. The consultant must have established backup resources who are available to handle emergencies when the consultant is not available. Establishing such resources at the beginning of the consultant's practice is essential. Consultees should always know whom to contact in the event of a clinical emergency.

Over time, the number of consultee-centered requests may increase. After the consultee establishes trust with the consultant, the consultee may feel more comfortable and able to focus on specific problems in the clinical situation. Over time, the consultee may be willing to examine lack of understanding, skill, or objectivity. Wonderful professional development can result from that level of self-examination, but trust usually needs to be firmly developed before such self-examination can take place with the consultant.

The consultant may find that the consultees' requests become more sophisticated over time. The consultee who initially requested basic assistance with care may develop skill, understanding, and confidence with basic issues such that future requests for consultation reflect more expert levels of concern and understanding. Such requests may involve more complex or unusual situations and can be catalysts for the consultant's ongoing professional growth. Experiencing the development of the consultee's professional practice is exciting and satisfying.

Conversely, boredom with requests may be an issue for the established consultant. Particularly in settings in which turnover of staff is high, the consultant may focus repeatedly on the same clinical concerns. Seeking support from a trusted colleague may help the consultant cope with frustration and avoid communicating frustration to consultees in inappropriate ways. Communicating a lack of interest with concerns presented by consultees is a sure way to derail both the specific consultation and the use of consultation as a means to address clinical problems. The consultant may also consider developing an educational program to address, in a different way, the needs commonly being expressed in consultation requests. If the problem is common, the consultant may also want to develop written guidelines, protocols, or care plans to share with consultees.

As the APN's consultation skills become widely appreciated in the system and in the community, the nature and types of consultation requests may change. Using different types of consultation, such as programmatic or administrative consultation, can be stimulating, and indeed, APN consultants have much to contribute in these areas. APNs should be careful to consider the impact of such shifts, however, because such requests move them away from their original purposes. Such requests can lead to job restructuring or new positions, which may or may not be advanced practice roles. Initially, the request to move into new professional areas can be seductive. The message that skills and perspectives are valued and that new avenues are available for exploration is gratifying. Developing new ideas and plans can be helpful to both the institution and the consultant; however, APNs should evaluate such shifts with care. Such changes can be time- and energy-consuming, leading the APN away from direct practice.

When APNs decide to apply their consultative skills in new areas and shift away from direct practice, recognizing the significance of new directions for consultees who have grown to rely on the consultant is critical. Planning with the consultees when such shifts occur can assure consultees that their concerns will continue to be considered even if the resource person changes temporarily or the response from the consultant is not going to be immediate.

EVALUATION OF THE CONSULTATION COMPETENCY

APNs evaluate individual consultations as the final step of the consultation process. Overall evaluation of the consultative process and skills is also important. Barron (1989) discussed both aspects of evaluation. APNs should consider strategies that will help them determine their overall effectiveness (see Chapter 25) and their specific effectiveness in relation to consultation. Data may be obtained from consultees, peers, administrators, review of the APN's documentation of consults, and the APN's self-evaluation.

Practices of individual APNs will vary considerably as to what questions and criteria are considered relevant to evaluation of consultation skills. (See Chapter 25 for a comprehensive discussion of evaluation of advanced practice nursing.) Some questions that may be useful in eliciting data regarding consultation have been suggested by Lewis and Levy (1982) and Barron (1989). Is the consultant re-contacted after the initial consultation? Are consultation requests becoming more sophisticated over time (Lewis & Levy, 1982)? Was the APN able to respond to all requests for consultation? Do glaring issues or needs seem to be going unaddressed? Do there seem to be patterns in terms of the theme, number, or location of consultations (Barron, 1989)? Are there delays in doing consultation triage?

The subjective experiences of the consultant are also important (Barron, 1989). Sensing openness and enthusiasm on the part of consultees can provide the APN with data. However, sensing resistance or unwillingness to implement consultation recommendations can also provide data. One would not want to rely solely on subjective data, but the feelings of the consultant can yield important information.

Clinical competency, competency in applying the consultation process, interpersonal skills, and professionalism are all areas to be considered in the evaluation process. Identifying the appropriate people to be involved in the evaluation and developing a systematic approach to data collection regarding the consultation aspects of an APN's practice are important. Evaluation can guide the APN's individual professional growth and can ultimately validate the need for the APN's service and skill in the specific work setting and beyond.

SUMMARY

APNs have had a long tradition of being involved in various aspects of direct and indirect patient care activities, including consultation. Consultation has the potential to improve care processes and patient outcomes. The power of consultative activities to inform and advance practice compels all APNs to consider consultation as an integral aspect of role performance. Consultation offers APNs the opportunity to both share and acquire the clinical expertise necessary to meet the increasingly challenging and diverse demands of patient care. This chapter has defined consultation; identified various types of consultation; and distinguished consultation from co-management, referral, and supervision. We have offered an ecological model of the APN consultation competency and have highlighted issues related to implementation of the consultative process. We encourage the reader to apply the model in practice and welcome input from APNs in all roles with regard to its utility. It remains imperative that the term *consultation* be used appropriately and that APNs participate in further defining this competency and understanding its impact on care processes and patient outcomes. We have attempted to clarify the concept of consultation because conceptual clarity will enhance its appropriate use in practice and in the literature.

We believe that APN consultation contributes to positive patient outcomes and may promote more appropriate use of scarce health care resources. These assumptions must be tested through quality improvement studies, cost-benefit studies, and research that examines the processes and outcomes of care. Outcomes of consultation activities can then be effectively measured. Ongoing discussion regarding this important topic will assist in the much-needed clarification of the other terms used to characterize relationships with other professionals. APNs can contribute to this discussion, as well as to the research, by sharing their experiences as both recipients and providers of consultation. We believe that consultation by and for APNs in all settings can enhance and extend quality nursing care and improve outcomes of care. Consultation can facilitate having comprehensive and specialty-related knowledge available to all patients who might need it and therefore should be an expected and integral aspect of APN role performance.

REFERENCES

American Association of Colleges of Nursing (AACN). (2006). *Essentials of doctorate education for advanced nursing practice.* Retrieved July 24, 2007, from www.aacn.nche.edu/DNP/pdf/Essentials.pdf.

American College of Nurse-Midwives (ACNM). (1992). *Clinical practice statement: Collaborative management in nurse-midwifery practice for medical, gynecological and obstetrical conditions.* Washington, DC: Author.

American College of Nurse-Midwives (ACNM). (1997). *Position statement—Clinical practice statement: Collaborative management in nurse-midwifery practice for medical, gynecological and obstetrical conditions.* Retrieved June 9, 2003, from www.midwife.org.

American College of Nurse-Midwives (ACNM). (2003). *Standards for the practice of midwifery.* Retrieved July 12, 2007, from www.acnm.org/display.cfm?id=485.

Barron, A.M. (1983). The clinical nurse specialist as consultant. In A.B. Hamric & J.A. Spross (Eds.), *The clinical nurse specialist in theory and practice* (pp. 91-113). New York: Grune & Stratton.

Barron A.M. (1989). The clinical nurse specialist as consultant. In A.B. Hamric & J.A. Spross (Eds.), *The clinical nurse specialist in theory and practice* (2nd ed., pp. 125-146). Philadelphia: Saunders.

Barron, A.M., & White, P. (1996). Consultation. In A.B. Hamric, J.A. Spross, & C.M. Hanson (Eds.), *Advanced nursing practice: An integrative approach* (pp. 165-183). Philadelphia: Saunders.

Barron, A.M., & White, P. (2000). Consultation. In A.B. Hamric, J.A. Spross, & C.M. Hanson (Eds.), *Advanced nursing practice: An integrative approach* (2nd ed., pp. 217-243). Philadelphia: Saunders.

Barron, A.M., & White, P. (2005). Consultation. In A.B. Hamric, J.A. Spross, & C.M. Hanson (Eds.), *Advanced practice nursing: An integrative approach* (3rd ed., pp. 225-255). Philadelphia: Saunders.

Birkholz, G., & Walker, D. (1994). Strategies for state statutory language changes granting fully independent nurse practitioner practice. *The Nurse Practitioner, 19,* 54-58.

Boyd, J.N., Stasiowski, S.A., Catoe, P.T., Wells, P.R., Stahl, B.M., Judson, E., et al. (1991). The merit and significance of clinical nurse specialists. *Journal of Nursing Administration, 21,* 35-43.

Calman, N.S. (1992). Variability in consultation rates and practitioner level of diagnostic certainty. *The Journal of Family Practice, 35,* 31-38.

Caplan, G. (1970). *The theory and practice of mental health consultation.* New York: Basic Books.

Caplan, G., & Caplan, R. (1993). *Mental health consultation and collaboration.* San Francisco: Jossey-Bass.

Critchley, D.L. (1985). Clinical supervision. In D.L. Critchley & J.T. Maurin (Eds.), *The clinical specialist in psychiatric mental health nursing* (pp. 495-510). New York: John Wiley & Sons.

Faut-Callahan, M., & Kremer, M. (2000). The certified registered nurse-anesthetist. In A.B. Hamric, J.A. Spross, & C.M.

Hanson (Eds.), *Advanced nursing practice: An integrative approach* (2nd ed., pp. 521-548). Philadelphia: Saunders.

Faut-Callahan, M., & Kremer, M. (2005). The certified registered nurse-anesthetist. In A.B. Hamric, J.A. Spross, & C.M. Hanson (Eds.), *Advanced practice nursing: An integrative approach* (3rd ed., pp. 583-616). Philadelphia: Saunders.

Forsyth, D., Rhudy, L., & Johnson, L. (2002). The consultation role of a nurse educator. *Journal of Continuing Education in Nursing, 33,* 197-204.

Gurka, A.M. (1991). Process and outcome components of clinical nurse specialist consultation. *Dimensions of Critical Care Nursing, 10,* 169-175.

Hanson, C.M. (2005). Understanding regulatory, legal, and credentialing requirements. In A.B. Hamric, J.A. Spross, & C.M. Hanson (Eds.), *Advanced practice nursing: An integrative approach* (3rd ed., pp. 781-808). Philadelphia: Saunders.

Hanson, C.M., & Spross, J.A. (1996). Collaboration. In A.B. Hamric, J.A. Spross, & C.M. Hanson (Eds.), *Advanced practice nursing: An integrative approach* (pp. 229-248). Philadelphia: Saunders.

Hanson, C.M., Spross, J.A., & Carr, D.B. (2000). Collaboration. In A.B. Hamric, J.A. Spross, & C.M. Hanson (Eds.), *Advanced practice nursing: An integrative approach* (2nd ed., pp. 315-347). Philadelphia: Saunders.

Hardin, S., & Langford, D. (2001). Telehealth's impact on nursing and the development of the interstate compact. *Journal of Professional Nursing, 17,* 243-247.

Hutcherson, C.M. (2001). Legal considerations for nurses practicing in a telehealth setting. (Electronic version). *Online Journal of Issues in Nursing, 6,* 3. Retrieved March 11, 2007, from www.nursingworld.org.

Ingersoll, G., & Jones, L. (1992). The art of the consultation note. *Clinical Nurse Specialist, 6,* 218-220.

Larson-Dahn, M. (2001). Tele-nurse practice: Quality of care and patient outcomes. *Journal of Nursing Administration, 31,* 145-152. Retrieved May 22, 2003, from www.80-gateway2.ovid.com.

Lewis, A., & Levy, J. (1982). *Psychiatric liaison nursing: The theory and clinical practice.* Reston, VA: Reston.

Lipowski, Z.J. (1974). Consultation-liaison psychiatry: An overview. *American Journal of Psychiatry, 131,* 623-630.

Lipowski, Z.J. (1981). Liaison psychiatry, liaison nursing and behavioral medicine. *Comprehensive Psychiatry, 22,* 554-561.

Lipowski, Z.J. (1983). Current trends in consultation-liaison psychiatry. *Canadian Journal of Psychiatry, 28,* 329-338.

Maddox, P.J. (2003). Ethics column: Ethics and the brave new world of e-health (Electronic version). *Online Journal of Issues in Nursing, 6,* 3. Retrieved March 11, 2007, from www.nursingworld.org.

Mahn-DiNicola, V.A., & Zazworsky, D.J. (2005). The advanced practice nurse case manager. In A.B. Hamric, J.A. Spross, & C.M. Hanson (Eds.), *Advanced practice nursing: An integrative approach* (3rd ed., pp. 617-675). Philadelphia: Saunders.

Manley, K. (1998). A conceptual framework for advanced practice: An action research project operationalizing an advanced practitioner/consultant role. In G. Rolfe & P. Fulbrook (Eds.), *Advanced nursing practice* (pp. 118-135). Boston: Butterworth Heinemann.

Minarik, P., & Price, L. (1999). Collaboration? Supervision? Direction? Independence? What is the relationship between the advanced practice nurse and the physician? States legislative and regulatory reform III. *Clinical Nurse Specialist, 13,* 34-37.

Monicken, D.R. (1995). Consultation in advanced practice nursing. In M. Snyder & M. Mirr (Eds.), *Advanced practice nursing* (pp. 183-195). New York: Springer-Verlag.

National Association of Clinical Nurse Specialists. (2004). *Statement on clinical nurse specialist education and practice* (2nd ed.). Harrisburg, PA: Author.

National Council of State Boards of Nursing (NCSBN). (2006). *NCSBN summit funded by federal grant to promote nurse licensure portability.* Retrieved March 11, 2007, from www.ncsbn.org.

Norwood, S.L. (1998). When the CNS needs a consultant. *Clinical Nurse Specialist, 12,* 53-58.

Ohler, L., & Daine, V. (2001). Potential telecommunication risks: Cautions and suggestions for the team. *Progress in Cardiovascular Nursing, 16,* 172-176. Retrieved May 22, 2003, from www.0-prpquest.umi.com.

Poteet, G.W. (1989). Consultation. *Clinical Nurse Specialist, 3,* 41.

Ricci, M., Cauto, M., Amour, M., Rogers, F., Sartorelli, K., Callas, P., et al. (2003). Telemedicine reduces discrepancies in rural trauma care. *Telemedicine Journal and e-Health, 9,* 3-11.

Roine, R., Ohinmaa, A., & Hailey, D. (2001). Assessing telemedicine: A systematic review of the literature. *Canadian Medical Association Journal, 165,* 765-773.

Sabatier, K. (2002). The Institute for Johns Hopkins Nursing: A collaborative model for nursing practice. *Nursing Education Perspectives, 23,* 178-182.

Safriet, B.J. (1992). Health care dollars and regulatory sense: The role of advanced practice nursing (special issue). *Yale Journal on Regulation, 9,* 417-488.

Scott, L., & Beare, P. (1993). Nurse consultant and professional liability. *Clinical Nurse Specialist, 7,* 331-334.

Sebus, M. (1994). Developing a collaborative practice agreement for the primary care setting. *Nurse Practitioner, 19,* 44-51.

Simmons, M.K. (1985). Psychiatric consultation and liaison. In D.L. Critchley & J.T. Maurin (Eds.), *The clinical specialist in psychiatric mental health nursing* (pp. 362-381). New York: John Wiley & Sons.

Skalla, K., & Hamric, A. (2000). The blended role of the clinical nurse specialist and the nurse practitioner. In A.B. Hamric, J.A. Spross, & C.M. Hanson (Eds.), *Advanced nursing practice: An integrative approach* (2nd ed., pp. 459-490). Philadelphia: Saunders.

Skalla, K., Hamric, A., & Caron, P. (2005). The blended role of the clinical nurse specialist and the nurse practitioner. In A.B. Hamric, J.A. Spross, & C.M. Hanson (Eds.), *Advanced practice nursing: An integrative approach* (3rd ed., pp. 515-550). Philadelphia: Saunders.

Solomons, N. (2006). Are home health agencies using telehealth and states with telehealth initiatives the little engine that could save Medicare? Unpublished manuscript, University of Southern Maine.

Spross, J.A. (1989). The clinical nurse specialist as collaborator. In A.B. Hamric & J.A. Spross (Eds.), *The clinical nurse specialist in theory and practice* (2nd ed., pp. 205-226). Philadelphia: Saunders.

Stichler, J. (2002). The nurse as consultant. *Nursing Administration Quarterly, 26,* 52-68.

Survillo, A.I., & Levine, A.T. (1993). Strategies to limit CNS malpractice liability exposure. *Clinical Nurse Specialist, 7,* 215-220.

Thede, L.Q. (2001). Overview and summary: Telehealth: Promise or peril? (Electronic version). *Online Journal of Issues in Nursing, 6,* 3. Retrieved March 11, 2007, from www.nursingworld.org.

Unnold, R. (2006). *Telehealth in homecare: Advanced practice implications.* Unpublished manuscript, University of Southern Maine.

INTRODUCTION

Research skills are a core competency for advanced practice nurses (APNs) (see Chapter 3) and are central to an APN's ability to fulfill his or her current and future roles. The need for APNs to be well prepared in implementing research findings has never been greater. Efforts to achieve Magnet status, national accreditation requirements, and local and national initiatives to improve the safety and quality of health care and minimize variation are driving the use of evidence-based practice (EBP) standards. The competencies are integral to the quality of an APN's individual practice and to the quality of care provided in any program or organization that employs APNs. In addition, the role of the APN is vital to any research endeavors being organized within a health care setting because of their clinical and leadership expertise. Ideally, APNs possess the essential qualities of clinical reasoning to be able to evaluate evidence and integrate evidence into practice (Debourgh, 2001; Munro, 2004; see also Chapter 5) and have sufficient understanding of the political environment of their health care setting to be able to work in a collaborative manner to initiate evidence-based practice changes (Aherns, 2005; Buonocore, 2004).

The ability to translate knowledge and evidence into practice and to role model that ability is crucial, and APNs are key to this activity, given their knowledge of the patient population, peer health care providers, and the organization (McKoen, Oswaks, & Cunningham, 2006). Unfortunately, the average time it takes for research findings to be translated into practice changes remains documented at 17 years (Balas & Boren, 2000), which is totally unsatisfactory from a quality-of-care perspective. APNs can decrease that delay time by fostering evidence-based, practice-friendly environments, but they need to be in positions of power (clinically or administratively) to impact the environment. APNs may have the power to change practice (the fundamental research competency), but they also need to be looking for opportunities to collaborate with other clinical leaders and administrators to use research to influence the larger practice environment (expanded competency).

The purpose of this chapter is to describe a set of three individual competencies that make up the core APN research competence. The individual competencies are (1) interpretation and use of research findings and other evidence in clinical decision making, (2) evaluation of practice, and (3) participation in collaborative research (Table 8-1). These research competencies are presented on two levels. The *fundamental level* includes activities that are reasonable to expect at graduation from a master's degree in nursing program and generally address an APN's individual practice (e.g., appraising scientific literature as a step to incorporating research findings into his or her own practice). The *expanded level* consists of activities that are acquired through experience and individual initiative while practicing in the APN role or through practice doctorate education (e.g., developing institutional mechanisms for implementing evidence-based practice to facilitate the attainment of Magnet status). The activities in the expanded level differ from those in the fundamental level in that they focus on a program or organizational level rather than on an individual practice level.

Recognition of these research competencies by clinicians, administrators, and educators can create the following advantages:

- APNs can use evidence in practice, role model research competencies, and take a leadership role in promoting the competencies with peers and colleagues across health care settings.
- Administrators can overtly promote the competencies in their hiring practices, job descriptions, performance evaluations, and reward systems. Their strategic and budgetary plans can provide resources to maintain a research-based practice environment (Stetler, 2003; Titler & Everett, 2006).

Table 8-1   OVERVIEW OF RESEARCH COMPETENCIES AND LEVELS

Competency	Fundamental Level	Expanded Level
I: Interpretation and use of research and other evidence in clinical decision making	Incorporate evidence-based practice (EBP) process into individual practice. Assist colleagues to incorporate EBP process into their individual practices.	Implement EBP process beyond own practice—at the unit, program, department, and/or organization level.
II: Evaluation of practice	Identify benchmarks appropriate for own practice. Design and implement a process to evaluate aspects of individual's advanced practice.	Design and implement a process to evaluate advanced practice nursing beyond the scope of individual practice (group of advanced practice nurses [APNs], unit, program, clinic, organization).
III: Participation in collaborative research	Function as a clinical expert/consultant in a collaborative knowledge-generating research project.	Function as an investigator or co-investigator in a collaborative knowledge-generating research project.

- Educators in master's and doctoral programs can develop curricula that promote research competencies as integral threads, thereby strengthening APN graduates' abilities in each area.

Consistency in the expectations of research competencies of APNs across health care settings or in the promotion of these competencies in formal education programs is limited. Practice settings seeking the American Nurses Credentialing Center's (ANCC's) Magnet Recognition (2004) status are most likely to have systems in place to promote integration of evidence into practice because it is a requirement. Graduate and doctoral programs prepare advanced clinicians for some level of research competency; the American Association of Colleges of Nursing's (AACN's) document on the Essentials of the Doctor of Nursing Practice (DNP) degree (AACN, 2006a) may be the first step in establishing agreement in the academic world as to what competencies align with levels of graduate education.

In spite of the growing emphasis on EBP, surveys of nurses indicate a continued need for education and resources; registered nurses (RNs) report inconsistent levels of knowledge and comfort with EBP. The results of the 2006 Evidence-Based Practice Research Study done by Sigma Theta Tau International (STTI) indicated the following:

- Of the RN respondents, 64% needed to access evidence at least weekly.
- Of the respondents, only 31% indicated a high level of familiarity with EBP; 24% rated their familiarity as low.

- Of the respondents, 27% considered resources to support EBP inadequate (Alspach, 2006; STTI, 2006).
- Of the respondents, 12% identified themselves as advance practice nurses (STTI, 2006). Findings were not reported by demographic subgroups.

In a descriptive survey of RNs (Pravikoff, Pierce, & Tanner, 2005) to determine nurses' readiness to implement EBP, the most frequent source of information was a colleague or peer. Almost half of the respondents were not familiar with EBP, and more than half did not believe that their peers use research findings in practice. Most did not do electronic literature searches, and only 27% stated they ever had instruction on how to do such searches. The most frequently mentioned barriers to EBP were lack of time, lack of value for research, and other goals with higher priority.

RESEARCH EXPECTATIONS OF ADVANCED PRACTICE NURSES

Historically, the APN role has included an expectation of some level of research competence (Hamric, 1989; McGuire & Harwood, 1989; see also Chapters 12-17). Published research from the early 1990s attests to the involvement of APNs in research (see Chapter 24). The relevance of research competencies to advanced practice nursing is supported by standards-of-practice documents developed by a variety of advanced practice professional organizations, AACN's *The Essentials of Doctoral Education for Advanced Nursing Practice* (2006a, 2006b), and the ANCC's Magnet Recognition Program (2004).

Many of the recent standards-of-practice documents released by various professional organizations emphasize integrating research findings into practice and evaluating practice. Specifically, documents published by APN professional organizations provide definitive support for research competence within APN roles. These standards-of-practice documents were reviewed for clear statements that reflected each of the three research competencies proposed in this chapter. Only two documents clearly referred to all three competencies. These were the *Scope of Practice & Standards of Professional Performance for the Acute & Critical Care CNS* developed by the American Association of Critical-Care Nurses (2002) and the *Standards of Professional Performance* for acute care nurse practitioners developed by the National Organization of Nurse Practitioner Faculties (NONPF) (2004). Competencies I (use of evidence) and II (evaluating practice) were evident in *Core Competencies for Basic Midwifery Practice* (American College of Nurse-Midwives [ACNM], 2007), *Domains and Core Competencies of Nurse Practitioner Practice* (National Organization of Nurse Practitioner Faculties [NONPF], 2006), and the *Statement on Clinical Nurse Specialist Practice and Education* (National Association of Clinical Nurse Specialists [NACNS], 2004). The American College of Nurse-Midwives (ACNM) further clarifies its position on research priorities in the *Research Agenda* (2005). Research competencies II (evaluation of practice) and III (participating in collaborative research) were apparent in the *Scope and Standards for Nurse Anesthesia Practice* (American Association of Nurse Anesthetists [AANA], 2005a).

The most current competencies for oncology nurse practitioners (NPs) (Oncology Nursing Society [ONS], 2007) list the use of evidence in planning and implementing patient care across the continuum and accomplishing quality improvement. NPs are also expected to identify recurrent problems and relevant research questions.

Three documents released by the AACN inform the description of APN research competencies according to level of education: the master's *Essentials* (AACN, 1996); the position statement on research (AACN, 2006b); and the DNP *Essentials* (AACN, 2006a) (see also Chapters, 2, 3, and 22 for more background on this latter document). The position statement (AACN, 2006b) indicated that master's degree programs should "…prepare nurses to critique research and to implement changes in practice based on research data. Their [master's prepared nurses] leadership skills enable them to form teams of professionals, and to initiate and evaluate new practice policies and programs within their agencies and professional groups" (p. 2). Further, the AACN noted that master's-prepared nurses "…identify practice and systems problems that need to be studied and collaborate with other scientists to generate new studies based on their expertise" (2006b p. 2).

The more recent DNP *Essentials* clarifies expectations of the DNP-prepared APN (AACN, 2006a). The third Essential, "Clinical Scholarship and Analytical Methods for Evidence-Based Practice," asserts that DNP graduates should provide leadership for evidence-based practice, develop evidence-based guidelines, evaluate their advanced practice, serve as clinical experts/consultants on collaborative research study teams, and disseminate findings of knowledge-generating and evidence-based projects (AACN, 2006a). These expectations are consistent with the APN research competency described in this chapter.

Another example of professional organizational support for a rich evidence-based environment is seen in the ANCC's Magnet Recognition Program. The Fourteen Forces of Magnetism include the nurses' autonomy to improve care and use of evidence to improve quality of care (ANCC, 2004).

NATIONAL INITIATIVES AND TRENDS

National initiatives and trends that most affect the need for APNs to be research-competent are national quality and safety initiatives, the increasing integration of information technology (IT) in health care practice, and the increasing emphasis on EBP.

Quality and Safety Initiatives

Trends addressed in the Institute of Medicine's (IOM) report, *Crossing the Quality Chasm* (2001), include the variable quality of care and the need for efforts to improve it and scientific and technological advances. These trends support the need for research competencies in APN roles. The IOM asserted that the health care delivery system needs to be redesigned to improve patient safety and quality of care. Health care leaders must focus attention on identifying the types of changes that will ensure well-designed care processes that contribute to safe, effective care (Richardson & Corrigan, 2003). Health care systems have not always tracked or rewarded quality, but recently, health care report cards have been published that facilitate the comparison of the quality of care across providers (Mehrotra, Bodenheimer, & Dudley, 2003).

The IOM (2001) recommended a partnership with the U.S. Department of Health and Human Services and professional and health care associations interested in quality to develop a program that supports clinicians' evidence-based decision making. According to the IOM report (2001), six aims on which to base quality improvement goals are safety, effectiveness (services based on scientific knowledge), timeliness, efficiency, equitable access and treatment, and a patient-centered emphasis. In partial response to these recommendations, various accrediting and regulating agencies have integrated quality measurement into their expectations. Examples include the ORYX initiative of The Joint Commission (TJC) (2007), the National Committee for Quality Assurance's (NCQA) health plan report card (2000), and Medicare's quality initiatives that track quality indicators by type of provider (Jencks, Huff, & Cuerdon, 2003).

Many organizations are involved in the Institute for Healthcare Improvement's (IHI) efforts to improve safety and quality. Particularly relevant to APN research competencies are selected white papers, such as "Execution of Strategic Improvement Initiatives to Produce System-Level Results" (Nolan, 2007) and "Transforming Care at the Bedside" (Rutherford, Lee, & Greiner, 2004). The IHI website (provided in Box 8-3 later in the chapter) also offers a selection of published literature about developing and using evidence-based protocols.

Information Technology and Telehealth

Access to the Internet and increasingly sophisticated information systems are transforming the delivery and evaluation of care. Information technology (IT) is an integral part of the APN research competency at all levels. In 2004, the first National Coordinator for Health Information Technology was appointed to advise the Secretary of Health and Human Services on the national 10-year initiative to have a secure and interoperable electronic medical record for each citizen (Health Information Technology, 2007). The Technology Informatics Guiding Education Reform (TIGER) initiative is designed to enable practicing RNs to meet the new challenges of IT in health care (Sensmeier, 2007). Using informatics is a core competency for clinicians emphasized in the IOM's quality reports, yet many nurses lack the skills they need to integrate IT into practice and evaluation

efforts. The goal of the TIGER vision and action plan is to align the practice and education of nursing with the national IT agenda. Electronically entered, stored, transported, and accessed information has the potential to improve the quality of care, increase the efficiency of clinical practice, and reduce human error (Masys, 2002). Electronic data allow for trending quality improvement processes and clinical outcomes and therefore can facilitate the evaluation of practice by both individual practitioners and the overall organization.

The DNP *Essentials* (AACN, 2006a) identifies "Information systems/technology and patient care technology for the improvement and transformation of health care" as Essential IV. The graduate of a DNP program will be prepared to design, use, and evaluate programs that monitor outcomes of care to develop and execute an evaluation plan using data extracted from information systems; evaluate consumer health information sources for accuracy, timeliness, and appropriateness; and teach the consumer how to evaluate websites (AACN, 2006a). These are new but appropriate roles for many APNs and are in keeping with the three research competencies proposed in this chapter. Access to evidence is accomplished primarily online with bibliographical databases and Internet websites (Competency I). Benchmarks and data for the evaluation of practice are also available for comparison via the Internet and information databases (Competency II).

Telehealth is the use of technology to provide health care over a distance using voice and video communication (Bowles & Baugh, 2007). Telehealth initiatives can facilitate access to health care services for vulnerable populations; however, the evidence of the impact of such care on outcomes (clinical, clinician, and health care organization) is limited (Gagnon, Lamothe, Hebert, Chanliau, & Fortin, 2006). Some studies of telehealth have determined a trend toward lower use of inpatient and outpatient health care services (Hopp et al., 2006), especially for patients with chronic pulmonary and cardiac diseases (Bowles & Baugh; Pare, Jaana, & Sicotte, 2007). Telehealth applications that are effective for cardiovascular health care include sensor technology, wearable monitors, videophones, and interactive voice response systems (Artinian, 2007), especially when the care is managed by APNs (Delgado-Passler & McCaffrey, 2006). These changes are creating new roles and opportunities for APNs as telehealth practitioners to consult electronically (Masys, 2002) with vulnerable and underserved patient populations. However, these new roles and activities will need to be based on evidence from studies that compare the outcomes of telehealth interventions with outcomes of traditional care.

Evidence-Based Practice

The term *evidence-based* was coined at McMaster University Medical School in Canada to describe a teaching-learning strategy designed to shape clinical decision making in medicine (Evidence-Based Medicine Working Group, 1992; Guyatt & Rennie, 2002; Sackett, Straus, Richardson, Rosenberg, & Haynes, 2000). The definition of Sackett and colleagues (1997) is often considered a classic for medicine and consists of three primary factors: (1) best research evidence, (2) applied with clinical expertise, and (3) applied with an appreciation of the patient's values and expectations. Despite Sackett's definition, the primary emphasis of evidence-based medicine (EBM) has continued to be the clinical application of medical research findings with little discussion of clinical expertise or adaptation for individual patient values and expectations. The term *evidence-based practice (EBP)* has evolved from EBM and acknowledges the interdisciplinary nature of health care, of which medical care is a part. Most definitions of EBP in nursing (Ledbetter & Stevens, 2000; Melnyk, 2005) refer to improving care and employing all three aspects that are included in the original definition by Sackett and colleagues (1997).

EBP is considered a total process, beginning with knowing what clinical question to ask, knowing how to find the best current evidence (which may or may not be research), and knowing how to critically appraise the evidence for validity and applicability to the particular care situation. The best evidence is then applied by the clinician and influenced by the clinician's knowledge drawn from experience as well as the interpretation of the needs and perspectives of the patient. The final aspect of the process is an evaluation of the effectiveness of care after implementation of the practice change and the continual improvement of the process from both the caregiver's and patient's perspectives (DePalma, 2000; Goode & Piedalue, 1999; Pearson & Craig, 2002).

Levels/Hierarchies of Evidence. Key differences in the definitions of EBM, evidence-based nursing, and EBP are (1) the range or levels of evidence that are inherent in each, that is, whether evidence other than results of research or randomized controlled trials (RCTs) is included and (2) whether any mention is made of patients and clinical expertise of the health care provider in the definition. To define levels or hierarchies of *evidence* is really to indicate the types of evidence that are deemed acceptable by an individual or group involved in the process of making clinical decisions based on evidence. Evidence hierarchies are classification schema for rank-ordering types of studies or evidence according to the credibility of methods used, the strength of research design, and/or the findings. Levels or hierarchies of evidence differ in the scope of evidence included. Some hierarchies rank-order the evidence on the basis of research design alone (Ball et al., 2001; Guyatt et al, 2000; Hadorn, Baker, Hodges, & Hicks, 1995; Harris et al., 2001). Others include non-research evidence such as quality or risk data, clinical experience, and expert opinion (Goode, 2000; Melnyk, 2004; Polit & Beck, 2008; Rutledge & Grant, 2002; Stetler, 2001). RCTs are considered the "gold standard" of research and are usually high in any hierarchy. Unfortunately, not all research areas have RCTs, and in fact, RCTs are not appropriate designs for some clinical questions. Rutledge and Grant's (2002) hierarchy of evidence differs from some other evidence hierarchies because it includes all types of research designs, systematic reviews, and non-research or practice-based evidence such as benchmark, quality, risk, and infection control data (see Box 8-1 for this particular hierarchy).

As seen in Rutledge and Grant's hierarchy, both research evidence and non-research evidence reflect nursing's broader view of the types of knowledge and information that comprise evidence. This may be because of nursing's tradition of using a variety of research methods, necessitated by "the concepts and situations that constitute the phenomena of interest to the nursing profession" (Pravikoff & Donaldson, 2001, p. 589). Because nursing involves a wide range of interventions and a perspective of care that focuses on the individual patient's experience with a disease or symptom, nurses draw on a diverse evidence base. This diverse evidence base spans the medical sciences, including the behavioral and social sciences, but also extends to public health, wellness, communications, and organizational change and management evidence (Pearson & Craig, 2002).

Only research evidence is discussed in this chapter, specifically individual research studies, systematic reviews of research studies, and evidence-based clinical guidelines. In making decisions about the application of findings to individuals or groups,

Box 8-1   LEVELS OF EVIDENCE

RESEARCH	**NON-RESEARCH**
Meta-analyses	Evidence-based consensus statements
Systematic reviews of research articles	Quality improvement data
Randomized controlled intervention studies	Risk or infection control data
Quasi-experimental studies	Program evaluation
Outcome studies	Case studies
Non-experimental and qualitative studies	Daily practice data
	Expert opinion

Adapted from Rutledge, D.N, & Grant, M. (2002). Introduction to evidence-based practice. *Seminars in Oncology Nursing, 18*(1), 1-2.

APNs are expected to integrate their clinical experiences, consider patients' preferences, and use quality improvement data (see Chapter 25). It is important to note that APN research competencies are often executed simultaneously or in conjunction with the leadership (Chapter 9) and collaboration competencies (Chapter 10).

Health Care Organizations and Evidence-Based Practice

Many health care organizations give verbal testament to the value of EBP, but not all provide the support and resources needed to successfully implement EBP changes. The culture and infrastructure of the organization will determine whether EBP can be implemented successfully (Collins, Phields, & Duncan, 2007; Cullen, Greiner, Greiner, Bombei, & Cumried, 2005; Stetler, 2003; Titler, 2007). The support of nursing leaders is essential for the success of EBP programs within health care organizations (Newhouse, 2007) because they influence the clinical environment. The ideal environment for EBP is one in which critical thinking, clinical inquiry, and challenging of current practice are fostered (Titler & Everett, 2006) and rewarded. Support for EBP needs to be overt in the organization and consistent across job descriptions, performance evaluations, committee structures, integration into the quality improvement system, and resources provided for those promoting EBP.

APNs are excellent facilitators of EBP in any clinical setting because they possess the necessary clinical expertise and have an awareness of patient, family, and health care provider needs. Because they are familiar with change processes and the health care system in which they practice, APNs can collaborate and negotiate with other clinical leaders and administrators for the support needed to truly implement EBP and change practice. As leaders in this process, APNs are often able to ensure the success of an initial evidence-based project by choosing one that will have the most impact on quality of care and cost. APNs' knowledge of the system allows a realistic assessment of the resources within the organization that can be employed to promote EBP. For example, total quality management (TQM) clinical groups may already exist within a system. Such groups are logical choices for leading and implementing EBP initiatives.

COMPETENCY I: INTERPRETATION AND USE OF RESEARCH AND OTHER EVIDENCE IN CLINICAL DECISION MAKING

As noted, clinical decisions ideally should be based on the best current evidence, applied with the expertise of the clinician, and individualized for the patient and family (DePalma, 2000; Sackett et al., 2000). The APN is a pivotal factor in promoting EBP in any clinical setting (Cooke et al., 2004; Klardie, Johnson, McNaughton, & Meyers, 2004; Melnyk & Fineout-Overholt, 2005; Munro, 2004). APNs promote EBP by the following:

- Promoting the value and usefulness of evidence in decision making
- Exercising systems leadership to effect change—especially related to barriers to EBP (Hockenberry, Wilson, & Barrera, 2006; Marshall, 2006)
- Serving as reliable sources of information (Thompson, Cullum, McCaughan, Sheldon, & Raynor, 2004)
- Demonstrating use of EBP in delivery of direct clinical care and clinical consultation (Munro, 2004)

- Fostering change in the organization to promote evidence-based care (Munro, 2004) while considering the political environment of the system (Aherns, 2005; Buonocore, 2004)

Fundamental and Expanded Levels of Research Competency I

As noted in Table 8-1, APNs demonstrate the fundamental level of Competency I by incorporating EBP into their individual practice and assisting colleagues to incorporate the EBP process into their practices. In order to demonstrate this competency, APNs must be able to identify reliable sources of evidence relevant to their practice, appraise/critique research, practice guidelines and other sources of evidence using an evidence hierarchy, and determine the applicability of findings and the feasibility of applying them in practice. This is a complex skill and is described in terms of phases.

Initially, APNs demonstrate the fundamental level of Competency I by demonstrating that, in the care of individual patients, they make practice decisions based on the best current evidence or help staff nurses and colleagues do the same. APNs also demonstrate the fundamental level of this competency when they function as preceptors for graduate students or begin a journal club with colleagues. APNs demonstrate the expanded level of Competency I when they develop and promote practice changes for patient populations at the system level based on evidence and when they advocate for the proper environment and resources to support EBP in a particular clinical setting or organization. This level of promoting EBP may occur in a clinical inpatient unit or outpatient clinic to which the APN is assigned; it may be done by a group of APNs employed in a particular setting; or it may be an initiative that involves the entire department of nursing or a total clinical organization. For example, a certified nurse-midwife (CNM) might distribute the evidence-based *Guide to Effective Care in Pregnancy and Childbirth* (Enkin et al., 2000). The clinicians within a birthing center could use this guide to evaluate current practices and determine whether changes are needed to improve the standard of care. By consensus, they could proceed to develop or revise an interdisciplinary critical pathway. It is important to note that graduate students must observe and/or participate with preceptors in the expanded level of this competency so they are prepared to develop and demonstrate the expanded competency in practice.

Phases of Competency I

EBP at both the fundamental and expanded levels requires a particular knowledge base and a set of core skills. There are numerous models of EBP and examples of implementing EBP in various practice settings (Brown, 1999; Hockenberry et al., 2006; Melynk & Fineout-Overholt, 2005; Rosswurm & Larrabee, 1999: Rycroft-Malone, 2004; Stetler, 2001; Vratny & Shriver, 2007), but they all contain similar phases or steps. The phases of the EBP process begin with understanding the clinical issues and being able to state a researchable problem or clinical question succinctly, followed by finding, evaluating, and synthesizing evidence; making a practice recommendation based on the level of available evidence; implementing appropriate practice changes; and, finally, evaluating those changes.

The APN's clinical expertise is critical in each phase of the competency, which requires an understanding of clinical care issues and processes within a particular clinical system. Each of the phases in Competency I are discussed from the viewpoint of a clinical group seeking an evidence-based answer to a clinical practice question, since this is the more common situation and is usually more complex than locating evidence for an individual patient problem. The APN frequently co-chairs such clinical groups in acute care settings and needs to be aware of how to facilitate the group through the steps of the competency. The same steps can be used by the individual APN seeking evidence to support quality practice in a particular patient-clinician situation. Table 8-2 lists the phases of Competency I and key activities appropriate to each.

Stating the Problem or Clinical Question.

A clearly stated clinical problem or question is critical to being able to focus the search for evidence and then selecting, appraising, and synthesizing evidence. When information about a particular treatment or intervention is being sought, the clinical problem or question is often easier to develop than in cases in which problems are more complex and involve both physical and psychosocial aspects of care (Glanville, Schirm, & Wineman, 2000). Two mnemonics/formats for structuring a problem statement or clinical question have been recommended: (1) "PICO"—population, intervention, condition/comparison, outcome (Craig, 2002), and (2) "PICOT"—population, intervention, condition/comparison, outcome, and time (Boswell & Cannon, 2007; Gibbs 2003).

The initial search for evidence may be brief and more informal as the APN tries to formulate the

Table 8-2   Competency I: Interpretation and Use of Research and Other Evidence in Clinical Decision Making

Component of the Process	Key Activities
Statement of the Problem	Facilitate a collaborative brainstorming with all stakeholders to list clinical issues and prioritize. Write a detailed problem statement with key words that can be searched.
Searching for and Retrieving Evidence	Conduct a computerized search of bibliographical databases. Conduct a computerized search of guideline resources. Focus and refocus the search.
Evaluating Evidence	Select a hierarchy of evidence. Create an evidence table to sort and compare studies Determine level of evidence or each evidence point accessed. Rate applicability and feasibility to clinical practice.
Synthesizing Evidence	Determine the status of current practice. Facilitate a collaborative multidisciplinary group to synthesize findings. Sort evidence by appropriate results. Identify key areas addressed across evidence. Compare results.
Making a Recommendation for Practice	Compare current practice with the evidence synthesis. Determine if evidence is sufficient to recommend practice change. Develop specific practice recommendations and rationales for each. Determine format for dissemination of practice change recommendations.
Implementing the Recommended Practice Change	Collect baseline data on current practice. Develop plan that includes implementation, maintenance, and evaluation of practice. Identify expected outcomes of the change. Determine costs and resources needed. Identify barriers and facilitators. Educate staff and other stakeholders. Monitor effects of practice changes on patient, staff, and organization.
Evaluating the Practice Change	Review the evaluation plan—revise if needed. Implement evaluation plan. Monitor process and outcomes. Compare outcomes with internal and external benchmarks. Facilitate ongoing review of data with continual improvement. Coordinate a process for dissemination of evaluation data to stakeholder at regular intervals. Coordinate ongoing education and periodic review of practice change.

clinical question. The quick initial search may lead the APN to change the question. Once a question has been formulated, it is wise to consult a librarian early in the process because both parties bring a wealth of different expertise to the search process (DePalma, 2005; Vrabel, 2005). When working with a librarian, a clear problem statement ensures that the most appropriate key words are used to direct the search. A quick scan of the search results—looking at titles and abstracts—may lead to refinement of the question and keywords as the APN continues to identify the research literature that is most relevant.

When a group of clinicians, such as a clinical quality improvement group, is seeking evidence, the process of developing and reaching consensus on the statement of the problem needs to be more formalized. Such groups often work to refine the question before starting the literature search. Ideally, an interdisciplinary group of stakeholders should ultimately develop the statement or clinical question and follow through with the remaining steps in the process. APNs are ideal leaders or co-leaders with a physician for such a planning group because of their clinical expertise, their knowledge of the systems

Box 8-2   Examples of Clinical Questions for Competency I

1. Do patients with chronic illnesses (PATIENTS/POPULATION) have fewer acute care admissions (OUTCOME) when they participate in telehealth home monitoring interventions (INTERVENTIONS) after discharge (TIME)?
2. Do cardiac patients (PATIENTS/POPULATION) managed by NPs (INTERVENTION) after discharge (TIME) have better outcomes than those patients managed by non-APN clinicians (COMPARISON)?
3. What are the key factors to include in education (INTERVENTION) of patients with cancer and their families (PATIENTS/POPULATION) in order

for patients to be able to self-management their pain (OUTCOME)?
4. Do husbands of women with ovarian cancer (POPULATION) who have participated in a peer support group experience (INTERVENTION) less hopelessness (OUTCOME)?
5. Which smoking cessation program (INTERVENTION) has the best cessation rate (OUTCOME) with pregnant women (POPULATION)?
6. Do family caregivers of patients with Alzheimer's disease (POPULATION) who participate in support groups (INTERVENTION) experience less caregiver burden (OUTCOME)?

APN, Advanced practice nurse; *.NPs*, nurse practitioners.

within the workplace, and their ability to facilitate group discussion and practice changes (Barnsteiner & Prevost, 2002).

For example, an interdisciplinary quality care work group met to discuss issues in respiratory care to identify and prioritize problems within the organization. A list of clinical issues was created and priorities established. The first priority was to improve weaning of ICU patients from ventilators. At first the question was broadly framed as the group brought different perspectives to the problem. The first search was driven by this question: What are the factors that influence weaning? After the results of the first search were reviewed, the question was narrowed to focus on two aspects of care that influence weaning and were problematic in current practice: nutrition and performing a tracheostomy. As a result, more focused questions could be formulated using the PICOT format:

- What particular range of serum albumin levels (INTERVENTION) in ventilator-dependent patients (PATIENT POPULATION) is most likely to facilitate weaning (OUTCOME) while the patient is in ICU (TIME)? The COMPARISON is implied in this question—different levels of serum albumin are compared.
- Is weaning (OUTCOME) of ICU ventilator-dependent patients (PATIENT POPULATION) more successful if a tracheostomy is performed (INTERVENTION) within the first 48 hours of admission (TIME) or if the patient remains intubated (COMPARISON)?

Box 8-2 provides additional examples of problem statements or clinical questions. Note that some questions in the box do not specify a comparison group, although one is often implied. Subjects who do not

receive the intervention are the implied comparison groups for questions 4 and 6; in the case of question 3, the comparison is likely to be "usual care" provided to the APN's patients.

Searching for/Retrieving Evidence. Before searching for evidence, the APN must be familiar with levels/hierarchies of evidence and understand that "evidence exists on a continuum of rigor" (Stevens & Ledbetter, 2000, p. 93). Ideally, the choice of a particular evidence hierarchy is determined before the search for evidence because this decision can help focus the search and inform the searching strategy. For example, if only RCTs are going to be acceptable, then the search needs to be limited to studies of that design.

Starting with broader evidence levels will ensure that research reviews, guidelines, and consensus statements—as well as individual published studies—are accessed (Rutledge & Grant, 2002). Evidence summaries such as evidence-based guidelines, meta-analyses, systematic reviews, and meta-syntheses should be the initial focus of the literature search. For many clinical questions there are no evidence summaries, and therefore the literature search is best concentrated on other types of review articles (e.g., comprehensive and clinically focused literature reviews) and individual studies. In addition to searching bibliographical databases such as MEDLINE and CINAHL, sites that offer systematic reviews, clinical guidelines, or specialty-specific standards are valuable resources and should be included in the search strategy (McSweeney, Spies, & Cann, 2001). (See Box 8-3 for a list of online evidence-based practice resources). Note that some of the

Box 8-3   EVIDENCE-BASED PRACTICE RESOURCES

SITE/URL	DESCRIPTION
SYSTEMATIC REVIEWS	
Cochrane Library Website: www.cochranelibrary.com/cochrane/	Systematic reviews and guidelines; rely strongly on RCTs; generally medically oriented but considered the gold standard of such reviews (can browse titles and get abstracts for free but need subscription or must pay fee for documents)
Database of Abstracts of Reviews of Effects (DARE) Website: www.nhscrd.york.ac.uk/welcome.htm	Systematic reviews produced and maintained by the National Health System's Centre for Reviews and Dissemination
ONS EBP Online Resource Center Website: www.ons.org	Integrated review area provides a list of integrated reviews pertinent to cancer care
CLINICAL PRACTICE GUIDELINES	
Agency for Healthcare Research and Quality (AHRQ) Website: www.ahcpr.gov/	Evidence report topics, evidence technical reviews, and clinical guidelines
National Guideline Clearinghouse (NGC) Website: www.guideline.gov/	Public resource for evidence-based clinical practice guidelines and measurement tools. NGC is sponsored by the AHRQ
Institute for Healthcare Improvement (IHI) Website: www.ihi.org	List of published articles about developing and using evidence-based protocols
SPECIALTY-SPECIFIC GUIDELINES	
American College of Chest Physicians Website: www.chestnet.org/education/guidelines/ currentGuidelines.php	Pulmonary guidelines, endorsed guidelines at other sites, and systematic reviews
National Comprehensive Cancer Network (NCCN) Website: www.nccn.org/index.html	Cancer care guidelines
Primary Care Clinical Practice Guidelines Website: www.medicine.ucsf.edu/resources/guidelines/	Guidelines and resources for primary care
Internet Stroke Center, Washington University Website: www.strokecenter.org/ebtcd-03/index.html	Evidence-based guides to specific aspects of stroke care
American Academy of Pediatrics Website: www.aap.org/ policy/ paramtoc.html	Guidelines for pediatric specialty
AGREE Collaboration *Website: www.agreecollaboration.org/*	*Guideline appraisal instrument and list of guidelines that have been appraised*
GENERAL SITES WITH EXCELLENT LINKS TO OTHER EBP SITES	
Academic Center for Evidence-Based Nursing (ACE), University of Texas Health Center, San Antonio Website: www.acestar.uthscsa.edu/	Comprehensive list of EBP resources

EBP, Evidence-based practice; *JAMA,* Journal of the American Medical Association; *ONS,* Oncology Nursing Society; *RCTs,* randomized controlled trials.

Box 8-3   EVIDENCE-BASED PRACTICE RESOURCES—cont'd

SITE/URL	DESCRIPTION
GENERAL SITES WITH EXCELLENT LINKS TO OTHER EBP SITES—CONT'D	
Centre for Health Evidence Canadian Office of Health Website: www.cche.net/che/home.asp	Users' guides for EBP series from JAMA; how to critique and use different types of evidence articles
Centre for Evidence-Based Nursing, University of York Website: www.york.ac.uk/healthsciences/centres/	Lists of pertinent systematic reviews and evidence research reports
Centre for Evidence-Based Medicine (CEBM) Website: www.cebm.net/	Links to evidence-based resources, tools, continuing education, and discussion groups
Evidence Network Economic & Social Research Council Website: http://evidencenetwork.org/index.html	Provides evidence-based resources to facilitate use of evidence in social policy fields Lists systematic reviews, examples of use of evidence in policy
Joanna Briggs Institute Website: www.joannabriggs.edu.au/about/home.php	Australia-based, privately owned EBP site—some free pages and some pages only by subscription; nursing and allied health topics Best practice information sheets and a systematic review database
Advanced Practice Nursing Website: www.enursescribe.com/	Privately owned site with links pertinent to evidence-based resources
ONLINE JOURNALS	
Bandolier Evidence-Based Health Care Website: www.jr2.ox.ac.uk/bandolier/	Independent journal about evidence-based health care, written by Oxford scientists
Evidence-Based Nursing (EBN) Online Website: www.ebn.bmjjournals.com/	Online version of the journal (requires subscription)
Online Journal of Clinical Innovations (OJCI), CINAHL Website: www.cinahl.com	Online journal of research reviews and clinical innovations (requires subscription)
New England Journal of Medicine Website: http://content.nejm.org/	Can subscribe to online. Search mechanism allows subscriber to search all issues for topics in online version.
WorldViews on Evidence Based Practice Website: www.nursingsociety.org/	New online journal as of 2004 (requires Sigma Theta Tau International subscription)

resources require that the user be a subscriber or pay a fee to either search or obtain a document.

Whenever possible, APNs should start by retrieving and reviewing evidence summaries. *Evidence-based clinical practice guidelines* are usually the most comprehensive type of summary—analysis and synthesis of individual studies, meta-analyses, systematic reviews, and other types of evidence result in a set of specific clinical recommendations. To facilitate implementation, these recommendations are often accompanied by tools such as algorithms, QI audit guidelines, and other resources. A *meta-analysis* can be thought of as a quantitative analysis and synthesis of quantitative research findings—a "study of studies." In a meta-analysis, statistical analyses are performed using data from already published studies (LoBiondo-Wood & Haber, 2002) to calculate a common statistic, such as an effect size, across studies. A comparison of multiple studies, even those with small sample sizes, using meta-analytic statistics permits conclusions to be drawn that may confirm existing findings from individual studies or clarify conflicting findings. An *integrative* or *systematic review* of the literature provides a narrative or qualitative synthesis of quantitative research findings about a clinical problem (Ropka & Spencer-Cisek, 2001). More recently, the terms *meta-synthesis* or *meta-summaries* have been used to describe narrative, qualitative syntheses of findings from qualitative studies (Dixon-Woods, Fitzpatrick, & Roberts, 2001;Whittemore, 2005). Well-done evidence summaries prepared by credible organizations or individuals can "jumpstart" an evidence-based project because the published synthesis may be all that is needed if it is current, comprehensive enough, and credible. The authors have done the work of reducing large quantities of information into a manageable form. If the evidence summary does not include the most recent research evidence then it can be used as a template. Current evidence can be added to the established categories identified in the original summary to update it (Melnyk & Fineout-Overholt, 2005).

APNs should become proficient and efficient in searching for evidence. With each search, APNs will become more skilled at focusing and refocusing the topic so that the most pertinent evidence is identified and retrieved. Basic searching strategies learned in undergraduate programs are reinforced and expanded for use in comprehensive searches through assignments in graduate-level programs. Given rapidly evolving information technology, APNs must plan to regularly update their knowledge and skills in searching for evidence. Familiar databases such as MEDLINE and CINAHL often revise existing menus or add new features that may change how the database is used or make search activities more efficient. In addition to taking advantage of updated, live, or on-line library and database tutorials, strategies for comprehensive searching can be found in the literature (Conn et al., 2003; Hockenberry, Wilson, & Barrera, 2006; Melnyk & Fineout-Overholt, 2002; Morrisey & DeBourgh, 2001; Vrabel, 2005). Searching strategies specific to finding systematic reviews have also appeared in the literature (McGowan & Sampson, 2005; Melnyk, 2003; Montori, Wilczynski,

Morgan, & Haynes, 2005; Shojania & Bero, 2001). Both MEDLINE and CINAHL offer a mechanism to limit a search to review articles.

If an interdisciplinary planning group is involved, the APN is frequently the most appropriate person to rework the search strategies because he or she has an expert view of the clinical topic and a clear focus on what is being sought. Again, this process should be a collaboration between the APN and a reference librarian (Burns & Grove, 2007; DePalma, 2005; Vrabel, 2005). Collaborative searching incorporates the expertise of each and can strengthen the process. If a librarian is not available in the clinical setting, the possibility of accessing a librarian at an affiliated university or another setting within the health care system should be explored. If there are no such affiliated sites with a librarian, the APN will need to develop his or her search skills and those of colleagues to ensure a group of health care providers with the needed expertise.

The body of literature that results from the search may range from a few individual studies to a very large body of evidence, including evidence summaries. If the body of literature is large, logical ways to focus and reduce the amount of literature need to be used in order to conduct a feasible evaluation. A group of APNs who did a synthesis project on sleep disturbances in patients with cancer for the Oncology Nursing Society used the following criteria to reduce 102 sources of evidence to the 52 that were synthesized for the final article (Clark, Cunningham, McMillan, Vena, & Parker, 2004):

- *Language:* English publications only
- *Time frame:* 1980-2003, with articles from past 5 years preferred; however, some classic citations should be considered
- *Sample:* adult patients (older than 17 years) diagnosed with neoplastic disease
- *Setting:* any setting
- *Measurement:* must have assessed sleep disturbances or sleep patterns as a primary variable
- *Types of evidence:* opinion articles omitted; had to be research or review

Final decisions regarding the body of literature or evidence to be reviewed and the criteria for evaluation need to be a consensus of the stakeholder planning group members so that all perspectives on the clinical issue are adequately represented.

Evaluating and Interpreting Evidence. This phase of Competency I is complex and time consuming and requires a variety of skills. Three factors must be considered when evidence is evaluated: the scientific merit, applicability to clinical practice, and feasibility for the setting.

Once individual research studies, reviews, guidelines, and other information have been retrieved, the evidence needs to be reviewed, rated, and compiled in a format that will facilitate the subsequent phases in Competency I: creation of a narrative synthesis and subsequent practice recommendations. The activities that need to be accomplished in this phase of the competency depend on the ability of the individual APN or the planning group members to critique different types of evidence, select a hierarchy of evidence, develop inclusion and exclusion criteria, and select available tools with which to organize information from the wide variety of evidence.

Inclusion and exclusion criteria need to be developed to guide decisions about which studies will be eliminated and which will be retained. Inclusion and exclusion criteria, informed by a clearly stated clinical question, ensures a focused and efficient search. This may have been done as part of the searching activity (see "Searching for and Retrieving Evidence" phase), but if such criteria have not been determined, they need to be identified in this phase. For example, the individual APN or clinical planning group interested in pain management may want to review only quantitative studies with adult samples in outpatient settings. Having established such criteria, it is easy to eliminate studies of children or inpatients.

If an individual APN is evaluating the evidence, he or she would be reading each publication, which can be a daunting task and makes focusing the evidence that much more important. If a planning group has the literature, the group needs to determine which members will read the literature collected. Some groups choose several people to read all of the literature; other groups divide the literature evenly among all members of the group. At least two people should read each item to allow for discussion and consensus (Papadopoulos & Rheeder, 2000).

Some type of recording tool, such as an evidence table, is essential for each person who reads the literature, thus ensuring that consistent information is reported on each publication. Such a table clearly highlights relevant features of individual research studies. Columns in the table may vary according to topic of interest but usually include such basic information as author(s), title, publication date, and key methodological issues and findings. Rosswurm and Larrabee (1999) designed a worksheet that can be used to evaluate individual studies that include all of the methodological and results factors plus a section on the quality of evidence, feasibility of making a practice change based on the findings, and what the benefit/risk would be for the patients if practice was changed (Figure 8-1). Examples of other such tables can be found in well-developed systematic reviews (Lyles et al., 2007; Ries et al., 2007).

Individual research studies, literature reviews, and guidelines require different evaluation processes and therefore are discussed separately.

Individual Research Studies. The evaluation of individual research studies for scientific merit is the same as the research critique process taught in undergraduate program research courses and reinforced in graduate programs. Guides for appraising individual research articles can be found in most research books (Burns & Grove, 2007; Melnyk & Fineout-Overholt, 2005; Polit & Beck, 2006) and address the basic steps in the research process, determining if the design and data analysis are appropriate for the research questions, whether the measurement instruments have a reliable and valid history, whether the sample is adequate to determine statistical significance, and what the major findings were. Some resources provide guides for critiquing specific types of individual studies, such as studies on prevention, diagnostic testing, or a therapy or intervention (Gibbs, 2003; Guyatt & Rennie, 2002).

Systematic Reviews and Meta-Analyses. The critique of a systematic review or a meta-analysis is unique because APNs may be less familiar with the statistical analyses used and because the feasibility and applicability of the recommendations to a particular population, clinical practice, or health care setting may be more difficult to assess. For example, a meta-analysis of the effect of complementary therapies on pain in cancer patients may include individual studies in which samples were drawn from both inpatients and outpatients, patients with early and late-stage disease, and patients with different cancer diagnoses. The APN is likely to be interested in complementary and alternative medicine (CAM) in a particular subset of cancer patients. The authors of such a meta-analysis may or may not make it clear that the heterogeneity of the samples does or does not affect the overall conclusions—a factor important to the determination about whether the findings can be applied to the APN's practice.

A Model for Change to Evidence-Based Practice _____

Title of Article: _____

Purpose/Research Questions/ Hypotheses	Research Variables	Design	Major Findings and Limitations
Purpose of Study: **Research Questions/ Hypotheses:**	**Independent:** **Dependent:**	**Level I:** Exploratory Descriptive **Level II:** Correlational survey Comparative survey **Level III:** Quasi-experimental Experimental	**Findings:** **Limitations:**

Sample	Setting	Major Tools	Quality of Evidence
Number: **Type:** **Age:** **Gender:** **Health status:** **Diagnosis:** **Other:**	**Type:** Acute care hospital Community Nursing home Other **Location:** Urban Rural	**Name(s):** #1 _____ #2 _____ #3 _____ **Reliability:** #1 _____ #2 _____ #3 _____ **Validity:** #1 _____ #2 _____ #3 _____	**Evidence rating:** I. a. Meta-analysis of randomized controlled trials b. One randomized controlled trial II. a. One well-designed controlled study without randomization b. One other type of well-designed quasi-experimental study III. Comparative, correlational, and other descriptive studies IV. Evidence from expert committee reports and expert opinions **Feasibility:** Could this practice change be implemented easily in your organization and with minimal resources? ❑ Yes ❑ No **Benefit/risk:** Would the benefits of this practice change outweigh the risks to patients? ❑ Yes ❑ No **Comments:**

FIGURE **8-1:** Worksheet for critique. (From Rosswurm, M.A., & Larrabee, J.H. [1999]. A model for change to evidence-based practice. *Image: The Journal of Nursing Scholarship, 31,* 320.)

Guides have been developed to facilitate the evaluations of systematic reviews (Boaz, Ashby, & Young, 2002; Johnston, 2005; Melnyk, 2003; Melnyk & Fineout-Overholt, 2005; Oxman, Guyatt, Cook, & Montori, 2002; Scanlon, 2006; Thomas, Ciliska, Dobbins, & Micucci, 2004; Whitney, 2004) and meta-analyses (Lam & Kennedy, 2005; Moher et al., 2000). An online guide to appraising systematic reviews is available through the Centre for Evidence-Based Medicine (CEBM) website (see Box 8-3).

These guides usually deal with methodological attributes of the review and evaluation of whether the findings apply to the particular clinical setting and the feasibility of implementing the findings in the particular clinical setting. The applicability of the findings to the particular clinical setting can be assessed with questions such as whether the sample, setting, and technology are comparable to those found in the planning group's agency. The feasibility of implementing the findings in a clinical setting is usually addressed with an assessment of the balance between benefit and risks to the patient, needed resources, cost, and clinical and administrative readiness and support for the adoption of the practice change (Melnyk, 2003; Melnyk & Fineout-Overholt, 2005; Stetler, 2001).

The step-by-step process employed to find and use systematic reviews of studies related to the care of patients with Alzheimer's disease demonstrates the phases of research Competency I in a specific nursing specialty (Forbes, 2003).

Clinical Guidelines. Clinical practice guidelines are systematically developed statements to assist practitioner and patient with decisions about what is the most appropriate heath care for specific clinical circumstances (IOM, 1990). Clinical guidelines can be displayed as an algorithm, a care pathway, or a protocol. Guidelines make explicit recommendations for a clinical situation, which may include screening or treatment interventions, symptom management, and education. Evaluating clinical practice guidelines is also unique and involves determining the credibility of the author or authoring organization, timeliness (Shekelle, Eccles, Grimshaw, & Woolf, 2001), validity of the evidence base and methods of development, cost-effectiveness in implementation (Thomas & Hotchkiss, 2002), and applicability to the particular practice setting. Questions to ask in evaluation of clinical practice guidelines are available in both the medical and nursing literature (AGREE Collaboration,

2001; Levin & Vetter, 2007; Luxford, Hill, & Bell, 2006; McSweeney et al., 2001; Thomas & Hotchkiss, 2002). Two formal instruments that can be used to evaluate a clinical guideline are the Appraisal of Guidelines Research and Evaluation (AGREE) Instrument (2001) and the Cluzeau Appraisal Instrument (Cluzeau, Littlejohns, Grimshaw, Feder, & Moran, 1999). Both of these instruments provide the person evaluating the guideline a rating system for key aspects of the guideline's development (stakeholders' involvement and rigor), presentation (clarity), and applicability to actual practice.

Synthesizing the Evidence. Synthesis is a high-level function that requires much thought and skill. In the typical literature review, each study's purpose, methods, and findings are described separately. A synthesis, informed by the clinical question, is organized based on key themes or categories that have been identified across all studies. In addition, important similarities and differences among studies, as well as conflicting findings, are highlighted (Garrard, 2007).

This phase requires a good deal of time with interaction of all members of the group. Time will be needed to present and discuss the evidence reviewed by individuals, and then the group will need to consider the evidence in total. One example of how time-consuming a formal literature synthesis can be involves review of oncology literature with the use of the Triad Model of Research Synthesis (Rutledge, DePalma, & Cunningham, 2004). Oncology APNs determined that to be successful in undertaking a practice-focused synthesis of evidence, they would need the expertise of an educator and a researcher. The total process took 1 year, which is too long for many clinically based groups looking to change practice, but the steps in the process are discussed, as well as situations that arose and how they were addressed in the different groups.

The actual synthesis product may resemble an outline for a systematic review article. General items to include are as follows:

- Statement of the clinical problem or question
- Details of the search strategy and results, including number of publications accessed and how these were focused to the ultimate number included in the synthesis
- Narrative summary of commonalities and differences across evidence, according to themes or categories derived from the studies reviewed

- Practice recommendations that can be made, based on the strength of the evidence, if the evidence is sufficient

The planning group needs to consider all of these items before a formal practice change recommendation is made.

Making a Recommendation for Practice. Having stakeholders that represent all aspects of care for the patient population addressed in the clinical question is especially important at this stage. Each stakeholder can see the clinical situation from his or her perspective and should be able to offer unique views and comments regarding the applicability of the evidence and the feasibility of making any practice changes.

The most important aspect of making any recommendation based on the reviewed evidence is to be true to the evidence. In other words, usually one of three decisions can be made from the evidence: (1) the group may conclude that sufficient evidence exists to justify a practice change recommendation, (2) the group may feel that the evidence in support of or negating existing practice is contradictory and therefore a clear recommendation cannot be made, or (3) the group may conclude that evidence is insufficient to be able to make a recommendation.

If a recommendation can be made from the evidence reviewed, then current practice should be compared with the recommendation to see if a practice change is needed. Sometimes the result of an evidence review is that current practice is validated as being consistent with "best" practice. If the recommendation would mean a practice change, for example, implementing a nutrition team for ventilator-dependent patients in the ICU, then questions must be asked about the value and feasibility of implementing such a change. The first thing to consider is whether the practice change would improve the quality of care significantly. In other words, would the outcomes of care be improved for a significant number of patients? If the practice change would greatly affect the quality of care provided for a significant number of patients, then questions of feasibility must be addressed, such as the following:

- What resources would be needed to implement this practice change?
- What support would administration and clinicians provide?
- How much time would it take to implement such a change?

- How much would the change cost the organization?

The planning group needs to consider all of these issues before formal recommendations are made. The members of the planning group should reach consensus about the practice changes they will recommend for adoption. Although a recommendation can be made based on evidence alone, the practice change may not be feasible if it would require many more resources than are available in the clinical setting. It may also take time to work with administration and key clinicians to convince them that such a change is both feasible and beneficial.

Examples of articles that describe the process of synthesizing evidence and making practice recommendations include a protocol for preventing opioid-induced constipation (Robinson et al., 2000), managing brain-injured patients (Fakhry, Trask, Waller, & Watts, 2004), managing patients with acute myocardial infarctions (Donohue, 2005), and using an evidence-based guideline to prevent pneumonia with ventilator-dependent patients (Dodek et al, 2004).

Implementing Recommended Evidence-Based Practice Change. APNs are vital to this phase of the competency because they understand the patient population and the organization. A realistic implementation plan must be based on an understanding of change theory and an understanding of what is possible within the organization. APNs understand the sources of power and levers of change in the organization, what the barriers and facilitators will be for a specific practice change, and how to design an implementation plan that is sensitive to the political environment of an organization.

Some practice changes may not require a formal implementation plan. For example, an APN-led unit-based clinical practice council evaluated the evidence on effective change-of-shift-reports and determined that they should change the way it was being done on their unit. The new report method was presented to staff on all three shifts, and the staff had adopted it within 2 weeks of this introduction. Although no change in policy and procedure was required, the implementation plan included evaluating care processes and staff satisfaction. However, many practice change recommendations require a formal population-wide and/or system-wide implementation plan.

If the practice change is going to be organization-wide and will require additional resources, then an implementation plan may be needed as a proposal to a clinical or administrative group that has the power to release such resources. If a formal implementation plan is needed, it should include a step-by-step strategy to accomplish a practice change and the resources needed to implement the change. A possible outline for such a plan is as follows:

- Current practice (based on internal data)
- Proposed change with evidence-based rationale and risks/benefits that can be anticipated
- Potential barriers and facilitators in the setting
- Necessary resources and costs to implement and monitor outcomes
- Step-by-step protocol for accomplishing the practice change
- Education of all involved with the practice change (content and timing)
- Potential timeline

When possible, a trial implementation (pilot testing) on one or two units should be done. A pilot provides concrete information on whether the implementation plan is reasonable and gives an opportunity for all practitioners to provide feedback on the implementation process. Involving the clinicians provides a sense of ownership of the change process and contributes to a smoother integration of the change (Rosswurm & Larrabee, 1999, Titler, 2004). An area, service, or unit should be chosen to initiate the implementation to offer the best opportunity for successful adoption. On the basis of the pilot evaluation, the practice change or the implementation plan or both can be modified and then rolled out across the institution.

Examples of implementation plans in the literature include the interdisciplinary implementation of evidence-based guidelines for the prevention of urinary tract infections (Reilly et al., 2006), the implementation of an evidence-based feeding protocol and aspiration risk–reduction algorithm in medical intensive care units (Bowman et al., 2005), and a new protocol to prevent brain hemorrhage and ischemic brain injury in very-low-birth-weight infants (McLendon et al., 2003). One example in the literature demonstrates the impact of the culture of the environment when teams from 11 medical center neonatal intensive care units attempted to implement family-centered care (Moore, DuBuisson, Swett, & Edwards, 2003). The differences in the degree of implementation depended on the unit culture and the ability to accept families as partners rather than only visitors.

Evaluating the Recommended Evidence-Based Practice Change. Evaluation of the impact of the practice change completes Competency I. Evaluation provides essential data for further decision making and assists staff and the planning group in determining whether the practice change is making a difference and should be continued. A practice change evaluation has many similarities to the evaluation of practice that is addressed in Competency II. Therefore understanding evaluation as it relates to Competency I will facilitate the APN's implementation of Competency II.

The evaluation plan should be developed in conjunction with the implementation plan once the team has identified the outcomes that will demonstrate that practice has been improved. To measure the outcomes, the team should establish a timeline that is realistic and allows enough time for staff to adopt the change. Findings should be reported to the appropriate clinical group. Progress in adopting the practice change plan should be reviewed by the planning group within the first quarter of implementation to identify and address any major issues that may have arisen. Significant differences in patients' clinical outcomes may not be apparent by that time. However, the process—including the extent to which the practice change is being accepted and used—can be evaluated, and the opinions of the clinicians concerning the practice change can be determined. If the practice change has not been adopted readily, additional measures may be needed to promote the change or the implementation plan may need to be revised.

The planning group should write an evaluation report when sufficient time for assessment of clinical outcomes has elapsed. In the interim, the administrative or clinical committees to whom the planning group reports may require quarterly reports that document evaluation activities. On the basis of the evaluation report, decisions may be made to continue monitoring outcomes or, in the face of disappointing outcomes, a new plan may need to be developed and implemented. Alternatively, if outcomes have exceeded expectations, the planning group may be asked to create a new plan to promote wider adoption of the recommendations. Finally, if there is significant variability in achieving expected outcomes, research projects may be undertaken to determine why some patients are achieving better outcomes than others or why certain areas in the setting are achieving better outcomes (Competency III).

The respiratory quality care work group (first described on p. 225) decided to adopt the policy of performing tracheostomies on ventilator-dependent patients within the first 48 hours after admission to the trauma unit. A formal implementation plan was not needed because the group had the power to change the policy temporarily until evaluation data were collected and analyzed. The evaluation plan was based on a comparison of weaning rates before and after the implementation of the new policy. Based on the average number of ventilator-dependent patients admitted to the trauma unit, it was decided that data would be collected at 3 months and 6 months to see if there was any trend toward improvement of weaning. The process would be assessed by the number of tracheostomies that were performed in the first 24 hours. After explaining the proposed change and eliciting clinician support at the weekly medical staff meeting, the respiratory quality care work group agreed to present the comparison between baseline data and the 3-month and 6-month results at two future staff meetings.

Exemplar 8-1 provides examples of fundamental and expanded levels of Competency I.

COMPETENCY II: EVALUATION OF PRACTICE

Competency II has both fundamental and expanded levels of activity (see Table 8-1). Advanced nursing practices should be evidence-based and fully evaluated. This is especially important in the current health care environment in which only roles that have a positive influence on patient care and are cost-effective and affordable can be continued in any clinical setting. Clinicians must demonstrate to the population being served and to those who pay for health care that they are providing the best, current practice, that their practice makes a difference in the quality of patient care, and that it is cost-effective. However, this is a daunting task for many busy APNs.

Fundamental and Expanded Levels of Competency II

Documenting the value and effectiveness of advanced practice nursing not only assists clinicians to improve their own practices but also provides valuable information for other stakeholders in the health care system, including consumers, administrators, insurers, health care systems, and regulatory and accrediting agencies. If employment of an individual APN or a group of APNs is cost-effective and results in improved clinical care, the APN role can be more easily justified when administrators make cost-cutting or quality-improvement decisions (see Chapter 23).

Assessment of the impact of advanced practice nursing on clinical outcomes and quality indicators is appearing more commonly in the professional literature (see Chapter 24 for a comprehensive list of studies). The positive impact of care provided by APNs has been demonstrated in specific settings such as home care (Neff, Madigan, & Narsavage, 2003) and tertiary care (Derengowski, Irving, Koogle, & Englander, 2000) or with specific patient

---

 EXEMPLAR 8-1   Competency I

These are examples of the improvement of practice by the application of research evidence to the development of evidence-based procedures, protocols, or programs. Some of these may exemplify one or more of the levels of Competency I—the *fundamental level* if applied to individual practice and the *expanded level* if the practice change was adopted by a group, unit, or entire clinical setting.

- Development of a guideline to change the practice of physical restraint use in acute care (Park & Tang, 2007). *Exemplifies the expanded competency because it is a protocol adopted by an entire setting.*
- Development of guidelines for cardiovascular disease prevention in women (Mosca et al., 2004). *Exemplifies the expanded competency because it is a protocol to be adopted by all health care providers in any setting.*

- Evidence-based approach to the prevention of work-related musculoskeletal injuries among nurses (Stetler, Burns, Sander-Buscemi, Morsi, & Grunwald, 2003). *Exemplifies the fundamental competency if it is applied to individual practice and the expanded competency if it is adopted by an entire setting.*
- A medication management intervention for frail, community-dwelling, older adult population (Alkema & Frey, 2006). *Exemplifies the fundamental competency if it is applied to individual practice and the expanded competency if it is adopted by an entire setting.*
- A systematic review of literature supporting a cardioversion service led by a nurse (Smallwood, 2005). *Exemplifies the expanded competency because it is a protocol to be adopted in a clinical setting.*

populations such as oncology patients (Cunningham, 2004) or outpatients with heart failure (Crowther, 2003; Delgado-Passler & McCaffrey, 2006; Kleinpell & Gawlinski, 2005; McCauley, Bixby, & Naylor, 2006; Naylor et al., 2004). Comparisons of care provided by APNs and traditional care (usually physician-driven) have demonstrated improved aspects of care with the APN-driven care for specific patient populations such as postoperative cardiovascular adults (Meyer & Miers, 2005) and patients with chronic hepatitis C (Ahern, Imperial, & Lam, 2004).

Implementing and maintaining an evaluation process, whether it be for an individual APN's practice (fundamental level of the competency) or for a total department of APNs (expanded level of the competency) are complex, requiring extensive planning, knowledge, and skills. A detailed discussion of the practice evaluation process and the integral relationship with performance evaluation and quality improvement is presented in Chapter 25. Also in that chapter are many resources to facilitate practice evaluation. Because of the thorough discussion in Chapter 25 about evaluation, this competency is addressed in a limited manner with emphasis on information that adds to what is presented in Chapter 25.

Identifying Key Aspects of Practice to Evaluate

APNs must be able to articulate the primary aspects of their practice that are essential to evaluate. Any of the following can serve as primary goals to drive an evaluation process:

- Scope, standards of practice, and competencies for the particular APN role
- Evidence-based guidelines and national quality indicators
- Role and job descriptions developed internally
- Program objectives

An evaluation of APN practice should include aspects of quality, access to care, and economic dimensions.

The *quality dimension* could be addressed by the fact that the practice is in keeping with the appropriate scope and standards of practice and evidence-based guidelines for the specialty. Quality of care could also address an improved outcome for the patient population demonstrated by quality indicators, such as fewer complications, fewer readmissions, improved patient self-management of care, increased wellness-promoting behaviors, and increased patient satisfaction. Improved access to care for a particular patient population, especially a vulnerable population, because of a particular APN's practice or APN-led program is another quality measure. Finally, the cost-effectiveness of APN practice should be addressed. APNs whose care results in reduced costs (e.g., reduction in hospital readmissions within 30 days of discharge) or increased revenue (e.g., increased reimbursements when clinical benchmarks are met) need to be sure this is included in evaluations of practice. In some cases, APN care may be revenue neutral—neither increasing nor decreasing costs—often a positive factor given the escalating costs of health care.

One example of standards of practice and competencies that have been developed and distributed by professional organizations is the NONPF consensus-based primary care competencies for adult, family, gerontological, pediatric, and women's health NPs (NONPF, 2006). Evidence-based guidelines can be found on the Internet (see Box 8-3). One example of a specialty-based evidence-based guideline is the *Senior Adult Oncology* guideline developed by the National Comprehensive Cancer Network (National Comprehensive Cancer Network [NCCN], 2007). This guideline deals with screening, assessment, and symptom management related to the various types of oncology treatment. The National Database of Nursing Quality Indicators (American Nurses Association [ANA], 2001) provides nursing-sensitive indicators that reflect the structure, process, and outcomes of nursing care. These indicators include characteristics of the nursing staff (the supply, the skill level, and the education/certification), basic care activities (assessment and intervention), and patient outcome indicators that are determined to be nursing-sensitive. Nurse-sensitive outcomes are those clinical conditions that improve if there is a greater quantity or quality of nursing care (e.g., pressure ulcers, falls, and intravenous infiltrations). An example of an illness-based source for quality indicators is the *National Healthcare Quality Report* (Agency for Healthcare Research and Quality [AHRQ], 2005). This source presents the effectiveness of health care for nine clinical conditions or care settings—cancer, diabetes, end-stage renal disease, heart disease, human immunodeficiency virus (HIV) and acquired immunodeficiency syndrome (AIDS), maternal and child health, mental health, respiratory diseases, and nursing home and home health care—as well as findings on patient safety, timeliness, and patient centeredness.

Job descriptions or key program objectives or services that involve APNs are also starting points for determining primary goals for practice evaluation, especially when evidence-based guidelines or national quality indicators cannot be found. The quality-of-care dimension of evaluation can include data on improved clinical care processes and patient outcomes.

Evaluation of the *access dimension* refers to assessment of direct care provided by APNs; this may include services made available, facilitated, or coordinated by APNs or information to facilitate patient decision making that is provided by APNs. APNs may be providing a level of care that would not be otherwise available or may be improving health care access by improving coordination of care. For example, an APN-led, community-based program of breast and cervical cancer screening for medically underserved, low-income women (Schulz, Ludwick, Cukr, & Kelly, 2002) improved access by removing barriers to care. The accessible, acceptable, and appropriate services that were provided resulted in an increased attendance rate with each screening program. Investigators attributed the high minority participation (20% of the screening programs' attendees were women of color from a predominantly white [96.1%] geographical area) to their emphasis on minority recruitment and the supportive informal network that emerged during the project (Schulz et al., 2002).

The *economy dimension* can include evaluation of institutional and population outcomes, such as costs; cost-effectiveness; the impact of underuse, overuse, or misuse of evidence-based interventions (IOM, 2001); and assessment of underuse of APNs. Cost-effectiveness may be demonstrated by reductions in lengths of stay, complications, or readmissions. Other cost savings may depend on specific patient populations. For example, CNMs' positive impact on costs of care might be measured by using data that demonstrate a decreasing number of cesarean deliveries and premature births. An annual cost analysis is another strategy for evaluating the economic dimension of advanced practice nursing (Vincent, 2002). A cost analysis of an academic-based nursing center was conducted and resulted in the identification of services that were profitable and those that were not (Vincent, 2002). On the basis of the analysis, recommendations were made to decrease administrative costs, increase the number of primary care visits, and decrease the variable costs of the Women, Infants, and Children (WIC) program to break even financially.

Ensuring Collection of Reliable and Valid Data

A key aspect of the data collection component of Competency II is determining what relevant data already exist internally and externally and whether they are sufficient to conduct a practice evaluation. Exactly what data should be collected can be determined by answering this question: "What information is needed to demonstrate that a particular goal has been met or an outcome achieved?" Review of external benchmarks from established standards of care, clinical guidelines, quality indicators, or published research can assist in validating appropriate and feasible data points.

The APN must plan and work closely with the information technology department in the clinical setting to ascertain what data are stored through the electronic medical record applications and what data are accessible for analysis and reporting. Data access must be done in accordance with Health Insurance Portability and Accountability Act (HIPAA) mandates (1996).

Knowledge and skills related to data analysis are similar regardless of whether data are collected for evaluation or for collaborative research projects. Such techniques are included among the skills necessary for research Competency III: "Participation in Collaborative Research," discussed in the next section. Because these techniques may be complex and require computer hardware and software with which many APNs may not be familiar, APNs should seek appropriate resources or consultants. For example, the institution may have quality improvement or data management personnel who can assist with the design of a data system for the evaluation project (see Chapter 25 for further discussion of data management).

Cost and feasibility of collecting the data must also be considered. Before selecting measures to collect data, APNs must be aware of data available through existing resources and databases to avoid unnecessary effort and duplication (Bozzo, 1999). Therefore APNs need an understanding of the types of data that are stored and retrievable from national and state databases as well as those within the particular clinical setting. They must also know how to plan for the development of additional databases, if needed.

Determining If Practice Change Is Necessary Based on Evaluation Results

Once a data collection process has been established, APNs need an adequate understanding of research methodology to interpret data appropriately and to recognize the potential for confounding variables. For example, when analyzing the impact of advanced practice nursing interactions on patients, it is important also to consider the influence of disease status over time. Decreasing functional status in a patient with stable disease has different implications than it would in a patient with progressive cancer.

The internal and external benchmark data that served as guides for establishing what data should be collected will also serve as comparison data. Internal reports can be requested on a regular basis (e.g., monthly or quarterly). External data, such as those received from Medicare and Medicaid, can also be used. Reports should be reviewed for what they reveal about current practice and compared with previous reports to identify trends.

As with Competency I, the next step is to determine what the data mean and whether practice needs to change. Data trended over a specific period will be most useful to indicate whether practice changes are needed. For example, if complication or readmission rates are increasing, an EBP change can be implemented and

then tracked for several months to look for improvement. Accomplishment of this step therefore requires the knowledge and skills of Competency I.

Also included in this phase of the competency is the effective dissemination of results, including cost and resource implications, to administrators and other key decision makers. Effective dissemination requires that the APN be able to clearly and comprehensively describe the process, explain the results, articulate how or why the results are related to his or her own practice or to advanced practice nursing in general, and link the findings with current practice or proposals for revised practice.

Table 8-3 outlines the components and key activities of Competency II. Exemplar 8-2 provides examples of practice evaluation.

COMPETENCY III: PARTICIPATION IN COLLABORATIVE RESEARCH

The third research competency relates to involvement in collaborative nursing or interdisciplinary research studies undertaken to generate knowledge

Table 8-3   COMPETENCY II: EVALUATION OF PRACTICE

Component of the Process	Key Activities
Identifying Key Aspects of Practice to Evaluate	Locate scope and standards of practice, evidence-based guidelines, and quality indicators that are relevant to practice as benchmarks. List major desired goals or impacts of practice on patients' clinical care, both short-term and long-term. List major desired goals or impacts of practice on the organization, both short-term and long-term. Ensure that the impacts are stated in a manner so that they are feasible and measurable.
Ensuring Collection of Reliable and Valid Data	Indicate what actual data will indicate proof of the achievement of desired practice goals. Review external benchmarks from established standards of care, clinical guidelines, quality indicators, or published research to validate what data points are appropriate and feasible. Review documentation for inclusion of all data points. Emphasize point-of-service data collection and not duplication. Identify and secure established data collection tools as needed. Design or revise current documentation tools to include all data points.
Determining if Practice Changes Are Necessary Based on Evaluation Results	Establish a process to compare data from individual or collaborative practice, ideally electronically, on a short-term and long-term basis. Establish a process that provides a periodic, user-friendly report of the benchmark comparisons. Establish a process that facilitates all appropriate stakeholders reviewing the data and making recommendations for practice changes based on the data. Disseminate process and results within clinical setting.

EXEMPLAR 8-2   Competency II

Published accounts of evaluation of practice are often within the activities described for Competency III because they tend to be formal studies evaluating a program or comparing advanced practice nursing outcomes with physician outcomes. Findings from such articles can be used by APNs, however, in designing their own practice evaluation projects related to standards, quality indicators, or outcomes of their care, which are the focus of Competency II activities.

- Evaluation of APN-directed versus RN-directed telemanagement programs for heart failure patients (Delgado-Passler & McCaffrey, 2006).
- Evaluation of a pediatric critical care NP role in a tertiary academic pediatric ICU: design, implementation, scope of practice, and outcomes

of the new role (Derengowski, Irving, Koogle, & Englander, 2005).
- Identifying differences in the rate of anesthesia complications when care administered by CRNA versus anesthesiologist (Simonson, Ahern, & Hendryx, 2007).
- APN-managed transitional care intervention for older adults hospitalized with heart failure: clinical and financial outcomes (Naylor et al., 2004).
- APN-managed transitional care for home care patients with chronic obstructive pulmonary disease (Neff, Madigan, & Narsavage, 2003).
- Evaluation of weekend on-call nurse anesthetist coverage—costs and risks/benefits (Dexter, Epstein, & Marsh, 2002).

APN, Advanced practice nurse; *CRNA*, certified registered nurse anesthetist; *ICU*, intensive care unit; *NP*, nurse practitioner; *RN*, registered nurse.

that enhances understanding of clinical phenomena, to define optimal nursing or other interventions for particular populations and specific clinical problems (Brooten & Naylor, 1995), or to examine formal outcomes of care (Whitman, 2002a, 2002b). This competency is consistent with the American Association of Critical Care Nurses' (2002) position that master's prepared nurses "…identify practice and systems problems that need to be studied and collaborate with other scientists to generate new studies based on their expertise" (p. 2). In addition to being consumers of research (Competency I) and users of the research process to examine their own practice (Competency II), APNs need to recognize the value of conducting research, understand the research process and their unique and essential contributions to this process, and make collaborative participation in knowledge-generating or outcomes research a priority (Martin, 1995).

This research competency for APNs is critical because it is through their direct participation in research studies that APNs can help to (1) ensure the clinical relevance of the research questions (Polit & Beck, 2008), (2) participate in selection of nursing-sensitive outcomes or outcomes that are critical components of quality patient care (Whitman, 2002a), and (3) ultimately influence the clinical applicability of the results (Polit & Beck, 2008). Two areas of research are vitally important for advanced practice nursing research collaboration:

knowledge-generating research that produces the evidence for new interventions that can be used in evidence-based clinical practice guidelines, and outcomes research that examines the quality of patient care or validates the role of selected personnel such as APNs (Clochesy, 2002; Jastremski, 2002; see also Chapter 24).

Regardless of an APN's work setting or responsibilities, this competency is essential rather than optional. However, it must be individualized, as with the other two competencies, to a particular APN's setting, position responsibilities, sociopolitical climate, and personal desires, goals, and values. Perhaps most important, this competency is a logical extension of research-related activity for APNs when Competency I reveals insufficient evidence in a given area or when Competency II does not yield the anticipated outcomes of one's practice, especially when the practice is based on existing research. In other words, when there is no evidence or when outcomes are less than optimal, it is likely that additional knowledge-generating research is necessary and the APN is the ideal clinician to participate in such research.

Fundamental and Expanded Levels of Competency III

Competency III has both fundamental and expanded levels of activity (see Table 8-1). At the fundamental level, defined as occurring on completion of a graduate program, the APN is capable of assuming a role as a consultant or clinical expert in a research study to ensure the clinical relevance of the study. Advanced education in the DNP program further develops the fundamental level of this competency. The expanded level, developed after much practical experience with a funded researcher or an established research team or after graduation from a PhD program, positions the APN as a principal investigator or co-investigator in knowledge-generating research. Again, the APN's work setting and position description may greatly influence his or her involvement in expanded-level Competency III activities because research may or may not be a major expectation in the clinical environment.

The ways in which APNs can participate in collaborative research are many, but two foundational elements are necessary. First, an APN must possess general knowledge about research paradigms and the phases of the research process, which should initially be acquired in a graduate program and continually developed over time. This basic research knowledge is thoroughly detailed in the typical nursing research textbooks used in most graduate nursing programs; two examples are those by Burns and Grove (2007) and Polit and Beck (2008). Other resources such as a network of professional colleagues knowledgeable about research (e.g., a professor from the APN's graduate program, an APN colleague who is active in research, or a practice partner who is engaged in research) and internal and external sources of information and materials on research (e.g., libraries, websites, professional organizations) are also helpful.

The second foundational element the APN needs is knowledge of how to identify, meet, and develop collaborations with active researchers who are studying areas of interest to the APN. This can be easy or challenging, depending on the APN's work setting, geographical area, and other factors such as motivation, interest, and support of administration. A detailed description of strategies is beyond the scope of this text, but several general suggestions may be helpful to the reader. If the APN works in an academic health center or academically affiliated setting, research may already be an integral component of the position description and collaborative participation may be a given. If APNs are not involved in research, there are likely to be clinical researchers in affiliated schools of nursing and medicine, some of whom may already be collaborating with others in the APN's setting. The APN can learn more about such individuals and their research from personal contacts; networking;

examining Web pages (e.g., research activities of faculty); or attending research presentations, journal clubs, and other research-related offerings. If the APN is not in an academic setting, he or she could explore potential collaborative opportunities with faculty and researchers in nearby academic settings or talk with local representatives of pharmaceutical or medical device companies, who are increasingly seeking research partners in the community, about participating in one or more of their studies. Other willing and useful collaborators might include rural health, migrant, and other federal, state, and local agencies that provide care to vulnerable populations.

Another tactic for identifying collaborative opportunities might be exploration of professional society research initiatives, such as the American Association of Critical-Care Nurses' Thunder I and II projects that assessed procedural pain behaviors during six common procedures (Puntillo, et al., 2004; Thompson et al., 2001) or the Association of Women's Health (Church-Balin & Damus, 2003; Sampselle et al., 2000). Federal or international projects also can be identified and joined. For example, the Communities of Practice endeavor across North America and Canada (McDonald & Viehbeck, 2007) is a consortium of Quitline Operators to enhance research capacity for tobacco control research. Technological advances in communication, computer support, and networking allow research partners to collaborate virtually; they do not all need to reside and work in the same geographical location. The bottom line is that it is important for the APN to "put out the word" about his or her interest in collaboration, because many researchers are interested in finding good clinical partners for their research projects and in having access to new clinical settings and will appreciate the involvement of interested APNs.

The scope of specific research activities in which APNs can become engaged within this research competency is wide-ranging. In most settings, the APN is the individual most likely to understand the clinical issues and questions in a given patient population and to be familiar with the routines and culture of the clinical setting. Thus the APN is ideally positioned to make meaningful contributions to all phases of the research process, regardless of whether the research is focused on generating descriptive knowledge, testing interventions, or examining outcomes of care.

Tables 8-4 and 8-5 outline the major phases of quantitative and qualitative research processes and

Table 8-4   Competency III: Selected Advanced Practice Nursing Activities in Collaborative Quantitative Research

Phase of the Research*	Selected Activities
1. Conceptual—formulating the problem, selecting a conceptual framework, developing study purposes, questions, and hypotheses	Identify nursing practice problems. Consult with researchers to translate problems into researchable questions. Help identify relevant clinical variables and nursing sensitive outcomes.
2. Design and Planning—deciding on the design and methods and developing procedures	Help determine appropriate study sample and selection criteria. Help ensure clinical feasibility of design and methods, assist in selecting appropriate instruments for the population, and minimize study burden to patients and staff. Help develop processes to ensure rigor, and participate in developing protocols or procedure manuals for study implementation. Help refine protocols for delivering interventions (if relevant) and collecting data, and assist with access to the site and study subjects. Help determine roles of staff and other relevant personnel, including self. Collaborate on preparation and submission of IRB materials.
3. Empirical—collecting the data and preparing it for analysis	Help ensure accurate and consistent collection of data, and participate in actual collection of data (if relevant). Assist researchers in cleaning and coding (if needed).
4. Analytic—analyzing the data and interpreting it	Work with investigators in reviewing the analyses and ensuring that they make sense clinically. Help provide clinical explanations for findings if needed. Put the findings into the real clinical context of the setting, comparing results with appropriate external benchmark data. Determine the implications for practice or the need for further research.
5. Dissemination—communicating research findings	Assist in identifying how and where results should be disseminated (both internal and external). Work with researchers to develop possible clinical, research, and methodological dissemination topics. Help develop abstracts, posters, slide shows, and manuscripts; take responsibility for arranging internal dissemination meetings.

*Adapted from Polit & Beck, 2006.
IRB, Institutional Review Board.

list, for each phase, specific activities in which APNs can become engaged. These activities are assumed to complement the solid foundation of general research knowledge mentioned previously. Further, they are not exhaustive because APNs engage in numerous additional activities, depending on the context of their work environment. The activities shown in Tables 8-4 and 8-5 are focused primarily at the fundamental level of activity for this research competency, namely participating as a clinical expert/consultant on a research team (see Table 8-1).

Participation in collaborative research is an essential competency for APNs, although clearly less critical to the quality and effectiveness of their own personal professional practices than are Competencies I and II. Participation by APNs in knowledge-generating research builds on Competencies I and II and contributes to the broader goal of evidence-based, high-quality care.

Exemplar 8-3 provides examples of Competency III.

ACQUIRING AND DEVELOPING RESEARCH COMPETENCIES

The acquisition and further development of research competencies generally depend on a combination of education and experience. APNs can be introduced to the required activities for each research competency in formal education programs, either at the master's or DNP level. What occurs in the practice

Table 8-5 COMPETENCY III: SELECTED ADVANCED PRACTICE NURSING ACTIVITIES IN COLLABORATIVE QUALITATIVE RESEARCH

Phase of the Research*	Selected Activities
1. Conceptualizing and Planning the Study—deciding on the focus, approach, site, and participants	Identify nursing practice problems. Consult with researchers to translate problems into researchable questions. Assist with access to the site and study participants. Help develop procedures that are compatible with the site. Collaborate on preparation and submission of IRB materials.
2. Conducting the Study (**NOTE:** in qualitative research, the conduct of the study and analysis of the data are often simultaneous or interrelated activities; thus this phase of "conducting the study" refers to both)	Assist researchers in identifying and contacting potential participants. Facilitate interviews or other data collection processes. Provide information to researchers in the ongoing process of data reduction and analysis. Provide expert clinical insight and knowledge to the interpretative phases of the study. Assist in identifying clinical implications.
3. Disseminating the Findings	Assist in identifying how and where results should be disseminated (both internal and external). Work with researchers to develop possible clinical, research, and methodological dissemination topics. Help develop abstracts, posters, slide shows, and manuscripts; take responsibility for arranging internal dissemination meetings.

*Adapted from Polit & Beck, 2006.
IRB, Institutional Review Board.

EXEMPLAR 8-3 Competency III

The following are examples of formal research studies in which APNs played key roles as clinical experts or co-investigators. The examples were chosen to illustrate the variety of ways APNs can participate in research.

- Survey of APNs to determine how frequently they assess and document risk factors for child abuse (Adams, 2005).
- RCT of vulnerable older adults with heart failure receiving APN-coordinated care (McCauley, Bixby, & Naylor, 2006).
- Challenges of implementing an APN-coordinated falls management program in long-term care and the specific influence APNs had on the behavior of the nursing staff (Capezuti, Taylor, Brown, & Strothers, 2007).
- National survey to determine whether CRNAs demonstrate gender bias in treating pain (Criste, 2003).
- Qualitative, phenomenological approach, interviewing women during pregnancy and 6 weeks postpartum with symphysis pubis dysfunction to determine their experience with pain. Implications for midwifery practice are discussed (Wellock & Crichton, 2007).
- Analysis of interaction logs created by APNs during five RCTs (very-low-birth-weight infants; women with unplanned cesarean deliveries or high-risk pregnancies; women who had undergone hysterectomy; and adults with cardiac medical and surgical diagnoses). Determined whether amount of APN time and contacts made a difference with clinical outcomes (Brooten, Youngblut, Deatrick, Naylor, & York, 2003).

APNs, Advanced practice nurses; *CRNAs,* certified registered nurse anesthetists; *RCT,* randomized controlled trial.

setting, after APNs complete their formal education, determines the extent to which expanded levels of the research competencies are achieved.

It is unrealistic to expect that any educational program can, with its temporal and structural constraints, prepare APNs for the full spectrum of possible research competency activities. The focus in APN programs is on acquiring the knowledge and skills to demonstrate fundamental levels of each competency, thus becoming a sophisticated consumer of research, and gaining the ability to evaluate one's own practice. APNs will continue to refine their fundamental research competencies throughout their careers. Achievement of the expanded levels of activity for the competencies will depend on the APN's own commitment and motivation and on opportunities that exist for research participation, mentoring experiences, and continuing education.

Post-Graduate Research Competency Development

Postgraduate development of research competencies that serve to move the APN toward the expanded levels of activity in all three research competencies (see Table 8–1) is highly individualized to the practice setting, specialty, position expectations, professional goals, and research opportunities. This discussion builds on what has been included under Competency III about finding opportunities to be involved in research projects.

APNs can use numerous vehicles to further develop their research competencies. The ones discussed here are limited to membership in professional societies that emphasize evidence-based practice and specialty-related research, continuing education programs, collaboration with experienced colleagues and/or mentorship, and independent self-study. Health care organizations that employ APNs should demonstrate support of research competencies by incorporating them into position descriptions and performance evaluations and providing resources to help APNs maintain, refine, and develop these skills. For example, institutions can develop and support a formalized program of EBP, complete with an organizational structure that provides personnel and resources to develop, implement, and evaluate EBP (Stricker & Sullivan, 2003). Similarly, they can provide resources for APNs to build on their knowledge of appropriate clinical research literature, appropriate benchmark measurement techniques, evidence-based practice, and research methodologies.

Membership in professional nursing specialty organizations is a good way to gain exposure to current thought and activities related to research competencies. For instance, many nursing specialty organizations such as the Association of Women's Health, Obstetrics and Neonatal Nurses, the Oncology Nursing Society, and the American Association of Critical-Care Nurses have active resources and programs for members that focus specifically on development and use of clinical practice guidelines, implementation and evaluation of EBP, and collaborative research aimed at improving practice. Often, the annual conferences of these organizations offer continuing education credit for participation in workshops related to expanded levels of research competencies. These workshops often provide examples of projects in which APNs are functioning at the expanded level.

APNs need to find a colleague or an interdisciplinary research team conducting research in an area of interest. Entering into a collaborative relationship with a colleague or a team establishes a mutually advantageous situation because such colleagues and teams are often academic-based and therefore welcome the involvement of more clinicians for their expertise and access to a patient population to study. From the APN's perspective, the researcher or team offers the APN a rich opportunity to be involved with funded, interdisciplinary, clinically relevant research.

The ideal relationship for an APN who is aspiring to develop research competencies at the expanded level is a mentor-protégé relationship with an experienced clinical researcher. APNs who are new in a role or new in an institution can seek out role models both within their organizations, their practice specialties, or academic sites. In one example, an APN who was a novice with EBP was mentored by the director of research and other experts to lead an oral care task force that developed, implemented, and evaluated an evidence-based oral care protocol for cancer inpatients (Stricker & Sullivan, 2003).

Regardless of the methods an individual APN chooses to advance his or her research competencies, self-study is essential to continued development. The multifaceted and increasingly interdisciplinary nature of clinical practice, research, and evidence-based practice will require any clinician to pursue in-depth knowledge and skills beyond his or her formal education to meet research competency needs and other practice requirements.

SUMMARY AND CONCLUSION

The core competency of research for APNs comprises three specific research competencies that are required for APNs to meet the various research-related demands of advanced practice nursing roles in the current and future health care delivery system: Competency I, integration and use of research and other evidence in practice decision making; Competency II, evaluation of practice; and Competency III, participation in collaborative research. These competencies are operationalized at two levels—fundamental activities learned through graduate education, and expanded activities acquired through postgraduate professional research development and doctoral study. These competencies are essential to APNs as they define, implement, refine, validate, and evaluate their practice, facilitate new knowledge generation to promote quality health care, and take visible leadership positions in the health care systems of the future.

REFERENCES

Adams, B.L. (2005). Assessment of child abuse risk factors by advanced practice nurses. *Pediatric Nursing, 31*(6), 498-502.

Agency for Healthcare Quality and Research (AHQR). (2005). *National Healthcare Quality Report—2005.* Retrieved August 17, 2007, from www.ahrq.gov/qual/nhqr05/nhqr05.htm.

AGREE Collaboration. (2001). *Appraisal of Guidelines Research and Evaluation (AGREE) Instrument.* Retrieved November 4, 2003, from www.agreecollaboration.org/instrument/.

Ahern, M., Imperial, J., & Lam, S. (2004). Impact of a designated hepatology nurse on the clinical course and quality of life of patients treated with REBETRON therapy for chronic hepatitis C. *Gastroenterology Nursing, 27*(4), 149-155.

Ahrens, T. (2005). Evidence-based practice: Priorities and implementation strategies. *AACN Clinical Issues, 16*(1), 36-42.

Alkema, G.E., & Frey, D. (2006). Implications of translating research into practice: A medication management intervention. *Home Health Care Services, 25*(1), 33-54.

Alspach, G. (2006). Nurses' use and understanding of evidence-based practice: Some preliminary evidence. *Critical Care Nurse, 26*(6), 11-12.

American Association of Colleges of Nursing (AACN). (1996). *The essentials of master's education for advanced practice nursing.* Washington, DC: Author.

American Association of Colleges of Nursing (AACN). (2006a). *The essentials of doctoral education for advanced nursing practice.* Washington, DC: Author.

American Association of Colleges of Nursing (AACN). (2006b). *Position statement on nursing research.* Retrieved August 7, 2007, from www.aacn.nche.edu/publications/positions/NsgRes.htm.

American Association of Critical-Care Nurses. (2002). *Scope of practice & standards of professional performance for the acute and critical care CNS.* Aliso Viejo, CA: Author.

American Association of Nurse Anesthetists (AANA). (2005). *Scope and standards for nurse anesthesia practice.* Park Ridge, IL: Author. Retrieved July 13, 2007, from www.aana.com/uploadedFiles/Resources/Practice_Documents/scope_stds_nap07_2007.pdf.

American College of Nurse-Midwives (ACNM). (2003). *Standards for the practice of midwifery.* Retrieved July 12, 2007, from www.acnm.org/display.cfm?id=4852005).

American College of Nurse-Midwives. (ACNM). (2005). *Research Agenda.* Retrieved December 20, 2007, from www.acnm.org/siteFiles/publications/ACNMResearchAgenda2005.pdf.

American College of Nurse-Midwives (ACNM). (2007). *Core competencies for basic midwifery practice.* Washington, DC: Author. Retrieved July 12, 2007, from www.acnm.org/site-Files/education/Core_Competencies_for_Basic_Midwifery_Practice_6_07.pdf.

American Nurses Association (ANA). (2001). *The National Database of Nursing Quality Indicators (NDNQI).* Retrieved August 17, 2007, from www.nursingworld.org/MainMenu-Categories/ThePracticeofProfessionalNursing/PatientSafetyQuality/NDNQI/NDNQI_1.aspx.

American Nurses' Credentialing Center (ANCC). (2004). *What is the Magnet Recognition Program?* Retrieved July 24, 2007, from www.nursingworld.org/ancc/magnet/index.html.

Artinian, N.T. (2007). Telehealth as a tool for enhancing care for patients with cardiovascular disease. *Journal of Cardiovascular Nursing, 22*(1), 25-31.

Balas, E.A., & Boren, S.A. (2000). *Managing clinical knowledge for healthcare improvements* (pp. 65-70). Germany: Schattauer Publishing.

Ball, C., Sackett, D., Phillips, B., Haynes, B., Straus, S., & Dawes, M. (2001). *Levels of evidence and grades of recommendations.* Retrieved March 21, 2004, from www.cebm.net/levels_of_evidence.asp.

Barnsteiner, J., & Prevost, S. (2002). How to implement evidence-based practice. *Reflections on Nursing Leadership, 28*(2), 18-21.

Boaz, A., Ashby, D., & Young, K. (2002). *Systematic reviews: What have they got to offer evidence based policy and practice?* London: ESTC UK Center for Evidence Based Policy and Practice.

Boswell, C., & Cannon, S. (2007). *Introduction to nursing research: Incorporating evidence-based practice.* Boston: Jones & Bartlett.

Bowles, K.H., & Baugh, A.C. (2007). Applying research evidence to optimize telehomecare. *Journal of Cardiovascular Nursing, 22*(1), 5-15.

Bowman, A., Greiner, J.E., Doerschug, K.C., Little, S.B., Bombei, C.L., & Comried, L.M. (2005). Implementation of an evidence-based feeding protocol and aspiration risk reduction algorithm. *Critical Care Nursing Quarterly, 28*(4), 324-333.

Bozzo, J. (1999). Databases and nursing outcomes. *American Journal of Nursing, 99*(4), 22.

Brooten, D., & Naylor, M.D. (1995). Nurses' effect on changing patient outcomes. *Image: The Journal of Nursing Scholarship, 27,* 95-99.

Brooton, D., Youngblut, J.M., Deatrick, J., Naylor, M., & York, R. (2003). Patient problems, advanced practice nurse (APN) interventions, time and contacts among five patient groups. *Journal of Nursing Scholarship, 35*(1), 73-79.

Brown, S. J. (1999). *Knowledge for health care practice: A guide to using research evidence.* Philadelphia: Saunders.

Buonocore, D. (2004). Leadership in action: Creating a change in practice. *AACN Clinical Issues, 15*(2), 170-181.

Burns, N., & Grove, S.K. (2007). *Understanding nursing research: Building an evidence-based practice* (4th ed.). Philadelphia: Saunders.

Capezuti, E., Taylor, J., Brown, H., & Strothers, H.S. (2007). Challenges to implementing an APN-facilitated falls management program in long-term care. *Applied Nursing Research, 20*(1), 21-29.

Church-Balin, C., & Damus, K. (2003). Preventing prematurity: A WHONN, March of Dimes partner for national campaign. *AWHONN Lifelines, 7,* 97-101.

Clark, J., Cunningham, M., McMillan, S., Vena, C., & Parker, K. (2004). Sleep-wake disturbances in people with cancer. Part II. Evaluating the evidence for clinical decision making. *Oncology Nursing Forum, 31*(4), 747-771.

Clochesy, J.M. (2002). Research designs for advanced practice nursing outcomes research. *Critical Care Nursing Clinics of North America, 14,* 293-298.

Cluzeau, F.A., Littlejohns, P., Grimshaw, J.M., Feder, G., & Moran, S.E. (1999). Development and application of a generic methodology to assess the quality of clinical guidelines. *International Journal for Quality in Health Care, 11*(1), 21-28.

Collins, C., Phields, M.E., & Duncan, T. (2007). An agency capacity model to facilitate implementation of evidence-based behavioral interventions by community-based organizations. *Journal of Public Health Management and Practice (Jan. Suppl.),* S16-S23.

Conn, V.S., Isaramalai, S., Rath, S., Jantarakupt, P., Wadhawan, R., & Dash, Y. (2003). Beyond MEDLINE for literature searches. *Journal of Nursing Scholarship, 35,* 177-182.

Cooke, L., Smith-Idell, C., Dean, G., Gemmill, R., Steingass, S., Sun, V., et al. (2004). "Research to practice": A practical program to enhance the use of evidence-based practice at the unit level. *Oncology Nursing Forum, 31*(4), 825-832.

Craig, J.V. (2002). How to ask the right question. In J.V. Craig & R.L. Smyth (Eds.), *Evidence-based practice manual for nurses* (pp. 21-44). Edinburgh: Churchill-Livingstone.

Criste, A. (2003). Do nurse anesthetists demonstrate gender bias in treating pain? A national survey using a standardized pain model. *AANA Journal, 71,* 206-209.

Crowther, M. (2003). Optimal management of outpatients with heart failure using advanced practice nurses in a hospital-based heart failure center. *Journal of the American Academy of Nurse Practitioners, 15*(6), 260-265.

Cullen, L., Greiner, J., Greiner, J., Bombei, C., & Comried, L. (2005). Excellence in evidence-based practice: Organizational and unit exemplars. *Critical Care Nursing Clinics of North America, 17*(2), 127-142.

Cunningham, R.S. (2004). Advanced practice nursing outcomes: A review of selected empirical literature. *Oncology Nursing Forum, 31*(2), 219-232.

Debourgh, G.A. (2001). Champions for evidence-based practice: A critical role for advanced practice nurses. *AACN Clinical Issues, 12,* 491-508.

Delgado-Passler, P., & McCaffrey, R. (2006). The influences of postdischarge management by nurse practitioners on hospital readmission for heart failure. *Journal of the American Academy of Nurse Practitioners, 18,* 154-160.

DePalma, J.A. (2000). Evidence-based clinical practice guidelines. *Seminars in Perioperative Nursing, 9,* 115-120.

DePalma, J.A. (2005). Using evidence in home care: The value of a librarian-clinician collaboration: the clinician's role. *Home Health Care Management & Practice, 17,* 302-307.

Derengowski, S.L., Irving, S.Y., Koogle, P.V., & Englander, R.M. (2005). Defining the role of the pediatric critical care nurse practitioner in a tertiary care center. *Critical Care Medicine, 28*(7), 2626-2630.

Dexter, F., Epstein, R.H., & Marsh, H.M. (2002). Costs and risks of weekend anesthesia staffing at 6 independently managed surgical suites. *AANA Journal, 70,* 377-381.

Dixon-Woods, M., Fitzpatrick, R, & Roberts, K. (2001). Including qualitative research in systematic reviews: Opportunities and problems. *Journal of Evaluation in Clinical Practice, 7*(2), 125-133.

Dodek, P., Keenan, S., Cook, D., Heyland, D., Jacka, M., Hand, L., et al. (2004). Evidence-based clinical practice guideline for the prevention of ventilator-associated pneumonia. *Annals of Internal Medicine, 141*(4), 305-313.

Donohue, M.A. (2005). Best-practice protocols: Evidence-based care for acute myocardial infarction. *Nursing Management, 36*(8), 23-27.

Enkin, M., Keirse, M., Neilson, J., Crowther, C., Duley, L., Hodnett, E., et al. (2000). *A guide to effective care in pregnancy and childbirth* (3rd ed.). London: Oxford Press. Retrieved July 25, 2007, from www.childbirthconnection.org/article.asp?ck=10218.

Evidence-Based Medicine Working Group. (1992). Evidence based medicine: A new approach to teaching the practice of medicine. *JAMA: The Journal of the American Medical Association, 268,* 2420-2425.

Fakhry, S.M., Trask, A.L., Waller, M.A., & Watts, D.D. (2004). Management of brain-injured patients by an evidence-based medicine protocol improves outcomes and decreases hospital charges. *The Journal of Trauma, 56*(3), 492-499.

Forbes, D.A. (2003). An example of the use of systematic reviews to answer an effectiveness question. *Western Journal of Nursing Research, 25*(2), 179-192.

Gagnon, M.P., Lamothe, L., Hebert, M., Chanliau, J., & Fortin, J.P. (2006). Telehomecare for vulnerable populations: The evaluation of new models of care. *Telemedicine Journal & E-Health, 12*(3), 324-331.

Garrard, J. (2007). *Health sciences literature review made easy.* Boston: Jones & Bartlett.

Gibbs, L.E. (2003). *Evidence-based practice for the helping professions.* Toronto, Ontario, Canada: Thomson Brooks/Cole.

Glanville, I., Schirm, V., & Wineman, N.M. (2000). Using evidence-based practice for managing clinical outcomes in advanced practice nursing. *Journal of Nursing Care Quality, 15,* 1-11.

Goode, C.J. (2000). What constitutes the "evidence" in evidence-based practice? *Applied Nursing Research, 13,* 222-225.

Goode, C.J., & Piedalue, F. (1999). Evidence-based clinical practice. *Journal of Nursing Administration, 29,* 15-21.

Guyatt, G.H., Haynes, R.B., Jaeschke, R.Z., Cook, D.J., Green, L., Naylor, C.D., et al. (2000). Users' guides to the medical literature: XXV. Evidence-based medicine: Principles for applying the users' guides to patient care. *JAMA: The Journal of the American Medical Association, 284,* 1290-1296.

Guyatt, G., & Rennie, D. (Eds.). (2002). Users' guides to the medical literature. Chicago: AMA Press.

Hadorn, D.C., Baker, D., Hodges, J.S., & Hicks, N. (1995). Rating the quality of evidence for clinical practice guidelines. *Journal of Clinical Epidemiology, 49,* 749-754.

Hamric, A.B. (1989). History and overview of the CNS role. In A.B. Hamric & J.A. Spross (Eds.), *The clinical nurse specialist in theory and practice* (2nd ed., pp. 3-18). Philadelphia: Saunders.

Harris, R.P., Helfand, M., Woolf, S.H., Lohr, K.N., Mulrow, C.D., Teutsch, S.M., et al. (2001). Current methods of the U.S. Preventive Services Task Force: A review of the process. *American Journal of Preventive Medicine, 20,* 21-35.

Health Information Technology. (2007). *Office of the national coordinator: Mission.* Retrieved August 17, 2007, from www.hhs.gov/healthit/onc/mission/.

Health Insurance Portability and Accountability Act (HIPAA). (1996). Public Law 104-191. Retrieved August 17, 2007, from http://aspe.hhs.gov/admnsimp/pl104191.htm.

Hockenberry, M., Wilson, D., & Barrera, P. (2006). Implementing evidence-based nursing practice in a pediatric hospital. *Pediatric Nursing, 32*(4), 371-377.

Hopp, F., Woodbridge, P., Subramania, U., Copeland, L., Smith, D., & Lowery, J. (2006). Outcomes associated with a home care telehealth intervention. *Telemedicine Journal & E-Health, 12*(3), 297-307.

Institute of Medicine (IOM). (1990). *Clinical practice guidelines: Directions for a new program.* Washington, DC: National Academy Press.

Institute of Medicine (IOM). (2001). *Crossing the quality chasm: A new health system for the 21st century.* Washington, DC: National Academy Press.

Jastremski, C.A. (2002). Using outcomes research to validate the advanced practice nursing role administratively. *Critical Care Nursing Clinics of North America, 14,* 275-280.

Jencks, S.F., Huff, E.D., & Cuerdon, T. (2003). Change in the quality of care delivered to Medicare beneficiaries, 1998-1999 to 2000-2001. *JAMA: The Journal of the American Medical Association, 289,* 305-312.

Johnston, L. (2005). Critically appraising quantitative evidence. In B. Melnyk & E. Fineout-Overholt, *Evidence-based practice in nursing & healthcare* (pp. 79-126). Philadelphia: Lippincott Williams & Wilkins.

The Joint Commission (TJC). (2003). *Health care at the crossroads: Strategies for addressing the evolving nursing crisis.* Oakbrook Terrace, IL: Author.

The Joint Commission (TJC). (2007). 2008 ORYX performance measure reporting requirements for hospitals and guidelines for measure selection. Retrieved December 18, 2007, from http://www.jointcommission.org/NR/rdonlyres/64C5EDF0-253A-42CE-9DE5-C8AFE6755267/0/oryx_hap_cm_req.pdf.

Klardie, K.A., Johnson, J., McNaughton, M.A., & Myers, W. (2004). Integrating the principles of evidence-based practice into clinical practice. *Journal of the American Academy of Nurse Practitioners, 16*(3), 98, 100-102.

Kleinpell, R., & Gawlinski, A. (2005). Assessing outcomes in advanced practice nursing practice. *AACN Clinical Issues, 16*(1), 43-57.

Lam, R.W., & Kennedy, S.H. (2005). Using meta-analysis to evaluate evidence: Practical tips and traps. *Canadian Journal of Psychiatry, 50*(3), 167-174.

Ledbetter, C.A., & Stevens, K.R. (2000). Basics of evidence-based practice. Part 2. Unscrambling the terms and processes. *Seminars in Perioperative Nursing, 9,* 98-104.

Levin, R.F., & Vetter, M. (2007). Evidence-based practice: A guide to negotiate the clinical practice guideline maze. *Research and Theory for Nursing Practice: An International Journal, 21*(1), 5-9.

LoBiondo-Wood, G., & Haber, J. (2002). *Nursing research: Methods, critical appraisal, & utilization* (5th ed.). St. Louis: Mosby.

Luxford, K., Hill, D., & Bell, R. (2006). Promoting the implementation of best-practice guidelines using a matrix tool. *Disease Management & Health Outcomes, 14*(2), 85-90.

Lyles, C.M., Kay, L.S., Crepaz, L.S., Herbst, J.H., Passin, W.F., Kim, A.S., et al. (2007). Bet-evidence interventions: Findings from a systematic review of HIV behavioral interventions from U.S. populations at high risk, 2000-2004. *American Journal of Public Health, 97*(1), 133-143.

Marshall, M.L. (2006). Strategies for success: Bringing evidence-based practice to the bedside. *Clinical Nurse Specialist, 20*(3), 124-127.

Martin, P.A. (1995). Finding time for research. *Applied Nursing Research, 8,* 151-153.

Masys, D.R. (2002). Effects of current and future information technologies on the health care workforce. *Health Affairs, 21,* 33-41.

McCaulcy, K.M., Bixby, M.B., & Naylor, M.D. (2006). Advanced practice nurse strategies to improve outcomes and reduce cost in elders with heart failure. *Disease Management, 9*(5), 302-310.

McDonald, P.W., & Viehbeck, S. (2007). From evidence-based practice making to practice-based evidence making: Creating communities of (research) and practice. *Health Promotion Practice, 8*(2), 140-144.

McGowan, J., & Sampson, M. (2005). Systematic reviews need systematic searches. *Journal of the Medical Library Association, 93*(1), 74-80.

McGuire, D.B., & Harwood, K.V. (1989). The CNS as researcher. In A.B. Hamric & J.A. Spross (Eds.), *The clinical nurse specialist in theory and practice* (2nd ed., pp. 169-203). Philadelphia: Saunders.

McKoen, L.M., Oswaks, J.D., & Cunningham, P.D. (2006). Safeguarding patients: Complexity science, high reliability organizations, and implications for team training in healthcare. *Clinical Nurse Specialist, 20*(6), 298-304.

McLendon, D., Check, J., Carteaux, P., Michael, L., Moehring, J., Secrest, J.W., et al. (2003). Implementation of potentially better practices for the prevention of brain hemorrhage and ischemic brain injury in very low birth weight infants. *Pediatrics, 111*(4 Pt 2), e497-503.

McSweeney, M., Spies, M., & Cann, C.J. (2001). Finding and evaluating clinical practice guidelines. *The Nurse Practitioner, 26*, 30, 33-34, 39 (passim), 43-47.

Mehrotra, A., Bodenheimer, T., & Dudley, R.A. (2003). Employers' efforts to measure and improve hospital quality: Determinants of success. *Health Affairs, 22*, 60-71.

Melynk, B.M. (2003). Finding and appraising systematic reviews of clinical interventions: Critical skills for evidence-based practice. *Pediatric Nursing, 29*(2), 125, 147-149.

Melynk, B.M. (2004). Integrating levels of evidence into clinical decision making. *Pediatric Nursing, 30*(4), 323-325.

Melynk, B.M. (2005). Advancing evidence-based practice in clinical and academic settings. *Worldviews on Evidence-Based Nursing, 2*(3), 161-165.

Melnyk, B.M., & Fineout-Overholt, E. (2002). Key steps in implementing evidence-based practice: Asking compelling, searchable questions and searching for the best evidence. *Pediatric Nursing, 22*(3), 262-266.

Melnyk, B.M., & Fineout-Overholt, E. (2005). *Evidence-based practice in nursing and healthcare.* Philadelphia: Lippincott Williams & Wilkins.

Meyer, S.C., & Miers. L.J. (2005). Cardiovascular surgeon and acute care nurse practitioner: Collaboration on postoperative outcomes. *AACN Clinical Issues, 16*(2), 149-158.

Moher, D., Cook, D.J., Eastwood, S., Olkin, I., Rennie, D., & Stroup, D. (2000). Improving the quality of reports of meta-analyses of randomized controlled trials: The QUOROM statement. *British Journal of Surgery, 87*(11), 1448-1454.

Montori, V.M., Wilczynski, N.L., Morgan, D., & Haynes, R.B. (2005). Optimal search strategies for retrieving systematic reviews from Medline: Analytical survey. *British Medical Journal, 330*(7482), 68-71.

Moore, K.A., DuBuisson, A.B., Swett, B., & Edwards, W.H. (2003). Implementing potentially better practices for improving family-centered care in neonatal intensive care units: Successes and challenges. *Pediatrics, 111*(4 Pt 2), e450-460.

Morrisey, L.J., & DeBourgh, G.A. (2001). Finding evidence: Refining literature searching skills for the advanced practice nurse. *AACN Clinical Issues, 12*, 560-577.

Mosca, L., Appel, L.J., Benjamin, E.J., Berra, K., Chandra-Strobos, N., Fabunmi, R.P., et. al. (2004). Evidence-based guidelines for cardiovascular disease prevention in women. *Circulation, 109*(5), 672-693.

Munro, N. (2004). Evidence-based assessment: No more pride or prejudice. *AACN Clinical Issues, 15*(4), 501-505.

National Association of Clinical Nurse Specialists (NACNS). (2004). *Statement on clinical nurse specialist practice and education* (2nd ed.). Harrisburg, PA: Author.

National Committee for Quality Assurance's (NCQA) Health Plan. (2000). *NCQA unveils free on-line consumer resource to rate health plans on clinical care, member satisfaction, overall quality.* Retrieved November 3, 2003, from www.ncqa.org/communications/news/hprcrel.htm.

National Comprehensive Cancer Network (NCCN). (2007). *Senior adult oncology guideline.* Retrieved August 18, 2007, from www.nccn.org/professionals/physician_gls/PDF/senior.pdf.

National Organization of Nurse Practitioner Faculties (NONPF). (2004). *Standards of professional performance for acute care nurse practitioners.* Retrieved August 15, 2007, from www.nonpf.org/ACNPcompsfinal20041.pdf.

National Organization of Nurse Practitioner Faculties (NONPF). (2006). *Domains and core competencies of nurse practitioner practice.* Retrieved July 13, 2007, from www.nonpf.com/NONPF2005/CoreCompsFINAL06.pdf.

Naylor, M.D., Brooten, D.A., Campbell, R.L., Maislin, G., McCauley, K.M., & Schwartz, J.S. (2004). Transitional care of older adults hospitalized with heart failure: A randomized controlled trial. *Journal of the American Geriatrics Society, 52*(5), 675-684.

Neff, D.F., Madigan, E., & Narsavage, G. (2003). APN-directed transitional home care model: Achieving positive outcomes for patients with COPD. *Home Healthcare Nurse, 21*(8), 543-550.

Newhouse, R.P. (2007). Creating infrastructure supportive of evidence-based nursing practice: Leadership strategies. *Worldviews on Evidence-Based Nursing, 4*(1), 21-19.

Nolan T.W. (2007). *Execution of strategic improvement initiatives to produce system-level results* (IHI Innovation Series white paper). Cambridge, MA: Institute for Healthcare Improvement. (Available on www.IHI.org)

Oncology Nursing Society (ONS). (2007). *Oncology nurse practitioner competencies.* Pittsburgh, PA: Author.

Oxman, A., Guyatt, G., Cook, D., & Montori, V. (2002). Summarizing evidence. In G. Guyatt & D. Rennie (Eds.), *Users' guides to the medical literature* (pp. 241-269). New York: American Medical Association.

Papadopoulos, M., & Rheeder, P. (2000). How to do a systematic literature review. *Journal of Physiotherapy, 56*, 3-6.

Paré, G., Jaana, M., & Sicotte, C. (2007). Systematic review of home telemonitoring for chronic diseases: The evidence base. *Journal of the American Medical Informatics Association, 14*(3), 269-277.

Park, M., & Tang, J.H. (2007). Changing the practice of physical restraint use in acute care. *Journal of Gerontological Nursing, 33*(2), 9-16.

Pearson, M., & Craig, J.V. (2002). In J.V. Craig & R.L. Smyth (Eds.), *Evidence-based practice manual for nurses* (pp. 3-20). Edinburgh: Churchill-Livingstone.

Polit, D.F., & Beck, C.T. (2006). *Essentials of nursing research: Method, appraisal and utilization* (6th ed.). Philadelphia: Lippincott Williams & Wilkins.

Polit, D.F., & Beck, C.T. (2008). *Nursing research: Generating and assessing evidence for nursing practice* (8th ed.). Philadelphia: Lippincott Williams & Wilkins.

Pravikoff, D.S., & Donaldson, N.E. (2001). Online journals: Access and support for evidence-based practice. *AACN Clinical Issues, 12*, 588-596.

Pravikoff, D.S., Pierce, S.T., & Tanner, A. (2005). Evidence-based practice readiness study supported by academy nursing informatics expert panel. *Nursing Outlook, 53*(1), 49-50.

Puntillo, K.A., Morris, A.B., Thompson, C.L., Stanik-Huff, J., White, C.A., & Wild, L.R. (2004). Pain behaviors observed during six common procedures: Results from Thunder Project II. *Critical Care Medicine, 32*(2), 421-427.

Reilly, L., Sullivan, P., Ninni, S., Fochesto, D., Williams, K., & Fetherman, B. (2006). Reducing Foley catheter device days in an intensive care unit: Using the evidence to change practice. *AACN Advanced Critical Care, 17*(3), 272-283.

Richardson, W.C., & Corrigan, J.M. (2003). Provider responsibility and system redesign: Two sides of the same coin. *Health Affairs, 22*, 116-118.

Ries, A.L., Bauldoff, G.S., Carlin, B.W., Casaburi, R., Emery, C.F., Mahler, D.A., et al. (2007). Pulmonary rehabilitation: Joint ACCP/AACVPR evidence-based clinical practice guidelines. *Chest, 131*(Suppl. 5), 4S-42S.

Robinson, C.B., Fritch, M., Hullett, L., Petersen, M.A., Sikkema, S., Theuninck, L., et al. (2000). Development of a protocol to prevent opioid-induced constipation in patients with cancer: A research utilization project. *Clinical Journal of Oncology Nursing, 4*, 79-84.

Ropka, M.E., & Spencer-Cisek, P. (2001). PRISM: Priority Symptom Management Project. Phase I: Assessment. *Oncology Nursing Forum, 28*, 1585-1594.

Rosswurm, M.A., & Larrabee, J.H. (1999). A model for change to evidence-based practice. *Image: The Journal of Nursing Scholarship, 31*, 317-322.

Rutherford P., Lee B., & Greiner A. *Transforming care at the bedside.* IHI Innovation Series white paper. Boston: Institute for Healthcare Improvement; 2004. (Available on www.IHI.org)

Rutledge, D.N., DePalma, J.A., & Cunningham, M. (2004). A process model for evidence-based literature syntheses. *Oncology Nursing Forum, 31*(3), 543-550.

Rutledge, D.N., & Grant, M. (2002). Evidence-based practice in cancer nursing: Introduction. *Seminars in Oncology Nursing, 18*, 1-2.

Rycroft-Malone, J. (2004). The PARIHS framework: A framework for guiding the implementation of evidence-based practice. *Journal of Nursing Care Quality, 19*, 297-304.

Sackett, D.L., Straus, S.E., Richardson, W.S., Rosenberg, W., & Haynes, R.B. (1997). *Evidence-based medicine: How to practice and teach EBM.* Edinburgh: Churchill Livingstone.

Sackett, D.L., Straus, S.E., Richardson, W.S., Rosenberg, W., & Haynes, R.B. (2000). *Evidence-based medicine: How to practice and teach EBM* (2nd ed.). Edinburgh: Churchill Livingstone.

Sampselle, C.M., Wyman, J.F., Thomas, K.K., Newman, D.K., Gray, M., Dougherty, M., et al. (2000). Continence for women: Evaluation of A WHONN's third research utilization project. *JOGNN: Journal of Obstetric, Gynecologic, & Neonatal Nursing, 29*, 9-17.

Scanlon, A. (2006). Critical appraisal of systematic review for nursing practice. *Australasian Journal of Neuroscience, 18*(1), 8-14.

Schulz, M.A., Ludwick, R., Cukr, P.L., & Kelly, D. (2002). Outcomes of a community-based three-year breast and cervical screening program for medically underserved, low income women. *Journal of the American Academy of Nurse Practitioners, 14*, 219-224.

Sensmeier, J. (2007). ANI connection. 2006 TIGER summit: Evidence and informatics transforming nursing. *CIN: Computers, Informatics, Nursing, 25*(1), 55-56.

Shekelle, P.G., Eccles, M.P., Grimshaw, J.M., & Woolf, S.H. (2001). When should clinical guidelines be updated? *British Medical Journal, 323*, 155-157.

Shojania, K.G., & Bero, L.A. (2001). Taking advantage of the explosion of systematic reviews: An efficient MEDLINE search strategy. *Effective Clinical Practice, 4*, 157-162.

Sigma Theta Tau International (STTI). (2006). *2006 EBP study: Summary of findings.* Retrieved July 24, 2007, from www.nursingknowledge.org/go/know.

Simonson, D.C., Ahern, M.M., & Hendryx, M.S. (2007). Anesthesia staffing and anesthetic complications during cesarean delivery: A retrospective analysis. *Nursing Research, 56*(1), 9-17.

Smallwood, A. (2005). Nurse-led elective cardioversion: An evidence-based practice review. *Nursing in Critical Care, 10*(5), 231-241.

Stetler, C.B. (2001). Updating the Stetler Model of Research Utilization to facilitate evidence-based practice. *Nursing Outlook, 49*(6), 272-279.

Stetler, C.B. (2003). Role of the organization in translating research into evidence-based practice. *Outcomes Management, 7*(3), 97-105.

Stetler, C.B., Burns, M., Sander-Buscemi, K., Morsi, D., & Grunwald, E. (2003). Use of evidence for the prevention of work-related musculoskeletal injuries. *Orthopaedic Nursing, 22*(1), 32-41.

Stevens, K.R., & Ledbetter, C.A. (2000). Basics of evidence-based practice. Part 1. The nature of the evidence. *Seminars in Perioperative Nursing, 9*, 91-97.

Stricker, C.T., & Sullivan, J. (2003). Evidence-based oncology care clinical practice guidelines: Development, implementation, and evaluation. *Clinical Journal of Oncology Nursing, 7,* 222-227.

Thomas, B.H., Ciliska, D., Dobbins, M., & Micucci, S. (2004). A process for systematically reviewing the literature: Providing the research evidence for public health nursing interventions. *Worldviews on Evidence-Based Nursing, 1,*176-184.

Thomas, L., & Hotchkiss, K. (2002). Evidence-based guidelines. In J.V. Craig & R.L. Smyth (Eds.), *Evidence-based practice manual for nurses* (pp. 187-210). Edinburgh: Churchill-Livingstone.

Thompson, C., Cullum, N., McCaughan, D., Sheldon, T., & Raynor, P. (2004). Nurses, information use, and clinical decision making: The real world potential for evidence-based decisions in nursing. *Evidence-Based Nursing, 7*(3), 68-72.

Thompson, C.L., White, C., Wild, L.R., Morris, A.B., Perdue, S.T., Stanik-Hutt, J., et al. (2001). Translating research into practice: Implications of the Thunder Project II. *Critical Care Nursing Clinics of North America, 13,* 541-546.

Titler, M. (2007). Translating research into practice: Models for changing clinician behavior. *American Journal of Nursing, 107*(Suppl. 6), 26-33.

Titler, M.G. (2004). Methods in translation science. *Worldviews on Evidence-Based Nursing, 1*(1), 38-48.

Titler, M.G., & Everett, L.Q. (2006). Sustain an infrastructure to support EBP. *Nursing Management, 37*(9), 14, 16.

Vincent, D. (2002). Using cost-analysis techniques to measure the value of nurse practitioner care. *International Nursing Review, 49,* 243-249.

Vrabel, M. (2005). Searching for Evidence—The value of a librarian-clinician collaboration: The librarian's role. *Home Health Care Management & Practice, 17*(4), 286-292.

Vratny, A., & Shriver, D. (2007). A conceptual model for growing evidence-based practice. *Nursing Administration Quarterly, 31*(2), 162-170.

Wellock, V.K., & Crichton, M.A. (2007). Understanding pregnant women's experiences of symphysis pubis dysfunction: The effect of pain. *Evidence Based Midwifery, 5*(2), 40-46.

Whittemore, R. (2005). Combining evidence in nursing research: Methods and implications. *Nursing Research, 54*(1), 56-62.

Whitman, G.R. (2002a). Outcomes research in advanced practice nursing: Selecting an outcome. *Critical Care Nursing Clinics of North America, 14,* 253-260.

Whitman, G.R. (2002b). Outcomes research: Getting started, defining outcomes, a framework, and data sources. *Critical Care Nursing Clinics of North America, 14,* 261-268.

Whitney, J.D. (2004). Reading and using systematic reviews. *Journal of Wound, Ostomy & Continence Nursing, 31*(1), 14-17

Clinical, Professional, and Systems Leadership

Judith A. Spross • Charlene M. Hanson

INTRODUCTION

More than ever before, the flattening of the world through global interactions (Friedman, 2006), the rate with which change occurs, and the unsettled status of health care make leadership skills a necessity for successful advanced practice nurses (APNs). Leadership is a core competency of advanced practice nursing, but the concept has some unique characteristics in the APN context. Our conceptualization of APN leadership involves three distinct defining characteristics: mentoring and empowerment, innovation and change agency, and activism. Calls for systems redesign and transformation (Institute of Medicine [IOM], 2000, 2001; Nolan, Resar, Haraden, & Griffin, 2004; Rutherford, Lee, & Greiner, 2004), changes in health professional education (American Association of Colleges of Nursing [AACN], 2006), and core interdisciplinary competencies for health professionals (Greiner & Knebel, 2003; HealthSciences Institute, 2005) have important implications for the leadership competency in APN education and practice. To provide leadership in individual patient care situations, APNs must be able to assess the clinical microsystems in which they provide care; understand the macrosystems that influence the smaller systems; determine the need for redesign to improve safety, quality, and reliability; and evaluate the results. In short, systems leaders must be able to identify the need for innovation and change and implement strategies to achieve it. In partnership with others, APNs craft approaches to evaluate, reassess, and implement systems redesign and innovation.

APNs exercise leadership in four key domains: in clinical practice environments, in the nursing profession, at the systems level, and in the health policy arena. APNs may exercise leadership activities at local, regional, and/or national levels; their activities may range from taking a stand on behalf of an individual patient to advocating for a change in national health policy. The leadership competency depends on and interacts with other APN competencies. Specific leadership skills should be discussed, nurtured, and developed during graduate education through refinement of communication skills, supported risk taking, reflective learning, and interactions with nurse leaders, mentors, and role models. The recommended movement of APN education to the Doctor of Nursing Practice (DNP) by 2015 has implications for the APN leadership competency (AACN, 2004). For example, the DNP essential requiring expertise in systems leadership means that the organizational and professional leadership components of advanced practice nursing curricula will need to expand (AACN, 2006).

The purposes of this chapter are to describe the defining characteristics and domains of the leadership competency, provide useful literature and resources on leadership and change, describe characteristics of effective leaders, identify obstacles to effective leadership, and discuss strategies for developing leadership skills. This chapter will help APNs define their need for leadership skills and develop a plan for acquiring the necessary skills appropriate to their particular positions and professional goals.

THE CONTEXT IN WHICH ADVANCED PRACTICE NURSES EXERCISE THE LEADERSHIP COMPETENCY

Leading in today's health care environment is a task of unprecedented complexity for APNs, administrators, and policymakers. To understand the need for APN leadership across the four domains, it is important to understand the factors that are shaping this competency in the twenty-first century. The Institute of Medicine (IOM) has issued a number of reports, all of which call for a radical redesign and transformation of the health care system; in addition, health professions education is being transformed. Such changes have not occurred quickly, in part because they require a significant rethinking of how care is delivered, the roles of patients and the education of providers, effective channels for diffusing innovation, how health care is financed, and what provider activities "count" and should be reimbursed (Greiner & Knebel, 2003; see also Chapter 22).

Health Care System Transformation

The IOM's call to transform the health care system is predicated on six national quality aims: safety, effectiveness, patient-centeredness, timeliness, efficiency, and equity (IOM, 2001). This far-reaching report has led to numerous assessments and initiatives. For example, the IOM noted that nursing homes are at high risk for the occurrence of adverse events, yet numerous institutional barriers to reporting such events exist, making institutional change unlikely (Wagner, Capezuti, & Ouslander, 2006). The Institute for Healthcare Improvement [IHI] launched a campaign to save 100,000 lives (from medical error) (Institute of Healthcare Improvement [IHI], 2007; Patient Safety and Quality Health Care, 2005). Many clinical systems are participating in efforts to improve safety and quality, such as Magnet recognition or participating in the IHI campaign. APNs represent nursing within an organization's culture and are well positioned to drive the safety process from within rather than through external regulatory dictates (Callahan & Ruchlin, 2003). APNs not only have a stake in these efforts but also have clinical expertise and leadership that can ensure success.

Redesign of Health Professional Education

Greiner and Knebel (2003), the HealthSciences Institute (2005), and the AACN (2006) have identified competencies that health professionals, including APNs, must have—many of which relate to the leadership competency. Although these recommendations affect primarily educators and the curricula they design, they have significant implications for APNs already practicing and for the environments in which APN students learn.

Interdisciplinary Competencies. The IOM identified five competencies that all health professionals must possess if the redesign and transformation of the U.S. health care system is to be realized: provide patient-centered care, work in interdisciplinary teams, employ evidence-based practices, apply quality improvement principles, and utilize informatics (Greiner & Knebel, 2003). The HealthSciences Institute (2005) published a model of Continuous Chronic Care™ and identified five levels of change. At the provider level of change, they identified three major competencies: promote health and prevent disease; manage diseases and disease impacts; and promote consumer independence and life quality. APN leaders will participate in creating environments in which these interdisciplinary competencies are not merely supported but can flourish. When APNs and others can implement these competencies fully, the transformation will be underway.

Advanced Practice Nurse Competencies. In the AACN's *The Essentials of Doctoral Education for Advanced Nursing Practice* (2006), several specific competencies relate to leadership for all DNP graduates, including APNs. Of the eight Essentials, four inform the leadership competency: organizational and system leadership for quality improvement and systems thinking; clinical scholarship and analytical methods; information systems/technology and patient care technology for the improvement and transformation of health care; and clinical prevention and population health for improving the nation's health. The reader will note that several of these Essentials are consistent with the competencies being expected of all health professionals just described.

In summary, numerous contextual and educational factors that require APN leadership have been identified in calls for the redesign and transformation of the health care system. Certain themes are apparent—in particular, patient-centeredness (see Chapter 5), teamwork (see Chapter 10, quality improvement and the use of information technology [IT]; see Chapter 25), and complexity. These factors must be considered in APN graduate and continuing education so that APNs acquire the knowledge and skills they need to lead effectively.

LEADERSHIP DOMAINS OF ADVANCED PRACTICE NURSES

Although the need for leadership in health care settings is well recognized (National Association of Clinical Nurse Specialists [NACNS], 2004; National Organization of Nurse Practitioner Faculties [NONPF] & AACN, 2002; Spencer & Jordan, 2001), the topic has not been well studied, and research on effective leadership is needed (Falk-Rafael, 2005; Vance & Larson, 2002). Not all APNs are comfortable with the idea of being leaders, but leadership is not an optional activity. As noted, the APN leadership competency can be conceptualized as occurring in four primary domains or areas: in clinical practice with patients and staff, within professional organizations, within health care systems, and in health policymaking arenas. The extent to which individual APNs choose to lead in each of these areas depends on patients' needs; APNs' personal characteristics, interests, and commitments; institutional or organizational priorities and opportunities; and priority health policy issues in nursing as a whole and within one's specialty Carroll, 2005; Leavitt, Chaffee, & Vance, 2007). There is considerable overlap in the knowledge and skills needed across the four domains; for example, developing skills in the clinical leadership domain will enable the APN to be more effective at the policy level.

Clinical Leadership

Clinical leadership focuses first on the patient and his or her needs and ensuring that quality patient care is achieved. It also occurs when APNs learn with and from others about how to build appropriate working relationships with health care team members, how to instill confidence in patients and colleagues, and how to problem-solve as part of a team (Bally, 2007; Engebretson & Wardell, 1997). APN leaders are role models and mentors who empower patients and colleagues. They propose and implement change strategies that improve patient care and enhance others' perceptions of the value of advanced practice nursing. Some clinical leadership skills are part of the competencies of consultation (see Chapter 7) and collaboration (see Chapter 10) and are portrayed in the exemplars in the role chapters (see Part III) as well. The most common clinical leadership roles APNs can expect to play are those of advocate (for patient, family, staff, or colleagues), group leader, and systems leader. APNs may advocate for a particular patient or family, as when an acute care nurse practitioner (ACNP) advocates with the attending physician about the need for a better explanation of the side effects of an elective surgery. Writing articles and presenting talks on clinical topics are other ways of expressing clinical leadership and influencing others.

Group leadership may be informal, as when an APN agrees to coordinate multiple referrals for a patient with complex care needs or when an APN has expertise in a particular clinical problem such as pain management and assumes a team leadership role because of this expertise. APNs may also have more formal leadership responsibilities; for example, an APN may lead a weekly team meeting or agree to convene a group and lead the development of a new practice protocol to bring care into line with new standards. One function of the APN leader is to motivate colleagues and facilitate their use of new knowledge and/or the adoption of new practices.

APNs often exercise leadership to ensure that clinical problems are addressed by administrative leaders at a systems level. Brown called this role the "shuttle diplomat" (1989), because APNs move between clinical and administrative arenas interpreting the needs of one to the other. APNs recognize the clinical problems related to their specialty that require attention or intervention from the larger (macro) system of which they are a part. For example, when a clinical nurse specialist (CNS) called a patient to learn why he had not kept his appointment at the heart failure clinic, she learned that he could not find parking nearby because of hospital construction, did not know that a shuttle would take him from the satellite lot to the clinic, and did not have the energy to walk from the satellite lot. The CNS knew that this could be a problem for other clinic patients and worked with administrators to make sure patients knew what to do. She understood the clinical (patients might experience more complications requiring readmission) and systems implications (e.g., lower quality, increased risks for patients, higher costs, missed appointments) of construction-related, missed appointments for her patient population.

APNs who lead patient care teams well and who perform well as shuttle diplomats find that their interdisciplinary leadership skills are in demand. Covey (1989) considers interdisciplinary leadership a high-level skill. For example, an APN who was successful in leading a quality improvement (QI) initiative to improve care of asthmatics admitted to the hospital was invited to chair a national task force of health care professionals developing practice guidelines for the treatment of asthma. The ability to provide clinical interdisciplinary leadership requires a firm grasp of both the clinical and the professional issues and differences within nursing while responding to the challenges of other disciplines and the larger society. As APNs gain skill in clinical leadership, they develop the attributes needed to lead in other domains.

Professional Leadership

Mentorship, empowerment, and active participation in organizations are particularly important within the professional domain. First, to be an effective leader, the APN must be able to collaborate with colleagues (see Chapter 10). Second, they must be able to recognize situations in which colleagues can benefit from being mentored and empowered. In the professional domain, APN leaders facilitate the growth of other nurses.

Novice APNs or experienced APNs seeking new challenges look for mentors who will foster their professional development. A prospective protégé may recognize and seek the APN's guidance on clinical or professional development issues. Sometimes it is the APN who recognizes a potential protégé and offers the person opportunities to learn and grow. APNs have a responsibility to mentor and prepare the next generation of advanced practice clinicians.

Professional leadership is also exercised by participation in professional organizations. Novice APNs may begin by seeking membership on a committee of a local or national nursing or interdisciplinary organization. As APNs become more experienced, they may seek opportunities to apply the leadership skills they have learned within their work organizations to their professional organizations. Most APNs are members of one or more nursing and interdisciplinary organizations. These memberships provide myriad leadership opportunities including organizing continuing education offerings, presenting at national conferences, chairing a committee, and running for the board of directors. In these situations, APNs exercise more choice as to whether and when they will participate in leadership activities than in their employee roles.

Professional leadership begins at the grassroots level and proceeds upward to state, national, and international levels. To acquire leadership skills and experience, novice APNs need to become involved in the leadership and committee work of local advanced practice nursing coalitions and organizations and move into state and regional leadership roles as they develop their style and strengths as APN leaders. The ability to place APN leaders in key local, state, and national positions is critical to the visibility and credibility of APNs and to the establishment of their roles within nursing and the larger health care community.

Systems Leadership

Systems leadership means leading at the organizational or delivery system level—a skill that requires a multidimensional understanding of systems. Within health care organizations, APNs may lead clinical teams, chair committees, chair or serve as members of boards, manage projects, and direct other initiatives aimed at improving patient care

and/or the clinical practice of nurses and other professionals. Systems leadership overlaps the professional domain in situations in which leaders are formally or informally elected or appointed to positions of authority or power within defined organizations and groups. For example, APNs may identify an increase in the rate of patient falls and create a task force to evaluate the problem and design corrective interventions. A critical care CNS or ACNP may initiate interdisciplinary rounds to monitor patients on mechanical ventilation and gather data on clinical variables such as complication rate and time to weaning. APNs may be asked to participate in or lead standing or ad hoc interdisciplinary committees (e.g., medical credentialing, ethics, institutional review board, pharmacy and therapeutics) to ensure that a nursing perspective will be articulated. APNs may be asked by administrators to participate in organizational reengineering or other activities aimed at improving the environment in which nurses practice (see Chapters 11, 23, and 25). APNs, whether in a line/supervisory position or not, should have the authority to provide systems leadership related to delivery of clinical care by virtue of their clinical credibility and specific APN job responsibilities.

Although most APNs will not be entrepreneurs, they need to be aware that the characteristics of successful entrepreneurs are desirable and valued in systems leaders. *Entrepreneurial leadership* refers to those leaders who go outside of traditional employment systems to create new opportunities to exercise their special abilities (Ballein, 1998; Shirey, 2004). When these leaders use the entrepreneurial skills of innovation and risk taking and assume responsibility for achieving specific targets within an organization, they are referred to as *intrapreneurs*. Because this leadership style is consistent with the call for health care system redesign, it is worth reviewing characteristics associated with entrepreneurial leadership. In a study of entrepreneurial leadership, corporate executive officers and senior nurse executives ranked high-level leadership and communication skills as most important, followed by the ability to build coalitions and to interact with political savvy (Ballein, 1998). Other entrepreneurial leadership characteristics were ranked as follows: confident, team player, persistent, innovative, risk taker, adjusts to change, decisive, strategic thinker, high integrity, and possesses vision. The ability to reach out to the community was also perceived as a core skill. The researcher concluded that nurse leaders must have strong entrepreneurial skills to succeed in the health care marketplace. Universities that prepare APNs are offering coursework on innovation, entrepreneurship, and "out of the box" thinking to prepare both entrepreneurial and intrapreneurial APN leaders (Shirey, 2007). Entrepreneurial leadership skills are illustrated in Exemplar 9-1, which also illustrates the evolving nature of the advanced practice nursing leadership competency and how it expands in breadth over time.

Health Policy Leadership

Although some APNs may not see themselves as being particularly interested in or talented at political advocacy, all APNs have a vested interest in policy-making that affects nursing generally and advanced practice nursing specifically. This domain is becoming increasingly important as more laws and regulations with implications for APN practice are enacted (see Chapters 21 and 22). APNs should be aware of and must often respond to local, state, and national policymaking efforts likely to affect these laws and regulations. To be a leader at the level of health policy requires an ability to analyze health care systems, an understanding of the personal qualities that are associated with effective leadership, and the skill to use these understandings to act strategically.

Across these four domains of leadership, APNs use their clinical expertise, coaching, and collaborative skills to build community around shared values such as patient-centeredness and commitment to quality. They also build the capacity of individuals and systems to respond promptly and efficiently to meet patient needs and improve outcomes (Spross, 2001). The defining characteristics of APN leadership—mentoring and empowerment, innovation and change agency, and activism—may be apparent in all four domains, but the emphasis accorded each one depends on the particular leadership demands. By outlining these various leadership domains early in the chapter, we want to encourage readers to reflect on the leadership opportunities they encounter, consider those that align with their clinical interests and personal characteristics, and begin to develop a leadership portfolio. We hope to challenge readers to rethink their ideas about leadership and to integrate a personally meaningful concept of leadership into their identities as APNs.

LEADERSHIP: DEFINITIONS, MODELS, AND CONCEPTS

The nursing, sociology, and business literatures are rich sources of leadership definitions, models, and concepts that help APNs develop as effective and dynamic leaders.

 EXEMPLAR 9-1   Entrepreneurial Leadership in Advanced Practice Nursing

Ellie's dream and goal upon entering a graduate family nurse practitioner (NP) program was to open a practice in the rural community where she and her family lived. She used her health policy course requirements to conduct a needs assessment and to set up interviews with the regional hospital to propose an outreach clinic that would be sponsored by the hospital. She planned to see patients independently and would contract with her physician preceptor to visit once a week for collaboration and to see patients who were beyond her scope of practice. Ellie's entrepreneurial leadership skills allowed her to negotiate with the managed care owner of the hospital and with the medical staff, and the outreach clinic was established. Over time, her community-based practice was viewed as a model of excellence for other NPs, and she served as a mentor and role model for many. As her clinic gained prominence, Ellie was nominated by the governor to represent advanced practice nurses (APNs) and rural interests

on the state board of nursing. She also wrote a column for the local weekly newspaper about prevention and wellness.

After 3 years in practice, Ellie wanted to use extra space in her clinic to broaden the services she offered, so she set up a meeting with members of a midwifery group in an adjoining town to invite them to use her office as a satellite clinic once a week. She also invited two clinical nurse specialists (CNSs) who were seeing mental health and oncology patients in the area to do the same. Her vision and excellent communication skills offered new alliances with other APNs and brought new services for rural patients. The visibility of her successful clinic led to her nomination to become a member of the National Rural Health Advisory Committee, which advises the Secretary of Health and Human Services on matters of rural health care. This nationally based committee work allowed Ellie to use her well-developed leadership skills to influence the health care system.

Definitions of Leadership

Contemporary definitions of leadership generally fit into one of two categories—transformational (Vance & Larson, 2002) or situational (Grohar-Murray & DiCroce, 1992). Barker (1994) defined *transformational leadership* as a process whereby "the purposes of the leader and follower become fused, creating unity, wholeness and a collective purpose" (p. 83). Transformational leadership can lead to changes in values, attitudes, perceptions, and/or behaviors on the part of the leader as well as the follower and lays the groundwork for further positive change. Thus transformational leadership occurs when people interact in ways that inspire higher levels of motivation and morality among participants. How do leaders do this? Transformational leaders analyze a situation to understand the particular leadership needs and goals; they use this information together with their interpersonal skills to motivate, stimulate, share with, conciliate, and satisfy their followers in an interdependent, interactional exchange. DePree (1989) described leadership as an art form that frees (empowers) people "to do what is required of them in the most effective and humane way possible" (p. 1). He contended that contemporary leadership may be viewed simply as a process of moving the self and others toward a shared vision that becomes a shared reality. Successful transformational leadership is relational, driven by a common goal or purpose, and satisfies the needs of both leader and follower. It is the leadership style often associated with effective change agents. Other authors who describe a transformational approach to leadership include Heifetz (1994), Secretan (1999, 2003), Senge, (2006), and Covey (1989). Some authors have suggested that transformation depends on the quality of team processes (Collins, 2001; Lencioni, 2005).

Some authors emphasize the community or organizational aspects of leadership aimed at transformation. For example, Wheatley (2005) maintains that it is in community that one gets a clear understanding of the needs or problems requiring leadership and that the person or people who can lead the effort to resolve the need or problem emerge from that community. Secretan (2003) helps leaders consider the alignment between a system's or organization's goals and the personal and professional goals of the individual(s) working within that organization. This alignment is based in large part on what inspires one to do his or her best work and, in turn, how one inspires others to do the same. Undertaking such an assessment can help leaders understand how and whether they can continue to lead within the particular system in ways that bring their personal and professional goals into alignment with organizational goals.

Situational leadership is defined as the interaction between an individual's leadership style and the features of the environment or situation in which he or she is operating. Leadership styles are not fixed and may vary based on the environment. Situational leadership depends on particular circumstances with leaders and followers assuming interchangeable roles according to environmental demands (Fiedler, Chermers, & Mahar, 1976; Stogdill, 1948). The role of follower is important to any discussion about APN leadership because APNs will find themselves in both roles at a given time. Grohar-Murray and DiCroce (1992) and DePree (1989) enlarged on this idea and used the term *roving leadership* to describe a participatory process that legitimizes the situational leadership of empowered followers through the support and approval of the hierarchical leader. This notion of leadership is relevant because APNs' work in collaborative health care teams requires that the roles of leader and follower be interchangeable to meet the complex needs of the patient.

Inherent in this discussion of transformational and situational leadership is the importance of vision. The APN as a leader with a vision of collaboration among health care team members may facilitate an atmosphere that supports individuals (followers) to assume leadership roles in various situations. The APN does not cease being the leader by empowering colleagues to appropriately assume a leadership role. In fact, across the domains of leadership, APNs must be capable of both sharing a vision and sharing power, issues discussed later in the chapter.

Leadership Models That Lead to Empowerment and Transformation

APNs can draw upon numerous models of leadership and change processes to inform their leadership development. Leadership models or frameworks that include the following concepts seem most applicable in these unsettled times:

- Empowerment of colleagues/followers
- Engagement of stakeholders within and outside nursing or one's agency in the change process
- Provision of individual and system support during change initiatives

Leadership models that informed this chapter are summarized in Table 9-1 (not all models in the table

Table 9-1 USEFUL MODELS OF TRANSFORMATIONAL LEADERSHIP AND CHANGE

Author	Title/Model	Relevant Concepts	APN Use
Senge (1990, 2006)	The Fifth Discipline	Describes five actions or processes that characterize effective teams and organizations that manage change well. • Personal mastery • Awareness of mental models • Shared vision • Team learning • Systems thinking	APNs can use these concepts to identify: • Personal leadership goals • Strengths and needs of the teams and organizations with whom they work • Strategies to enhance team development and collaboration
Secretan (2004)	Values-Centered Leadership Model™	Describes key elements of transformational leadership: • Power • Direction • Accelerators • Alignment of individual and organizational destiny, cause, and calling is central • CASTLE principles	APNs can use the available tools to assess: • Alignment of personal values/mission and goals with those of the organization • The culture of an organization
Collins (2005)	Good to Great	Describes five levels of leadership: • Executive • Effective leader • Competent manager • Contributing team member • Highly capable individual	Levels of leadership help APNs: • Formulate a "strategic plan" for their own leadership development (e.g., novice APNs are likely to focus on being highly capable team members) • Understand the different types of leaders with whom they work
Nelson, Batalden et al. (2002)	Microsystems in Health Care: High-Performing Clinical Units	Studied 20 varied microsystems; identified nine common success characteristics associated with delivery of high-quality, cost-efficient care: • Leadership • Culture • Organizational support • Patient focus • Staff focus • Interdependence of care team • Information and information technology • Process improvement • Performance patterns	APNs can use these characteristics to assess one's system and identify gaps in and opportunities for leadership
Massoud et al. (2006)	A Framework for Spread	Model evolved by the Institute for Healthcare Improvement to understand phases of successful system change. Key elements: • Prepare for spread • Establish aim for spread • Develop an initial spread plan • Execute and refine plan Presents a case study of model application in the VA system	APNs can use ideas for each phase of spread. Also useful for: • Understanding importance of leadership in planning for spread • Detailing elements of the aim and initial plan for spread (addresses the who, what, when, where)

Continued

Author	Title/Model	Relevant Concepts	APN Use
Greenhalgh et al. (2004)	Diffusion of Innovation in Service Organizations	Proposes a complex model of diffusion of innovation: Identifies three "mechanisms" of spread of innovation: • "Let it happen" • "Help it happen" • "Make it happen"	APNs can use the model to: • Inform an institutional assessment of factors likely to facilitate or impede diffusion • Anticipate and influence the likely trajectory of diffusion based on assessment
Cain, M & Mittman, R. (2002)	Diffusion of Innovation in Health Care	Based on Rogers' Diffusion of Innovation theory, authors identified "ten critical dynamics of diffusion innovation" Particularly focused on diffusion of technology innovation (e.g., computerized order entry or electronic medical records)	APNs can use the dynamics of diffusion innovation when they are involved in: • Diffusion of technology • Institutional planning for disseminating other technology or new products that require change in practice
Kimball (2005)	Cultural Transformation in Health Care	Based on literature review and 40 interviews with health care executives, proposed that institutional transformation is: • Not linear but fluid and unpredictable • An adventure	APNs can use to assess institution prior to or during system redesign initiatives to: • Develop or modify implementation plans, especially when there is considerable unpredictability • Identify strategies for helping staff reinterpret experiences of uncertainty and unpredictability related to change

are described in the chapter). Models are organized by their focus on transformational leadership or change. The numerous national initiatives calling for system redesign means that change, transformation, and uncertainty are constants. We believe the models in Table 9-1 have the most promise for helping APNs survive and thrive under these circumstances because both individuals and the organizations in which they work are considered. Table 9-1 highlights elements of each model that relate to APN leadership. Readers are encouraged to consult original sources for full descriptions of each model.

The Fifth Discipline (Senge). *The Fifth Discipline* (Senge 1990; 2006) includes concepts that will be useful to APNs as they strive to master the APN leadership competency. Whereas certain people may have innate gifts for leadership, others can develop these proficiencies through practice and commitment to the task. To become an effective leader, Senge's definition implies that one must practice and commit to lifelong learning. In this case, APN leaders are constantly striving to become effective team members who empower others and facilitate change to create effective learning organizations.

Senge outlines five disciplines or practices associated with leadership; the framework provides a structure APNs can use to understand leadership and change within complex structures and environments. The five disciplines (Senge, 1990, 2006) are as follows:

- *Personal mastery* is the act of continually redefining and clarifying one's personal vision, refocusing energies, maintaining objectivity, and committing to personal goals and objectives. The importance of personal growth and development is vital to attaining the leadership competency.
- *Mental models* are the images that influence how one views the world and attains new insights. Leaders must be aware of their mental models and be willing to examine them and hold them up for inquiry and scrutiny by others. This discipline speaks to the need for clear vision about advanced practice nursing and the ability to defend this viewpoint.
- *Shared vision* refers to the leader's ability to help a team develop and sustain a common image of what the team seeks to create in the future—it

is the ability to share a vision with others rather than to dictate that vision. The ability to empower others to share the dream and implement change is critical to this discipline.

- *Team learning* is the ability to suspend one's own assumptions, listen to other viewpoints, and genuinely think together.

- *Systems thinking* is the fifth discipline—a framework for leadership based on the ability to see the whole picture rather than the isolated parts. It helps us see how our own actions influence what is happening in the larger system (health care). This discipline is an important concept for APNs, who must be able to view advanced practice within the overall context of health care as one member of a team of professionals and patients.

Senge and colleagues (1999) noted that challenges are inherent in the change process—challenges such as delays, competition, and fragmented management that thwarts new, productive relationships. By nature, change is dynamic, nonlinear, and characterized by complexity. Senge defines *systems citizens* as persons who have a perspective and an awareness of the entire world rather than just the local areas in which they live. Catastrophes such as Hurricane Katrina and bridge collapses may not touch us directly, but they do influence our thinking about how to make changes in health care and safety. Unexpected and unplanned events, both large and small, can make it difficult to predict the trajectory a change initiative will take and highlight the importance of a flexible, responsive leadership style. Such a style fosters cohesion, collaboration, and communication among team members, enabling them to approach problem identification and solving with candor, commitment, and creativity.

The Values-Centered Leadership Model™ (Secretan). Secretan's Values-Centered Leadership Model™ is a spiritual and transformational one; he believes organizations thrive from a "soulful" place—a place where leaders and followers inspire each other (Secretan, 2003, 2004). Using a bicycle as a metaphor, he explains that the back wheel is the power, the front wheel is the direction, and the shifts are the accelerators—the actions that ensure the power is going in the right direction. The "power" concepts are mastery (high standards, best work), chemistry (effective relational skills), and delivery (meeting the needs of others). The "direction" concepts are learning, empathizing, and listening. The "shifts" or "accelerators" reflect specific changes that

are required to have the values and direction move as one. There are five "shifts"—from self to other; from things to people; from breakthrough to "kaizen" (not simply celebrating doing things better but celebrating doing them differently); from weaknesses to strengths; and from competition and fear to love. APNs will find this model and the associated tools useful for several different circumstances: assessing the impact of a change in organizational leadership (e.g., new executive or a merger), trying to understand why an individual or system is "stuck" and how one might move forward, and determining whether one's values are still compatible with the organization's. For example Secretan describes six principles using the acronym *CASTLE* that form the basis of an assessment tool *(www.secretan.com/castle/)*. The CASTLE principles are courage, authenticity, service, truthfulness, love, and effectiveness. He believes organizations thrive when their values are aligned with those of the individuals working within them; ideally, individuals and organizations are in alignment with regard to destiny, cause, and calling (Secretan, 1999). Defining individual and organizational destinies answers this question: "Why are we here?" Articulating a cause answers these questions: "How will we be?" and "What will we stand for?" Defining *calling* answers this question: "How will we use our gifts and talents to serve?" Extensive resources are available on his website for individual and organizational assessment *(www.secretan.com/freetools.php)*.

The Seven Habits of Highly Effective People (Covey). Stephen Covey's 1989 best-seller presented both personal and interdependent characteristics that foster acquisition of leadership skills. In creating a personal view of leadership, Covey suggested that the most effective way to "keep the end in mind" is to create a personal mission statement that becomes a standard to live by as one progresses to new levels of independence and subsequent interdependence. In Covey's model, interdependence is achieved only after one has defined and integrated this personal mission/standard into one's practice. He described attributes of those who lead from a philosophy of interdependence: listening twice as much as you speak, remaining trustworthy by never compromising honesty, maintaining a positive attitude, and keeping a sense of humor. Interdependence allows one to hear and understand the other person's viewpoint, leading to a synergistic or win-win level of communication. Covey expanded on his leadership ideas in light of managing people in the Information

Age (Covey, 2006). A key concept in this update is that leaders must be aware that the ways in which they lead will influence workers' choices. He described five choices ranging from *rebel* or *quit* to *creative excitement*. This can be considered an empowerment model: leadership of knowledge workers "will be characterized by those who find their own voice and who, regardless of their formal position, inspire others to find theirs" (p. 15).

Leadership Models That Address Systems Change and Innovation

Change is a constant in today's clinical environments. Efforts to transform the health care system are generally focused in three areas: diffusion of innovation, clinician behavior change, and patient behavior change. The reality is that change is "messy" and not always welcome, even when it seems straightforward. Leaders must be able to stay focused, listen, and manage multiple and changing contingencies. Since the call for redesign and transformation of the health care system, efforts to understand the messiness of systems redesign and transformation have redoubled. For example, an integrative review of diffusion and dissemination of innovations reveals why redesign and transformation are messy—they are exceedingly complex (Greenhalgh, Robert, MacFarlane, Bate, & Kyriakidou, 2004)!

Diffusion of Innovation in Service Organizations (Greenhalgh and Colleagues). The conceptual model developed by Greenhalgh and colleagues (2004) identifies several key characteristics that must be considered by change agents:

- The nature of the innovation—What change is being sought?
- Adoption by individuals—How will members (staff) be brought on board?
- Assimilation by the system—How will the organization incorporate the change?
- Diffusion and dissemination—How will the change be implemented?
- System antecedents—What current system policies and activities will affect implementation?
- System readiness for change—Is the system poised to change or reluctant to change?
- Outer context—What other considerations in the environment will affect the change?
- Implementation and routinization—How long and how difficult will it be to fully implement change?

While there is considerably more for APNs to learn from this work, these key concepts can be used to assess the readiness to change within a unit, practice, or organization. Such an in-depth assessment can enable APNs and colleagues to design a successful innovation implementation plan. Greenhalgh and colleagues' findings illustrate the challenges and complexities inherent in changing clinician behavior and clinical practice.

The Tipping Point (Gladwell). Another perspective on change and leadership is offered by Gladwell (2000). Gladwell posited social change as the "biography of an idea" (p. 7) and explored specific social changes using questions such as these: How does something catch on and become popular? What "tips" a phenomenon from being uncommon to common, unpopular to popular? Using the public health notion of epidemics, he helps readers understand how phenomena as diverse as health problems (e.g., teenage smoking, acquired immunodeficiency syndrome [AIDS]), successful products [Hush Puppies shoes], and programs [Sesame Street]) arise. Three elements seem to push an event or phenomenon to the tipping point: the *law of the few*, the *stickiness factor*, and the *power of context*. The *law of the few* refers to the fact that it does not take many people to move things forward, but building the momentum for change requires exceptional people who are persuasive—people he describes as *mavens*. Mavens can be described as experts or self-appointed leaders who have charisma. Thus within nursing, one might think of Florence Nightingale or Loretta Ford, who has spoken for APNs with a clear voice, as mavens. The *stickiness factor* refers to the fact that one can package a message, a program, or a product to make it "irresistible" (p. 132); the challenge is to find what makes it stick. For example, although pain continues to be undertreated, pain assessment has improved; thus one might consider the initiative to make pain the fifth "vital sign" as a good illustration of the *stickiness factor*. The *power of context* is the third element. Social and physical environments shape thought and behavior to a significant degree, so that what we see and hear around us defines what decisions we make. Epidemics are a good example—at the height of the AIDs epidemic, when people were dying of the effects of unprotected sex, a radical change in sexual practices occurred; contaminated food scares changed the way we shop for groceries. It may take many small movements to create "one contagious movement" (Gladwell, 2000, p. 192). The three elements defined by Gladwell are important to developing the leadership potential of APNs. It takes only a few APN mavens whose understanding of stickiness and context enable them to make changes in health care.

When considering these models of leadership and change, several common themes emerge that inform the remainder of this chapter: effective leadership requires sound knowledge of oneself and one's organization with regard to values, strengths, and weaknesses, as well as expert communication and relationship-building skills and the ability to think and act strategically.

Concepts Related to Change

In this section, *change* is used to refer to any of the various types of initiatives aimed at improving the quality and safety of practice whether by revising policies or helping clinicians master new knowledge and change behavior. In other words, change is seen as any clinical or systems effort to encourage the adoption and diffusion of innovation, including but not limited to quality improvement, product rollouts, clinician education, and skill development. Change does not have a discrete beginning and ending but, instead, appears to be a series of continuous transitions that overlap one another. Because of this, change agency must be woven into the fabric of an APN's everyday life and work. As with patient assessment to effect individual behavior change, to be effective change agents APNs must be skilled at assessing and reassessing their organizations and the complex forces that drive the health care system. Systems innovation requires leadership that is continuous and flexible and demands ongoing attention to and redefinition of appropriate strategies (Greenhalgh et al., 2004; Klein, Gabelnick, & Herr, 1998; Massoud, Nielsen, Nolan, Schall, & Sevin, 2006).

Opinion Leadership. One specific change strategy associated with leading a change initiative is "opinion leadership" (Greenlhalgh et. al., 2004; Locock, Dopson, Chambers, & Gabbay, 2001; Oxman, Thomson, Davis, & Haynes, 1995; Soumerai et al., 1998; Thomson et al., 1999). Opinion leaders are clinicians who are identified by their colleagues as likeable, trustworthy, and influential (Doumit, Gattellari, Grimshaw, & O'Brien, 2007; Oxman et al., 1995) A clinician is likely to listen to the opinion leader and might make a change in practice based on

what he or she learned from the opinion leader. The role of an opinion leader parallels that of the maven described by Gladwell (2000). One study of opinion leaders in several different clinical settings indicated that contextual factors influenced the ability of an opinion leader to promote guideline adoption by colleagues (Locock et al., 2001). As APNs become recognized for their accurate clinical decision making, they become opinion leaders. They are sought out by others, and when the APN speaks, others listen. Thus a staff nurse may ask a CNS to look at a wound and advise, or an NP returns to her practice from a conference and when she shares what she learned, colleagues are eager to try the new information. This finding suggests the importance of attending to environmental cues when change is planned. Although studies of opinion leaders have been done, findings about their effectiveness are mixed, in part, because the activities of opinion leaders are not well described (Oxman et al., 1995). How opinion leaders and their activities fit into diffusion and adoption of innovations is a component of the model evolved by Greenhalgh and colleagues (2004).

Driving and Restraining Forces. Driving and restraining forces are useful concepts for APNs as they plan for change and evaluate both planned and unplanned changes. For example, as APNs extend their practices across state lines, the movement toward multistate licensure is gaining momentum (see Chapter 21). Depending on existing policies and procedures for reimbursement and prescriptive authority within states, these forces can serve as driving or restraining influences for APNs. As multistate licensure for APNs evolves, telehealth may be considered a driving force, and states' rights may be a restraining force. Driving and restraining forces are also useful for analyzing the organizational settings in which APNs work. For example, an organizational assessment of these various forces is useful in determining an institution's level of commitment to diversity.

At times, physicians have been perceived as restraining forces for change. Experienced APNs know that one of the challenges in system redesign and transformation has been engaging physicians in the work of improving quality, an observation confirmed by health services research (Shortell, Bennett, & Byck, 1998). Physicians themselves have begun to recognize this and have made specific recommendations that administrators and APNs can use for engaging physicians in this important work (Reinertsen, Gosfield,

Rupp, & Whittington, 2007). For example, physicians and APNs together can request support through workshops and on-site experts in making an institutional change to electronic medical records.

Pace of Change. A major concern for health care stakeholders at all levels is the rapidity with which change is occurring in health care. Even when one develops detailed plans for a change, events may occur that reshape process and progress so that what gets implemented may not be exactly the same as the original proposal. As the rapidity of change increases, the time frame to accomplish change strategies shortens. This phenomenon makes change more difficult for individuals and organizations to manage. As a consequence, many of the traditional models still being used to implement change do not work. Planned versus unplanned change is based predominantly on issues of time (Senge, 2006)—time to plan for and think through the desired change, time to orient and allow stakeholders to become comfortable with change, and time to educate and allow the change process to occur. In most health care systems, people perceive a poverty of time; this barrier requires creativity to transcend.

O'Connell (1999) questioned whether health care organizations can sustain fast-paced change unless a "culture of change" is in place that assists and supports adaptation to new systems and ways of knowing and doing. A culture of change requires several components including learning about change and change strategies, encouraging dialogue, valuing collaboration, and being committed to enacting change. O'Connell proposed the following strategies for promoting a culture of change within an organization:

- Maintain momentum toward change.
- Emphasize managerial support in the process of changing work flow and practice patterns.

- Encourage the question "why," and exercise tolerance for the results.
- Emphasize the importance of personal concerns and address them.
- Find new and different ways to demonstrate administrative support.

The Greenhalgh and colleagues' model (2004) cited earlier could be used as a basis for assessing whether an institution has a culture of change. APNs can also use one or more of the models of leadership described here to assess their systems. Knowing where one's system is in terms of readiness for change and identifying the forces that will support or restrain adoption of an innovation can help the APN design strategies that will work. It is also helpful to consider the techniques used for implementing change, such as building alliances, creating a shared vision, being assertive, negotiating conflict (Norton & Grady, 1996), and managing transitions (see Chapter 6) as they relate to providing a positive culture for change. Senge's (1990) analogies, in which leading is compared with athletic coaching or playing in a jazz ensemble, speak to the importance of individuality, sensitivity, and conviction in leading change efforts. Most important, leaders need to understand the personal implications of change if a culture of change is to be realized. Box 9-1 provides a useful set of strategies for APN leaders who are helping their organizations and colleagues work through change transitions.

DEFINING CHARACTERISTICS OF THE ADVANCED PRACTICE NURSE LEADERSHIP COMPETENCY

The three defining characteristics of APN leadership—mentoring and empowerment, innovation and change agency, and activism—are listed along with their core elements in Table 9-2. These characteristics

---

Box 9-1 LEADERSHIP STRATEGIES FOR MOVING THROUGH THE TRANSITION OF CHANGE

- Spark a passion; believe in what you are doing; shine a light on activities that inspire and excite.
- Understand the organizational culture.
- Create a vision.
- Get the right people involved.
- Hand the work over to the champions of change.

- Let values serve as the compass for where you are headed.
- Change people first; organizations evolve.
- Seek and provide opportunities for professional renewal and regeneration.
- Maintain a healthy balance.

Adapted from Kerfoot, K., & Chaffee, M.W. (2007). Ten keys to unlock policy change in the workplace. In D.J. Mason, J.K. Leavitt, & M.W. Chaffee (Eds.), *Policy and politics in nursing and health care* (pp. 482-484). Philadelphia: Saunders; and Kerfoot, K. (2005). On leadership: building confident organizations by filling buckets, building infrastructures, and shining the flashlight. *Dermatology Nursing, 17*, 154-156.

Table 9-2   Defining Characteristics and Core Elements of the Leadership Competency for Advanced Practice Nurses

Defining Characteristic	Core Elements (Knowledge and Skills)
Mentoring and empowerment	Shared vision Seeks mentors and serves as a mentor Willing to share power Self-reflection
Innovation and change agency	Knowledge of models of leadership and change Systems thinking Systems assessment skills Flexibility Risk taking Expert communication Credibility
Activism	Knowledge and understanding of factors driving change in the health care system Involvement in policy arenas, whether local, regional, national, or global Advocacy for patients, advanced practice nurses, and the nursing profession

are discussed separately to help readers grasp the differences among them. However, there is considerable overlap in the knowledge and skills needed for each characteristic. Experienced APNs are able to demonstrate these characteristics in all four leadership domains. Although they have beginning competence in leading within each domain, novice APNs tend to exercise leadership in the clinical domain. Over time, they expand their leadership activities into other arenas.

Mentoring and Empowerment

Mentoring. The responsibility to mentor is central to all of the definitions of leadership and change outlined earlier and is a key element of the APN leadership competency. The ability to help others grow and to encourage them toward self-actualization requires competent, caring leaders who are interested in the success and well-being of their followers. Mentoring bridges the gap between education and real-world experience (Barker, 2006). Coaching and guiding, leading by example, and role modeling with an awareness and attentiveness to the needs and concerns of followers are basic characteristics of successful leaders. The ideas behind the colloquial statements "taking someone under your

wing" or "giving a colleague a leg up" are grounded in the mentoring process. Mentors have been defined as being competent and self-confident, as having qualities that epitomize success in their own careers, and as having the ability and desire to help others succeed. Most important, mentors are role models who help those with less experience gain expertise through example (Fawcett, 2002) by shared learning and commitment to each other's professional growth (Tourigny & Pulich, 2005). Protégés (or mentees) are viewed as individuals who exhibit a desire to learn, are committed to the long course of events, and are open to the process of trial and error. Successful protégés have high self-esteem, are able to self-monitor, and are resilient risk takers (Tourigny & Pulich, 2005). The reward for the mentor is to step back and enjoy the success and achievements of the protégé.

Two types of mentoring are described in the literature. The first, *formal mentoring,* has the approval and support of the organization with objectives, a selection process, and a mentoring contract. Mentors are chosen from the ranks of experienced clinicians and provide exposure to clinical situations that offer opportunities to demonstrate competence, coaching, and role modeling and afford protection in controversial situations (Tourigny & Pulich, 2005). Many professional organizations, such as Sigma Theta Tau, offer formal mentoring programs. Readers can consult their professional and specialty organizations' websites for information on formal mentoring programs. Another example of formal mentoring is the APN/physician relationship in preceptorships during graduate education. Such preceptorships tend to be shorter, have educational objectives for learning new skills, and are driven by state or federal regulation; some are more like supervision than true mentorship (Barker, 2006).

Informal mentoring has been described as a mutual attraction (akin to love), which is unstructured and mutually beneficial; the experiences usually last longer and are self-selected (Tourigny & Pulich, 2005). Good mentors foster growth rather than dependency and instill the internal strengths to enable protégés to traverse rough spots in career development. As mentoring relationships progress, the protégé is given more freedom to try new behaviors and develops confidence in trying new skills, always with the knowledge that someone is behind them.

It is important to note that there are two parts to the APN mentorship equation: APNs who are seeking to be mentored by those they aspire to emulate, and APNs who can serve as mentors. Unfortunately, some APN leaders are reluctant to mentor, perhaps thinking that the protégé will compete with them, will overshadow their expertise, or will not work as hard as they did to be successful. However, Vance (2003) asserted that the current chaotic health care environment makes mentoring support more important than ever. She suggested that mentors and protégés adopt a mentoring philosophy that encourages collaboration with others, not competition. Novice APNs are fortunate if they can find a mentoring relationship that lasts over time. The APN mentor creates a safety net in which the protégé can expose vulnerabilities and be coached to develop confidence in new skills (Davis, Little, & Thornton, 1997). Mentoring is a gift that allows new APN leaders to emerge.

An interrelationship exists between the concepts of mentoring, organizational culture, and leadership. Bally (2007) described *organizational culture* as the values, norms, and rituals that make up an organization and set the rules for its members. A positive organizational culture offers social support and a sense of well-being and empowerment that fosters the mentoring process (Bally, 2007; Shirey,

2004). Thus APNs should seek opportunities to mentor or be mentored and articulate the benefits of mentoring activities to their organization.

Empowering Others. As the word implies, *empowerment* is defined as giving power to another, encouraging, or giving authority. APNs operationalize empowerment by sharing power with other nurses, colleagues, and patients or by enabling them to access or assert their own power. Empowerment as a leadership strategy is guided by the shared vision of the leader and follower and a willingness of the leader to delegate authority to others. Visionary leaders who empower their followers greatly increase the influence of APNs both within nursing and beyond nursing's boundaries.

Empowerment requires more than just giving others permission to act on their own. Empowerment is a developmental process that a good leader fosters over time; it encourages constituents to feel competent, responsible, independent, and authorized to act. Rajotte (1996) offered a useful six-step method for advanced practice nursing leaders to use to empower others, whether patients, nurses, or members of other disciplines.

- Educate to empower through increasing the individual's knowledge base
- Use inspiration, motivation, and encouragement
- Provide structure that offers protection and security as one moves into new territory
- Provide resources to support others' growth and development
- Mentor to give the support and direction necessary for change toward empowerment
- Foster actualization, empowering others to evoke change

For example, CNMs empower pregnant women by putting them in control of the birthing process through education, mentoring, and providing resources for parenting that nurture self-esteem and enhance family structure.

Innovation and Change Agency
As the prior discussion suggests, initiating change and diffusing and sustaining innovations are critical elements of the APN leadership competency. Covey's work (1989) with interdisciplinary groups is instructive to APNs who are learning change agent skills. Change occurs at both the system and the personal

level, and one must deal with core values to successfully change or serve as an agent for change. Covey contends that people have a changeless core inside them that they need if they themselves are to be able to change. Thus one key to the ability of people to change is a changeless sense of who they are, what they are about, and what they value. Real change comes from the inside out. This observation is relevant to APNs. First, APNs need to identify their own core values to become effective in leading change. Second, Covey's insight can help APNs who encounter resistance to change initiatives, especially when it persists. The resistance may come from a sense that a core value is being threatened.

There is an affective dimension to change (Greenhalgh et al., 2004). Although many people are excited by the prospect of change, some changes are difficult and painful, and any change contains an element of loss. Senge (2006) described this feeling as an emotional tension associated with holding a vision that differs from the current reality. Mastering emotional tension during change requires perseverance, patience, and compassion. At best, change can be described as challenging and invigorating (Norton & Grady, 1996). To understand change within today's health care environment, APNs must explore the dynamics of change and the culture in which it occurs.

Taken together, this discussion suggests that APNs must consider several factors when they are experiencing or trying to introduce change: the relevance of power and influence, stakeholders' concerns and interests, contextual factors, individuals' values, and the affective dimensions of change. Understanding these important factors is integral to the APN leadership competency.

Political Activism

As doctorally prepared APNs hone their skills for systems leadership and change, political activism and advocacy will become even more important. Many of the skills needed to successfully navigate in political waters are closely associated with good leadership. The core elements that define contemporary leadership—such as shared vision, systems thinking, and the ability to engage in high-level communication within the context of a changing environment—are all basic to political effectiveness. Again, change is the common denominator that drives APNs to advocate for advanced practice

and patient issues. In fact, there is little room for discussion about whether APNs need to take on the mantles of policymaker and patient advocate as part of their leadership role (see Chapter 22). For many, this falls within the context of a moral imperative: "Nurses practice at the intersection of public policy and personal lives (of their patients); they are, therefore, ideally situated and morally obligated to include sociopolitical advocacy in their practice" (Falk-Rafael, 2005, p. 222). Indeed, working for social justice is seen as part of the ethical decision-making competency of APNs (see Chapter 11). APNs must position themselves strategically at the policy table to advocate for access to care and appropriate interventions for everyone. There is also little question about whether APNs are up to the task. Great strides have been made in developing nurses' skill and acuity as policymakers (see Chapter 22, Exemplar 22-2). Rapidly evolving policy situations mean that APNs are often faced with "trial by fire" learning when it comes to activism and advocacy. Identifying trusted mentors with whom to debrief and develop a plan of action can help APNs develop the poise and skills needed to respond effectively in unexpected, chaotic, and tense political situations.

ATTRIBUTES OF EFFECTIVE ADVANCED PRACTICE NURSE LEADERS

Several personal attributes are deemed necessary for successful leadership (Box 9-2). These qualities are very broad; all leaders should demonstrate these qualities since they are needed in the interdisciplinary context of today's health care. No longer do nurse leaders have the luxury of leading only in nursing circles. The history of advanced practice nursing (see Chapter 1) demonstrates that nurse leaders have led outside the realm of organized nursing education and practice. Certified registered nurse anesthetist (CRNA) leaders played a role in improving care for anesthetized patients early in the century. The multifaceted roles that APNs have played during times of war and natural disasters also exemplify the interdisciplinary nature of APN leadership.

Vision

Vision, the ability to anticipate the future and communicate that image to others, is often perceived as the most important component of leadership and the

Box 9-2   ATTRIBUTES OF NURSE LEADERS

EXPERT COMMUNICATION SKILLS
Articulate in speech and in writing
Able to get one's point across
Uses excellent listening skills
Desires to hear and understand another's point
    of view
Stays connected to other people

COMMITMENT
Gives of self personally and professionally
Listens to one's inner voice
Balances professional and private life
Plans ahead; makes change happen
Engages in self-reflection

DEVELOPING ONE'S OWN STYLE
Gets and stays involved
Sets priorities

Manages boundaries
Uses technology
Engages in lifelong learning
Maintains a good sense of humor

RISK TAKING
Gets involved at any level
Demonstrates self-confidence and assertiveness
Uses creative and big picture thinking
Willing to fail and begin again
Has an astute sense of timing
Copes with change

WILLINGNESS TO COLLABORATE
Respects cultural diversity
Desires to build teams and alliances
Shares power
Willing to mentor

Adapted from Hanson, C., Boyle, J., Hatmaker, D., & Murray, J. (1999). *Finding your voice as a leader.* Washington, DC: American Academy of Nursing.

talent that is most coveted (Carroll, 2005). Vision encompasses a long-range view of both personal and collective goals that can be shared and that empower others to move forward. Innovation is associated with and closely linked to vision. It is the ability to "think big" or to "think outside the box"—the capacity to see alternatives to the current thinking on a given issue. In fact, in some graduate schools, teaching APNs innovation and thinking outside the box is a program goal (Shirey, 2004). Vision is also grounded in a deep knowledge of the subject and brings with it the responsibility to stay abreast of trends and issues in the field. However, having vision is not enough. A leader must be able to articulate and develop a shared vision, one that others can embrace as their own (Christopher, Miller, Beck, & Toughill, 2002; Senge, 2006). To do this well, a visionary leader must not get too far out in front of his or her followers because teamwork is critical to shared vision. Tornabeni (1996), a nurse leader, noted that she would not have been able to "hold onto the vision" (p. 65) had she not broadened her scope of influence to include others outside of the discipline of nursing. Another important element of vision is the ability to set priorities so that there is a clear path to the ultimate goal.

Leaders are involved with change at many points in the change process. Anticipating and preparing for change can help ensure success. Visionary change

makers intervene early in the change process, before change occurs, and set the stage for the events that follow. They provide the guiding principles and assumptions for the proposed change and begin to introduce themes that position the organization and its members in a positive direction toward the new events. Change implementers—as defined by Kantor, Stein, and Jick (1992)—have the difficult task of making it happen.

Timing

A good sense of timing may be an inherent gift, but for most people it requires painstaking development and practice. APN leaders know when to act and when to hold back. They recognize the need for urgency at times as, for example, during an unexpected legislative vote in Congress; they also know to take the time to develop a carefully thought-out plan with deliberate strategy when a change in scope of practice is being considered. The notion of timing is apparent when APNs use mandated change as opportunities to introduce other changes. For example, institutions applying for accreditation by The Joint Commission (TJC) are expected to demonstrate compliance with TJC's current evidence-based standards for specific health care problems (TJC, 2000). Many institutions use these mandated changes to launch a variety of initiatives aimed at improving care management.

Self-Confidence and Risk Taking

Taking risks is inherent in the leadership process and is tied inextricably to self-confidence and vision. The willingness to take a chance, to try, and to fail occasionally is the mark of a true leader. The mantra "take a risk, make a decision, pay the price," coined by Helen Mannock in 1959, is worth keeping in mind (cited in Norton & Grady, 1996). Risk-taking behaviors differentiate APNs who will be recognized as leaders and change drivers from other capable nurses. By learning to take risks, APNs enhance their leadership repertoire, allowing for more spontaneity and flexibility in response to conflict, resistance, anger, and other reactions to change and high-risk situations (Norton & Grady, 1996). Motivation, which can be described as the desire to move forward, can also be viewed as a component of risk. Wheatley (2005) affirmed that another component of risk taking is the willingness to be disturbed. Certainty is more comfortable. Staying put is rarely as risky as taking the chance to move ahead.

It is not accidental that several of the key attributes in Box 9-2 incorporate some form of the word *willingness*. The abilities to be open and willing, to take what comes, and to work through differences are key to all levels of leadership. Leadership is about negotiation and interactions with others to reach common goals. To do this may mean failing and trying again and again to reach the desired outcome. This quality of personal hardiness—the ability to pick oneself up and start again—is seen repeatedly in biographies of successful leaders who have made change happen in difficult times.

Expert Communication and Relationship Building

The relevance of expert communication skills and collegial relationships to quality health care has received significant attention in the past few years (Houghton, 2003; King, 2002; Rider, 2002). APNs must be able to communicate effectively to collaborate with other professionals (see Chapter 10) and participate in the identification and resolution of clinical and ethical conflicts among team members (see Chapter 11). The successful leader must have superb communication skills to build the trust and cooperation necessary to negotiate difficult intraprofessional and interprofessional issues. The ability to understand another's viewpoint and respect opposing views is key to effective communication and ultimately to reaching a mutually satisfactory outcome.

Covey (1989) suggested that one should "seek first to understand and then to be understood" (p. 235). Good leaders listen and really try to hear the other person's viewpoint before they speak. The charisma that is associated with many natural-born leaders is often simply outstanding listening and communication skills. The ability to influence, a key power strategy used to gain the cooperation of others, is an outcome of excellent communication.

A second part of expert communication is relationship building. The art of building strong alliances and coalitions with others and staying connected with colleagues and groups is basic to the sense of community needed to lead effectively. Building relationships within the work environment can minimize the impact of organizational structures that hinder one's ability to collaborate and solve problems (Wheatley, 2005). Such alliances are important whether at the highest levels of international policy-making or at the local level in building coalitions to address a recurring patient issue. Building relationships is central to the effectiveness of a team who cares for patients. Not only must APNs establish effective relationships with their co-workers, they are often in a position to strengthen relationships among other members of the team through role modeling and mediation.

Building relationships is also central to another advanced practice nursing communication skill—conflict negotiation (see Chapter 10). Advanced practice nursing students may come to their graduate programs having been socialized to be silent or to suppress their opinions in situations of conflict. Specific approaches to identifying conflicts and resolving them successfully have been identified and used successfully in business (Fisher, Ury, & Patton, 2002) and in health care (Longo & Sherman, 2007). Readers are referred to the following websites for resources and information on conflict negotiation: The Conflict Resolution Network *(www.crnhq.org/)*; and The Program on Negotiation at Harvard Law School *(www.pon.org/)*.

Boundary Management

Managing boundaries refers to the ways in which APNs limit or extend various aspects of advanced practice nursing such as scope of practice, workload, and interpersonal boundaries. Sometimes APNs are in the position of "guarding" the boundary such as when they are approached to undertake a task that is not within their scope of practice. Managed care productivity requirements mean that APNs must be clear about the numbers and kinds of patients that they care for on a given day. Often, managing boundaries means extending them—building a bridge that enables the APN to partner with other groups or expanding a boundary as other patient or health care needs are identified, an idea increasingly recognized in calls for core health professional competencies (Greiner & Knebel, 2003; HealthSciences Institute, 2005). For example, although CRNAs may not need prescriptive authority in a given state, they assist their colleague NPs in their quest for state prescriptive authority. Extending a boundary may also mean expanding one's scope of practice at an agency level so that patient needs can be better met. Knowing where the current boundaries of nursing practice are and making strategic decisions about going beyond them are other ways to define risk taking.

As boundary managers, APNs recognize communications and behaviors that breach or enhance interpersonal relationships (see the later section, "Horizontal Violence and Dysfunctional Leadership Styles"). APN leaders also teach others how to collaborate with colleagues in other disciplines, build coalitions, and set limits while maintaining their own boundaries—a fine distinction, but strategically important. For example, a CNM may delicately negotiate the boundaries or responsibility among the neonatologist, the obstetrician, and the nurse-midwifery staff. Both clinical leadership and professional leadership require the negotiation of boundaries, regardless of whether the borders are drawn around professional roles, patient populations, or organizations.

Self-Reflection

Self-reflection is an important activity for APNs who aspire to be leaders. Self-reflection enables APNs to make sense of and learn from experience. One must recognize that often a chasm exists between the rhetoric and the reality of nursing. Self-reflection helps one to step back and evaluate what has happened before moving ahead. Self-reflection as a strategy for refining direct care and coaching competencies is addressed in Chapters 5 and 6 and also by Longo and Sherman (2007). For one to lead successfully, it is especially instructive to reflect on previous experiences of socialization and acculturation as a member of a particular family, peer group, and discipline. For example, the need to group together along some continuum of sameness is the basis of family structure, as well as the basis for stereotyping. As a consequence, self-assessment of one's history with

and valuing of diversity needs to be a continuous, evolving activity for APNs.

Respect for Cultural Diversity

Cultural competence and valuing diversity are significant attributes of APN leaders. These attributes require awareness of one's own biases and the awareness of damaging attitudes and behaviors that surface at all levels of interaction and in all settings. An APN leader needs to serve as role model by demonstrating respect for the cultural, racial, and ethnic differences of individuals and constituencies in any given situation. When a systems framework is used for understanding a complex concept such as culturally competent leadership, four levels can be identified: societal, professional, organizational, and individual. For the APN, the responsibility for culturally competent care includes all four of these levels. Culturally competent care is delivered with knowledge, sensitivity, and respect for the patient's and family's cultural, racial, and ethnic background and practices. Cultural competence is an ongoing process that involves accepting and respecting differences and not letting personal beliefs get in the way (Giger et al., 2007). This definition is built on the assumption that care providers are fully aware of and sensitized to their own cultural, racial, and ethnic backgrounds and that they are able to integrate this sensitivity into their delivery of care. The interactive nature of caregiving requires the authentic engagement of the provider with the patient in order to appreciate and respond to differences that may affect giving or receiving care. A good example of the challenge that culturally competent care presents is provided by Wheatley (2005). A group practice offered free car seats and training in their use to parents but no one took advantage of the gift. On debriefing, the providers learned that for Asian parents, using a car seat was an invitation to God to cause a car accident. Differences are issues for every member of the human race, and they become even more important when one becomes a leader and role model. Working with colleagues who are different gives APNs opportunities for soliciting information about others' experiences. Box 9-3 provides strategies for enhancing cultural awareness.

Balance in Personal and Professional Life

Most people know when they have overextended themselves—their bodies give clues such as fatigue, stress signals, feelings of frustration, and even physical illness. One of the negative aspects of being a

Box 9-3   Strategies to Achieve Cultural Competence

• Explore and learn about your own racial/ethnic culture and background.	• Take advantage of training opportunities to increase your cultural awareness and sensitivity.
• Explore and learn about the different racial/ethnic cultures most frequently encountered in your practice.	• Be able to identify personal biases and develop strategies to manage, eliminate, or sublimate those potentially damaging attitudes and behaviors.
• Read ethnic newspapers, magazines, and books.	
• Listen to the music from a different culture.	• When faced with a difficult patient, consider whether unconscious biases may be operating for you or your colleagues.
• Learn the language of a different culture. Become bilingual with the verbal and the nonverbal behavior of the culture.	

Adapted from Hanson, C.M., & Malone, B. (2000). Leadership: Empowerment, change agency, and activism. In A.B. Hamric, J.A. Spross, & C.M. Hanson (Eds.), *Advanced nursing practice: An integrative approach* (2nd ed., pp. 279-313). Philadelphia: Saunders.

good leader is the provocative realization that one is being asked to play many important cutting-edge roles at the same time. Such invitations are exciting and seductive because they open new opportunities and speak to the high regard others have for the leader. For these reasons, it is very easy for good leaders to overextend their activities well beyond manageable, realistic boundaries. The skills of being able to delegate tasks, mentor others to take on some of the load, and enlarge the circle of leaders, strategists, and followers are integral to effective leadership. Unfortunately, the inability to set realistic personal boundaries paves the way for stress, frustration, and burnout. It is not easy to be both a leader and a competent APN provider, but it can be done.

The process of self-reflection is useful for APNs to see what personal and work characteristics seem to set off imbalances. We offer three strategies, which are simple in concept but can be complicated in execution. First, expecting perfection is often a setup for imbalance. Keeping in mind the axiom, "Perfect is the enemy of good," may help APNs establish realistic expectations. Another strategy is for APNs to examine what makes them say "yes" or "no." It is easy to think, "If I just do this one more thing, everything will be fine." One APN kept a Post-it note on her phone that read, "The answer is no." This reminded her to either decline something that would tip the scales to overcommitment or to buy time by asking, "Can I think about it and call you tomorrow?" One colleague avoids commitments that are perceived as distant elephants; these are invitations for activities months or even years in the future. Such activities may not appear to threaten one's usual commitments and deadlines. However, as the time to fulfill the

commitment approaches, distant elephants can become as threatening as an impending stampede. The challenge for the APN is to ensure that adequate time to plan for, develop, and organize the work is budgeted well in advance of the due date. The third strategy is to make appointments with oneself for important personal and professional activities. By putting such appointments on a calendar, APNs can lessen the risk of giving away time that they need to maintain balance.

DEVELOPING SKILLS AS ADVANCED PRACTICE NURSE LEADERS

In considering a leadership development plan, there are formal and informal strategies. Students must have formal and informal opportunities to develop leadership skills in each domain. These can occur in the classroom, in clinical practica, in student leadership, and in health-related service projects. In general, lessons learned in one domain will apply to leadership situations in other domains. Health policy leadership is discussed separately because it has specific features that are somewhat different from the APN's everyday leadership activities.

Factors Influencing Leadership Development

Power Resources. A common myth is that leaders are born and not made. Trent (2003) asserted that this is not true and that individuals can learn to lead by understanding and using "power resources" as described by Rost (1993). Power resources include many of the attributes described in this chapter such as education, experience, expert communication, networking, assertiveness, and collaboration and are clearly demonstrated in the studies of leadership discussed in the following sections. Recent work by Zaccaro (2007) argues that with increases in conceptual and methodological resources, combinations of both inborn traits and learned attributes are more likely to predict leadership than once was believed. Leadership represents complex patterns of behavior explained in part by multiple leader attributes (Zaccaro, 2007). In this section we explore leadership traits and attributes that are innate and those that can be learned as APNs develop their leadership competence.

Personal Characteristics/Experiences.

Allen (1998) explored perceptions of 12 nurse leaders regarding the primary factors and individual characteristics that influenced their leadership development. Self-confidence, traced to childhood and subsequent risk-taking behaviors, was perceived as a critical factor. Feedback from significant others led to enhanced self-confidence over time. The nurse leaders also spoke about having innate qualities and tendencies of leaders, such as being extroverted or bossy and wanting to take charge, and about having roles as team captains and officers in organizations. They were seen as people who rise to the occasion. A third important factor was a progression of experiences and successes that were pivotal in moving them forward. Being at the right place at the right time and taking advantage of opportunities that were presented in those situations allowed them to grow as leaders. Closely aligned with this factor was the influence of significant people such as mentors, role models, faculty, and parents who had the ability to encourage and provide opportunities for advancement. A final set of factors identified in this study were personal life factors, defined as situations in which time, family, health, and work schedules influenced their development to a greater or lesser degree. For example, study participants who had supportive spouses and relatives who assisted with family and home responsibilities and employers who were flexible found these factors to be important to the leadership development process.

Zaccaro, Kemp, and Bader (2004) developed a model that described distal attributes (personality, cognitive abilities, motives, values) and proximal attributes (social appraisal skills, problem-solving skills, expertise, tacit knowledge) as they relate to a leader's

emergence, effectiveness, and advancement. In this model, the leader's operating environment influenced the trajectory toward success, which supports the importance of organizational culture described by Bally (2007) in the mentoring section. Carroll (2005) identified six factors that were present in women leaders and nurse executives: personal integrity; strategic vision/action orientation; team building/communication skills; management and technical competencies; people skills (collaboration, empowering others, valuing diversity); and personal survival skills. The reader will note the similarity with the attributes in Box 9-2.

Strategies for Acquiring Competency as a Leader

Formal educational opportunities such as those experienced during graduate school fit well into the process of leadership development. Opportunities to work with role models and mentors help students acquire leadership skills and further reinforce their self-confidence. Running for graduate student office or local leadership positions in professional organizations and serving on local and national coalitions are other good strategies for developing this competency (Grossman, 2006, Sandrick, 2006). Also, leadership conferences that foster effective communication and interaction are beneficial. Exemplar 9-2 shows how students can practice their leadership development during graduate education.

Leadership skills are developed and perfected over time and in myriad ways. Communication is one of the strengths often attributed to nurses, and it is a skill that can be augmented through practice. Many other skills and attributes listed in Box 9-2 are familiar to APNs and just need to be framed within the context of leadership. For example, the notion of staying connected is important for busy APNs and can be operationalized in a variety of ways, from electronic mailing lists and shared projects to attending conferences that allowed for time to interact and problem solve with colleagues about similar professional issues (Hanson, Boyle, Hatmaker, & Murray, 1999). A sense of timing was described by one leader in the study by Hanson and colleagues as negotiating childcare duties with her spouse for time to lobby for prescriptive authority, with the understanding that she would increase her family responsibilities at the end of the legislative session. For faculty and students in graduate programs to become involved in raising the visibility of advanced practice nursing roles in

EXEMPLAR 9-2   Mentoring an APN Student to Develop Health Policy Skills

Joan was beginning her second year as a student advanced practice nurse (APN). She had completed her core courses, which gave her a good foundation in the theoretical concepts related to role development, health policy, and research. Now she was ready to move on to the clinical component of her program and to complete her scholarly project. Joan had thought carefully about this and wanted to focus her project on developing her leadership skills in the policy arena. She knew that one of her faculty, Dr. Wesson, who had taught her health policy course, was a respected state and national leader who was actively engaged in the process of gaining primary care provider (PCP) status for APNs. Joan made an appointment to talk with Dr. Wesson about how she could help with the PCP issue and at the same time complete her scholarly project. Dr. Wesson suggested three things: Joan should use the Internet to become familiar with and articulate about the proposed legislation; she could accompany Dr. Wesson to the next statewide meeting of APNs and offer to carry out the phone survey of APNs that was needed by this group; and she could develop the research proposal, implement the survey methodology, and present the findings as part of

testimony at the hearing at the state capitol in the spring. These activities would allow Joan to interact with leader role models, try out her new leadership skills, and complete her research assignment. Dr. Wesson also suggested that Joan apply for the student scholarship offered by a national advanced practice nursing organization to attend the Washington, D.C.–based APN Summit.

Throughout the fall and winter, Joan implemented the phone survey with the advanced practice nursing community. She interacted with many practicing APNs and learned a great deal about advanced practice nursing. The APN leaders at the state meeting were excellent role models, and Dr. Wesson served as an excellent mentor throughout the year. Joan was extremely proud of her contribution to advanced practice nursing when she presented her findings at the hearing. Throughout the process, she had used many of the skills that she had read about in her leadership class, such as communication, networking, vision, and timing. Because Joan has a husband and a 4-year-old child, she also learned about balance and boundary management. Her most lasting recollection was how important it was to have a mentor to guide her through the process.

their institutions and communities is extremely important to building a community of advanced practice nursing leaders.

To acquire leadership skills and experience, novice APNs need to become involved in the leadership and committee work of local advanced practice nursing coalitions and organizations and move into state and regional leadership roles as they develop their style and strengths as APN leaders. The ability to place nurse leaders in key positions is critical to the visibility and credibility of APNs and to the establishment of roles for APNs within nursing and within the larger health care community.

DEVELOPING LEADERSHIP IN THE HEALTH POLICY ARENA

Health policy issues affecting APNs and their patients and including strategies for political advocacy are explored in Chapter 22. The following section describes how APNs can develop skills to influence health policy through creative leadership and political advocacy, whether by means of local grassroots endeavors or directly through congressional

involvement. *Advocacy* can be defined as the act of pleading another person's cause; it is multifaceted with diverse activities (Halpern, 2002, Kendig, 2006); "the endpoint of advocacy is the health and welfare of the public" (Leavitt et al., 2007, p. 37). APNs are being called on, collectively and individually, to make their voices heard as the nation and individual states struggle with budget constraints and difficult decisions about health policies and the funding of health care programs.

Becoming an Astute Political Activist: The Growth Process

In the political arena, developing power and influence is an imperative that tests one's leadership skills. Leadership strategies used by APNs in the political arena include developing influence with policymakers, influencing contacts, motivating colleagues to stay abreast of current issues, and providing bridges to other leaders who have access to important resources. Mentoring APNs to understand their power and influence in the health policy arena is a key role for the APN leader. The developmental process for becoming a political activist can begin as early as primary school when children are first introduced to government and the political system. However, serious involvement often begins in graduate school, when health policy is offered as one of the core courses in the curriculum (see Exemplar 9-2). During master's education, APN students are coached to better understand the power inherent in policymaking, the power of policies to influence practice, and the ways that they can influence the system, both individually and collectively, to better their own practice and to be high-level patient advocates. Faculty need to serve as resource persons to keep students informed about key legislative issues and to introduce them, through role modeling, to the role of political advocacy. Inviting APNs to accompany faculty who are giving testimony at a legislative hearing is an appropriate way to model the advocacy role.

Depth of Involvement. There is no question that influencing policy is costly in terms of commitment, time, and energy. Timing is an important consideration. It is important for APNs to ask themselves several personal and professional questions to determine the degree of involvement and level of sophistication at which advocacy is to be undertaken. These questions include the following:

- What are my personal responsibilities related to wage earning, small children, dependent parents, single parenthood, health issues, school, and gaining initial competence as an APN?
- How can I best serve the APN community at this time?
- What learning opportunities will help me be an effective APN advocate?
- How can I develop a short-term and long-term plan for becoming a more politically astute advocate for myself, for my patients, and for nursing?
- What am I able to commit to, based on the response to these questions?

Once APNs have made a decision about the depth of involvement to which they can commit, they need to find an appropriate mentor. Advanced practice nursing has a wealth of effective nursing leaders and advocates who are willing and able to move new advocates into positions to make positive changes in health policy. Opportunities for input and influence exist at various levels of the legislative process (Larson, 2004; Winterfeldt, 2001; see also Chapter 22).

Using Professional Organizations to the Best Advantage. For APNs, close contact with their professional organizations is an important link for staying abreast of national and state policy agendas, for finding a support network of like-minded colleagues, and for accessing information about changes in credentialing and practice issues. Box 9-4 presents a list of useful websites. Unfortunately, in today's complex world, this means being an active member of more than one affiliate organization to stay on the cutting edge of pertinent issues. Most APNs are aligned with at least one nursing organization; those APNs who aspire to an active role in influencing policy will need to have membership in several. As new graduates move from the educational milieu into diverse practice settings, they must align with the advanced practice nursing organizations that best meet their needs and offer the strongest support, choosing to actively engage in some and remain on the periphery in others.

Choosing the "right" organizations to belong to is a very personal decision based on particular needs, comfort level, specialty, and experience. Many APNs belong to one organization that meets their particular clinical needs (e.g., the Oncology Nursing Society [ONS] or the American Association of Nurse Anesthetists [AANA]) and to another that offers cutting-edge access to pressing professional issues (e.g., the National Organization of Nurse Practitioner Faculties [NONPF] or the American Nurses Association [ANA]). Others use the local, regional, or state affiliate of a professional organization as a support group that offers nurturing and professional sustenance, a group that understands local advanced practice nursing concerns.

The critical factor in interfacing with organizations is getting and staying involved in a definitive way. At a minimum, APNs will need to stay current on the issues by reading the organization's publications. Reading newsletters and journals, being part of an electronic mailing list or chat room, attending meetings and conferences, participating on committees or expert panels, and working up the ladder to leadership positions represent different levels of involvement. Professional organizations offer an important source of leadership and collective wisdom necessary to stay the course in today's political and policy arena. The notions of strength in numbers and speaking with one strong voice are not new concepts but are essential to the success of advanced practice nursing.

Box 9-4   Websites Useful to Advanced Practice Nurse Leaders

Agency for Healthcare Research and Quality:
   www.ahrq.gov
American Academy of Nurse Practitioners:
   www.aanp.org
American Association of Colleges of Nursing:
   www.aacn.nche.edu
American Association of Nurse Anesthetists:
   www.aana.com
American College of Nurse-Midwives:
   www.acnm.org
American College of Nurse Practitioners:
   www.nurse.acnpweb.org
American Medical Association: www.ama-assn.org
American Nurses Association: www.ana.org
American Nurses Credentialing Center:
   www.nursingworld.org/ancc
Fast Company: www.fastcompany.com
Leader to Leader Institute: www.leadertoleader.org
National Association of County and City Health
   Officials: www.naccho.org
National Association of Neonatal Nurses:
   www.nann.org
National Association of Pediatric Nurse Practitioners:
   www.napnap.org

National Certification Board of Pediatric Nurse
   Practitioners/Nurses: www.pnpcert.org
National Council of State Boards of Nursing:
   www.ncsbn.org
National Institute of Nursing Research:
   www.ninr.nih.gov
National Institutes of Health: www.nih.gov
National League for Nursing: www.nln.org
National Organization/Nurse Practitioner Faculties:
   www.nonpf.org
National Rural Health Association:
   www.nrharural.org
Oncology Nurses Society: www.ons.org
Reuters Health Information Services:
   www.reutershealth.com
State Government:
   www.state.(insert abbreviation).us
Thomas: Legislative Information on the Internet:
   www.thomas.loc.gov
U.S. Government Printing Office:
   www.access.gpo.gov
U.S. House of Representatives: www.house.gov
U.S. Senate: www.senate.gov
World Health Organization: www.who.int

Political Action Committees. A political action committee (PAC) is the arm of an organization that finances political campaigns. Federal guidelines dictate how donations and funds are raised and administered (Malone & Chafee, 2007). PACs are structured as a separate entity. PAC contributions do not buy votes, but they do buy access to candidates and visibility in a campaign, which is critical to the advocacy process (Malone & Chafee, 2007). Decisions about endorsements are complex and are made at the national professional organization level based on careful research and candidates' past support for nursing and health care interests that align with the organization's professional priorities and values. Fund-raising to support candidates is a major function of PACs and requires nursing support at every level. PACs are important to APN leaders both nationally and at state levels because the decisions about Medicare and Medicaid that undergird APN reimbursement are at stake.

Internships and Fellowships. One excellent way to develop the necessary skills to move into the role of advanced practice nursing policy advocate is to apply for a national or state policy internship or

fellowship. These appointments, which last from several days to 1 or 2 years, offer a wide range of health policy and political experiences that are targeted to both novice and expert APNs. For example, the Nurse in Washington Internship (NIWI), sponsored by the Nursing Organizations Alliance, is a 4-day internship that introduces nurses to policymaking in Washington, D.C. *(www.nursing-alliance.org/niwi.cfm)*. This internship serves as an excellent beginning step in learning the APN policy role. The National Rural Health Association also offers fellowships from time to time. Federal fellowships and internships that link nurses to legislators or to the various branches of federal and state government are invaluable in assisting APNs to understand how leaders are developed and how the system for setting health policy operates. Currently two NPs, sponsored by supporters of the Nurse Practitioner Healthcare Foundation (NPHF), are completing internships in the U.S. Surgeon General's Office.

Raising Awareness Through Communication

The ability of APNs to influence public policy rests with the individual nurse, as well as with collective groups of APNs. The ability to communicate with others accurately, efficiently, and in a timely manner is a driving force in the world of policy and politics. Never before have people had such an opportunity to share information in its original form and to engage with others at a distance (Wakefield, 2003). Face-to-face, one-on-one interaction and on-site networking are always the best ways to ensure successful communication that satisfies all parties. However, time and distance make these modes of communication a luxury rather than a reality.

The Internet, E-Mail, Fax, and Telephone Communication. Today's communication networks are wonderful resources for gaining awareness and keeping current on policy initiatives and concerns from a wide variety of perspectives. Probably the most useful tool available to APNs is the World Wide Web, which makes it possible for APNs to influence policy change from their own homes. It is possible to follow committee sessions in Congress via television or computer as they happen or later the same day via networks such as CNN. Conference calls save countless hours on the road or in the air. Often, APNs at the grassroots level must push for this type of interaction with major policy activists and organizations. It is important for APNs in busy practices to press for distance access to engage directly in policy activities without disruptions in delivering patient care.

The Media. The media in all forms—whether newsprint, television, the Internet, books, or journals—serve as a springboard for policy initiatives, information, opinions, and a means to communicate with policymakers, stakeholders, and constituents. Basic media communication strategies are shown in Box 9-5. APNs need to consider how to present themselves effectively and comfortably. Is it easier to conceive of doing a speech or a radio or television spot or writing an article or letter to the editor for the newspaper? In which mode are you best able to communicate your point using the strategies in Box 9-5? What venue will get the most visibility at the best time? How controversial is the issue? Is it important to pave the way with other stakeholders, in and outside of nursing, before you make a public statement? Is it important to reach many people (the public), or do you need to focus on educating a particular legislator or committee? If you are speaking publicly, are you ready to see your remarks in print the next day? Can you back up what you say? (deVries & Vanderbilt, 1992; Hassmiller, 1995). The Center for Nursing Advocacy is a website that helps nurses stay abreast of media directed toward nursing, to design nurse-driven media, and to search media resources *(www.nursingadvocacy.org).*

Educating Policymakers and Legislators. Educating busy, influential leaders and policymakers requires special consideration. Often issues are assigned to staffers and aides who stay abreast of the issues. The staff members' work is structured around specific committees, and so they are much closer to and often more informed about the issues than is the policymaker. Legislators have personal goals, as well as responsibilities to their constituents. They are bombarded on every side by multiple special interest groups who want their attention and their vote. The *sine qua non* of educating and influencing busy policymakers can be summed up in the following four basic strategies:

- Use staff to the fullest degree possible. The staffers follow the legislation and have the best insight about the strengths and weaknesses of your ideas and strategies for getting what you want.
- Be clear; understand the issue fully; know what you hope to gain and what you are willing to give up.
- Use multiple strategies, such as face-to-face communication, letter writing, e-mail campaigns, fact sheets, and meeting on home turf.
- Garner support from others who have a like mission; build coalitions of constituents.

Box 9-5   BASIC MEDIA COMMUNICATION STRATEGIES

- Understand how the system works.
- Make your point.
- Get the facts straight.
- Use data to back up your statements.
- KISS it (Keep It Short and Simple).

- Do your homework.
- Ask for what you want.
- Tell the truth.
- Personalize the message.

Educating the Public. A common misconception among APNs is that the public in general is aware of the roles and issues surrounding health care and advanced practice nursing. APNs are often amazed to discover that physicians, legislators, and their patients really have very little understanding of what APNs are about, what they can do, and how they fit into the overall scheme of health care. Each APN has a primary responsibility for educating people he or she encounters and for conducting this education in a clear and articulate manner. This may seem to be an easy task, but in fact, it is fraught with political complexities and varying levels of sophistication. Using the strengths of professional associations is key to getting out a unified message to the public that is clear and appropriate. Most APN organizations have packaged materials and references that APNs at the grassroots level can access from the Internet.

The ways in which APNs gain visibility with the public are based on personal style. One APN may write a weekly column in the local newspaper, another may be very visible on local planning and advisory boards, and a third may host a radio talk show. Volunteering for community service or as a member of the local or state speakers' bureau also works well. Written materials or videotapes in office waiting rooms provide patients and families with an important introduction to advanced practice nursing services. In addition, personal visits to legislators, policymakers, and health care leaders are critical components for gaining needed visibility for advanced practice nursing. The epitome of gaining public visibility is to run for professional or public office.

Special Interest Groups. One way to offer advocacy and become more visible with the public is to align with and keep abreast of issues that have high priority with special interest groups. Special interest groups or key stakeholders are often the deciding factor in policy decisions. For example, using the American Association of Retired Persons' (AARP's) website is a good way to track the policy and legislative agenda of senior citizens and to share the expertise of APNs with senior citizens. A feature story on the role of the NP in retirement communities or offering information about polypharmacy problems in *AARP The Magazine,* the journal for the AARP, can provide needed visibility for advanced practice nursing as well as educate the public about a serious health issue. Likewise, exploring the linkages for the American College of Nurse-Midwives online can lead one to the issues surrounding home births or birthing center care provided by APNs.

Special interest groups have important connections to legislators and high-ranking policymakers, and these groups can serve as allies to ensure that APNs are positioned to influence policy.

General Political Strategies

APNs have come a long way in demonstrating their political acumen at both state and national levels and have considerable power to achieve positive change if they capitalize on their newfound status. An important cohesiveness within nursing has emerged recently in response to health care system changes. The nursing profession as a whole is beginning to recognize its strength at the policy table (see Chapter 22). Politics and ethics are inherent in relationships at all systems levels and most obviously in policy development. Therefore nursing's ethical stance on social mandates that support poor and underserved populations needs to be clearly articulated (Falk-Rafael, 2005; Sarikonda-Woitas, 2002). Advanced practice nursing leaders have a responsibility to bring their views and perspectives to decision-making and policy forums. They need to turn competitors into partners to make changes that will result in a less fragmented and more interdisciplinary system.

Unfortunately, dialogue about health care reform and managed care initiatives has caused some physicians and other important health care stakeholders to retrench, leading to a heightened perception of APNs as a threat. This has made the current political arena extremely sensitive. The political agenda that is carried out at the professional level (American Nurses Association/American Medical Association [ANA/AMA]) and among APN specialty organizations is much different from the agenda played out at the grassroots level. There is evidence that locally practicing physicians and nurses have strong collaborative relationships and that they are frustrated by the lack of cohesion among professional organizations when it comes to policymaking. APNs must closely monitor policy issues through phone trees, newsletters, and regional meetings. There is no question that an important strategy for the removal of barriers is enlisting support from physician and APN teams who are practicing successfully in a collegial manner.

Creating local networks of APNs and close interaction with collaborating physicians and leaders of local health care entities is crucial to removing barriers and developing workable practice guidelines. States that have made the greatest strides in removing practice barriers need to help states that continue to have serious constraints on advanced practice.

Nurses have a formidable voting power base of more than 2.2 million. This is an incredible strength for nurses but requires cohesiveness within the ranks to make positive change for advanced practice nursing. The notion that someone else will carry the flag is not realistic. Developing political acumen and competence is a required skill for all practicing APNs, and most certainly for APN leaders, that is nurtured through time and experience. Peters (2002) asserted that nursing is facing an important "policy window" triggered by the nursing shortage, decreased access to care, and skyrocketing health care costs that provides an opportunity for nurses to gain leverage in the policy arena. Because all these factors are still problems, one author (C.M.H.) believes this window is still open. It will be important for APNs to take advantage of this opportunity.

OBSTACLES TO LEADERSHIP DEVELOPMENT AND EFFECTIVE LEADERSHIP

Professional and System Obstacles

There are several obstacles to achieving competence as an APN leader. Most of the obstacles result from conflict or competition among individuals, groups, or organizations. Professional turf issues have plagued APNs since the early days of their clinical practice. A lack of legal empowerment to practice to the fullest extent of knowledge and skills has been a dominant barrier to the optimal practice of NPs (Dempster, 1994). CNMs and CRNAs have the longest track record in dealing with these issues and have many successes to their credit. Competition can be both intraprofessional, as between APN groups, and interprofessional, as between physicians and nurses. Grensing-Pophal (1997) identified several barriers to good leadership and offered this advice: Being respected rather than being "liked" is one desired criterion for leadership; for most people, this is a difficult reality because being accepted and popular with others is important. Trying to "do it all" rather than delegating to others is a common trap that plagues busy leaders. As noted earlier, a good leader is able to encourage a shared workload that recognizes the talents and abilities of followers.

Horizontal Violence and Dysfunctional Leadership Styles

Horizontal violence in nursing is described as an aggressive act that is carried out by one nursing colleague toward another (Longo & Sherman, 2007).

This type of behavior is often seen among oppressed groups as a way for individuals to achieve a sense of power. Although there are many barriers to leading effectively and creating community, several constellations of behaviors that are particularly destructive have been identified. Nurses may be vulnerable to these destructive behaviors because of the profession's historical marginalization as a female and relatively powerless group within health care. The culture of an organization as described earlier is also a factor in the development of these dysfunctional styles. These behaviors undermine successful APN leadership. APNs must avoid engaging in such behaviors and intervene assertively when instances occur. Three manifestations of horizontal violence in workplace culture limit the ability of APNs to lead: the *star complex,* the *queen bee syndrome,* and *failure to mentor* ("eating one's young"). These behaviors are of particular concern when the profession needs to recruit and mentor younger nurses to help them create satisfying careers and pass on the legacy of a satisfying career to future generations of nurses. Faculty and advanced practice nursing preceptors need to be alert to the appearance of such behaviors in students and coach the students to understand their destructive impact on patients and colleagues. Readers are referred to the articles by King (2002), Rider (2002), Longo and Sherman (2007), and Bally (2007) for specific suggestions on strategies for communicating with students and colleagues who demonstrate these negative interpersonal styles.

Abandoning One's Nursing Identity: The Star Complex. An effective APN leader is proud of his or her identity as a nurse. Those with the star complex deny their nursing identity or minimize their affiliation with nursing when being identified as a nurse might diminish their influence (e.g., some nurse authors use only their academic credentials in publications within and outside of nursing). The star complex is a condition that is seen in some experienced APNs or in APNs who have not been well socialized into nursing as a profession. Although the psychology of this phenomenon is beyond the scope of this chapter, individuals with the star complex are those whose sense of self and identity depend a great deal on the opinions of powerful others. Acknowledging or promoting their identity as nurses is seen to diminish their power or the opinions powerful others hold about them. As an example, consider

Janice, an expert APN who provides superior patient-focused care. Physician colleagues considered her to be a partner in the delivery of care, but staff and other APNs gave up consulting with her because her self-promotion often interfered with patient and colleague interactions. In a recent conversation, a well-respected physician colleague told her how impressed he was with her practice. "In fact," he stated, "you're really not a nurse. You're different from all the other nurses I know." Janice graciously accepted this compliment, knowing that stardom, although overdue, had finally arrived. She had ascended to the heights of provider status and crashed through the nursing ceiling into a zone beyond nursing. Clearly, Janice's understanding of herself as an APN was dormant.

APNs are particularly vulnerable to being seduced into believing they are something other (more) than a nurse. Advanced practice nursing specialties that have expanded roles may seek the status of medicine. This vulnerability stems from the historical lack of recognition of nursing by physicians, other disciplines, and even other nurses; the need for approval; and a lack of personal mastery.

A primary strategy for the management of this obstacle is effective mentoring by a powerful APN with an intact nursing identity. An APN with the star complex may have been mentored exclusively by individuals outside of nursing. The affirmation of the APN's expert clinical skills and even personal mastery are thus validated by a reference group outside of nursing. An additional essential strategy is to use clear and concise communication skills to provide an appropriate response to a colleague who believes that it is a compliment to be identified as other than a nurse. An appropriate response for Janice to have made would have been, "Thank you, but I'm proud to be an APN. It is good that we can work together to help our patients." The existence of the star complex may represent a more fundamental problem for the APN than good communication skills can address. The issue is whether the APN truly desires to be identified as a nurse, performing at the boundaries of nursing practice and accepted by other nurses as a valued member of the nursing profession. As APNs are increasingly recognized as valued members of the health care team and as mentoring and empowerment become understood as core elements of leadership, star complex behavior will become unnecessary and less frequent.

Hoarding or Misusing Power: The Queen Bee Syndrome. An effective leader is generous, looking for opportunities to lift colleagues up by sharing opportunities, knowledge, and expertise and acknowledging the contributions of others. Queen bees hoard all of the visible leadership tasks for themselves. Like those with the star complex, the effort to garner power is a theme. In this case, power derives not from powerful others but from the queen bee's own knowledge and expertise. Such APNs are threatened by strong individuals and tend to denigrate them instead of sharing power. This type of leader prefers to be surrounded by servile individuals who will not challenge his or her authority. For example, Jackie, an experienced wound and ostomy APN, makes sure she sees every patient and that patients know she is the authority on wounds and ostomies. Staff nurses who are competent in these skills report that Jackie undermines them with patients by saying the care should have been done a certain way. Jackie was not happy when the staff on a surgical unit, who had tried unsuccessfully to involve her in a unit project, conducted a quality improvement project during which both physicians and patients identified some service delivery issues relative to ostomy care. These staff members had the support of an assertive new CNS and a nurse manager and, over time, slowly changed the way wound and ostomy services were managed.

The antidote to the queen bee syndrome is to use knowledge and expertise to move away from hoarding power toward collaborative, empowered leadership. Queen bee behavior is the antithesis of good leadership and, unfortunately, is not uncommon among women and nurses. As advanced practice nursing leaders become more confident in their leadership abilities and as more APNs join the circle of leaders, queen bees will have more difficulty remaining as leaders and keeping positions of stature. All effective leaders empower others.

Failure to Mentor. The most distressing form of horizontal violence is, unfortunately, the most common. "Nurses eat their young" is an epithet that characterizes the experience of many novice nurses and APNs, as well as of some older, experienced nurses (Baltimore, 2006). Nurses who advance in their profession may forget their roots and leave novice nurses behind or, worse, actively undermine their advancement. For example, nurses are often criticized by other nurses for continuing their education and moving into APN roles. This denigration of important values and goals by colleagues is dispiriting and discouraging; it can hamper nurses from moving forward in their careers. In another example, the orientation process for a new position may become a survival test to see whether the new APN can survive without mentoring or a supportive network. Because perceived powerlessness is at the root of this behavior, an important antidote is empowerment. The common practice of mentoring, apprenticing, and "giving a leg up" to the least experienced is not as common in nursing as it is in many other professions.

Failure to mentor may be evident in the following behaviors (Baltimore, 2006; Longo & Sherman, 2007):

- Gossiping or bad mouthing
- Criticizing
- Failure to give assistance when needed
- Setting up road blocks by withholding information
- Bullying
- Scapegoating
- Undermining performance

Bullying is a severe form of horizontal violence attributed to oppressed group behavior. Hutchinson, Vickers, Jackson, and Wilkes (2005), Longo and Sherman, (2007), and Keefe (2007) suggest that horizontal violence is a more complex phenomenon and includes those external to nursing who make up the organization's culture and add to stress in the work setting. Curran (2006) reports that with the baby boomer generation, there will be more career nurses vying for leadership positions and that forms of horizontal violence such as bullying will worsen. Bullying is not a one-time event but, instead, is a subtle, deliberate, ongoing behavior that accumulates over time and leaves the victim feeling hurt, vulnerable, and powerless (Hutchinson et al., 2005; Longo & Sherman, 2007).

Personal and organizational symptoms of horizontal violence are job dissatisfaction, increased stress levels, and physical and psychological illness. If the broader cause is a negative organizational culture, then the most effective leadership strategy to prevent its occurrence is to adopt a zero-tolerance policy and a shared set of values with the staff (Longo & Sherman, 2007) that support positive behaviors. For example, fostering mentoring opportunities and enhancing the transition of colleagues into new positions of leadership can create a positive culture that does not tolerate horizontal violence. See Box 9-6 for suggested leadership strategies to eliminate horizontal violence.

Negative behaviors that are expressed as failure to mentor, bullying, and disenfranchising others may continue to be present in an increasingly stressful health care environment (McAvoy & Murtagh, 2003; Thomas, 2003). It is not an overstatement to claim that the future health of the profession depends on overcoming this barrier and relegating it to history. It is the role of APN leaders as role models to create a more empowering and humane work environment for their colleagues and those who follow them (see the discussion of healthy work environments in Chapter 5).

STRATEGIES FOR IMPLEMENTING THE LEADERSHIP COMPETENCY

Developing a Leadership Portfolio

Throughout the chapter, definitions, attributes, and components of leadership and key strategies for developing competency in APN leadership have been presented. These approaches will help new APNs

---

Box 9-6 LEADERSHIP STRATEGIES TO STOP THE CYCLE OF HORIZONTAL VIOLENCE

- Examine the organizational culture for symptoms of horizontal violence.
- Name the problem as horizontal violence when you see it.
- Educate staff to break the silence.
- Allow victims of horizontal violence to tell their stories.
- Enact a process for dealing with issues that occur.

- Provide training for conflict and anger management skills.
- Empower victims to defend themselves.
- Engage in self-reflection to ensure that your leadership style does not support horizontal violence.
- Encourage a culture of zero tolerance for horizontal violence.

Adapted from Longo, J., & Sherman, R.O. (2007). Leveling horizontal violence. *Nursing Management, 38*(3), 34-37, 50-51.

acquire leadership skills. Developing a leadership component as part of a marketing portfolio is helpful to novice APNs who desire to individualize continuing development of the leadership competency consistent with their personal vision, goals, timeline, and APN role in the practice setting. Falter (2003) suggested the use of a strategy map that includes vision, goals, and objectives that outline steps to achieve a particular strategy. Portfolios are designed to meet the needs of individual APNs and should be consistent with clinical and personal interests and professional goals and provide a timeline that allows for personal and professional balance and boundary setting. Chapter 20 provides the elements of a marketing portfolio.

Promoting Collaboration Among Advanced Practice Nursing Specialties

At different times, each subgroup of APNs has emerged as a leader for the nursing profession. Psychiatric CNSs were among the first entrepreneurial APNs to hang out their shingles, despite the litigious climate in which they could be threatened with lawsuits for "practicing medicine." CNMs and CRNAs have led the way in using data effectively to justify their practice and attain appropriate scopes of practice. Early in their history, both groups began to record the results of their practices, showing the quality and suitability of their care (see Chapter 1). In the 1990s, NPs, with their flexible, community-based primary care practices, stood at the forefront of the changing health care delivery system. Although these subgroups of APNs have made impressive strides for advanced practice nursing, an obstacle to effective leadership is the tendency for APN specialty groups to separate and establish rigid boundaries that distinguish them from one another, thereby fragmenting APN groups and blocking opportunities for the increased power that unity would bring.

The tension and fragmentation created by rigid boundaries require leaders who can transcend APN roles and specialties. APNs must both manage and bridge boundaries among other nursing groups and within the ranks of the various APN constituencies. Although the uniqueness of each type of APN must be protected, a professional structure that provides a forum for discussing issues pertinent to all types of APNs also needs to be created. This structure may be simply an annual meeting for APNs, or it may be a permanent entity residing within an existing or new professional organization. Consensus groups at the national level are meeting to discuss policy issues in which the power of collective numbers of all APN groups speaking with one voice cannot be overemphasized (see Chapters 2, 10, and 21). APN specialty groups have joined to speak out collaboratively about state regulations regarding reimbursement, prescriptive authority, and managed care empanelment.

It is critical that each APN, regardless of specialty, take on the responsibility of moving toward an integrative and unified understanding of advanced practice nursing. Creating community in the current health care environment is particularly challenging because of the realignment of clinical decision making, scopes of practice for APNs and physicians, and new roles that blur boundaries between nursing and medicine.

An understanding of change, effective communication, coalition building, shared vision, and collaborative practice leads to the development of structures on which unity is built. These five building blocks form the foundation of interdisciplinary leadership and practice.

Motivating and Empowering Others

Motivation and empowerment are core elements of the APN leadership competency. Earlier in the chapter, empowerment was defined as the ability of the leader to give followers the freedom and authority to act. However, truly empowering others requires more than just giving them permission to act on their own. Empowerment is a developmental process; over time, a good leader encourages their constituents' sense of responsibility and competence, thus reinforcing their autonomy and authority to act. Wheatley affirms the importance of motivation and empowerment in developing innovators. She attests that older notions of power and control are things of the past, as does Senge (Senge, 2006; Wheatley, 2005). APN leaders of today need to use the tools of empowerment and motivation to mentor future leaders who can lead with creativity, innovation, and caring.

Networking

Networking is an essential technique used by leaders to stay informed and connected regarding APN issues. Networking, both formal and informal, is not a new strategy for APN leaders. Formal networks take the form of committees, coalitions, and consortia of people who come together to share information, collaborate, and plan strategy regarding mutual issues. Formal networks open doors to new opportunities and provide shared resources that ensure a competitive edge in the organization (Carroll, 2005). Informal networking is a behind-the-scenes strategy that allows for contact with APNs and others who "speak the same language," have the same viewpoints, and can offer support and feedback at critical times. The ability of APNs to stay connected to important practice and education issues through networking is key to the leadership competency. The most effective strategy for becoming an insider is networking with colleagues within the circle of APN peers and with other health care providers who have a stake in the outcomes of a particular issue.

Engaging Others in Planning and Implementing Change

The skills outlined in the "Attributes of Effective Advanced Practice Nurse Leaders" section on personal attributes of successful leaders (p. 263) are integral to leading innovation and change. However, other strategies also assist in the process. It is important to analyze the situation and explore the need for change. If change is warranted, one must craft an implementation plan that involves everyone. Box 9-1 provides a list of leadership strategies that are useful for moving through these transitions. Bonalumi and Fisher (1999) suggested that an important component of leadership during times of change is the ability to foster and encourage resilience in change recipients. O'Connell (1999) defined the characteristics of resilient people as follows: being positive and self-assured in the face of life's complexities; having a focused, clear vision of what they want to achieve; and having the abilities to be organized but flexible and proactive rather than reactive. Helping colleagues and followers develop resilience should be a major focus for advanced practice nursing leaders who seek to facilitate the growth of their followers.

The second DNP Essential for advanced nursing practice education addresses the provision of sophisticated leadership that "emphasizes practice, ongoing improvement of health outcomes and ensuring patient safety"; to accomplish these goals, APNs will need "expertise in assessing organizations, identifying systems issues and facilitating

organization-wide changes in practice delivery" (AACN, 2006, p. 10).

Institutional Assessment

With the emphasis on evidence-based practice and the knowledge that evidence-based guidelines and therapies are underused (IOM, 2001; McGlynn et al., 2003), overused, or misused (IOM, 2001), APNs have an important systems leadership role in improving care. This can be accomplished by leading and collaborating with nurses and interdisciplinary colleagues to ensure the adoption of best practices (Duffy, 2002; Spencer & Jordan, 2001; Spross & Heaney, 2000). An institutional assessment of specific factors will help the APN identify facilitators of and barriers to change. These data can then be used to design a plan for change in collaboration with others. Box 9-7 lists key assessment questions to consider.

SUMMARY

The health care system is constantly changing. Despite the challenges of change, the future is bright for APNs as clinical, professional, and systems leaders. APNs can define the scope of their leadership influence in far-reaching ways, from the bedside to the White House. The evolution of APNs in all the various roles has had significant influence on this country's health care system, as well as on nursing itself—at every level. APNs exercise leadership when they present ideas or dilemmas and offer solutions to colleagues, whether on an electronic mailing list or at a national meeting. As Gladwell (2000) noted, many small changes contribute to a big change, so APNs should not underestimate the impact of leadership exercised at the bedside or in the clinic and with patients, colleagues, and administrators. It is important for all APNs to consider the ways in which they can lead, make a difference, and commit to doing so, knowing that they can redefine the scope of their leadership influence in response to opportunities or changing life circumstances.

Nursing care is based on an interactive style that empowers patients and colleagues. This foundation holds APN leaders in good stead as they move into the interdisciplinary paradigm of the future. As APNs contemplate the demands and opportunities for leadership that the future holds, they must work toward identifying, clarifying, and demystifying the health care system of today, for within today's reality lies the basis of tomorrow's change. APNs are change specialists who operate at the boundary between

Box 9-7   Institutional Assessment Questions

- What is the nature of the change (e.g., a policy, procedure, new skill or behavior)?
- Is the issue significant? For all stakeholders or just one group?
- Is a national policy, guideline, or standard the focus of the change? Is it a mandate with which the agency must be in compliance?
- Is the change simple or complex? Will different stakeholders perceive its simplicity or complexity differently?
- Do you foresee major problems associated with change, such as an increase in errors or resistance on the part of a group?
- Will it be possible to address these major problems?

- Are there vested interests—who is likely to gain from the change, who will view the change as a loss (e.g., of power)?
- Are there opinion leaders who will promote the change? Do you anticipate strong opposition?
- Have you observed a gap between public statements and private actions? (For example, a colleague agrees to serve on a committee but never shows up or participates in the committee's work.)
- Are there resource implications? What are the costs (e.g., staffing, materials, lost revenue)?

Adapted from The University of York National Health Centre for Reviews and Dissemination. (1999). Getting evidence into practice. *Effective Health Care Bulletin, 5*(1): 1-16.

today's health care system and tomorrow's. Kerfoot (2005) suggested it will take the ability to "pay attention" in ways never done before to manage change effectively. In a health care future that is fraught with instability, past success of a leader, especially in traditional hierarchical settings, may not be a good predictor of future leadership success. "The 21st century may need new methods and new criteria for developing and selecting leaders" (Carroll, 2005, p. 152). The attributes and goals of APNs put them at the forefront of this leadership frontier.

REFERENCES

Allen, D.W. (1998). How nurses become leaders: Perceptions and beliefs about leadership development. *Journal of Nursing Administration, 28,* 15-20.

American Association of Colleges of Nursing (AACN). (2004). *Position statement on the practice doctorate in nursing.* Washington, DC: Author.

American Association of Colleges of Nursing (AACN). (2006). *The essentials of doctoral education for advanced nursing practice.* Washington, DC: Author

Ballein, K.M. (1998). Entrepreneurial leadership characteristics of Senior Nurse Executives [SNEs] emerge as their role develops. *Nursing Administration Quarterly, 22,* 60-69.

Bally, J.M.G. (2007). The role of nursing leadership in creating a mentoring culture in acute care environments. *Nursing Economic$, 25*(3), 143-148.

Baltimore, J. (2006). Nurse collegiality: Fact or fiction. *Nursing management, 37*(5), 28-36.

Barker, A. (1994). An energy leadership paradigm: Transformational leadership. In E.I. Hein & M.J. Nicholson (Eds.), *Contemporary leadership* (4 ed., pp. 81-86). Philadelphia: Lippincott.

Barker E.R. (2006). Mentoring: A complex relationship. *Journal of the American Academy of Nurse Practitioners, 18*(2), 56-61.

Bonalumi, N., & Fisher, K. (1999). Health care change: Challenge for nurse administrators. *Nursing Administration Quarterly, 23,* 69-73.

Brown, S.J. (1989). Supportive supervision of the CNS. In A.B. Hamric & J.A. Spross (Eds.), *The clinical nurse specialist in theory and practice* (2nd ed., pp. 285-298). Philadelphia: Saunders.

Cain, M., & Mittman, R. (2002). *Diffusion of innovation in health care.* Retrieved November 21, 2007, from http://www.chcf.org/documents/ihealth/Diffusion of Innovation.pdf.

Callahan M., & Ruchlin, H. (2003). The role of nursing leadership in establishing a safety culture. *Nursing Economic$, 21*(6), 296.

Carroll, T.L. (2005). Leadership skills and attributes of women and nurse executives: Challenges for the 21st century. *Nursing Administration Quarterly, 29*(2), 146-153.

Christopher, M.A., Miller, J., Beck, T., & Toughill, E. (2002). Working with the community for change. In D. Mason, J. Leavitt, & M. Chaffee (Eds.), *Policy and politics in nursing and health care* (4 ed., pp. 933-946). Philadelphia: Saunders.

Collins, J. (2001). *Good to great: Why some companies make the leap . . . (and others don't).* New York: Harper Business.

Collins, J. (2005). *Good to great and the social sectors: A monograph to accompany Good to Great.* Boulder, CO: Jim Collins.

Covey, S. (1989). *The seven habits of highly effective people: Powerful lessons in personal change.* New York: Simon & Schuster.

Covey, S. (2006). Leading in the knowledge worker age. *Leader to Leader Journal, 41,* 11-15.

Curran, C. (2006). Boomers: Bottlenecked, bored, and burned out. *Nursing Economic$, 24*(2), 57, 93.

Davis, L.L., Little, M.S., & Thornton, W.L. (1997). The art and angst of the mentoring relationship. *Academic Psychiatry, 21,* 61-71.

Dempster, J.S. (1994). Autonomy: A professional issue of concern for nurse practitioners. *Nurse Practitioner Forum, 5,* 227-232.

DePree, M. (1989). *Leadership is an art.* New York: Doubleday/Currency.

deVries, C.M., & Vanderbilt, M.W. (1992). *The grassroots lobbying handbook: Empowering nurses through legislative and political action.* Washington, DC: American Nurses Association.

Doumit, G., Gattellari, M., Grimshaw, J., & O'Brien, M. (2007). Local opinion leaders: Effects on professional practice and health care outcomes. [Electronic Version]. *Cochrane Database of Systematic Reviews.* Retrieved August 12, 2007 from http://www.cochrane.org/reviews/en/ab000125.html.

Duffy, J.R. (2002). The clinical leadership role of the CNS in the identification of nursing-sensitive and multidisciplinary quality indicator sets. *Clinical Nurse Specialist, 16*(2), 70-76.

Engebretson, J., & Wardell, D.W. (1997). The essence of partnership in research. *Journal of Professional Nursing, 13*(1), 38-47.

Falk-Rafael, A. (2005). Speaking truth to power: Nursing's legacy and moral imperative. *Advances in Nursing Science, 28*(3), 212.

Falter, E. (2003). Successful leaders map and measure. *Nurse Leader, 1*(4), 40-42, 45.

Fawcett, D. (2002). Mentoring: What it is and how to make it work. *AORN Journal, 75,* 950-954.

Fiedler, F.E., Chermers, M.M., & Mahar, L.C. (1976). *Improving leadership effectiveness: The leader match concept.* New York: John Wiley & Sons.

Fisher, R., Ury, W., & Patton, B. (2002). *Getting to yes: How to negotiate an agreement without giving in* (2nd ed.). New York: Penguin Putnam.

Friedman, T.L. (2006). *The world is flat* (expanded and updated). New York: Farrar, Straus, & Giroux.

Giger, J., Davidhizar, R., Purnell, L., Taylor-Harden, J., Phillips, J., & Strickland, O. (2007). Understanding cultural language to enhance cultural competence. *Nursing Outlook, 55*(4), 212-213.

Gladwell, M. (2000). *The tipping point: How little things can make a big difference.* New York: Little Brown.

Greenhalgh, T., Robert, G., Macfarlane, F., Bate, P., & Kyriakidou, O. (2004). Diffusion of innovation in service organizations: Systematic review and recommendations. *The Millbank Quarterly, 82,* 581-629.

Greiner, A., & Knebel, E. (Eds.). (2003). *Health professions education: A bridge to quality.* Washington, DC: Institute of Medicine.

Grensing-Pophal, L. (1997). Improving your leadership skills: Seven common pitfalls to avoid. *Nursing, 27,* 41-42.

Grohar-Murray, M.E., & DiCroce, H.R. (1992). *Leadership and management in nursing.* Norwalk, CT: Appleton & Lange.

Grossman, D. (2006). *Fostering leadership through collaboration: Move over physicians. Nurses belong on health care boards too,* Third Quarter 2006, Sigma Theta Tau International. Retrieved October 2, 2006, from www.nursingsociety.org.

Halpern, I.M. (2002). Reflections of a health policy advocate: The natural extension of nursing activities. *Oncology Nursing Forum, 29,* 1261-1263.

Hanson, C.M., Boyle, J., Hatmaker, D., & Murray, J. (1999). *Finding your voice as a leader.* Washington, DC: American Academy of Nursing.

Hassmiller, S. (1995). *Legislative logistics for leaders.* Washington, DC: Health Resources and Services Administration.

HealthSciences Institute. (2005). *Chronic care competency model.* Chicago, IL. Author. Retrieved August 21, 2007 from www.chroniccare.org/documents/FullCCPCompetencyModel.pdf.

Heifetz, R. (1994). *Leadership without easy answers.* Cambridge, MA: Belknap Press.

Houghton, A. (2003). Bullying in medicine. *British Medical Journal, 326,* S125.

Hutchinson, M., Vickers, M., Jackson, D., & Wilkes, L. (2005). Workplace bullying in nursing: Toward a more critical organizational perspective. *Nursing Inquiry, 13*(2), 118-126.

Institute for Healthcare Improvement (IHI). (2007). *Protecting 5 million lives.* Retrieved August 12, 2007, from www.ihi.org.

Institute of Medicine (IOM). (2000). *To err is human: Building a safer health system.* Washington, DC: National Academy Press.

Institute of Medicine (IOM). (2001). *Crossing the quality chasm: A new health system for the 21st century.* Washington, DC: National Academy Press.

The Joint Commission (TJC). (2000). *Joint Commission focuses on pain management.* Retrieved April 7, 2004, from www.jcaho.org.

Kantor, R.M., Stein, B.A., & Jick, T.D. (1992). *The challenge of organizational change: How companies experience it and leaders guide it.* New York: The Free Press.

Keefe, S. (2007). Bullying among nurses. *Advance for Nurses, July 16,* 36-38.

Kendig, S. (2006). *Advocacy, action, and the allure of butter: A focus on policy.* Medscape article 523631. Retrieved July 18, 2007, from www.medscape.com/viewarticle/523631.

Kerfoot, K. (2005). On leadership: Attending, questioning, and quality. *Medsurg Nursing, 14*(4), 263-266.

Kerfoot, K., & Chaffee, M.W. (2007). Ten keys to unlock policy change in the workplace. In D.J. Mason, J.K. Leavitt, & M.W. Chaffee (Eds.), *Policy and politics in nursing and health care* (pp. 482-484). Philadelphia: Saunders.

Kimball, B. (2005). *Cultural transformation in health care.* Princeton, NJ: The Robert Wood Johnson Foundation. http://www.rwjf.org/files/publications/Nursing Cultural Trans.pdf.

King, J. (2002). Dealing with difficult doctors. *British Medical Journal, 325,* S43.

Klein, E., Gabelnick, F., & Herr, P. (1998). *The psychodynamics of leadership.* Madison, CT: Psychosocial Press.

Larson, L. (2004). Telling the story: Trustees and grassroots political advocacy. *Trustee, 57*(7), 6-11.

Leavitt, J.K., Chaffee, M.W., & Vance, C. (2007). Learning the ropes of policy, politics, and advocacy. In D.J. Mason, J.K. Leavitt, & M.W. Chaffee (Eds.), *Policy and politics in nursing and health Care* (5 ed.). Philadelphia; Saunders

Lencioni, P. (2005). *Overcoming the five dysfunctions of a team: A field guide for leaders, managers, and facilitators.* San Francisco: Jossey-Bass.

Locock, L., Dopson, S., Chambers, D., & Gabbay, J. (2001). Understanding the role of opinion leaders in improving clinical effectiveness. *Social Science and Medicine, 53*, 745-757.

Longo, J., & Sherman, R.O. (2007). Leveling horizontal violence, *Nursing Management, 38*(3), 34-37, 50-51.

Malone, P., & Chafee, M. (2007). Interest groups: Powerful political catalysts in health care. In D.J. Mason, J.K. Leavitt, & M. Chaffee (Eds.), *Policy and politics in nursing and health care* (5 ed., pp. 766-770). Philadelphia: Saunders.

Massoud M.R., Nielsen G.A., Nolan K., Schall M.W., & Sevin C. (2006). *A framework for spread: From local improvements to system-wide change.* IHI Innovation Series white paper. Cambridge, MA: Institute for Healthcare Improvement. Retrieved August 12, 2007, from www.ihi.org/IHI/Results/WhitePapers/AFrameworkforSpreadWhitePaper.htm.

McAvoy, B., & Murtagh, J. (2003). Workplace bullying: The silent epidemic (Letter). *British Medical Journal, 326*, 776-777.

McGlynn, E.A., Asch, S.M., Adams, J., Keesey, J., Hicks, J., DeCristofaro, A., et al. (2003). The quality of health care delivered to adults in the United States. *New England Journal of Medicine, 348*(26), 2635-2645.

National Association of Clinical Nurse Specialists (NACNS). (2004). *Statement on clinical nurse specialist practice and education.* Harrisburg, PA: Author.

National Organization of Nurse Practitioner Faculties (NONPF) & The American Association of Colleges of Nursing (AACN). (2002). *Nurse practitioner primary care competencies in specialty areas: Adult, family, gerontological, pediatric, and women's health.* Washington, DC: U.S. Department of Health and Human Services. (HRSA Contract 00-0532[P])

Nelson, E.C., Batalden. P.B., Huber, T.P., Mohr, J.J., Godfrey, M.M., Headrick, L.A., et al. (2002). Microsystems in health care: Part I. Learning from high-performing front-line clinical units, *Journal on Quality Improvement, 28*, 472-493.

Nolan, T., Resar, R., Haraden, C., & Griffin, F.A. (2004). *Improving the reliability of healthcare.* Cambridge, MA: Institute for Healthcare Improvement.

Norton, S.F., & Grady, E.M. (1996). Change agent skills. In A. B. Hamric, J.A. Spross, & C.M. Hanson (Eds.), *Advanced nursing practice: An integrative approach* (pp. 249-271). Philadelphia: Saunders.

O'Connell, C. (1999). A culture of change or a change of culture. *Nursing Administration Quarterly, 23*, 65-68.

Oxman, A.D., Thomson, M.A., Davis, D.A., & Haynes, R.B. (1995). No magic bullets: A systematic review of 102 trials of interventions to improve professional practice. *Canadian Medical Association Journal, 153*, 1423-1431.

Patient Safety and Quality Health Care. (2005). IHI launches national campaign to save 100,000 lives in U.S. hospitals. Retrieved August 12, 2007, from www.ihi.org.

Peters, P.M. (2002). Nurse administrators' role in health care policy: Teaching the elephant to dance. *Nursing Administration Quarterly, 26*, 1-8.

Rajotte, C.A. (1996). Empowerment as a leadership theory. *Kansas Nurse, 71*, 1.

Reinertsen, J., Gosfield, A., Rupp, W., & Whittington, J. (2007). *Engaging physicians in a shared quality agenda.* Cambridge, MA: Institute for Healthcare Improvement.

Rider, E. (2002). Twelve strategies for effective communication and collaboration in medical teams. *British Medical Journal, 325*, S45.

Rost, J.C. (1993). *Leadership for the 21st century.* Westport, CT: Praeger.

Rutherford, P., Lee, B., & Greiner, A. (2004). Transforming care at the bedside. Retrieved June 24, 2007, from www.ihi.org.

Sandrick, K. (2006). The new political advocacy. *Trustee, 59*(7), 6-10.

Sarikonda-Woitas, C. (2002). Ethical health care policy: Nursing's voice in allocation. *Nursing Administration Quarterly, 26*, 72-80.

Secretan, L. (1999). *Inspirational leadership: Destiny, cause and calling.* Canada: the Secretan Center.

Secretan, L. (2003). *Reclaiming higher ground: Creating organizations that inspire the soul.* Canada: the Secretan Center.

Secretan, L. (2004). *Inspire: What great leaders do.* Canada: The Secretan Center.

Senge, P. (1990). *The Fifth Discipline: The art and practice of the learning organization.* New York: Doubleday.

Senge, P. (2006). *The Fifth Discipline: The art and practice of the learning organization* (revised edition). New York: Currency/Doubleday.

Senge, P., Kleiner, A., Roberts, C., Ross, R., Roth, G., & Smith, B. (1999). *The dance of change: The challenges of sustaining momentum in learning organizations.* New York: Doubleday/Currency.

Shirey, M.R. (2004). Social support in the workplace: Nurse leader implications, *Nursing Economic$, 22*(6), 313-319.

Shirey, M.R. (2007). AONE leadership perspectives. Competencies and tips for effective leadership: from novice to expert. *Journal of Nursing Administration, 37*(4), 167-170.

Shortell, S.M., Bennet, C.L., & Byk, G.R. (1998). Assessing the impact of continuous quality improvement on clinical practice: What will it take to accelerate progress. *The Milbank Quarterly, 76*(4), 593-624.

Soumerai, S.B., McLaughlin, T.J., Gurwitz, J.H., Guadagnoli, E., Hauptman, P.J., Borbas, C., et al. (1998). Effect of local medical opinion leaders on quality of care for acute myocardial infarction: A randomized controlled trial. *JAMA: The Journal of the American Medical Association, 279*, 1358-1363.

Spencer, J., & Jordan, R. (2001). Educational outcomes and leadership to meet the needs of modern health care. *Quality and Safety in Health Care, 10*(Suppl. 2), 38-45.

Spross, J.A. (2001). Harnessing power and passion: Lessons from pain management leaders and literature. *Innovations in End-of-Life Care, 3*(1). Retrieved August 12, 2007, from www.edc.org/lastacts.

Spross, J.A., & Heaney, C.A. (2000). Shaping advanced nursing practice in the new millennium. *Seminars in Oncology Nursing, 16*(1), 12-24.

Stogdill, R.M. (1948). Personal factors associated with leadership in a survey of the literature. *Journal of Psychology, 25,* 35-71.

Thomas, S.P. (2003). Anger: The mismanaged emotion. *Dermatology Nurse, 15*(4), 351-357.

Thomson, M.A., Oxman, A.D., Haynes, R.B., Davis, D.A., Freemantle, N., & Harvey, E.L. (1999). *Local opinion leaders to improve health professional practice and health care outcomes.* Oxford: The Cochrane Library.

Tornabeni, J. (1996). Changes in the advanced practice of administration: A personal perspective of the changes affecting the role. *Advanced Practice Nursing Quarterly, 2,* 62-66.

Tourigny, L., & Pulich, M. (2005). A critical examination of formal and informal mentoring among nurses. *The Health Care Manager, 24*(1), 68-76.

Trent, B.A. (2003). Leadership myths. *Reflections on Nursing Leadership, 29*(3), 8.

The University of York National Health Service Centre for Reviews and Dissemination. (1999). Getting evidence into practice. *Effective Health Care Bulletin, 5*(1), 1-16.

Vance, C. (2003). Mentoring at the edge of chaos. *Nurse Leader,* 42-43.

Vance, C., & Larson, E. (2002). Leadership research in business and health care. *Journal of Nursing Scholarship, 34,*165-171.

Wagner L.M., Capezuti E., & Ouslander J.G. (2006). Reporting near-miss events in nursing homes. *Nursing Outlook, 54*(2), 85-93.

Wakefield, M.K. (2003). Change drivers for nursing and health care. *Nursing Economic$, 21,* 150-151.

Wheatley, M.J. (2005). *Finding our way: Leadership for uncertain times.* San Francisco: Berrett-Koehler.

Winterfeldt, E. (2001). Influencing public policy. *Topics in Clinical Nutrition, 16,* 8-16.

Zaccaro, S.J. (2007). Trait-based perspectives of leadership. *American Psychologist. 62*(1), 6-16.

Zaccaro, S.J., Kemp, C., & Bader, P. (2004). In J. Antonakis, A.T. Cianciolo, & R.J. Sternberg (Eds.), *The nature of leadership* (p. 122). Thousand Oaks, CA: Sage.

Collaboration

Charlene M. Hanson • Judith A. Spross

INTRODUCTION

Collaboration works. This simple statement belies the complexity of the phenomenon and the significant interpersonal commitment involved in building collaborative relationships. Broome (2007) suggests that "magic happens" as each individual in a collaborative group brings his or her unique perspective and skill to bear on a problem. Readers who have experienced this "magic" know exactly what Broome means. Her characterization of collaboration as magic illuminates the elusiveness of this particular process. The fact that good collaboration feels like magic speaks to the complexity of this competency and the relative dearth of research on a process that is essential to quality care. Our goal is to define collaboration and to try to make more explicit the values, behaviors, structures, and processes we believe facilitate effective collaboration—the "magic"—so that advanced practice nurses (APNs) can implement this core APN competency and demonstrate the impact of this process on patient and institutional outcomes.

The presence or absence of collaborative relationships affects patient care. Patients assume that their health care providers communicate and collaborate effectively. Patient dissatisfaction with care, unsatisfactory clinical outcomes, and clinician frustration can often be traced to a failure to collaborate. Collaboration depends on clinical and interpersonal expertise and an understanding of factors that can promote or impede efforts to establish collegial relationships. The primary focus of this chapter is on collaboration between and among individuals and work groups within organizations and across larger health care delivery systems.

A paradox of the contemporary health care system is that both incentives and disincentives exist for members of different disciplines, work groups, and organizations to collaborate. Incentives and disincentives may be equally powerful, so that motivation to collaborate can be diminished or eliminated by a compelling counterforce. An understanding of this paradox can help APNs and their colleagues approach opportunities for collaboration strategically and build and sustain clinical environments that support collaboration. Numerous clinical initiatives aimed at improving quality and safety, the need to eliminate health care inequities, and an increasing proportion of non-physician health care professionals underscore that interdisciplinary collaboration at educational, clinical, and institutional levels is essential (American College of Graduate Medical Education, 2002; Cramer, 2002; Disch, 2002; Lindeke, 2005; Zwarenstein & Reeves, 2002). In fact, the ability to collaborate is essential if future APNs are to implement interdisciplinary practice models and to analyze complex health problems in an interactive environment (American Association of Colleges of Nursing [AACN], 2006).

Research, although far from definitive, supports the premise that collaboration results in better patient outcomes, including patient satisfaction, and provides personal and professional satisfaction for clinicians. APNs must have or acquire interpersonal communication skills and behaviors that make collaboration possible among a broad range of professionals and patients.

Historically, discussions about collaboration in the health field have focused on the relationship between physicians and nurses because that is where the most serious tensions have occurred. However, it is increasingly important that any discussion of collaborative relationships address intradisciplinary collaboration among nurses, collaboration between nurses and members of other disciplines, and collaboration among work groups and agencies.

Although collaboration is recognized by many as central to improving the quality and effectiveness of health care, publications about implementing collaborative processes have not kept pace with the number of national initiatives that require effective collaboration. Only a few publications that address interdisciplinary collaboration (particularly with physicians) and advanced practice specifically have appeared since the last edition. However, important ideas about collaboration from thought leaders in other disciplines inform this discussion of collaboration. The absence of a growing body of literature on collaboration, as well as organized efforts to discredit APNs at a time when national initiatives related to quality and safety have been undertaken, are of serious concern because of the negative effects of failure to collaborate on patients and clinicians. In addition to updating the literature, our aim is to help readers understand what collaboration "looks like" in practice, to strengthen this competency in their practices, to enhance their leadership of collaborative teams and initiatives, and to increase the motivation of clinicians and institutions to adopt structures and processes that support the collaboration competency.

A CONCEPTUALIZATION OF COLLABORATION

In this section we cover domains of collaboration, our definition of collaboration and its background, assumptions we make about the collaboration competency, and other less-sophisticated interactive processes that are frequently confused with collaboration.

Domains of Collaboration in Advanced Practice Nursing

APNs execute the collaboration competency in several domains—between or among individuals, work groups, and organizations. The collaboration competency is often executed at the same time as other competencies, as the description of the domains illustrates. It is a dynamic competency, shifting as the particulars of a situation change.

Collaboration with Individuals. Collaboration with patients, families, and colleagues in the delivery of direct care is the primary domain in which collaboration is practiced. For example, in forming partnerships with patients (see Chapter 5), APNs aim to understand how the patient wants to work with the APN and other providers. APNs collaborate with patients when they set and revise goals and determine barriers to adherence—such activities are aimed at uncovering a common purpose, a hallmark of collaboration. APNs also collaborate with individual clinicians. For example, the diabetes clinical nurse specialist (CNS) may collaborate with the cardiac CNS and a staff nurse to determine who will do which aspects of patient education for a patient. The collaborative process may include determining the

order and timing of content to be taught. In this case, the APN is also executing the direct care (interacting with the patient to assess learning needs) and coaching (coaching the staff nurse in the diabetes content) competencies.

Collaboration with Teams/Groups. Another common domain in which APNs implement collaboration is in their work with clinical teams and on departmental and institutional committees. Such groups may comprise individuals from one or more disciplines. A key function of the collaborative competency is the facilitation of teamwork to ensure the delivery of effective, high-quality care. The literature and our experience suggest that APNs play key roles in facilitating and leading interdisciplinary teams. As APNs become more experienced, their skill in facilitating collaboration in groups grows. Thus APNs often lead interdisciplinary performance improvement teams, an activity that requires integration of the collaboration and leadership competencies (see Chapters 9 and 25).

Collaboration in the Organizational and Policy Arenas. In this domain, the focus of collaboration extends beyond the delivery of care to individuals and groups. The organizational and policy forces shaping advanced practice nursing and clinical care require that even novice APNs attend to collaboration in this area. Initiatives aimed at clarifying credentialing requirements, making it easier to practice across state lines, and improving reimbursement for APNs require APNs to use their status as clinicians, citizens, and members of professional organizations to collaborate with organizational leaders and policymakers.

Collaboration in Global Arenas. Global or international collaboration is becoming an essential collaborative domain within the APN collaboration competency. Friedman (2005) argued that global communication and collaboration will be the keys to successful living, working, and economic success over the next century—we believe this is true for health care. There is evidence that globalization is already affecting practice—the APN covering the emergency room at night may be communicating with a radiologist in Australia about a diagnostic image that was sent electronically to be interpreted in "real time." In addition, APNs' experiences with volunteerism in other countries (e.g., Doctors without Borders) are shaping APN goals and opportunities.

Definition of Collaboration

Some background on our definition of collaboration is warranted. When we began writing about collaboration, extant definitions of collaboration were inadequate to describe the process we experienced as clinicians (Hanson & Spross, 1996; Spross, 1989). According to the dictionary, collaboration means "to work together, especially in a joint intellectual effort"; it also means to cooperate with the enemy (McKechnie, 1983). The term *collaboration* is often associated with teamwork and partnership. The description of collaboration in the American Nurses Association's (ANA's) *Social Policy Statement* (American Nurses Association [ANA], 1995, 2003) and the American College of Nurse-Midwives' (ACNMs') definitions of collaboration, consultation, and referral (American College of Nurse-Midwives [ACNM], 1997; see also Chapters 7 and 16) have informed our conceptualization and definition of collaboration. The ANA recognized that the boundaries of each health care professional's practice change and that high-quality care depends on a common focus, a recognition of each other's expertise, an appreciation for the skills and knowledge shared across disciplines, and the collegial exchange of ideas and knowledge. Yet none of these meanings in these resources adequately represented the concept of collaboration as it exists or should exist in the provision of health and illness care.

On the basis of a review of the literature and our experiences, we developed this definition of collaboration as a dynamic, interpersonal process for the first edition (Hanson & Spross, 1996):

> Collaboration is a dynamic, interpersonal process in which two or more individuals make a commitment to each other to interact authentically and constructively to solve problems and to learn from each other to accomplish identified goals, purposes, or outcomes. The individuals recognize and articulate the shared values that make this commitment possible. (Hanson & Spross, 1996, p. 232).

This definition captures the complexity and challenge of collaboration and affirms that collaborators are interdependent in setting and achieving goals (Hughes & Mackenzie, 1990; Tjosvold, 1986). Characterizing collaboration as an interaction is intended to convey both the communicative and behavioral aspects of this competency. Our definition implies partnership, shared values, commitment, and goals and yet allows for differences in opinions and approaches. It also acknowledges that collaboration requires individuals to interact holistically (strengths, weaknesses, emotions) and authentically, to share power, and to remain open to the possibilities for personal and professional transformation that exist within a collaborative relationship. Including the notions of shared values and commitment makes it clear that collaboration is a process that evolves over time. Collaboration engages the head, the heart, and the will (Senge, Scharmer, Jaworski, & Flowers, 2004). These three "thresholds" are the essence of collaboration and are consistent with our definition.

The ability to commit to authentic and constructive interaction suggests that prospective partners must bring certain characteristics and qualities to initial and ongoing encounters. To interact authentically means that partners do not leave some part of themselves behind. For example, partners share the emotional satisfactions and frustrations of clinical work and develop ways of supporting each other. Although not discussed in the literature, we have observed that successful collaboration can lead to an intimacy that arises from working closely together over time. In her sixth year in a collaborative practice, one nurse practitioner (NP) compared the relationship to a marriage in terms of the interpersonal ups and downs that occurred and the challenge of dealing with the same person daily over matters of great or negligible, albeit clinical, import. Thus mature collaboration can be both rewarding and challenging. This phenomenon has been characterized in the business literature as having an "office spouse" (Weiss, 2007).

By definition, collaboration describes relationships that are positive and work well for professionals and patients. There is room for disagreement in collaborative relationships; partners develop strategies for dealing with disagreement that are mutually satisfactory and enhance collaboration. The other types of interactions described in the following sections do not always require collaboration as it is described here, although a collaborative relationship is likely to enhance many of these interactions. It is important to note that collaboration is an interpersonal and developmental process that demands a fairly sophisticated level of communication; collaboration cannot be mandated.

Collaboration: What It Is Not

Collaboration can be thought of as one of several modes of interaction that occur between and among clinicians during the delivery of care—it is probably the most sophisticated and complicated interaction that occurs in practice. In addition to collaboration, we have observed other interactions between clinicians in practice. We assume that these interactions represent a hierarchy that proceeds from simple to complex and from less effective to more effective. Thus parallel communication may be the simplest form of communication but is likely to be the least effective for facilitating optimal outcomes, and collaboration is the most complex and most effective:

Parallel communication: Providers interact with a patient separately; they do not talk together before seeing a patient, nor do they see the patient together. There is no expectation of joint interactions. For example, the staff registered nurse, the medical student, and the attending physician all ask the patient about his or her medications. In this example, the three different interactions are burdensome, if not frustrating, to the patient. At best, the patient is inconvenienced; at worst, an error may occur because each clinician elicits different information and subsequent clinical decisions are made on information that may be incomplete or inaccurate.

Parallel functioning: Providers care for patients, addressing the same clinical problem, but do not engage in any joint or collaborative planning. For example, nurses, physical therapists, and physicians document their interventions for pain in separate parts of the patient record. The effect of such interactions is the same as for parallel communication.

Information exchange: Informing may be one-sided or two-sided and may or may not require action or decision making. If action is needed, the decision is unilateral—not a result of joint planning. Information exchange may be sufficient and exert a neutral or beneficial effect on care processes and outcomes. If the situation actually requires joint planning and decision making, then there is a risk of miscommunication.

Coordination: Structures communication and actions to minimize duplication of effort. The charge nurse role is an example.

Consultation: The clinician who is caring for a patient seeks advice regarding a patient concern but retains primary responsibility for care delivery (see Chapter 7).

Co-management: Two or more clinicians provide care, and each professional retains accountability and responsibility for defined aspects of care. This process usually arises from consultation in which a problem requires management that is outside the scope of practice of the referring clinician (see Chapters 7 and 16). Providers must be explicit with each other about their responsibilities. Co-management may also be a process used by interdisciplinary teams.

Referral: The APN directs the patient to a physician or another practitioner for management of a particular problem or aspect of the patient's care when the problem is beyond the APN's expertise (see Chapter 7).

With the exceptions of parallel communication and parallel functioning, the processes just described require some level of interaction and communication among providers but may not involve collaboration. For particular situations, information exchange, coordination, consultation, co-management, and referral may be sufficient for the purposes of achieving clinical goals. For these processes to work to benefit patients and minimize errors, clinicians must engage in effective and timely communication. By comparing these types of communication with our definition of collaboration, readers should be able to appreciate the complexity of collaboration and the exquisite interpersonal skills needed to be a collaborator.

Types of Collaboration: Multidisciplinary, Interdisciplinary, Transdisciplinary

The terms *multidisciplinary, interdisciplinary,* and *transdisciplinary* collaboration are often used interchangeably. We believe there are subtle but important differences among these terms—that the prefix actually indicates the level and depth of interactions to which the term refers. The differences were best expressed in early work by Garland, McGonigel, Frank, and Buck (1989). A key difference among the terms is reflected in the philosophy of team interaction. In a multidisciplinary team, the philosophy of team interaction is a simple recognition of the importance of contributions of other disciplines. In an interdisciplinary team, members willingly share responsibility for providing care or services to patients. In a transdisciplinary team, members are committed to teaching each other, learning from each other, and working across boundaries to plan and provide integrated services to clients (Garland, McConigel, Frank, & Buck).

We believe APNs should aspire and help teams achieve transdisciplinary collaboration. According to Kuhlman (2005), the first use of the term *transdisciplinary* was attributed to Dorothy Hutchinson; transdisciplinary teams share information, knowledge, and skills across disciplinary boundaries. This notion of transcending boundaries is reflected in more recent philosophical work (Boix, Mansilla, & Gardner, 2003; Nowotny, 2001) on transdisciplinary knowledge. Transdisciplinary work fosters the development of new understandings and new fields of inquiry, and in clinical care, we propose that this level of interaction leads to new insights in interpretation of assessments and creative and effective clinical problem solving.

There is a heightened urgency to ensure that collaboration occurs. We believe that efforts to transform the health care system to improve reliability of care, safety, quality, efficiency, and cost-effectiveness will fail if clinicians, teams, and administrators do not undertake the important collaborative work necessary to effect this transformation.

CHARACTERISTICS OF EFFECTIVE COLLABORATION

The definition of collaboration proposed in this chapter demands a radical rethinking of how APNs, physicians, and others are prepared for their roles and how clinicians interact to ensure positive patient outcomes. The definition also invites exploration of the characteristics that make up a successful collaborative relationship and the personal and setting-specific attributes that are pivotal to successful professional collaborations. As noted, collaboration involves a bond, a union, a commitment to caring for patients that goes beyond a single approach to care and represents a synergistic alliance that maximizes the contributions of each participant (Evans, 1994).

Some characteristics of collaboration have long been recognized and promulgated, but too often clinicians and organizations have resisted adopting the philosophy, commitment, and behaviors necessary to develop collaborative practices. Steele's (1986) analysis of collaboration among NPs and physicians revealed several characteristics: mutual trust and respect, an understanding and acceptance of each other's disciplines, positive self-image, equivalent professional maturity arising from education and experience, recognition that the partners are not substitutes for each other, and a willingness to negotiate. In their program of research, Baggs (1989), Baggs and Schmitt (1988, 1997), and Baggs and colleagues (1999) noted the following characteristics of collaboration between registered nurses and physicians: assertiveness, shared decision making, communication, planning together, and coordination. Hughes and Mackenzie (1990) outlined four characteristics of NP-physician collaboration: collegiality, communication, goal sharing, and task interdependence. Spross (1989) described three essential elements of collaboration: a common purpose, diverse and complementary professional knowledge and skills, and effective communication processes. Although this is not an exhaustive summary of the literature on collaboration, it is clear that certain core elements characterize collaboration; these elements are listed in Box 10-1.

The discussion of characteristics of collaboration that follows elaborates on each of these elements. However, the reader will notice their overlapping and interlinked nature, because many are mutually dependent on others for full collaboration to be realized. Collaboration requires clinical competence, common purpose, and effective interpersonal and communication skills (or a willingness to learn them). Trust, mutual respect, and valuing each other's knowledge and skills are equally important but develop fully only over time. For these characteristics to develop, prospective partners must approach encounters with a willingness to trust, a commitment to respect each other, and an assumption that the other's knowledge and skills are valuable. In one sense, these characteristics are thus prerequisites, but in another sense they are fully realized only after many constructive and

Box 10-1 ESSENTIAL CHARACTERISTICS OF COLLABORATION

- Clinical competence and accountability
- Common purpose
- Interpersonal competence and effective communication, including assertiveness
- Trust
- Mutual respect
- Recognition and valuing of diverse, complementary knowledge and skills
- Humor

productive interactions. Collaboration is facilitated when prospective partners recognize that a problem can be solved only when each party's input, expertise, and participation are solicited (Stichler, 1995). Finally, a sense of humor among team members serves many functions in helping team members stay committed to each others' collaborative practice.

Clinical Competence and Accountability

Clinical competence is perhaps the most important characteristic underlying a successful collaborative experience among clinicians; without it, the trust and desire needed to work together are not possible. Trust and respect are built on the assurance that each member is able to carry out his or her role, function in a competent manner, and be accountable for his or her practice. That clinical competence is a critical element of collaboration has been validated in research (Cairo, 1996; Hanson, Hodnicki, & Boyle, 1994; Prescott & Bowen, 1985), yet stereotyped views of nursing and medical practice may interfere with collaborative efforts. Physicians are sometimes perceived as all-knowing and as having ultimate responsibility for patient care, whereas nurses may be viewed as nonintellectual, second-best substitutes for excellent health care (Cairo; Fagin, 1992; Sands, Stafford, & McClelland, 1990) who have little authority or responsibility for patient care outcomes (Larson, 1999). The status of advanced practice nursing is still such that nurses must prove their competence to the profession and to society (Fagin; Hodnicki, Dietz, McNeil, & Miles, 2004; Prescott & Bowen, 1985).

When collaborating clinicians can rely on each other to be clinically competent, mutual trust and respect develop. Partners recognize that leadership is problem-based, not team-or role-based, and are open to sharing power. Instead of one person always being the team leader, leadership can shift among partners in a departure from the traditional "captain of the team" approach. Thus the person with the most expertise, interest, or talent can respond to the particular demands of the situation or problem. The trust and respect among collaborators are such that they can count on satisfactory resolution of the problem even when they know as individuals that they might have approached the issue differently. In fact, this openness to shared leadership and alternative solutions allows partners to learn from each other. For example, APNs usually have expertise in educating patients about their illnesses and lifestyle choices.

Physicians are often expert diagnosticians. Thus collaboration offers APNs and physicians opportunities to model their varied assessment and intervention strategies, which fosters mutual learning and appreciation for the contributions of each to the care of patients and families. Because consumers and physicians may underestimate the expertise, competence, and authority of nurses, APNs need to showcase their exemplary practice to build nursing's reputation for competence (Drenning, 2006; Fagin, 1992; see also Chapter 24).

Being accountable for practice also enhances collaboration. APNs who share in planning, decision making, problem solving, goal setting, and assuming responsibility are modeling full partnership on caregiving teams (Baggs & Schmitt, 1988).

Common Purpose

The notion that a common purpose must be the basis for collaboration is well supported in the literature (Alpert, Goldman, Kilroy, & Pike, 1992; King, 2002; Nolan, Resar, Haraden, & Griffin, 2004; Rider, 2002; Senge, 2006; Spross, 1989). Even if partners have not discussed the purposes and goals of their interactions, the organizations in which they work usually have an explicit mission and goals. These can be the starting point for identifying the goals and purposes of clinical collaboration. Common purpose may range from ensuring that an underserved patient gains access to preventive services to creating an ambitious quality improvement agenda to improve the management of heart failure patients across settings.

One of the paradoxes of collaboration is that the partners are autonomous (self-governing, accountable) but interdependent, reflecting a reciprocal reliance on each other for support in carrying out their responsibilities. Recognizing their interdependence, team members can combine their individual perceptions and skills to synthesize care plans that are more complex and comprehensive than they could have created working alone (Covey, 1989; Forbes & Fitzsimmons, 1993). Like other characteristics, the common purpose that initially brought partners together may change over time. The organizational goal or situation that brought two clinicians together may become subordinate to the deep, personal commitment to work together in ways that improve patient care and are interpersonally and professionally satisfying. Reinertsen, Gosfield, Rup, and Whittington (2007) noted that the difficulties physicians and administrators have in identifying a common purpose can be traced to "damaged relationships, which are often the elephant in the room in conversations about engaging physicians in quality" (p. 10).

Besides a common purpose, partners who are guided by a shared vision of the possibilities inherent in collaboration, who believe in the value of collaboration, and who are committed to achieving the relationship's potential (Krumm, 1992; Lindeke, 2005) will be most able to move toward transdisciplinary collaboration. Developing a shared vision does not negate the differences among partners' ideas, opinions, and actions. On the contrary, it permits—and may even value—such differences. Conger and Craig (1998) suggested that shared vision and collaboration between NPs and CNSs could be used to implement a cost-effective model of community-based health care.

Interpersonal Competence and Effective Communication

Interpersonal competence is the ability to communicate effectively with colleagues in a variety of situations, including uncomplicated, routine interactions; disagreements; value conflicts; and stressful situations. It is imperative that nurses understand and articulate to team members the skills and knowledge they bring. The key to demonstrating interpersonal competence is the APN's ability to communicate openly, clearly, and convincingly, both orally and in writing. The ability to communicate well with physicians, other staff members, the patient, and the patient's family was highly regarded by physicians in a study by Hanson and colleagues (1994). Physicians reported that they valued the NPs' communication skills in enhancing patient interactions and facilitating communication amongst office staff.

In light of corporate, governmental, and research scandals, the concept of transparency of communication and behavior has emerged in health care today. The Institute of Medicine's (IOM's) *Crossing the Quality Chasm* lists transparency as one of the "rules" for the twenty-first century health care system (IOM, 2001). *Transparency* can be defined as the honest and open sharing of information and ideas. It includes open communication among parties—keeping everyone in the loop. It also means that one does not dissemble or pretend that everything is fine when it is not. The concept of transparency underlies the current wisdom that the patient and family are advised as soon as possible when a clinical error has been made. Transparent communications are closely linked to accountability; transparency engenders trust and thus is an underlying requisite for collaboration. After clinical competence, interpersonal competence and effective communication may be the most important characteristics needed for APNs to establish collaborative relationships.

Assertiveness is a key element of interpersonal competence, and APN students need to learn and practice assertiveness skills. APNs must have the fortitude to challenge disconfirming or aggressive encounters with colleagues (Coeling & Wilcox, 1994). A range of qualities may be required for APNs to be able to take risks; discuss honest disagreements in clinical judgment and agree to criteria for resolving such conflicts; be able to avoid a "near miss" such as an error in prescribing or interpretation of clinical data; admit that a mistake, a miscommunication, or an oversight has happened; or report a colleague's incompetence. Assertiveness is not sufficient in certain situations and environments, and in these cases courage will be required to confront the problem. Trust and assertiveness seem to act reciprocally in collaboration—as individuals trust each other more, their ability to engage in difficult communications increases. Responding assertively in situations of risk and keeping the focus on the patient's welfare can enhance trust. Over time, experience and confidence increase an APN's interpersonal competence. Environments in which courage rather than assertiveness is routinely required for an APN to practice with integrity need to be evaluated and changed (see Chapter 11).

Trust and Mutual Respect

Implicit in discussions of collaboration is the presence of mutual trust, mutual respect, and personal integrity—qualities evinced in the nature of interactions between partners. In fact, distrust is often cited as a major barrier to successful collaborative relationships (Alpert et al., 1992; Cairo, 1996; Evans, 1994). The development of trust and respect depends on clinical competence; it is very difficult to trust and respect a colleague whose clinical competence is questionable. This does not mean that novice APNs cannot establish collaborative relationships. However, the environments in which advanced practice nursing students and new graduates work must support their "novicehood" so they can learn and mature clinically.

In a conversation with a group of psychiatric APNs, one APN reported that the medical director of psychiatry "loved APNs"; and apologizing in advance for how it might sound, the director said he thought of APNs as "discount physicians." Although such a perspective may be intended as a compliment, it diminishes advanced practice nursing contributions and impedes the development of the mutual respect that we view as essential. Respect for others' practice and knowledge is key to successful collaboration because it enhances shared decision making. Respect extends to acknowledgment and appreciation for each other's time and competing commitments.

Recognition and Valuing of Diverse, Complementary Knowledge and Skills

There must be a belief, at a very personal level, that the complementary knowledge other team members have will enhance one's own personal plan for patient care. Appreciation for the diverse and complementary knowledge each party brings to the work, a commitment to quality and patient-centeredness, and a willingness to invest in the partnership or team are all necessary for collaboration to become the normative process in team interactions.

A lack of knowledge about another's discipline is thought to be a barrier to developing effective teamwork (Gilbert et al., 2000). Partners must recognize and value the overlapping and diverse skills and knowledge that each discipline brings to the team (Spross, 1989; Stichler, 1995) so that mutual trust and respect can develop and deepen over time. Partners observe that patients benefit from their combined talents and efforts. They come to depend on each other to use good clinical judgment and to take appropriate actions.

Initially, collaborators have limited knowledge of each other as individuals and as professionals; collaboration is a "conscious, learned behavior" that improves as team members learn to value and respect one another's practice and expertise (Alpert et al., 1992; Moeller, Vezeau & Carr, 2007). The first step is to recognize these differing contributions. Medicine and nursing, although overlapping disciplines, are culturally distinct and have diverse goals for patient care. In many cases, they complement each other in their quest to restore patients to health. These complementarities extend to other disciplines as well. Collaboration is built on the respect and valuing of the contributions of each profession to the common goal of optimal health care delivery (Sloand & Groves, 2005; Stichler, 1995).

Humor

A final important aspect of the collaborative process is humor. Humor in which the intent is positive and non-threatening is a creative way to set the stage for effective communication and problem solving among members of different disciplines (Balzer, 1993). In collaborative practice, humor serves to decrease defensiveness, invite openness, relieve tension, and deflect anger. It helps individuals keep perspective and acknowledge the lack of perfection, and it sets the tone for trust and acceptance among colleagues so that difficult situations can be reframed (Balzer). The use of humor helps defuse the need for persons to argue their own point of view and allows them to refocus on how they can work together to meet common goals (Hill & Hewlett, 2002). Graduate students can be encouraged to observe the ways in which humor is used by preceptors and colleagues and identify those uses that seem effective in improving communication and defusing conflict situations.

• • •

Although this list of characteristics may seem daunting to the novice, a consistent commitment to and practice of collaboration can develop this competency over time in an APN's practice. Exemplar 10-1 showcases the elements of collaboration in an individual APN's practice. Italicized text in the exemplar affirms many of the characteristics and processes required for effective collaboration. APNs and their professional colleagues need to recognize that an important component of clinical practice is investing the time and energy to build such relationships. The high levels of interchange of ideas and expertise possible when all of these characteristics come together is one of the great satisfactions of collaborative practice.

IMPACT OF COLLABORATION ON PATIENTS AND CLINICIANS

Experience and evidence suggest that collaboration works, yet effective collaboration eludes many clinicians. Why? Some authors link barriers to the history of the health care professions, traditional gender roles, disciplinary heritage, ineffective communication, and hierarchical relationships (Christman, 1998; Larson, 1999; Martin, O'Brien, Heyworth, & Meyer, 2005; Reuben et al., 2004; Rosenstein & O'Daniel, 2005; Zwarenstein & Reeves, 2002). Over the years, there have been many reports of successful collaborative relationships involving APNs (Brooten et al., 2005; Cowan et al., 2006; Hales, Karshmer, Montes-Sandoval, & Fiszbein, 1998; Lindeke, 2005; Litake et al., 2003; Siegler & Whitney, 1994a; Steele,

EXEMPLAR 10-1   **Elements of Collaboration in One Advanced Practice Nurse's Practice**

A national organization instituted a program to honor NPs who had achieved high levels of success in their practice. Letters requesting nominations were sent to physicians and nurses, inviting them to nominate an NP colleague. The letters returned by the physicians and nurses who nominated successful NPs for the award all appeared to say the same thing: "The individual exhibits a high level of collaboration." The following composite of the nomination letters received from physician nominators exemplifies several of the characteristics of successful collaboration put forth in this chapter.

"I would like to tell you about Mary Q., a nurse practitioner who is a member of our group primary care practice. Mary is an extremely *competent* nurse practitioner and an *able* diagnostician. I would *trust* her to care for my own wife and children. She is totally *committed* to her patients, strives to give them the best possible care, and

has many of the *same values and ideas about good patient care* that my physician partner and I do. Although Mary carries her own panel of patients very successfully, she seems to *want to consult* with me and our other physicians if she is concerned about a complex patient. We all *function as a team,* and we have all *learned from Mary's nursing expertise,* as she has from ours. All of us *work together* to give high-quality care. Most important, Mary is a *team player;* all the members of our group practice enjoy her *quick wit* and *willingness to share* her expertise. At first, one of the partners did not want a nurse practitioner to join the group, but Mary won him over with her *professional and interpersonal competence.* I guess that the most important quality that I would share is that Mary is *a people person;* she works hard to *communicate at a high level,* and it pays off. We *trust* her as a *professional colleague and a friend."*

1986). The importance of collaboration in various aspects of advanced practice nursing continues to be recognized (Arford, 2005; Ingersoll, McIntosh, & Williams, 2000; Jackson et al., 2003; Kleinpell et al., 2002; Sheer, 2007).

Although few studies of collaboration have measured patient outcomes systematically (Litaker et al., 2003; Sullivan, 1998; Torres & Dominguez, 1998; see also Chapter 24), both patient and provider benefits have been documented. Patients are sensitive to the relationships among caregivers and are quick to pick up on the lack of respect or trust among their providers. Some research suggests that collaborative relationships among interdisciplinary health care providers can ameliorate some of these negative effects (Afflitto, 1997; Weinstein, McCormack, Brown, & Rosenthal, 1998). Successful collaborative practices are those in which patients easily move back and forth between providers as their care and situations dictate. Collaboration requires an ability to transform competitive situations into opportunities for working together that are mutually beneficial and in which all parties can imagine the possibility of creating a win-win situation.

Studies of the impact of APNs on disease management and care transition interventions indicate that there are positive outcomes for patients. Collaboration is implied based on the fact that the APNs

in these studies typically communicated with other providers, but collaboration is rarely identified or measured (these studies are discussed in Chapters 6 and 24). Table 10-1 illustrates the types of patient and provider benefits that have been ascribed to clinical collaboration. Competencies required by the American College of Graduate Medical Education (ACGME) for participants in medical residency programs include behaviors related to interdisciplinary teamwork, group problem solving, and communication across boundaries. These collaborative expectations were adopted in 2002 by the ACGME. Over time, these behaviors may lead to improved physician collaboration with other clinicians, as seen in Exemplar 10-2.

Evidence That Collaboration Works

The National Joint Practice Commission. In the 1970s, the ANA and the American Medical Association (AMA) formed the National Joint Practice Commission (NJPC) (1979). The committee was created to respond to tension and conflict between physicians and nurses, believed to be caused by increased patient loads and cost constraints that were placing excessive demands on both groups. The NJPC funded several demonstration projects to implement joint practice arrangements within four

Table 10-1   BENEFITS OF COLLABORATION

For Patients	For Providers
Improved quality of care	Increased sharing of responsibility
Increased patient satisfaction	Increased sharing of expertise
Lower mortality rate	More mutually satisfying problem solving
Improved patient outcomes	Improved communications
Patients feel more secure, cared for, closer to nurses	Increased personal satisfaction
	Increased quality of professional life
	Enhanced mutual trust and respect
	Bridges care-cure dichotomy
	Expands horizons of providers
	Avoids redundant care and ensures coverage
	Empowers providers to influence health policy

Adapted from Sullivan, T.J. (1998). *Collaboration: A health care imperative* (pp. 26-27). New York: McGraw-Hill Health Professionals Division.

 EXEMPLAR 10-2   **Collaboration Works for Patients and Clinicians**

While a clinical nurse specialist (CNS) at a tertiary hospital, one of the authors (JS) noted that patients who were admitted directly from the oncology clinic for a short admission were receiving their chemotherapy late at night because members of the house staff were not taking the patients' histories and performing physical examinations until last. Lengths of stay were longer, treatments that could have been prepared and given during the better-staffed day shift were burdening the evening and night staff, and patients were dissatisfied. House staff left these admissions until last because the patients tended to be clinically stable, and to the interns, this was an appropriate way of triaging their workload. The CNS and nurse manager met with the physician director of hematology/oncology to propose that short-stay chemotherapy admissions be handled differently from other admissions—an idea for which there was no precedent. The physician direc-

tor had also recognized the problem and willingly collaborated with the nursing leaders to craft a solution. Previously, all admissions had been done by the interns and residents. Under the new arrangement, patients came to the unit directly from the clinic with their admission orders written by the attending physician. Intravenous lines were initiated immediately, prescriptions were filled by the pharmacy as the orders came down, and nurses were able to initiate teaching and other interventions in a timely fashion.

The outcomes of this new plan included increased patient, nurse, and house staff satisfaction, and decreased time from admission to beginning chemotherapy. Patient length of stay also decreased. Perhaps most importantly, the success of the joint problem solving in this case provided a precedent for increased interdisciplinary collaboration on the hematology/oncology service.

different hospital settings that were attempting to improve nurse-physician relationships. The NJPC identified five critical elements of collaborative practice in hospital settings: primary nursing, integrated patient records, encouragement of nurse decision making, a joint practice committee, and a joint record review (Devereux, 1981; NJPC, 1979). The NJPC demonstration project was one of the earliest studies to document that collaboration benefited clinicians and patients. Although the data from these NJPC projects indicated improved communication and improved patient care outcomes,

the work was never completed. Unfortunately, there has not been widespread implementation of the NJPC's recommendations (Crowley & Wollner, 1987; Fagin, 1992). Efforts to improve collaboration stalled; broad initiatives were not undertaken again until the 1990s.

Outcomes of Intensive Care Unit Stays.
One of the first studies to identify the impact of nurse-physician communication on patient outcomes indicated that the most significant factor associated with decreased mortality rates in intensive

care units (ICUs) was effective nurse-physician communication patterns (Knaus, Draper, Wagner, & Zimmerman, 1986). The investigators reported that another factor associated with lower mortality rates was the presence of a comprehensive nursing education support system in which CNSs had responsibility for staff development. Hospitals with lower mortality rates had systems that ensured excellent nurse-physician communication.

In an extension of this research, a study of 17,440 patients in 42 ICUs provided additional evidence that interactions among caregivers affect patient care (Shortell et al., 1994). Effective caregiver interactions were associated with lower risk-adjusted length of stay, lower nurse turnover, better quality of care, and greater ability to meet family member needs. In the analytical model the investigators used, caregiver interaction included the culture, leadership, coordination, communication, and conflict management abilities of the unit's staff. Greater technological availability, a measure of state-of-the-art treatments, was also associated with lower risk-adjusted mortality rates. Hospitals that were more profitable, that were involved in teaching activities, and in which the unit leaders were more involved in quality improvement activities had greater technological availability.

Effect of Hospitalist Physician and Advanced Practice Nurse Collaboration on Hospital Cost. A study was conducted that compared 627 control patients who received usual care with 1207 hospitalized medical patients who received care from MD/NP teams. The researchers compared multidisciplinary team-based planning, expedited discharge, and assessment after discharge with usual patient management. The study found that multidisciplinary care management reduced the length of hospital stay, reduced hospital stay costs, and improved hospital care without altering readmissions or mortality (Cowan et al., 2006).

Primary Care: Impact on Chronic Disease Management. Efforts to improve the management of chronic diseases such as diabetes, heart failure, and hypertension often involve an APN, usually an NP or a CNS. For example, Litaker and colleagues (2003) conducted an experiment to compare the care provided to diabetics and hypertensive patients by a physician–NP team with usual care provided by primary care physicians. Despite higher costs, the investigators found

statistically and clinically significant improvements in hemoglobin A_{1c} (HbA$_{1c}$) levels and high-density lipoprotein (HDL) levels, as well as increased satisfaction (general satisfaction, communication with provider, and interpersonal care). There were no observed significant differences in total cholesterol and quality of life. The authors observed that the increased costs of care (usual care was about one-third less than that of the MD-NP team) may be justified because the improved clinical indicators are associated with better longer-term outcomes such as reduction in disease complications, re-hospitalizations, and mortality. The investigators noted that the benefits of team treatment disappeared within 12 months of study completion, leading them to conclude the following (Litaker et al., 2003):

> The potential value of an ongoing interaction with the team is substantiated by the rapid return of HbA$_{1c}$ levels to pre-study ranges once team contact was terminated. Therefore, if one were to consider the study results in terms of health care *value* (quality of care divided by costs of care), the disease management strategy presented may be preferable to usual care. (p. 233)

Similarly, an integrative review of the impact of transdisciplinary teams on the care of the underserved demonstrated benefits for underserved populations (Ruddy & Rhee, 2005).

Bourbonniere and Evans (2002), in an integrative review of the impact of APN outcomes on care, affirmed that interdisciplinary collaboration is an important function of APNs. Readers are encouraged to stay abreast of literature on chronic disease management since this is an area in which APNs are practicing and participating in research. Results from such studies will continue to shape our understanding of both collaboration and coaching competencies of APNs (see Chapter 6).

Other Evidence. In studies of clinical expertise in nurses, Benner, Hooper-Kyriakidis, and Stannard (1999) identified the myriad ways in which expert nurses, including APNs, contribute to collaboration and teambuilding. Box 10-2 lists the behaviors of expert nurses that represent collaborative activities within specific domains of nursing practice. Wells, Johnson, and Salyer (1997) examined interdisciplinary collaboration in seven inpatient units over time. They hypothesized that (1) staff in units using different interdisciplinary strategies would report different levels of collaboration and (2) staff who perceived

Box 10-2 COLLABORATIVE ACTIVITIES USED BY EXPERT CRITICAL CARE NURSES

DIAGNOSING AND MANAGING LIFE-SUSTAINING PHYSIOLOGICAL FUNCTIONS IN UNSTABLE PATIENTS
- Coordinating and managing multiple, instantaneous therapies

THE SKILLED KNOW-HOW OF MANAGING A CRISIS
- Organizing the team and orchestrating their actions during a crisis
- Exhibiting experiential leadership when a physician is present
- Taking necessary medical action to manage a crisis when a physician is absent
- Recognizing clinical talent and skilled clinicians and marshaling these for the particular situation
- Modulating one's emotional responses and facilitating the social climate

COMMUNICATING MULTIPLE CLINICAL, ETHICAL, AND PRACTICAL PERSPECTIVES
- Teambuilding: developing a community of attentiveness, skill, and collaboration

MONITORING QUALITY AND MANAGING A BREAKDOWN
- Front-line quality improvement, monitoring, and risk management
- Teambuilding in the context of breakdown
- Minimizing health care system failures in destabilized work environments

THE SKILLED KNOW-HOW OF CLINICAL LEADERSHIP AND THE COACHING AND MENTORING OF OTHERS
- Facilitating the clinical development of others
- Building and preserving collaborative relationships
- Transforming care delivery systems

Data from Benner, P., Hooper-Kyriakidis, P., & Stannard, D. (1999). *Clinical wisdom and interventions in critical care* (p. 3). Philadelphia: Saunders.

high physician involvement in collaborative practice would report greater collaboration than staff who perceived low physician involvement. Although perceived collaboration differed based on critical pathway use, the findings suggested that physician involvement was more strongly associated with degree of collaboration than with the type of strategy used.

Collaboration has also been associated with decreased costs of care. Lassen, Fosbinder, Minton, and Robins (1997) reported that the complex diagnosis and treatment of neonates with sepsis were enhanced by collaborative nurse-physician relationships and that cost of care was reduced while quality was improved. The frequency of urgent care visits to a geriatric primary care clinic were decreased through collaborative care provided by NPs and physicians (Sears, Maxwell, & Townsend, 2003). Jackson and colleagues (2003) reported that fewer fiscal resources were required when obstetricians and certified nurse-midwives (CNMs) worked within a collaborative care birth center model.

Some commentators have noted that collaboration may actually cost more in the short run (Litaker et al., 2003). Kinnaman and Bleich (2004), from an administrative perspective, observed that collaboration is a more complex and labor/resource–intensive problem-

solving strategy. One of the challenges of evaluating cost-effectiveness when it comes to clinical collaboration is to measure change over an appropriate time-horizon. As the Litaker study suggested, a 1-year collaborative intervention was enough to change patient behaviors in ways that reduced important clinical markers but was not sufficient to assess and measure the impact of complications and disease-related comorbidities on the disease trajectory over time. The fact that the 1-year intervention was insufficient to sustain the behavior changes that led to the reduced clinical markers supports our conceptualization of collaboration as a process that evolves and matures over time and suggests that our understanding of long-term changes in patient behavior and clinical outcomes may depend on a more complete empirical understanding of collaborative processes.

The importance of collaboration to effective, accessible health care has been recognized by several philanthropies that support health care initiatives. The report of the Pew Health Professions Commission identified collaborative care core competencies needed for future health professionals (Gelman, O'Neil, Kimmey, & the Task Force on Accreditation of Health Professions Education, 1999; Pew Health Professions Commission, 1995). The

Pew-Fetzer Task Force (1994) described three dimensions of such care—the patient-practitioner relationship, the community-practitioner relationship, and the practitioner-practitioner relationship—and described the requirements for relationship-centered care:

> Effective, empathic care requires a community of practitioners who commit themselves to working together to serve the complex matrix of individuals' needs in health and illness…. Such relationships serve the needs of practitioners as well as patients: building communities enables health care providers to care for one another and give and receive the support and encouragement that produces personal and professional maturation and more effective patient care. (p. 27)

The Robert Wood Johnson Foundation (RWJF) has supported projects that provide further evidence that collaboration works. RWJF's Partnerships for Quality Education (PQE) Project, conducted from 1998 to 2003, included a program that helped NPs and medical residents learn how to work together (Johnson-Pawlson, Posey, Dalal, & Page, 2003).

More recently, the Institute for Health Care Improvement (IHI) has published a series of white papers, a number of which relate to collaboration, including "Transforming Care at the Bedside" (TCAB; note that RWJF partnered with IHI on this project) (Rutherford, Lee, & Greiner, 2004) and "Engaging Physicians in a Shared Quality Agenda" (Reinertsen et al., 2007). Although specific recommendations from these documents are woven throughout this chapter, a few points are worth making here. The TCAB recommendations are built on a framework of four main themes: safety and reliability, patient-centeredness, *care team vitality* (emphasis ours), and increased value. The goal for vitality as described in TCAB is the following: "Within a joyful and supportive environment that nurtures professional formation and career development, effective care teams continually strive for excellence" (Rutherford et al., p. 7). There is also evidence that institutions can create structures to facilitate collaboration. While much has been made of the application of "Crew Resource Management" [CRM] principles to facilitate collaboration and cooperation among health care team members, Zwarenstein and Reeves (2002) point out that health care organizations are bigger, more complex, and more widely dispersed geographically than many of the industries, such as aviation, in which they have been tested. Even so, there is evidence that

organizationally supported teams, such as rapid response teams, can improve patient outcomes (Nolan et al., 2004).

Although efforts to improve collaboration between nurses and physicians stalled after the NJPC project, recent initiatives demonstrate a renewed interest in creating collaborative environments—in large part because of the evidence that collaboration works and that failure to collaborate is costly for patients, clinicians, and organizations.

Effects of Failure to Collaborate

For Organizations. Failure to collaborate has implications for organizations and individuals. The anthrax scare after the events of 9/11 provided health care professionals with a compelling example of the failure of organizations and agencies to collaborate. The Centers for Disease Control and Prevention (CDC) and other parts of the U.S. Public Health Service failed to share data and resources with other agencies that would have ensured timely, broad-based solutions to the anthrax problem. Conversely, in February 2003, effective collaboration and coordination between the World Health Organization and several nations in dealing with the severe acute respiratory syndrome (SARS) outbreak received worldwide acclaim (Hotez, 2003). Numerous studies and initiatives are aimed at understanding the impact of organizational processes such as teamwork, "handoffs," continuity of care, and disruptive behaviors. Rosenstein and O'Daniel (2005) noted that more is known about the impact of disruptive behaviors on job satisfaction but that the impact of work relationships on patient outcomes has not been well studied. Although a review of this body of work is beyond the scope of the chapter, we see this as evidence that accrediting organizations, health care executives, administrators, and researchers are paying attention to the collaborative and communication processes that undermine institutional bottom lines—positive patient *and* financial outcomes. Indeed, the most important result of failure to collaborate is its negative effect on patient care.

For Individuals. The failure to communicate and collaborate s individual patients and clinicians. Failure to collaborate may contribute to inefficiencies in the delivery of patient care (Cooper, Henderson, & Dietrich, 1998; Grumbach & Coffman, 1998; Nolan et al., 2004). Alpert and colleagues (1992) found that job satisfaction and attitude were negatively affected when collaboration failed and that territoriality and competitiveness increased. The absence of collaboration has been identified as a source of distress to nurses (Aiken, Smith, & Lake, 1994; Fagin, 1992). Lack of collaboration and the diminished autonomy that often accompanies it may contribute to job dissatisfaction and staff turnover and more recently is believed to contribute to the nursing shortage (Rosenstein & O'Daniel, 2005). Job dissatisfaction and turnover among staff nurses are serious concerns, especially during a nursing shortage, and are particularly relevant to CNSs and blended-role APNs. Although APNs may experience these effects of failure to collaborate, APNs usually have more autonomy and advanced communication skills than staff nurses and can work within the work setting to improve collaboration.

IMPERATIVES FOR COLLABORATION

We believe that organizations and individual clinicians have a moral obligation to collaborate, yet collaboration cannot be mandated. The following are a set of imperatives we believe clinicians must consider as they make decisions about collaboration and collaborative relationships. The effects of collaboration or failure to collaborate can be seen in the way that we resolve ethical and institutional dilemmas and in the way we conduct research. Providers must be willing to negotiate and transcend their disciplinary boundaries in all activities aimed at improving the quality, safety, and reliability of care for individuals and populations.

The Ethical Imperative to Collaborate

Some writers have suggested that the failure to collaborate is an ethical issue. The clinical imperative to collaborate is embedded within the ethical imperative. Compassionate, ethical patient care that provides a healing environment requires collaborative working relationships between physicians and nurses (Larson, 1999; Smith, Hiatt, & Berwick, 1999). As noted in Chapter 11, communication and collaboration problems are often components of ethical dilemmas. Thus environments that foster collaboration may also create a more supportive context for addressing ethical issues.

Larson (1999) identified key beliefs about collaboration on which nurses and physicians differ: the importance of relationships, what constitutes effective and desirable communication, the degree to which communication and shared decision making occur, the authority nurses have to make decisions, and what

strategies would improve communication. The failure of physicians and nurses to understand each other's perspectives, a prerequisite for collaboration, results in a difficult work environment and contributes to uncoordinated, unsafe care (Larson, 1999).

Gianakos (1997) identified three reasons for nurses and physicians to collaborate and asserted that the *ethical imperative to collaborate* is the most important. Collaboration is a moral imperative—good patient care requires it; collaboration reinforces commitment to a common goal and reaffirms the message that patient welfare is the goal; and collaboration enhances shared knowledge as physicians and nurses educate each other repeatedly about the patient.

The Institutional Imperative to Collaborate

The evidence that collaboration works suggests that there are structural as well as interpersonal dimensions to collaboration. That is, although institutional policies or standards do not guarantee collaboration, they can establish expectations for communication and collaboration. Such institutional expectations can provide a structure that facilitates interpersonal communication and relationship-building (Knaus et al., 1986). The mutual goal of good patient care and the ethical imperative to collaborate should be at the center of any interdisciplinary effort to plan care or resolve conflicts in approaches to care (Pellegrino, 1996). Institutions that apply for Magnet Status are expected to have a structure in place for effective communication among nurses, physicians, and administrators as one of five key characteristics (McClure & Hinshaw, 2002; North Shore Long Island Jewish Health System, 2001). The incentive for hospitals to move to Magnet Status has never been higher with the current emphases on nurse retention, quality, and safety. Institutions that have applied for the American Nurses Credentialing Center (ANCC) Magnet credential must demonstrate that they meet 14 characteristics (McClure & Hinshaw, 2002). These criteria have been associated with the ability to attract and retain nurses. Of the 14 criteria, several relate to collaboration such as interdisciplinary relationships and professional models of care. APNs are usually intimately involved in efforts to seek Magnet Status: they have led quality improvement initiatives, facilitated professional development of staff, and contributed to the establishment of policies and procedures that support nurses' autonomy—efforts that shape an environment in which effective collaboration can occur.

Finally, incentives and mandates to reduce error and increase the reliability of care by adopting evidence-based practices constitute another significant institutional imperative to foster collaboration; improvements that result from such initiatives are often tied to reimbursement (e.g., pay-for-performance).

An example of the institutional imperative to collaborate is the rapid progression of the Doctor of Nursing Practice (DNP). The national concerns about the quality and safety of health care (Institute of Medicine [IOM], 2001) informed the development of the DNP and helped form consensus among schools, faculty, and other stakeholders (AACN, 2004). The DNP *Essentials* (AACN, 2006) affirm the importance of collaboration as a core competency. The document includes numerous mentions of the words *collaboration* and *collaborative* in the competencies that will need to be met by all who seek DNP education, including APNs. Examples of situations from the DNP *Essentials* that require collaborative competencies include the ability to create change in health care delivery systems, the need to collaborate across boundaries to enhance population-based health care, and the need for interprofessional collaboration to implement practice guidelines and peer review processes (AACN, 2006).

The Research Imperative to Study Collaboration

Schmitt (2001) suggested that collaboration be examined as an intermediate outcome when health care is evaluated. In a review of the literature, Schmitt cited a number of challenges health services researchers face in trying to understand collaboration and its impact on outcomes. Methodological challenges include the need for more robust, well-designed studies, including clinical trials to provide more conclusive evidence about the impact of collaboration on patient outcomes. In addition, sample selection, measurement of collaboration, and outcome measurement pose dilemmas for those interested in studying the phenomenon. A major limitation of existing knowledge is that much of it comes from hospital-based practice, and according to Schmitt, studies of collaboration and its outcomes are underdeveloped. Schmitt noted: "If there is an important place for interprofessional collaboration in health care delivery then it is a high priority task to get on with the research, difficult as it is, that demonstrates what mix of collaborators, for what purposes, for whom, with what outcomes and at what costs matters" (p. 63).

Institutional imperatives to collaborate and the research imperative to study collaboration are becoming more closely aligned. For example, the Agency for Healthcare Research and Quality (AHRQ) has become an important resource for funding and disseminating the results of research on quality improvement, patient safety, the adoption of evidence-based practices, and other issues associated with the delivery of safe and reliable health care (see, e.g., *www.ahrq.gov/QUAL/advances/*). In addition, the National Institutes of Health's (NIH's) "Road Map Initiative" *(http://nihroadmap.nih.gov/)* is changing the structure of funding and the conduct of clinical research by requiring collaboration among clinical investigators. Drenning (2006) urged collaboration among nurses, APNs, and nurse researchers to understand and implement evidence-based practice (EBP) changes that are likely to improve patient care.

Collaboration among providers with different perspectives results in a creative and multidimensional intelligence that is emotionally rewarding because patients do better and clinicians derive personal and professional gratification from this work. This conclusion has implications for APNs, administrators, physicians, researchers, and others. APNs and their administrative and clinical colleagues need to assess the collaborative climate, determine facilitators and barriers, and work together to strengthen relationships and build an organizational culture that values collaboration. Researchers must help APNs and administrators understand the structures and processes that are associated with collaboration and the extent to which collaboration affects patient and utilization outcomes. This work is essential and should be a priority for institutions and individuals.

THE CONTEXT OF COLLABORATION IN CONTEMPORARY HEALTH CARE

The pressures on APNs, physicians, and others to improve quality, work more efficiently, and allow others (e.g., insurers) to be involved in decisions about patient care could be expected to foster collaboration among clinicians. Paradoxically, these same factors may undermine collaboration. As APNs have acquired more education and have become better prepared to practice autonomously and collaboratively, physicians have experienced multiple pressures, including the increasing supply of APN providers (Cooper, Henderson, & Dietrich, 1998; Cooper, Laud, & Dietrich, 1998; Phillips, Harper, Wakefield, Green & Fryer, 2002), which apparently or actually encroach on the physicians' autonomy and willingness to collaborate. The mounting pressures on physicians may lead them to fear "undifferentiation"—that no one will be able to tell them from physician assistants, APNs, or other providers—which could underlie turf battles. These same pressures generate concern about relinquishing authority and power—fears that may cause individuals to withdraw from or sabotage efforts to collaborate. Thus the transition to a (presumably) more effective, accessible, and efficient health care system may actually undermine collaboration, a process many leaders believe is central to achieving the goal of a health care system that is accessible, effective, and affordable.

In addition, confusion about scope of practice can be damaging to collaboration for all involved. Physicians may ask themselves: What's in it for me to collaborate? What areas of my work do I get to expand because other providers can do things I have traditionally done (Cairo, 1996)? APNs may be uncertain about their scope of practice when a physician or institution asks them to assume responsibility for a new skill, such as performing an invasive procedure. The reality is that managed care and regulatory initiatives are rearranging practice boundaries almost daily. These changes are often at the heart of the tension associated with collaboration among players as roles and boundaries of disciplines blur and expand.

Incentives and Opportunities for Collaboration

Efforts to reduce costs and improve quality of health care actually provide APNs, physicians, and administrators with common goals toward which to work and with opportunities for learning from each other. Medicare guidelines that are used to document care for coding and billing purposes are structured to encourage physicians and nurses to work together to provide the appropriate level of care necessary to meet the standards for reimbursement. National interdisciplinary guidelines and standards of care are intended to reduce unwarranted, often expensive, variation in health care. Many guidelines specify interdisciplinary collaboration as a critical component of effective care. Standards and guidelines developed and agreed upon by interdisciplinary groups, whether at the local (office or institution) or national level, offer a sound starting point for jointly determining patient care goals, processes, and outcomes. Accreditation activities offer another opportunity to build collaborative relationships. The Joint Commission

(TJC) (2007) requires documentation that demonstrates collaborative, interdisciplinary practice. The requirement to document these activities can help providers develop stronger interdisciplinary approaches to care. The need for a highly coordinated system of chronic care management led the Health-Sciences Institute to develop and promulgate interdisciplinary competencies. The goals for chronic illness care that include promoting health and preventing disease, managing disease and disease impacts, and promoting consumer independence and life quality are centered around a model of interdisciplinarity in which all players are valued for their contributions and collaborative effort (Health-Sciences Institute, 2005, 2007).

The move toward a more community-based, health promotion/disease prevention model of care is also creating new opportunities for collaborative practice in primary care (Bodenheimer & Grumbach, 2007). As well, the use of telehealth and electronic medical records offers creative opportunities for interaction (Waldo, 2003). For these systems to work, APNs, physicians, and other clinicians need to be involved in selecting, piloting, modifying, and implementing new technologies. From selection of vendors to full deployment of the technology, the adoption of new technologies offers opportunities for clinicians to develop collaborative, learning communities. In the current global market, innovative new alliances, both among advanced practice nursing groups and between advanced practice nursing groups and physician groups, need to be developed and nurtured.

Barriers to Collaboration

It is easier to discuss professional liaisons and draw up collaborative arrangements on paper than to actually implement effective collaborative professional relationships in the workplace. Sands and colleagues (1990) suggested that team members see themselves primarily as representatives of their own discipline rather than as members of a collaborative team, an observation affirmed by Reuben and colleagues (2004). Several barriers to collaboration exist and can be characterized as professional, sociocultural, organizational, and regulatory.

Disciplinary Barriers. *Silos in medical and nursing education* have long been barriers to successful collaboration. Each profession is a culture with its own values, knowledge, rules, and norms (Lindeke, 2005; Reuben et al., 2004). Often, clinicians differ in their basic philosophy of care based on how they have been socialized into the system. For example, medicine is oriented toward biomedical research, technical solutions, hierarchical relationships, and a strong sense of personal responsibility for patient outcomes (Bray & Rogers, 1997). This sense of responsibility is apparent even among physicians who support APNs but imply or explicitly indicate that physician oversight of APNs' practice is necessary (American Medical Association [AMA], 2006; Cairo, 1996). Fagin (1992) asserted that the stance preferred by physicians is not to collaborate with anyone. This is a strong statement and might seem inflammatory. Yet the Pew-Fetzer Task Force (1994) (the majority of whose members were physicians) also acknowledged that collaboration was a particular challenge for physicians. Current efforts to place certified registered nurse anesthetists (CRNAs) under physician supervision (see Chapter 17) also suggest that collaboration is difficult for physicians. In an evaluation of the Hartford Foundation initiative to strengthen interdisciplinary team training in geriatrics, faculty and students in advanced practice nursing, medicine, and social work were influenced by disciplinary attitudes and cultural factors that were obstacles to teamwork—a phenomenon the authors termed *disciplinary split* (Reuben et al.). They observed that disciplinary heritage and a differential willingness to participate in teamwork characterized disciplinary split and constituted significant obstacles to implementing effective interdisciplinary teamwork in geriatrics training.

There are *few opportunities for interdisciplinary education* as health care providers learn their professions. The RWJF Partnerships for Training initiative (RWJF, 2003) identified many of the stresses inherent in building and sustaining interdisciplinary, academic-community partnerships. Stresses encountered by participants as they developed partnerships centered on money, differing agendas, systems that were not integrated, varying philosophies, and long-held beliefs about "how things should be done."

The *nursing shortage*, especially in hospital-based nursing, may be exacerbated by a lack of collaboration in the workplace (Rosenstein & O'Daniel, 2005). Tensions between physicians and nurses and between nurses and other nurses rank high in reasons that nurses are dissatisfied with their work environment (Hanson & Beverly, 2001; Hamric & Blackhall, 2006). The nursing shortage and the negative effects of failure to collaborate suggest that the need for productive

models of collaboration that benefit patients, nurses, and physicians is urgent.

Collaboration at the community *"grassroots" level* is easier to implement and maintain than at the *professional organizational level*. Although collaboration happens daily among practicing clinicians, at national levels, where it is really needed, collaboration may be nonexistent, impeding efforts to move toward a coordinated health care system. The positions espoused by "old guard" policymakers from all disciplines may be based on stereotyped beliefs about disciplinary roles and responsibilities, rather than reflective consideration of the issues or what is best for consumers. These factors make it increasingly important for APNs and physicians practicing at local levels who have learned the art of collaboration to take an active role in bringing their perspectives and experiences to policymaking at institutional, community, state, and national levels that foster collaboration. According to Gianakos (1997), "[f]or physicians and nurses to become more collegial, major medical and nursing organizations must make interdisciplinary collegiality a priority" (p. 58). A broader statutory definition of professional autonomy for APNs than exists in many states is necessary if the more complex autonomy of interdependent collaborators is to be exercised effectively (Forbes & Fitzsimmons, 1993; Lugo, O'Grady, Hodnicki, & Hanson, 2007).

Despite these existing challenges to collaboration, there is evidence of progress. The U.S. Preventive Services Task Force, which is part of the federal AHRQ, is made up of an interdisciplinary group of providers and researchers who develop, disperse, and revise evidence-based recommendations on screening and prevention for a variety of health care concerns (U.S. Preventive Services Task Force, 2003).

Ineffective Communication and Team Dysfunction. Communication styles may also be a barrier to collaboration. Dysfunctional styles of interactions among health care professionals that particularly undermine collaboration have been identified. These styles have been characterized as follows: being difficult, bullying, or abusive (Anonymous, 2001; Houghton, 2003; King, 2002; McAvoy & Murtagh, 2003; Rider, 2002). More recently, the term *disruptive behavior* has been used to include these and other intimidating behaviors. Clinicians whose behavior is disruptive display the attitudinal and behavioral problems (e.g., arrogance, rudeness, and poor communication) of those who are unable to work as part of a team (King, 2002; Rosenstein & O'Daniel, 2005). Although such individuals may be clinically competent, if their behavior is harassing, coercive, or abusive, they put patients at risk, in part because other clinicians may be unwilling to deal with these individuals around nonclinical behaviors or actions (King, 2002; Rosenstein & O'Daniel, 2005). We encourage APN readers to recognize disruptive behavior as risks to collaboration and safe patient care and to develop a repertoire of interpersonal and system strategies with which to address such behaviors directly and promptly.

Lencioni, a business consultant on team effectiveness, proposed a model of team dysfunction (2005). The field guide (Lencioni, 2005) will be of practical use to APNs. In his model, the first four of the five dysfunctions reflect the absence of key components of our conceptualization of collaboration: (1) absence of trust; (2) fear of conflict; (3) lack of commitment; (4) avoidance of accountability; and (5) inattention to results. The fifth dysfunction, inattention to results, is consistent with the observation that efforts within health care to improve safety, reliability, and quality represent an opportunity to foster teamwork and collaboration by examining the processes and outcomes of care—attending to results.

Sociocultural Issues. Tradition, role, and gender stereotypes are obstacles to collaboration (Rafferty, Ball, & Aiken, 2001). Safriet (1992, 1998) suggested that the field of medicine staked out broad turf early on and considered any movement into this turf by nurses at any level to be unacceptable. Thus turf issues have been a major stumbling block to successful interactions between nurses and physicians. Although nurses are highly valued for the physical care, nurturing, and psychosocial support they provide for patients, it is clear that the physician is perceived and valued as the decision maker about treatment. Many people think of APNs as second-best providers or as caregivers for the unfortunate or indigent. Such attitudes perpetuate the view that the physician is the supervisor and the nurse is the subordinate.

Nursing remains a predominantly female profession and, despite the influx of women into medicine and efforts to recruit men into nursing, gendered role stereotypes still exist and affect collaboration. Gender stereotypes dominate images of staff nurses in the media, and APNs are rarely portrayed on television. Media bias and the nursing profession's inability to market itself adequately make nursing and advanced practice nursing invisible (Fagin, 1992). The "doctor-nurse game," a phenomenon that is influenced by roles and gender and was first described in the 1970s, continues to operate in many institutions; however, it is apparent that the rules are changing and nurses do not want to play anymore (Rafferty et al., 2001; Rosenstein & O'Daniel, 2005; Stein, Watts, & Howell, 1990). Stereotypical images and the invisibility of APNs influence how nursing is viewed by both health care professionals and consumers: at best, nurses are viewed as kind and nice; at worst, as unintelligent and incompetent. Thus APNs often find that they must actively counter low expectations with interactions and practices that convey their intelligence, competence, confidence, and trustworthiness.

Organizational Barriers. Competitive situations arise that can interfere with collaboration among APNs and between APNs and other disciplines at the level of systems and organizations. In her extensive work in the field of health policy, one of the authors (CH) has observed one group of APNs who aligned around a common viewpoint early in a debate, while members of other advanced practice nursing groups used precious time debating fine points, delaying or eliminating the possibility of unity on a policy issue that would affect all advanced practice nursing groups. Competitive stances and polarizing statements, whether they occur within or between disciplines, are barriers to collaboration.

The inability of APNs to be part of managed care panels, in many settings, makes collaboration difficult at best and may contribute to unproductive competition. The intent of Medicare billing requirements is to foster cooperation between clinicians, but they also discourage collaborative relations between health care providers and may actually serve as disincentives. For example, "Incident-to" billing (see Chapter 19) requires that patient care services provided by APNs be directly supervised by physicians, severely hampering a collaborative environment (Wolf, 2003).

Regulatory Barriers. Legislation and regulation have been barriers to the implementation of collaborative roles (Fagin, 1992; Minarik & Price, 1999). In the early days of advanced practice nursing, the overlap in APNs' and physicians' scopes of practice was often addressed by requiring "physician supervision" of aspects of an APN's practice (see Chapter 22). An outcome of this historical "accident" is that supervision of APNs by physicians is often mentioned explicitly or implicitly in some advanced practice nursing literature on collaboration as well as in state practice acts and regulations. In the past 15 years, there has been a slow but steady movement away from language requiring physician supervision and reference to protocols and toward emphasizing consultation, collaboration, peer review, and use of referral (Lugo et al., 2007).

In addition, some state statutes and regulations support a hierarchical structure that impedes collaboration between nurses and physicians (Hodnicki et al., 2004; Lugo et al., 2007). A scope of APN practice that is based on joint purposes and the public's interest is more likely to foster collaboration between the professions (Safriet, 2002). The view advanced here is that a supervision requirement precludes the development of a collaborative relationship and that physicians cannot truly supervise advanced practice nursing.

Addressing regulatory barriers to collaboration will become more important for several reasons. As telehealth technologies expand, consumers and clinicians will be interacting across state lines—whether it is via e-mail, telephone, or some other type of remote monitoring. In addition, consumers are becoming increasingly likely to consult quality scorecards, licensing boards, websites, blogs, and other Internet resources to identify those agencies and individual clinicians who provide the best health care. Adopting a multi-state licensure compact for APNs will become important to ensure that collaboration and continuity of care can occur (Philipsen & Haynes, 2007).

Opportunities to create collaborative relationships can be lost in the morass of money, political power, and control issues that arise when too-rapid changes in health care delivery systems occur (Dziabis & Lant, 1998). Furthermore, nurses and other stakeholders who are confronting their own professional concerns may not fully appreciate the stresses physicians experience in today's volatile market. This factor is a serious deterrent to collaborative relationships.

While conflicts with the medical community regarding regulation can make collaborative practice difficult for APNs, collaboration within the APN nursing community is at times problematic as well. Overall, there are four dimensions of APN regulation: education, certification, accreditation, and licensure. Often, language and policy barriers make it

difficult for the groups responsible for each of these dimensions to collaborate. These groups are making a concerted effort to enter into a truly collaborative network that allows them to match their individual organizational priorities to the priorities for APNs overall. Exemplar 10-3 describes this current effort; it illustrates how an initial failure to collaborate turned into a win-win situation for all involved.

PROCESSES ASSOCIATED WITH EFFECTIVE COLLABORATION

Recurring Interactions

In addition to the characteristics discussed previously, several processes enable effective collaboration. A theme implicit in the reports of those who have written about their positive experiences with collaboration is that establishing a trusting and collaborative relationship is a developmental process that depends on recurring, meaningful interactions (Alpert et al., 1992; Bray & Rogers, 1997; Krumm, 1992; Wells et al., 1997). Although this notion of development over time is relevant to all aspects of collaboration, it is particularly important to establishing trust. The fact that effective collaboration is developmental and time dependent explains why collaborative relationships are difficult to develop in organizations in which a high staff turnover or frequent rotation of clinicians occurs, such as with house physicians. A physician wrote that the process seemed to be related to how well the nurse and physician know each other (Alpert et al., 1992). Thus it seems likely that a series of less-complicated interactions, such as information exchange and coordination, that have been meaningful and satisfactory clinically or personally contribute to the development of collaborative relationships. Team members need recurring interactions to acquire an understanding of each other's backgrounds, roles, and functions and to develop patterns of interaction that are constructive, productive, and supportive. Several reports illustrate the developmental aspects of interactions that lead to collaborative relationships (Alpert et al., 1992; Bray & Rogers, 1997). Redmond, Riggleman, Sorrell, and Zerull (1999) and Sloand and Groves (2005) suggest that projects focused on quality and outcomes of care that involve joint collection and analysis of data build collegiality and foster collaboration. In our experiences, membership on such interdisciplinary committees as pharmacy and therapeutics, performance improvement, institutional review boards, ethics, and others

EXEMPLAR 10-3   A Shared Vision for the Future Education and Regulation of Advanced
Practice Nurses

For more than 3 years, two groups of advanced practice nursing leaders (the APRN Consensus Group, made up of representatives of educators, certifiers, accreditors, and professional groups; and the National Council of State Boards of Nursing APRN Advisory Committee) have been working to create a new vision for APRN regulation. Early on, both of these groups had very disparate beliefs about how the process and vision for APRN regulation should unfold. Two markedly diverse papers were under development. Two years ago, after a great deal of conflict, the two groups decided to meet as a Joint Dialogue Group with representation from both groups. Ground rules of conduct were developed, which included several tenets of collaboration—respect, transparency, trust, coming to common ground, a common purpose. The goal was to establish a vision of the future that was complementary and not divisive and to promote effective communication among the four regulatory bodies (licensure, accreditation, certification, education—termed *LACE*). The group met several times over the next 2 years. Members were faithful to the process, and few, if any, missed a meeting. The work began by establishing areas of agreement and consensus about APN regulation. This was the easy part. After each joint dialogue meeting, the decisions were brought back to the constituent groups for validation. As time progressed, areas of disagreement surfaced and were negotiated until agreement was reached. Over time, members of the group began to "hear" the concerns voiced by committee members from other organizations. They began to view the issue from a stance that was above what was right for themselves and see how a collaborative decision was needed to embrace all four APN roles (NP, CNM, CRNA, CNS) and LACE. At times this was very difficult work, but the commitment to collaborate to achieve a successful outcome carried the group along. The process is still unfolding, but great strides have been made in developing a new vision for regulation of APNs—the most important being that the group has decided that one collaborative vision for APN regulation is needed rather than the two visions that were originally planned.

APN, Advanced practice nurse; *APRN,* advanced practice registered nurse; *CNM,* certified nurse-midwife; *CNS,* clinical nurse specialist; *CRNA,* certified registered nurse anesthetist; *NP,* nurse practitioner.

with a patient-care focus also fosters communication and collegiality.

Effective Conflict Negotiation and Resolution Skills

As individuals, teams, and organizations work more closely together on their shared goals, inevitably, conflict will arise. APNs need to have some general approaches to conflict negotiation and resolution. As they work with particular partners with whom they will have relationships over time, it is wise to anticipate and discuss the criteria the partners, team, or organization will use to address conflicts and disagreements. Box 10-3 lists some key conflict resolution skills (The Conflict Resolution Network, 2003). Extensive detail on these skills and how to apply them is available on *www.crn.org.*

Bridging and Consensus Building

Krumm (1992) noted that bridging is a component of collaboration. She did not define *bridging* but implied that it is the ability to develop connections that support positive outcomes for individuals and populations of patients. She described one bridging skill as the "ability to recognize and rearrange boundaries within the practice setting" (p. 24). Appreciative inquiry is another strategy for building bridges and may keep conflict from escalating. Partners and teams work together to identify what is working in the situation and what needs to improve (notice—the focus is not on what is "wrong") (see, for example, *www. appreciativeinquiry.org/* and *http://appreciativeinquiry. case.edu/intro/whatisai.cfm*).

A current groundbreaking example of bridging and of how the early work of the NJPC has fostered collaboration is the regulatory document entitled "Changes in Health Care Professions Scope of Practice: Legislative Considerations" (National Council of State Boards of Nursing [NCSBN] et al., 2006). This document is the outcome of a collaborative effort of the disciplines of social work, physical therapy, nursing, medicine, pharmacy, and occupational therapy to remove turf battles from scope statements and focus on patient safety. These six disciplines

Box 10-3   THE CONFLICT RESOLUTION NETWORK'S 12 SKILLS SUMMARY*

- The win/win approach (identify attitude shifts to respect all parties' needs)
- Creative response (transform problems into creative opportunities)
- Empathy (develop communication tools to build rapport. Use listening to clarify understanding)
- Appropriate assertiveness (apply strategies to attack the problem, not the person)
- Co-operative power (eliminate "power over" to build "power with" others)
- Managing emotions (express fear, anger, hurt, and frustration wisely to effect change)

- Willingness to resolve (name personal issues that cloud the picture)
- Mapping the conflict (define the issues needed to chart common needs and concerns)
- Development of options (design creative solutions together)
- Introduction to negotiation (plan and apply effective strategies to reach agreement)
- Introduction to mediation (help conflicting parties to move towards solutions)
- Broadening perspectives (evaluate the problem in the broader context)

*Source: ©The Conflict Resolution Network, PO Box 1016 Chatswood, NSW Aust; Fax +61 2 9413-1148; PH +61 2 9419-8500; e-mail: crn @crnhq. org; website: www.crnhq.org/twelveskills.html.

have collaborated to develop guidelines to assist legislators and regulatory bodies to make decisions about scope of practice that focus on the provision of safe health care to patients rather than perpetuate clinician boundaries. Their ability to do this work is a fine example of the progression of collaboration across disciplines and portrays our collaboration conceptualizations of shared goals and partnering to reach mutual outcomes.

Consensus building goes beyond bridging. Leaders identify any one who has a stake in the outcome (as many as possible) to participate in the process. Stakeholders work together to identify the common ground in issues that cross disciplinary boundaries and may or may not have been divisive.

Partnering and Teambuilding

It is only recently that health care leaders have begun to examine ways to improve the functioning of teams (Moeller et al., 2007; Rutherford et al., 2004). Effective models of teamwork have been used in subspecialties in psychology and health care (e.g., child development and rehabilitation). As health care leaders engage in the redesign and transformation of health care delivery, APNs can draw on the lessons learned in these fields. Some of the processes that have been associated with effective teambuilding and conflict negotiation that are listed in Box 10-3 are further illustrated in Exemplar 10-3.

IMPLEMENTING COLLABORATION

APNs may feel as if they are the only ones with an active commitment to collaboration (Spross, 1989). Of all the competencies required for advanced

practice, collaboration may be the most difficult to accomplish because it is mediated by social processes (Siegler & Whitney, 1994b) and attitudinal and cultural factors that are ingrained in their professions or society in general. Efforts to change the environment to one that is more collaborative involve proving oneself over and over and challenging colleagues' behaviors that restrain attempts to work together. These intrapersonal demands, along with the clinical demands of one's job, can be exhausting. Therefore APNs need to evaluate the potential for collaboration when seeking employment opportunities. Questions about how clinicians work together—the interpersonal climate as well as organizational structures that support collaboration—should be a high priority. A realistic appraisal of the existence of or potential for collaboration is needed to determine whether APNs can provide the standard and quality of care that are characteristic of advanced practice nursing and whether they can expect a reasonable level of job satisfaction.

Assessment of Personal, Environmental, and Global Factors

APNs bring many personal attributes to a professional partnership. Assessment of their current attributes against the characteristics of collaboration listed in Box 10-2 can help beginning APNs to see the areas in most need of development.

In *The Fifth Discipline: The Art and Practice of the Learning Organization*, Senge (1990, 2006) used the metaphors of a superlative basketball team and a fantastic jazz ensemble to illustrate the power of people working in collaboration. Senge discussed the energy and power that are produced when teams become aligned to purpose, when they are able to combine energies and harmonize to produce a synergistic effect. Although individuals may come to the team with great skills and expertise, it is the shared vision and the commonality of purpose that lead to success and improved outcome (Senge, 1990, 2006). These ideas can inform the work of teams who want to improve collaboration and achieve targeted patient outcomes. Successful professional relationships—regardless of whether they are formed within a basketball team, a team of primary care physicians and nurses, a birthing center group, or a team of anesthesiologists and CRNAs—need continued work and practice to grow and succeed. According to Senge (1990); Senge, Kleiner, Roberts, Ross, and Smith (1994); and Senge and colleagues (1999), practice is the hallmark of teamwork. For a synopsis of Senge's work on teambuilding and leadership, readers are referred to the following website: *www.infed.org/ thinkers/senge.htm.*

Covey (1989) offered another perspective on moving toward a higher level of interdependence with colleagues. He portrayed interdependence as a higher level of performance than independence. Only individuals who have gained competence and confidence in their own expertise are able to move beyond autonomy and independence toward the higher synergistic level of collaboration. Collaboration appears to have the same meaning as interdependence in Covey's work. This view is provocative when one considers the hierarchical context that often frames clinical collaboration. The notion that interdependence is the higher level of performance is supported in the evolution of advanced practice nursing. A number of clinical specialties are evolving to such a stage as disciplines mature and identify a shared interdisciplinary component to their work. For

example, in the specialty of diabetes, advanced diabetes management involves transdisciplinary collaboration and is recognized by a certification examination open to multiple disciplines (see Chapter 18).

It must not be forgotten that teams collaborate with patients and their families; this collaborative relationship can be problematic for clinicians or for patients. When patients are abrasive or ill-equipped to deal with conflict, Crocker and Johnson (2006) suggested that clinicians remember to treat patients with dignity and respect even when disagreeing with them and to remember that a patient is more than his or her illness. In addition, illness can interfere with or diminish patients' normal/effective communication skills. When patients have difficulty because their clinicians lack compassion, are abrasive, or otherwise fail to communicate with and care for them, Crocker and Johnson suggested that patients assert themselves by honoring their bodies' wisdom and firing noncompassionate caregivers. Self-assessment is one important component to consider when one is embarking on a new professional relationship or evaluating the success or failure of current or potential collaborative relationships. The self-directed questions in Box 10-4 may help individuals identify their personal strengths and weaknesses vis-à-vis collegiality. In addition to understanding personal characteristics that affect collaboration, APNs should consider contextual factors in the systems in which they practice.

Administrative leadership plays a key role in the development of collaborative relationships between organizational members. Administrators who support team and interdisciplinary administrative models and who are good communicators themselves can do a great deal to increase the momentum of new collaborations. Differing philosophies and standards of care within organizational settings can cause conflict between team members and need to be resolved early (Spross, 1989). The common vision of quality patient care and staff satisfaction

---

Box 10-4　PERSONAL STRENGTHS AND WEAKNESSES QUESTIONNAIRE

- Am I clear about my role in the partnership?
- What values do I bring to the relationship?
- What do I expect to gain or lose by collaborating?
- What do others expect of me?
- Do I feel good about my contribution to the team?

- Do I feel self-confident and competent in the collaborative relationship?
- Are there anxieties causing repeated friction that have not been addressed?
- Has serious thought been given to the boundaries of the collaborative relationship?

that makes collaboration possible should bring APNs and nursing administrators together to create administrative structures that support collaboration (Krumm, 1992; see also Chapter 23).

One environmental factor that needs to be understood is the loci of formal and informal power. Understanding and addressing power differences between groups can equalize the hierarchical differences among members, making collaboration possible if there is sufficient expertise among players (Stichler, 1995).

Global interactions require high levels of individual and organizational collaboration beyond what we can envision. "Systems citizenship refers to seeing the systems we have shaped and in turn, how they shape us and our decisions" (Senge, 2006, p. 343). APNs who recognize the need for global participation and collaboration at the personal, organizational, and systems level are more likely to become the systems citizens of which Senge speaks.

STRATEGIES FOR SUCCESSFUL COLLABORATION

Individual Strategies

The abilities to listen to and encourage others, to experience someone else's success or failure, and to have the capability to know a colleague well foster the ability to work successfully as an interactive team (Dziabis & Lant, 1998). Box 10-5 provides a list of strategies (Rider, 2002) that are thought to promote collaboration. Students and practicing APNs can examine their interactions for opportunities to implement these ideas and strengthen their interpersonal competence.

One strategy is for APNs to promote their exemplary nursing practices to help other health professionals and consumers better understand the strengths of APNs as health care providers (Fagin, 1992; see also Chapter 24). Participating in interdisciplinary quality improvement initiatives and development and evaluation of evidence-based practice guidelines (see Chapter 8) are other ways to engage with colleagues within and across disciplines. It is useful for APNs to role model their practice strategies for other nurses to facilitate intranursing collaboration and consultation. One way to share excellence in practice is to include in grand rounds or team conferences the opportunity for each care team member to describe his or her own decision making about patients and suggest new strategies for care to the team.

Working together on joint projects is another way to facilitate good collaboration. Collaborative research and scholarly writing projects, as well as community service projects that tap into the strengths of various members, open people's eyes to the benefits of collaboration. Federal and private agencies are currently supporting interdisciplinary collaborative studies. Reporting the results in the literature will illustrate the considerable advantages of collaborative interactions. In addition, social opportunities at conferences and receptions allow camaraderie to grow and help reinforce the bond between members of the partnership (Fitzpatrick, Wykle, & Morris, 1990; Hanson, 1993). These strategies move across lines from personal life to organizational settings and from education to practice arenas. New models that foster joint medical and nursing care are needed in primary care, as well as within specialty practice in all settings.

Box 10-5   Strategies to Promote Effective Communication and Collaboration

- Be respectful and professional.
- Listen intently.
- Try to understand the other person's viewpoint.
- Model an attitude of collaboration, and expect it.
- Identify the bottom line. Decide what is negotiable and non-negotiable.
- Acknowledge the other person's thoughts and feelings.
- Pay attention to your own ideas and what you have to offer to the group.
- Be cooperative.
- Be direct.

- Identify common, shared goals and concerns.
- State your feelings using "I" statements.
- Do not take things personally.
- Learn to say "I was wrong" or "You could be right."
- Do not feel pressure to agree instantly.
- Think about possible solutions before meeting, and be willing to adapt if a more creative alternative is presented.
- Think of conflict negotiation and resolution as a helical process, not a linear one; recognize that negotiation may occur over several interactions.

Adapted from Rider, E. (2002). Twelve strategies for effective communication and collaboration in medical teams. *British Medical Journal, 325,* S45.

More important, collaboratively developed practice guidelines improve communication and clarify clinicians' roles in patient treatment (Cooper, 2007; U.S. Preventive Services Task Force, 2003; Weinstein et al., 1998).

Team Strategies

A primary focus for groups is to develop effective teams—the development of effective teams was one of the IOM's recommendations for improving health care quality (2001). Cooper, Laud, and Dietrich (1998) suggest that medicine and nursing are all in the same "leaky boat" and would do well to pull together. Lencioni's field guide (2005) provides activities aimed at helping team members overcome the team dysfunctions described earlier. Lencioni notes that there are two important questions team members must ask themselves: Are we really a team? Are we ready to do the heavy lifting that will be required to become a team? If a group of collaborators can respond affirmatively to both questions, they will be able to use the field guide to advantage. The activities are aimed at helping teams address each of the five dysfunctions by helping them build trust, master conflict, achieve commitment, embrace accountability, and focus on results.

One serious challenge to collaboration is team members who are uninterested in developing collaborative teams. In this situation, APNs must step up and operate from a stance and expectation of collaboration; that is, APNs should model collaboration in all interactions and expect the same from all other members of the team. Building a group of like-minded colleagues can also increase the momentum toward collaboration as the expected style of interaction within a team. APNs should understand that collaboration as defined here is not routinely taught in health professions schools. Consequently, they must be prepared to teach this process to others.

As early as 1997, Kaiser Permanente in Georgia developed primary care teams with goals of higher patient satisfaction and lower cost. Several teams made up of physicians, APNs, physician assistants (PAs), and other health care professionals provided care to a panel of patients using communication and collaborative skills training to improve outcomes (Bodenheimer & Grumbach, 2007). An integrative review of communications skills training for oncology professionals found that such training improved the ability of clinicians to provide high level patient

care (Kennedy Sheldon, 2005). Team approaches that are collaborative lighten the load of providers and enhance care to patients (Arford, 2005).

A recent concept is the idea of a "group visit" by a collaborative group of providers. The group visit can be understood as an extended office visit during which not just physical and medical needs are met but also educational, psychological, and social concerns are addressed by a collaborative group of caregivers who are all invested in caring for the patient. A suggested starter group kit might include ways to plan ahead before starting collaborative group visits, how to let patients know about the new change, who needs to be part of the collaborative provider group, who does what, and an agenda for the visit (Bodenheimer & Grumbach, 2007). An example of a new group visit practice that includes an NP, a CNS and a CNM is "Centering Pregnancy: a New Program for Adolescent Prenatal Care" (Moeller, Vezeau, & Carr, 2007). The beauty of the group visit is the inclusion of the patient as part of the group and the cost-effective use of resources to address multiple aspects of the patient's care.

Organizational Strategies

The numerous initiatives to improve safety and quality that evolved from the IOM reports in the past 10 years help health administrators and leaders create organizational structures that will facilitate collaboration while attending to important quality and safety goals. The IHI's white papers, TJC and Magnet requirements for evidence of interdisciplinary collaboration in patient care, toolkits for interdisciplinary education such as Faculty Leadership in Interprofessional Education to Promote Patient Safety (FLIEPPS; Mitchell, Robins & Schaad, 2005), and clinical and organizational toolkits to facilitate the adoption of evidence-based practice guidelines (e.g., the Registered Nurses Association of Ontario [rnao.org]) are available. These toolkits often include assessments that can be done to identify where the barriers are and where the opportunities for improvement lie. APNs, physicians, and other clinical colleagues and leaders can use these assessments to develop strategic plans for improving the collaborative environment. Depending on the results of the assessment, clinicians may need professional development to enable them to collaborate.

Organizational leaders must take seriously reports of disruptive behavior and take actions to eliminate such behavior (Rosenstein & O'Daniel, 2005). It is incumbent upon APNs to report these and other organizational factors that impede collaboration and expect action. Kinnaman and Bleich (2004) observed that collaboration is "the highest developmentally, and most complex and resource-intensive interdisciplinary behavior" (p. 316). The authors posited that collaboration requires more resources and suggested that the type of problem-solving behavior should be matched to the degree of complexity and uncertainty inherent in the problem. As APNs practice and collaborate with administrators and physicians, it will be useful to pay attention to the costs (time, money, resources, patient outcomes) of collaborating and not collaborating, or coordinating (or delegating coordinating functions). Documenting positive and negative patient and institutional outcomes of collaboration or its absence can contribute to identifying what clinical resources are needed to achieve clinical and institutional goals.

Fagin (1992) and Hanson (1993) identified several strategies that foster successful collaboration at all levels. As noted previously, there needs to be a move toward interdisciplinary educational programs that allow for face-to-face interaction between medical and nursing students. Definitive changes in the structure of clinical hours and sequencing of content will be required. Given the entrenched bureaucracies involved, this will be a difficult task requiring stronger interactions between schools of medicine and schools of nursing. Health care providers need to be learning about health policy issues from a perspective that offers broad-stroke solutions to health care issues. Faculty in both nursing and medicine need to be evaluating and treating patients and supervising students together. It is important to introduce joint appointments of nursing faculty to medical schools (and medical faculty to nursing schools) to give faculty opportunities to role model advanced practice nursing care and build rapport (Fitzpatrick et al., 1990). Although not focused on APNs or APN education particularly, the process and outcomes of the FLIEPPS curriculum development project will be of interest to APNs and APN educators alike (Mitchell, Robins, & Schaad, 2005). In addition to being a case study of curriculum development to teach interdisciplinary collaboration as it relates to patient safety, this AHRQ-funded project is, itself, an example of organizational collaboration around a clinical issue.

National and state medical and nursing organizations must endorse the shift toward a more collaborative model (Fagin, 1992; Hanson, 1993, NCSBN et al., 2006). Strategies that facilitate this shift—such as retreats, social interactions, communication workshops, joint practice committees, and sensitivity training sessions aimed at consensus building—are imperative. As noted earlier, there are some successful models of consensus building in some sectors of health care. Models of successful consensus building across diverse stakeholders must be replicated more widely in health care if barriers to successful interprofessional collaboration are to be reduced.

Exemplar 10-4 provides an example of an APN's efforts to develop a collaborative approach to addressing the institutional issue of pain management. In an analysis of why this collaborative effort worked, several organizational and professional factors were found to be facilitators. Organizationally, the support provided by the director of nursing and the neurologist, who also had administrative responsibilities, was central. The neurologist's "buy-in", occurring about 6 months after the CNS was hired, resulted from a combination of her personal commitment to improve patient care and the knowledge she acquired at the pain management conference. The fact that she chaired the quality improvement committee was also useful. The interdisciplinary team came together as a team about 18 months after the CNS had begun to work at the hospital. A structural factor that facilitated the development of the pain management program was the weekly team meetings held to discuss each patient. The team meetings provided an opportunity for the CNS to identify pain management issues and report progress on decreasing pain for particular patients. This structure enabled the team, as a team, to see that managing pain well actually improved patients' participation in therapy, contrary to the widely held belief that patients in rehabilitation should not be receiving analgesics. This shift in attitude occurred over several months. In addition, the CNS could identify those staff members who had a particular interest in pain management and were open to being coached regarding pain management, thus building a community commitment to relieving pain.

Another structural factor was the presence of an NP on each of the patient care units. Units were organized such that an internist and an NP were responsible for the medical management of the patients. In fact, some of the internists were among the last to buy in to the institutional efforts to improve pain management. NPs, because of their close collaboration with internists facilitated the

EXEMPLAR 10-4   Collaboration in Quality Improvement: Pain Management

One of the authors (JS) was hired as a clinical nurse specialist (CNS) to start a cancer rehabilitation program. The director of nursing made it clear that she also wanted to improve pain management for all patients in the rehabilitation hospital, not just oncology patients. The CNS began by developing collaborative relationships with the staff on the unit for which she had primary responsibility. As the staff on the unit got to know the CNS's skills, they began to consult her for pain management problems. As the CNS worked with patients, she learned that one of the full-time pharmacists was very interested in pain management, and the two began to work together regularly—jointly evaluating patients and proposing pharmacological interventions to physicians. This collaboration was particularly beneficial for patients and staff because the CNS worked only half-time. Over time, the head nurse, the unit physician, and the consulting neurologist and physiatrist with whom the CNS and pharmacist had worked on some difficult pain issues began to ask the two clinicians to see patients in other units. The neurologist, in particular, seemed interested in learning more about pain management. The neurologist was also the chairperson of the quality improvement committee. At the CNS's suggestion, the neurologist attended an all-day seminar on pain management that was being offered locally by a nationally known nurse leader in pain management. When the neurologist came back from the conference, where she learned about the clinical problems associated with using meperidine, she immediately sent a memo to clinical staff about its dangers. She then worked with the CNS, the quality improvement committee, and the pharmacy and therapeutics committee to limit the use of the drug for pain management by creating a policy and making the prescription of meperidine a sentinel event, to be evaluated by the CNS, the pharmacist, or the neurologist.

Over time, the CNS, with the support of the director of nursing, the neurologist, and the pharmacist, created an interdisciplinary team for pain management that included—in addition to the initial three disciplines of nursing, medicine, and pharmacy—two nurse educators, a head nurse, a psychologist, a physical therapist, a physical therapy assistant, an occupational therapist, a social worker, and a nurse case manager. Staff from all disciplines learned techniques to assess and treat pain. The team learned more about each other's skills and developed a "transdisciplinary" consultation model so that, regardless of discipline, each member knew the critical elements of patient and chart assessment. An interdisciplinary assessment tool and core interventions that could be initiated by any member of the team were developed. This meant that any team member could do an initial evaluation of the patient to determine what steps needed to be taken. In situations where the initial evaluation revealed the need for a formal pain diagnosis, team members would recommend to the internist or nurse practitioner (NP) that a neurology consult be made if the primary physician or NP could not make such a diagnosis. All team members learned how to look at a medication Kardex to evaluate how well prescribed analgesics were being used. If undertreatment was evident from the Kardex review, the psychologist or physical or occupational therapist would involve the CNS or pharmacist. All team members knew some simple non-drug pain management techniques and the criteria for using them.

CNS's collaboration with these same physicians to address patients' pain management issues.

From a process standpoint, the hospital philosophy and staff behavior reflected a commitment to patients. The fact that team meetings were "institutionalized" enabled clinicians to maintain a patient-centered focus even when there were disagreements about how to manage pain. In the beginning of the CNS's tenure, there was great reluctance to use opioids for relief of non-cancer pain. Both experiences with patients and discussion of results of pain management efforts in team meetings reinforced the emphasis on patient comfort and progress in therapy as outcomes. Repeated experience with the CNS, in which her competence and the positive results for patients were observed, served to modify the attitudes of many of the staff members. One internist's buy-in occurred after the CNS effectively used relaxation, guided imagery, and therapeutic touch to treat the physician's own chronic back pain. (He was against use of medication for his own pain, although he had come to prescribe analgesics more frequently for patients because of the advocacy of the staff nurses for their patients.)

This was a situation that evolved to an unusually high level of collaboration. Had the team never evolved, the pharmacist and CNS would have still made a contribution to improving pain management. However, the level of transdisciplinary collaboration that ultimately resulted would not have occurred without the administrative, professional, and personal factors that contributed to the success of the initiative.

CONCLUSION

Many of the barriers to successful collaboration occur because of values, beliefs, and behaviors that have, until recently, gone unchallenged in society and in the organizations in which nurses practice. Radical change is needed if the conditions conducive to collaboration are to become the norm. Collaborative relationships not only are professionally satisfying but also improve access to care and patient outcomes. Although APNs collaborate with many individuals within and outside of nursing and do so successfully, APNs may find that one of their most important collaborative relationships—that with physicians—may also be the most challenging. Despite the fact that there are many successful individual APN-physician collaborative practices, including many with data that demonstrate their beneficial effects on health care, tradition and stereotypes are often powerful negative influences on policymaking and in health care and professional organizations.

To meet the demands for cost-effectiveness and quality, clinicians from all disciplines are meeting together to discuss the care they provide and to define ways to deliver it so as to maximize quality and minimize duplication of effort. These interactions foster the trust and respect required for mature collaboration. They enable collaborators to recognize their interdependence and value the input of others, thus creating a synergy that improves the quality of clinical decision making (HealthSciences Institute, 2005; Lassen et al., 1997; Stichler, 1995; Weinstein et al., 1998). APNs will find that their success as clinicians and leaders often depends on their proficiency as collaborators.

Margaret Wheatley (2007) noted that broad-based commitment to participation is not optional. "No one person is smart enough to design anything for the whole system. No one of us will know what will work inside the dense networks we call organizations" (p. 79). That is how "Google" took over the world market and how Wikipedia works so that everyone who desires has input into the definitions they publish on the Web. Wikipedia is an open system. Systems citizenship starts with seeing the systems we have shaped and which in turn shape us (Friedman, 2005). Collaboration becomes a priority as the interconnectedness of the world enters our everyday interactions in the complex health care arena in which APNs practice. Both Friedman's *The World is Flat* (2005) and Senge's revision of *The Fifth Discipline* (2006) and his reference to "systems citizens" assure us that globalization through interactive technologies will force collaborative relationships worldwide.

In the current health care environment, collaboration may flourish regardless of the barriers identified in this chapter. However, the need is urgent to better understand the organizational structures, communications, and interactive styles that enable clinicians to collaborate in ways that benefit clinical processes and outcomes. APNs can contribute to this understanding in several ways: (1) by documenting and analyzing their experiences with collaboration in published case studies, (2) by precepting students and helping them develop the skills essential for collaboration, and (3) by working with researchers who are studying the characteristics and clinical implications of collaboration. Effective collaboration must be at the heart of any redesign of the health care delivery system, whether that redesign occurs in a unit, in a clinic, within and between organizations, or globally.

REFERENCES

Afflitto, L. (1997). Managed care and its influence on physician-patient relationship: Implications for collaborative practice. *Plastic Surgical Nursing, 17,* 217-218.

Aiken, L.H., Smith, H.L., & Lake, E.T. (1994). Lower Medicare mortality among a set of hospitals known for good nursing care. *Medical Care, 32,* 771-787.

Alpert, H., Goldman, L., Kilroy, C., & Pike, A. (1992). 7 Gryzmish: Toward an understanding of collaboration. *Nursing Clinics of North America, 27,* 47-59.

American Association of Colleges of Nursing (AACN). (October 2004). *AACN position statement on the practice doctorate in nursing.* Washington, DC: Author.

American Association of Colleges of Nursing (AACN). (2006). *The essentials of doctoral education for advanced nursing practice.* Washington, DC: Author.

American College of Graduate Medical Education. (2002). *ACGME outcome competencies.* Retrieved September 20, 2003, from www.ACGME.org.

American College of Nurse-Midwives (ACNM). (1997). *Collaborative management in nurse-midwifery practice for medical, gynecological, and obstetrical conditions.* Retrieved September 20, 2003, from www.midwife.org/prof/display.cfm?id=117.

American Medical Association (AMA). (2006). AMA adopts measure to promote quality and safety at store based clinics. Retrieved June 9, 2007, from www.ama-assn.org/ama/pub/category/16463.html.

American Nurses Association (ANA). (1995). *Nursing's social policy statement.* Washington, DC: Author.

American Nurses Association (ANA). (2003). *Nursing's social policy statement (new draft language)* (2nd ed.). Washington, DC: Author.

Anonymous. (2001). Bullying in medicine. *British Medical Journal, 323,* 1314.

Arford, P. (2005). Nurse-physician communication: An organizational accountability. *Nursing Economic$, 23*(2), 72-77.

Baggs, J.G. (1989). Intensive care unit use and collaboration between nurses and physicians. *Heart & Lung: The Journal of Acute and Critical Care, 18,* 332-338.

Baggs, J.G., & Schmitt, M.H. (1988). Collaboration between nurses and physicians. *Image: The Journal of Nursing Scholarship, 20,* 145-149.

Baggs, J.G., & Schmitt, M.H. (1997). Nurses' and resident physicians' perceptions of the process of collaboration in an MICU. *Research in Nursing & Health, 20,* 71-80.

Baggs, J.G., Schmitt, M.H., Mushlin, A.L., Mitchell, P.H., Eldredge, D.H., Oakes, D., et al. (1999). Association between nurse-physician collaboration and patient outcomes in three intensive care units. *Critical Care Medicine, 27,* 1991-1998.

Balzer, J. (1993). Humor: A missing ingredient in collaborative practice. *Holistic Nursing Practice, 7,* 28-35.

Benner, P., Hooper-Kyriakidis, P., & Stannard, D. (1999). *Clinical wisdom and interventions in critical care: A thinking-in-action approach.* Philadelphia: Saunders.

Bodenheimer, T., & Grumbach, K., (2007). *Improving primary care.* New York: McGraw-Hill Lange.

Boix Mansilla, M., & Gardner, H. (2003). Assessing interdisciplinary work at the frontier: An empirical exploration of the "symptoms of quality" (electronic version). *Rethinking Interdisciplinarity.* Retrieved September 14, 2005, from www.interdisciplines.org/interdisciplinarity/papers/6.

Bourbonniere, M., and Evans, L. (2002). Advanced practice nursing in the care of frail older adults. *Journal of the American Geriatrics Society, 50,* 2062-2076.

Bray, J.H., & Rogers, J.C. (1997). The Linkages Project: Training health professionals for collaborative practice with primary care physicians. *Families, Systems & Health, 15,* 55-62.

Broome, M. (2007). Collaboration: The devil's in the detail. *Nursing Outlook, 55*(1), 1-2.

Brooten, D., Youngblut, J., Blais, K., Donahue, D., Cruz, I., & Lightbourne, M. (2005). APN-physician collaboration in caring for women with high risk pregnancies. *Journal of Nursing Scholarship, 37*(2), 178-184.

Cairo, J.M. (1996). Emergency physicians' attitudes toward the emergency nurse practitioner role: Validation versus rejection. *Journal of the American Academy of Nurse Practitioners, 8,* 411-417.

Christman, L. (1998). Advanced practice nursing: Is the physician's assistant an accident of history or a failure to act? *Nursing Outlook, 46,* 56-59.

Coeling, H., & Wilcox, J. (1994). Steps to collaboration. *Nursing Administration Quarterly, 18,* 44-55.

The Conflict Resolution Network. (2003). *12 Skills summary: Conflict resolution skills.* Retrieved October 5, 2003, from www.crnhq.org/ twelveskills.html.

Conger, M., & Craig, C. (1998). Advanced nurse practice: A model for collaboration. *Nursing Case Management, 3,* 120-127.

Cooper, R.A. (2007). New directions for nurse practitioners and physician assistants in an era of physician shortages. *Academic Medicine, 82*(9): 827-828.

Cooper, R.A., Henderson, T., & Dietrich, C.L. (1998). Roles of nonphysician clinicians as autonomous providers in patient care. *JAMA: The Journal of the American Medical Association, 280,* 795-800.

Cooper, R.A., Laud, P., & Dietrich, C.L. (1998). Current and projected workforce of nonphysician clinicians. *JAMA: The Journal of the American Medical Association, 280,* 788-794.

Covey, S.R. (1989). *The seven habits of highly effective people.* New York: Simon & Schuster.

Cowan M.J., Shapiro M., Hays R.D., Afifi A., Vazirani S., Ward C.R., et al. (2006). The effect of multidisciplinary hospitalist/physician/advanced practice nurse collaboration on hospital costs. *Journal of Nursing Administration, 36*(2), 79-85.

Cramer, M.E. (2002). Factor influencing organized political participation in nursing. *Policy, Politics, and Nursing Practice, 3*(2), 97-107.

Crocker, L., & Johnson, B. (2006). *Privileged presence: Personal stories of connections in health care.* Boulder, CO: Bull Publishing.

Crowley, S.A., & Wollner, I.S. (1987). Collaborative practice: A tool for change. *Oncology Nursing Forum, 14,* 59-63.

Devereux, P. (1981). Nurse/physician collaboration: Nursing practice considerations. *Journal of Nursing Administration, 9,* 37-39.

Disch, J. (2002) Collaboration is in the eye of the beholder. *The Joint Commission Journal on Quality Improvement, 28*(5), 233-234.

Drenning, C. (2006). Collaboration among nurses, advanced practice nurses, and nurse researchers to achieve evidence based practice. *Journal of Nursing Care Quality, 21*(4), 298-301.

Dziabis, S.P., & Lant, T.W. (1998). Building partnerships with physicians: Moving outside the walls of the hospital. *Nursing Administration Quarterly, 22,* 1-5.

Evans, J.A. (1994). The role of the nurse manager in creating an environment for collaborative practice. *Holistic Nursing Practice, 8,* 23-31.

Fagin, C. (1992). Collaboration between nurses and physicians: No longer a choice. *Nursing and Health Care, 13,* 354-363.

Fitzpatrick, J., Wykle, M., & Morris, D. (1990). Collaboration in care and research. *Archives of Psychiatric Nursing, 4,* 53-61.

Forbes, E., & Fitzsimmons, V. (1993). Education: The key for holistic interdisciplinary collaboration. *Holistic Nursing Practice, 7,* 1-10.

Friedman, T.L. (2005). The world Is flat: A brief history of the 21st century. New York: Farrar, Straus and Giroux.

Garland, C.G., McGonigel, J.J., Frank, A., & Buck, D. (1989). *The transdisciplinary model of service delivery.* Lightfoot, VA: Child Development Resources.

Gelman, S., O'Neill, E., Kimmey, J., & The Task Force on Accreditation for Health Professions Education. (1999). *Strategies for change and improvement: The report of the Task Force on Accreditation of Health Professions Education.* San Francisco: Center for the Health Professions, University of California at San Francisco.

Gianakos, D. (1997). Physicians, nurses and collegiality. *Nursing Outlook, 45,* 57-58.

Gilbert, J.H.V., Camp, R.D., Cole, C.D., Bruce, C., Fielding, D.W., & Stanton, S.J. (2000). Preparing students for interprofessional teamwork in health care. *Journal of Interprofessional Care, 14,* 223-235.

Grumbach, K., & Coffman, J. (1998). Physicians and nonphysician clinicians. *JAMA : The Journal of the American Medical Association, 280,* 825-826.

Hales, A., Karshmer, J., Montes-Sandoval, L., & Fiszbein, A. (1998). Preparing for prescriptive privileges: A CNS-physician collaborative model. Expanding the scope of the psychiatric-mental health clinical nurse specialist. *Clinical Nurse Specialist, 12,* 73-80.

Hamric, A.B., & Blackhall, L.B. (2007). Nurse-physician perspectives on the care of dying patients in intensive care units: collaboration, moral distress, and ethical climate. *Critical Care Medicine, 35,* 422-429.

Hanson, C.M. (1993). Our role in health care reform: Collegiality counts. *American Journal of Nursing, 93,* 16A-16E.

Hanson, C.M., & Beverly, K.B. (May 2001). *Code blue: Workforce in crisis.* Atlanta: Georgia Department of Community Health, State of Georgia Health Strategies Council.

Hanson, C.M., Hodnicki, D.R., & Boyle, J.S. (1994). Nominations for excellence: Collegial advocacy for nurse practitioners. *Journal of the American Academy of Nurse Practitioners, 6,* 471-476.

Hanson, C.M., & Spross, J.A. (1996). Collaboration. In A.B. Hamric, J.A. Spross, & C.M. Hanson (Eds.), *Advanced nursing practice: An integrative approach* (pp. 229-248). Philadelphia: Saunders.

Hanson, C.M., Spross, J.A., & Carr, D.B. (2000). Collaboration. In A.B. Hamric, J.A. Spross, & C.M. Hanson, (Eds.), *Advanced nursing practice: An integrative approach* (2nd ed., pp. 315-347). Philadelphia: Saunders.

HealthSciences Institute. (2005). *Chronic Care Competency Model.* HealthSciences Institute, Chicago, IL. Retrieved July 25, 2007, from www.chroniccare.org/documents/FullCCPCompetencyModel.pdf.

HealthSciences Institute. (2007). *Chronic Care Professional Certification Program.* HealthSciences Institute, Chicago, IL. Retrieved July 25, 2007, from www.chroniccare.org/profdev_CCcert.html.

Hill, M.N., & Hewlett, P.O. (2002). Getting to the top: Martha Hill, President American Heart Association. In D.J. Mason, J.K. Leavitt, & M.W. Chaffee. (Eds.), *Policy and politics in nursing and health care* (pp. 621-625). Philadelphia: Saunders.

Hodnicki, D.R., Dietz, A., McNeil, F., & Miles, K. (2004). Prescriptive authority: Medication-ordering patterns of advanced practice registered nurses in Georgia. *American Journal for Nurse Practitioners, 8*(1), 9-24.

Hotez, P. (April 13, 2003). For the latest disease, a faster response. *The Washington Post,* pp. B1, B4.

Houghton, A. (2003). Bullying in medicine. *British Medical Journal, 326,* S125.

Hughes, A., & Mackenzie, C. (1990). Components necessary in a successful nurse practitioner–physician collaborative practice. *Journal of the American Academy of Nurse Practitioners, 2,* 54-57.

Ingersoll, G.L., McIntosh, E., & Williams, M. (2000). Nurse-sensitive outcomes of advanced practice. *Journal of Advanced Nursing Practice, 32,* 1272-1281.

Institute of Medicine (IOM), Committee on Quality Health Care in America. (2001). *Crossing the quality chasm: A new health system for the 21st century.* Washington, DC: National Academies Press.

Jackson, D.J., Lang, J.M., Swartz, W.H., Ganiats, T.G., Fullerton, J., Ecker, J., et al. (2003). Outcomes, safety, and resource utilization in a collaborative care birth center program compared with traditional physician-based perinatal care. *American Journal of Public Health, 93,* 999-1006.

Johnson-Pawlson, J., Posey, L., Dalal, A., & Page, J. (2003). *Educating primary care practitioners in their home communities: Partnerships for training.* Washington, DC: Partnerships for Training, Association for Academic Health Centers.

Kennedy Sheldon, L. (2005). Communication in oncology care: The effectiveness of skills training workshops for healthcare providers. *Clinical Journal of Oncology Nursing, 9*(3), 305-312.

King, J. (2002). Dealing with difficult doctors. *British Medical Journal, 325,* S43.

Kinnaman, M.L.R., & Bleich, M.R.P. (2004). Collaboration: Aligning resources to create and sustain partnerships. *Journal of Professional Nursing, 20,* 310-322.

Kleinpell, R.M., Faut-Callahan, M., Lauer, K., Kremer, M., Murphy, M., & Sperhac, A. (2002). Collaborative practice in advanced nursing in acute care. *Critical Care Nursing Clinics of North America, 14,* 307-313.

Knaus, W.A., Draper, E.A., Wagner, D.P., & Zimmerman, J.E. (1986). An evaluation of outcome from intensive care in major medical centers. *Annals of Internal Medicine, 104,* 410-418.

Krumm, S. (1992). Collaboration between oncology clinical nurse specialists and nursing administrators. *Oncology Nursing Forum, 19*(Suppl. 1), 21-24.

Kuhlman, M.E. (2005) Transdisciplinary teams: An evolving approach in rehabilitation. *UTMB Graduate School of Biosciences Alumni Newsletter.* DOI: 830067.

Larson, E. (1999). The impact of physician-nurse interaction on patient care. *Holistic Nursing Practice, 13,* 38-46.

Lassen, A.A., Fosbinder, D., Minton, S., & Robins, M. (1997). Nurse/physician collaborative practice: Improving health care quality while decreasing cost. *Nursing Economic$, 15,* 87-91.

Lencioni, P. (2005). *Overcoming the five dysfunctions of a team: A field guide for leaders, managers, and facilitators.*San Francisco: Jossey-Bass.

Lindeke, L. (2005). Nurse-physician workplace collaboration. *Online Journal of Issues in Nursing, 10*(1), 1-7.

Litaker, D., Mion, L.C., Planavsky, L., Kippes, C., Mehta, N., & Frolkis, J. (2003). Physician–nurse practitioner teams in chronic disease management: The impact on costs, clinical effectiveness, and patients' perception of care. *Journal of Interprofessional Care, 17*(3), 223-237.

Lugo, N.R., O'Grady, E.T., Hodnicki, D.R., & Hanson, C.M. (2007). Ranking state NP regulation: Practice environment and consumer health care choice. *American Journal for Nurse Practitioners, 11*(4), 8-23.

Martin, D.R., O'Brien, J.L., Heyworth, J.A., & Meyer, N.R. (2005). The collaborative health care team: Intensive issue warranting ongoing consideration. *Journal of the American Academy of Nurse Practitioners, 17*(8), 325-330.

McAvoy, B., & Murtagh, J. (2003). Workplace bullying: The silent epidemic (letter). *British Medical Journal, 326,* 776-777.

McClure, M., & Hinshaw A. (Eds.). (2002). *Magnet hospitals revisited: Attraction and retention of professional nurses.* Washington, DC, American Nurses Association.

McKechnie, J.L. (Ed.). (1983). *Webster's new universal unabridged dictionary.* New York: Simon & Schuster.

Minarik, P.A., & Price, L.C. (1999). Collaboration? Supervision? Direction? Independence? What is the relationship between the advanced practice nurse and the physician? States' legislative and regulatory forum III. *Clinical Nurse Specialist, 13,* 34-37.

Mitchell, P., Robins, L., & Schaad, D. (2005). *Advances in patient safety: From research to implementation* (Vol. 4). AHRQ Publication No. 050021 (4). Retrieved July 7, 2007, from www.ahrq.gov/qual/advances/.

Moeller, A.H., Vezeau, T.M., & Carr, K.C. (2007). Centering pregnancy: A new program for adolescent prenatal care. *American Journal for Nurse Practitioners, 11*(6), 48-56.

National Council of State Boards of Nursing (NCSBN), Association of Social Work Boards, Federation of State Boards of Physical Therapy, Federation of State Medical Boards, National Association of Boards of Pharmacy, and the National Board for Certification in Occupational Therapy. (2006). *Changes in the healthcare professions scope of practice: Legislative considerations* (brochure). Chicago. Authors.

National Joint Practice Commission (NJPC). (1979). *Brief description of a demonstration project to establish collaborative or joint practice in hospitals* (pp. 2-6). Chicago: Author.

Nolan, T., Resar, R., Haraden, C., & Griffin, F.A. (2004). *Improving the reliability of health care.* Cambridge, MA: Institute for Healthcare Improvement. Retrieved July 7, 2007, from www.ihi.org/IHI/Results/WhitePapers/ ImprovingtheReliabilityofHealthCare.htm.

North Shore Long Island Jewish Health System. (2001). *Magnet award.* Retrieved May 3, 2004, from www.northshorelij. edu/body.cfm?id=1081.

Nowotny, H. (2001). The potential of transdisciplinarity. *Interdisciplines* Volume 5, DOI. Retrieved July 7, 2007, from www.interdisciplines.org/interdisciplinarity/papers/5.

Pellegrino, E.D. (1996). What's wrong with the nurse-physician relationship in today's hospitals? A physician's view. *Hospitals, 40,* 70-80.

Pew Health Professions Commission. (1995). *Critical challenges: Revitalizing the health professions for the twenty-first century* (3rd report). San Francisco: University of California—San Francisco Center for the Health Professions.

Pew-Fetzer Task Force on Advancing Psychosocial Health Education. (1994). *Health professions education and relationship-centered care.* San Francisco: Pew Health Professions Commission.

Philipsen, N.C., & Haynes, D.R. (2007). The multi-state nursing licensure compact: Making nurses mobile. *Journal for Nurse Practitioners, 3*(1), 36-40.

Phillips, R.L., Harper, D.C., Wakefield, M., Green, L.A., & Fryer, G.E. (2002). Can nurse practitioners and physicians beat parochialism into plowshares? *Health Affairs, 21*(5), 133-142.

Prescott, P., & Bowen, S. (1985). Physician-nurse relationships. *Annals of Internal Medicine, 103,* 127-133.

Rafferty, A.M., Ball, J., & Aiken, L.H. (2001). Are teamwork and professional autonomy compatible and do they result in improved hospital care? *Quality in Health Care, 10* (Suppl. II), ii32-ii37.

Redmond, G., Riggleman, J., Sorrell, J.M., & Zerull, L. (1999). Creative winds of change: Nurses collaborating for quality outcomes. *Nursing Administration Quarterly, 23,* 55-64.

Reinertsen, J., Gosfield, A., Rupp, W., & Whittington, J. (2007). *Engaging physicians in a share quality agenda.* Boston: Institute for Healthcare Improvement. Retrieved July 7, 2007, from www.ihi.org/IHI/Results/WhitePapers/ EngagingPhysiciansWhitePaper.htm.

Reuben, D.B., Levy-Storms, L., Yee, M.N., Lee, M., Cole, K., Waite, M., et al. (2004). Disciplinary split: A threat to geriatrics interdisciplinary team training. *Journal of the American Geriatrics Society, 52*(6), 1000-1006.

Rider, E. (2002). Twelve strategies for effective communication and collaboration in medical teams. *British Medical Journal, 325,* S45.

Robert Wood Johnson Foundation (RWJF). (2002). Partnerships for training: Educating primary care practitioners in their home communities. Retrieved May 3, 2004, from www.pftweb.org/pft_brochure_web.pdf.

Rosenstein, A.H, & O'Daniel, M. (2005). Disruptive behaviors and clinical outcomes: Perceptions of nurses and physicians, and administrators say that clinicians' disruptive behavior has negative effects on clinical outcomes. *Nursing Management, 36*(1), 18-28.

Ruddy, G., & Rhee K. (2005). Transdisciplinary teams in primary care for the underserved: A literature review. *Journal of Health Care for the Poor and Underserved, 16*(2), 248-256.

Rutherford, P., Lee B., & Greiner A. (2004). *Transforming care at the bedside.* Cambridge, MA: Institute for Healthcare Improvement. Retrieved June 24, 2007, from www.ihi.org/IHI/Results/WhitePapers/TransformingCareattheBedsideWhitePaper.htm.

Safriet, B.J. (1998). Still spending dollars, still searching for sense: Advanced practice nursing in an era of regulatory and economic turmoil. *Advanced Practice Nursing Quarterly, 4,* 24-33.

Safriet, B.J. (1992). Health care dollars and regulatory sense: The role of advanced practice nursing. *Yale Journal on Regulation, 9,* 417-487.

Safriet, B.J. (2002). Closing the gap between "can" and "may" in health care providers' scopes of practice: A primer for policymakers. *Yale Journal on Regulation, 19,* 301.

Sands, R., Stafford, J., & McClelland, M. (1990). "I beg to differ": Conflict in the interdisciplinary team. *Social Work in Health Care, 14,* 55-72.

Schmitt, M.H. (2001). Collaboration improves the quality of care: Methodological challenges and evidence from U.S. health care research. *Journal of Interprofessional Care, 15*(1), 47-66.

Sears, L., Maxwell, W., & Townsend, C. (2003). Urgent-care visits to a geriatric primary care clinic. *American Journal for Nurse Practitioners, 7,* 15-18.

Senge, P.M. (1990). *The Fifth Discipline: The art and practice of the learning organization.* New York: Doubleday.

Senge, P.M. (2006). *The Fifth Discipline (revised and updated): The art and practice of the learning organization.* New York: Currency/Doubleday.

Senge, P., Kleiner, A., Roberts, C., Ross, R., Roth, G., & Smith, B. (1999). *The dance of change: The challenges of sustaining momentum in learning organizations.* New York: Doubleday/Currency.

Senge, P., Kleiner, A. Robert, C., Ross, R., & Smith, B.J. (1994). *The Fifth Discipline field book: Strategies and tools for building a learning organization.* New York: Doubleday.

Senge, P.M., Scharmer, C.O., Jaworski, J., & Flowers, B.S., (2004). *Presence: An exploration of profound change in people, organizations, and society.* New York: Currency/Doubleday.

Sheer, B. (2007). ICN advanced practice nurses network meets in Japan. *Nurse Practitioner World News, 12*(8), 1, 10-11.

Shortell, S.M., Zimmerman, J.E., Rousseau, D.M., Gillies, R.R., Wagner, D.P., Draper, E.A., et al. (1994). The performance of intensive care units: Does good management make a difference? *Medical Care, 32,* 508-525.

Siegler, E.L., & Whitney, F.W. (Eds.). (1994a). *Nurse physician collaboration: Care of adults and the elderly.* New York: Springer-Verlag.

Siegler, E.L., & Whitney, F.W. (1994b). Social and economic barriers to collaborative practice. In E.L. Siegler & F.W. Whitney (Eds.), *Nurse-physician collaboration: Care of adults and the elderly* (pp. 21-32). New York: Springer-Verlag.

Sloand, E., & Groves, S. (2005). A community oriented primary care nursing model in an international setting that emphasizes partnerships. *Journal of the American Academy of Nurse Practitioners, 17*(2), 47-50.

Smith, R., Hiatt, H., & Berwick, D. (1999). Shared ethical principles for everybody in health care: A working from the Tavistock group. *British Medical Journal, 318,* 248-251.

Spross, J.A. (1989). The CNS as collaborator. In A.B. Hamric & J.A. Spross (Eds.), *The clinical nurse specialist in theory and practice* (2nd ed., pp. 205-226). Philadelphia: Saunders.

Steele J.E. (Ed.). (1986). *Issues in collaborative practice.* Orlando, FL: Grune & Stratton.

Stein, L.I., Watts, D.T., & Howell, T. (1990). The doctor-nurse game revisited. *New England Journal of Medicine, 322,* 546-549.

Stichler, J.F. (1995). Professional interdependence: The art of collaboration. *Advanced Practice Nursing Quarterly, 1,* 53-61.

Sullivan, T.J. (1998). *Collaboration: A health care imperative.* New York: McGraw-Hill Health Professions Division.

The Joint Commission. (2007). Setting the standards for quality health care. Retrieved November 30, 2007, from www.rogershospital.org/documents/joint_commission_brochure.pdf.

Tjosvold, D. (1986). The dynamics of interdependence in organizations. *Human Relations, 39,* 517-540.

Torres, S., & Dominguez, L.M. (1998). Collaborative practice: How we get from coordination to the integration of skills and knowledge. In C.M. Sheehy & M.C. McCarthy (Eds.), *Advanced practice nursing: Emphasizing common roles* (pp. 217-240). Philadelphia: F.A. Davis.

U.S. Preventive Services Task Force. (2003). *About USPSTF* (AHRQ Publication No. 00-P046). Retrieved May 3, 2004, from www.ahrq.gov/ clinic/uspstfab.htm.

Waldo, B. (2003). Telehealth and electronic medical records. *Nursing economic$, 21*(5), 245-246.

Weinstein, M.E., McCormack, B., Brown, M.E., & Rosenthal, D.S. (1998). Build consensus and develop collaborative practice guidelines. *Nursing Management, 29,* 48-52.

Weiss, T. (2007). *The 9-to-5 marriage.* April 17, 2007. Forbes.com. Retrieved July 7, 2007, from www.forbes.com/2007/04/17/office-spouses-workplace-lead-careers-cx_tw_0417bizbasics.html.

Wells, N., Johnson, R., & Salyer, S. (1997). Interdisciplinary collaboration. *Clinical Nurse Specialist, 12,* 161-168.

Wheatley, M.J. (2007). *Finding our way: Leadership for an uncertain time.* San Francisco: Berrett-Koeller Publishers.

Wolf, A. (2003). Collaborative APN practice. In J.J. Fitzpatrick, A. Glascow, & J.N. Young (Eds.), *Managing your practice: A guide for advanced practice nurses.* New York: Springer.

Zwarenstein, M., & Reeves, S. (2002). Working together but apart: Barriers and routes to nurse-physician collaboration. *The Joint Commission Journal on Quality and Patient Safety, 28*(5), 1-7.

Ethical Decision Making

Ann B. Hamric • Sarah A. Delgado

INTRODUCTION

Various factors, including changes in interprofessional roles, advances in medical technology, availability of information online, revisions in patient care delivery systems, and heightened economic constraints, have increased the complexity of ethical issues in the health care setting. Nurses in all areas of health care routinely encounter disturbing moral issues, yet the success with which these dilemmas are resolved varies significantly. Because nurses have a unique relationship to the patient and family, the moral position of nursing in the health care arena is distinct. As the complexity of issues intensifies, the role of the advanced practice nurse (APN) becomes particularly important in the identification, deliberation, and resolution of difficult moral problems. Although all nurses are moral agents, APNs are expected to be leaders in resolving moral problems, working to create ethical practice environments, and promoting social justice in the larger health care system. It is a basic tenet of the central definition of advanced practice nursing (see Chapter 3) that skill in ethical decision making is one of the core competencies of all APNs. In addition, the Doctor of Nursing Practice (DNP) essential competencies emphasize leadership in developing and evaluating strategies to manage ethical dilemmas in patient care and organizational arenas (American Association of Colleges of Nursing [AACN], 2006). This chapter explores the distinctive ethical decision-making competency of advanced practice nursing, the process of developing and evaluating this competency, and barriers to ethical practice that APNs can expect to confront.

CHARACTERISTICS OF ETHICAL DILEMMAS IN NURSING

In this chapter, the terms *ethics* and *morality* or *morals* are used interchangeably (see Beauchamp and Childress [2001] for a discussion of the distinctions between these terms). A problem becomes an ethical or moral problem when issues of core values or fundamental obligations are present. An *ethical* or

moral dilemma occurs when obligations require or appear to require that a person adopt two or more alternative actions but the person cannot carry out all the required alternatives. The agent experiences tension because the moral obligations resulting from the dilemma create differing and opposing demands (Beauchamp & Childress, 2001; Purtilo, 2005). In some moral dilemmas, the agent must choose between equally unacceptable alternatives; that is, both may have elements that are morally unsatisfactory. For example, a family nurse practitioner (FNP) may suspect, based on her evaluation, that a patient is a victim of domestic violence although the patient denies it. The FNP is faced with two options that are both ethically troubling: connect the patient with existing social services and possibly bring unnecessary strain into the family, or avoid intervention and allow the possibility of violence to persist. As described by Silva and Ludwick (2002), honoring the FNP's desire to prevent harm (the principle of beneficence) justifies reporting the suspicion, whereas respect for the patient's autonomy justifies the opposite course of action.

Jameton (1984, 1993) distinguished two additional types of moral problems in nursing from the classic moral dilemma, which he called *moral uncertainty* and *moral distress*. In situations of moral uncertainty, the nurse experiences unease and questions the right course of action. In moral distress, nurses believe they know the ethically appropriate action but feel constrained from carrying out that action because of institutional obstacles such as lack of time or supervisory support, physician power, institutional policies, or legal constraints. The phenomenon of moral distress has received increasing attention in nursing as well as medical literature (Corley, 2002; Elpern, Covert, & Kleinpell, 2005; Hamric, 2000; Hamric & Blackhall, 2007; Hamric, Davis, & Childress, 2006) as a potentially negative influence on nurses' decisions to remain in clinical practice. APNs play an important role in decreasing the incidence of both moral uncertainty and moral distress among nursing staff through education, empowerment, and problem solving.

Although the scope and nature of moral problems experienced by nurses, and more specifically APNs, reflect the varied clinical settings in which they practice, three general themes emerge when ethical issues in nursing practice are examined. These themes are problems with communication, the presence of interdisciplinary involvement, and nurses' difficulties with managing multiple commitments and obligations.

Communication Problems

The first theme encountered in many ethical dilemmas is the erosion of open and honest communication. Clear communication is an essential prerequisite for informed and responsible decision making. In fact, some ethical disputes reflect inadequate communication rather than a difference in values (Hamric & Blackhall, 2007; LaMear-Tucker & Friedson, 1997). The APN's communication skills are applied in several arenas. Within the health care team, discussions are most effective when members are accountable for presenting information in a precise and succinct manner. In patient encounters, disagreements between the patient and a family member or within the family can be rooted in faulty communication, which then leads to ethical conflict. The skill of listening is just as crucial in effective communication as having proficient verbal skills. Listening involves recognizing and appreciating various perspectives. To listen well is to allow others the necessary time to form and present their thoughts and ideas.

It is also the case that understanding the language used in ethical deliberations helps the APN frame the concern. This framing can help parties see the components of the ethical problem rather than be mired in their own emotional responses. When ethical dilemmas arise, effective communication is the first key to negotiating and facilitating a resolution. Jameson (2003) noted that the long history of conflict between certified registered nurse anesthetists (CRNAs) and anesthesiologists influences how these providers communicate in practice settings. In interviews with members of both groups, Jameson found that some transcended role-based conflict whereas others became mired in it, particularly in the emotion around perceived threats to role fulfillment. She recommended enhancing communication through focus on the common goal of patient care rather than on the conflicting opinions about supervision and autonomous practice. In other words, focusing on

shared values rather than the values in conflict can promote effective communication.

Multidisciplinary Involvement

Most ethical dilemmas that occur in the health care setting are multidisciplinary in nature—the second theme. Issues such as refusal of treatment, end-of-life decision making, cost containment, and confidentiality all have multidisciplinary elements interwoven in the dilemmas; therefore an interdisciplinary approach is necessary for successful resolution of the issue. Health care professionals bring varied viewpoints and perspectives into discussions of ethical issues (Shannon, 1997). These differing positions can lead to creative and collaborative decision making or to a breakdown in communication and lack of problem solving. Thus a multidisciplinary theme is prevalent in both the presentation and resolution of ethical problems.

For example, a clinical nurse specialist (CNS) is writing discharge orders for an older woman who is terminally ill with heart failure. The plan of care, agreed upon by the interdisciplinary team, the patient, and her family, is to continue oral medications but discontinue intravenous (IV) inotropic support and all other aggressive measures. Just before discharge, the social worker informs the CNS that medical coverage for the patient's care in the long-term care facility will be covered by the insurer only if the patient has an IV line in place. The attending cardiologist determines that the patient can be discharged to her daughter's home because she no longer requires skilled care, and the social worker agrees to proceed with this plan. However, the CNS is concerned that the patient's need for assistance with activities of daily living will overwhelm her daughter, and she believes that the patient is better off returning to the long-term care facility. Although each team member shares responsibility to ensure that care is provided consistent with the patient's wishes and to minimize the cost burden to the patient, they differ in how to achieve these goals. Such legitimate but differing perspectives from various team members can lead to ethical conflict.

Multiple Commitments

The third theme that frequently arises when ethical issues in nursing practice are examined is the issue of balancing commitments to multiple agents. Nurses have numerous and, at times, competing fidelity obligations to various stakeholders within the health care and legal systems (Chambliss, 1996; Hamric, 2001; Saulo & Wagener, 1996). Fidelity is an ethical concept that requires persons to be faithful to their commitments and promises. For the APN, these obligations start with the patient and family but also include physicians and other colleagues, the institution or employer, the larger profession, and oneself. Ethical deliberation involves analyzing and dealing with the differing and opposing demands that occur as a result of these commitments. An APN may face a dilemma if encouraged by a specialist consultant to pursue a costly intervention on behalf of a patient while the APN's hiring organization has established cost containment as a key objective and does not support use of this intervention (Donagrandi & Eddy, 2000). In this and other situations, APNs are faced with an ethical dilemma created by multiple commitments and the need to balance obligations to all parties.

The general themes of communication, multidisciplinary involvement, and balancing multiple commitments are prevalent in most ethical dilemmas. Although these characteristics emerge as common elements, specific ethical issues may be unique to the specialty area and clinical setting in which the APN practices.

ETHICAL ISSUES AFFECTING ADVANCED PRACTICE NURSES

Primary Care Issues
Situations in which personal values contradict professional responsibilities often confront nurse practitioners (NPs) in a primary care setting. Issues such as abortion, teen pregnancy, patient nonadherence to treatment, childhood immunizations, regulations and law, and financial constraints that interfere with care were cited as ethical issues frequently encountered in one study (Turner, Marquis, & Burman, 1996). Ethical problems related to insurance reimbursement, such as when a patient is unable to fill a prescription because of restrictive prescription plan formularies, are a growing issue for APNs. The problem of inadequate reimbursement can also arise when transparency is lacking regarding the specifics of services covered by an insurance plan. For example, a patient who received diagnostic testing during an inpatient stay may later be informed that the test is not covered by insurance because it was done on the day of discharge. Had the patient and the NP known of this policy, the testing could have been

scheduled on an outpatient basis with prior authorization from the insurance company and thus be a covered expense.

More recently, Laabs (2005) found that the issues most often noted by NP respondents as causing moral dilemmas were those of being required to follow policies and procedures that infringed upon personal values, needing to bend the rules to ensure appropriate patient care, and patients refusing appropriate care. Issues leading to moral distress included pressure to see an excessive number of patients, clinical decisions being made by others, and a lack of power to effect change (Laabs). In another study, primary care NPs interpreted their moral responsibilities as balancing obligations to the patient, family, colleagues, employer, and society (Viens, 1994). Often APNs in a rural setting have fewer resources to assist with resolution of ethical dilemmas than do their acute care colleagues. Studies of primary care NPs suggest that the quality of the patient-practitioner relationship is the central feature in facilitating or hindering ethical decision making (Turner et al., 1996; Viens, 1994, 1995).

Issues of quality of life and symptom management traverse primary care and acute health care settings (Omery, Henneman, Billet, Luna-Raines, & Brown-Saltzman, 1995; Solomon et al., 1993). Pain relief and symptom management can be problematic for both nurses and physicians (Oberle & Hughes, 2001). APNs must confront the various and sometimes conflicting goals of the patient, family, and other health care providers regarding the plans for treatment, symptom management, and quality of life. The APN is often the individual who coordinates the plan of care and thus is faced with clinical and ethical concerns when participants' goals are not consistent or appropriate.

In addition, conflict between agency demands and patient needs can create problems for APNs in any setting. Increasing expectations to care for more patients in less time are routine in all types of health care settings as pressures to contain costs escalate.

Acute and Chronic Care
In the acute care setting, APNs struggle with moral dilemmas involving pain management, end-of-life decision making, advance directives, assisted suicide, and dealing with medical errors (Hall, 1996; Hebert, Levin, & Robertson, 2001; O'Connor, 1996; Robichaux & Clark, 2006; Schlenk, 1997). One survey of registered nurses (RNs) practicing in the

northeastern United States found that although some issues were commonly encountered in hospital settings, certain infrequently experienced issues were more personally troubling. Respondents reported that the most frequently encountered ethical problems involved feeling unable to protect patients' rights, inadequate informed consent, and providing care that may harm the nurses' health. The most troubling ethical issues faced by these respondents were staffing levels that compromised patient care delivery, prolonging the dying process, and implementing care without considering quality of life (Fry & Riley, 1998).

More recently, Rajput and Bekes (2002) identified ethical issues faced by hospital-based physicians, including obtaining informed consent, establishing a patient's competence to make decisions, maintaining confidentiality, and transmitting health information electronically. APNs in acute care settings who blend expert nursing care with medical decision making may experience ethical dilemmas similar to those of both physicians and nurses. Recent studies have revealed that feeling pressured to continue aggressive treatments that respondents believed were not in the patients' best interest or were situations in which the patient was dying; working with physicians or nurses who were not fully competent; inadequate informed consent; and inadequate pain control were all issues that engendered moral distress (Elpern et al., 2005; Gordon & Hamric, 2006; Hamric & Blackhall, 2007).

APNs bring a distinct perspective to collaborative decision making and often find themselves bridging communication between the medical team and patient or family. For example, the neonatal nurse practitioner (NNP) is responsible for the day-to-day medical management of the critically ill neonate and may be one of the first providers to respond in emergency situations (Juretschke, 2001). While at the bedside, the NNP is able to observe the family's interactions with the infant. The NNP establishes a trusting relationship with the family and becomes aware of the values, beliefs, and attitudes that shape the family's decisions. Thus the NNP has insight into the perspectives of both the health care team and family. This in-the-middle position, however, can be accompanied by moral distress (Hamric, 2001), particularly when the treatment decision carried out by the NNP is not congruent with the NNP's professional judgment or values. Waltman and Schenk (1999) conducted an informal survey of NNPs who felt inadequately prepared to deal with ethical issues that arise in the neonatal intensive care unit (NICU). Knowing the best interests of the infant and balancing those obligations to the infant with the emotional, cognitive, financial, and moral concerns that face the family struggling with a critically ill neonate is a complex undertaking. Care must be guided by an NNP and health care team who understand the ethical principles and decision making related to issues confronted in NICU practice.

Societal Issues

The arrival of managed care organizations (MCOs) and ongoing cost-containment pressures in the health care sector have significantly changed the traditional practice of delivering health care. Managed care goals of reduced expenditures and services and increased efficiency may compete with enhanced quality of life for patients and improved treatment and care, creating conflict and tension among nurses, physicians, and employers with diverse goals (Rowdin, 1995). Ulrich and colleagues (2006) surveyed NPs and physician assistants (PAs) to identify their ethical concerns in relation to MCOs. They found that over two thirds of respondents reported ethical concerns related to limited access to care, and more than half reported concerns related to the quality of care. An earlier study of 254 NPs, some of whom were affiliated with MCOs, revealed that 80% of the sample perceived that it was sometimes necessary to bend managed care guidelines to help patients (Ulrich, Soeken, & Miller, 2003). The majority of respondents in this study reported being moderately to extremely ethically concerned with managed care, with

> …concerns ranging from practitioners' personal values and ethics being compromised by managed care practices (67%) to indicating their concern for patients' needs being overridden by the business decisions of MCOs (86%). Moreover, 78% of the sample perceived that they were becoming agents for the health plan instead of agents for their patients with more than three-quarters (78%) indicating their concern for the potential of unethical practices associated with this system of care. (pp. 171-172)

An example of how managed care goals can create conflict is a situation in which a certified nurse midwife (CNM) practices in a MCO in which a routine obstetrical ultrasound examination is not approved unless performed in a tertiary care setting. This decision by the organization was based on a cost-benefit analysis that found that second trimester ultrasonography done in non-tertiary settings was not associated with a net cost benefit (Vintzileos, Ananth, Smulian, Beazoglou, & Knuppel, 2000). Although this decision meets the objective of cost-effective care, limiting options for women conflicts with the goals of improving access and quality of care (Chervenak & McCullough, 1995). In some cases, a woman's decision to continue a pregnancy is based on the presence or absence of serious fetal anomalies detected on routine ultrasound examination. In a managed care environment, the CNM may be faced with several alternatives. The CNM could simply not offer a woman routine ultrasound and thus exclude the option for early detection of fetal anomalies by this test. Another option would be to offer in-office ultrasound examination but state at the outset that this diagnostic test would not be covered by the managed care plan. A third option involves dishonesty on the part of the CNM and would require devising some reason for the woman to be considered at high risk for carrying a fetus with congenital anomalies, thereby sanctioning the use of and reimbursement for ultrasound examination in a tertiary setting. Each option places the CNM in conflict with some other party, either the patient or the MCO.

Technological advances, such as the rapidly expanding field of genetics, are further challenging APNs. The completion of the Human Genome Project ushered in a new era in biomedical research and clinical medicine (Collins & Mansoura, 2001; Harris, Winship, & Spriggs, 2005). As Hopkinson and Mackay (2002) noted, while the potential impact of this information is immense, the challenge of how to rapidly translate genetic data into improvements in prevention, diagnosis, and treatment of disease remains. To effectively counsel patients on the risks and benefits of genetic testing, APNs need to stay current in this rapidly changing field (Horner, 2004). Issues such as inadvertent detection of nonpaternity, expanded reproductive choices, denial of reimbursement for genetic testing, loss of eligibility for insurance, and the potential for discrimination may surface as the use of genetic technology increases (Dwyer, 1998; Williams & Lea, 1995). In addition, genetic testing poses a unique challenge to the informed consent process; patients may feel pressured by family members to undergo or refuse testing and may require intensive counseling to understand the complex implications of such testing (Erlen, 2006). APNs are also involved in post-test counseling, which raises ethical concerns that include whether to disclose test results

to other family members (Erlen, 2006). Because genetic information is crucially linked to the concepts of privacy and confidentiality and the availability of this information is increasing, it is inevitable that APNs will encounter legal issues and ethical dilemmas related to the use of genetic data.

APNs engage in research as principal investigators, co-investigators, or data collectors for clinical studies and trials. In addition, leading quality improvement (QI) initiatives is a key expectation of the DNP-prepared APN (AACN, 2006). Ethical issues abound in clinical research, including recruiting and retaining patients in studies, ensuring informed consent, protecting vulnerable populations from undue risk, ensuring fair access to research, and ensuring study subjects' privacy (Grady, 1991; Sadler, Lantz, Fullerton, & Dault, 1999). As APNs move into QI and research initiatives, they may experience the conflict between the clinician role (in which the focus is on the best interests of an individual patient) and that of the researcher (in which the focus is on ensuring the integrity of the study) (Edwards & Chalmers, 2002).

Access to Resources and Issues of Justice

Issues of access to and distribution of resources create powerful dilemmas for APNs, many of whom care for underserved populations. Issues of social justice and equitable access to resources present formidable challenges in clinical practice. Trotochard (2006) described how the growing number of uninsured individuals lack access to routine health care, experience worse outcomes from acute and chronic diseases, and face higher mortality rates than those with insurance. A recent study confirms this association between lack of insurance and morbidity. McWilliams, Meara, Zaslavsky, and Ayanian (2007) found that previously uninsured Medicare beneficiaries required significantly more hospitalizations and office visits when compared with those with similar health problems who, before Medicare eligibility, had private insurance. In 1994, Viens found that NPs in primary care experienced distress in witnessing the injustice of inadequate access to care for patients who lacked insurance. As the proportion of Americans who are uninsured has risen to 15% (Trotochard), the associated distress among APNs has likely become more widespread.

The allocation of scarce health care resources also creates ethical conflicts for providers (Bodenheimer & Grumbach, 2005; Trotochard, 2006). Allocation issues are often described in the area of organ transplantation, but dilemmas related to scarce resources arise in day-to-day decisions as well (e.g., a CNS guiding the assignment of patients in a staffing shortage or an FNP finding that a specialty consultation for a patient is not available for several months). Whether in community or acute care settings, APNs must daily balance their obligation to provide holistic, evidence-based care with pressures to contain costs and the reality that some patients will not receive needed health care. As Bodenheimer and Grumbach (2005) noted, "Perhaps no tension within the U.S. health care system is as far from reaching a satisfactory equilibrium as the achievement of a basic level of fairness in the distribution of health care services and the burden of paying for those services" (p. 189).

One value-added component that APNs bring to any practice setting is creativity in the use of a wide range of patient management strategies, which is a crucial skill in caring for large numbers of uninsured and underinsured persons. It is not uncommon for an APN to encounter a patient who has been forced to omit medications for financial reasons. Although many practitioners prescribe generic forms of medications if they are available, some patients still face exorbitant prices for their medications. For example, an acute care nurse practitioner (ACNP) managing an underinsured patient with chronic lung disease and heart failure discovers that the patient is unable to pay for all the medications prescribed and has elected to forego the diuretic and angiotensin-converting enzyme inhibitor (ACE-I). Because the ACNP knows the reduced morbidity and mortality rates associated with benefits of the ACE-I and the importance of the diuretic in symptom management and preventing rehospitalization, these choices are discouraged. Instead, the ACNP helps the patient make more suitable choices when altering his medications, such as dosing some medications on an every-other-day basis. The ACNP has helped the patient cope with the situation but must face the morally unsettling fact that this plan of care is medically inferior.

Finally, as APNs broaden their perspectives to encompass population health and increased policy activities—(both essential competencies of the DNP-prepared APN) (AACN, 2006)—they will experience the tension between caring for the individual patient and the larger population (Emanuel, 2002). Caregivers are increasingly being asked to incorporate population-based cost considerations into individualized clinical decision making (Bodenheimer & Grumbach,

2005), as noted in the earlier example of the CNM and the ultrasound test.

Legal Issues

Over the past 30 years, the complexity of ethical issues in the health care environment and the inability to reach agreement among parties have resulted in participants turning to the legal system for resolution. A body of legal precedents has emerged, reflecting changes in society's moral consensus. Ideally, moral rights are upheld or protected by the law. For example, the Patient Self-Determination Act (part of the Omnibus Budget Reconciliation Act of 1990) upholds the rights of patients to enact an advance directive to guide future medical treatments. More recently, the Culturally and Linguistically Appropriate Services (CLAS) Standards established by the U.S. Department of Health and Human Services mandate that health care institutions receiving federal funds provide services that are accessible to patients regardless of their cultural background (USDHHS, 2001). These standards provide a legislative and regulatory voice for the ethical obligation to respect all persons, regardless of their cultural background and primary language. The APN must understand the relevance of current laws and regulations to clinical practice and the repercussions that exist for failure to meet set guidelines.

In some cases, public policies and legal guidelines may infringe on the process of ethical decision making. The APN must recognize that the law is open to interpretation, and current laws surrounding an issue in conflict may be overemphasized or misinterpreted. For example, an APN in Virginia may be involved with a case of withdrawing nutrition and hydration. Parties involved in the case may misunderstand the U.S. Supreme Court ruling in the case of Nancy Cruzan (*Cruzan v. Missouri Department of Health et al.,* 1990) and incorrectly assume that nutrition and hydration cannot be withdrawn. Or, they may be concerned about the Terri Schiavo case and the issues raised about surrogate decision making in the withdrawal of nutrition and hydration (Gostin, 2005). In the Schiavo case, the legal guidelines were clear; the Florida court system repeatedly upheld her spouse's right to refuse nutrition and hydration on her behalf. However, advocacy groups and Ms. Schiavo's parents used the media to offer a variety of interpretations of the case and wielded political power to prevent the removal of Ms. Schiavo's feeding tube and to twice have it replaced after it was removed. If the APN is familiar with these highly publicized cases, general misconceptions can be explained and clarified. APNs who are knowledgeable about relevant case law and pertinent state and federal policies are better able to take moral action when dilemmas arise.

Unfortunately, in the current health care climate, there is an increasing tendency to look to the law for the final word. The tendency to resort to the courts for guidance in ethical decision making is troubling because clinical understanding may be absent from the judicial perspective. Involvement of the media further confuses the situation, as was evident in the Schiavo case (Gostin, 2005). APNs must use caution and not conflate legal perspectives with ethical decision making. In many cases, there is no relevant law, and thoughtful deliberation on the ethical issues offers the best hope of resolution.

The Health Insurance Portability and Accountability Act (HIPAA) offers a clear example of the limitations of the law in determining the ethical course of action. HIPAA regulates the transmission of patient information for reimbursement, research, and education. In addition, the privacy act in HIPAA provides specific guidelines for how patient information is handled, such as locking patient records when they are not in use (USDHHS, 2003). With the increased use of electronic communication, NPs in outpatient settings may communicate with their patients more quickly by e-mail. Similarly, APNs may use e-mail as a mechanism for consulting with providers whom they do not regularly see in person. These electronic communications may include private patient information. HIPAA legislation does address the need for safeguards but does not explicitly regulate the use of e-mail between patient and provider or between providers (USDHHS, 2003). Thus, legally, the APN can use-email in this way; however, the ethical obligation to safeguard the patient's privacy means the electronic transmission of identifiable patient information must be carefully limited.

THE ETHICAL DECISION-MAKING COMPETENCY OF ADVANCED PRACTICE NURSES

There are a number of reasons why ethical decision making is a core competency of advanced practice nursing. As noted, clinical practice gives rise to numerous ethical concerns, and APNs must be able to address these concerns. Also, ethical involvement follows and evolves from clinical expertise (Benner, Tanner, & Chesla, 1996). Ethical involvement requires

APNs to extend beyond the technical demands of clinical practice and enter the patient's world (Dreyfus, Dreyfus, & Benner, 1996). As experienced clinicians, APNs relinquish an exclusive focus on clinical skills and blend clinical knowledge with humanistic and spiritual knowledge (Dreyfus et al., 1996; Leavitt, 1996).

Another reason that ethical decision making is a core competency can be seen in the expanded collaborative skills that APNs develop (see Chapter 10). APNs practice in a variety of settings and positions, but in most cases the APN is part of an interdisciplinary team of caregivers. The team may be loosely defined and structured, as in a rural setting, or more definitive, as in the acute care setting. Regardless of the structure, APNs need the knowledge and skills to avoid power struggles, broker interdisciplinary communication, and facilitate consensus among team members in ethically difficult situations.

Phases of Core Competency Development

The core competency of ethical decision making for APNs can be organized into four phases. Although progression in phases is not entirely linear, competence in each phase depends to a large extent on the acquisition of the knowledge and skills embedded in the previous level. Thus the competency of ethical decision making is understood as an evolutionary process in an APN's development. Phase 1 and beginning exposure to Phase 2 should be explicitly taught in the APN's graduate education. In addition, the concepts important in enacting Phases 3 and 4 should also be introduced. Phases 3 and 4 evolve as APNs mature in their roles and become comfortable in the practice setting; these phases represent leadership behavior and the full enactment of the ethical decision-making competency. Phase 4 relies on competencies required of DNP-prepared APNs, and the knowledge and skills needed for Phases 3 and 4 should be incorporated into DNP programs. Although an expectation of the practice doctorate, all APNs should develop their ethical knowledge and skills to include elements of all four phases of this competency. The essential elements of each phase are described in Table 11-1.

Phase 1: Knowledge Development

The first phase in the ethical decision-making competency is developing core knowledge in both ethical theories and principles and the ethical issues common to specific patient populations or clinical

Table 11-1   PHASES OF DEVELOPMENT OF CORE COMPETENCY FOR ETHICAL DECISION MAKING

Phase	Knowledge	Skill/Behavior
Phase 1: Knowledge Development— Moral Sensitivity	Ethical theories Ethical issues in specialty Professional code Professional standards Legal precedent Moral distress	Sensitivity to ethical dimensions of clinical practice Values clarification Sensitivity to fidelity conflicts Gather relevant literature related to problems identified Evaluate practice setting for congruence with literature Identify ethical issues in the practice setting and bring to the attention of other team members
Phase 2: Knowledge Application— Moral Action	Ethical decision-making frameworks Mediation/facilitation strategies	Apply ethical decision-making models to clinical problems Use skilled communication regarding ethical issues Facilitate decision making by using select strategies Recognize and manage moral distress in self and others
Phase 3: Creating an Ethical Environment	Preventive ethics Awareness of environmental barriers to ethical practice	Role model collaborative problem solving Mentor others to develop ethical practice Address barriers to ethical practice through system changes Use preventive ethics to decrease unit-level moral distress
Phase 4: Promoting Social Justice Within the Health Care System	Concepts of justice Health policies affecting specialty population	Ability to analyze the policy process Advocacy, communication, and leadership skills Involvement in health policy initiatives supporting social justice

settings. This dual knowledge enables the advanced practice nursing student to integrate philosophical concepts with contemporary clinical issues. The emphasis in this initial stage is on cognitive mastery, in which the APN learns the theories, principles, codes, paradigm cases, and relevant laws that influence ethical decision making. With this knowledge, the APN begins to compare current practices in the clinical setting with the ethical standards described in the literature.

Phase 1 is the beginning of the APN's personal journey toward developing a distinct and individualized ethical framework. The work of this phase includes developing sensitivity to the moral dimensions of clinical practice (Weaver, 2007). A helpful initial step in building moral sensitivity is values clarification, in which students clarify the personal and professional values that inform their care (Raines, 1993; Uustal, 1987). Values clarification uncovers personal values that may have been internalized and not openly acknowledged and is particularly important in our multicultural world.

Another key aspect of this phase is developing the ability to distinguish a true ethical dilemma from a situation of moral distress or other clinically problematic

situation. This requires a general understanding of ethical theories, principles, and standards that help the APN define and discern the essential elements of an ethical dilemma. Novice APNs should be able to recognize a moral problem and seek clarification and illumination of the concern. The APN identifies ethical issues and formulates the concerns about which others are uneasy. This step earns credibility and enables the APN to gain self-confidence by bringing the issue to the awareness and attention of others. If the issue remains a moral concern after clarification, the APN should pursue resolution and may seek additional help if needed.

Formal education in ethical theories and concepts should be included in graduate education programs for APNs. Although some beginning graduate students will have had significant exposure to ethical issues in their undergraduate programs, most have not. Graduate education builds upon the ethical foundation of professional practice emphasized at the undergraduate level. Moreover, the graduate nursing student brings a knowledge of ethical issues that is blended with clinical experience. The AACN (1996) proposed that graduate nursing programs provide ethics education and experience for graduate students to understand and analyze the role of personal and professional values in systems of health care. The more recent DNP *Essentials* (AACN, 2006) contains explicit ethical content in six of eight major Essentials of DNP practice. Exposure to ethical theories, principles, and concepts allows the APN to develop the language necessary to articulate ethical concerns in an interdisciplinary environment. It is important that knowledge development extend beyond classroom discussions. Clinical practicum experiences also need to explicitly build in discussions of ethical dimensions of practice rather than assume that such discussions will naturally occur. In one study of the clinical experiences in managed care settings of graduate students from four graduate programs, only 4 of 20 students identified having experience with an ethical dilemma and only 2 of 22 preceptors noted any exposure to ethical dilemmas for students (Howard & Steinberg, 2002). The authors concluded that this apparent void in clinical education may have been a function of limited recognition of ethical decision-making processes by both APN students and preceptors. More recently, Laabs (2005) noted that 67% of her NP respondents claimed to never or rarely encounter ethical issues. Some respondents showed confusion regarding the language of ethics and related principles. Both studies provide compelling commentary on the need for Phase 1 content and experience in graduate curricula.

The core knowledge of ethical theories should be supplemented with an understanding of issues central to the patient populations with whom the APN works. As APNs assume positions in specific clinical areas or with particular patient populations, it is incumbent upon them to gain an understanding of the applicable laws, standards, and regulations, as well as relevant paradigm cases in their specialty. This information may be garnered from current literature in the field, continuing education programs, or discussions with colleagues. Information on legal and policy guidelines should be offered during graduate practicum experiences in the area of clinical concentration.

While Phase 1 is the building block for the other phases of this competency, it is also an ongoing process. APNs will gain core knowledge in graduate education, but as societal issues change and new technologies emerge, new dilemmas and ethical problems emerge. The ability to be a leader in creating ethical environments involves a commitment to lifelong learning about ethical issues, of which professional education is just the beginning.

Developing an Educational Foundation. As noted, education in ethical theories, principles, rules, and moral concepts provides the foundation for developing skills in ethical reasoning. Through graduate education, the APN studies models of ethical decision making and is introduced to the importance of understanding value systems. Because the APN will apply the theoretical principles in actual encounters with patients, it is imperative that consideration of the contextual factors in specific situations be strengthened. A portion of graduate ethics education should involve discussion of typical issues encountered by APNs rather than issues that receive extensive media attention yet occur infrequently. Howard and Steinberg (2002) maintained that graduate curricula preparing APNs to deal with managed care ethics needed to go beyond traditional ethical issues to encompass building trust in the APN-patient relationship, professionalism and patient advocacy, resource allocation decisions, individual versus population-based responsibilities, and managing tensions between business ethics and professional ethics. The latter three areas are crucial for developing the Phase 4 level of the ethical decision-making competency.

Continuing education programs are also effective and necessary forums in which current information can be provided in a rapidly changing health care environment. Ethical issues are dynamic and re-emerge in altered forms. As technology changes and new dilemmas confront practitioners, the APN must be prepared to anticipate conditions that erode an ethical environment. Knowledge and skills in all phases of this competency depend on the application of current ethical knowledge in the clinical setting. Ethical reasoning and clinical judgment share a common process, and each serves to teach and inform the other (Dreyfus et al., 1996; Leavitt, 1996; Solomon et al., 1991). Therefore the importance of clinical practice (see Chapter 5) cannot be overemphasized.

Overview of Ethical Theories
Principle-Based Model. Although ethical decision making in health care is extensively discussed in the bioethics literature, two dominant models are most often applied in the clinical setting. The first model of decision making is a principle-based model (Box 11-1) in which ethical decision making is guided by principles and rules (Beauchamp & Childress, 2001). In cases of conflict, the principles or rules in contention are balanced and interpreted with the contextual elements of the situation. However, the final decision and moral justification for

Box 11-1   Principles and Rules Important to Professional Nursing Practice

Principle of Respect for Autonomy	The duty to respect others' personal liberty and individual values, beliefs, and choices
Principle of Nonmaleficence	The duty not to inflict harm or evil
Principle of Beneficence	The duty to do good and prevent or remove harm
Principle of Formal Justice	The duty to treat equals equally and treat those who are unequal unequally
Rule of Veracity	The duty to tell the truth and not to deceive others
Rule of Fidelity	The duty to honor commitments
Rule of Confidentiality	The duty not to disclose information shared in an intimate and trusted manner
Rule of Privacy	The duty to respect limited access to a person

Adapted from Beauchamp, T.L., & Childress, J.F. (2001). *Principles of biomedical ethics* (5th ed.). New York: Oxford University Press.

actions are based on an appeal to principles. In this way, the principles are both binding and tolerant of the particularities of specific cases (Beauchamp & Childress, 2001; Childress, 1994). The principles of respect for persons, autonomy, beneficence, nonmaleficence, and justice are commonly applied in the analysis of ethical issues in nursing. The American Nurses Association's *Code of Ethics for Nurses* (ANA, 2001) endorses the principle of respect for persons and underscores the profession's commitment to serving individuals, families, and groups or communities. The emphasis on respect for persons throughout the *Code* implies that it is not only a philosophical value of nursing but also a binding principle within the profession.

Although ethical principles and rules are the cornerstone of most ethical decisions, the principle-based approach has been criticized as too formalistic for many clinicians and as lacking in moral substance (Clouser & Gert, 1990). Other critics argue that a principle-based approach conceals the particular person and relationships and reduces the resolution of a clinical case to simply balancing principles (Gudorf, 1994). Because all the principles are considered of equal moral weight, this approach has been seen as inadequate to provide guidance when choice is necessary (Childress, 1994; Clouser & Gert, 1990). In spite of these critiques, appeal to bioethical principles remains the most common ethical "language" used in clinical practice settings.

Casuistry. Box 11-2 lists alternatives to principle-based ethical decision making. The second common

approach to ethical decision making is the casuistic model, in which current cases are compared with paradigm cases (Beauchamp & Childress, 2001; Jonsen & Toulmin, 1988; Toulmin, 1994). The strength of this approach is that a dilemma is examined in a context-specific manner and then compared with an analogous earlier case. The fundamental philosophical assumption of this model is that ethics emerges from human moral experiences. Casuists approach dilemmas from an inductive position and work from the specific case to generalizations rather than from generalizations to specific cases (Beauchamp & Childress; Gaul, 1995).

Concerns have also been raised regarding the use of a casuistic model for ethical decision making. As a moral dilemma arises, the selection of the paradigm case may differ among the decision makers, and thus the interpretation of the appropriate course of action will vary. In nursing, there are few paradigm cases of ethical issues on which to construct a decision-making process. Furthermore, other than the reliance on previous cases, casuists have no mechanisms to justify their actions. The possibility that previous cases were reasoned in a faulty or inaccurate manner may not be fully considered or evaluated (Beauchamp & Childress, 2001). In spite of these concerns, the case-based moral reasoning employed in casuistry appeals to clinicians because it mimics clinical reasoning, in which providers often appeal to earlier similar cases to make clinical judgments. Artnak and Dimmitt (1996) applied the casuistic model to an analysis of a complex case, concluding that the use of this approach allowed fuller consideration of the

Box 11-2 ALTERNATIVE ETHICAL APPROACHES

Casuistry	Direct analysis of particular cases
	Uses previous "paradigm" cases to infer ethical action in a current case
	Analogs in common law and case law
	Values "practical" knowledge rather than theory—"pretheoretical"
	Privileges experience
Narrative Ethics	Supplements principles by emphasizing importance of full context
	Gathering views of all parties provides more complete basis for moral justification
	Story and narrator substitute for ethical justification, which emerges naturally
	Privileges stories
Virtue-based Ethics	Emphasizes the moral agent, not the situation or the action
	Maintains that right motives and character reveal more about moral worth than do right actions
	Character is more important than conformity to rules
	Right motives make for right actions
	Privileges the actor's values and motives
Feminist Ethics	Views women as embodied, fully rational, and having experiences relevant to moral reasoning
	Emphasizes view of the disadvantaged: women and other underrepresented groups
	Emphasizes importance/value of openness to different perspectives
	Concerned with power differentials that create oppression
	Importance of attention to the vulnerable and to the inequalities that result
	Privileges power imbalances
Care-based Ethics	Emphasizes creating and sustaining responsive connection with others
	Importance of context and subjectivity in discerning ethical action
	Sees individuals as interdependent rather than independent; focuses on parties in relationship
	Privileges relationships

contextual particulars of the case and provided a systematic approach for organizing and analyzing the facts of the case.

Narrative Ethics. Because neither of these theoretical approaches has been seen as fully satisfactory, other alternatives have emerged (see Box 11-2). Narrative approaches to ethical deliberation have evoked considerable interest (Charon, 1994; Nelson, 1997; Rorty, Werhane, & Mills, 2004). Narrative ethics emphasizes the particulars of a case or story as vehicles for discerning the meaning and values embedded in ethical decision making. The argument is that all knowing is bound up in a narrative tradition and that "all participants in an ethical deliberation—the medical ethicist, the health professionals, the patient, and the patient's family—require that which only narrative knowledge can give: the coherence, the resonance, and the singular meaning of particular human events" (Charon, 1994, p. 261). Narrative ethics begins with a

patient's story and has some similarities with casuistry in its inductive, particularistic approach. Critics of this approach have argued that, although narrative is a necessary element in ethical analysis, it cannot supplant principle- or theory-based ethics (Arras, 1997; Childress, 1997). There is, however, growing recognition that careful consideration of patients' stories can enlarge and enrich ethical deliberations; in commenting on narrative versus principle-based approaches, Childress noted, "We need both in any adequate ethics" (p. 268). As with casuistry, narrative-based approaches appeal to nurses, who find much of the meaning in their work through entering into the stories of their patients' lives.

Care-Based Ethics. Other approaches such as virtue-based ethics, feminist ethics, and care-based ethics provide alternative processes for moral reflection and argument (Beauchamp & Childress, 2001). In particular, the ethics of care has emerged as relevant to nursing (Cooper, 1989). The care perspective constructs the central moral problem as sustaining responsive connections/relationships with important others and consequently focuses on issues surrounding the intrinsic needs and corresponding responsibilities that occur within relationships (Cooper, 1989; Gilligan, 1982). In this approach, moral reasoning requires empathy and emphasizes responsibilities rather than rights. The response of an individual to a moral dilemma emerges from the affiliate relationship and the norms of friendship, care, and love (Beauchamp & Childress; Cooper, 1991). Viens (1995) found that NPs she interviewed used a moral reasoning process that mirrored Gilligan's model in the major themes of caring and responsibility.

Although every ethical theory has some limitations and problems, an understanding of contemporary approaches to ethics and bioethics enables the APN to appeal to a variety of perspectives in achieving a moral resolution. In the clinical setting, ethical decision making most often reflects a blend of the various theories rather than the application of a single theory (Ahronheim, Moreno, & Zuckerman, 2000). A more thorough discussion of ethical theory is beyond the scope of this chapter, but the reader is referred to the references cited for more detail on these approaches.

Professional Codes and Guidelines. The ANA's (2001) *Code of Ethics for Nurses* describes the profession's philosophy and the general ethical obligations of the professional nurse. The *Code* describes broad guidelines that reflect the profession's conscience more than they provide specific directions for particular clinical situations. The *Code* provides a framework that delineates the nurse's overriding moral obligations to the patient, family, community, and profession.

Professional organizations delineate standards of performance that reflect the responsibilities, obligations, duties, and rights of the members. These standards also can serve as guidelines for professional behavior and define desired conduct. Although the general principles are relatively stable, professional organizations often reflect on contemporary issues and take a proactive position on pivotal concerns. For example, the American Association of Critical-Care Nurses (2000) issued a position statement on maintaining patient-focused care in environments with nursing shortages and fiscal constraints. APNs must be familiar with the profession's position on topics relevant to their areas of practice. Some degree of involvement with professional and specialty organizations is necessary to strengthen the APN's voice in guiding the profession's moral accountability to the public.

Personal and Professional Values. During graduate education, the APN should be introduced to the concept of value systems and undergo a process of values clarification. Individuals' interpretations and positions on issues are a reflection of their underlying personal value systems. Value systems are enduring beliefs that guide life choices and decisions in conflict situations (Ludwick & Silva, 2000; Uustal, 1987). Viens (1995) found that values were an essential feature of the everyday practice of the 10 primary care NPs she interviewed. Values of caring, responsibility, trust, justice, honesty, sanctity/quality of life, empathy, and religious beliefs were articulated by study participants. According to Viens (1995):

> Values were ideals that motivated the nurse practitioners as persons and as nurses. Values, therefore, played a part in the NP role, and this nursing role in turn played a part in defining values…the relationship between the environment, the NP role, and values was interlinked." (p. 280)

An awareness of personal values generates more consistent choices and behaviors and can also assist APNs to be aware of the boundaries of their personal and professional values so they can recognize when their own positions may be unduly influencing patient and family decision making (Mahon, Deatrick, McKnight, & Mohr, 2000). Values clarification enables students to define and analyze their personal and professional beliefs, attitudes, and value systems (Saulo & Wagener, 1996). Uustal (1987) developed a number of interesting exercises in values clarification.

Values awareness should include an understanding of the complex interplay between cultural values and ethical decision making (Buryska, 2001; Long, 2000; Ludwig & Silva, 2000; Wright, Cohen, & Caroselli, 1997). When patient/family decisions contradict traditional Western medical practice, health care providers may resort to coercive or paternalistic measures to influence patients' choices to be more consistent with providers' values. APNs and other health care providers must understand the assumptions they make based on their own cultural values and biases and how these assumptions may influence their recommendations of particular treatments. As health care professionals gain an understanding of factors that guide a person's decisions, treatment plans that reflect the patient's value preferences are more easily developed. For example, a patient from a Southeast Asian culture may show respect to authority figures by obeying the APN's treatment suggestions, even if he or she disagrees with the plan. In this situation, the APN could assure the patient that questions about the plan of care are welcomed and are not disrespectful (Wright et al., 1997).

By the same token, claims made in the name of religious and cultural beliefs are not absolute (Buryska, 2001; Orr & Genesen, 1997). Buryska (2001) offers a number of helpful guidelines for clinicians to consider in assessing the defensibility of patient and family claims made in the name of cultural or religious considerations. For example, he maintains that spiritual or cultural claims grounded in an identifiable and established community are more defensible than those that are idiosyncratic to the person making the claim. While it is critical for caregivers to respond with respectful dialogue, support, and compassionate care, patient/family demands for treatment must be considered in relation to other claims that also have ethical weight: the professional integrity of providers, legal considerations, economic realities, and issues of distributive justice.

Professional Boundaries. In their professional capacity, APNs have access to personal and private patient information and may develop long-term therapeutic relationships with many of their patients. The atmosphere of intimacy in the nurse-patient relationship coupled with the need to touch the patient during a physical examination sets up a power differential that accentuates the patient's vulnerability (Holder & Schenthal, 2007). Boundaries must be established that acknowledge the appropriate and necessary use of this patient information and intimacy to meet the patient's needs and provide care. While the obligation to maintain professional boundaries within a therapeutic relationship is shared with all nurses (ANA, 2001), APNs must be sensitive to this issue given their expanded roles. They are also in a position to observe for boundary violations by others and to intervene when they occur.

Boundary violations, in which the APN or another health care professional either inadvertently or purposely breaches the limits and expectations of the relationship, may profoundly alter the foundation of a therapeutic relationship. Such transgressions may be subtle, such as sharing excessive personal information, or blatant, as in sexually seductive behavior. Regardless of the magnitude of the violation, the behavior must be confronted immediately and the culpable individual must be removed from interaction with the patient. Other members of the health care team should strive to restore the patient's integrity and trust, involving the help of others as necessary (National Council of State Boards of Nursing, 1996).

Phase 2: Knowledge Application

The second phase of the core competency is applying the knowledge developed in the first level to the clinical practice arena. Phase 2 continues the APN's journey in assessing ethical problems and being actively involved in the process of resolving ethical dilemmas. As APNs acquire core ethical decision-making knowledge, the responsibility to take moral action becomes more compelling. Rather than retrospectively analyzing ethical dilemmas, the APN takes moral action, which implies that the APN recognizes, pursues, and responds to ethical issues. Moral action requires dedication to work until a resolution is achieved or options are exhausted and courage to pursue emotionally charged and complex ethical problems. Often, the inequities toward or infringements on other persons are enough to motivate moral action, and a timely response can change the course in present, as well as future, situations. Therefore the importance of moral action should not be underestimated as a core APN skill, and it should be recognized, fostered, and valued by others. Experience in the practice setting and the courage of the APN to openly discuss sensitive issues enable the APN to assume an active role in dispute resolution. The success and speed with which the APN gains these behavioral skills are related to the presence of mentors in the clinical setting and the willingness of the APN to become immersed in ethical discussions. *Once an advanced nursing role is assumed, however, the APN accepts the responsibility to be a full participant in the resolution of moral dilemmas rather than simply an interested observer or one of many parties in conflict.*

Institutional resources such as ethics committees and institutional review boards provide valuable opportunities for APNs to participate in the discussion of ethical issues. Typically, hospital ethics committees serve three functions: policy formation, case review, and education (Spencer, 1997). As a member of the ethics committee, the APN exchanges ideas with colleagues and gains an understanding of ethical dilemmas from a variety of perspectives. In addition, the APN is informed of current legislation, regulations, and hospital policies that have ethical implications. This is an extremely valuable experience that can accelerate the development of ethical decision-making skills.

Unfortunately, the majority of APNs do not have the opportunity to serve on an interdisciplinary ethics committee and in some cases may have few professional colleagues available to mentor and develop the skills of ethical decision making. Thus the APN must advance this phase by actively seeking opportunities to engage in ethical dialogue with professional colleagues. Professional organizations offer materials (American Association of Critical-Care Nurses, 2004) and workshops in which case studies are discussed and analyzed. This format is helpful to the inexperienced APN who needs guidance in applying knowledge to clinical cases.

Ethical Decision-Making Frameworks. Several authors have proposed a stepwise approach to ethical decision making (Challey & Loriz, 1998;

McCormick-Gendzel & Jurchak, 2006; Purtilo, 2005; Spencer, 2005; Weuste, 2005). In Box 11-3, the steps suggested by Purtilo (2005) are listed as an example. Purtilo's process of ethical decision making is intended for all allied health professionals and thus is applicable to a wide variety of situations.

Most frameworks for ethical decision making include information gathering as a key step. Generally, information about the clinical situation, the parties involved and their obligations and values, and legal, cultural and religious factors are needed. However, this factual information is not sufficient unless tempered with the contextual features of each case. Identifying the cause of the problem and determining why, where, and when it occurred, as well as who or what was affected, will help clarify the nature of the problem.

Problem identification is also a common step in most frameworks. Strong emotional responses to a situation can be the first signal that ethical conflict exists. However, many conflicts that arise in the clinical setting generate powerful emotional responses but may not be ethical issues. As noted, ethical issues are those that involve some form of controversy

---

Box 11-3 SAMPLE ETHICAL DECISION-MAKING FRAMEWORK

GATHER INFORMATION
Clarify the additional information needed.
Categories of information to consider include clinical indications, patient preferences, quality of life, and contextual factors.
Caution is advised not to make this step an end in itself.

IDENTIFY THE TYPE OF ETHICAL PROBLEM
Locus of authority: conflict involves determining who should make a decision.
Ethical dilemma: conflict in which two opposing courses of action are both ethically justifiable but cannot both be satisfied.
Moral distress: conflict in which the ethical course of action is perceived but the agent feels unable to carry it out.

USE ETHICAL THEORIES OR APPROACHES TO ANALYZE THE PROBLEM
A utilitarian approach would focus on the consequences of potential actions.
A deontological approach would focus on the duties of involved parties.

Various ethical theories provide additional perspectives.

EXPLORE THE PRACTICAL ALTERNATIVES
Imagination is required to ensure that a wide range of alternatives are identified.
Diligence in assessing the feasibility of identified actions is also essential.

COMPLETE THE ACTION
Once determined, motivation to carry out the ethical action is essential.
To not act at this point is a conscious choice with consequences.

EVALUATE THE ACTION
What went well and why?
To what other situations might this experience apply?
What do the patient, family, and other providers say about the course of action taken?

Adapted from Purtilo, R. (2005). *Ethical dimensions in the health professions* (4th ed.). Philadelphia: Saunders.

about conflicting moral values and/or fundamental duties or obligations (Ahronheim et al., 2000). The APN must distinguish and separate moral dilemmas from other issues such as administrative concerns, communication problems, or lack of clinical knowledge. For instance, a communication problem between a staff nurse and a physician may be resolved if an APN acts as a facilitator ensuring that each understands the perspective of the other. In this case, ethical decision making may not be needed; the conflict does not result from a difference in values but rather a failure to communicate. As noted, effective and compassionate communication skills undergird this competency.

Although a framework provides structure and suggests a method of examining and studying the ethical issues, the essential component of resolution of ethical dilemmas is moral action. Simply knowing the right course of action does not guarantee that a person has the motivation or courage to act (Rest, 1986).

Strategies for Resolution of Ethical Conflict. When the APN is directly involved in a conflict situation, the skills of negotiation are most useful in moving toward a satisfactory settlement. However, in cases in which resolution is not easily achieved, it is best to solicit help from a member of the ethics committee or another professional colleague not involved in the case. The challenge in most cases of ethical dispute is to have all involved listen to each other's perspectives to understand the basis of the disagreement and to work together to create a collaborative solution (Saulo & Wagener, 1996). In many cases, the APN must serve as a facilitator for the parties in dispute and apply the strategies involved in mediation and conflict negotiation (see Chapter 9 for further discussion of conflict negotiation). The key difference between these roles is the level of active involvement in deciding the goals and strategies for resolving the dilemma. As a negotiating party, the APN suggests solutions and identifies acceptable plans (Beare, 1989). In the role of a mediator, the APN guides the process but does not offer opinions or solutions (Ostermeyer, 1991). The process and steps used in negotiation and mediation overlap in many ways, and in both approaches the parties in conflict discover and determine the acceptable solutions (Beare, 1989; Dubler & Marcus, 1994; Ostermeyer, 1991). The objective of successful negotiation and mediation in ethical disputes is to achieve an integrity-preserving solution that is satisfactory to all parties. In reality,

however, that is not always possible. The issues of time, cost, available resources, level of moral certainty, and perceived value of the relationship play important roles in the strategy used and likelihood of reaching a desired outcome (Spielman, 1993).

Strategies for resolving ethical conflicts (Spielman, 1993) are listed in Box 11-4, in order of desirability. Collaboration is the preferred approach to achieving moral resolution. As described in Chapter 10, APNs develop skills in collaboration through graduate education and clinical practice. In ethical conflicts, a collaborative approach is the most likely one to result in a solution that preserves the integrity of all involved parties. Compromise is an appropriate approach to ethical decision making when the parties involved are committed to preserving their relationship and each possesses a high moral certainty about their positions. Alternatively, accommodation occurs when one party is more committed than the other to preserving the relationship; the committed party defers to the other with the result that only one perspective directs the outcome. Accommodation is unlikely to promote the integrity of all involved parties and should be used only when time is limited or the issue is trivial. Coercion is also a strategy unlikely to result in an integrity-preserving outcome. In this strategy, the more powerful party, who has a strong commitment to a particular position, determines the outcome of the conflict through an aggressive stance. Avoidance is the most dangerous of the strategies considered by Spielman, because the less powerful party does not articulate their ethical concerns. Exemplar 11-1 provides examples of each of these strategies in a situation that evoked considerable ethical conflict.

An additional dynamic may be operating in environments in which avoidance is the norm in dealing with ethical conflict. In a series of observational, qualitative studies of hospital-based nurses, Chambliss (1996) documented a phenomenon he called "routinization of the world." In routinization, nurses became enmeshed in the tasks and routines of care delivery and, over time, became accustomed and desensitized to the ethical conflicts around them. The routine blunted the nurses' moral sensitivity and moral agency, and therefore moral difficulties were not recognized; nurses commented, "You just get used to it." Chambliss noted that nurses were aware of problems but often did not see them as "ethics problems," nor did those in authority. The

Box 11-4   Strategies for Resolution of Ethical Conflict in Order of Desirability

COLLABORATION (MOST DESIRABLE)
Step 1: Understand both cognitive and emotional perspectives
Nonjudgmental listening
Must deal with power imbalances if they exist
Establish ground rules of mutual respect and shared decision making

Step 2: Engage all involved parties in active interaction and consensus building
Focus on interests rather than positions
Acknowledge varying perspectives
Move toward identifying consensus positions

Step 3: Make a decision and develop a plan by:
Reframing
Identifying shared interests/needs/goals
Openly examining differences

COMPROMISE
Appropriate when:
- Parties in conflict are committed to maintaining their relationship
- Parties each possess high moral certainty about opposing courses of action
- There is time before action is needed
- Each party relinquishes some control
- Trade-offs are made
- An integrity-preserving compromise can be achieved

ACCOMMODATION
Appropriate when:
- The issue is seen as trivial

- Only one party is committed to preserving the relationship
- Time is limited
- Outcome is determined by one party; the other party relinquishes control

Can be used as a negotiating tactic to decrease friction
Monitor use of this strategy because it may not preserve the integrity of all parties

COERCION
Occurs when time is short, as in an emergency
Reflects strong commitment to a particular position
One party adopts an aggressive posture; can be damaging to relationships
Monitor use of this strategy because it generates or perpetuates a power imbalance

AVOIDANCE
Occurs when:
- Moral issue is seen as trivial OR situation is highly charged emotionally
- Time is short
- The conflict is not addressed or discussed, and no deliberate course of action is decided

May represent general conflict avoidance or abdicating moral accountability
Monitor use of this strategy because repeated use generates insensitivity to moral issues

Adapted from Spielman, B.J. (1993). Conflict in medical ethics cases: Seeking patterns of resolution. *Journal of Clinical Ethics, 4,* 212-218.

great ethical danger in such an environment is not that nurses would make the wrong choice when faced with an important decision but, rather, that they would never realize that they were facing a decision at all. APNs must be alert for signs of routinization of the moral dimension of practice in the environments in which they practice. Identifying and addressing features of the system that blunt or dismiss the moral sensitivity of any care provider are critical parts of APN leadership and move the APN into Phase 3 of the ethical decision-making competency.

Phase 3: Creating an Ethical Environment
As the APN becomes more skilled in the application of ethical knowledge, the third phase of competence begins to develop. The quality of the ethical environment is a critical factor in whether ethical problems are productively addressed. In one study of NPs, the participants' perception of the ethical environment was the strongest predictor of ethical conflict in practice; the more ethical the environment, the lower was the ethical conflict (Ulrich et al., 2003). The APN's level of influence needs to extend beyond the individual patient encounter to create

EXEMPLAR 11-1 A Case of Ethical Conflict: Strategies for Resolution

An ACNP in a hospital-based clinic provides comprehensive care to patients with HIV/AIDS. T.D., a 44-year-old female patient, has an additional history of diabetes mellitus, hypertension, cigarette smoking, and depression. She arrives at the clinic after missing multiple appointments. In the interval since her last visit, she has been placed on house arrest because of pleading guilty to fraud. T.D. accepted government aid without reporting a change in income that rendered her ineligible for this support.

At this visit, the patient reports that she has not taken medications for diabetes or hypertension because she ran out of pills and had no mechanism for refilling them. She is depressed, hyperglycemic, and dehydrated and is given 2 liters of intravenous fluids in the clinic because she refuses hospital admission. She is fearful of violating the conditions of her house arrest; she is permitted to leave her home only for prescheduled medical appointments. She is scheduled to return in 1 week and is given prescriptions for an antidepressant, an oral hypoglycemic, and glucose monitoring supplies.

The following day, a pharmacist calls the clinic to report that the prescriptions given to him by T.D. have been altered. The frequency of the antidepressant has been changed from once a day to twice a day, and the number of refills for the hypoglycemic agent has been changed from 3 to 18. Furthermore, the pharmacist is annoyed with the patient because her behavior in the pharmacy was disruptive. He states that he plans to refuse to dispense medications for her if this continues. On hearing about this incident, the clinic nurse, who has worked with the patient over a long period, becomes angry and states her view that this is consistent with the patient's past behavior in the clinic. She suggests that the ACNP tell the patient that her alteration of the prescriptions can be reported to the Department of Corrections (even though there is no legal obligation to do so). She asks that the patient be told that further incidents like this will result in termination from care at this clinic. The social worker, whose ongoing contact with the patient was instrumental in getting her to return to the clinic after a long absence, advises the ACNP that a report to the correction officer is not required. She states her belief that to even mention this to the patient would result in the patient ceasing to come to the clinic.

The ACNP notes the emotional responses of the interdisciplinary team members, which signal an ethical conflict. Her initial thought is to wait until T.D.'s scheduled return visit to identify a course of action. This strategy is an example of avoidance. Another option considered that would fit with this strategy is to send the patient to another provider for her medications. For instance, an endocrinologist could be consulted for the diabetes medication. The ACNP considers, but does not select, these courses of action.

In communications with the pharmacist, the ACNP employs accommodation as a strategy for managing ethical conflict. She validates his concern about the negative impact of the patient's behavior on his other customers, and she agrees that he can refer her to another pharmacy if her behavior continues to be inappropriate. The pharmacist agrees to accept corrected prescriptions faxed directly from the ACNP and to dispense these to the patient if she is not disruptive when she returns the next day. He also agrees to notify the ACNP if she is disruptive and therefore does not get her medications.

The strategy favored by the social worker is also an example of accommodation. She believes that the obligation of the clinic staff is the delivery of patient care, not upholding the legal regulations around the handling of prescriptions. She suggests not providing prescriptions to T.D. again but, instead, adopting a policy of calling or faxing all prescriptions for her directly to a pharmacy. Direct communication with the pharmacy would ensure that T.D. has no opportunity for altering them. In this way, T.D.'s unethical behavior is accommodated by a change in clinic practice.

The clinic nurse's strategy is an example of coercion. In coercive strategies, the ethical decision maker resolves the conflict by exerting a controlling influence on another party whose actions or values are fueling the conflict. Suggesting to the patient that her actions will be reported and that these actions may decrease her access to health care can be expected to influence her behavior. The disadvantage of this kind of strategy is the powerlessness it imposes. If this course of action is implemented, T.D. will not make an autonomous decision to be more careful in handling her prescriptions but may avoid altering them simply because she feels she has no choice.

When the patient arrives for her follow-up appointment the next week, the ACNP uses collaboration to manage the ethical conflict. She informs the patient that the pharmacist called about the prescriptions and that this created concern among

ACNP, Acute care nurse practitioner; AIDS, acquired immunodeficiency syndrome; HIV, human immunodeficiency virus.

Continued

EXEMPLAR 11-1   A Case of Ethical Conflict-Strategies for Resolution—cont'd

the providers at the clinic. She tells the patient, "I do not want you to be in trouble, and changed prescriptions can get you in trouble. I want to work with you to help you stay well." She asks the patient for her story. The patient then explains her fear of again running out of the hypoglycemic agent she knows she needs and of being unable to afford medication refills. T.D. mistakenly thought that by altering the prescriptions, she would get a larger supply of the medicines. The ACNP agrees to help T.D. identify strategies to obtain her medications through prescription assistance programs, and the patient agrees not to alter prescriptions she is given.

Another conflict evident in this case is between the nurse and the social worker. Compromise is needed to maintain an effective working relationship as the two provide care to the same patient population. Compromise can be achieved in an ethical conflict if the two parties focus on a common goal and relinquish control of some elements of the final decision. In this case, the ACNP meets with both parties and they identify that their common goal is efficient delivery of quality health care. Through compromise, the nurse recognized the value that the social worker places on keeping the patient in care and relinquished her desire to report the patient to the Department of Corrections. Similarly, the social worker recognized that the nurse wanted to avoid disruptive behavior that is upsetting to other clinic patients. She agreed to relinquish her accommodating approach to the patient's behavior if it negatively affected the clinic's operation in the future.

ACNP, Acute care nurse practitioner; AIDS, acquired immunodeficiency syndrome; HIV, human immunodeficiency virus.

a climate in which ethical concerns are routinely addressed.

Role modeling and mentoring others regarding ethical decision making and creating an ethical environment are leadership behaviors seen in the practice of the mature APN. Once the APN transforms ethical knowledge into moral action, the role of mentoring others emerges. Too often, other nurses and members of the health care team remain silent about ethical issues (Gordon & Hamric, 2006). In a mentoring capacity, the APN helps colleagues deal with moral uncertainty and develop the ability to voice ethical concerns. In this way, the APN supports and empowers other team members to develop confidence and fosters an environment in which diverse views are expressed and problems are moved toward resolution. The experienced APN also initiates informal learning opportunities for nurses and other professional colleagues. Ethics rounds and case review are two ways to engage colleagues in the discussion of moral issues.

The roots of interdisciplinary conflict in the clinical setting are often based on preconceived stereotypes of the moral viewpoints of other disciplines and perceptions of the moral superiority of one's own discipline (Shannon, 1997). The APN can help professionals from other disciplines understand the perspectives and socialization of nurses. In addition, the APN models successful negotiation with other disciplines. Teaching and mentoring activities of the mature APN often focus on other professional colleagues to proactively prepare them to openly communicate with patients about ethical concerns. Indeed, one way for APNs to maintain the trust and respect of professional colleagues is to acquire ethical knowledge and expertise in their specialty area.

This phase also encompasses aspects of coaching and teaching patients and families in ethical decision making. It is not sufficient for the APN to simply provide information to patients and families facing difficult moral choices and expect them to arrive at a comfortable decision. The ethical competency is linked closely with the ability to mobilize patients, families, and the APN's colleagues so that those who need help move through the necessary steps to reach resolution.

APNs should strive to develop environments that encourage patients and caregivers to express diverse views and raise questions about the ethical elements of clinical care. Thoughtful ethical decision making arises from an environment that supports and values the critical exchange of ideas and promotes collaboration among members of the health care team, patients, and families. A collaborative practice environment, in turn, supports shared decision making, shared accountability, and group participation, fostering relationships based on equality and mutuality (Pike, 1991). The APN is integral to the development and preservation of a collaborative culture that inspires and empowers individuals to respond to moral dilemmas.

The current nature of health care delivery in both inpatient and outpatient settings creates a climate in which many workers feel overwhelmed, stressed, and discouraged by the lack of time to care for patients and their increased acuity levels. Combined with a sense of powerlessness and routinization (Chambliss, 1996), these factors can result in nurses retreating from a stance of moral agency. An ethically sensitive environment is one in which providers are encouraged to acknowledge when they feel overwhelmed and seek help when they need it (Scott, Aiken, Mechanic, & Moravcsik, 1995). The *Code of Ethics for Nurses* (ANA, 2001) affirms the importance of nurses contributing to an ethically sensitive health care environment, as well as preserving personal integrity. Indeed, one new provision of the *Code* states, "The nurse owes the same duties to self as to others, including the responsibility to preserve integrity and safety ..." (p. 4). Only when care providers recognize and attend to their personal needs will they be better able to detect and nurture the needs of others.

As APNs become more competent and capable in ethical reasoning, they are able to anticipate situations in which moral conflicts will occur and recognize the more subtle presentations of moral dilemmas. The ability to look beyond the immediate situation and foresee potential issues directs the APN down a path of preventive ethics.

Preventive Ethics. In learning Phase 2 knowledge and skills, APNs concentrate on resolving current and ongoing issues rather than preventing the recurrence of moral dilemmas (Forrow, Arnold, & Parker, 1993). In Phase 3, APNs extend the concept of ethical decision making beyond problem solving in individual cases and move toward a paradigm of preventive ethics, assuming an important leadership role in creating an ethical environment. Preventive ethics is derived from the model of preventive medicine (Forrow et al.) and emphasizes developing effective organizational policies and practices that prevent ethical problems from developing (McCullough, 2005). The ability to predict areas of conflict and develop plans in a proactive, rather than reactive, manner will avert some potentially difficult dilemmas (Benner, 1991; Forrow et al; McCullough). When value conflicts arise, resolution becomes more difficult because one value must be chosen over another. Preventive ethics emphasizes that all important values should be reviewed and examined before a conflict arises so that situations in which values may differ can be anticipated (Forrow et al.). In

other words, the goals of the health care team should be articulated as clearly as possible to avoid potential misinterpretations. For example, a CRNA should have an understanding of a terminally ill patient's values regarding aggressive treatment if a cardiopulmonary arrest occurs during surgery. However, the CRNA's moral and legal obligations should be openly discussed so that both patient and professional appreciate and recognize each other's values and moral and legal positions. Modeling this preventive approach in ethical deliberations encourages the early identification of values and beliefs that may influence treatment decisions and allows time to resolve impending issues before problems arise. In much the same way, early anticipation of potential complications in patient trajectories can lead to proactive discussions of ethical issues and restructuring of the care environment to anticipate and avoid ethical conflict.

In addition to the early examination and ongoing dialogue regarding values, a conscientious inspection of other factors that influence the evolution of moral dilemmas is required. Numerous environmental factors can become barriers to ethical practice. Chambliss (1996) makes the important point that features of the work setting and their role as employees often create moral problems for nurses. The roles and responsibilities of all parties must be clearly defined to expose any existing power imbalance. During this process, issues of powerlessness and collaborative practice surface as areas in which the APN can influence change. By providing knowledge, promoting a positive self-image, and preparing others for participation in decision making, the APN empowers individuals. The skill of the APN is used not to resolve moral dilemmas single-handedly but to mentor others to assume a position of moral accountability and engage in shared decision making. This process of enhancing others' autonomy and providing opportunities for involvement in reaching resolution is a key concept in preventive ethics (Forrow et al., 1993). The Veteran's Administration has prepared some excellent materials on preventive ethics (see www. ethics.va.gov/IntegratedEthics).

Preventive ethics environments are enhanced by a process of ongoing, rather than episodic, ethical inquiry. Throughout this process, the APN incorporates the skills, ethical expertise, and clinical background on issues necessary to facilitate dialogue, mediate disputes, analyze options, and design optimal solutions. In this phase, the ethical decision-making skills of the APN move the resolution of moral dilemmas beyond individual cases

EXEMPLAR 11-2 Addressing Staff Moral Distress Through Preventive Ethics*

Dea, a CNS in a neuroscience ICU seeks to change the management of patients with TBI. She and other members of the staff have noted that the care of this population is inconsistent, and many staff members have a fatalistic attitude about these patients' hope of recovery. She is also aware of recent research on the use of a new technology, brain tissue oxygen monitoring, that has shown promise in improving outcomes for these patients. As an initial step, she invites a CNS from another state, an expert in the management of TBI whom she knows to be an inspiring speaker, to give a presentation on brain tissue oxygen monitoring. Dea arranges for staff coverage so that all neuroscience ICU RNs can attend the presentation in which the speaker describes how the technology is used to prevent progressive injury in patients with TBI. Members of the respiratory therapy team, staff in the emergency room, and nurses from the trauma ICU are also invited to the presentation, which is highly successful. Dea then collaborates with the nurse manager and administration to implement brain tissue oxygen monitoring in the neuroscience ICU. She obtains key physician support, provides training sessions, supports the staff when the technology is introduced into patient care, and develops algorithms for acting on the information this technology provides. Dea also creates a "Wall of Fame" highlighting all unit patients who have recovered, to help staff celebrate successes in caring for this challenging patient population.

As staff members develop skills and knowledge related to the management of TBI patients, they notice the improved outcomes in monitored patients because the technology detects changes in cerebral oxygen level and these data promote early aggres-

sive intervention. However, Dea begins to realize that this success itself is creating a new source of moral distress. Although patients with TBI are often managed in the neuroscience ICU, they are also admitted to other ICUs where this technology is not available. In addition, the application of the technology varies depending on the preferences of the attending physician and the residents assigned to manage TBI patients. Although some of the medical staff members are open to the use of the brain tissue oxygen monitor, others do not agree that it is a valid tool. Because the nurses see the better-than-expected outcomes of monitored patients as compared with those who do not receive monitoring, they think that all patients should receive this technology. The staff's moral distress heightens after a particularly troubling case of a young TBI patient who was never monitored with the new technology and subsequently died.

Recognizing an ethical conflict with the potential to reoccur with increasing frequency, Dea takes action using a preventive ethics approach. She consults a nurse with expertise in ethics to meet with the staff. In that meeting, their moral distress is articulated. The nurses value their growing expertise in brain tissue oxygen monitoring and note that this new technology has served as the impetus for improving the care of TBI patients. However, the nurses are not empowered to maximize its application because decisions about the admission of patients with TBI to an ICU are made without nursing input and because the medical staff, not the nursing staff, makes the final decision to apply the brain tissue oxygen monitor.

During the meeting, the staff members identify a number of strategies for decreasing their moral distress. One is directing admission of TBI patients

*The authors gratefully acknowledge Dea Mahanes, MSN, RN, Charlottesville, VA, for sharing this exemplar.
CNS, Clinical nurse specialist; *ICU,* intensive care unit; *RNs,* registered nurses; *TBI,* traumatic brain injury.

toward the cultivation of an environment in which the moral integrity of individuals is respected. Development and preservation of this ethical environment are the key contributions of the APN. Although ethical issues may develop with little warning, the practice of preventive ethics greatly improves a team's ability to handle these issues in a morally responsible, innovative, and humanistic manner. Exemplar 11-2 provides an example of preventive ethics in addressing staff moral distress.

This case highlights how the ethical decision making competency of APNs can lessen the reoccurrence of

moral problems. In this situation, Dea's actions went beyond resolving a single conflict and focused on the features of the system that were contributing to the distress of the staff. As this exemplar shows, ethical problems are sometimes a result of the structure of care delivery systems in institutions and are not confined to interpersonal interactions. Dea's case demonstrates that applying a preventive ethics approach to the system requires perseverance and ongoing identification of new strategies in order to change complex and interrelated system features.

EXEMPLAR 11-2   Addressing Staff Moral Distress Through Preventive Ethics*—cont'd

to the neuroscience ICU, recognizing at the same time that patients with thoracic and abdominal trauma as well as TBI would still be admitted to the trauma ICU; in addition, many TBI patients are first admitted to the trauma ICU while these other problems are ruled out. Better communication between ICU charge nurses was considered as a means to improve nursing input into bed assignment. Another strategy discussed in the meeting was advocacy for patients' needs on the part of the neuroscience nurses with the medical staff. The staff is encouraged to use Dea as a resource when they encounter resistance from their medical colleagues. A final strategy identified at this meeting was to track the outcomes of patients who receive brain tissue oxygen monitoring and thus develop a database to support the value of this tool. Dea agreed to collect the data as well as review each case and follow up on quality-of-care issues.

Dea then works with a colleague in the trauma ICU to improve communication between the neuroscience ICU, trauma ICU, and neurosurgical team. They arrange a meeting with nurses from both ICUs and surgeons from the neurosurgery and trauma teams. At that meeting, the use of aggressive measures including brain tissue oxygen monitoring in patients with TBI are discussed. In follow-up, Dea and her physician colleagues in neurosurgery and neurocritical care develop algorithms for management of TBI, identifying patients who may benefit from brain tissue oxygen monitoring and facilitating their admission to the neuroscience ICU. These algorithms are reviewed by the trauma service for incorporation into the trauma manual, a document all trauma residents use.

Dea also continues to encourage and support her staff to be proactive advocates. She coaches the nurses toward effective advocacy and role models collaboration and information sharing

in her own communications with residents and attending physicians. Over time, Dea begins to see an increased acceptance of the new technology and of an aggressive approach to managing TBI among the neurosurgery teams.

Two members of the nursing staff, with Dea's encouragement and guidance, developed a poster about their moral distress and steps to address it. The poster was accepted and presented at a national conference (Pracher, Moss, & Mahanes, 2006). The nurses attending the conference to present the poster learned that their situation is not unique; other conference attendees noted similar conflicts in their own units and validated the distress experienced as a result.

While closer connection between the neuroscience and trauma ICUs is a secondary benefit, concerns about inconsistencies in care continue. Patients with TBI continue to be admitted to both the neuroscience ICU and the trauma ICU and are not always transferred quickly if they need monitoring. Through a collaborative process with the CNS in the trauma ICU, a new approach to standardizing the care of TBI patients is identified and plans are made to incorporate brain tissue oxygen monitoring in the trauma ICU. The database Dea has maintained demonstrates positive patient outcomes that support this change. Dea lends support to the CNS in that unit as she begins to train the staff in the use of the technology and the algorithms for responding to the information it provides. Two years after the initial educational session on this technology, Dea notes that "there is still work to do to optimize the care of these patients." However, because of her proactive response to the staff's distress, champions for this technology now exist on both units and an environment for effecting positive change has been created.

Phase 4: Promoting Social Justice Within the Health Care System

The final phase in the ethical decision making competency is seen in mature APNs who have expanded their focus of concern to incorporate the needs of their larger specialty population within the health care system. This phase again builds on the previous ones, as APNs move their sphere of involvement beyond their institution into the societal sector. Moving into

the arena of social justice is both an historical legacy and a current imperative. Falk-Rafael (2005) noted that Nightingale's work bequeathed to professional nursing "a legacy of justice-making as an expression of caring and compassion" (p. 212). The AACN's *Essentials of Doctoral Education for Advanced Nursing Practice*" (2006) strongly supports APNs moving into a larger arena of ethical decision making. The need for nursing to speak to mounting concerns regarding the quality of patient care delivery and outcomes in policy and public forums is one justification for doctoral-level education for APNs. Most of the DNP Essentials address the need for systems leadership in these larger forums; one Essential in particular, "Health Care Policy for Advocacy in Health Care" (AACN, 2006), advocates for DNP graduates to:

> …design, implement and advocate for health care policy which addresses issues of social justice and equity in health care. The powerful practice experiences of the DNP graduate can become potent influencers in policy formation." (p. 13)

In a number of hallmark reports, the Institute of Medicine (IOM, 1999, 2001, 2003) highlighted the fragmentation and systems failures in health care and called for restructuring efforts to achieve safe, effective, and equitable care. Equity is primarily an issue of justice; as noted, concerns about access to and distribution of health care resources are key justice concerns of APNs. In this phase, APNs work as agents of change for justice in the health care system on behalf of their specialty populations.

Nurses in many roles are increasingly concerned about the current health care system, its business rather than caring orientation, and the gaps in care provision to many of the neediest members of society. Some authors assert that all nurses should include sociopolitical advocacy in their practice if the profession is to fulfill its social mandate (Falk-Raphael, 2005). This is a tall order, and most undergraduate nursing programs do not include the requisite skills needed for this level of advocacy. Even APN curricula may not include such content, so the APN must commit to continued skill development and involvement in national organizations to reach this phase. One distinguishing feature of the APN's activities in this arena as compared with other nurses is the clinical expertise of the APN. The central competency of direct clinical practice and the APN's cutting-edge understanding of the clinical needs of his or her patient population provide the platform from which the APN speaks to social justice issues. Indeed, nurses in policy, research, or other non-APN roles often call upon APNs to provide expert information on the policy and larger system issues that confront their specialty populations.

To enact this level of the ethical decision-making competency requires sophisticated use of all of the core competencies of advanced practice nursing. In particular, advocacy, communication, collaboration (see Chapter 10), and leadership (see Chapter 9) are

required. APNs active in this phase are often consultants to policymakers or serve on expert panels crafting policies for specialty groups. Essential knowledge needed for this phase includes an understanding of the concepts of justice, particularly distributive justice (the equitable allocation of scarce resources) and restorative justice (the duty owed to those who have been systematically disadvantaged through no fault of their own). Also, to move into this level of activity, APNs need knowledge of the health policy process in general (see Chapter 22) and specific health policies affecting their specialty population.

Although this phase of the ethical decision-making competency may sound daunting to the novice, beginning activities in this arena, such as involvement in institutional or community policymaking groups and sustained efforts to build knowledge in the areas discussed, can lay the foundation for larger policy involvement. Many graduate programs and most DNP programs have courses dedicated to the development of policy skills. Frequently the experience of moral outrage over the unethical treatment of patients propels the APN into the policy arena as the APN sees the consequences of the gaps in current health care. Examples of Phase 4 activities are seen in many of the situations discussed in Chapter 22.

EVALUATION OF THE ETHICAL DECISION-MAKING COMPETENCY

The evaluation of ethical decision making should focus on two areas: the process and the outcome. Process evaluation is important because it provides an overview of the moral disagreement, the interpersonal skills employed, the interactions between the parties in conflict, and the problems encountered during the phases of resolution. Whether the APN was the facilitator or a party in conflict, a deliberate and reflective evaluation of the process of resolution should occur. It is useful for the APN to assess the type of issue, the interrelational and situational variables, the conceptual shifts that occurred during the process, and the strategies used by both parties during the negotiation phase (Olczak, Grosch, & Duffy, 1991). As the APN reflects on the process, attention should be given to how similar situations could be anticipated and resolved in the future. Debriefing situations with the affected parties is also an important process evaluation strategy. To avoid the session becoming simply a venting of emotions, the APN must keep the focus on preventive ethics and what needs to change in the environment to avoid or minimize future problems.

Deliberate and consistent review of the process will help the APN assess various approaches to the resolution of ethical dilemmas and identify the onset of moral conflict earlier. This ongoing evaluation of process is particularly important in Phase 4, as changes in system-wide health policies to support social justice require years in the making. Evaluating grassroots and legislative efforts as they occur will help identify strategies likely to be successful versus those that ought to be abandoned.

Evaluation of the outcome is also critical because it acknowledges creative solutions and celebrates moral action. Components of the outcome evaluation include the short-term and long-term consequences of the action taken and the satisfaction of all parties with the chosen solution (Olczak et al., 1991). Unfortunately, a successful process does not always result in a satisfactory outcome. Occasionally, the outcome reveals the need for changes within the institution or health care system. The APN may need to become involved in advancing these desired changes or identifying appropriate resources to pursue them. The goal of outcome evaluation is to minimize the risks of a similar event by identifying predictable patterns and thereby averting recurrent and future dilemmas. The questions "What do we want to happen differently if we are confronted with a similar situation?" and "What first steps can we take to achieve this change?" can be helpful in framing the discussion.

Evaluation of the ethical problem is an important step in preventing future dilemmas and building ethically sensitive environments; however, in some situations, tension and uneasiness will remain. In true ethical dilemmas, even the best process may still result in a course of action that is not seen positively by all participants. It is important for the APN to acknowledge that many issues leave a "moral residue" that continues to trouble participants involved in the conflict (Webster & Baylis, 2000). Part of the outcome evaluation must address the reality of these lingering feelings and the related tensions they create.

BARRIERS TO ETHICAL PRACTICE AND POTENTIAL SOLUTIONS

A number of factors influence how moral issues are addressed and resolved in the clinical setting. Some barriers, once identified, can be corrected and eliminated. Others may require attention at institutional,

state, or national levels. Regardless of type, the APN must identify and respond to the barriers that inhibit the development of a morally responsive practice environment.

Intraprofessional Barriers

The APN often relies on other nurses and caregivers to recognize ethical issues and initiate dialogue with professional colleagues. In some situations, nurses are uncertain, fearful, insecure, unable to articulate their moral concern, or incapable of taking moral action (Gordon & Harmic, 2006; Pike, 1991). Nurses who do not feel secure with their ethical knowledge may dismiss an issue as insignificant or discount and minimize their perceptions of the dilemma. Unfortunately, too many ethical issues are "swept under the rug" because of this moral uncertainty and inaction. It is far better for nurses to raise a concern that may be viewed as insignificant than to wait for the problem to erupt with chaos and conflict. Often, others are also concerned about the issue but have not voiced their perspective for fear of having their viewpoint invalidated.

Conflict between a nurse's personal values and the professional values of nursing as articulated in the *Code of Ethics* (ANA, 2001) may be a source of moral distress. For example, an emergency room NP may be faced with providing care for a criminal injured in a gunfight that killed innocent bystanders. Although it is disturbing and difficult to provide care for an individual who has caused harm to others, the NP's personal views should not interfere with the quality of the care provided. The process of values clarification is helpful in preparing for this situation. Once personal values are realized, the nurse can more easily anticipate situations in which such conflicts will arise and either avoid becoming part of the problem or develop a defined strategy to deal with the issue.

Perceptions of powerlessness influence how active nurses become in the resolution of ethical dilemmas (Ceci, 2004; Erlen & Frost, 1991; Gaul, 1995; Gordon & Hamric, 2006). Powerlessness can be both an intraprofessional and an interprofessional barrier. Power issues between the APN and bedside nurse may evolve because the bedside nurse views the APN as having enhanced decision-making authority and a more direct line of communication to the physician. Certainly, in some cases, the sense of powerlessness is a reality. For example, both staff nurses and APNs may encounter situations in which their clinical judgment is contradicted by administrative policy (Austin, 2007).

Feelings of powerlessness can result in individuals feeling vulnerable and defenseless. The APN's role encompasses overcoming one's own destructive feelings of vulnerability, empowering professional staff and patients, and working to change policies that do not support quality patient care. One of the most effective strategies for empowering others is that of role modeling and teaching from a stance of mutual respect and professional accountability. Fostering respect and collegiality among all members of the nursing staff and holding nurses accountable for their actions are potent antidotes to powerlessness (see Chapter 9). Through role modeling, APNs demonstrate critical thinking as they identify and clarify moral problems and guide others through the process. Including ethical aspects of a patient's case in interdisciplinary rounds, scheduling debriefing sessions after a particularly difficult case, reading and discussing ethics articles specific to the specialty patient group in a journal club, or using simulation activities in which caregivers role play different scenarios are additional strategies the APN can propose to cultivate skills in critical reflection and the ability to consider alternate interpretations of a situation. Such activities provide both education and support for other nurses in examining ethical issues and working toward collaborative problem solving. Nurses must be able to express diverse views without fearing ridicule or rejection from peers. An environment that supports ethical reasoning and judgment will foster action.

Interprofessional Barriers

Nurses and physicians define, perceive, analyze, and reason through ethical problems from distinct and sometimes opposing perspectives (Curtis & Shannon, 2006; Shannon, 1997). Although the roles are complementary, these differing approaches may create conflict between a nurse and a physician, further separating and isolating the perspectives. A physician may be unaware of the nurse's differing opinion or may not recognize this difference as a conflict (Gramelspracher, Howell, & Young, 1986; Hamric & Blackhall, 2007; Shannon, Mitchell, & Cain, 2002). Conflicts are intensified when the physician does not agree with the nurse that certain details and specifics of the situation are important or simply does not feel accountable to resolve the conflict with the nurse (Gramelspracher et al.). One study indicated that physicians and nurses dealt with the same ethical problems and used similar moral reasoning but that differences were related

to professional roles, the kinds of responsibilities each group had in the situation, and the resulting different questions each group raised (Oberle & Hughes, 2001). The APN must first deal with any interprofessional communication problems between a nurse and physician before seeking resolution of ethical problems.

Although open communication is a necessary component of a collaborative environment, it is not sufficient. Physicians and other members of the health care team must understand the nurse's role and responsibilities and vice versa. In the traditional hospital setting, some physicians may still view the nurse as a subordinate who functions primarily to carry out their orders (Gramelspracher et al., 1986). In some cases, physicians perceive their authority as threatened when nurses expand their education and assume more autonomous roles as APNs (Haddad, 1991). They may also feel threatened by the level of expertise that the APN demonstrates in his or her clinical area. However, respect generally increases as the physician realizes the APN's competence and accountability and recognizes that physician and nurse roles are very complementary in improving patient care.

Successful collaboration between nurses and physicians is grounded in communication, cooperation, competence, respect, accountability, and trust (Baggs & Schmitt, 1988; see also Chapter 10). These factors may be influenced negatively or positively by the professional relationship that exists between the physician and the APN. Important questions in understanding this relationship include the following: For whom does the APN work—the physician, the department, the institution? Who pays the APN's salary? Are APNs able to bill for their services, or are they paid from physician or institutional billings? These factors certainly influence the issue of power in the relationship. What role did the physician have in hiring the APN? Was the physician professionally invested in working with APNs initially, or did the institution mandate that physicians work with APNs? Has the physician had experience working with an APN, and what was the nature of the experience? Obviously, a physician who actively seeks to work with an APN is more likely to have a successful and collaborative interaction. However, even in this case, the intention may not necessarily be to improve patient care by adding another discipline's expertise but, rather, to make the physician's job easier by bringing an APN on the team. Do the physician and APN work as a team or as two independent agents?

What is the level of interaction between APN and physician: constant, side-by-side interaction; or once a day or once a week?

Physicians can influence patients' perceptions of APNs. If the patient sees early on that the APN has a role and the physician recognizes and reinforces that role, then in fact the APN will have a more significant and clinically important role. Conversely, if the physician does not refer APN-specific issues to the APN but attempts to handle them himself or herself or does not define for the patient the importance of the APN's role, the patient is unlikely to see the APN as important to his or her health care. The patient's perception of the APN's role and influence in his or her care will in turn influence the professional interaction, balance of power, and level of collaborative behavior between physician and APN. All of these factors will either enhance or constrain the quality of ethical decision making that occurs.

Again, open communication, cooperation, demonstrated competence, accountability for both role and actions, and developing trust by both the physician and the APN will facilitate overcoming these barriers to successful collaboration. Time and ongoing interactions in this relatively new (for many physicians) arena will also aid in improving the professional relationship. Physicians and APNs need to engage in moral discourse to understand and support the ethical burden each professional carries (Curtis & Shannon, 2006; Hamric & Blackhall, 2007; Oberle & Hughes, 2001; Shannon, 1997). One of the encouraging indications of interdisciplinary activity is the work of the Tavistock Group, who proposed a set of five ethical principles to guide all health professionals who deliver and affect health care (Smith, Hiatt, & Berwick, 1999). More recently, the American Association of Critical-Care Nurses (2005) issued a document entitled *Standards for Establishing and Sustaining Healthy Work Environments* and identified skilled communication and true collaboration as two of the six elements that foster an environment for excellence in patient care. Among the collaborative partners endorsing these standards are the American College of Chest Physicians, the American Thoracic Society, and the Society of Critical Care Medicine. These endorsements indicate an interdisciplinary commitment to improving patient care through enhanced communication and attention to collaboration.

Although this discussion has focused on physician/APN interactions, similar barriers can arise with other professional groups as well. Building collaborative interdisciplinary teams that emphasize preventive ethics is the key strategy for eliminating interprofessional barriers.

Patient/Provider Barriers

Health care providers, employees of the health care institution, and patients and families make up the multicultural clinical settings in which most APNs practice. As noted earlier, APNs may encounter a conflict when they are confronted with a cultural practice that they regard as harmful (Kikuchi, 1996; Linnard-Palmer & Kools, 2004). For example, parents may inform an NP in a pediatric outpatient setting that because of cultural and religious reasons, they do not want their child immunized. In this case, the NP is faced with a cultural belief that places both the child and community at risk (Kikuchi, 1996). The NP wants to preserve the parent's rights and preferences but is concerned about the child's best interests and the potential harm to other children if they are exposed to an illness from a non-immunized child. Issues that result from cultural diversity are difficult to resolve without help from others more familiar with the specific cultural practices and beliefs. Occasionally, contact with the language department of a local university can direct the APN to helpful resources for understanding more about the culture. In troubling cases, when the risk of harm is great, the APN should consult with ethics consultants, clergy, and other resources to help identify some reasonable, culturally sensitive options that preserve the rights and dignity of the patient and family without harming others.

The absence of an advance directive may be a barrier to upholding the patient's wishes regarding end-of-life care. Advance directives are legal documents that support the rights of patients to determine in advance their wishes for future end-of-life treatment. The two types of advance directives are the living will and the durable power of attorney for health care (DPAHC) or health care proxy. The DPAHC is the more flexible and legally binding advance directive, and all patients should be encouraged to have one. It allows the patient to appoint an individual who will make treatment choices for the patient in the event the patient becomes incapacitated. For patients who have executed an advance directive, the APN should discuss with the patient and family how the advance directive would guide end-of-life decision making. If no advance directive is executed, the decision maker for the incapacitated patient is determined according to state statute. It is entirely possible that an estranged relative may be assigned this responsibility, adding to the moral complexity of the situation. APNs in primary care settings have a particular responsibility to encourage patients and families to consider the DPAHC before an emergency renders the patient incapable of stating his or her wishes.

Another barrier to ethical practice that challenges many APNs is the issue of patient nonadherence. Patients may choose not to be actively involved in their care or resist an APN's attempts to improve their well-being, which raises both clinical and ethical questions. Once clinical reasons for nonadherence (e.g., inadequate assessment of patient goals, lack of resources, literacy issues, inadequate communications) have been explored and addressed, the APN has several choices. The first response is to determine whether the underlying problem can be rectified, such as by obtaining financial support to assist in purchasing medications. However, if the patient simply chooses to ignore the agreed-upon plan of care, the APN may be faced with terminating the patient-provider relationship, maintaining the relationship with less optimal objectives for care, or continuing to try to persuade the patient to adhere to the best treatment plan. Often, APNs spend a disproportionate amount of time with nonadherent patients, attending to preventable exacerbations of their illness or in follow-up conversations attempting to convince them to follow the recommended treatment plans. These patients are unsettling to the APN because other patients, who are more amenable to the plan of care, receive less time than do nonadherent patients. There are no easy solutions to managing the nonadherent patient (Resnick, 2005), and full consideration of this issue is beyond the scope of this chapter. In many cases, patients do not intentionally choose to ignore the provider's recommendations. Other factors, such as impaired thinking and concentration, financial issues, and emotional disorders, can impede the patient's ability to follow the prescribed treatment plan (Bishop & Brodkey, 2006). Members of the health care team often view patient adherence as a direct responsibility of the APN, and APNs may feel pressure from the team when efforts to enhance patient adherence are unsuccessful. In these cases, the APN should solicit help from other resources, such as social workers or home health nurses, to uncover the underlying causes and find solutions.

In some cases, the health care team, including the APN, has one perspective based on common values and beliefs. When the team presents a unified perspective that challenges the patient's and family's values, feelings of intimidation surface and the patient and family may become silent. Rather than first trying to elicit the patient's and family's perspectives, the health care team often states the plan of care and goal of treatment without a clear understanding of the patient's wishes. This process of intimidation is subtle and unintentional. The health care team does not strive to repress the patient's autonomy. However, the act of presenting information in an authoritative, direct, and straightforward manner can be interpreted as the only right way to manage the patient's condition. This practice is often seen in fast-paced environments with significant time constraints on providers.

It is often easier for patients and families to express diverse views when someone first solicits their position, preferences, and goals for care and genuinely listens to their perspectives. The APN can help patients and families overcome feelings of intimidation by asking what they think should be done, clarifying any misconceptions, and accepting their understanding and interpretation of the situation. Nonjudgmental acceptance can break down barriers and lead to communication that is open and honest and facilitates shared decision making. This is not to suggest that providers must always agree with or act on the patients' and families' interpretations. Instead, listening carefully to another's perspective engenders trust and indicates respect. This creates an atmosphere in which the positions of the providers and family can more easily be aligned with a common goal of balancing best interests with patient autonomy. In a study of families of intensive care unit (ICU) patients, Ahrens, Yancey, and Kollef (2003) found that 42 of 43 families receiving support and enhanced communication from a CNS-physician team were able to make decisions to withhold or withdraw care at the end of life. The authors noted, "This finding underscores the importance of intentional and well-designed communication and support systems for families making medical and moral decisions" (Ahrens et al., 2003, p. 322).

Organizational/Environmental Barriers

Lack of support for nurses who speak up regarding ethical problems in work settings is a potent barrier to ethical practice. Unfortunately, both early research and recent findings reveal disturbing examples of environments in which nurses' concerns were minimized or ignored by physicians, administrators, and even by other nurses (Ceci, 2004; Erlen & Frost, 1991; Hamric & Blackhall, 2007; Klaidman, 2007). These findings lend urgency to the need for APNs to provide leadership in building ethical practice environments. The ongoing nursing shortage has lent importance to nurses as a key stakeholder group within health care organizations, but that has not always translated to support and respect for all nurses within an organization. APNs need to assess the level of support nurses receive from others and work to create environments that are "morally habitable places" (Austin, 2007, p. 86). Consideration should be given to organizational ethics programs, which focus on building structures and processes to deal with conflicts of roles and expectations (Mills, Spencer, & Werhane, 2001; Rorty et al., 2004).

In environments where moral distress persists, health professionals' moral integrity may suffer and result in compromised patient care quality (Hamric et al., 2006). While the consequences of moral distress are just beginning to be studied, mounting data implicate moral distress in RN turnover and burnout (Corley, 1995; Elpern, et al., 2005; Hamric & Blackhall, 2007; Meltzer & Huckaby, 2004). APNs need to develop skills in collaborative conflict resolution and preventive ethics to build ethical practice environments in which moral distress is minimized and the moral integrity of all caregivers is respected and protected.

The unfortunate reality in many health care settings is that time is so limited that the benefits of collaboration or compromise are seldom realized. To overcome this barrier, the APN may need to resolve a presenting dilemma in stages, with the most central issue addressed first. The APN also needs to enlist the aid of administrative and physician colleagues in recognizing the ongoing consequences of lack of time for team deliberations. For example, if a patient is not receiving adequate pain management because the bedside nurse is concerned about hastening death in a terminally ill patient and is unaware of the full treatment plan, the CNS should first focus on relieving the patient's pain. Once the immediate need is addressed, the CNS can help the nurse understand the natural course of the disease (whose outcome is death), identify nonpharmacological interventions to promote comfort, and educate the nurse about the dosage and timing of medications to prevent wide fluctuations in pain management. At this point, the administrative leadership may need to be approached about supporting ongoing staff education in end-of-life care. An additional strategy such as arranging for the nurse to rotate to a hospice unit represents a preventive approach to avert similar dilemmas in the future.

Providing continuity of care and the ability to know the patient and family over time are significant problems in acute care settings. Many institutions continue to push for shorter lengths of stay and more streamlined and "efficient" management of patients. In primary care settings, similar pressures to see more patients in less time can decrease the APN's time for individualized problem solving for patients and families. Ironically, some nurses have moved into APN roles specifically because they desire to spend more time with patients. Typically, these time-pressured environments do not embrace the concept of "knowing the patient" (Radwin, 1996). Tanner, Benner, Chesla, and Gordon (1993) found that knowing the patient was central to expert clinical judgment and facilitated patient and family advocacy. Whittemore (2000) argued that resolving ethical dilemmas requires knowing the patient as a person to be able to recognize the salient aspects of a situation that are important for resolution. However, care in too many acute care settings is based on knowing the expected response to illness and rapid and episodic treatment of a select population of patients. In other words, individualized care is not standard practice. Although this philosophy has numerous financial advantages, the patient and family may lose the necessary individualized attention that can greatly enhance their recovery. APNs struggle in such environments to balance the needs of individuals with generalized treatment approaches and productivity targets.

Thomas, Finch, Schoenhofer, and Green (2004) interviewed seven NP/patient dyads and identified attributes of the caring relationship established between them. One theme, the enhanced personhood of the patient, was related to the NPs' interpersonal skills and their ability to address patients' needs in a holistic fashion. Pressure to see more patients may impede the development of this caring relationship. While APNs must continue to advocate for providing individualized care to patients and families, this position may be difficult and risky when it contradicts the objectives of the institution or third-party payers. Despite these objectives, APNs are morally obligated to work toward improving the work environment if current conditions are not in the patients' best interests. Fortunately, many institutions are willing to make some concessions in the delivery of patient care if clear outcome data support a change in practice.

APNs should identify and build resources both within and outside the institution to assist with the resolution of ethical problems. Internal resources may include chaplain staff, liaison psychiatry staff, patient representatives, social work staff, ethics committees and their members, and ethics consultation services. Resources outside the institution include the ANA's Center on Ethics and Human Rights (*www.nursingworld.org/ethics*), ethics groups within national specialty organizations, and ethics centers in universities or large health care institutions. The recognition of a moral dilemma does not commit the APN to individually conducting and managing the process of resolution. APNs should engage appropriate resources to address the identified needs and work toward agreement. However, in many situations, such as in rural clinics, resources within the organization are not available. Without another professional colleague to help decipher the problem, the APN is sometimes left with little more than intuition. Guidelines from professional organizations regarding the APN's moral obligations (see "Websites with Ethics Policy Statements or Guidelines" and "Ethics and Legal Search Sites" provided on the Evolve website) are helpful in providing some direction for action. APNs practicing in isolation should network with colleagues and establish contact with resources such as community religious leaders or ethicists in nearby institutions for providing direction in ethical reasoning.

Finally, nursing's ethical obligations to maintain a competent and caring relationship with patients and their families can be challenged with the implementation of cost-containment practices. Taylor (2001) identified six challenges for nurse case managers, which apply to all APNs: fidelity to the unique needs of individual patients, competing loyalties, resolving role conflict, owning responsibilities to underserved populations, identifying personal biases, and balancing care for others with appropriate self-care. In addition to personal reflection and values clarification, nurses should assess their competence to provide effective care and address any deficiencies that are exposed. Because patients have shorter hospital stays, open communication and collaboration with the health care team, patients, and families are essential behaviors for optimal planning. In addition, as described in Phase 4 of the ethical decision-making competency, APNs should maintain and affirm patients' rights by questioning and challenging changes in the health care system that negatively affect the quality of care delivered. Finally, there is a need to consistently review patient outcomes and quality of nursing care provided (see Chapters 24 and 25), because these data can be powerful in building the case for change. These strategies empower the APN to act—initially, on smaller and more manageable parts of the problem; and over time, in widening circles of influence.

CONCLUSION

The changing health care environment has placed extraordinary demands on nurses in all care settings. The limitations of time, reimbursement, and resources conflict with nursing's moral imperatives of involvement, connection, and commitment. Ethical decision-making skills involve four phases of progressively complex knowledge and skills in moving patient care, caregiving environments, and the larger system toward ethical practices. As a core competency for the APN, ethical decision making reflects both the art and science of nursing. The APN is in a key position to assume a more decisive role in managing the resolution of moral issues and helping create ethically responsive health care environments. The identification of patterns in the presentation of moral issues enables the APN to engage in preventive strategies to improve the ethical climate in patient care environments. Ethical decision-making skills together with clinical expertise and leadership empower the APN to critically analyze and assume leadership roles in public policy processes that promote social justice within the larger health care arena. Preparation for this competency begins in graduate education, but it continues throughout the APN's career.

REFERENCES

Ahrens, T., Yancey, V., & Kollef, M. (2003). Improving family communications at the end of life: Implications for length of stay in the intensive care unit and resource use. *American Journal of Critical Care, 12,* 317-323.

Ahronheim, J.C., Moreno, J., & Zuckerman, C. (2000). *Ethics in clinical practice* (2nd ed.). Gaithersburg, MD: Aspen.

American Association of Colleges of Nursing (AACN). (2006). *The essentials of doctoral education for advanced nursing practice.* Washington, DC: Author.

American Association of Critical-Care Nurses. (2000). *Maintaining patient-focused care in an environment of nursing staff shortages and financial constraints* (position statement). Aliso Viejo, CA: Author.

American Association of Critical-Care Nurses (2004). *The 4 A's to rise above moral distress.* Aliso Viejo, CA: Author.

American Association of Critical-Care Nurses (2005). *Standards for establishing and sustaining healthy work environments.*

Aliso Viejo, CA: Author. Retrieved November 19, 2007, from http://www.aacn.org/aacn/hwe.nsf/vwdoc/HWEHomePage.

American Nurses Association (ANA). (2001). *Code of ethics for nurses with interpretive statements.* Washington, DC: Author.

Arras, J.D. (1997). Nice story, but so what? In H.L. Nelson (Ed.), *Stories and their limits: Narrative approaches to bioethics* (pp. 65-88). New York: Routledge.

Artnak, K., & Dimmitt, J.H. (1996). Choosing a framework for ethical analysis in advanced practice settings: The case for casuistry. *Archives of Psychiatric Nursing, 10,* 16-23.

Austin, W. (2007). The ethics of everyday practice: Healthcare environments as moral communities. *Advances in Nursing Science, 30*(1), 81-88.

Baggs, J.G., & Schmitt, M.H. (1988). Collaboration between nurses and physicians. *Image: The Journal of Nursing Scholarship, 20,* 145-149.

Beare, P.G. (1989). The essentials of win-win negotiation for the clinical nurse specialist. *Clinical Nurse Specialist, 13,* 138-141.

Beauchamp, T.L., & Childress, J.F. (2001). *Principles of biomedical ethics* (5 ed.). New York: Oxford University Press.

Benner, P. (1991). The role of experience, narrative and community in skilled ethical comportment. *Advances in Nursing Science, 14,* 1-21.

Benner, P., Tanner, C.A., & Chesla, C.A. (1996). *Expertise in nursing practice: Caring, clinical judgment, and ethics.* New York: Springer.

Bishop, G., & Brodkey, A.C. (2006). Personal responsibility and physician responsibility: West Virginia's Medicaid plan. *New England Journal of Medicine, 355,* 756-758.

Bodenheimer, T.S., & Grumbach, K. (2005), *Understanding health policy: A clinical approach* (4th ed.). New York: Lange Medical Books/ McGraw Hill.

Buryska, J.F. (2001). Assessing the ethical weight of cultural, religious and spiritual claims in the clinical context. *Journal of Medical Ethics, 27,* 118-122.

Ceci, C. (2004). Nursing, knowledge and power: A case analysis. *Social Science and Medicine, 59,* 1879-1889.

Chally, P.S., & Loriz, L. (1998). Ethics in the trenches: Decision making in practice. *The American Journal of Nursing, 98*(6), 17-20.

Chambliss, D.F. (1996). *Beyond caring: Hospitals, nurses, and the social organization of ethics.* Chicago: University of Chicago Press.

Charon, R. (1994). Narrative contributions to medical ethics. In E.R. DuBose, R. Hamel, & L.J. O'Connell (Eds.), *A matter of principles?* (pp. 260-283). Valley Forge, PA: Trinity Press International.

Chervenak, F.A., & McCullough, L.B. (1995). The threat of the new managed practice of medicine to patients' autonomy. *Journal of Clinical Ethics, 6,* 320-323.

Childress, J.F. (1994). Principles-oriented bioethics: An analysis and assessment from within. In E.R. DuBose, R. Hamel, & L.J. O'Connell (Eds.), *A matter of principles? Ferment in U.S. bioethics* (pp. 72-98). Valley Forge, PA: Trinity Press International.

Childress, J.F. (1997). Narrative(s) versus norm(s): A misplaced debate in bioethics. In H.L. Nelson (Ed.), *Stories and their limits: narrative approaches to bioethics* (pp. 252-271). New York: Routledge.

Clouser, K.D., & Gert, B. (1990). A critique of principlism. *Journal of Medicine and Philosophy, 15,* 219-236.

Collins, F.S., & Mansoura, M.K. (2001). The Human Genome Project: Revealing the shared inheritance of all humankind. *Cancer, 91*(Suppl. 1), 221-225.

Cooper, M.C. (1989). Gilligan's different voice: A perspective for nursing. *Journal of Professional Nursing, 5,* 10-16.

Cooper, M.C. (1991). Principle-oriented ethics and the ethic of care: A creative tension. *Advances in Nursing Science, 14,* 22-31.

Corley, M.C. (1995). Moral distress of critical care nurses. *American Journal of Critical Care, 4,* 280-285.

Corley, M.C. (2002). Nurse moral distress: A proposed theory and research agenda. *Nursing Ethics, 9,* 636-650.

Cruzan v. Missouri Department of Health, et al., 110 S. Ct. 2841 (1990).

Curtis, J.R., & Shannon, S.E. (2006). Transcending the silos: Toward an interdisciplinary approach to end of life care in the intensive care unit. *Intensive Care Medicine, 32,* 15-17.

Donagrandi, M.A., & Eddy, M. (2000). Ethics of case management: Implications for advanced practice nursing. *Clinical Nurse Specialist, 14*(5), 241-249.

Dreyfus, H.L., Dreyfus, S.E., & Benner, P. (1996). Implications of the phenomenology of expertise for teaching and learning everyday skillful ethical comportment. In P. Benner, C.A. Tanner, & C.A. Chesla (Eds.), *Expertise in nursing practice: Caring, clinical judgment, and ethics* (pp. 258-279). New York: Springer.

Dubler, N.N., & Marcus, L.J. (1994). *Mediating bioethical disputes.* New York: United Hospital Fund.

Dwyer, M.L. (1998). Genetic research and ethical challenges: Implications for nursing practice. *AACN Clinical Issues, 9,* 600-605.

Edwards, M., & Chalmers, K. (2002). Double agency in clinical research. *Canadian Journal of Nursing Research, 34*(1), 131-142.

Elpern, E.H., Covert, B., & Kleinpell, R. (2005). Moral distress of staff nurses in a medical intensive care unit. *American Journal of Critical Care, 14,* 523-530.

Emanuel, E.J. (2002). Patient v. population: Resolving the ethical dilemmas posed by treating patients as members of populations. In M. Danis, C. Clancy, & L.R. Churchill (Eds.). *Ethical dimensions of health policy* (pp. 227-245). New York: Oxford University Press.

Erlen, J.A. (2006). Genetic testing and counseling: Selected ethical issues. *Orthopaedic Nursing, 25*(6). 423-426.

Erlen, J.A., & Frost, B. (1991). Nurses' perceptions of powerlessness in influencing ethical decisions. *Western Journal of Nursing Research, 13,* 397-407.

Falk-Raphael, A. (2005). Speaking truth to power: Nursing's legacy and moral imperative. *Advances in Nursing Science, 28,* 212-223.

Forrow, L., Arnold, R.M., & Parker, L.S. (1993). Preventive ethics: Expanding the horizons of clinical ethics. *Journal of Clinical Ethics, 4,* 287-294.

Fry, S.T., & Riley, J.M. (1998). *Ethical issues in clinical practice: A multi-state study of practicing registered nurses.* Retrieved June 20, 2007, from http://jmrileyrn.tripod.com/nen/research.html#anchor195458.

Gaul, A.L. (1995). Casuistry, care, compassion, and ethics data analysis. *Advances in Nursing Science, 17,* 47-57.

Gilligan, C. (1982). *In a different voice.* Cambridge, MA: Harvard University Press.

Gordon, E.J., & Hamric, A.B. (2006). The courage to stand up: The cultural politics of nurses' access to ethics consultation. *Journal of Clinical Ethics, 17*(3), 231-254.

Gostin, L.O. (2005). Ethics, the constitution, and the dying process: The case of Theresa Marie Schiavo. *Journal of the American Medical Association, 293*(19), 2403-2407.

Grady, C. (1991). Ethical issues in clinical trials. *Seminars in Oncology Nursing, 7,* 288-296.

Gramelspracher, G.P., Howell, J.D., & Young, M.J. (1986). Perceptions of ethical problems by nurses and physicians. *Archives of Internal Medicine, 146,* 577-578.

Gudorf, C.E. (1994). A feminist critique of biomedical principlism. In E.R. DuBose, R. Hamel, & L.J. O'Connell (Eds.), *A matter of principles? Ferment in U.S. bioethics* (pp. 260-283). Valley Forge, PA: Trinity Press International.

Haddad, A.M. (1991). The nurse/physician relationship and ethical decision making. *AORN Journal, 53,* 151-154, 156.

Hall, J.K. (1996). Assisted suicide: Nurse practitioners as providers? *Nurse Practitioner, 21,* 63-66, 71.

Hamric, A.B. (2001) Reflections on being in the middle. *Nursing Outlook, 49,* 254-257.

Hamric, A.B. (2000). Moral distress in everyday ethics. *Nursing Outlook, 48,* 199-201.

Hamric, A.B., & Blackhall, L.J. (2007). Nurse-physician perspective on the care of dying patients in intensive care units: Collaboration, moral distress, and ethical climate. *Critical Care Medicine, 35*(2), 422-429.

Hamric, A.B., Davis, W.S., & Childress, M.D. (2006). Moral distress in health care professionals: What is it and what can we do about it? The *Pharos of Alpha Omega Alpha–Honor Medical Society, 69*(1), 16-23.

Harris, M., Winship, I., & Spriggs, M. (2005). Controversies and ethical issues in cancer-genetics clinics. *Lancet Oncology, 6*(7), 301-310.

Hebert, P.C., Levin, A.V., & Robertson, G. (2001). Bioethics for clinicians: Disclosure of medical error. *Canadian Medical Journal, 164*(4), 1-12.

Holder, K.V., & Schenthal, S.J. (2007). Watch your step: Nursing and professional boundaries. *Nursing Management, 38*(2), 24-29.

Hopkinson, I., & Mackay, J. (2002). The clinical impact of the Human Genome Project: Inherited variants in cancer care. *Annals of Oncology, 13*(Suppl. 4), 105-107.

Horner, S.D. (2004) Ethics and genetics: Implications for CNS practice. *Clinical Nurse Specialist, 18*(5), 228-231.

Howard, E.P., & Steinberg, S. (2002). Evaluations of clinical learning in a managed care environment. *Nursing Forum, 37,* 12-20.

Institute of Medicine (IOM). (1999). *To err is human: Building a safer health system.* Washington, DC: National Academies Press.

Institute of Medicine (IOM). (2001). *Crossing the quality chasm: A new health system for the 21st century.* Washington, DC: National Academies Press.

Institute of Medicine (IOM). (2003). *Health professions education: A bridge to quality.* Washington, DC: National Academies Press.

Jameson, J.K. (2003). Transcending intractable conflict in health care: An exploratory study of communication and conflict among anesthesia providers. *Journal of Health Communications, 8,* 563-581.

Jameton, A. (1984). *Nursing practice: The ethical issues.* Englewood Cliff, NJ: Prentice Hall.

Jameton, A. (1993). Dilemmas of moral distress: Moral responsibility and nursing practice. *AWHONN's Clinical Issues in Perinatal and Women's Health Nursing, 4,* 542-551.

Jonsen, A.R., & Toulmin, S. (1988). *The abuse of casuistry: A history of moral reasoning.* Berkeley: University of California Press.

Juretschke, L.J. (2001). Ethical dilemmas and the nurse practitioner in the NICU. *Neonatal Network, 20,* 33-38.

Kikuchi, J.F. (1996). Multicultural ethics in nursing education: A potential threat to responsible practice. *Journal of Professional Nursing, 12,* 159-165.

Klaidman, S. (2007). *Coronary: A true story of medicine gone awry.* New York: Scribner.

Laabs, C.A. (2005). Problems and distress among nurse practitioners in primary care. *Journal of the American Academy of Nurse Practitioners, 17*(2), 76-84.

LaMear-Tucker, D., & Friedson, J. (1997). Resolving moral conflict: The critical care nurse's role. *Critical Care Nurse, 17,* 55-63.

Leavitt, F.J. (1996). Educating nurses for their future role in bioethics. *Nursing Ethics, 3,* 39.

Linnard-Palmer, L., & Kools, S. (2004). Parents' refusal of medical treatment based on religious and/or cultural beliefs: The law, ethical principles, and clinical implications. *Journal of Pediatric Nursing, 19,* 351-356.

Long, S.O. (2000). Living poorly or dying well: Cultural decisions about life-supporting treatment for American and Japanese patients. *Journal of Clinical Ethics, 11,* 236-237.

Ludwig, R., & Silva, M.C. (2000). Nursing around the world: Cultural values and ethical conflicts. *Online Journal of Issues in Nursing.* Retrieved September 1, 2003, from www.nursingworld.org/ojin/ethicol/ethics_4.htm.

Mahon, M.M., Deatrick, J.A., McKnight, H.J., & Mohr, W.K. (2000). Discontinuing treatment in children with chronic, critical illnesses. *Nurse Practitioner Forum, 11,* 6-14.

McCormick-Gendzel, M., & Jurchak, M. (2006). A pathway for moral reasoning in home healthcare. *Home Healthcare Nurse, 24*(10), 654-661.

McCullough, L.B. (2005). Practicing preventive ethics: The keys to avoiding ethical conflicts in health care. *Physician Executive, 31*(2), 18-21.

McWilliams, J.M., Meara, E., Zaslavsky, A.M., & Ayanian, J.Z. (2007). Use of health services by previously uninsured Medicare beneficiaries. *New England Journal of Medicine, 357*(2), 143-153.

Meltzer, L.S., & Huckaby, L.M. (2004). Critical care nurses' perceptions of futile care and its effect on burnout. *American Journal of Critical Care, 13*, 202-208.

Mills, A.E., Spencer, E.M., & Werhane, P.H. (Eds.). (2001). *Developing organization ethics in healthcare: A case-based approach to policy, practice and compliance.* Frederick, MD: University Publishing Group.

National Council of State Boards of Nursing. (1996). *Professional boundaries: A nurse's guide to the importance of appropriate professional boundaries.* Chicago: Author.

Nelson, H.L. (Ed.). (1997*). Stories and their limits: Narrative approaches to bioethics.* New York: Routledge.

Oberle, K.R., & Hughes, D. (2001). Doctors' and nurses' perceptions of ethical problems in end-of-life decisions. *Journal of Advanced Nursing, 33*, 707-715.

O'Connor, K.F. (1996). Ethical/moral experiences of oncology nurses. *Oncology Nursing Forum, 23*, 787-794.

Olczak, P.V., Grosch, J.W., & Duffy, K.G. (1991). Toward a synthesis: The art with the science of community mediation. In K.G. Duffy, J.W. Grosch, & P.V. Olczak (Eds.), *Community mediation* (pp. 329-343). New York: The Guilford Press.

Omery, A., Henneman, E., Billet, B., Luna-Raines, M., & Brown-Saltzman, K. (1995). Ethical issues in hospital-based nursing practice. *Journal of Cardiovascular Nursing, 9*, 43-53.

Omnibus Budget Reconciliation Act of 1990, PL, 101-508, 42 U.S.C. § 4206.

Orr, R.D., & Genesen, L.B. (1997). Requests for "inappropriate" treatment based on religious beliefs. *Journal of Medical Ethics, 23*, 142-147.

Ostermeyer, M. (1991). Conducting the mediation. In K.G. Duffy, J.W. Grosch, & P.V. Olczak (Eds.), *Community mediation* (pp. 91-104). New York: The Guilford Press.

Pike, A.W. (1991). Moral outrage and moral discourse in nurse-physician collaboration. *Journal of Professional Nursing, 7*, 351-362.

Pracher, T., Moss, B., & Mahanes, D. (April 2006). *Moral distress in the care of patients with traumatic brain injury.* Poster presentation, American Association of Neuroscience Nurses, San Diego, CA.

Purtilo, R. (2005). *Ethical dimensions in the health professions* (4th ed.). Philadelphia: Saunders.

Radwin, L.E. (1996). "Knowing the patient": A review of research on an emerging concept. *Journal of Advanced Nursing, 23*, 1142-1146.

Raines, D.A. (1993). Values: A guiding force. *AWHONN's Clinical Issues, 4*, 533-541.

Rajput, V., & Bekes, C.E. (2002). Ethical issues in hospital medicine. *Medical Clinics of North America, 86*, 869-886.

Resnick, D.B. (2005). The patient's duty to adhere to prescribed treatment: An ethical analysis. *Journal of Medicine and Philosophy, 30*, 167-188.

Rest, J.R. (1986). *Moral development: Advances in research and theory.* New York: Praeger.

Robichaux, C.M., & Clark, A.P. (2006). Practice of expert critical care nurses in situations of prognostic conflict at the end of life. *American Journal of Critical Care, 15*(5), 480-489.

Rorty, M.V., Werhane, P.H., & Mills, A.E. (2004). The Rashomon effect: Organization ethics in health care. *HEC Forum, 16*(2), 75-94.

Rowdin, M.A. (1995). Conflicts in managed care. *New England Journal of Medicine, 332*, 604-607.

Sadler, G.R., Lantz, J.M., Fullerton, J.T., & Dault, Y. (1999). Nurses' unique roles in randomized clinical trials. *Journal of Professional Nursing, 15*, 106-115.

Saulo, M., & Wagener, R.J. (1996). How good case managers make tough choices: Ethics and mediation. *Journal of Care Management, 2*, 10-16, 35-38, 42.

Schlenk, J.S. (1997). Advance directives: Role of nurse practitioners. *Journal of the American Academy of Nurse Practitioners, 9*, 317-321.

Scott, R.A., Aiken, L.H., Mechanic, D., & Moravcsik, J. (1995). Organizational aspects of caring. *The Milbank Quarterly, 73*, 77-95.

Shannon, S.E. (1997). The roots of interdisciplinary conflict around ethical issues. *Critical Care Nursing Clinics of North America, 9*, 13-28.

Shannon, S.E., Mitchell, P.H., & Cain, K.C. (2002). Patients, nurses, and physicians have differing views of quality of critical care. *Journal of Nursing Scholarship, 34*, 173-179.

Silva, M.C., & Ludwick, R. (2002). Domestic violence, nurses and ethics: What are the links? *Online Journal of Issues in Nursing.* Retrieved January 3, 2007, from nursingworld. org/ojin/ethicol/ethics_8.htm.

Smith, R., Hiatt, H., & Berwick, D. (1999). Shared ethical principles for everybody in health care: A working draft from the Tavistock group. *British Medical Journal, 318*, 248-251.

Solomon, M.Z., Jennings, B., Guilfoy, V., Jackson, R., O'Donnell, L., Wolf, S.M., et al. (1991). Toward an expanded vision of clinical ethics education: From individual to the institution. *Kennedy Institute of Ethics Journal, 1*, 225-245.

Solomon, M.Z., O'Donnell, L., Jennings, B., Guilfoy, V., Wolf, S.M., Nolan, K., et al. (1993). Decisions near the end of life: Professional views on life-sustaining treatments. *American Journal of Public Health, 83*, 14-23.

Spencer, E.M. (1997). A new role for institutional ethics committees: Organizational ethics. *Journal of Clinical Ethics, 8*, 372-376.

Spencer, E.M. (2005). A case method for consideration of moral problems. In J.C. Fletcher, E.M. Spencer, & P.A. Lombardo (Eds.), *Fletcher's introduction to clinical ethics* (3rd ed., pp. 339-347). Hagerstown, MD: University Publishing Group.

Spielman, B.J. (1993). Conflict in medical ethics cases: Seeking patterns of resolution. *Journal of Clinical Ethics, 4*, 212-218.

Tanner, C.A., Benner, P., Chesla, C., & Gordon, D.R. (1993). The phenomenology of knowing the patient. *Image: The Journal of Nursing Scholarship, 25,* 273-280.

Taylor, C. (2001). Ethical issues in case management. In E.L. Cohen & T.G. Cesta (Eds.), *Nursing case management* (pp. 369-386). St. Louis: Mosby.

Thomas, J., Finch, L.., Schoenhofer, S., & Green, A. (2005). The caring relationships created by nurse practitioners and the ones nursed: Implications for practice. *Topics in Advanced Practice Nursing e-Journal, 4*(4). Retrieved November 27, 2007, from www.medscape.com/viewarticle/496420.

Toulmin, S. (1994). Casuistry and clinical ethics. In E.R. DuBose, R. Hamel, & L.J. O'Connell (Eds.), *A matter of principles?* (pp. 310-318). Valley Forge, PA: Trinity Press International.

Trotochard, K. (2006). Ethical issues and access to healthcare. *Journal of Infusion Nursing, 29*(3), 165-170.

Turner, L.N., Marquis, K., & Burman, M.E. (1996). Rural nurse practitioners: Perceptions of ethical dilemmas. *Journal of the American Academy of Nurse Practitioners, 8,* 269-274.

Ulrich, C., Soeken, K., & Miller, N. (2003). Predictors of nurse practitioners' autonomy: Effects of organizational, ethical and market characteristics. *Journal of the American Academy of Nurse Practitioners, 15*(7), 319-325.

Ulrich, C.M., Danis, M., Ratcliffe, S.J., Garrett-Mayer, E., Koziol, D. Soeken, K., et al. (2006). Ethical conflicts in nurse practitioners and physician assistants in managed care. *Nursing Research, 55*(6), 391-401.

U.S. Department of Health and Human Services, Office of Minority Health. (2001). *National standards for culturally and linguistically appropriate services in health care.* Rockville, MD: IQ Solutions. Retrieved June 19, 2007, from www.omhrc.gov/assets/pdf/checked/executive.pdf.

U.S. Department of Health & Human Services (USDHHS), Office of Civil Rights. (2003). *Summary of the HIPAA privacy rule.* Retrieved June 19, 2007, from www.hhs.gov/ocr/privacysummary.pdf.

Uustal, D. (1987). Values: The cornerstone of nursing's moral art. In M.D. Fowler & J. Levine-Ariff (Eds.), *Ethics at the bedside* (pp. 136-153). Philadelphia: Lippincott.

Viens, D.C. (1994). Moral dilemmas experienced by nurse practitioners. *Nurse Practitioner Forum, 5,* 209-214.

Viens, D.C. (1995). The moral reasoning of nurse practitioners. *Journal of the American Academy of Nurse Practitioners, 7,* 277-285.

Vintzileos, A.M., Ananth, C.V., Smulian, J.C., Beazoglou, T., & Knuppel, R.A. (2000). Routine second-trimester ultrasonography in the United States: A cost-benefit analysis. *American Journal of Obstetrics and Gynecology, 182*(3), 655-660.

Waltman, P.A., & Schenk, L.K. (1999). Neonatal ethical decision making: Where does the NNP fit in? *Neonatal Network, 18,* 27-32.

Weaver, K. (2007). Ethical sensitivity: State of knowledge and needs for further research. *Nursing Ethics, 14*(2), 141-155.

Webster, G.C., & Baylis, F.E. (2000). Moral residue. In S.B. Rubin & L. Zoloth (Eds.), *Margin of error: the ethics of mistakes in the practice of medicine* (pp. 217-230). Hagerstown, MD: University Publishing Group.

Whittemore, R. (2000). Consequences of not "knowing the patient." *Clinical Nurse Specialist, 14,* 75-81.

Williams, J.K., & Lea, D.H. (1995). Applying new genetic technologies: Assessment and ethical considerations. *Nurse Practitioner, 20,* 16, 21-26.

Wright, F., Cohen, S., & Caroselli, C. (1997). Diverse decisions: How culture affects ethical decision making. *Critical Care Nursing Clinics of North America, 9,* 63-74.

Wueste, D.E. (2005). A philosophical yet user friendly framework for ethical decision making in critical care nursing. *Dimensions of Critical Care Nursing, 24*(2), 70-79.

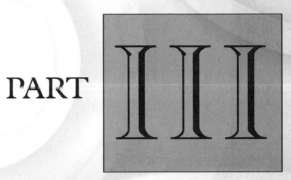

PART III

Advanced Practice Roles: The Operational Definitions of Advanced Practice Nursing

The Clinical Nurse Specialist

Patricia S. A. Sparacino • Cathy C. Cartwright

INTRODUCTION

The CNS role was created (1) to provide direct care to patients with complex diseases or conditions, (2) to improve patient care by developing the clinical skills and judgment of staff nurses, and (3) to retain nurses who are experts in clinical practice. Expert clinical practice is the essence, the core value, of the clinical nurse specialist (CNS) role. Historically, the role has been versatile, evolving, "flexing," responsive, and adaptable to patient populations and health care environments. Consider Exemplar 12-1, which might be a typical day in the life of a critical care CNS.

The activities of CNSs are as varied as their individual specialty practices. The diversity of CNS specialties, the differences in their individual practices, and the practice differences among CNSs in the same institution often mask what CNSs do. Unlike other advanced practice nurses (APNs) whose primary role is to deliver direct patient care, the multifaceted CNS delivers direct patient care, improves the care delivered by nurses and nursing personnel to larger patient populations, provides leadership to specialty practice program development, and influences health care delivery systems.

The variability in CNS practice, even within the same institution, has defined the role since its creation. The definition of the CNS role is deliberately broad so that CNSs can respond to changing clinical environments. Consequently, the practice of a critical care CNS with an experienced, certified specialty staff will differ noticeably from his or her work with staff who may be new to critical care nursing. Similarly, if an intensive care unit (ICU) population is homogeneous (e.g., mostly cardiac patients), a CNS's activities will be different than if the population were heterogeneous. Several clinical, staff, and system variables must be weighed when planning for CNS positions and implementing the role, including the number, type, and background of nurses and other clinical staff; the clinical, educational, or institutional resources; and the patient population, acuity, outcomes, and quality data.

In the 1990s, CNS practice was poorly understood, and its impact on clinical outcomes and costs of care lacked convincing data, resulting in the loss of CNS positions in many parts of the country and a call to merge CNS and NP roles (see Chapters 1 and 15). Some of the difficulty in defining succinctly the advanced practice of CNSs can be traced to the role's inherent flexibility and responsiveness and its retrenchment in the 1990s. However, clarifying the work of CNSs and their competencies was further delayed because other specialty organizations established educational, competency, and practice standards for CNSs (e.g., critical care, oncology, or neuroscience specialties). The National Association of Clinical Nurse Specialists (NACNS) was not established until 1995 (see Chapter 1). The NACNS itself acknowledged that the other advanced practice organizations had a significant head start in defining competencies and influencing health policies related to advanced practice nursing (NACNS, 2004b). The American Nurses Association, many specialty organizations, and APN leaders have worked hard to define CNS practice, define standards and competencies, and develop CNS curricula (see Chapters 1 and 2). More work, however, is required to educate colleagues, administrators, and the public about the CNS role. For reasons outlined later in this chapter and discussed in Chapter 21, we believe that CNSs and the nursing profession are at a critical juncture—for the purposes of licensure, accreditation, credentialing, and education, the work and contributions of CNSs as APNs must be made unambiguously clear.

In the past 25 years, market forces have radically changed health care, making it more difficult to define CNS practice for the marketplace, but CNSs have been responsive. Successful CNSs have consistently delivered care that improves patient care quality and outcomes, patient safety, and nursing practice and that ensures efficient use of resources, cost efficiency, cost savings, and revenue generation (NACNS, 1998, 2004b; see also Chapter 24). CNSs' clinical acumen and expertise are not limited to their patients' physiological and

EXEMPLAR 12-1   A Day in the Life of a Clinical Nurse Specialist

Sophie is a unit-based CNS at an academic medical center. She arrives at the unit at 6 AM in time to check in with the nursing staff who work 7 PM to 7 AM. She listens to them as they wrap up their work and get ready for report and change-of-shift nursing rounds. She learns that some of the staff who attended a certification review in which she taught passed the Critical Care Registered Nurse examination. She congratulates them and makes a note to share the news. (The unit leaders have a goal of having a certain percentage of nursing staff certified.) On rounds she identifies a patient who began to be weaned from the ventilator yesterday and whose progress is not smooth. She can tell from the report that the nurse could use some coaching, not only in intervening with the patient, but in communicating with the hospitalist about appropriate next actions. After rounds she returns to this patient, speaks with the nurse, and assesses the patient with the nurse. Together they discuss the next actions—nursing interventions that are likely to decrease the patient's agitation and a discussion with the hospitalist about adjusting the weaning schedule and medications. The staff nurse seems more confident and knows how to reach Sophie if she needs help with the patient or communicating with the physician. She and Sophie agree to talk by phone in an hour to evaluate the outcome of the nurse's interventions. Sophie determines that the charge nurse and staff have no immediate needs for her and

returns to her office. She spends the next hour reviewing notes for an in-service she is giving on metabolic syndrome and getting ready for an 11 AM organ donation advisory committee (ODAC) meeting she co-chairs. The agenda includes a review of two recent organ donation cases, one of which went well and one in which staff members were concerned about the way the family was approached about donation. Just before she leaves for the meeting, she checks in with the staff nurse, who says that the patient being weaned seems a little better and the conversation with the hospitalist went well. Some adjustments in the treatment plan were made and she will confer with Sophie after lunch.

After the ODAC meeting, Sophie heads to the cafeteria for lunch with a colleague; she is paged. It is a call for the Rapid Response Team, of which she is a member. Staff on a telemetry unit have a patient whose condition is deteriorating. Sophie excuses herself and rushes to the telemetry unit. The team evaluates the patient, and the patient is transferred to the Critical Care Unit. Sophie does a short debriefing with the staff. As the day goes on, Sophie does get lunch and responds to a consult from the oncology CNS about a patient's chemotherapy-induced cardiotoxicity. She later talks to the gerontology and psychiatric CNS about the status of plans to open an Acute Care for the Elderly (ACE) unit and what her involvement will be so they can identify the clinical resources needed.

psychological needs. Their clinical expertise permeates the other elements of their multifaceted responsibilities: education, research, health policy, organizational factors, and political change.

Historically, the CNS's multidimensional practice and the failure of organizations and administrators to appreciate CNS contributions to clinical and institutional outcomes meant that CNS positions were vulnerable in times of cost containment. The nursing shortage and the emphasis on knowledge, quality, safety, and interdisciplinary communication have led to a renewed recognition of the importance of CNS practice: providing direct care, improving quality of care, and retaining nurses. Evidence-based practice, Magnet accreditation, and other initiatives to improve health and illness care require the CNS's clinical expertise and leadership skills. CNSs are integral to such efforts, designing and implementing practice guidelines

and innovative practice models, evaluating the cost efficiency and fiscal impact of technology, and assessing its impact on patient care, quality of care, continuity of care, and patient satisfaction. The CNS role has survived and seems destined to thrive. The need for CNSs who can care for complex patients and specialty populations; educate and mentor nurses; build interdisciplinary teams; assess, implement, and evaluate evidence-based practices; and lead other quality and safety initiatives is as pressing as ever.

The purposes of this chapter are (1) to provide a profile of the CNS role, (2) to review the role's core elements in light of evolving conceptualizations about it, (3) to describe the role with an integrated conceptualization of CNS practice (Hamric's model of advanced nursing practice; see Chapter 3) and the NACNS model, and (4) to identify contemporary issues and challenges common to all CNSs.

Although the CNS role exists in other countries, international practice will not be discussed in this chapter. Some countries do not require a graduate nursing degree. In other countries, advanced practice nursing may refer only to nurse practitioners. These interpretations of advanced practice nursing conflict with the definition of advanced practice nursing in this text and with the characteristics of CNS practice in the United States.

PROFILE OF THE ROLE

Definition

The nursing profession, specialty nursing organizations, and nurse authors have developed and gradually refined the definition of the CNS role. In 1976, the American Nurses Association (ANA) was the first entity to define the role of a CNS (ANA, 1976). The 1980 edition of *Nursing: A Social Policy Statement* (ANA, 1980) was the first document to differentiate between a nurse with a baccalaureate degree and a specialist in nursing practice prepared at the graduate level who is also "a generalist in providing the full range of nursing practice." This ANA document promulgated the classic CNS definition: a registered nurse "who, through study and supervised practice at the graduate level (master's or doctorate), has become expert in a defined area of knowledge and practice in a selected clinical area of nursing" (ANA, 1980, p. 23). In 1983, Hamric refined the definition by making the distinction between direct care functions (e.g., expert practitioner, role model, and patient advocate) and indirect care functions (e.g., change agent, consultant/resource person, clinical teacher, supervisor, researcher, liaison, and innovator) (Hamric, 1983b). In 1986, the ANA's Council of Clinical Nurse Specialists expanded the established definition further to delineate the multifaceted dimensions of the role (expert clinical practice, education, consultation, research, and administration) and to define the flexible boundaries dictated by the needs of complex patients, evolving nursing specialties, and the needs of the health care market. Current CNS practice reflects this conceptual evolution. Prepared at the master's or doctorate level, a CNS is an expert clinician in a specialized area of nursing practice. The specialty may be defined by a population (e.g., children or women), a setting (e.g., a critical care unit), a disease or medical subspecialty (e.g., oncology or cardiovascular disease), a type of care (e.g., rehabilitation or psychiatric care), or a type of problem (e.g., wounds or pain) (NACNS, 1998, 2004b).

Distribution and Utilization

Data about graduate APN students pursuing CNS education is relatively easy to find. However, determining how many APNs are practicing as CNSs in the United States is an elusive goal. The number of students graduating from CNS programs is increasing. From 2003 to 2005, the percentage of CNSs who graduated increased by 14.9% and blended CNS/NPs by 50.8%, compared with a 3.6% increase in NPs who graduated from a master's program (American Association of Colleges of Nursing [AACN], 2006a). These changes do not reflect post-master's completion of CNS education or certification requirements. Between 2003 and 2005, the number of CNS programs at the master's level increased by 11.6% (AACN, 2006a); this modest increase followed a significant 28% increase in the number of CNS-only programs between 1997 and 2001 (Walker et al., 2003). Adult health nursing (formerly medical-surgical) has remained the most popular area of specialization for master's level graduates, with community health, adult acute and critical care, and psychiatric/mental health following in descending order. More than 10% of CNS graduates cannot obtain CNS certification because an examination does not exist for their area of specialization (AACN, 2006a).

The number of CNSs currently practicing is more difficult to ascertain. Between 1984 and 1985, the ANA's database listed 19,070 nurses who identified themselves as CNSs, but only 5,245 of that number were prepared at the graduate level (ANA, 1985). By 2004, a Health Resources and Service Administration's (HRSA) survey estimated that there were 72,521 master's-prepared CNSs, which is roughly 30% of the RNs prepared for advanced practice. This estimate includes 14,689 CNSs with dual preparation as NPs; these individuals were more likely to be functioning with an NP title. CNSs were the second largest group of advanced practice nurses after NPs, but only 16.5% were practicing under the title of *clinical nurse specialist* (HRSA, 2005). The low percentage of practicing CNSs using the CNS title may be the result of some specialty nursing organizations and many health care organizations using the generic term *APN* for CNSs, NPs, CNSs also trained as NPs, and other APN roles. Foregoing use of the CNS title is problematic, however, because it makes tracking data about CNS practice, outcomes, and impact a challenging enterprise.

Graduate Education and Programs

The goal of graduate level education is to prepare a nurse to think critically and abstractly, to assess patient and clinical situations at an advanced level, and to use and integrate research into clinical practice (National Council of State Boards of Nursing [NCSBN], 2002a). The knowledge, skills, and clinical experience acquired in a graduate program should prepare a CNS to practice at an advanced level, regardless of setting or patient population. Experience in direct patient care is desirable before entering a CNS program because it provides a foundation on which to develop advanced clinical expertise. Identifying and reaching consensus on a core body of knowledge for practice has been the dilemma in defining appropriate CNS education. The intent of developing a core curriculum is standardization. Without common standards for the educational preparation of a CNS, it is difficult to define uniform standards of practice, to provide uniform certification at the advanced level, and to define standards for credentialing. Early efforts to standardize CNS education arose within specialties; the focus in this chapter is on the profession's efforts to address this issue of standardization.

The ANA's Council of Clinical Nurse Specialists, and subsequently its Council for Advanced Practice Nursing, the NACNS, and the AACN, have consistently worked toward standardizing a curriculum. For many years, the AACN's *The Essentials of Master's Education for Advanced Practice Nursing* (AACN, 1996) was *the* blueprint for APN education. The NACNS (1998, 2004b) also recommended the inclusion of 13 core content areas necessary for developing CNS competencies and 18 guidelines for evaluating CNS programs (NACNS, 2004c). More recently, the process for elucidating CNS competencies was described (Baldwin et al., 2007).

CNS graduate students must complete a minimum of 500 clinical hours (NACNS, 2004b). This recommendation coincides with the requirements for other APN master's programs and for CNS certification. Clinical practice that offers sufficient opportunities to master and apply knowledge and skills and begin the maturation from competency to expertise in a selected area of clinical practice is a critical and integral part of CNS educational preparation. The NACNS specifies further that a student's experience should be "consistent with

the conceptual framework of the three spheres of influence" (NACNS, 2004b, p. 53). The NCSBN has indicated that clinical experience should be directly related to a graduate student's specialty and that supervision should be provided by a person licensed for the same APN role (NCSBN, 2002a, 2002b).

Despite these efforts to standardize CNS graduate preparation, programs vary substantially (NACNS, 2004b). To ensure that the CNS continues to be a recognized advanced practice nursing role, the need is urgent to clarify competencies, to standardize CNS curricula, and to reach a rational consensus on how to credential CNSs from multiple specialties. Many initiatives are underway and will directly or indirectly affect future CNS preparation, credentialing, and practice. Many of these initiatives are detailed in Chapters 2, 3, and 21, and some examples are summarized here. In late 2003, the NACNS, the American Association of Colleges of Nursing (AACN), and the National Organization of Nurse Practitioner Faculty initiated a data collection program to better identify CNS data and educational issues (AACN, 2006b). In May 2006, representatives from the ANA and the American Board of Nursing Specialties (ABNS) initiated a consensus-building project with representatives of specialty nursing organizations to develop CNS core competencies that would apply to all specialties in all practice domains. Asked to respond to the AACN credentialing process, the NACNS made recommendations to strengthen the process as it relates to CNS programs (NACNS, 2007).

The AACN has mandated that the DNP will be the required practice-focused degree by 2015. Restructuring doctoral education and creating the DNP requirement is expected to facilitate the application of scientific knowledge to patients with complex care needs in complicated health care systems and to ensure quality patient care and outcomes. *The Essentials of Doctoral Education for Advanced Nursing Practice* (AACN, 2006b) outlines the competencies expected of DNP-prepared APNs. The DNP *Essentials* includes eight foundational competencies (see Chapter 2) that are the basis for specialized advanced nursing practice and are meant to complement the competencies, content, and practica that are defined by national APN and specialty organizations (AACN, 2006b), such as the NACNS, the Oncology Nursing Society (Jacobs, Scarpa, Lester, & Smith, 2004), and the American Association of Critical-Care Nurses (2002). In 2006, the NACNS convened meetings with national specialty organizations to discuss the implications of the DNP for CNS practice (NACNS, 2006). The NACNS "White Paper on the Nursing Practice Doctorate" (NACNS, 2005a) details its position on the DNP and is available at *http://www.nacns.org/nacns_dnpwhitepaper2.pdf*. The AACN's DNP initiative and the goal of requiring new APNs to have a clinical doctorate has engendered considerable debate and discussion within the CNS community. As this effort unfolds, CNSs can expect direct and indirect impacts on their competencies, curricula, and credentialing.

CLINICAL NURSE SPECIALIST ROLE: A CONCEPT IN EVOLUTION

The evolution of the CNS role has been dynamic (see Chapter 1). The CNSs who pioneered the role were specialists in psychiatry and mental health. The CNS was initially conceptualized as an expert clinician, consultant, educator, and researcher. Direct care, although central, was not the only focus. Integrating these role manifestations was difficult but essential to sustain the role's effectiveness, yet differentiating these elements was not sufficient to describe what CNSs do.

In 1989, Hamric (1989a) proposed a three-dimensional model (Figure 12-1) to delineate the role's defining characteristics and the relationships among its primary criteria (i.e., graduate study in a specialty, certification, and dedicated practice to the

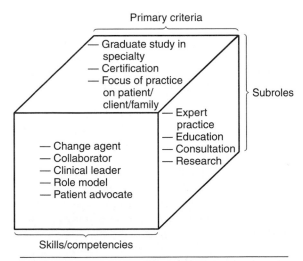

FIGURE 12-1: Defining characteristics of the CNS role. (From Hamric, A.B. [1989a]. History and overview of the CNS role. In A.B. Hamric & J.A. Spross [Eds.], *The clinical nurse specialist in theory and practice* [2nd ed.]. Philadelphia: Saunders.)

patient/client/family unit), its four subroles (clinical expert, consultant, educator, and researcher), and its skills or competencies (i.e., change agent, collaborator, clinical leader, role model, and patient advocate). This important development helped to clarify CNS practice. Subsequently, Hamric elucidated seven competencies that characterize all advanced practice nursing roles: direct clinical practice, expert coaching and guidance, consultation, research, clinical and professional leadership, collaboration, and ethical decision making (Hamric, 1996; see Chapters 2 and 3). This conceptualization was informed by and is consistent with the CNS competencies that were being described by professional nursing organizations (American Nurses Association [ANA], 1986; NACNS, 1998, 2004b).

The NACNS's *Statement on Clinical Nurse Specialist Practice and Education* (NACNS, 1998, 2004b) also helped to clarify CNS practice. The most recent edition (NACNS, 2004b) addresses CNS characteristics, including clinical expertise, specific skills, and attributes; a conceptual model (Figure 2-1, Chapter 2); eight core competencies and associated outcomes organized according to the nursing process; and recommendations for graduate education. The NACNS conceptual model articulates a critical concept: spheres of influence (discussed in the next section). CNSs have often been challenged to explain their work, especially elements that are not direct care. Delineating spheres of influence was intended to diminish perceived or experienced role ambiguity and to distinguish CNSs from other APNs (NACNS, 1998).

CLINICAL NURSE SPECIALIST PRACTICE: SPHERES OF INFLUENCE AND ADVANCED PRACTICE NURSING COMPETENCIES

Although other models of CNS practice have been described (see Chapter 2), the NACNS's three spheres of influence and Hamric's seven competencies (see Chapter 3 and Chapters 5 through 11) will be used to organize and explain CNS practice in this chapter. The CNS characteristics, attributes, skills, and competencies outlined in the NACNS *Statement* (2004b) are consistent with Hamric's seven competencies of advanced practice nursing. CNS students are encouraged to familiarize themselves with the NACNS *Statement* (2004b) and with specialty-specific standards (e.g., the American Association of Critical-Care Nurses' integration of the Synergy Model with CNS competencies and the three spheres of influence (Becker, Kaplow, Muenzen, & Hartigan, 2006) to better understand the discussion of spheres and competencies. To be successful, a CNS must understand and apply the seven competencies of advanced practice nursing across the three spheres of influence, regardless of setting or specialty (ANA, 1986; Hamric, 1996; NACNS, 1998, 2004b).

Advanced practice competencies are categories of proficient performance and include specific knowledge and skill sets. According to Hamric's model (Chapter 3), there are seven competencies: direct care; expert guidance and coaching; consultation; research; collaboration; clinical, professional, and systems leadership; and ethical decision making. The direct care of patients and families is the *central* competency in Hamric's model (see Figure 2-10) and informs every other competency. According to the NACNS's model, the impact and influence of CNSs are felt within three spheres of influence: *Direct Care of Patients or Clients,*[1] *Nurses and Nursing Practice, and Organizations and Systems* (NACNS, 1998, 2004b) (see Figure 2-1). Both the Hamric and NACNS models emphasize the importance of direct care; clinical expertise and direct care are basic to CNS practice. For this reason the *Direct Care of Patients or Clients* sphere of influence is the largest sphere in the NACNS's model and encompasses the other two spheres.

CNSs demonstrate all seven competencies across the three spheres of influence and often execute some competencies simultaneously. They exert influence in the *Nurses and Nursing Practice* sphere by caring for patients directly and by serving as coaches, guides, and role models for nursing staff and other caregivers. They provide consultation. They demonstrate research competencies by working with staff to develop, implement, and evaluate evidence-based practices. They may collaborate in clinical research—an activity likely to affect all three spheres of influence. Similarly, they collaborate and facilitate team development, assess and intervene to alleviate the moral distress inherent in clinical care, and create environments that support clinicians' ethical decision making. They exert influence in the *Organizations and Systems* sphere by providing clinical and systems leadership in many ways, whether it is articulating nursing issues to team members, advocating for a patient, taking a stand on behalf of nurses, or evaluating the quality and cost-effectiveness of technologies and care processes. Interventions and activities in the other two spheres are intended to affect the care of patients; therefore these two spheres are encompassed by the *Direct Care of Patients or Clients* sphere in the NACNS's model. Throughout all three spheres, CNSs apply the nursing process; assessment, planning, implementation, and evaluation activities are designed to improve the care of patients, to develop nurses, and to improve the systems in which nurses work and care is delivered. Experienced CNSs understand that activities in each sphere of influence and their advanced practice competencies exert reciprocal influences on each other.

The variety of activities, the challenge of in-the-moment problem solving that characterizes clinical work, and intermediate and long-rage planning efforts to improve the care of patients attracts CNSs to this work. Throughout the history of CNS practice and despite the changes in health care, reimbursement, and credentialing that have affected advanced practice nursing, CNSs have remained focused on championing excellence in nursing practice and on improving clinical care and the systems in which the care is delivered.

The reader can imagine that, without sustained engagement in direct care (*Direct Care of Patients or Clients* sphere), it would be difficult, if not impossible, to continue to be effective in the other two spheres since they depend on the CNS's clinical credibility. However, because CNSs provide more than just direct care, maintaining their commitment to patient care is often challenged as organizational priorities change. Direct care is the *central competency;* many texts (Gawlinski & Kern, 1994; Hamric & Spross, 1989; Hamric, Spross, & Hanson, 1996, 2000, 2005; Shea, Pelletier, Poster, Stuart, & Verhey, 1999; Sparacino, Cooper, & Minarik, 1990; Zuzelo, 2007) and the professional journal *Clinical Nurse Specialist* offer practical suggestions for successfully implementing the CNS role. In the following sections the ways in which CNSs implement the seven competencies across three spheres of influence are described.

Direct Clinical Practice

Specialization was the genesis of the CNS role, but expert clinical practice—and direct patient care—is its heart. The central competency of direct clinical practice is explicitly linked to the patient/client

---

[1]In the NACNS document, this sphere is called *Client Direct Care.* For clarity in this chapter, this sphere is referred to as *Direct Care of Patients or Clients.*

sphere of influence; the insights and outcomes of providing direct care influence the CNS's work in the other two spheres of nursing practice and systems. Implementing competencies across the three spheres results in improvements in clinical outcomes, patient safety, patient/family satisfaction, resource allocation, professional nursing staff knowledge and skills, health care team collaboration, and organizational efficiency.

CNS practice includes advanced assessment skills and the integration of "biophysical, psychosocial, behavioral, sociopolitical, cultural, economic, and nursing science" into specialized, expert nursing practice (AACN, 2006b, p. 16). Skills (clinical, advanced communication, and relational) and knowledge (theoretical, practical, and particular) are essential, but practical wisdom is a hallmark of advanced practice nursing (Oberle & Allen, 2001). Many authors have described strategies for successfully implementing the expert clinician dimension, building on the conceptual foundations of previous authors (Felder, 1983; Koetters, 1989; Sparacino & Cooper, 1990). Each strategy is highly dependent on the individual CNS and his or her practice setting, and can fluctuate from year to year in relation to the prevailing health care environment. It is easy for the direct care component of the role to be either overemphasized or underemphasized due to institutional priorities and competition for CNS expertise. The unique skill set of CNSs may result in them being continually pulled away from direct care to lead projects that are of high priority for the institution. Conversely, if an institution recognizes value only in the revenue generation component of direct care, the CNS may be required to focus exclusively on that component of the role. The CNS role is optimally enacted when there is the opportunity to use what they've learned from direct clinical practice to improve care for individual patients and families and patient populations, whether that occurs at the patient-CNS interface, through nursing personnel, or through organizational improvements.

Although clinical expertise is the cornerstone of CNS practice, a CNS's success will not be measured by clinical knowledge or technical expertise alone. Providing regular and consistent direct patient care is essential for the CNS:

- To evaluate the quality, effectiveness, efficiency, and safety of patient care and to determine if inadequacies are the result of a lack or ineffective use of nursing resources, insufficient equipment and supplies, or systems' inefficiencies—this assessment by CNSs has been characterized as surveillance (see Chapter 5)
- To demonstrate one's clinical competency and maintain clinical expertise, thereby role modeling clinical behaviors, establishing credibility, and maintaining team relationships and collegial trust
- To identify nursing staff learning needs, including knowledge and skill development
- To refine one's clinical expertise and reflective abilities
- To maintain CNS credentials/certification

Direct care, or direct clinical practice, refers to CNS activities and responsibilities that occur within the patient-nurse interface (see Chapter 5). For many years, a CNS's direct clinical practice was embedded in a hospital's interdisciplinary care and was not linked to patient outcomes or resource utilization (Hamric, 1995). Thus little data were available to justify the role and correlate its expense with the cost avoidance and quality improvement aspects of the role when health care institutions were restructuring their operating systems. However, most of the patients requiring the expertise of a CNS are sicker, more frail, and in need of specialized, expert care. Clinical studies with high-risk patients, including very-low-birth-weight infants, women with a high-risk pregnancy, and older adults with cardiac diagnoses, have consistently shown improved patient outcomes and reduced health care costs when CNSs and other APNs were directly involved with patient care, including assessing, teaching, counseling, and negotiating systems (Brooten, Youngblut, Deatrick, Naylor, & York, 2003).

A CNS is most likely to care directly for a patient whose diagnosis or care is complex, unique, or problematic. Examples of complex or problematic patients include an infant with very low birth weight, a frail older person with multiple hospital readmissions, a child with complex congenital heart disease, a young pregnant woman with a transplanted organ, or a man diagnosed with bipolar disorder who has survived a suicide attempt but who requires prolonged physical rehabilitation. Examples of unique situations are the care of a patient with the rarely used Eloesser flap for the treatment of a tuberculous empyema; the evaluation and implementation of a new intervention, such as teletechnology to assess the efficacy of preventive interventions for pressure ulcers; or the introduction of an experimental chemotherapeutic agent. CNSs have the advanced skills to care for these challenging patients by incorporating a holistic perspective, forming therapeutic partnerships, and using expert clinical thinking and skillful performance to optimize outcomes. The CNS has the access and ability to evaluate the latest evidence and apply it in diverse ways to manage complex cases.

Direct care also affords a CNS the opportunity to assess the quality of care for a specific patient population. This qualitative assessment enhances the interpretation of quantitative data and directs changes in care processes. For example, a CNS might notice a pattern of frequently missed clinic appointments for a heart failure patient. Through the therapeutic partnership, the CNS may determine that a lack of clinic parking results in a barrier for this patient to keep appointments. The outcome is not one of a noncompliant patient but a logistical failure that requires immediate resolution for the benefit of all clients with heart failure. When a home care nurse notes that older patients are not taking medications consistently, a CNS's engagement with those patients can provide a more detailed and complex assessment. The result of such an assessment may be that the older patients are cognitively impaired and forget to take their medications; the medication regimen may be too complex, causing a patient to miss doses; or the medication may be too expensive and not covered by supplemental insurance or Medicaid, causing a patient to halve or skip doses and to let prescriptions go unfilled. The CNS's evaluation might integrate advanced assessment skills, such as cognitive screening, into the admission assessment of all older patients; might identify therapeutic alternatives, such as a simpler or more economical medication regimen, to improve compliance; or might introduce other creative interventions to promote health and quality of life.

A CNS's clinical practice interventions may be (1) continuous, in which the CNS carries a consistent caseload; or (2) time-limited, regular, or episodic, in which the CNS cares for complex cases as they arise (Koetters, 1989). Examples of regular care include providing care for all patients with newly diagnosed diabetes in a community clinic; providing psychotherapy, medication management, and other specialized nursing care for patients requiring mental health care; delivering total patient care to the first patients in an innovative surgery program; or visiting all patients with congestive heart failure in a home care

agency who have had more than one hospital readmission within 60 days of their initial hospital admission. Episodic care helps a CNS assess and intervene in a particular problem. Examples of episodic care include planning and coordinating a patient's complex hospital discharge, facilitating a support group for patients with primary pulmonary hypertension, and providing total patient care (similar to a staff nurse but with a different lens) to determine the feasibility of proposed changes in patient care or other system changes. Involvement in regular or episodic care enables CNSs to identify systems' problems that interfere with care and require CNS intervention. Examples include lack of staff knowledge, the need for clinical policies or procedures, and the need for conflict mediation among team members. For each clinical situation, a CNS takes a comprehensive approach, using discriminative judgment, advanced knowledge, and expert skill, including expertise in the technical, humanistic, and organizational aspects of care. In these situations, CNSs are particularly skilled at the use of surveillance, quickly identifying both patient and system issues and intervening to avoid further complications. A CNS intervention may be as simple as assisting a patient and family to navigate a hospital's bureaucracy. A CNS knows how and when to break the rules and when to bypass organizational or philosophical roadblocks, thus ensuring the focus on the patient and family and a successful outcome.

If clinical skills (e.g., particularly psychomotor ones, such as administering chemotherapy and troubleshooting ventricular assist devices) are not used periodically, CNSs become less proficient. Regular clinical practice helps a CNS maintain the expertise and clinical competence needed to practice and to develop the skills of other nurses. Besides maintaining and refining clinical skills, direct clinical practice is imperative at two pivotal points: during a CNS's orientation to establish credibility; and before and occasionally throughout the implementation of organizational change to assess the impact of the change on patient care. CNSs must weigh the benefits and costs of different ways to implement direct care. Advantages, such as developing credibility with staff or maintaining one's skills, are evaluated against potential disadvantages, such as competing demands or time pressures. For example, the critical care CNS may need to prioritize responsibilities, such as meeting with a hospital's administration to design a new ICU, teaching a critical care class, and remaining at the bedside to assess the effectiveness of new staff orientation. Besides episodic involvement with particular patients, a critical care CNS could schedule 8 hours of staff nursing per month to maintain clinical skills, to assess staff needs and the quality of teamwork and communication, and to identify obstacles to the delivery of care. This hands-on involvement helps a CNS understand the conditions under which nurses are expected to implement standards of care and ensure quality.

Clinical practice can also occur indirectly. For example, a CNS may delegate direct care to a staff nurse but still guide the care. A CNS's goal is always to improve the direct care skills and knowledge of staff nurses. A CNS may select a patient population in which there are recurrent problems, poor outcomes, or recidivism and then collaborate with members of the health care team to develop and implement standards of care, clinical pathways, clinical procedures, or quality or performance improvement plans. Implementation of and adherence to recommended practice changes should be evaluated to assess the impact of the change on outcomes, to refine algorithms or guidelines, to improve clinical management, and to promote consistent adherence. Algorithms and guidelines are rarely self-sustaining and require a champion who continuously facilitates their implementation, constantly evaluating new evidence that may result in the need for revisions. This role is imperative if the algorithm or guideline is to be successful and achieve its intended outcome. A CNS is often the person to fulfill the champion role.

System responsibilities for evaluating technology and its impact on patients and resources is another facet of the CNS's indirect clinical practice. Technological advances have accelerated changes in health care delivery. Such advances, however, coupled with the pressure of cost containment, increased competition, heightened consumer expectations, and capped budgets, create conflicting demands and priorities. Technological advances have provided the objective data necessary to make clinical judgments (e.g., medication titration based on hemodynamic indices), devices to remotely assess a patient (e.g., telemonitoring of vital signs and weights), and interventional alternatives to treat disease (e.g., fiberoptic, robotic, and virtual reality surgery). Yet technology warrants close scrutiny, for with it comes a responsibility to evaluate its impact on budgets, quality of care, the environment, risk-versus-benefit, staff, and patients.

Patient safety is integral to all aspects of both direct and indirect clinical practice, including CNS availability to and support of novice nurses (Ebright, Urden, Patterson, & Chalko, 2004). It is this direct clinical practice that empowers a CNS to assume a leadership role in evaluating patient safety and preventing adverse events. As a change agent who influences others, a CNS builds trust and defuses the atmosphere of blame surrounding safety issues and adverse event investigations (Ebright, Patterson, & Render, 2002).

Although providing direct care to patients is a core competency, how CNSs provide direct care varies across CNS specialties and practice settings, is determined by population needs, is influenced by the expertise of other nursing personnel, and is affected by regulatory designations of CNSs as APNs and their scopes of practice. When, how, for whom, and with whom direct care is given are fluid and are negotiated and renegotiated with professional nursing staff and organizational leadership, based on patient needs and the knowledge and clinical skill of nursing personnel.

Exemplar 12-2 illustrates how the second author (C.C.), a pediatric CNS, uses her professional competencies to provide expert care to a specific patient population and demonstrates the importance of direct care to execution of the other CNS competencies. This pediatric CNS coordinates health care services for a large pediatric craniofacial population, specifically infants with craniosynostosis. The pediatric neurosurgeon with whom C.C. works developed a new, less invasive technique to correct craniosynostosis in young infants. To inform families and referring health care providers about craniosynostosis treatment within her hospital, C.C. has developed and maintains a craniosynostosis link on the institution's website. This new surgical treatment—and its follow up—has drawn patients from all over the United States and the world.

Expert Coaching and Guidance

The nursing literature describes the essential components of the CNS role as expert coach, guide, and educator (Sparacino & Cooper, 1990; Spross, Clarke, & Beauregard, 2000). The expert coaching and guidance competency depends on the interaction of technical, clinical, and interpersonal competencies and self-reflection (see Chapter 6), and its development is also influenced by scholarly inquiry and the use, interpretation, and application of relevant research. CNSs use both formal and informal coaching and teaching strategies with patients and families, nurses and nursing personnel, graduate nursing students, clinical nurse

EXEMPLAR 12-2   Direct Clinical Practice of the Clinical Nurse Specialist

I (author C.C.) perform the preoperative history and physical examination in the clinic; order appropriate radiographs, laboratory tests, and consultations; and obtain cephalometric measurements and photographs. Because surgery is the next day, staff nurses who will be caring for the patient postoperatively are notified of pertinent findings and specific needs. Postoperatively, I assess the patient for adequate pain control, dietary needs, vital sign changes, incisions, swelling, and neurological function. These findings, the staff nurses' concerns, and the plan of care are discussed. Standing orders, developed in collaboration with the neurosurgeon, are adapted for each patient.

CONSULTATION
I am frequently consulted by staff nurses, referring physicians, or other advanced practice nurses to assess misshapen heads, either by physical assessment or reviewing radiographs. These consultations provide opportunities to teach health care professionals how to recognize the differences between positional plagiocephaly and craniosynostosis, leading to earlier referrals for improved outcomes.

EXPERT COACHING AND GUIDANCE
The World Wide Web can be an excellent resource for families seeking health care information about medical conditions and treatment options. To help families learn more about craniosynostosis, I created a website (no longer available) that described the various types of craniosynostosis and treatment options, including a new less-invasive technique. As a result, I received 20 to 30 e-mails or telephone calls each day from families seeking information about this new technique for their babies. Providing accurate information on the website was critical so that families could make informed decisions about surgery. Much of the preoperative teaching was done by telephone or e-mail in preparation for the first preoperative visit, the day before surgery. Before the craniofacial website was available, only three or four patients a year were candidates for the less-invasive technique. After the website was initiated, we saw as many as 70 patients in 1 year.

Educating nurses about the early recognition of craniosynostosis, surgical options, and positional plagiocephaly has been done through professional journal articles, presentations at national nursing conferences, the school of nursing, and in-service

education programs to the staff nurses. Mentoring graduate students provided additional opportunities for role modeling.

RESEARCH
Collaboration on research with the pediatric neurosurgeon yielded data that demonstrated that the new surgical technique decreased patients' hospital stays, decreased costs, and improved patient outcomes. When parents noticed a sharp decrease in fussiness in their babies immediately after surgery, I developed a questionnaire to survey parents' perceptions of fussiness and irritability in their babies before and after surgery. Statistically significant decreases in fussiness and irritability were found postoperatively, suggesting that babies with craniosynostosis experienced increases in intracranial pressure.

CLINICAL AND PROFESSIONAL LEADERSHIP
In this unique role, I can provide care throughout the continuum, using clinical pathways to help the families navigate the hospital system in an efficient manner. Bringing a baby to an unfamiliar city for surgery by surgeons they have never met is a daunting experience for most parents. My leadership skills are put to the test coordinating preoperative donor-directed blood, arranging lodging at the Ronald McDonald House, scheduling preoperative workups and follow-up appointments with the neurosurgeon, plastic surgeon, ophthalmologist, and anesthesiologist, and coordinating the helmet molding.

COLLABORATION
Collaboration occurs at many levels. First, I have a collaborative practice agreement with the pediatric neurosurgeon as required by hospital policy and the state board of nursing. I collaborate with the staff nurses who care for these babies with craniosynostosis, providing in-service educational programs about the disorder and conducting rounds with them on the postoperative patients. Collaboration also occurs with other members of the craniofacial team, such as ophthalmologists, genetic counselors, plastic surgeons, and orthotic designers. I confer with referring health care providers to provide continuity after the patients leave the hospital and between follow-up visits.

ETHICAL DECISION MAKING
Although this new surgical treatment for craniosynostosis results in minimal blood loss, an infant will occasionally present with a low

EXEMPLAR 12-2   Direct Clinical Practice of the Clinical Nurse Specialist—cont'd

hemoglobin or experience excessive intraoperative blood loss. Some families refuse blood transfusions for religious reasons, requiring more intensive preoperative preparation to minimize the need for a blood transfusion. A protocol for preoperative erythropoietin injections was sent to the patient's pediatrician in an attempt to increase the hemoglobin. Other families have religious symbols they want placed on the baby during surgery. These requests are also accommodated. The CNS must obtain a thorough history, noting religious preferences and beliefs, so that the families' wishes can be known to all who care for the child.

A great deal of preparation is required for a family to bring their baby to another state or country for a new kind of surgery. The CNS is instrumental in facilitating this process, using the core competencies and spheres of influence.

specialists, health professionals, consumer groups, and organizations or systems (see Chapter 6).

Patients and Families. A CNS's expert coaching and guidance are pivotal in providing or influencing patient and family education. CNS coaching and teaching complements the care given to a patient and family by other nurses and health professionals. CNSs continually seek better ways to coach patients and families using combinations of cognitive, educational, and behavioral strategies to improve patient education and adherence to interventions. However, a CNS cannot teach every patient and family and so must assess whom to teach. For example, a CNS could mentor a case manager or presurgical program educator to provide routine preoperative teaching for cardiac surgical patients. A CNS could then allocate more time to coach high-risk, complex, unusual, or "difficult" patients, such as an octogenarian who is undecided about an aortic valve replacement or a young adult with a bicuspid aortic valve, leukemia, and endocarditis who requires intravenous chemotherapy. A CNS may demonstrate how to facilitate difficult conversations with patients and their families by supporting the parents of a newborn who died, working with a patient and family on end-of-life decisions, or "translating" a physician's technical explanation into lay terms.

As health care systems are restructured, there is increasing emphasis on patients' accountability for their own health. This means that, in addition to coaching individuals, CNSs are even more likely to be involved in educational program planning and implementation aimed at helping groups of patients manage chronic illnesses and associated symptoms. Many patients know that they need to be better informed and educated about health risk determinants, preventive self-care, treatment options, and the risks and benefits of treatments, but their health care behaviors are influenced by many personal, psychological, and sociocultural factors. Because a patient is not always able or willing to change his or her lifestyle or to adhere to health care recommendations, a CNS must determine which patient or patient population is most appropriate for CNS coaching, such as a prenatal patient with poor social support living in an economically depressed community, an African-American woman at risk of contracting human immunodeficiency virus (HIV), or a teenager who is newly diagnosed with type I diabetes. With many consumers seeking health care from nontraditional providers (Tindle, Davis, Phillips, & Eisenberg, 2005), CNSs often help patients and providers integrate conventional and integrative therapies into care plans.

Nurses and Nursing Personnel. A CNS is a role model for nurses, demonstrating the practical integration of theory and evidence-based practice. Whereas NPs and certified nurse-midwives (CNMs) primarily coach patients and families, a CNS strives to continuously improve clinical practice and to integrate new knowledge into practice, thereby influencing the further development of the proficient and expert nurse and enhancing the staff nurse's accountability and self-sufficiency. A CNS cannot be effective when he or she is or is perceived to be territorial, omnipotent, or omniscient (see Chapter 9). A CNS's time is often better spent by teaching others the why, what, and how of common patient care interventions than repeatedly providing those same interventions. For example, a well-developed, standardized nursing care plan that details the assessment of different wound types and stages with stage-specific interventions will enable nursing staff to provide consistent and evidence-based care to patients with the simpler types of wounds. The CNS is appropriately consulted for the complex wounds. Developing standards for patient education and providing resources to ensure that it is consistent across populations are equally important CNS educational activities (see Chapter 6 for more about health literacy and patient coaching). As a staff nurse applies the new knowledge and skills taught by a CNS, the CNS can attend to new or more complex responsibilities. A staff nurse can become the role model for the skill mastered or the knowledge gained, and so a CNS's influence will continue to improve patient care. This notion of extending the "reach" of the CNS's expertise can be considered a defining characteristic of the coaching competency of CNS practice. The cycle of enrichment and growth is never complete. Whenever major staff turnover occurs or a CNS enters a new practice setting, the cycle must begin anew.

Students. A CNS has a professional responsibility to educate graduate nursing students and, when the opportunity arises, to be their mentor. In working with graduate nursing students in the classroom or in a clinical setting, a CNS shares knowledge, models the integration of practical and scientific knowledge into expert clinical practice, and demonstrates the level of advanced practice nursing to which a student can aspire. A CNS can provide opportunities for a graduate nursing student to do a clinical practicum or residency; the reward of working with an excellent student is being able to do more, to extend one's influence more broadly, and to make advanced practice expertise more widely available. Besides providing patient care, a student completes projects (e.g., writing patient education materials or clinical procedures) or tasks (e.g., a literature review to support proposed changes in clinical practice) that benefit the practice setting as well. A CNS may also be involved in the education of undergraduate nurses and other health professionals.

Other Health Care Providers and the Public. A CNS has many opportunities to educate other health care providers and consumer groups—usually more than one can reasonably fulfill. When considering such an opportunity, a CNS must determine if the topic is within his or her specialty, the size of the audience or the number who can be reached, visibility (internal or external to the institution), and the potential for cost savings or revenue. Sometimes

such requests are opportunities to expand one's area of expertise. When the content is outside a CNS's specialty, however, the CNS has to prepare extensively to compensate for inexperience and risks overcommitment. In any case, a CNS must carefully balance teaching obligations within his or her practice setting with teaching requests outside of the practice setting or the immediate community. The more a CNS is pulled away from the practice setting, the higher the risk of becoming an invisible and, therefore, an unnecessary health care provider.

Consultation

The nursing literature offers classic descriptions of the essential components of consultation and strategies for ensuring the success of a CNS as a consultant (Barron, 1983, 1989; Gurka, 1991; Hamric, 1983b; Noll, 1987; Sneed, 1991; Sparacino & Cooper, 1990). Skill as a consultant cannot be assumed although it is an expected CNS competency, and each CNS's consultative proficiency and the need to use this competency vary (see Chapter 7).

The consultation competency affects all three spheres of CNS influence (see Chapter 7). As a content expert, a CNS can suggest a wide range of alternative approaches or solutions to clinical or systems problems, whether internal or external to the practice setting. As a consultant, the CNS often directs staff to other resources (e.g., other colleagues, community resources, practice guidelines) that enable nurses and others to make decisions based on relevant and appropriate alternatives. A CNS is a process consultant and facilitates change so that decisions can be made for immediate and future situations (Sparacino & Cooper, 1990). Process activities and outcome achievement are two critical and measurable elements of the CNS consultation competency. Documenting consultations and linking them to outcomes are important. An example of this connection is described by Gurka (1991), who used four consultative process activities (the fact finder, educator, informational expert, and advocate modes) from Lippitt and Lippitt's consultation model and measured three major outcomes (prevention of complications, maintenance or development of standards of care, and improvement in staff nurses' clinical judgment skills).

A CNS is both an internal and external consultant.

Internal Consultation. Internal consultation includes assisting staff and facilitating organizational development in one's own practice setting, especially the creative use of resources and alternative strategies to overcome or eliminate perceived system obstacles. A CNS may determine that a request for internal consultation requires the collaboration of multiple consultants, including other CNSs and members of other disciplines. A CNS often initiates the plan, mobilizes the resources, convenes team meetings, defuses the politics, and facilitates the resolution. Examples of CNS consultation from the literature and our own experiences include:

- A liaison psychiatric CNS consults with an obstetrical/gynecological department to screen and provide treatment for mental health problems in women (D'Afflitti, 2004)
- A behavioral health CNS and a critical care CNS collaborate and lead a multidisciplinary team to implement a standardized assessment tool and treatment protocol for alcohol withdrawal (Phillips, Haycock, & Boyle, 2006)
- An oncology CNS who rarely cares for patients with brain tumors consults a neurology or neurosurgery CNS when brain tumor patients are admitted for assistance in developing a care plan that addresses neurological deficits and that ensures the effective monitoring of potential complications
- A neurologist consults with a cardiovascular surgery CNS for assistance in preparing a patient, admitted with a brain abscess and a previously undiagnosed congenital cardiac anomaly, for urgent cardiac surgery

External Consultation. External consultation occurs apart from the CNS's practice or employment setting. External consultation offers approaches or solutions to specific problems to assist the nursing profession, a specialty organization, other health care providers, and health systems. External consultation may require ongoing, intensive interaction to effect significant change (Rantz et al., 2001). Examples of external consultation include:

- A geropsychiatric CNS provides consultation to a nursing unit or a nursing home about psychological issues associated with caring for an older population (Kennedy, Covington, Evans, & Williams, 2000)
- A geriatric care CNS consults with nursing homes about the clinical decision-making processes involved in preventing falls and reducing restraint use (Wagner et al., 2007)

Unless internal or external consultation is a CNS's primary responsibility (e.g., the internal consultation provided by a psychiatric liaison CNS), problems may arise if a CNS's time is used more for consultations than for direct care. The impact on patient care is less visible unless the content and process of consultations are well documented and the outcomes are measured. See Chapter 7 for further discussion of documenting and evaluating the consultation competency.

Research

In implementing the research competency, CNSs aim to evaluate and improve nursing practice and activities may range from scholarly inquiry to formal scientific investigation. The three specific research competencies, each of which has basic and advanced levels of activity, are interpretation and use of research findings (evidence- or research-based practice), participation in collaborative research, and evaluation of practice (see Chapter 8).

Nurse-sensitive indicators have been defined that capture nursing's unique contributions to patient outcomes. Assuming responsibility for identifying nursing-sensitive and multidisciplinary quality indicators (Duffy, 2002; Kleinpell & Gawlinski, 2005) and using outcome data to improve patient care delivery are prime opportunities for a CNS to assess patient care strategies and community systems, analyze interdisciplinary communication and collaboration, coordinate care, and monitor patient and system progress. Much work has yet to be done, however, to develop the science linking nursing, health care processes, available measures, and quality outcomes (Naylor, 2007). All CNSs must demonstrate the research competency and have ongoing accountability for monitoring and improving their practice and the practice of other nurses (NACNS, 1998, 2004b). CNSs implement this competency in a variety of ways depending on experience, expertise, circumstances, setting, and resources. The following discussion illustrates how CNSs implement the research competency.

Interpretation and Use of Research and Evidence in Practice. *Evidence-based practice* has become an umbrella term for *research utilization, research-based practice,* or *outcomes research* (Jennings, 2000; see also Chapter 8). Integration of new scientific findings and science-based knowledge influences the development and evaluation of new approaches to clinical practice (AACN, 2006b).

For CNSs, interpretation and use of research often begins with a clinical question identified by the CNS or the staff with whom he or she works. Knowledge is the basis for practice, and yet, too frequently, routine practice may not be based on research findings. The foundation of improved quality of care and patient outcomes is the analysis of research-based evidence and consensus-dependent practice changes to ensure best practice and achieve quality patient care. When research is systematically evaluated for its applicability, informed decisions about providing patient care and achieving optimal patient outcomes are made and nursing practice is documented (McPheeters & Lohr, 1999). Inherent in the CNS role is the evaluation of the appropriateness of research and the application of its findings to clinical practice. A CNS is the ideal clinician to assess those factors that are barriers and facilitators to change and to develop, implement, and evaluate evidence-based practice. Evidence-based practice is integrated into clinical procedures, administrative policies, educational materials for patients and staff, and clinical pathways. A CNS's involvement in developing clinical pathways and procedures means that evidence informs clinical processes and standards. A CNS who develops an evidence-based guideline of care for a patient population promotes improved patient outcomes throughout the three spheres of influence. The patient's physical or mental function improves, treatment is safer and with fewer complications, there is continuity of care across the health care continuum, and nursing practice improves (McCabe, 2005). Multiple examples of CNS-led evidence-based practice can be found in the literature. CNS contributions to improving patient outcomes by providing evidence-based care include implementation of an intensive intravenous insulin protocol for critically ill patients (Ward & Clark, 2006), reduction of CNS prescribing errors (O'Malley, 2007), the design of a weight management program for African-Americans (Walker-Sterling, 2005), and participation with other APNs as facilitators for the Nurses Improving Care for Health-system Elders project (Fulmer et al., 2002).

The Center for Advanced Nursing Practice (Soukup, 2000), BryanLGH Medical Center, in Lincoln, Nebraska, exemplifies a collective effort of APNs to use research. The Center's purposes are to advance scholarly clinical practice, to develop a practice model that includes four interactive phases (evidence-triggered, evidence-supported, evidence-observed, and evidence-based), and to promulgate evidence-based practice across the care continuum. Some of the Center's representative initiatives include improving chest pain management by linking staff at tertiary care institutions with those in rural areas (Rasmussen & Barnason, 2000), a mental health prevention intervention (Adams, 2000), an interdisciplinary approach to a total knee replacement program (Seemann, 2000), and selection and implementation of a transparent dressing for central vascular access devices (Woods, Nass, & Deisch, 2000).

Evaluation of Practice. At the most basic level, this competency requires that a CNS evaluate his or her practice across spheres of influence. Several authors have discussed CNS evaluation from a variety of perspectives, including self-evaluation, staff evaluation, and peer review (Cooper & Sparacino, 1990; Girouard, 1996; Girouard & Spross, 1983; Hamric, 1983a, 1989b). Peer review is not institutional performance evaluation. In the former, the key participants are other practicing CNSs and essential elements are clinical practice, leadership, and professional behaviors (Briggs, Heath, & Kelley, 2005). Although each CNS specialty develops practice-setting-specific evaluation tools, a standardized tool should be developed for expected competencies and the ensurance of outcome quality. Lunney, Gigliotti, and McMorrow (2007) designed a tool for graduate students to use for self-evaluation of CNS competency development, which could be adapted for practicing CNSs.

CNSs may document the components of their clinical practice, including the numbers of patients seen, types and frequencies of interventions, and outcomes achieved; educational activities for staff, including one-on-one coaching, in-service programs, orientation, and continuing education; and system initiatives, such as quality improvement activities and interdisciplinary rounds (AACN, 2006b). To evaluate one's ability and effectiveness in exercising influence, a CNS may ask nursing and interdisciplinary colleagues to comment on his or her communication and collaboration skills. CNSs may use these data for self-assessment to determine whether the allocation of activities is consistent with personal, professional, and institutional goals; to prepare quarterly reports; or to assemble a portfolio for one's annual evaluation. Tracking such data enables CNSs to identify recurring events that may require an intervention at the staff or system level and midcourse corrections if schedule demands require a shift in goals or a realignment of expectations.

In the early days of CNS practice, few studies documented the impact of CNSs on patient and family outcomes. The evidence is mounting, however, and the positive impact on patient outcome is irrefutable (see Chapter 24). One should expect optimal patient outcomes when CNS competencies complement patient needs or characteristics (Becker et al., 2006). Outcome studies can help CNSs document their activities and their effects on patient and family outcomes. Classic studies include evaluation of the impact of CNS interventions on low-birth-weight infants and older patients in the hospital (Brooten et al., 1986; Neidlinger, Kennedy, & Scroggins, 1987). More recent studies have shown the impact of CNS interventions on patients who received transitional care services and were discharged from a hospital earlier than the norm (Brooten et al., 2002). Patients with congestive heart failure whose care was managed by CNSs had significantly shorter lengths of hospital stay and lower hospital expenses than those patients receiving customary care (McCauley, Bixby, & Naylor, 2006; Naylor et al., 2004; Topp, Tucker, & Weber, 1998;). Patients who had surgery for a solid, late-stage malignancy and who received specialized home care from APNs had 2-year survival rates twice those of patients who received usual care in an ambulatory setting (McCorkle et al., 2000). As these topics suggest, CNSs can identify relevant structure, process, and outcome variables that can be used to assess the CNSs' contributions to quality patient care. How CNSs use clinical practice guidelines and their effect on clinical outcomes should also be evaluated. The relationship between implementation and outcomes may depend on the recency of the scientific evidence (Cunningham, 2006) and the sensitivity of outcomes to nursing practice, such as symptom experience, functional status, prevention of adverse events, and psychological distress (Gobel, Beck, & O'Leary, 2006). See Chapters 8 and 25 for further discussion of evaluation strategies.

Evaluation of CNS practice often includes outcomes management (AACN, 2006b). One component of outcomes management is the analysis of data regarding care efficiency and cost-effectiveness, the results of which guide systematic and continuous process and performance improvement. Examples include the use of an outcome-driven clinical pathway developed by an interdisciplinary team to improve patient outcomes and reduce cost of care (Patton & Schaerf, 1995); initiation of an evidence-based, falls-prevention program in an acute care setting (Stetler, Corrigan, Sander-Buscemi, & Burns, 1999); and creation and implementation of a new central venous catheter procedure, application of research findings to practice, and an evidence-based practice construct (Newell-Stokes, Broughton, Guiliano, & Stetler, 2001).

Practice evaluation must be integrated into one's daily work. Although researchers have begun to identify the interventions most often used by APNs, most of this work has been done in the evaluation of primary care or as part of programs evaluating the interventions of CNSs and NPs providing transitional care to discharged patients (Brooten et al., 1986; Brooten et al., 2002; see also Chapters 24 for additional research evidence of APN impact and Chapter 25 for evaluation strategies).

Participation in Collaborative Research. Collaborative research between a CNS and a researcher facilitates the application of research findings to clinical practice. Researchers provide CNSs with new evidence for patient care practices and the assessment of their impact. In turn, CNSs stimulate researchers to investigate the science that explains their observations of patients and populations. Typically, novice CNSs are not involved in collaborative research because the competencies that are directly related to patient care should be mastered first.

For experienced CNSs, collaborative research is often a realistic CNS goal. Whether novice or experienced CNSs become involved in research depends on the setting, pregraduate and graduate school experience, resources within the setting, and access to research expertise. Many CNSs find satisfaction with involvement in research as a consultant or co-investigator. A CNS is the clinical expert, understands clinical issues, has access to patients, and can anticipate clinical and system challenges that may occur throughout the research process. A nurse researcher is a research expert, knows research methodology, and has access to the resources that support the research. The CNS is optimally positioned to stimulate a researcher's interest because of his or her direct clinical association with patients or participant populations (Nelson, Holland, Derscheid, & Tucker, 2007). Before participating in a research project, a CNS must determine if there is readiness and receptiveness in the practice setting, if there is administrative support, and if research activities are a realistic performance goal. Evaluating outcomes of nursing practice to assess and improve the quality of care is an important element of the research competency (see Chapter 8).

Interdisciplinary collaborative research offers opportunities and benefits, including an enriched practice environment, examination of clinically relevant issues, and policy and practice improvements (Disch et al., 2006). CNSs know the organizational and social facilitators and barriers to clinical research, are able to bridge the academic-clinical gap, and can assist in recruiting and retaining research participants (Fitzgerald, Tomlinson, Peden-McAlpine, & Sherman, 2003; Nelson et al., 2007).

Whatever the model, a CNS is a key player in developing and implementing relevant nursing-sensitive and multidisciplinary quality indicators for measuring patient and system outcomes. Besides applying research findings to clinical practice, CNSs must use research to influence public policy. Although conducting prospective research to address statutory or regulatory initiatives is rare, research results can provide substantive and objective facts that are more powerful and meaningful than impassioned pleas. The research literature is extensive, and professional, state, and national agencies have extensive data banks. This research must be used wisely, translating the findings to commonly understood and generally applicable language (Hamric, 1998).

Clinical, Professional, and Systems Leadership

The CNS uses advanced communication and leadership skills to evaluate practice and to effect change in complex health care delivery systems (AACN, 2006b). There are different domains and types of leadership and different attributes of leadership (see Chapter 9). Leadership is integral to the role because a CNS has responsibility for clinical innovation and change within the patient care system. A CNS has significant formal and informal impact; a CNS must be visionary yet practical. Through a CNS's clinical and systems leadership, change strategies are implemented and nursing practice and patient care improve systems. A CNS is the link between many disciplines and resources and asserts clinical and professional leadership in the practice setting or health care system, in health care policy and delivery decisions, and in the administration of direct care programs. A CNS identifies the need for practice changes and leads the development and implementation of clinical procedures, practice guidelines, and clinical pathways; designs and directs performance improvement initiatives; chairs interdisciplinary committees or manages clinical projects; and influences or guides

institutional health care policy decisions. Clinical and professional leadership competencies are integrated with the other CNS competencies to support an organization's purpose and goals.

Most health care organizations are a bureaucratic maze. A CNS works with and advocates for staff, patients, and families to help them understand the complexities and wend their way through the system. A CNS can be an advocate, or "shuttle diplomat," between administrators and clinical staff, helping both groups understand the vagaries of organizational change, listening and supporting when appropriate, and explaining decisions when needed (Brown, 1989). A CNS can facilitate the design, implementation, and evaluation of a clinical information system, leading the collaboration between computer designers and users, integrating the needs of clinicians and patients, and facilitating innovative practice changes (Roggow, Solie, & Tracy, 2005). As leaders, CNSs also help the members of one discipline understand the priorities of another discipline and often negotiate agreements that bring diverse perspectives into alignment. Such mediation benefits patients, promotes communication, and creates an environment that fosters collaboration, as discussed in the next section.

Collaboration

CNSs must be skilled at collaboration because so many people regularly work and interact with a CNS (see Chapter 10). A CNS collaborates with nurses, physicians, other health care providers, and patients and their families. A CNS provides an interface between patient, family members, staff, and physician (AACN, 2006b). Many patients have such complex health care needs that no one health care professional can manage them all. CNSs understand the knowledge and skills of other team members and actively participate in or lead interdisciplinary teams and rounds. A CNS can assist a patient and family members determine their needs; help them ask questions and assess treatment options; and facilitate timely referrals to other disciplines to ensure a positive outcome. Throughout his or her interactions with patients and colleagues, a CNS models the communication and collaboration skills that help teams mature.

A CNS can be thought of as a nurse attending, a teacher, and a role model for nursing staff. CNSs often identify potential or actual conflicts. CNS advocacy often prevents adversarial situations and their negative sequelae. A CNS must be skilled in helping team members address and negotiate conflicts to optimize patient care. The outcome of CNS-coordinated collaboration is the empowerment of nurses and the recognition of the nurse as a critical member of the health care team (Boyle, 1996; see Chapters 9 and 10). This results in team building, synergy, and integrative solutions. CNSs and physicians also collaborate, although some practice settings and working relationships are more conducive to partnership than others. Some CNSs and physicians have written collaborative practice agreements that outline CNS responsibilities, including state-approved prescriptive authority, lines of communication, and when to seek medical consultation if a health care issue is beyond the CNS's scope of practice. Further descriptions of collaborative practice agreements are found in Chapter 20. When boundary issues are put aside, the differences in physician and CNS practice are complementary, afford integrative solutions, and further strengthen collaboration (Minarik & Sparacino, 1990). The outcome is high-quality and cost-efficient patient care (Baggs et al., 1999). Integrated care management, especially in controlling capitated risk in health care delivery systems, is best achieved by a collaborative team approach (Moss, Steiner, Mahnke, & Cohen, 1998). Collaboration between a CNS and organizations outside of the health care realm, such as academia and industry, can be mutually beneficial and improve patient care (Benedict, Robinson, & Holder, 2006; Kerfoot, Rapala, Ebright, & Rogers, 2006).

Collaboration between a CNS and other health care professionals leads to effective and efficient health care, especially for complex patient populations. CNSs can integrate the insights of many individuals with different perspectives, each providing theoretical and applied knowledge. Collaboration is an essential competency—the well-earned result of clinical competence, effective communication, mutual trust, the valuing of complementary knowledge and skills, collegiality, and a favorable organizational structure (Benedict et al., 2006; D'Afflitti, 2004; Hughes & Mackenzie, 1990; Phillips et al., 2006; see also Chapter 10). For example, a pediatric CNS for neurosurgery collaborated with the pediatric hospitalist in the care of a 16-year-old adolescent with a recently resected pituitary tumor and a history of anorexia; their goal was to maintain her independence yet still provide optimum nutrition. Further collaboration with the pediatric CNS for endocrinology was essential to coordinate hormone replacement therapy with other therapies.

Blurring of boundaries can occur as the CNS role develops. These boundaries can overlap between the CNS and the staff nurse or even between the CNS and another APN. As a pediatric CNS teaches the mother of a child with traumatic brain injury how to comfort him without raising his intracranial pressure, she is delivering direct patient care and role modeling for the orientee caring for that child. Blurred boundaries are also evident when a pediatric neurosurgery CNS and a pediatric oncology CNS collaborate to plan the comprehensive discharge care for a 10-year-old child with a recently resected brain tumor who required radiation therapy, chemotherapy, and a plan for reintegration into his school. Such collaboration with others in the health care system enables a CNS to influence their colleagues to improve patient care across specialties, not just of the particular patient but in future situations in which patients' needs are similar. CNSs must avoid being "territorial"; this limits their effectiveness and they are unlikely to develop positive relationships that could help patients and families efficiently navigate the health care system.

Ethical Decision Making

CNSs often identify or consult on ethical issues and facilitate their resolution. In some cases, a CNS is consulted on what staff perceive is a clinical issue but really turns out to be an ethical concern. Being able to recognize, name, and address the moral distress and ethical concerns that are inherent in clinical care is a crucial part of CNS practice. A CNS can significantly influence the negotiation of moral dilemmas, the direction of patient care, access to care, and the allocation of resources. CNSs consider numerous factors when making ethical decisions, including professional and religious codes, cultural values, bioethical principles, and ethical theories (see Chapter 11). CNSs play critical roles in preventive and applied ethics. In promoting preventive ethics, a CNS is responsible for anticipating ethical conflicts when possible, for using ethical theories to analyze and explain ethical issues, for helping staff and patients clarify values, for serving as a role model in discussions with patients about treatment preferences and options, for demonstrating critical thinking in the analysis of moral dilemmas, and for enhancing others' autonomy (Forrow, Arnold, & Parker, 1993).

CNSs have similar responsibilities when applying ethical decision-making skills to patient and organizational issues. They recognize clinicians' experiences of moral distress and articulate moral dilemmas, often serving as advocates for patients, families, and staff. They interpret and mediate patient, family, and team members' views to ensure as complete a discussion of the dilemma as possible. They recognize the need to consult an ethics committee and often initiate that consult. When necessary, CNSs validate staff nurses' concerns and help nurses present their concerns to other team members, ensuring that the nursing perspective is considered when ethical issues are discussed. When CNSs are excluded from interdisciplinary ethical decisions, opportunities for effective nursing care are minimized and outcomes, such as timely and appropriate end-of-life care, are compromised (Oddi & Cassidy, 1998). As CNSs facilitate optimal care for frailer and sicker patients, the ethical challenge is to balance the expectations for quality care with the limitations of appropriate care and to articulate the moral dilemmas for patients, nursing personnel, and organizations.

Exemplar 12-3 (from C.C.'s practice) demonstrates the CNS's ethical decision making competency and shows how C.C. integrated clinical leadership and collaborative skills to facilitate a morally and clinically acceptable resolution. Consideration of the three spheres of influence is also reflected in the actions taken by the CNS.

Exemplar of CNS Practice: An Integrative Perspective on CNS Competencies and Spheres of Influence

Exemplar 12-4, a composite case taken from the practice of one of the authors (P.S.A.S.), illustrates the multidimensional and complex nature of CNS practice—implementing seven competencies across three spheres of influence. Exemplar 12-4 discusses a critically ill woman with complex medical problems, her distraught and divided family, a concerned but overwhelmed physician, and many caring but inexperienced nursing staff. Key elements, including pragmatic implementation of CNS competencies and the impact of the CNS in a complex and uncertain situation, are emphasized. The commentary explains the ways in which the author applied the competencies across the spheres of influence.

ISSUES AND CHALLENGES

Patient care has always been and will continue to be the very essence of the CNS role. A CNS's flexibility is well suited to adapt to systems changes while keeping the patient and direct patient care as the central focus. A number of issues continue to challenge the CNS role. These issues include but are not limited to factors influencing CNS practice, such as the balance between direct care focus and organizational priorities; organizational placement; standardization of

 EXEMPLAR 12-3   Ethical Decision Making

Mr. B. was a 60-year-old developmentally disabled man who resided in a skilled nursing facility longer than anyone could remember. With no living relatives, his legal decisions were made by a court-appointed guardian. Although not able to speak, the patient was able to get around in a wheelchair and feed himself. He was referred to a neurosurgeon when he experienced a decline in mental status and motor function. Once the physician surmised that an arachnoid cyst causing hydrocephalus could be the reason for the patient's decline, the guardian gave permission for a third ventriculostomy in hopes that Mr. B. would return to his previous state of health. Postoperative complications required intubation and mechanical ventilation. Several attempts to wean him from the ventilator failed, and placement of a tracheostomy and gastrostomy tube was considered. The clinical nurse specialist (CNS) and a staff nurse in the neuro intensive care unit (ICU) were

concerned about the nursing staff experiencing moral distress if further procedures were performed. The guardian wanted to do what the physicians wished and did not have an advanced directive for the patient. The CNS organized a meeting that included two members of the hospital ethics committee, the staff nurse caring for the patient, the attending neurosurgeon, and the guardian. The discussion that followed helped to clarify issues such as the patient's long-term prognosis and quality of life. It was agreed that a tracheostomy and gastrostomy tube would be less burdensome for the patient than continuous mechanical ventilation and nasogastric feedings and that further decisions could be made at a later date based on the patient's status. This discussion was extremely helpful for the staff nurse, neurosurgeon, guardian, and CNS, who all believed they had reached a decision that would improve the patient's outcome.

Box 12-1   A Selection of Internet Resources for the Clinical Nurse Specialist

American Association of Critical-Care Nurses:
www.aacn.org

American Association of Colleges of Nursing:
www.aacn.nche.edu

American Nurses Association:
www.nursingworld.org

American Nurses Credentialing Center:
www.nursingworld.org/ancc/

Oncology Nursing Society:
www.ons.org

National Association of Clinical Nurse Specialists:
www.nacns.org

National Council of State Boards of Nursing:
www.ncsbn.org

National Guideline Clearing House:
www.guideline.gov

education, certification, and practice requirements; and legal and regulatory challenges, including prescriptive authority, titling and title protection, and reimbursement. See Box 12-1 for a list of Internet resources for the CNS.

Clinical Practice: Visibility and Viability

Role Entry and Role Development. Role development of advanced practice nurses, including CNSs, is discussed in detail in Chapter 4; therefore only a few points are made here. Certain elements of role development are the same whether a CNS is a novice or is an experienced CNS assuming a new position. For example, the greatest amount of time and energy in the first 4 to 12 months is spent establishing credibility, especially through providing direct patient care and building key organizational or system relationships. The key strategy in this early stage is clear identification of and agreement about the CNS role and its responsibilities. This strategy is particularly important if there are multiple and conflicting expectations. Trust, acceptance, and interdependence are evident as the CNS becomes established; the result is that the CNS becomes more effective, flexible, and recognized and with time and experience is able to exercise all competencies across the three spheres.

It is worth noting that experienced CNSs often re-experience some of the emotions and stages that novice CNSs typically experience. For example, when a CNS assumes a new position, he or she may be surprised to feel like a novice at times; the new position requires new skills or their prior CNS experience does not automatically confer clinical credibility. CNSs may also re-experience earlier stages of role development when significant changes in organizational leadership occur. Finally, some experienced CNSs are at risk for becoming settled ("frozen") or complacent (see Chapter 4), which may affect their productivity and, ultimately, their employability. Self, peer, and administrative evaluations can help experienced CNSs recognize when they might be at risk for becoming too complacent to be effective.

Focus on Direct Care. Unlike other APNs who spend the majority of their time providing direct care, the CNS role is threatened when competing system demands and other organizational needs are deemed more important than the CNS's patient care responsibilities, downgrading the value of direct patient care. An administrator may argue that the organization cannot afford having a CNS providing direct patient care but, in fact, it cannot afford not to. A CNS who cannot provide direct patient care will lose his or her credibility and the ability to influence patient care quality and outcomes and will lose the flexibility to care for patients across the continuum of care.

If there are repeated pressures to relinquish direct patient care, a CNS may wonder if preparation as an acute care nurse practitioner (ACNP) or as a NP or blended CNS/NP will help him or her retain patient care responsibilities and ensure job security in the changing environment. When a nurse relinquishes his or her CNS role, however, the decision should be based on an assessment of personal, clinical, institutional, and statutory factors and the understanding that an ACNP has fewer opportunities to exercise a CNS's influence in areas such as staff education and development, nurse mentorship, leadership, consultation, research, and organizational or systems changes.

The most compelling argument for the value of the CNS role will result when CNS effectiveness is evaluated in a way that focuses on patient care and the CNS's role in delivering that care. Evaluation must link CNS practice to structure, process, and outcome variables to estimate CNS impact on cost,

EXEMPLAR 12-4   Advanced Practice Competencies and Spheres of Influence: CNS Practice with a Complex Patient

Mrs. H. was an 82-year-old woman brought by paramedics to the emergency department with acute abdominal pain and severe pulmonary congestion. For the past few weeks, Mrs. H. had been experiencing dyspnea on exertion and was unable to walk more than a few steps. These symptoms progressively worsened. She was having severe respiratory distress at rest and slept elevated on three pillows.

Mrs. H's medical history included insulin-dependent diabetes mellitus, hypertension, atrial fibrillation, coronary artery disease, critical aortic stenosis, severe heart failure, mild chronic obstructive pulmonary disease (COPD), chronic renal insufficiency, chronic urinary tract infections, and obesity. On admission, Mrs. H. was alert and oriented but somnolent, and she had labored breathing. Pertinent diagnostic results from the chest x-ray examination showed mild cardiac enlargement, pulmonary edema, left pleural effusion, and calcification of the aortic valve. A cardiac catheterization showed severe calcification of the aortic valve not amenable to valvuloplasty.

In discussing the results of the examinations with Mrs. H., it became clear that she wanted the valve replaced surgically despite the extensive risks of the surgery at her age and in her condition. The surgeon and staff nurses expressed discomfort with the patient's request; therefore the CNS (author P.S.A.S.) was consulted.

P.S.A.S. met the patient and her family to assess the situation. Mrs. H. seemed withdrawn and had poor eye contact and limited interaction. P.S.A.S. also recognized that English was the patient's second language. The son was very vocal about preferences for his mother's care, but the older daughter had multiple personal crises and tended to defer to her two sons (Mrs. H.'s grandsons). The younger daughter was hesitant to voice opinions about medical decisions. Mrs. H. stated that she did not want to continue living as a "cardiac cripple" and continued to demand the surgery.

P.S.A.S. believed that several interventions needed to occur to ensure that Mrs. H. was making an informed decision and that appropriate consideration of risks had been taken by everyone involved. P.S.A.S. facilitated a health team care conference with all disciplines to review the case and clarify the risks of proceeding with the surgery. Because there was concern about the language barrier, P.S.A.S. also facilitated a care conference with the health care team, Mrs. H.,

her family, and an interpreter. This satisfied the health care team that Mrs. H. clearly understood her options.

P.S.A.S. performed a literature search and spoke with the surgeon to clarify the risks vs. benefits of this surgery in an octogenarian. She initiated an Ethics Committee consult with the staff to discuss concerns related to moral distress about performing surgery in an older patient with such high risk for a poor outcome. She held multiple in-services to discuss the literature search results and the ethical principles involved in proceeding with the surgery. She used the expertise of her psychiatric CNS colleague to help staff identify communication techniques for maintaining optimal relationships with the patient and family.

P.S.A.S. also recognized that Mrs. H. had not completed an advance directive. She initiated a consult with the Palliative Care Team, who discussed with Mrs. H. how she envisioned her postoperative care. As a result, Mrs. H. completed an advance directive and made her wishes known to not be indefinitely dependent on external life support.

Mrs. H. had the surgery to replace her aortic valve with a tissue valve. Her postoperative course was complicated by another surgery to control bleeding, hypotension requiring pharmacological and pacemaker support, complete heart block, and low urine output. Because of her COPD, Mrs. H. was difficult to wean from the ventilator and required a percutaneous tracheostomy placement. Because of her diabetes, her sternal wound failed to heal. An episode of sepsis resulted in renal failure requiring continuous renal replacement therapy (CRRT). P.S.A.S. was active in assisting both the novice and experienced nurses to provide direct care to this challenging patient and in teaching them new procedures, such as placing a tracheostomy at the bedside, managing fluid balance in a cardiac patient with CRRT, and managing skin care needs for the sacral pressure wound.

Mrs. H.'s family continued to have difficulty reaching a consensus and showed frustration with the situation. They had unrealistic expectations related to the likelihood of Mrs. H.'s recovery and believed that staff should "cure her" despite the extensive discussions before surgery regarding the high surgical risks and poor prognosis. P.S.A.S. facilitated multiple care conferences with the health care team and family to keep communication lines open.

EXEMPLAR 12-4   Advanced Practice Competencies and Spheres of Influence: CNS Practice with a Complex Patient—cont'd

Approximately 6 weeks after surgery, it became clear that Mrs. H. would likely never be weaned from the ventilator and would need to be placed in a long-term care facility. P.S.A.S. facilitated one final care conference with the health care team and the family to discuss Mrs. H.'s poor likelihood of improvement and to review her advance directive. With assistance from the health care team, the family decided that, in accordance with Mrs. H.'s wishes, she should be transitioned to comfort care and have the ventilator removed and dialysis discontinued. P.S.A.S. reassured the family that the patient's pain would be well managed, and she spoke with them about the rituals important to them in facilitating end-of-life care. P.S.A.S. ensured that Mrs. H.'s wishes were honored, such as having spiritual music played in the room, a bedside prayer service led by her pastor, and her extended family present. Mrs. H. died several days after the transition to comfort care.

COMMENTARY
Direct Care
P.S.A.S. demonstrated skill in performing direct care for Mrs. H., including tracheostomy care, complex sternal wound care, and CRRT; in expert communication skills in the original assessment of patient and family needs; and in ongoing discussions of difficult issues with the family, staff, and interdisciplinary team. (*Direct Care of Patients or Clients* sphere)

Expert Coaching and Guidance
P.S.A.S. was active in role modeling and coaching staff nurses in the complex care required by Mrs. H. and her family. She tailored her coaching interventions to the experience level of the nurse. She also coached the family as they worked to make decisions about Mrs. H's care. (*Direct Care of Patients or Clients* sphere, *Nurses and Nursing Practice* sphere)

Consultation
P.S.A.S. maintained good communication with the staff nurses and interdisciplinary team, creating an environment in which they felt comfortable

consulting in a difficult situation. P.S.A.S. sought consultation from colleagues to ensure optimal care. (All three spheres)

Research
P.S.A.S. used her skills in searching and evaluating the literature to clarify the risks of this type of surgery in an octogenarian. She used evidence to support implementation of new treatments. (*Direct Care of Patients or Clients* sphere, *Nurses and Nursing Practice* sphere)

Leadership
P.S.A.S. demonstrated leadership across several competencies and spheres of influence. She knew when and how to bring consultants into the case. She made certain that the nurses' concerns were represented in discussions with the physician, and she facilitated team meetings so that staff felt empowered to participate and communicate with colleagues. She ensured continuity of care and communication during Mrs. H.'s prolonged hospital stay, demonstrating both clinical and systems leadership. (*Organization and Systems* sphere)

Collaboration
P.S.A.S. facilitated interactions with multiple individuals—patient, family members, staff, physicians, and consultants. The case demonstrates aligning multiple, conflicting perspectives to maintain appropriate care as everyone's central purpose. (*Nurses and Nursing Practice* sphere, *Organization and Systems* sphere)

Ethical Decision Making
P.S.A.S.'s expertise in ethical decision making enabled her to remain objective and to elicit and discuss staff nurses' moral distress, interpret their concerns to team members, and explain the ethical principles underlying all decisions. This enabled the staff to provide good care and to respect Mrs. H.'s autonomy. (All three spheres)

quality, and patient safety and outcomes (Benedict et al., 2006; Brooten, et al., 2003; McCauley et al., 2006; Rapp, 2003; Topp et al., 1998). CNS effectiveness is measured or evaluated in various ways, such as appraisal of competencies or activities, including self-evaluation and database analysis of consults and

interventions, administrative and peer review, and program and outcomes evaluation (Cooper & Sparacino, 1990; Girouard, 1996; see also Chapters 24 and 25). Evaluation strategies are planned, and routine evaluation is at least annual, with periodic interim reports. CNSs should not wait until a practice setting experiences a reorganization or financial exigency to document their value to an organization. From day 1, CNSs should establish some system (or use the agency's) to document their activities and their impact on structures, processes, and patient and institutional outcomes, and these data should be incorporated into annual evaluations. In a financial crisis, the CNS can retrieve the information, providing more detail, if necessary, about their impact on outcomes, especially those related to quality of patient care, patient safety, cost avoidance, and revenue generation. The more directly CNS interventions are linked to patient and institutional outcomes, the less likely administrators are to limit CNSs clinical practice or eliminate CNS positions altogether. Consumer demand for quality of care and patient safety will make it easier to maintain direct patient care as a CNS priority.

Balancing Clinical Nurse Specialist Responsibilities. Balancing CNS competencies across the three spheres of CNS influence and honoring professional and personal commitments are challenges. Maintaining control over priorities and equitably allocating time to each can be achieved by continuous evaluation of needs, outcomes, effectiveness, and congruence between CNS and organizational expectations. Patient/client, nurse, and organizational needs far exceed what one CNS can provide, but a CNS is in a pivotal influential position. By role modeling expert patient care, demonstrating the practical integration of theory and evidence-based practice, teaching nurses knowledge and skills for common patient care interventions, and working with the organization to influence system changes, a CNS can address new patient problems, program implementation, and other new and complex responsibilities. CNSs must also attend to their own needs for continuing education and skill development in their specialties. The trajectory of growth never plateaus, the cycle of enrichment is never complete, and the need for CNSs in clinical settings remains.

Even without organizational or financial crises, the focus of a CNS's role will change over time. A CNS rarely focuses on all three spheres at any one time or to the same degree. For example, if a setting has an influx of new staff nurses, the CNS is likely to collaborate with staff development colleagues and focus on the nursing sphere, providing specialty-related education. For a new surgical technique or procedure, the CNS

may spend more time providing direct care to that population and develop the nursing staff's expertise at the same time. For an organizational priority to improve pain management across units and disciplines, the CNS may focus on the organizational sphere. In addition, a CNS's own expertise and interests may change. For example, a CNS may decide to acquire subspecialty certification or an additional advanced practice certification. An adult health CNS may decide to become certified as a diabetes educator because of the increase in diabetics and an organizational emphasis on chronic illness self-management, or a gerontology CNS may decide to pursue advanced education and certification in palliative care to provide better end-of-life care to nursing home residents.

Organizational Placement. The constant emphasis on organizational redesign and other critical elements, including organizational structure and climate, administrative justification, and required changes in role focus and role titling, can significantly threaten a CNS's practice. A classic but recurring debate is whether a CNS should be in a staff or a line position (Baird & Prouty, 1989; Prouty, 1983; see Chapter 23). In a staff position, a CNS is freed from more administrative responsibilities and allowed to focus on patient care delivery and related issues and the less-threatening consultative capacity. The disadvantage of such a position is a lack of formal authority, such that power is referent or exercised by virtue of clinical expertise and knowledge. The advantage for a CNS in a line position is formal authority, but the distinct disadvantage is that administrative responsibilities may dominate his or her activities and erode the time available for clinical issues and patient care. Regardless of organizational placement, CNSs must be able to exercise clinical and systems leadership.

Where a CNS is listed on an organizational chart and to whom he or she reports in the management chain of command may reveal the value of the CNS role. Strategic maneuvering to improve a CNS's position in the organizational hierarchy may afford greater visibility and better opportunities to manage the unexpected and to influence a preferred future. Changing systems, priorities, reimbursement mechanisms, and hierarchies also can make CNS positions vulnerable. Data on the nature and the impact of CNSs' work can provide information on logical placement in times of reorganization. The biggest risks of reorganization are removing CNSs from direct care or eliminating positions. CNSs who document and analyze their practice data are in a better position to negotiate changes that keep the patient a primary focus of their work.

Standardization: Education, Certification, and Practice

Education. A major weakness in current CNS education preparation is the huge variability in CNS graduate programs. Walker and colleagues (2003) surveyed 139 schools and found that only 56.1% used the NACNS *Statement* and only 67.3% prepared CNS graduates for prescriptive authority. There were ten important content areas that were least likely to be integrated into the CNS curriculum, including advanced physiology; advanced pathophysiology; advanced pharmacology; consultation theory; teaching and coaching; and selection, use, and evaluation of technology and devices.

Recent initiatives are challenging traditional CNS education and practice. The AACN has called for a change in education for advanced practice nursing, with the DNP degree required for all APN specialties by 2015 (AACN, 2006b). Although the DNP is considered by many to be a fait accompli, there is debate about its consequences, some of which may be unintended (Chase & Pruitt, 2006; NACNS, 2005a). Concerns that may affect preparing a sufficient number of CNSs to meet the current shortage include the length of the DNP curriculum, further exacerbation of disparities in health care and its providers, whether the curriculum is innovative or additive, the focus on disease management at the expense of philosophy of science or metatheoretical issues, the separation of the profession's practice and research missions, the inability of some programs to offer doctorates, the differences in master's-prepared and doctoral-prepared CNS competencies, the acronym's suggestion that a DNP is an NP, and regulatory considerations (Chase & Pruitt, 2006; Fulton & Lyon, 2005; Meleis & Dracup, 2005; NACNS, 2005). Another concern about the DNP degree is that the focus on disease management displaces the significance of wellness management and the CNS-sensitive impact on human responses to health and illness. Despite the increase in DNP programs, the range of concerns expressed by some nursing leaders and APN organizations suggests the jury is still out regarding the appropriateness of DNP preparation for APNs, including CNSs (see Chapter 2).

The positive effect of *The Essentials of Doctoral Education for Advanced Nursing Practice* (AACN, 2006b) may be improved standardization of CNS graduate education and inclusion of essential curriculum content, specifically advanced health and physical assessment, advanced physiology and pathophysiology, and advanced pharmacology.

Certification and Credentialing. Resolution of differing views on APN certification is essential if the profession is to retain control over APN licensing and credentialing and to ensure the protection of the public. Certification for CNSs by examination is available through the American Nurses Credentialing Center (ANCC) or through the certification boards of specialty organizations (e.g., Oncology Nursing Society, American Association of Critical-Care Nurses, Orthopaedic Nurses Association). However, certification examinations are not available for many CNS specialties. The lack of certification is a major regulatory barrier for many CNS specialties in those states that require CNS certification for second licensure (Minarik, 2005). In developing national standards for credentialing APNs (see Chapter 21), creating a universal CNS certification examination that all CNSs can take has become more urgent. Several stakeholder organizations are examining the possibility of a core CNS examination that would evaluate core knowledge and competencies and would use portfolio documentation to document specialty knowledge when specialty certification is not available (e.g., NACNS, 2005).

The profession's requirements for APN certification and credentialing notwithstanding, it is likely that future CNSs will require credentialing in the institutions in which they work. That is, they will need to undergo a formal process (as many NPs, CRNAs, and CNMs do) of submitting documentation to an institution's credentialing committee to demonstrate, among other requirements, that they are appropriately credentialed and eligible for reimbursement.

Emerging Clinical Nurse Specialist Specialties. Historically, CNSs concentrated on direct patient care and the systems within which care was given. As complex patient or population needs are identified and organizational priorities are marketed, new specialties and roles emerge. When an APN role is developed in an emerging specialty, it is critical not only that the role be appropriate for the patient population and setting but also that direct care be a significant part of the role (Spross & Heaney, 2000). A nursing specialty may not evolve into an APN role if standardization of graduate level educational preparation and APN competencies is lacking (Hanson & Hamric, 2003).

Because CNS roles are usually very specialized, CNS practice is most likely to be affected by emerging specialties as compared with other APN roles. Will existing competencies, educational programs, and certification be sufficient to prepare CNSs for new specialties? What changes will need to occur and in what arenas? Will such changes affect other CNS specialties and scopes of practice? Can the profession address these issues in a systematic and collaborative way? These and other challenges associated with the development of new specialties are particularly relevant to CNSs (see Chapter 18).

Legislative and Regulatory Challenges

CNSs confront the same legislative and regulatory barriers as other APNs: restrictions on scope of practice, withholding authority to prescribe drugs, and reimbursement. The current debate about regulating CNS and APN practice—professional control versus legislative-mandated scope of practice and standardization—is centered primarily within the nursing profession. Statutory requirements for physician supervision or formalized APN-physician collaboration should be eliminated. Stakeholder organizations, including those representing APN groups, are actively seeking a consensus on the credentialing requirements for APNs, including CNSs. Because this work is still in progress (see Chapters 2 and 21), readers should consult the websites of the stakeholder organizations (www.nacns.org, www.aacn.nche.edu, www.ncsbn.org) and the websites for state nursing organizations.

Prescriptive Authority. Prescriptive authority is an aspect of CNS practice that has generated much discussion. Prescriptive authority is a skill set, and like any other skill set, the question is whether it is needed for a particular practice. Some CNSs may not need or desire to prescribe drugs or may not have the opportunity to prescribe drugs with sufficient frequency to do it safely. Nonetheless, educational programs should include content that prepares the CNS to be eligible for prescriptive authority, and CNS advocates should support legal efforts to obtain CNS prescriptive authority for those who can or must prescribe. For example, at the time of this writing, APNs are lobbying the Missouri legislature (the state in which the second author lives) to allow all APNs to expand prescriptive authority to include controlled substances.

Prescriptive authority may encompass prescribing not only medications but also treatments and medical equipment. Not all CNSs want prescriptive authority. Other CNSs do not need prescriptive authority because of the nature their practice. The NACNS considers prescriptive authority to be optional for the CNS (NACNS, 2004b; Phillips, 2006, 2007). Although, to date, prescriptive authority is not a requirement for practice, it is very beneficial in direct clinical practice in certain specialties; CNS students are expected to learn the content that will prepare them for prescriptive authority.

All states provide prescriptive authority to some extent for APNs, but the degree of independence allowed varies greatly (O'Malley & Mains, 2003). However, some states do not have laws or regulations that recognize the CNS as an APN or that permit CNSs to obtain prescriptive authority (NACNS, 2003; see also Chapter 21). Prescriptive authority usually depends on scope of practice and often requires the CNS to have a collaborative practice agreement with a physician. This legal agreement usually consists of the following mutually agreed upon elements: (1) guidelines or protocols, (2) responsibilities, (3) evaluation, and (4) periodic reviews of protocols or guidelines (NACNS, 2003; see also Chapter 26). In fact, prescriptive authority has been a major issue for psychiatric APNs since the 1990s.

Some states provide that a physician may delegate to an APN (including a CNS) the authority to administer, dispense, or prescribe drugs pursuant to a collaborative practice agreement. Other states promulgate collaborative practice agreements that provide that APNs (CNSs) may be authorized to prescribe all drugs except controlled substances. In other states, CNSs may prescribe only durable medical equipment, whereas NPs may obtain independent prescriptive authority for controlled substances. Readers are advised to consult their own state regulatory bodies to understand the scope of prescriptive authority for CNSs.

When considering obtaining prescriptive authority, the CNS needs to determine how that will enhance his or her practice. For the CNS who manages complex or specialty populations, prescriptive privileges allow flexibility in providing care, expedite treatments, increase patient satisfaction, and may decrease length of stay. Although prescriptive authority is often thought of as prescribing medications, the CNS may prescribe nonpharmacological treatments such as physical therapy, occupational therapy, dressing changes, activity levels, diet changes, radiographs, and orthotic devices and may request consultation from other specialists. For example, CNSs with a neurosurgical population could advance the diet as tolerated for a postoperative craniotomy patient, order physical and occupational therapy to assist with ambulation, discontinue the Foley catheter when the patient's neurological status improves, and consult social services for nursing home placement or rehabilitation. This expedites the patient's recovery by ordering advanced levels of care as the patient recovers. CNSs are in a unique position to make these decisions because of the advanced knowledge they possess about their specialty populations.

Titling and Title Protection. Although the flexibility and responsiveness of the CNS role to systems change has made it extremely effective, it has also made it vulnerable to organizational restructuring and position retitling. The role was established before the development of a coherent educational curriculum, criteria for certification, consistent use of competencies, agreement about regulatory control, and implementation of third-party reimbursement. In the past decade, regulatory forces and organizational or systems priorities have reshaped contemporary CNS practice. As noted earlier many CNS positions were eliminated in the past for financial reasons. When CNSs and administrators do not understand the CNS role, disparate and arbitrary utilization dissipates its impact. CNS positions may have been eliminated in part because few CNSs and administrators linked CNS activities to patient or institutional outcomes, such as reduced turnover of staff nurses, cost avoidance (e.g., evaluation that leads to selection of a less expensive but equally effective product or fewer expenditures associated with lower turnover), improved patient safety, or increased revenue.

Some critics thought that merging CNS and NP roles would ensure job security. Singular titling for CNSs and NPs as APNs was first proposed in the 1980s to bring a measure of uniformity and efficiency to educational, regulatory, and related issues. Although the feasibility and acceptability of singular titling generated widespread debate and opposition (Cronenwett, 1995; Fenton & Brykczynski, 1993; Soehren & Schumann, 1994; Sparacino & Durand, 1986; Spross & Hamric, 1983), the APN designation became a widely accepted term that included the CNS, NP, CNM, and certified registered nurse anesthetist (CRNA). Although the CNS and NP roles

share many similarities, they are distinctly different in ideology, role, and practice (Lincoln, 2000; Mick & Ackerman, 2002). The merging or blending of these roles is addressed in Chapters 3 and 15.

Whereas one legislative approach favors fewer references to specific titles, emphasizing similarities rather than the uniqueness of the various APN roles, another legislative approach advocates the statutory and regulatory recognition of the different contributions and scope of practice of each role, such as the CNS (Davidson et al., 2001). Significant variability exists among states in terms of their approach to titling, and this includes recognition of the CNS title by state boards of nursing. *Model Rules and Regulations for CNS Title Protection and Scope of Practice* (NACNS, 2004a) includes the NACNS definition of the CNS and offers positions and language on scope of practice, standards for practice, and optional prescriptive and dispensing authority. NACNS also states that the CNS title should be protected in statute but that the scope of CNS practice should be defined in rules and regulations (NACNS, 2004a, 2007). In 2006, the National Council of State Boards of Nursing (NCSBN) challenged CNS titling in their *Vision Paper: Future Regulation of Advanced Practice Nursing* (NCSBN, 2006), in which they proposed to assume control of educational requirements, certification programs, and licensure. In 2006 the NCSBN proposed to exclude CNSs from regulatory oversight as APNs because it viewed CNS practice as occurring within the scope of nursing practice and therefore not needing separate regulation (NCSBN, 2006). This proposal provoked significant controversy and has been essentially withdrawn, with NCSBN and CNS consensus groups agreeing that CNSs are indeed APNs with the requisite education and certification required for APN licensure. The critical lesson learned from this proposal was that excluding the CNS from regulatory oversight would not only threaten the existence of the CNS role but also allow anyone to use the title without the necessary graduate education and clinical expertise. Even though the purpose of a regulatory model is to guide licensure, its language influences the entire nursing profession.

However, the Standard Occupational Classification System, used by the U.S. Department of Labor's Bureau of Labor Statistics to develop its Occupational Employment Statistics Classification System lacks APN specificity and therefore challenges CNS title protection. The Standard Occupational Classification System lists Registered Nurses as a single occupation under the subset of Healthcare Practitioners and Technical Occupations. The description for Registered Nurse does include "advance (sic) practice nurses such as nurse practitioners, clinical nurse specialists, certified nurse midwives, and certified registered nurse anesthetists." There are separate categories for the occupations of Dentists, Physicians and Surgeons, and Therapists, however. Because the Occupational Employment Statistics are used to track occupational data and are used to determine economic trends, it has been recommended that a subset of four APN categories (i.e., CNS, NP, CNM, and CRNA) be added, mirroring the current subset designations for Physicians and Surgeons (Goudreau, 2007).

Reimbursement. Legislative and regulatory barriers still prevent many CNSs from billing for their services. Many regulatory requirements and nonlegislative policies dictate if and how APNs are to be reimbursed, including collaborative practice agreements (e.g., physician supervision of APNs) and national certification. Medicare regulations require collaboration for an APN to be reimbursed, even if a state's law allows independent CNS practice. Some private insurance companies require national certification, even if a state's law does not require it for APN practice (Minarik & Price, 1999).

CNS reimbursement also may be influenced by practice site. APNs in acute and critical care may not be reimbursed in a prospective payment system but may be reimbursed in a physician payment system. However, even when an APN is eligible for reimbursement, barriers exist including, but not limited to, overlapping provider services and the nonbillable aspects of care that are often provided by APNs (Buppert, 2005). The current pay-for-performance reimbursement demonstration projects have not yet included APNs, but they should (see Chapter 25). As evidence of CNSs' impact on outcomes accumulates (e.g., providing transitional care to older adults at high risk for hospital readmission, thus reducing readmissions and care costs), reimbursement mechanisms will likely change. Contemporary graduate education ensures that APNs can meet clinical standards for care, helping agencies retain a competitive edge in the health care marketplace (Kennerly, 2007).

CONCLUSION

Amid the current emphasis on quality and safety and concern for nursing shortages, the CNS role is thriving. CNSs have long been recognized for their contributions in creating a healthy work environment (Disch, Walton, & Barnsteiner, 2001) and improving patient outcomes. Although the future of health care is uncertain, advancing the CNS position and its influence is imperative. CNSs have weathered many challenges during the past several decades, including forced changes in role responsibilities and title, increased responsibility for directing other health care providers, and constant organizational redesign oblivious to the CNS's diverse contributions. To dispel the institutional notion that CNSs are expendable in times of fiscal crisis, CNSs must ensure that their practice is measured across all three spheres and that the data demonstrate their impact on clinical and institutional processes and outcomes. The contemporary focus on transforming the health care system also is creating exciting opportunities for CNS and other APNs.

A CNS plays an indispensable, collaborative role in any health care delivery system by ensuring a comprehensive focus on quality nursing care and extensive documentation to facilitate and measure quality patient outcomes. Health care reform in the past decade has provided CNSs with an opportunity to quantify what has always been their purpose: linking advanced practice nurse interventions and influence to patient outcomes and resource utilization. The impact of CNSs has been evident in patient and family outcomes, evidence-based practice, quality care outcomes, care efficiency, and cost-effectiveness. Further study is needed to substantiate which CNS competencies are most critical in ensuring optimal patient care and in improving clinical processes and patient outcomes. The three purposes for which the role was established remain relevant today: to provide direct care, to improve the direct care of other nurses, and to retain nurses.

This chapter has described how a CNS executes competencies and operates in the three spheres of influence. Like other APNs, CNSs have unique talents and skills, and the central focus of every CNS remains the patient. The CNS's multifaceted focus on patients, nurses, and system makes her or him unique among other APNs. Although the link between CNS practice and patient and institutional outcomes must be reinforced, important advances have been made. With the powerful analytic capabilities of health care information systems and the availability of national, regional, and institutional databases, CNSs are well positioned to demonstrate their impact on improved quality, patient outcomes, and financial benefits, including cost efficiency, cost savings, and revenue generation. With the emphasis on evidence-based practice, performance improvement, and quality and safety of patient care, CNSs can take the lead on clinical and systems improvement. CNSs will thrive as they integrate new knowledge into practice and influence and implement practice guidelines and innovative practice models.

REFERENCES

Adams, P. (2000). Insight: A mental health prevention intervention. *Nursing Clinics of North America, 35,* 329-338.

American Association of Colleges of Nursing (AACN). (1996). *The essentials of master's education for advanced practice nursing.* Washington, DC: Author.

American Association of Colleges of Nursing (AACN). (2006a). *Enrollment and graduations in baccalaureate and graduate programs in nursing.* Washington, DC: Author.

American Association of Colleges of Nursing (AACN). (2006b). *The essentials of doctoral education for advanced nursing practice.* Retrieved February 12, 2007, from www.aacn.nche.edu/DNP/pdf/Essentials.pdf.

American Association of Critical-Care Nurses. (2002). *Scope of practice and standards of professional performance for the acute and critical care clinical nurse specialist.* Aliso Viejo, CA: Author.

American Nurses Association (ANA). (1980). *Nursing: A social policy statement.* Kansas City, MO: Author.

American Nurses Association (ANA). (1985). *Facts about nursing 84–85* (p. 27). Kansas City, MO: Author.

American Nurses Association (ANA). (1986). *The role of the clinical nurse specialist.* Kansas City, MO: Author.

American Nurses Association (ANA). (1976). The scope of nursing practice. In *Congress of Nursing Practice, Description of Practice: Clinical Nurse Specialist.* Kansas City, MO: Author.

Aroskar, M.A. (1998). Administrative ethics: Perspectives on patients and community-based care. *Online Journal of Issues in Nursing, Topic 8.* Retrieved January 22, 2007, from www.nursingworld.org/ojin/topic8/topic8_4.htm.

Baggs, J.G., Schmitt, M.H., Mushlin, A.I., Mitchell, P.H., Eldredge, D.H., Oakes, D., et al. (1999). Association between nurse-physician collaboration and patient outcomes in three intensive care units. *Critical Care Medicine, 27,* 1991-1998.

Baird, S.B., & Prouty, M.P. (1989). Administratively enhancing CNS contributions. In A.B. Hamric & J.A. Spross (Eds.), *The clinical nurse specialist in theory and practice* (2nd ed., pp. 261-284). Philadelphia: Saunders.

Baldwin, K., Lyon, B., Clark, A., Fulton, J., Davidson, S., & Dayhoff, N. (2007). Developing clinical nurse specialist practice competencies. *Clinical Nurse Specialist, 21,* 297-303.

Barron, A. M. (1983). The clinical nurse specialist as consultant. In A.B. Hamric & J.A. Spross (Eds.), *The clinical nurse specialist in theory and practice* (pp. 91-113). New York: Grune & Stratton.

Barron A. M. (1989). The clinical nurse specialist as consultant. In A.B. Hamric & J.A. Spross (Eds.), *The clinical nurse specialist in theory and practice* (2nd ed., pp. 125-146). Philadelphia: Saunders.

Becker, D., Kaplow, R., Muenzen, P.M., & Hartigan, C. (2006). Activities performed by acute and critical care advanced practice nurses: American Association of Critical-Care Nurses Study of Practice. *American Journal of Critical Care, 15,* 130-148.

Benedict, L., Robinson, K., & Holder, C. (2006). Clinical nurse specialist practice within the Acute Care for Elders interdisciplinary team model. *Clinical Nurse Specialist, 20,* 248-252.

Boyle, D.M. (1996). The clinical nurse specialist. In A.B. Hamric, J.A. Spross, & C.M. Hanson (Eds.), *Advanced nursing practice: An integrative approach* (pp. 299-336). Philadelphia: Saunders.

Briggs, L.A., Heath, J., & Kelley, J. (2005). Peer review for advanced practice nurses: What does it really mean? *AACN Clinical Issues, 16,* 3-15.

Brooten, D., Kumer, S., Brown, L.P., Butts, P., Finkler, S.A., Bakewell-Sachs, S., et al. (1986). A randomized clinical trial of early hospital discharge and home follow-up of very-low-birth-weight infants. *New England Journal of Medicine, 315,* 934-939.

Brooten, D., Naylor, M.D., York, R., Brown, L.P., Munro, B.H., Hollingsworth, A.O., et al. (2002). Lessons learned from testing the Quality Cost Model of Advanced Practice Nursing (APN) Transitional Care. *Journal of Nursing Scholarship, 34,* 369-375.

Brooten, D., Youngblut, J.M., Deatrick, J., Naylor, M., & York, R. (2003). Patient problems, advanced practice nurse (APN) interventions, time and contacts among five patient groups. *Journal of Nursing Scholarship, 35,* 73-79.

Brown, S.J. (1989). Supportive supervision of the CNS. In A.B. Hamric & J.A. Spross (Eds.), *The clinical nurse specialist in theory and practice* (2nd ed., pp. 285-298). Philadelphia: Saunders.

Buppert, C. (2005). Capturing reimbursement for advanced practice nurse services in acute and critical care. *AACN Clinical Issues, 16,* 23-35.

Chase, S.K., & Pruitt, R.H. (2006). The practice doctorate: Innovation or disruption? *Journal of Nursing Education, 45,* 155-161.

Cooper, D.M., & Sparacino, P.S.A. (1990). Acquiring, implementing, and evaluating the clinical nurse specialist role. In P.S.A. Sparacino, D.M. Cooper, & P.A. Minarik (Eds.), *The clinical nurse specialist: Implementation and impact* (pp. 41-75). Norwalk, CT: Appleton & Lange.

Cronenwett, L.R. (1995). Molding the future of advanced practice nursing. *Nursing Outlook, 43,* 112-118.

Cunningham, R.S. (2006). Clinical practice guideline use by oncology advanced practice nurses. *Applied Nursing Research, 19,* 126-133.

D'Afflitti, J.G. (2004). A psychiatric clinical nurse specialist as liaison to OB/GYN practice. *Journal of Obstetric, Gynecologic, and Neonatal Nursing, 34,* 280-285.

Davidson, S.B., Beardsley, K., Busch, A.H., Garner, A., Heresa, S., Hodges, N.D., et al. (2001). Statutory and regulatory recognition for clinical nurse specialists in Oregon. *Clinical Nurse Specialist, 15,* 276-279.

Disch, J., Chlan, L., Mueller, C., Akinduoto, T., Sabo, J., Feldt, K., et al. (2006). The Densford Clinical Scholars Program: Improving patient care through research partnerships. *Journal of Nursing Administration, 36,* 567-574.

Disch, J., Walton, M., & Barnsteiner, J. (2001). The role of the clinical nurse specialist in creating a healthy work environment. *AACN Clinical Issues, 12,* 345-355.

Duffy, J.R. (2002). The clinical leadership role of the CNS in the identification of nursing-sensitive and multidisciplinary quality indicator sets. *Clinical Nurse Specialist, 16,* 70-76.

Ebright, P.R., Patterson, E.S., & Render, M.L. (2002). The "new look" approach to patient safety: A guide for clinical nurse specialist leadership. *Clinical Nurse Specialist, 16,* 247-253.

Ebright, P.R., Urden, L., Patterson, E., & Chalko, B. (2004). Themes surrounding novice nurse near-miss and adverse-event situations. *Journal of Nursing Administration, 34,* 531-538.

Felder, L. (1983). Direct patient care and independent practice. In A.B. Hamric & J. Spross (Eds.), *The clinical nurse specialist in theory and practice* (pp. 59-72). New York: Grune & Stratton.

Fenton, M.V., & Brykcyznski, K.A. (1993). Qualitative distinctions and similarities in the practice of clinical nurse specialists and nurse practitioners. *Journal of Professional Nursing, 9,* 313-326.

Fitzgerald, M., Tomlinson, P.S., Peden-McAlpine, C., & Sherman, S. (2003). Clinical nurse specialist participation on a collaborative research project: Barriers and benefits. *Clinical Nurse Specialist, 17,* 44-49.

Forrow, L., Arnold, R.M., & Parker, L.S. (1993). Preventive ethics: Expanding the horizons of clinical ethics. *Journal of Clinical Ethics, 4,* 287-294.

Fulmer, T., Mezey, M., Bottrell, M., Abraham, I., Sazant, J., Grossman, S., et al. (2002). Nurses Improving Care for Healthsystem Elders (NICHE): Using outcomes and benchmarks for evidence-based practice. *Geriatric Nursing, 23,* 121-127.

Fulton, J.S., & Lyon, B.L. (2005). The need for some sense making: Doctor of Nursing Practice. *Online Journal of Issues in Nursing, 10.* Retrieved October 18, 2005, from www.nursingworld.org/ojin/topic28/tpc28_3.htm.

Gawlinksi, A., & Kern, L.S. (Eds.). (1994). The clinical nurse specialist role in critical care. Philadelphia: Saunders.

Girouard, S.A. (1996). Evaluating advanced nursing practice. In A.B. Hamric, J.A. Spross, & C.M. Hanson (Eds.), *Advanced nursing practice: An integrative approach* (pp. 569-600). Philadelphia: Saunders.

Girouard, S.A., & Spross, J. (1983). Evaluation of the clinical nurse specialist: Using an evaluation tool. In A.B. Hamric & J. Spross (Eds.), *The clinical nurse specialist in theory and practice* (pp. 207-218). New York: Grune & Stratton.

Gobel, B.H., Beck, S.L., & O'Leary, C. (2006). Nursing-sensitive patient outcomes: The development of the Putting Evidence into Practice resources for nursing practice. *Clinical Journal of Oncology Nursing, 10,* 621-624.

Goudreau, K.A. (2007). National Association of Clinical Nurse Specialists responds to Office of Management and Budget regarding standard occupational classification. *Clinical Nurse Specialist, 21,* 124-125.

Gurka, A.M. (1991). Process and outcome components of clinical nurse specialist consultation. *Dimensions of Critical Care Nursing, 10,* 169-175.

Hamric, A.B. (1983a). A model for developing evaluation strategies. In A.B. Hamric & J.A. Spross (Eds.), *The clinical nurse specialist in theory and practice* (pp. 187-206). New York: Grune & Stratton.

Hamric, A.B. (1983b). Role development and functions. In A.B. Hamric & J. Spross (Eds.), *The clinical nurse specialist in theory and practice* (pp. 39-56). New York: Grune & Stratton.

Hamric, A.B. (1989a). History and overview of the CNS role. In A.B. Hamric & J.A. Spross (Eds.), *The clinical nurse specialist in theory and practice* (2nd ed., pp. 3-18). Philadelphia: Saunders.

Hamric, A.B. (1989b). A model for CNS evaluation. In A.B. Hamric & J.A. Spross (Eds.), *The clinical nurse specialist in theory and practice* (2nd ed., pp. 83-104). Philadelphia: Saunders.

Hamric, A.B. (1995). Creating our future: Challenges and opportunities for the clinical nurse specialist. *Oncology Nursing Forum, 22,* 547-553.

Hamric, A.B. (1996). A definition of advanced nursing practice. In A.B. Hamric, J.A. Spross, & C.M. Hanson (Eds.), *Advanced nursing practice: An integrative approach* (pp. 42-56). Philadelphia: Saunders.

Hamric, A.B. (1998). Using research to influence the regulatory process. *Advanced Practice Nursing Quarterly, 4,* 44-50.

Hamric, A.B., & Spross, J.A. (Eds.). (1989). *The clinical nurse specialist in theory and practice* (2nd ed.). Philadelphia: Saunders.

Hamric, A.B., Spross, J.A., & Hanson, C.M. (Eds.). (1996). *Advanced nursing practice: An integrative approach.* Philadelphia: Saunders.

Hamric, A.B., Spross, J.A., & Hanson, C.M. (Eds.). (2000). *Advanced nursing practice: An integrative approach* (2nd ed.). Philadelphia: Saunders.

Hamric, A.B., Spross, J.A., & Hanson, C.M. (Eds.). (2005). *Advanced practice nursing: An integrative approach* (3rd ed.). Philadelphia: Saunders.

Hanson, C.M., & Hamric, A.B. (2003). Reflections on the continuing evolution of advanced practice nursing. *Nursing Outlook, 19,* 262-268.

Health Resources and Services Administration (HRSA). (2005). *The registered nurse population: Findings from the 2004 National Sample Survey of Registered Nurses. Chapter 111: The registered nurse population 2004.* Rockville, MD: Author. Retrieved November 26, 2007, from http://bhpr.hrsa.gov/healthworkforce/rnsurvey04/3.htm#apn.

Hughes, A., & Mackenzie, C. (1990). Components necessary in a successful nurse practitioner–physician collaborative practice. *Journal of the American Academy of Nurse Practitioners, 2,* 54–57.

Jacobs, L.A., Scarpa, R., Lester, J., & Smith, J. (2004). Oncology nursing as a specialty: The education, scope, and standards for advanced practice nursing in oncology. *Oncology Nursing Forum, 31.* Retrieved January 22, 2007, from www.ons.org/ Publications/journals/ONF/Volume 31/Issue3/3103507.asp.

Jennings, B.M. (2000). Evidence-based practice: The road best traveled? *Research in Nursing & Health, 23,* 343-345.

Kennedy, B., Covington, K., Evans, T., & Williams, C.A. (2000). Mental health consultation in a nursing home. *Clinical Nurse Specialist, 14,* 261-266.

Kennerly, S. (2007). The impending reimbursement revolution: How to prepare for future APN reimbursement. *Nurse Economics, 25,* 81-84.

Kerfoot, K.M., Rapala, K., Ebright, P., & Rogers, S.M. (2006). The power of collaboration with patient safety programs. *Journal of Nursing Administration, 36,* 582-588.

Kleinpell, R., & Gawlinski, A. (2005). Assessing outcomes in advanced practice nursing: The use of quality indicators and evidence-based practice. *AACN Clinical Issues, 16,* 43-57.

Koetters, T.L. (1989). Clinical practice and direct patient care. In A.B. Hamric & J.A. Spross (Eds.), *The clinical nurse specialist in theory and practice* (2nd ed., pp. 107-124). Philadelphia: Saunders.

Lincoln, P.E. (2000). Comparing CNS and NP role activities: A replication. *Clinical Nurse Specialist, 14,* 269-277.

Lunney, M., Gigliotti, E., & McMorrow, M.E. (2007). Tool development for evaluation of clinical nurse specialist competencies in graduate students. *Clinical Nurse Specialist, 21,* 145-151.

McCabe, P.J. (2005). Spheres of clinical nurse specialist practice influence evidence-based care for patients with atrial fibrillation. *Clinical Nurse Specialist, 19,* 308-317.

McCauley, K.M., Bixby, B., & Naylor, M.D. (2006). Advanced practice nurse strategies to improve outcomes and reduce cost in elders with heart failure. *Disease Management, 9,* 302-310.

McCorkle, R., Strumpf, N.E., Nuamah, I.F., Adler, D.C., Cooley, M.E., Jepson, C., et al. (2000). A specialized home care intervention improves survival among older post-surgical cancer patients. *Journal of the American Geriatrics Society, 48,* 1707-1713.

McPheeters, M., & Lohr, K.N. (1999). Evidence-based practice and nursing: Commentary. *Outcomes Management for Nursing Practice, 3,* 99-101.

Meleis, A.I., & Dracup, K. (2005). The case against the DNP: History, timing, substance, and marginalization. *Online Journal of Issues in Nursing, 10.* Retrieved October 18, 2005, from www.nursingworld.org/ojin/topic28/tpc28_2.htm.

Mick, D.J., & Ackerman, M.H. (2002). Deconstructing the myth of the advanced practice blended role: Support for role divergence. *Heart & Lung, 31,* 393-398.

Minarik, P.A. (2005). Issue: Competence assessment and competency assurance of healthcare professionals. *Clinical Nurse Specialist, 19,* 180-183.

Minarik, P.A., & Price, L.C. (1999). Collaboration? Supervision? Direction? Independence? What is the relationship between the advanced practice nurse and the physician? States' Legislative and Regulatory Forum III. *Clinical Nurse Specialist, 13,* 34-37.

Minarik, P.A., & Sparacino, P.S.A. (1990). Clinical nurse specialist collaboration in a university medical center. In P.S.A. Sparacino, D.M. Cooper, & P.A Minarik (Eds.), *The clinical nurse specialist: Implementation and impact* (pp. 231-260). East Norwalk, CT: Appleton & Lange.

Moss, J.K., Steiner, K., Mahnke, K., & Cohen, R. (1998). A model to manage capitated risk. *Nursing Economics, 16,* 65–68.

National Association of Clinical Nurse Specialists (NACNS). (1998). *Statement on clinical nurse specialist practice and education.* Glenview, IL: Author.

National Association of Clinical Nurse Specialists (NACNS). (2003). Regulatory credentialing of clinical nurse specialists. *Clinical Nurse Specialist, 17,* 163-169.

National Association of Clinical Nurse Specialists (NACNS). (2004a). *Model rules and regulations for CNS title protection and scope of practice.* Harrisburg, PA: Author.

National Association of Clinical Nurse Specialists (NACNS). (2004b). *Statement on clinical nurse specialist practice and education.* Harrisburg, PA: Author.

National Association of Clinical Nurse Specialists (NACNS). (2004c). Guidelines for clinical nurse specialist education. *Clinical Nurse Specialist, 18,* 285-287.

National Association of Clinical Nurse Specialists (NACNS). (2005a). *White paper on the nursing practice doctorate.* Harrisburg, PA: Author.

National Association of Clinical Nurse Specialists (NACNS). (2005b). *White paper on certification of clinical nurse specialists.* Harrisburg, PA: Author. Retrieved January 31, 2008, from http://www.nacns.org/NACNS_certification_wp_9_05.pdf.

National Association of Clinical Nurse Specialists (NACNS). (2005c). *White paper on advanced pharmacology: Practice, curricular and regulatory recommendations.* Retrieved January 31, 2008, from http://www.nacns.org/NACNS_certification_wp_9_05.pdf.

National Association of Clinical Nurse Specialists (NACNS). (2006). Executive summary: 2006 CNS summit, July 21-22, Indianapolis, IN. *Clinical Nurse Specialist, 21,* 50-51.

National Association of Clinical Nurse Specialists (NACNS). (2007). Legislative update: Assuring the public's access to CNS services: Model statutory/regulatory language to regulate CNS practice. Retrieved January 2007 from http://www.nacns.org/legislative.shtml.

National Council of State Boards of Nursing (NCSBN). (2002a). *Regulation of advanced practice nursing: 2002 National Council of State Boards of Nursing position paper.* Retrieved July 20, 2003, from www.ncsbn.org/public/regulations/res/APRN_Position_Paper2002.pdf).

National Council of State Boards of Nursing (NCSBN). (2002b). *Requirements for accrediting agencies and criteria for APRN certification programs.* Retrieved April 24, 2004, from www.ncsbn.org/pdfs/ APRN_approved_criteria_requirements_04.pdf.

National Council of State Boards of Nursing (NCSBN). (2006). *Vision paper: Future regulation of advanced practice nursing.* Chicago: Author. Retrieved March 20, 2006, from www.ncsbn.org/Draft_APRN_Vision_Paper.pdf.

Naylor, M.D. (2007). Advancing the science in the measurement of health care quality influenced by nurses. *Medical Care Research and Review, 64,* 144S-169S.

Naylor, M.D., Brooten, D.A., Campbell, R.L., Maislin, G., McCauley, K.A., & Schwartz, J.S. (2004). Transitional care of older adults hospitalized with heart failure: A randomized, controlled trial. *Journal of the American Geriatric Society, 52,* 675-684.

Neidlinger, S., Kennedy, L., & Scroggins, K. (1987). Effective and cost efficient discharge planning for hospitalized elders. *Nursing Economic$, 5,* 225-230.

Nelson, P.J., Holland, D.E., Derscheid, D., & Tucker, S. J. (2007). Clinical nurse specialist influence in the conduct of research in a clinical agency. *Clinical Nurse Specialist, 21,* 95-100.

Newell-Stokes, V., Broughton, S., Guiliano, K.K., & Stetler, C.B. (2001). Developing an evidence-based procedure: Maintenance of central venous catheters. *Clinical Nurse Specialist, 15,* 199-204.

Noll, M. (1987). Internal consultation as a framework for clinical nurse specialist practice. *Clinical Nurse Specialist, 1,* 46-50.

Oberle, K., & Allen, M. (2001). The nature of advanced practice nursing. *Nursing Outlook, 49,* 148-153.

Oda, D.S. (1985). Community health nursing in innovative school health roles and programs. In S.E. Archer & R.P. Fleshman (Eds.), *Community health nursing.* Boston: Jones & Bartlett.

Oddi, L.F., & Cassidy, V.R. (1998). The message of SUPPORT: Change is long overdue. *Journal of Professional Nursing, 14,* 165-174.

O'Malley, P. (2007). Order no harm: Evidence-based methods to reduce prescribing errors for the clinical nurse specialist. *Clinical Nurse Specialist, 21,* 68-70.

O'Malley, P., & Mains, J. (2003). Update on prescriptive authority for the clinical nurse specialist. *Clinical Nurse Specialist, 17,* 191-193.

Patton, M.D., & Schaerf, R. (1995). Thoracotomy, critical pathway, and clinical outcomes. *Cancer Practice, 3,* 286-294.

Phillips, S.J. (2006). Legislative update: A comprehensive look at the legislative issues affecting advanced nursing practice. *The Nurse Practitioner, 31,* 6-38.

Phillips. S.J. (2007). Legislative update: A comprehensive look at the legislative issues affecting advanced nursing practice. *The Nurse Practitioner, 32,* 14-17.

Phillips, S., Haycock, C., & Boyle, D. (2006). Development of an alcohol withdrawal protocol: CNS collaborative exemplar. *Clinical Nurse Specialist, 20,* 190-198.

Prouty, M.P. (1983). Contributions and organizational role of the CNS: An administrator's viewpoint. In A.B. Hamric & J. Spross (Eds.), *The clinical nurse specialist in theory and practice.* New York: Grune & Stratton.

Rantz, M.J., Popejoy, L., Petroshki, P.F., Madsen, R.W., Mehr, D.R., Zwygart-Stauffacher, M., et al. (2001). Randomized clinical trial of a quality improvement intervention in nursing homes. *Gerontologist, 41,* 525-538.

Rapp, M.P. (2003). Opportunities for advanced practice nurses in the nursing facility. *Journal of the American Medical Directors Association, 4,* 337-343.

Rasmussen, D., & Barnason, S. (2000). Chest pain management: Liking tertiary and rural settings. *Nursing Clinics of North America, 35,* 321-328.

Roggow, D.J., Solie, C.J., & Tracy, M.F. (2005). Clinical nurse specialist leadership in computerized provider order entry design. *Clinical Nurse Specialist, 19,* 209-214.

Seemann, S. (2000). Interdisciplinary approach to a total knee replacement program. *Nursing Clinics of North America, 35,* 405-415.

Shea, C.A., Pelletier, L.R., Poster, E.C., Stuart, G.W., & Verhey, M.P. (Eds.). (1999). *Advanced practice nursing in psychiatric and mental health care.* St. Louis: Mosby.

Sneed, N.V. (1991). Power: Its use and potential for misuse by nurse consultants. *Clinical Nurse Specialist, 5,* 58-62.

Soehren, P.M., & Schumann, L.L. (1994). Enhanced role opportunities available to the CNS/nurse practitioner. *Clinical Nurse Specialist, 8,* 123-127.

Soukup, M. (2000). The Center for Advanced Nursing Practice evidence-based practice model. *Nursing Clinics of North America, 35,* 301-309.

Sparacino, P.S.A., & Cooper, D.M. (1990). The role components. In P.S.A. Sparacino, D.M. Cooper, & P.A. Minarik (Eds.), *The clinical nurse specialist: Implementation and impact* (pp. 11-40). Norwalk, CT: Appleton & Lange.

Sparacino, P.S.A., Cooper, D.M., & Minarik, P.A. (Eds.). (1990). *The clinical nurse specialist: Implementation and impact.* Norwalk, CT: Appleton & Lange.

Sparacino, P.S.A., & Durand, B.A. (1986). Editorial on specialization in advanced nursing practice. *Momentum, 4,* 2-3.

Spross, J., Clarke, E.B., & Beauregard, J. (2000). Expert coaching and guidance. In A.B. Hamric, J.A. Spross, & C.M. Hanson (Eds.), *Advanced nursing practice: An integrative approach* (2nd ed., pp. 183-215). Philadelphia: Saunders.

Spross, J., & Hamric, A.B. (1983). A model for future clinical nurse specialist practice. In A.B. Hamric & J. Spross (Eds.), *The clinical nurse specialist in theory and practice* (pp. 291-306). New York: Grune & Stratton.

Spross, J.A., & Heaney, C.A. (2000). Shaping advanced nursing practice in the new millennium. *Seminars in Oncology Nursing, 16,* 12-24.

Stetler, C.B., Corrigan, B., Sander-Buscemi, K., & Burns, M. (1999). Integration of evidence into practice and the change process: Fall prevention program as a model. *Outcomes Management for Nursing Practice, 3,* 102-111.

Tindle, H.A., Davis, R.B., Phillips, R.S., & Eisenberg, D.M. (2005). Trends in use of complementary and alternative medicine by U.S. adults. *Alternative Therapies in Health and Medicine, 11,* 42-49.

Topp, R., Tucker, D., & Weber, C. (1998). Effect of a clinical case manager/clinical nurse specialist on patients hospitalized with congestive heart failure. *Nursing Case Management, 3,* 140-147.

Wagner, L.M., Capezuti, E., Brush, B., Boltz, M., Renz, S., & Talerico, Kutu (2007). Description of an advanced practice nursing consultative model to reduce restrictive siderail use in nursing homes. *Research in Nursing & Health, 30,* 131-140.

Walker, J., Gerard, P.S., Bayler, E.W., Coeling, H., Clark, A.P., Dayhoff, N., et al. (2003). A description of clinical nurse specialist programs in the United States. *Clinical Nurse Specialist, 17,* 50-57.

Walker-Sterling, A. (2005). African- Americans and obesity: Implications for clinical nurse specialist practice. *Clinical Nurse Specialist, 19,* 193-198.

Ward, S., & Clark, A.P. (2006). Improving patient outcomes with intensive insulin therapy. *Clinical Nurse Specialist, 20,* 170-174.

Woods, S.S., Nass, J., & Deisch, P. (2000). Selection and implementation of a transparent dressing for central vascular access devices. *Nursing Clinics of North America, 35,* 385-394.

Zuzelo, P.R. (2007). *Clinical nurse specialist handbook.* Sudbury, MA: Jones & Bartlett.

CHAPTER 13

The Primary Care Nurse Practitioner

Ann Reid Anderson • Eileen T. O'Grady

INTRODUCTION

This chapter provides an overview of the primary care nurse practitioner (NP) role. The primary care NP provides care for patients in acute, long-term, and community-based settings. This chapter explores the historical context and evolution of primary care NP roles and settings and relates the NP role to the Institute of Medicine (IOM) definition of primary care. Advanced practice nurse (APN) competencies of direct clinical practice, expert coaching and guidance, consultation, collaboration, leadership, research, and ethical decision making as operationalized in primary care NP practice are described. Exemplars of pediatric and family NPs practicing in urban and rural settings are provided to demonstrate the integration of NP competencies in diverse primary care settings. Finally, information about role implementation and key issues confronting primary care NPs is presented.

HISTORICAL ROOTS OF PRIMARY CARE IN THE UNITED STATES

Before Word War II, The U.S. health care system was almost exclusively a "primary care" model in that each patient was under the care of a family physician and would see specialists only if referred. Throughout the 1930s and 1940s, primary care expanded to include pediatricians, internists, and public health nurses (Institute of Medicine [IOM], 1996). *Primary care* as a term was not seen until the 1960s; at the same time, there was a growth in specialist physician care.

The triad of circumstances in the 1960s—President Kennedy's assassination, President Johnson's "War on Poverty," and the women's movement—sparked a widespread commitment to public service and instigated a re-valuing of nursing that encompassed women's work, caring, ethics, and knowledge. These social forces coupled with a physician workforce maldistribution provided a powerful social context to lay the groundwork for a demonstration project at the University of Colorado to build on and reclaim the role of the public health nurse. Thus the role of NPs was birthed and historically rooted in primary care. This emerging NP model was quite distinct from the medical model in that it focused on prevention, health and wellness, patient education, and informing patients of all cost-benefit alternatives so that they were empowered to weigh treatment options.

The 1970s brought a rapid influx of capitated group practice models, or health maintenance organizations (HMOs), which emphasized primary care and lower hospitalization rates. The expansion of the HMO grew out of the Health Maintenance Organization Act of 1973, which intended to control expenditures for employee benefits. Despite these efforts, primary care did not flourish for a number of reasons, one of which was that the role of primary care as "gatekeeper" was perceived as a barrier for patients' access to specialty care by physicians. Today, patients who enroll in HMOs are assigned to a primary care physician. Each physician is assigned or "empanelled" approximately 1500 patients to care for (Murray, Davies, & Boushon, 2007). Some HMOs do not empanel NPs, rendering NPs' contribution to primary care invisible. NP empanelment would provide a basis for more accurately measuring the effectiveness of NPs, whose services are often now significantly underestimated because they are recorded as being provided by their collaborating physicians (Health Resources and Services Administration [HRSA], 2004).

Most of primary care practice can be considered a "cottage industry," with many small businesses (physician practices that employ NPs) that are not integrated vertically with other sectors of the health care system. Many NPs work as employees in group physician practices who operate in a fee-for-service delivery system. Some primary care NPs are associated with academic/medical center primary care services. This relationship of NPs as employees of private, physician-owned businesses further adds to the lack of data on NP primary care practice.

Since the first primary care NP role focused on the care of children, a variety of primary care NP roles have emerged over four decades, emphasizing care to specific populations such as families, adults, older adults, and women. All of these roles were conceived to increase access to primary care and address the needs of underserved populations, and NPs have been acknowledged as cost-effective providers of quality primary care (Brown & Grimes, 1993; Clawson & Osterweis, 1993; Cook & Nolan, 1996; Kane et al., 1991; Mundinger et al., 2000).

THE FEDERAL GOVERNMENT AND PRIMARY CARE

The Health Resources and Services Administration (HRSA), an agency of the U.S. Department of Health and Human Services, is the primary Federal agency for improving access to health care services for people who are uninsured, isolated, or medically vulnerable. HRSA's Bureau of Primary Care funds grants that build a safety net infrastructure in high-poverty counties, such as health centers that provide primary health care regardless of the ability to pay for care. It is argued that these programs are helping reduce health care disparities because health professions graduates are 3 to 10 times more likely to practice in underserved areas and be minorities themselves (Coalition for Health Funding, 2007).

HRSA's Shortage Designation Branch

About 20% of the U.S. population reside in primary medical care Health Professional Shortage Areas (HPSAs). One of the criteria for this shortage designation is a community that has a population of 3500 to one full-time primary care physician (in one of the four primary care specialties—general or family practice, general internal medicine, pediatrics, and obstetrics and gynecology) (HRSA, 2007). Currently, NPs, certified nurse-midwives (CNMs), and physician assistants (PAs) are not included in the counts of primary care providers for designation purposes. There are several reasons for this resolve, and they are critically important for the APN community (see Chapter 22). First, there is concern that counting NPs and CNMs would render communities ineligible for shortage designation because they would raise the eligibility ratio higher for communities that had APN(s) to more than the population-to-provider ratio of 3500:1, thus creating a catch-22. Second, the outdated state practice acts governing NP and CNM practice vary widely, as some state laws permit independent APN practice whereas others are highly restrictive. This variability across states

introduces systematic bias in counting them as full-time equivalent primary care providers, as an APN in a restrictive state is not able to practice to full capability because of restrictive laws. Finally and perhaps most important, there is a substantial lack of data on the location and practice patterns of NPs. HRSA intends to include NPs and CNMs in the designation methodology in the future but only in the states that have adequate data and whose laws permit them to independently provide services traditionally considered "physician services" (Gaston, 1997). Without a zip-code level census of all practicing NPs, this provider group will remain invisible in the shortage designation methodology.

Primary Care Access and the Health Care Home

New research is demonstrating the critical role that care coordination plays in patient outcomes and speaks strongly to the skills of the primary care NP (Naylor et al., 2007). Care coordination, a key dimension of primary care, refers to the delivery of a wide application of care and case management principles to health care services. This effort uses health informatics, disease management, and telehealth technologies to facilitate access to care and improve the health of designated individuals and populations; the intent is to provide the right care in the right place at the right time (Veterans Administration [VA], 2007). These services are carried out within the context of a health care home and are clearly within the NPs' scope of practice. A health care home is not a building, house, or hospital but, rather, a longitudinal, cost-effective and prevention-based approach to providing comprehensive primary care. A health care home provides a structure for the longitudinal relationship between a patient and NP provider to grow. It promotes a strong partnership with the patient to ensure that all of the current and anticipated needs of the patient are met. Through this partnership, the nurse practitioner can help the family/patient access and coordinate specialty care, educational services, out-of-home care, family support, and other public and private community services that are important to the overall health of patients. Care coordination has been integral to primary care but has not typically been reimbursable, largely because this service has been invisible and undervalued. Emerging pay-for-performance demonstrations are providing evidence that care coordination improves efficiency and health outcomes (Centers for Medicare and Medicaid Services [CMS], 2007). Nurse practitioners need to be part of these pay-for-performance activities.

Primary Care Workforce Composition

The National Sample Survey of Registered Nurses in 2004 (Table 13-1) estimated the number of NPs at 141, 209 (HRSA, 2004). This number is only an estimate of the NP primary care workforce because no national data break down the practicing NPs by specialty (e.g. acute care, gerontology, family). A survey of NPs in New York State (n = 8208), however, found that almost 50% were employed in the primary care sector (Center for Health Workforce Studies, 2004). This estimate may reflect the trend nationally as more NPs enter specialty practices. The

2006 graduation data depicted in Table 13-2 suggests that the majority of all NP graduates (84%) selected primary care specialties. Although these graduation data do not fully inform the current workforce composition, they do suggest that the majority of NPs entering the workforce are entering primary care. These estimates and the dearth of data on the NP workforce make a compelling case for more robust data on NP practice patterns, distribution, and impact on outcomes. Policymakers at both the state and federal levels have cited the difficulty in obtaining accurate information on NPs in the workforce (National Advisory Council on Nurse Education and Practice [NACNEP], 2002; Virginia General Assembly, 1999). Overlapping of specialty areas, clinical nurse specialist (CNS)/NP blended and dual NP specialty practice roles, and varied titling by states make it difficult to determine the number of primary care NPs in the nation. While the overall number of NPs continues to grow and the number of Doctor of Nursing Practice (DNP) level NP programs expands, it is difficult to predict whether the growth will occur in primary care or in specialty settings.

Table 13-1   COMPOSITION OF THE PRIMARY CARE WORKFORCE

The Primary Care Workforce	Estimated Number
Nurse Practitioners (2004)[*]	141,209
Physician Assistants (2007)[†]	63,609
Family Medicine Physicians (2006)[‡]	100,152
General Internal Medicine Physicians (2006) [‡]	99,913
General Pediatric Physicians (2006) [‡]	51,915
TOTAL	**456,798**

[*]From U.S. Department of Health and Human Services (USDHHS), Health Resources and Service Administration (HRSA). (2004). *The registered nurse population: Findings from the March 2004 national sample survey of registered nurses.* This survey is a sample of the registered nurse population, not the subpopulation of nurse practitioners (NPs), making the accuracy of the NP estimate less reliable. Moreover, this estimate reflects all NPs in all specialties and settings, making it an overestimate for the primary care workforce. There are no national workforce data on NPs by specialty certification.

[†]American Academy of Physician Assistants. (2007). *Projected number of people in clinical practice as PAs as of January 2007.* This number is an overestimate because it includes all physician assistants (PAs) practicing in all specialties and settings. Website: www.aapa.org/research/06number-clinpractice06.pdf.

[‡]American Association of Colleges of Medicine, Center for Workforce Studies. (2006). *Physician specialty data: A chart book.* Website: https://services.aamc.org/Publications/showfile.cfm?file=version67.pdf&prd_id=160&prv_id=190&pdf_id=67.

Table 13-2   2006 GRADUATES OF MASTER'S-LEVEL NURSE PRACTITIONER PROGRAMS[*]

Clinical Track/ Certificate Examination	Graduates
Family NP	3442 (53%)
Adult NP	1015 (16%)
Pediatric NP	543 (8%)
Gerontological NP	99 (2%)
Women's Health NP	294 (5%)
The above primary care specialties account for 84% of all specialties selected by graduates in 2006.	
Acute care NPs	321 (11%)
Psych/mental health NP	211 (4%)
NP dual track/other NP	197 (3%)
TOTAL	**6504 NP graduates in 2006**

From American Association of Colleges of Nursing and National Organization of Nurse Practitioner Faculties. (2007). *Annual survey.* Washington, DC: Authors.

NP, Nurse practitioner.

*Percentages may not total 100 due to rounding.

PROFILE OF THE PRIMARY CARE NURSE PRACTITIONER ROLE

Primary Care Nurse Practitioner Practice

The IOM defines primary care as "the provision of integrated, accessible health care services by clinicians who are accountable for addressing a large majority of personal health needs, developing a sustained partnership with patients, and practicing in the context of family and community" (IOM, 1996). Box 13-1 summarizes the defining characteristics of the key terms, which are explained in detail in the IOM report. Among the NP roles there are five primary care specialties: adult, family, gerontological, pediatric, and women's health (National Organization of Nurse Practitioner Faculties [NONPF], 2002). The IOM definition of primary care encompasses much of the essence of advanced practice nursing and APN competencies with its emphasis on accountability, a holistic approach to direct patient care, inclusion of health promotion and disease prevention activities, and description of a patient-clinician relationship "predicated on the development of mutual trust, respect, and responsibility" (IOM, 1996, p. 37). A primary care NP certainly brings these attributes and activities to the primary care setting. The APN's use of professional caring with patients as partners in health care sets nursing's contributions to primary care apart from other providers' practice (Green-Hernandez, 1997). In Chapter 5, the use of a holistic framework and the forming of partnerships with patients are identified as two of the major characteristics of the APN. By engaging in the nursing process in the primary care setting (i.e., data collection, assessment, planning, implementation, and evaluation) with defined advanced practice skills and competencies, an NP can effectively provide primary care. The population of patients for which the NP is prepared to provide care (e.g., families, adults, neonates, children, women, older adults) serves to differentiate the types of primary care NPs' practice. The American Nurses Association (ANA) "Scope and Standards of Advanced Practice Registered Nursing" reflects the integration of primary care delivery and the nursing process in this APN role (ANA, 1996).

The concept of integrated, accessible health care services described by the IOM (1996) also underscores the importance of a team approach in primary care delivery. An important APN competency is collaboration among the professionals providing health services (see Chapter 10). Nursing models of care have emphasized developmental and systems theories in considering human responses to illness (i.e., caring over time or finding deep meaning

---

Box 13-1   Institute of Medicine Terms Used to Define Primary Care

INTEGRATED
Comprehensive, coordinated care throughout the life cycle
Focused on particular needs of patients
Clinician continuity
Effective communication of information
Patient record continuity

ACCESSIBILITY
Ease with which care is attained
Elimination of geographic, cultural, language, reimbursement, and administrative barriers

CLINICIAN
Uses recognized scientific knowledge base
Authority to direct the delivery of care

ACCOUNTABLE
Clinician and system accountability for services provided

MAJORITY OF PERSONAL HEALTH CARE NEEDS
Competency to manage majority of health problems
Use of consultation or referral as needed
Sustained partnership
Relationship between patient and clinician over time

CONTEXT OF FAMILY AND COMMUNITY
Understanding of the circumstances and facts surrounding the patient (socioeconomic status, family dynamics, work issues)
Awareness of public health trends
Need for specific health promotion and disease prevention strategies

From Institute of Medicine. (1996). *Primary care: America's health in a new era.* Washington, DC: National Academies Press.

through illness). Using a holistic approach to assessment and treatment, the primary care NP addresses illness, promotes health, and prevents disease. Developing trusting relationships through strong interpersonal skills, patient and family education, and coaching and guidance is a critical element of practice. APNs integrate elements of care from nursing and medical models in a collaborative approach to clinical practice that enhances the comprehensiveness and quality of care rendered. Many of the skills and competencies in primary care NP practice are based on the knowledge and skills needed to manage common acute and chronic health problems encountered in primary care settings. By employing expert clinical reasoning and using diverse management approaches, the NP provides appropriate cost-effective primary care (see Chapter 5).

Nurse Practitioner Practice and the Nursing Process. Primary care NP practice meets the criteria for advanced practice nursing as described in Chapter 3: graduate nursing education, national certification, and practice focused on the patient/family. Primary care NPs develop skills and competencies in their practices that build on a foundation of basic nursing education. NP competencies are continually developed through clinical experience and ongoing professional education. In Chapter 3, the synergistic impact of graduate education and clinical practice experience on APN development is described and a set of core competencies in each APN role is identified. An overview of each of the APN competencies in primary care NP practice follows.

Primary care services encompass the entire life span of patients. Primary care NPs may be broadly prepared to care for patients at any stage of life (e.g., family NPs) or may have a particular population focus in their practice (e.g., pediatric NPs). No matter what the focus, primary care NPs are involved in the management of health and illness status using the nursing process, graduate core competencies, and the APN competencies.

Assessment. Advanced patient history taking and physical assessment skills are critical tools for primary care NPs. Effective communication skills and the ability to establish partnerships with patients enhance the NP's ability to obtain a comprehensive history and tailor interventions most appropriate for the patient. A working knowledge of cultural diversity provides an important foundation for this process.

Particular attention is paid to personal health habits, stressors, genetics, and an assessment of health risk factors to identify appropriate health promotion and disease prevention strategies. The DNP *Essentials* identify these same components but acknowledge that with specialization comes the need for a more sophisticated understanding of the complexity of issues facing the individual patient or group.

Diagnosis. Evaluating the subjective and objective data collected using advanced assessment skills requires critical thinking and diagnostic reasoning skills on the part of the primary care NP. These aspects of clinical decision making are required not only in the identification of problems but also in the further evaluation and management of health needs of primary care patients. Specific health promotion needs based on stages of physical and psychosocial development may be assessed. Much of primary care NP practice involves the diagnosis and management of acute, self-limiting, minor illnesses and stable chronic diseases. However, NPs in primary care practice must be able to recognize signs and symptoms of complex and unstable health problems requiring medical or other consultation. They must also recognize emergency situations and be able to initiate effective emergency care. Graduate nursing preparation provides the APN with additional skills to make these sometimes subtle distinctions.

Planning. After the initial assessment phase of the nursing process, the primary care NP's plan for care may include additional diagnostic studies, specific therapeutic measures, and coaching and guidance strategies. Clinical practice guidelines such as those cited on the websites for the Agency for Healthcare Research and Quality (AHRQ) *(www.ahrq.gov/clinic/cpgonline.htm)* and the National Guideline Clearinghouse *(www.guideline.gov/)* help guide the clinician in planning appropriate interventions. Age-specific screening examinations are useful as outlined in the "Guide to Clinical Preventive Services" (Agency for Healthcare Research and Quality [AHRQ], 2007). Specific therapeutic measures may encompass both pharmacological and nonpharmacological therapies. If pharmacological therapy is initiated, the NP determines the appropriate treatment and counsels the patient about drug regimens and side effects. For example, the JNC 7 report from the Joint National Committee on Prevention, Detection, Evaluation and Treatment of High Blood Pressure outlines management of high blood pressure that includes both pharmacological and nonpharmacological interventions *(www.nhlbi.nih.gov/guidelines/hypertension/)*. These guidelines are based on the review of medical literature and recommendations of experts in the field of cardiovascular medicine. In addition, the NP would review the literature for other approaches to reduce cardiovascular risk. Evidence-based practice allows the NP to "evaluate the quality and consistency of the vast literature available and more effectively assist patients with health care decision-making" (Kania-Lachance, Best, McDonah, & Ghosh, 2006, p. 46). For example, a conversation about risk reduction with a person experiencing cardiovascular disease would certainly include the appropriate use of statin and antihypertensive medication, weight reduction, and other modifiable risk factors. The NP would also link the mind-body connection and address the issues of stress and depression and their role in cardiovascular health. The NP might introduce the concept of meditation, tai chi, or other mindfulness-based disciplines aimed at reducing stress.

Intervention. By critically evaluating nursing, medical, and other scientific literature, the NP builds a strong foundation on which to base interventions, recommendations, and counseling. As previously mentioned, the primary care NP's therapeutic recommendations may be nonpharmacological (e.g., specific dietary or activity recommendations, stress management strategies). In fact, primary care NPs are more likely to use nonpharmacological therapies than are traditional medical practitioners (Moody, Smith, & Glenn, 1999). Patient education and counseling strategies in the management of health and illness status include anticipatory guidance related to normal growth and development for patients and families, as well as potential changes they may experience as a result of specific health problems. Additional coaching and guidance competencies used in NP practice are discussed in the following section. *Healthy People 2010* (U.S. Department of Health and Human Services [USDHHS], 2000) identifies Leading Health Indicators or specific health concerns of individuals and communities across the United States *(www.Healthy People.gov)*. Current Leading Health Indicators include issues addressed frequently in primary care such as physical activity, obesity, tobacco and substance abuse, mental health, sexual behavior, and immunizations. Strategies to improve national health are based on these Leading Health Indicators.

Evaluation. Once plans of care are developed and implemented, the primary care NP uses expected outcomes criteria to evaluate the effectiveness of interventions. Scheduling phone or office follow-up visits to appropriately monitor patients is an important aspect of ongoing evaluation. When outcome criteria are not achieved, the plan of care is revised accordingly and further consultation may be indicated (NONPF, 2002). Careful documentation of all services provided is necessary for third-party reimbursement. Outcome data for groups of patients are a critical measure of practice safety and efficacy. These data are closely monitored by the payers of health care and help validate professional practice. NPs should incorporate quality measurement tools to measure practice outcomes. The Healthcare Effectiveness Data and Information Set (HEDIS) is one example of performance measures used to evaluate primary care practice (Buppert, 2004; National Committee for Quality Assurance, 2007; see also Chapter 25).

The Doctor of Nursing Practice

In response to the need to support the advanced educational needs of the APN, the practice doctorate is the expected requirement for APN preparation in the future. Endorsed by the American Association of Colleges of Nursing (AACN), the DNP is a practice-focused doctorate designed to "prepare experts in specialized advanced nursing practice" (AACN, 2004). Foundational competencies as well as competencies in an area of specialization and role are part of DNP preparation. The APN competencies for DNP-prepared APNs both expand and refine the existing clinical knowledge and leadership capacity of the APN. The central and core APN competencies remain unchanged and are woven into DNP preparation. The DNP *Essentials* (AACN, 2004) outline specific foundational competencies and learning experiences in a variety of settings so that the broad consequences of decision making can be identified. These competencies are central to current APN practice and particularly salient to primary care advanced practice.

ADVANCED PRACTICE NURSE COMPETENCIES IN PRIMARY CARE NURSE PRACTITIONER PRACTICE

In the following section, the APN competencies are interspersed with exemplars that describe typical primary care NP practice. The reader is referred to the specific competency chapters in Part II for further clarification of the APN competencies.

Direct Clinical Practice

As with other advanced practice roles, direct clinical practice is the heart and soul of the work of the primary care NP. The work of the primary care NP unfolds around the premise that individuals seek care for a broad range of health care concerns over time and across the life span. Relationships evolve over time, which facilitates a sense of mutual respect and trust. Within that relationship, a deep understanding of the patient's life and the meaning of the illness or health issue at hand develops. Knowing patients and their family members, their jobs and careers, and their challenges in raising children and caring for aging parents is part of walking with patients through the transitions of life. Spross (2005) describe these transitions as "paradigms for life and living," and it is during these times that the APN can provide support and guidance. Exemplars follow that illustrate the central competency of direct clinical practice, as well as the core competencies of expert coaching and guidance, consultation, and collaboration.

For primary care NPs, one day is as varied as the next. Some days are filled with episodic visits, and some days are spent predominantly on health care maintenance and education. The day described in Table 13-3 illustrates a typical day for Carol, a primary care NP, that this narrative explains. The complexity of care and the NP's familiarity with patients are cultivated over a series of encounters. While the hallmark of the primary care NP's practice is the breadth of health issues encountered, the privilege of patient/NP relationships occurs over time. This enables the NP to tailor evidence-based interventions to the individual and sustain a holistic practice. Characteristics of direct clinical practice and strategies for enacting them are outlined in Chapter 5.

Reflective Practice: A Component of Direct Patient Care. Expert clinical thinking and skillful performance are cultivated through repeatedly evaluating similar sets of health and illness scenarios and formulating plans of care based on patient expectations, standards of care, experience, clinical judgment, and current research. APNs continuously synthesize knowledge and experience so that, over time, they acquire *practical wisdom*, which Oberle and Allen (2001) define as "knowing when a particular action ought to be taken" (p. 151). Experienced APNs incorporate this practical wisdom into their decision making, taking actions that they may have been unlikely to take as novice practitioners.

Practical wisdom involves knowing what to do and when. When is a patient ready to begin home glucose monitoring? When is it time to suggest respite care or home health? What is the right time to address sexuality issues with a preteen or teen? What is the right time to address an issue directly, and when is it time to back off from confronting difficult issues?

Often an assessment of the chief complaint unearths a multitude of issues, some of which the patient may not be aware. The skilled practitioner helps the patient sift and sort through the issues, establish priorities, and understand the interconnectedness of these priorities. Practical wisdom guides the practitioner to use expert clinical thinking and skillful interviewing to develop a plan of care that is likely to improve health and quality of life and be carried out by the patient (see Chapter 5). For example, in Carol's typical day practice, understanding the acute and potentially serious nature of G.J.'s (patient 1) pneumonia and bronchospasm led to swift evaluation, treatment, and a plan for close follow-up within 24 hours. Knowing the complexity of glycemic control enabled the APN to approach L.B.'s (patient 11) hyperglycemia both pharmacologically and socially. When D.T. (patient 5) exhibited presenting symptoms of upper respiratory infection (URI) the APN distinguished between symptoms of a viral infection and one of bacterial etiology. The experienced practitioner knew when otitis media with effusion would not clear with another round of antibiotics and knew when to refer the patient to an otolaryngologist, as in the case of J.M. (patient 6). NPs are expert clinical thinkers who listen carefully to the story the patient tells them.

Partnerships with patients and families develop over time. Relationships with patients should be therapeutic regardless of whether the encounter is the first or the hundredth. As partnerships deepen, the relationship becomes an even more important clinical tool. For example, F.B. and L.B. (patients 10 and 11) are an older adult woman and her mentally handicapped daughter in Carol's practice. When the issue of transitioning to assisted living from their apartment surfaced, Carol drew on a relationship of trust developed over several years to approach the challenge cooperatively with L.B. and F.B. Carol explored the losses associated with the move and the meaning of the change for both of them. Acknowledging the grief associated with this major life change and identifying positive, unexplored aspects of assisted living helped them accept this transition.

Table 13-3   Typical Day for Carol: A Primary Care Nurse Practitioner

Patient	Age	Sex	Chief Complaint	Complexity	Competency
1 G.J.	50	F	Acute bronchitis Lupus Hypertension	Moderate	Direct clinical practice Expert coaching and guidance
2 T.Y.	35	F	Back pain Carpal tunnel syndrome Situational stress	Moderate	Direct clinical practice Expert coaching and guidance Collaboration
3 J.D.	46	F	Hypertension Weight gain Grief reaction	Moderate	Direct clinical practice Expert coaching and guidance Collaboration
4 S.D.	87	M	Hypertension follow-up	Low	Direct clinical practice Expert coaching and guidance
5 D.T.	40	M	Viral upper respiratory infection (URI)	Low	Direct clinical practice Expert coaching and guidance
6 J.M.	50	M	Sinusitis Bilateral otitis media with effusion	Moderate	Direct clinical practice Expert coaching and guidance Research skills Consultation
7 M.W.	35	M	Knee pain Psoriasis	Moderate	Direct clinical practice Expert coaching and guidance Consultation
8 K.L.	26	F	Contraception/annual examination Chlamydia	Moderate	Direct clinical practice Expert coaching and guidance
9 M.N.	37	F	Depression Annual examination	Moderate	Direct clinical practice Expert coaching and guidance
10 F.B.	82	F	Hypertension Reflux Skin avulsions	Moderate	Direct clinical practice Expert coaching and guidance Collaboration
11 L.B.	55	F	Type 2 diabetes Hypertension Obesity Asthma Mental retardation	High	Direct clinical practice Expert coaching and guidance Consultation Ethical decision making
12 J.P.	39	M	Hypertension New-onset type 2 diabetes Diabetes teaching	Moderate	Direct clinical practice Expert coaching and guidance Research skills Collaboration
13 P.M.	22	M	Human immunodeficiency virus (HIV) screening	Moderate	Direct clinical practice Ethical decision making Expert coaching and guidance
14 L.R.	38	F	Orthostatic hypotension Dehydration Gastroenteritis	High	Direct clinical practice Consultation

Patients are more likely to comply with medical recommendations if they are given a part in the decisions about their care. The primary care NP worked to form a partnership with S.D. (patient 4) as a means of improving his compliance with his antihypertensive medication. A partnership with K.L. (patient 8) is described in Exemplar 13-1. The annual examination is an opportunity to nurture the APN/patient relationship with the patient, assess health status, perform appropriate health screening, identify risky behaviors, and evaluate developmental issues. For some women, this is their only access to health care so it must be time wisely spent. The APN is especially qualified to provide this service using a holistic approach.

The development of a holistic perspective is another characteristic of direct clinical practice. Understanding the relationship among poor ergonomics in the workplace, the responsibility to take care of a handicapped child, and the development of chronic pain reflects the NP's holistic view of symptoms and etiology and the implications for treatment in the case of T.Y. (patient 2). Issues of independence and dependence play into the success of caring for mother and daughter F.B. (patient 10) and L.B. (patient 11). Understanding functional and cognitive abilities is critical in the management of L.B.'s diabetes.

In practice, APN core competencies (see Chapter 3) are often executed simultaneously to achieve the best outcome. However, for purposes of didactic discussion, specific competencies are discussed within the individual exemplars for clarity. The exemplars reflect the extent to which the core competencies enhance direct clinical practice: the core of primary care.

Expert Coaching and Guidance

The relationship of the primary care NP and the patient creates a strong foundation for the coaching and guidance competency (see Chapter 6). Carol's ongoing relationship with K.L. in Exemplar 13-1 allows her to encourage her to make wise choices and lead a healthier lifestyle and to anticipate K.L.'s needs as she continues in young adulthood. Patient

---

 EXEMPLAR 13-1   **Direct Clinical Practice of the Primary Care Nurse Practitioner**

Carol is a primary care APN working in a university-affiliated internal medicine practice. She has practiced in this setting for 9 years with six internists and a variety of specialists from the university medical center. Although her focus is primary care, she has access to several subspecialists for consultation purposes. For Carol, scheduling patients occurs in several ways. Telephone triage nurses screen patient calls of an acute nature. The triage nurse makes a brief telephone assessment of the patient's symptoms and then schedules the patient to see either Carol or a physician, depending on availability. Visits are typically 15 minutes for acute and follow-up visits. Educational, counseling, and annual examination visits are 20 to 30 minutes. Follow-up visits are also scheduled with the APN as appropriate. Physicians refer patients to the APN for follow-up of chronic medical problems such as hypertension, diabetes, and asthma. Assessment of additional problems, counseling, education, and medication management may occur during these visits. Patients are also free to self-schedule appointments with Carol or another APN. Some patients use Carol's services on an intermittent basis, and others receive the majority of their primary care from her. Many women in the practice see Carol for their annual examination.

Table 13-3 provides a sampling of patients whom Carol may see in her primary care practice during an 8-hour day and illustrates the range of competencies used throughout a typical day. The case of K.L (patient 8) illustrates the core competency of direct clinical practice and coaching and guidance.

K.L. is a 26-year-old female presenting for her annual examination. Carol first met K.L. when K.L.'s mother, an existing patient, brought her daughter in to discuss contraception. K.L. was 19 years old at the time and was considering becoming sexually active. During that initial visit, Carol started to develop a trusting relationship that would be the foundation of their relationship for subsequent years. The first visit focused on contraception education, emotional readiness to begin a sexual relationship, safe sex, and a brief screening for any type of high-risk behavior. There were no contraindications for hormonal contraception so K.L. was given a prescription for a 3-month supply of birth control pills and instructed to return after 3 months of use for follow-up. She was given written instructions about oral contraception including signs and symptoms of clotting problems related to estrogen use. Phone availability for questions was also offered to K.L.

During K.L.'s college years, Carol continued to see her for her annual examination. During those years, K.L. engaged in some high-risk sexual behavior, some of which was related to excessive alcohol use. Carol used each annual visit to continue to raise awareness of the consequences of high-risk sexual behavior and alcohol use and to reaffirm safe sex practices. K.L. kept her annual visit appointment during those tumultuous years. Each visit included screening for chlamydia, gonorrhea, syphilis, and HIV; screening for HPV was not available at that time.

K.L. finished college and took a job teaching kindergarten in a near-by school district. She is now in her fourth year of teaching and has been dating a young man for 2 years. She takes birth control pills and calcium supplements. She has no major concerns during this visit except a question about a mole on her right leg. K.L. is satisfied with her teaching job, and she and her partner have recently talked about getting married. Carol noted during the interview that K.L.'s exposed skin is tanned.

K.L.'s annual examination focused on wellness and prevention issues. She has no current weight issues and reports a negative history for eating disorders. She has no current or remote symptoms of depression. Her diet includes some red meat and regular servings of chicken and fish. She eats a variety of fruits and vegetables, does not drink milk, and eats cheese or yogurt about three times a week. She drinks two to four glasses of wine per week and does not smoke. She does not get any regular exercise outside of her job. Now that she has settled in to her teaching position, she has developed an interest in gardening and scrapbooking. She happily reports that her relationship with her boyfriend is steady and mutually loving. She denies any physical or emotional abuse. She and her partner have decided to forego condom use since they are monogamous and eventually plan to be married. K.L. reports a normal libido and is satisfied with her sex life. A brief overview of newer contraceptive options was given, but K.L. is satisfied with the 20-mcg oral contraceptive pill prescribed 3 years ago. She has no new contraindications for estrogen use and denies any side effects from taking the hormone. Serious side effects from taking estrogen are reviewed. There is no change in her family history and since her last visit. Significant family history includes mother's diagnosis of melanoma 5 years ago for which she has been disease-free for 5 years. K.L. denies family history of early heart disease, breast cancer, colon cancer, skin cancer (other than mother's melanoma), or diabetes. She does admit to several "bad" sunburns as a teenager. Immunizations are up-to-date, and she receives an annual flu shot through the school system.

Her review of symptoms is negative except for a reported increase in the size of a mole on her right leg. The physical examination includes skin, thyroid, cardiovascular, respiratory, breast, abdominal, and pelvic examination. Findings were normal except for a 10 millimeter mole on her right lateral knee with a slightly irregular border and bathing suit tan lines. Emphasis was given to skin and breast self-examination instruction as part of the examination. Thin-layer pap testing was done along with chlamydia, gonorrhea, and KOH and saline wet prep. Blood glucose and cholesterol testing are normal from the previous year and are not repeated.

The opportunity for teaching and counseling occurs at the conclusion of the visit. K.L. is offered the opportunity to ask questions, and she expresses interest in the new HPV vaccine, GARDASIL. Carol provides a handout with information about the vaccine. Carol explains that the vaccine immunizes a young woman against the strains of HPV that are implicated in cervical cancer. Because of her age, she is eligible for the vaccine. She will check with her insurance company about coverage and consider starting the series.

Carol reviews the need for adequate calcium and provides a list of calcium-rich foods. Options for exercise that fit with K.L.'s lifestyle were reviewed. The health benefits of exercise were reinforced. Current recommendations for daily sunscreen use are reviewed, and a sunscreen handout is provided. The importance of protective clothing including hats and sunglasses is emphasized. Carol realizes that a more in-depth discussion of sun-related issues will occur with the dermatologist, so she chooses to limit her counseling at this time.

A referral is made to a nurse practitioner colleague specializing in dermatology. This is the same colleague who follows K.L.'s mother since her melanoma diagnosis. K.L. will be notified of her laboratory results in writing in about 2 weeks. Recommended follow-up is in 1 year.

After direct care responsibilities, Carol spends the remainder of her day completing documentation, returning phone calls, reviewing laboratory reports, writing letters, refilling prescriptions, and authorizing referrals. The telephone triage nurse consults with Carol on several patient calls, and appropriate disposition is discussed. Carol's final call of the day is to a nurse practitioner student to arrange a start date for her adult health practicum.

APN, Advanced practice nurse; *HIV*, human immunodeficiency virus; *HPV*, human papillomavirus; *KOH*, potassium hydroxide; *pap*, Papanicolaou.

teaching is also a function of the coaching role. This occurs in every patient encounter when NPs routinely review medications and individualize self-care recommendations. NPs participate in or lead health information classes in areas such as diabetes, women's health, and prepared childbirth, in which groups of patients are coached regarding common health issues.

A challenge for the primary care provider is to identify serious illness and involve other disciplines in the care of the complex patient. Exemplar 13-2 with L.M. illustrates the coaching competency as described by Spross in Chapter 6. It also shows how the NP collaborates with other health care professionals to provide comprehensive care to complex patients. In this case, L.M.'s NP may be the first provider to see the young adult with an eating disorder.

Primary care NPs weave multiple competencies throughout their practice. These competencies enable the APN to achieve positive results in caring for patients. APNs would like to fill their days with successful, fulfilling patient encounters as described earlier, but this sometimes is not the case. Some patients exhibit ambivalence and inconsistency in their approach to their health, and despite mobilizing all of one's competencies, a positive outcome may be elusive. For example, patients such as H.B., a 35-year-old noncompliant male patient with type 2 diabetes, described in Exemplar 13-3, often struggle with not only the reality of the illness but also assuming self-care for its management. NPs need to develop skill in understanding and handling such situations, not only to facilitate patient care but also to manage their own feelings of frustration or failure when patients are unable to make lifestyle changes that promote health and reduce the risk of complications.

Therapeutic success depends on the patient's acceptance of the disease and his or her willingness to enter into a coaching relationship with the NP that fosters and supports the needed changes. It is hard to understand why a patient seems to "choose" illness over health. Sometimes patients are simply not ready to make changes because they understand that such lifestyle changes will increase the complexity of their lives, routines, or relationships. There are times when, despite the best efforts to offer a coaching relationship or to match a particular patient with a provider who can be an effective coach, the APN's efforts are rebuffed.

A multitude of issues could be explored in Exemplar 13-3: individual response to chronic illness, the role of denial in chronic illness, and nonadherence,

to name a few. The NP must be prepared for the frustration and disappointment that comes when, despite the best of efforts, the desired outcome is not achieved. What distinguishes the APN from other nurses and practitioners is the tenacity to continue to use diverse approaches to problem solving, to look for other explanations, and to continue to develop the partnership with the patient. NPs have a deep knowledge of the change process and a menu of tools to use depending on where the patient is in the cycle of change. Time is another tool for the primary care NP. As in the case of H.B., the primary care NP will be available to him on his journey with diabetes, either through a direct encounter about his diabetes or by way of another primary care issue. Each encounter may supply a piece of the puzzle about his nonadherence and an opportunity for H.B. to become an active participant in his care. A collaborative and supportive relationship with other primary care providers will sustain the APN in times of frustration. Tenacity and commitment will also sustain the primary care NP as he or she journeys with a reluctant H.B. through his transitional challenge, a diagnosis of diabetes. In this situation, the fact that the patient continued to return to the NP for monitoring and care and that he did bring his wife to learn more about the illness were, for the NP, indicators of modest success and sustained her hope that a breakthrough might yet occur.

Consultation

Consultative relationships are critical to primary care NP practice. Relationships with NPs, physicians, nurses, and other health care providers ensure that patients have access to comprehensive care. The direct clinical practice exemplars illustrate different consultative relationships. Throughout the day, Carol informally consults with the primary care physicians (PCPs) in the practice about problematic cases or clarification of a treatment plan. She sees the patients of all of the PCPs in the practice and updates them if a new problem is identified or if a specific concern needs to be addressed in follow-up. This informal consultation style is a frequent part of the daily rhythm of the practice and includes elements of the collaboration competency. NPs in smaller or solo practices would not have easy access to this consultation style and would have to seek a style that suited their practice (see Chapter 7).

Formal consultations with specialists are also initiated for complex medical problems. J.M. (patient 6)

EXEMPLAR 13-2   Coaching, Guidance, and Collaboration in Primary Care Practice*

L.M. is a 21-year-old male college student who sees Cindy, a family NP. L.M. was referred to the NP after multiple meetings with the college nutritionist revealed significant, progressive, and rapid weight loss. L.M. is an otherwise healthy Caucasian male who wanted to lose weight so that he had more energy and endurance for soccer. The nutritionist reported that L.M. lost about 20 pounds by exercising, eating healthier choices, and reducing portion sizes. After successfully losing 20 pounds, L.M. exhibited signs of anxiety (i.e., heart palpitations and sweaty palms) when faced with eating. L.M. reports the anxiety is caused by the fear he will gain the weight back. He reports feeling fatigued but otherwise feels well. L.M. denies laxative or diuretic use and purging. His vital signs on initial presentation are as follows: weight, 112 pounds; height, 5'7"; BMI, 17.5; BP, 90/60 with no evidence of orthostatic hypotension. He appears pale, has sunken temples, and is very thin for his stature. The rest of his examination is unremarkable. L.M. is talkative, is well groomed, and exhibits good eye contact with a broad affect.

Blood specimens are drawn for basic laboratory studies (CBC, phosphate, magnesium, CMP, TSH), and an appointment is made for L.M. to see university counselors and the student health psychiatrist. L.M. and Cindy talk openly and expressed their concerns and thoughts on his weight loss. L.M. reports that he is doing better and that he will not lose more weight if given one more week. L.M. and Cindy develop a plan as to what he can do this week to ensure that he maintains his weight. L.M. reports he is agreeable to the plan and is scheduled for follow-up in 1 week. The next visit reveals another 6-pound weight loss in 6 days despite reporting sufficient caloric intake. Clinical examination reveals a cachectic young male with clothes that hang on him, temporal wasting, gaunt features, and a flat affect with slight psychomotor retardation. The rest of the examination was unremarkable except for bradycardia. Because of L.M.'s physical state and psychomotor retardation from his nutritional deficiencies, it was decided with the patient, psychiatrist, nutritionist, counselor, and family that L.M. needed to be admitted to a local hospital for nutritional supplementation, as well as tests to rule out possible malignant causes of weight loss. Cindy had tried throughout her relationship with L.M. to use touch, validation, active listening, and encouragement; however, L.M.'s physical and mental well-being continued to decline. At this visit, L.M. pleads and bargains to not go to the hospital, but Cindy explains that the clinical significance of his weight loss is too profound at this time to wait any longer. The admission would improve his physical status (i.e., gain weight, normalize all laboratory values) and mental health status (improve his altered mental status, monitor anti-anxiety medication).

L.M.'s father and L.M.'s girlfriend of 5 years came to the clinic to accompany L.M. to the hospital. Cindy and the nutritionist met with L.M.'s father to explain the urgent medical and psychological situation. They actively listened to his questions and answered them with an open and honest manner. Their intention was to decrease the family's anxiety, stress, and uncertainty regarding the diagnosis of anorexia nervosa and the pending hospital admission. L.M. and his family were concerned about the impact of a hospitalization on L.M.'s college courses. With the help of the psychiatrist and L.M.'s girlfriend, Cindy was able to involve L.M.'s professors by writing them a letter explaining his current medical condition. In doing this, L.M. and his family were able to focus on his physical and mental health instead of worrying about missed classes or falling grades.

L.M.'s hospital stay lasted several days, during which time the hospital staff ruled out other causes of rapid weight loss. L.M.'s diagnosis of anorexia nervosa was confirmed, and his health was stabilized. L.M. and his family decided inpatient treatment for anorexia nervosa was not appropriate for them at this time. Therefore the university psychiatrist, Cindy, the physician, the nutritionist, and university counseling agreed to attempt to monitor L.M.'s mental and physical status through an outpatient team approach. L.M. was involved in developing this plan, and he agreed that if his weight decreased or if he missed follow-up appointments, inpatient treatment would become the only option. L.M. was agreeable to this plan.

It has been 1 year since this crisis for L.M., and he continues to maintain the weight he gained. L.M. continues to see his counselor and psychiatrist on a regular basis. His visits with Cindy have stopped because he is medically stable, but they can resume at any time. The lines of communication remain open between L.M. and his "team."

*The author gratefully acknowledges Courtney Bickett, FNP, for assistance with this exemplar.
BMI, Body mass index; *BP,* blood pressure; *CBC,* complete blood count; *CMP,* complete metabolic panel; *NP,* nurse practitioner; *TSH,* thyroid-stimulating hormone.

EXEMPLAR 13-3   The Nonadherent Patient in Primary Care

H.B. is a 35-year-old male whom Paul, the primary care NP, has known for several years. H.B was initially referred by his PCP for diabetes education. He was diagnosed with diabetes a few years earlier by a physician in another state and was not on medication when he first visited Paul's practice. His glycemic control eroded over the next several years despite triple drug oral therapy. He made no significant changes in his diet and did not exercise regularly despite participation in a diabetes education program. Paul would periodically see H.B. for episodic issues and would take the opportunity to check on the status of his diabetes. H.B. would always say that he felt fine; thus he did not need to check his blood sugars. During these visits, Paul would search for barriers to adherence, assess for symptoms of depression, and offer support and encouragement for H.B. to take a more proactive approach in the care of his diabetes. Approximately 1 year elapsed during which Paul did not see H.B. His HbA$_{1c}$ level continued to rise, and his physician determined that the addition of insulin was necessary to improve glycemic control. Several more months elapsed before H.B. finally made an appointment with Paul for insulin teaching. During that visit, H.B. admitted that he was not performing home glucose monitoring because sticking himself was too painful. He voiced serious reservation about daily insulin injections but felt pressured by his physician to keep the appointment. Paul could not determine any other mitigating factor except fear of pain and an apparent inability to grasp the seriousness of his illness. H.B. reluctantly agreed to proceed with the teaching program but refused to inject himself. He conceded that he might permit his wife to administer the insulin and agreed to bring her in for an educational session. When Paul realized that teaching

was not going to happen during the visit, the focus shifted to assessing current stressors or other barriers to accepting his diabetes. H.B reported that he is happily married and feels successful and satisfied in his work. He does not discuss his diabetes with his wife, family, or co-workers. Because H.B. generally feels well, he has difficulty accepting the fact that his diabetes control has deteriorated. He has no history of depression, anxiety, or substance abuse. He was not interested in any counseling to explore his issues with diabetes. He eventually agreed to ask his wife to learn how to give his insulin. Paul encouraged follow-up and tried to be positive and supportive so that H.B. would return. Paul followed up with a reminder note 2 weeks later. A month elapsed, and H.B. had not scheduled any follow-up.

Paul consults with the PCP and shares his concern about the lack of follow-up and proactive behaviors H.B. demonstrates in the care of his diabetes. The PCP is equally puzzled about H.B.'s adherence issues. The NP is unable to elicit from H.B. any insight as to his unwillingness to adopt the self-care skills and lifestyle changes required for effective disease management. Eventually, H.B. and his wife return for instructions on insulin use. H.B. still vigorously refuses to inject or perform home glucose monitoring, although his wife learns to inject insulin and perform finger sticks and is willing to perform these tasks for her husband. He agrees to the plan, and a schedule for bedtime insulin was prepared. Paul then negotiates with H.B. the minimum number of times each week he is willing to perform home glucose monitoring, and a schedule for this is also suggested. H.B. agreed to send or call in blood sugar results in 2 weeks, with follow-up in 1 month. Paul receives no results, and a follow-up appointment was not made.

HbA1c, Hemoglobin A$_{1c}$; *NP,* nurse practitioner; *PCP,* primary care physician.

was referred to an ear, nose, and throat (ENT) specialist for evaluation of his bilateral otitis media with effusion. The case of M.W. (patient 7) involved consultation with the PCP and the rheumatologist (Exemplar 13-4). Carol regularly provides consultation to the clinic nurses, who are the first line of communication with patients. Their assessments of patient problems and the patients' responses to treatment are valuable information for the NP.

Other APNs in the outpatient and inpatient setting can provide consultations in their specialty areas. For example, the primary care NP might ini-

tiate a consultation with a psychiatric CNS to evaluate depression in a hospitalized patient. A referral for consultation with a CNM for preconception counseling provides valuable information to the woman ready to start a family. Newly diagnosed patients with type 2 diabetes benefit from consultation with a CNS whose specialty is diabetes management, and the expertise of home health nurses is critical in discharge planning. Community health nurses have a wealth of knowledge regarding other community resources and insurance coverage for home care services. NPs often initiate consultations

EXEMPLAR 13-4   Consultation: The Complex Patient in Primary Care

M.W. is a 35-year-old male (patient 7) whose presenting symptoms include a protracted case of right knee pain. He was diagnosed with gout by his PCP, and after several flare ups over the past 7 years, he was prescribed allopurinol. M.W. remained on the allopurinol until 1 month ago, at which time he had acute onset of right knee pain and swelling. He was initially treated with colchicine, with minimal improvement in his symptoms. His PCP changed his medication to indomethacin, with some improvement in his symptoms. M.W. was scheduled for follow-up with Carol, the primary care NP, at the request of the PCP. On physical examination, M.W was pleasant though discouraged by the lack of resolution of his symptoms. His right knee was mildly edematous and without warmth or erythema. He had pain on full flexion and full extension. There was no evidence of instability or meniscal or ligamentous involvement. Carol also noted several large psoriatic plaques on the extensor surfaces of his forearms and legs. M.W. was diagnosed with psoriasis 10 years ago. The first episode of gout was 5 years ago. He noted that the gout flares up in the winter months, which often disrupts his vacation plans. M.W. owns a landscaping business and maintains a brisk commercial business in the spring, fall, and summer. He usually schedules vacation in January to meet friends in the Florida Keys. This is now the second consecutive year that his vacation plans have been thwarted by gout symptoms. In the course of further discussion, M.W. commented that he had also had painful swelling of his right index finger about 1 year ago and that the x-ray film had shown some arthritis. Hand symptoms had not recurred. Carol reviewed the chart and read a radiology report indicating degenerative changes in the PIP joint of the right second digit. Physical examination of the right hand shows enlargement of the PIP joint. M.W. also reported two episodes of bilateral ankle pain that were never evaluated. A sedimentation rate and uric acid were ordered, as well as a two-view x-ray film of his right knee. M.W. is advised to stay on the indomethacin until test results are received. Laboratory and x-ray studies are within normal limits. Later that week Carol discussed the case with M.W.'s PCP, and they decided to refer M.W. to a rheumatologist for further evaluation of possible psoriatic arthritis. Carol called the patient and discussed the test results and the recommendation for a specialty evaluation. M.W agreed and was transferred to the referral coordinator to set up the rheumatology appointment and obtain insurance preauthorization.

PCP, Primary care physician; *PIP,* proximal interphalangeal; *NP,* nurse practitioner.

with physical therapists, occupational therapists, speech therapists, nutritionists, and social workers based on a home health nurse's evaluation. (Lindeke & Sieckert, 2005).

Research

Clinical practice in this "age of information" offers exciting opportunities and challenges for the primary care NP. Health care knowledge resources in electronic form, especially on the Internet, are increasingly available. Health care informatics have facilitated the development of clinical practice guidelines based on current research and the consensus of clinical experts (Anderko, Bartz, & Lundeen, 2005; Fonteyn, 1998). Today's primary care NPs must be able to retrieve evidence-based information and appraise important practice innovations for their relevance and appropriateness to practice (Goolsby, 2004; Kania-Lachance et al., 2006).

Evidence-based clinical practice guidelines can be used to improve primary care. With the advent of managed care systems, practice guidelines are used to reduce costs, standardize practice, and decrease medical liability. NPs can evaluate clinical practice guidelines and work to adopt those that will ensure that best practices are used in primary care delivery. The Agency for Healthcare Research and Quality (AHRQ), the Healthcare Effectiveness Data and Information Set (HEDIS), the National Guideline Clearinghouse (NGC), and the National Quality Measures Clearinghouse are reliable resources for evidence-based clinical guidelines and performance measures (Box 13-2). These guidelines can also be used in conjunction with agency outcomes and performance measures to provide feedback to clinicians about the extent to which best practices are used (Goolsby, 2004; see also Chapters 24 and 25).

AHRQ has identified potentially preventable hospitalizations as a critical area of health care quality and has developed indicators for health care problems that afford a high risk for hospitalization. For example, bacterial pneumonia, chronic obstructive pulmonary disease, and low birth weight fall into this category. These ambulatory care sensitive outcomes

Box 13-2   Useful Websites for Primary Care

Organization	Website	Content
Association of Colleges of Graduate Medical Education	www.acgme.org	Medical education Competencies
Agency for Healthcare Research and Quality	www.ahrq.gov/clinic	Clinical practice guidelines
National Quality Measures Clearinghouse	www.qualitymeasures. ahrq.gov/	
Preventive Services	www.ahrq.gov/clinic/ prevenix.htm	Age-specific screening examination recommendations
National Guideline Clearinghouse	www.guideline.gov/	
National Advisory Council on Nurse Education and Practice (NACNEP)	www.bhpr.gov/nursing/ nacnep	APNs in the workforce data
National Organization of Nurse Practitioner Faculties (NONPF)	www.nonpf.com	APN competencies APN education data APNs in the workforce data
American Association of Colleges of Nursing (AACN)	www.aacn.nche.edu	APNs in the workforce data
National Sample Survey of Registered Nurses	www.bhpr.hrsa.gov/ nursing	RNs in the workforce data
Healthcare Effectiveness and Data Information Set (HEDIS)	www.ncqa.org/Programs/ HEDIS	Performance measures for primary care practice
Robert Wood Johnson Foundation	www.rwjf.org	Health policy
Division of Nursing, Bureau of Health Professions, Health Resources and Services Administration, Department of Health and Human Services	www.bhpr.hrsa.gov/ nursing	
Health Insurance Portability and Accountability Act (HIPAA)	www.hrsa.gov/website.htm	

APNs, Advanced practice nurses; *RNs,* registered nurses.

relate directly to quality in primary care in that these are conditions in which a primary care NP can prevent the need for hospitalization (AHRQ, 2007). Primary care NPs should take an active role in clinical practice research, the development of clinical practice guidelines, and review of outcome and performance measures. AHRQ (2007) cites opportunities for interdisciplinary collaboration in primary care research and the creation of primary care research centers. These activities require a mastery of basic research skills, as discussed in Chapter 8.

Collaboration and Leadership

Each of the competencies in primary care NP practice discussed so far requires the development of collaborative relationships and leadership skills with patients and with other health care professionals.

Collaboration and leadership are closely related and so are discussed together here. Direct clinical practice in primary care with expert coaching and guidance exemplifies a collaborative relationship between patient and NP. The IOM definition of primary care (1996) implies the use of professional collaboration to deliver "integrated" and "accessible" care. Effective collaboration results in more comprehensive, patient-focused care (Bodenheimer & Grumbach, 2007) that promotes high-quality, cost-effective outcomes (Cowan et al., 2006; Lindeke & Sieckert, 2005). Expert coaching and guidance also require the establishment of a collaborative relationship between patient and provider (Dick & Frazier, 2006). Professional consultation and research entail collaborative relationships among a variety of health care providers with common goals and purposes (Drenning, 2006; Kania-Lachance et al., 2006).

At the local practice level, NPs enact the leadership role when they guide and support staff, when they triage patients, and when they oversee appropriate utilization of resources. NPs must ensure that primary care practices have an evidence base and have meaningful, systematic quality improvement initiatives. On a broader level, primary care NPs engaged in clinical and professional leadership must also use effective collaborative skills to assist groups and organizations to envision preferred futures, achieve consensus, and implement change. The essence of primary care is the sustained continuity of health care for the patient and family. As the long-term member of the team that provides continuity and stability in the care and management of patients over long periods, primary care NPs often emerge as leaders in primary care teams in health care settings. Furthermore, the primary care NP's role as a leader in the community through membership on boards of health and education and as an influential policymaker cannot be underestimated (see Chapters 9 and 10).

Ethical Decision Making

The primary care NP may encounter patient care concerns that raise ethical issues. Examples include reproductive issues, informed consent, and conflicting health care goals among family members. NPs have opportunities to engage in preventive ethics by initiating discussions about advance directives and organ donation with patients in a relaxed and thoughtful manner before they become pressing issues. In addition, NPs identify and address ethical conflicts that arise when clinical goals conflict with institutional goals (ANA, 2001; Johnson, 2005; McCaughan, Thompson, Cullum, Sheldon, & Raynor, 2005; Ulrich, Soeken, & Miller, 2003; see also Chapter 11).

Primary care NPs are accountable first and foremost to their patients, with patient confidentiality honored at all times. This professional value has recently become the focus of more intense government regulation and scrutiny with the implementation of the Health Insurance Portability and Accountability Act (HIPAA) regulations (see Chapters 19 and 21). Primary care NPs must be vigilant in their protection of confidential patient information in whatever form it takes. In an era of managed health care, the primary care clinician's accountability to the health care system in which he or she practices may create tension, especially where the use of resources for patient care is concerned. Primary care NPs must always be ethically accountable for their actions, especially where financial incentives related to resource utilization are involved (Bodenheimer & Grumbach, 2007; Laabs, 2005).

EXEMPLARS OF PRIMARY CARE NURSE PRACTITIONER PRACTICE

The role of the primary care NP in the interface of direct clinical practice with patients has been discussed in earlier exemplars. However, the influence and skill of the primary care NP can extend beyond that basic relationship to assist in meeting the primary care needs of a particular community. Exemplars 13-5 and 13-6 illustrate how NPs engage in the delivery of primary care and provide leadership to underserved populations in two very different settings—a low-income urban community and a rural health center. In community-based practices such as these, the importance of community assessment has been recognized as a way for primary care practitioners to more effectively meet the needs of the population they serve (George Washington University Medical Center, 2006; NONPF, 2003). A community needs assessment can identify existing and potential health problems as well as health promotion needs. Once these needs are identified, collaboration with other health care professionals, educators, and community leaders can provide a critical link in empowering individuals, families, and communities to improve their health status. Primary care NPs can serve a leadership role in these situations.

ADVANCED PRACTICE NURSE CHALLENGES AND THE FUTURE OF PRIMARY CARE

Overcoming Invisibility

Although nurse practitioners have made great strides over the past several years in establishing stable independent and collaborative practices, there is still work to be done (Arford, 2005; Mundinger et al., 2000; Sears, Maxwell, & Townsend, 2003). Negotiating the evolving health care marketplace and moving from an "invisible" provider status in many managed care systems and private physician practices to recognized members of provider panels and PCPs of record are two major challenges facing primary care NPs today. NPs have long been recognized as providers of cost-effective, high-quality care. These attributes are in keeping with today's emphasis on prevention, quality, and cost savings. However, access to

EXEMPLAR 13-5   Urban Pediatric Nurse Practitioner Primary Care Practice

Jane is a pediatric NP caring for children in a low-income urban community. This community once thrived as part of a major industrial center but was devastated by factory closings and a declining local economy. Recent health status indicators for this urban area reveal increasing rates of teen pregnancy. Concern is growing in the community about substance abuse, school drop-out rates, and community violence.

This setting is a challenging one, but Jane believes that, by working with children and families through the community child health clinic, she might be able to help them deal with the risks that poverty introduces to their health and wellness. The clinic is a public-private venture jointly funded by the local health department, the community hospital, and various charitable organizations in the greater metropolitan area. It serves as a source of primary care to many of the community's children, whose health care is subsidized by Medicaid and who are now enrolled in a statewide managed care program. The clinic also provides services to non-Medicaid recipients using a sliding-scale fee. Jane sees a variety of infants, children, and adolescents who come to the clinic for both well-child visits and acute/episodic health problems. Her care entails thorough health assessments using history-taking, physical assessment, and appropriate diagnostic studies or screening examinations. She then recommends appropriate interventions (both pharmacological and nonpharmacological) for the child. These are in keeping with established clinical guidelines used in the clinic. Much of Jane's time is spent discussing with parents normal childhood growth and development and effective parenting skills, nutritional needs, immunizations, and age-specific injury prevention guidelines. If the child is ill, Jane describes ways to monitor the child's health status. Jane's days take on a busy pace as she sees children for regularly scheduled well-child visits and manages a variety of episodic health problems during the clinic's walk-in hours.

At times, Jane may consult with the clinic pediatrician about acute health problems or abnormal health screening findings. For children and families with complex health problems, she may also consult with other members of the clinic team for further evaluation and management. Public health nurses are available for home assessment and case management services, and the clinic social worker provides additional outreach services. A nutritionist and eligibility worker from the WIC nutrition program are on-site to address nutritional needs in depth.

Jane also engages with this community outside the walls of the clinic. Involvement with community activities enhances her credibility and acceptance among this low-income population. On occasion she is asked to assist with health screening examinations for the local Head Start program. Recently, concern has been growing about unmet needs for child health services in the greater urban area. Inappropriate use of local emergency rooms for episodic health care and a rising incidence of asthma and lead poisoning have contributed to a renewed commitment to pediatric primary care. Jane works closely with the school nurses to follow high-risk children and to provide backup for emergency situations. As a respected primary care provider for an underserved community, Jane has been asked to serve on a local child health task force. She will work with other health care providers and community leaders to identify ways to more effectively use public and private resources in addressing children's health needs. Together, they hope to promote a healthier future for the community at large.

NP, Nurse practitioner; *WIC,* Women, Infant and Children.

primary care NPs continues to be controlled by organized health agencies in the private sector. In most cases, physicians who employ NPs are responsible for NP performance and compensation. This invisible provider status makes it difficult for health care consumers to gain direct access to NP care, and it is equally challenging to evaluate the impact of NP services on costs and outcomes in capitated systems of care (American College of Physicians, 2006; Johnson, 2005; Kendig, 2002).

Managed care organization (MCO) executives have reported a high degree of satisfaction with NPs serving as primary care providers and recognize their value in providing expert coaching and guidance (Mason, Cohen, O'Donnell, Baxter, & Chase, 2002). NPs are regularly being empanelled on MCO provider panels and gaining designation as PCPs on a more regular basis (Buppert, 2004). However, NPs must continue to educate administrators, payers, and patients about their role in primary care delivery. The

EXEMPLAR 13-6   Rural Nurse Practitioner Primary Care Practice

With 3 years of experience as an FNP at the Mountain Breeze Rural Health Center, Mary realized how well she had developed as a primary care provider. She had worked as a public health nurse for 10 years in this coal-mining and industrial community of Appalachia and was familiar with its poverty and limited access to health care. In fact, the mountains themselves, with their narrow, winding roads, posed one of the major barriers to care in this area—transportation.

Before the long-time local family physician retired, Mary had been able to pursue her NP education through a master's degree program offered by the state university satellite program on the community college campus 40 miles away. The 1-hour commute to school seemed long, but that trip was short compared with the additional 300 miles she would have had to travel if teleconferencing with faculty on the main campus were not available. Mary was the recipient of a state scholarship for her graduate education, and in return, she agreed to practice in a medically underserved area of the state that had been her home during her entire life.

Anticipating the loss of their beloved physician, the community had worked hard to support the establishment of a rural health center in the area. Mary was well known to the local citizens as a public health nurse, and they readily accepted her in her new role as an FNP. The nearest hospital, 30 miles away, had recently been engaged in the development of rural health networks and provided physician coverage in the center 3 days per week. The retiring family physician had been an important professional asset for Mary in her first year after graduation as she made the transition to her new role. Now, on the 3 days per week that physicians were on-site to collaborate, she could be sure that patients requiring more complex medical management were scheduled. These days also provided an opportunity to review and discuss other patient management issues and to develop skills and knowledge related to the medical issues in her practice.

Mary's days at the center were always full but never predictable. As an FNP, she provided care for a wide range of episodic health concerns for patients across their life spans. She cared for many adults with chronic health problems such as diabetes and hypertension. She devoted much of her effort to working with patients and their families on improved nutritional status and other health promotion strategies. One of her diabetic patients had recently started insulin therapy. After teaching him how to monitor his glucose at home, she was able to adjust his initial insulin therapy over the phone. The phone proved to be a valuable tool for her practice because many families had no regular source of transportation to the clinic. As the only female primary care provider in the area, Mary found much of her time devoted to women's health care. Women found it easy to share their concerns with her, and Mary frequently discussed family health problems with them during these visits. She also followed many children from infancy through childhood for well-child and episodic visits.

One afternoon a week, Mary left the clinic and made rounds to visit patients in the local nursing home. She worked closely with the staff there to identify ways to assist this older adult population in maintaining as much independence as possible. She also enjoyed occasional trips to the local high school to assist with sports physicals. From time to time she was invited to be a speaker at the employee health seminars held at the nearby packaging plant.

Her work was rewarding, and many challenges were ahead. She had recently discussed the area's low childhood immunization rates with local leaders. They were now developing a proposal for a mobile health unit to increase access to immunizations and other primary preventive services to remote sections of the tri-county area. Mary was asked to portray some of this Appalachian community's health needs to a contingent of state and federal legislators visiting the area. She hoped to make a compelling case for a mobile health unit so that funding for the project could be secured.

FNP, Family nurse practitioner.

---

development of sound marketing strategies that clearly define NP care and its benefits is essential in negotiating with managed care plans and other stakeholders (Kendig, 2002; Kennedy, 2003). Kendig, a practicing primary care NP, suggests three important strategies for defining NP care (2002):

- Maintain your nursing identity.
- Remember that true collaboration is the key.
- Focus on a unique skill set as an advanced practice nurse, rather than demonstrating how APN practice is similar to physician practice. (p. 271)

Identifying a "professional niche" that contributes to decreased costs and improved outcomes may be of particular benefit in marketing efforts (see Chapter 20). To be successful in today's health care marketplace, NPs must also have a proficient understanding of accounting, finance, economics, and reimbursement practices (Frakes & Evans, 2006; Kennerly, 2007; see also Chapter 19). Whether paid by Medicare, Medicaid, indemnity insurers, or MCOs, the primary care NP must be familiar with the reimbursement policies of third-party payers including documentation and billing guidelines (Buppert, 2004; Reel & Abraham, 2007).

The development of more formal contracting, credentialing, and privileging processes for NPs in a variety of health systems is likely as the health care system evolves. The primary care NP must be familiar with organizational credentialing measures and follow them. It is likely that NPs will need to provide data on the outcomes of care they have provided. The HEDIS has specific performance measures for primary care. An understanding of HEDIS measures and how HEDIS scores will affect clinicians is critical to the future of all primary care providers (HEDIS, 2004; see also Box 13-2).

Removing Regulatory Barriers

Removing regulatory barriers for APN practice will be required in order for the full impact of the APN in primary care to be realized. State practice acts that restrict patients' access to NPs, prescription writing, diagnostic test ordering, and referral to specialty care will directly impede the APNs' capacity to impact health outcomes favorably. Practice opportunities and perceived differences in NP scope of practice are largely related to arbitrary state regulations and the practice environments they create (Cooper, Henderson, & Dietrich, 1998; Lugo, O'Grady, Hodnicki, & Hanson, 2007; Mason et al., 2002; Safriet, 2002; Sekscenski, Sansom, Bazell, Salmon, & Mullan, 1994). NPs must continue to remove restrictions on their scope of practice, prescriptive authority, and eligibility for reimbursement that create barriers to patient care. The committed efforts of NP leaders at state and national levels, combined with support from nursing organizations to educate policymakers and effect change in these areas, have been commendable. However, much remains to be done to remove remaining legal and regulatory restrictions to practice (see Chapter 21). Furthermore, ongoing professional vigilance is necessary to protect the gains of the past. Professional unity with APNs, coalition building, and strong leadership at state and national levels are critical to achieve these goals. NPs in primary care practice must be willing to invest in these organizations and activities to protect and promote their professional futures.

Caring for the Chronically Ill and Aging

The number of persons 65 years of age and older in the United States will nearly double—from 42 million to 80 million—over the next three decades. The average lifespan for Americans is rising, and the fastest growing segment of our population is older than 80 years. Ninety percent of seniors have at least one chronic disease and 77% have two or more chronic diseases, and 85% of Medicare payments go toward treating chronic illness. It is estimated that in 2030, 46 million Americans will be diabetic (American Hospital Association [AHA], 2007). Managing chronic illness requires a complex set of skills and continuous management, which is an integral part of primary care NP education and practice. Many of these chronic illnesses are brought on by lifestyles that are not conducive to robust health. This exploding age and chronicity demography creates challenges for the primary care NP to develop best practices for preventing complications in those with chronic illnesses and coaching seniors in healthy lifestyle changes that will minimize the risks and burdens of chronic illness. This segment of NP primary care practice offers unlimited opportunity for NPs to engage in community-based care.

Reinventing the Primary Care Infrastructure

Our current health care delivery system, even in managed, integrated delivery systems, is not organized or structured to manage chronic illness in the primary care setting. The United States has built a specialty-oriented care delivery system since the first medical specialty board was created in 1916 (Starfield, 2006). Chronic care delivery has shown promising results for improved patient outcomes in the primary care setting. Effective interventions to improve primary care outcomes fall into one of five areas: the use of evidence-based, planned care; reorganization of practice systems and provider roles; improved patient self-management support; increased access to expertise; and greater availability of clinical information (Bodenheimer, Wagner, & Grumbach, 2002). All of these interventions are part of the Essentials of APN and DNP education. The challenge for primary care NPs is to organize these components into an integrated primary care system designed to manage chronic illness. Our current lack of delivery system integration across settings is amplified by the growth of hospitalists, which puts primary care providers including NPs on the periphery of managing acute, episodic illness. Moreover, restrictive state practice acts and discriminatory hospital policies prevent APNs, in some instances, from following patients into the different delivery systems such as hospice, hospitals, and skilled nursing facilities. Primary care is the cornerstone of a modern high-quality health care system, and NPs will need to use their clinical expertise and leadership skills to link primary care with data systems and quality measurement on a foundation of patient safety.

Convenient Care Clinics

Convenient care clinics (CCCs) have emerged as a response to unmet consumer needs for affordable and convenient primary care. These express clinics employ NPs as the primary caregiver and are housed in nontraditional settings such as drugstores, "big box" stores, airports, and grocery chains across the United States. They offer a low-cost, low-overhead approach to addressing needs not well met by today's primary care system. Convenient care clinics are attracting two diverse segments of the population—the higher-income insured who are willing to pay for convenient basic health care, and the uninsured whose only other alternative is the emergency department. Convenient care clinics offer basic primary care services only; they do not bill nor do they offer the full complement of services that require expensive technology and personnel. Yet, these clinics are hugely successful because they are focused on consumer needs and convenience. The rapid expansion of these clinics is a direct result of the poor access to care that patients of all types experience. Over time, these clinics will either compete directly with physician office practices or develop a mutually beneficial model that best meets patient needs. In the meantime, they are vastly enhancing the visibility and recognition of primary care NPs as viable health care providers (see Chapter 19).

THE NURSE PRACTITIONER AS DISRUPTIVE INNOVATOR

APNs are a disruptive innovation to the traditional medical model of primary care delivery. It is to be expected that stakeholders who have dominated an industry would resist a disruptive innovator who has the potential to overturn the status quo. While NPs have worked within the medical system as collaborative partners, more must be done to meet the primary care needs of the United States. Enhancing the supply of APNs, specifically primary care NPs, through expansion of DNP programs will be required. As DNP graduates in primary care stream into the workforce, it is expected that the primary care system will be substantially strengthened with nursing leaders who have the clinical credibility to influence change and create policy that builds a population-based health care system.

Global issues, such as bioterrorism and international political and economic unrest, are forces that require new models of care delivery and affect the future practice of primary care (Bodenheimer & Grumbach, 2007; Persell et al., 2001). Primary care NPs will require a more in-depth understanding and awareness of biological and chemical agents and the appropriate evidence-based interventions. NPs can provide leadership and collaboration in planning a public health response to bioterrorism.

The advent of telehealth offers exciting possibilities for primary care NPs to expand the breadth and scope of their education and practice. With these developments come new professional challenges related to interstate licensure and professional reimbursement for telehealth services (Boodley, 2006; Connors, 2002; Jenkins & White, 2001; Schoen et al., 2006). NPs (as well as patients) will have untold opportunities available to them via the Internet and other evolving modalities. NPs will need to become familiar with the new sources of electronic health care information available to their patients and counsel them about reliable resources to use. Useful websites for primary care NPs are found in Box 13-2.

Future models of primary care delivery need to serve as a roadmap for primary care policy (Showstack, Lurie, Larson, Rothman, & Hassmiller, 2004a; Showstack, Rothman, & Hassmiller, 2004b). Primary care must move from a cottage industry to a practice-integrated system that manages the health of the population. Primary care NPs can lead the way in this effort. They must move toward a model of primary care that empowers patients to minimize their direct care challenges and behavioral risk factors. The future of primary care will likely involve *more* personalized care through the use of genetics and strategic targeting of high-risk patients. This care will be delivered by APNs with an orientation toward disease management and behavior change and will incorporate expanded use of communication technology and lay-led group visits.

CONCLUSION

Primary care NPs have been recognized as pioneers in APN practice, and they are emerging as ideal providers of primary care for all patient populations. A description of the APN core competencies as used by the primary care NP has been described and illustrated by the exemplars. As with other APN roles, the continued professional development of NPs will lead to greater proficiency in each of the competencies over time. The traditional period from student to professional primary care NP with deep and broad expertise provides an important time to expand knowledge and strengthen clinical practice. NPs will assume a critical role in the primary care workforce of the future. Both professional unity and interdisciplinary collegiality must undergird their efforts as they take an active role in developing stable health policy and care delivery systems that will allow for patient access to primary care services provided by NPs.

REFERENCES

Agency for Healthcare Research and Quality (AHRQ). (2007). *Preventable hospitalization: Window into primary and preventive care.* Retrieved May 14, 2007, from www.ahrq.gov/data/hcup/factbk5.

Agency for Healthcare Research and Quality (AHRQ). (2007). U.S. preventive services task force. Retrieved December 5, 2007, from *www.ahrq.gov/clinic/uspstf/uspstopics.htm*.

American Association of Colleges of Nursing (AACN). (October 2004). *AACN position statement on the practice doctorate in nursing.* Washington, DC: Author.

American Association of Colleges of Nursing (AACN) and National Organization of Nurse Practitioner Faculties (NONPF). (2007). *Annual survey.* Washington, DC: Authors.

American College of Physicians. (2006). *Impending collapse of primary care medicine and its implications for the state of the nation's health care: A report from the American College of Physicians.* Retrieved May 14, 2007, from www.acponline.org/hpp/statehc06_1.pdf - 2006-01-31.

American Hospital Association (AHA). (2007). *When I'm 64: How boomers will change health care.* Retrieved May 14, 2007, from www.aha.org/aha/content/2007/pdf/070508-boomerreport.pdf.

American Nurses Association (ANA). (1996). *The scope and standards of practice of advanced practice registered nursing.* Washington, DC: Author.

American Nurses Association (ANA). (2001). *Code of ethics for nurses with interpretive statements.* Washington, DC: Author.

Anderko, L., Bartz, C., & Lundeen, S. (2005). Practice based research networks: Nursing centers and communities working collaboratively to reduce health disparities. *Nursing Clinics of North America, 40*(4), 747-758.

Arford, P. (2005). Nurse-Physician communication: An organizational accountability. *Nursing Economic$, 23*(2), 72-77.

Bodenheimer, T., & Grumbach, K. (2007). *Understanding health policy: A clinical approach.* New York: Lange/McGraw/Hill.

Bodenheimer, T., Wagner, E.H., & Grumbach, K. (2002). Improving primary care for patients with chronic illness: The chronic care model, Part II. *JAMA, 288*(15), 1909-1914.

Boodley, C.A. (2006). Primary care telehealth practice. *Journal of the American Academy of Nurse Practitioners, 18*(8), 343-345.

Brown, S.A., & Grimes, D.E. (1993). *Nurse practitioners and certified nurse midwives: A meta analysis of process of care, clinical outcomes, and cost-effectiveness of nurses in primary care roles* (#NP-85). Washington, DC: American Nurses Association.

Buppert, C. (2004). *Nurse practitioner's business practice and legal guide* (2nd ed.). Boston: Jones & Bartlett.

Center for Health Workforce Studies, Albany. (2004). *Nurse practitioners in New York State: A profile of the profession in 2000.* Retrieved May 14, 2007, from http://chws.albany.edu/index.php?nps_nys.

Centers for Medicare and Medicaid Services (CMS). (2007). *Pay for performance initiatives.* Retrieved May 14, 2007, from www.cms.hhs.gov/apps/media/press/release.asp?Counter=1343.

Clawson, D.K., & Osterweis, M. (Eds.). (1993). *The roles of physician assistants and nurse practitioners in primary care.* Washington, DC: Association of Academic Health Centers.

Coalition for Health Funding. (March 28, 2007). *Statement to the House Labor-HHS-Education Appropriations Subcommittee on the FY 2008 Funding Recommendations for the U.S. Public Health Services Agencies and Programs.* Retrieved May 14, 2007, from www.aamc.org/advocacy/healthfunding/start.htm-6k.

Connors, H.R. (2002). Telehealth technologies enhance children's health care. *Journal of Professional Nursing, 18,* 311-312.

Cook, T., & Nolan, W. (1996). A nurse practitioner–led, collaborative, out-patient practice: A case study in outcomes management. *Seminars for Nurse Managers, 4,* 154-162.

Cooper, R.A., Henderson, T., & Dietrich, C.L. (1998). Roles of nonphysician clinicians as autonomous providers of patient care. *Journal of the American Medical Association, 280,* 795-802.

Cowan, M.J., Shapiro, M., Hays, R., Afifi, A., Vazirani, S., Ward, C.R., et al. (2006). The effect of a multidisciplinary hospitalist/physician and advanced practice nurse collaboration on hospital costs. *Journal of Nursing Administration, 36*(2), 79-85.

Dick, K., & Frazier, S.C. (2006). An exploration of nurse practitioner care to homebound frail elders. *Journal of the American Academy of Nurse Practitioners, 18*(7), 325-334.

Drenning, C. (2006). Collaboration among nurses, advanced practice nurses, and nurse researchers to achieve evidence-based practice. *Journal of Nursing Care Quality, 21*(4), 298-301.

Fonteyn, M. (1998). The Agency for Health Care Policy and Research guidelines: Implications for home health care providers. *American Association of Colleges of Nursing Clinical Issues, 9,* 338-354.

Frakes, M.A., & Evans, T. (2006). An overview of Medicare reimbursement regulations for advanced practice nurses. *Nursing Economic$, 24*(2), 59-65.

Gaston, M. (February 13, 1997). *Testimony on safety net health care programs by Marilyn H. Gaston, M.D.,* Director, Bureau of Primary Health Care. Health Resources and Services Administration. U.S. Department of Health and Human Services. Before the House Committee on Government Reform and Oversight, Subcommittee on Human Resources. Retrieved May 14, 2007, from www.hhs.gov/asl/testify/t970213b.html.

George Washington University Medical Center/Faculty resources. (2006). *Building a practice in your home community.* Retrieved May 15, 2007, from www.gwumc.edu/healthsci/faculty_resources/health_science_learning_objects.cfm.

Goolsby, M.J. (2004). Integrating the principles of evidence-based practice into clinical practice. *Journal of the American Academy of Nurse Practitioners, 16*(3), 98-105.

Green-Hernandez, C. (1997). Application of caring theory in primary care: A challenge for advanced practice. *Nursing Administration Quarterly, 21,* 77-82.

Health Resources and Services Administration (HRSA). (2004). *A comparison of changes in the professional practice of nurse practitioners, physician assistants, and certified nurse midwives: 1992 and 2000.* Retrieved May 14, 2007, from bhpr.hrsa.gov/healthworkforce/reports/nursing/changeinpractice/default.htm.

Health Resources and Services Administration (HRSA). (2007). Guidelines for Medically Underserved Area and Population Designation. Retrieved December 11, 2007, from http://bhpr.hrsa.gov/shortage/muaguide.htm.

HEDIS 2004. (2004). *What's in it and why it matters* (Vol. 1). Retrieved September 25, 2003, from www.ncqa.org/programs/HEDIS.

Institute of Medicine (IOM). (1996). *Primary care: America's health in a new era.* Washington, DC: National Academies Press.

Jenkins, R.L., & White, P. (2001). Telehealth: Advancing nursing practice. *Nursing Outlook, 49*(2), 100-105.

Johnson, R. (2005). Shifting patterns of practice: Nurse practitioners in a managed care environment. *Research Theory in Nursing Practice, 19*(4), 323-340.

Kane, R.L., Garrard, J., Buchanan, J.L., Rosenfeld, A., Skay, C., & McDermott, S. (1991). Improving primary care in nursing homes. *Journal of the American Geriatrics Society, 39,* 359-367.

Kania-Lachance, D.M., Best, P.J., McDonah, M.R., & Ghosh, A.K. (2006). Evidence-based practice and the nurse practitioner. *The Nurse Practitioner, 31*(10), 46-54.

Kendig, S. (2002). Managing managed care: A nurse practitioner response to barriers to direct third-party reimbursement. In D.J. Mason, J.K. Leavitt, & M.W. Chaffee (Eds.), *Policy and politics in nursing and health care* (4 ed., pp. 265-272). Philadelphia: Saunders.

Kennedy, B.L. (2003). Negotiation: Getting what you need. In J.J. Fitzpatrick, A. Glasgow, & J.N. Young (Eds.), *Managing your practice: A guide for advanced practice nurses.* New York: Springer.

Kennerly, S. (2007). The impending reimbursement revolution: How to prepare for future APN reimbursement. *Nursing Economic$, 25*(2), 81-83.

Laabs, C.A. (2005). Moral problems and distress among nurse practitioners in primary care. *Journal of the American Academy of Nurse Practitioners, 17*(2), 76-78.

Lindeke, L.L., & Sieckert, A.M. (April 6, 2005). Nurse-physician workplace collaboration. *The Online Journal of Issues in Nursing, 10*(1), 1-7. Retrieved March 31, 2007, from www.medscape.com/viewarticle/449286.

Lugo, N.R., O'Grady, E.T., Hodnicki, D.R., & Hanson, C.M. (2007). Ranking state NP regulation: Practice environment and consumer health care cost. *American Journal for Nurse Practitioners, 11*(4), 8-23.

Mason, D.J., Cohen, S.S., O'Donnell, J.P., Baxter, K., & Chase, A.B. (2002). Managed care organizations' arrangements with nurse practitioners. *Nursing Economic$, 15,* 306-314.

McCaughan, D., Thompson, C., Cullum, N., Sheldon, T., & Raynor, P. (2005). Nurse practitioner and practice nurses' use of research information in clinical decision making: Findings from an exploratory study. *Family Practice, 22,* 490-497.

Moody, N.B., Smith, P.L., & Glenn, L.L. (1999). Client characteristics and practice patterns of nurse practitioners and physicians. *Nurse Practitioner, 24*(3), 94-96, 99-100, 102-103.

Mundinger, M.O., Kane, R.L., Lenz, E.R., Totlen, A.M., Tsai, W., Cleary, P.D., et al. (2000). Primary care outcomes in patients treated by nurse practitioners or physicians: A randomized trial. *Journal of the American Medical Association, 283,* 59-68.

Murray, M., Davies, M., & Boushon, B. (2007). Panel size: How many patients can one doctor manage, *Family Practice Management 14*(4), 44-51.

National Advisory Council on Nurse Education and Practice. (2002). *Nurse practitioner workforce report executive summary.* Washington, DC: Author.

National Committee for Quality Assurance. (2007). *The Healthcare Effectiveness and Data Information Set (HEDIS).* Retrieved December 5, 2007, from *www.ncqa.org/Programs/HEDIS.*

National Organization of Nurse Practitioner Faculties (NONPF) and the American Association of College of Nursing (AACN). (April 2002). *Nurse practitioner primary care competencies in specialty areas: Adult, family, gerontological, pediatric, and women's health.* Washington, DC: Authors.

National Organization of Nurse Practitioner Faculties (NONPF). (2003). *Community health in family nurse practitioner education.* Washington, DC: Author.

Naylor, M.D., Hirschman, K.B., Bowles, K.H., Bixby, M.B., Konick-McMahan, J., & Stephens C. (2007). Care coordination for cognitively impaired older adults and their caregivers. *Home Health Care Services Quarterly, 27*(4), 57-58.

Oberle, K., & Allen, M. (2001). The nature of advanced practice nursing. *Nursing Outlook, 49,* 148-153.

Persell, D.J., Arangie, P., Young, C., Stokes, E.N., Payne, W.C., Skorga, P., et al. (2001). Preparing for bioterrorism. *Nurse Practitioner, 26,* 12-29.

Reel , S.J., & Abraham, I.L., (2007). *Business and legal essentials for nurse practitioners: From negotiating your first job through owning a practice* (Chapter 19). St Louis: Mosby.

Safriet, B.J. (2002). Closing the gap between can and may in health care providers' scopes of practice: A primer for policymakers. *Yale Journal of Regulation, 19,* 301-334.

Schoen, C., Osborn, R., Huynh, P.T., Doty, M., Peugh, J., & Zapert, K. (2006). On the front lines of care: Primary care doctors' office systems, experiences, and views in seven countries. *Health Affairs, 25*(6), w555-w571.

Sears, L., Maxwell, W., & Townsend, C. (2003). Urgent-care visits to a geriatric primary care clinic. *American Journal for Nurse Practitioners, 7,* 15-18.

Sekscenski, E.S., Sansom, S., Bazell, C., Salmon, M.E., & Mullan, F. (1994). State practice environments and the supply of physician assistants, nurse practitioners, and certified nurse-midwives. *New England Journal of Medicine, 331,* 1266-1271.

Showstack, J., Lurie, N., Larson, E.B., Rothman, A.A., & Hassmiller, S.B. (2004a). Primary care, the next renaissance. In J. Showstack, A.A. Rothman, & S.B. Hassmiller (Eds.), *The future of primary care.* San Francisco: Jossey-Bass.

Showstack, J., Rothman, A.A., & Hassmiller, S.B. (2004b). *The future of primary care.* San Francisco: Jossey-Bass.

Spross, J.A., (2005). Expert coaching and guidance. In A.B. Hamric, J.A. Spross, & C.M. Hanson (Eds.), *Advanced practice nursing: An integrative approach* (3rd ed., pp. 187-223). Philadelphia: Saunders.

Starfield, B. (2006). *AAMC Third Annual AAMC Physician Workforce Research Conference examines trends in the supply of U.S. doctors.* Retrieved May 14, 2007,from www.aamc.org/workforce/pwrc/start.htm.

Ulrich, C.M., Soeken, K.L., & Miller, N. (2003). Ethical conflict associated with managed care: Views of nurse practitioners. *Nursing Research, 52,* 168-175.

U.S. Department of Health and Human Services (USDHHS). (2000). *Healthy People 2010* (2nd ed.). Washington, DC: U.S. Government Printing Office.

Veterans Administration (VA). (2007). Office of Care Coordination. Retrieved July 11, 2007, from www.va.gov/occ/.

Virginia General Assembly. (1999). *Directing the Joint Commission on Health Care to study the need to collect workforce data on nurse practitioners, clinical nurse specialists, registered nurses, licensed practical nurses, and certified nurse aides* (House Joint Resolution No. 682).

The Acute Care Nurse Practitioner

Marilyn Hravnak • Ruth M. Kleinpell
• Kathy S. Magdic • Jane Guttendorf

INTRODUCTION

The purpose of the acute care nurse practitioner (ACNP) is to diagnose and manage disease and promote the health of patients with acute, critical, and complex chronic health conditions across the continuum of acute care services. The ACNP provides comprehensive care in a collaborative model with physicians, staff nurses, and other health care providers, as well as with patients and their families. The ACNP not only shares common functions and skills with the other nurse practitioner (NP) subspecialties but also applies unique knowledge and skills in caring for very complex and vulnerable patient populations. Although all ACNPs share specialty role attributes, there may be intra-role variability based on the nature of the care delivery system or location in which they practice (e.g., private practice group vs. hospital employee; intensive care unit vs. hospital ward or ambulatory care facility) and physiological specialty (e.g., cardiac, pulmonary, orthopedic, oncology). This chapter presents an overview of the ACNP role, including scope of practice, core and role-specific competencies, the move toward doctoral education, reimbursement, and future challenges.

EMERGENCE OF THE ACUTE CARE NURSE PRACTITIONER ROLE

Although the role of NPs in primary care has been well documented since the 1960s (see Chapter 13), the newer role of the ACNP in secondary and tertiary care has not been as extensively described or studied. As early as the 1970s, neonatal NPs (NNPs) first began caring for infants in secondary and tertiary care settings because of cutbacks in pediatric residencies coupled with increased neonatal patient acuity and complexity. Changes in the delivery of care to acutely and critically ill adults in the 1970s and 1980s similarly predated the adult ACNP role. Advances in medical care increased patient longevity and consequently produced a larger pool of fragile older adults with multiple co-morbidities who were more apt to

require hospitalization during acute illness or exacerbation of chronic illness. Simultaneously, increased availability of technological monitoring and life support further advanced the complexity of patient care and the need for specially trained providers. Conversely, at this very time when acuity and technological support of hospital inpatients were increasing, a paradigm shift among health systems toward primary care decreased the preparation of physician specialists and medical trainee coverage for both pediatric and adult patients with acute and critical illness (Daly & Gent, 1997). Silver and McAtee (1988) proposed using NPs in the hospital setting to provide high-quality acute care in the face of physician reductions, particularly in teaching hospitals. ACNPs were to be educated to identify health risks and health promotion needs and to manage acute, critical, and complex chronic illness in collaboration with and under the supervision of a physician (e.g., intensivist, internist, cardiologist). Silver and McAtee envisioned that these NPs would develop specialized clinical decision-making and technical skills necessary to admit patients to the hospital, complete the history and physical examination, and assess and manage rapidly changing patient conditions. They envisioned ACNPS also writing inpatient medical orders, performing a variety of diagnostic and therapeutic tests, ordering and interpreting laboratory studies, and counseling patients and their families in collaboration with physicians.

Initially, primary care NPs (family NPs and adult NPs) were recruited to care for adult patients in hospital-based settings, with on-the-job training to provide secondary and tertiary care skills (an example of advanced practice nurse [APN] evolution is described in Chapter 18). By the late 1980s, NPs were increasingly used in tertiary care centers (Barber & Burke, 1999). It became apparent that a new adult NP specialty was emerging. Education specifically designed to meet the needs of vulnerable adult patients with acute, critical, and complex chronic illness that ensured consistency in the knowledge, training, and quality of care provided by NP graduates in this new specialty was required. Master's level graduate adult ACNP programs began to emerge in the late 1980s, and in 1995, the first national certification examination for ACNPs was administered. As of 2005, there are 70 adult ACNP educational programs in the United States (Kleinpell, Perez, & McLaughlin, 2005).

Because of these same historical forces, a need for pediatric NPs specifically educated to meet the needs of acutely ill children also emerged. In 2004, the National Association of Pediatric Nurse Practitioners (NAPNAP) expanded their pediatric nurse practitioner (PNP) "Scope of Practice" to reflect the acute care role (National Association of Pediatric Nurse Practitioners [NAPNAP], 2004). An acute care pediatric nurse practitioner (PNP-AC) examination from the Pediatric Nursing Certification Board (PNCB) became available in 2005, and as of 2005, approximately 20 PNP-AC programs are in existence (Clinton & Sperhac, 2005).

Numerous studies support that the ACNP provides both safe and effective care. The National Nurse Practitioner Database of the American Academy of Nurse Practitioners (AANP) indicates that of approximately 97,000 NPs in the United States in 2003, 4365 (4.5%) were ACNPs (Goolsby, 2005). This NP specialty continues to grow as the continued need for the unique services that ACNPs offer is recognized. Furthermore, recent constraints in graduate medical trainee work hour restrictions also provide a growing need for inpatient coverage—a need that can be met by the ACNP (Lundberg, Wali, Thomas, & Cope, 2006). The ACNP role has now spread outside of the United States and is being implemented to meet the needs of acutely and critically ill patients in the health care systems of other countries (Chang, Mu, & Tsay, 2006; Kaan & Dunne, 2001; Norris & Melby, 2006; van Soeren & Micevski, 2001).

SHAPING THE SCOPE OF PRACTICE FOR THE ACUTE CARE NURSE PRACTITIONER

The scope of ACNP practice is influenced from five levels: national (professional organizations), state (government), health care institution, service related, and individual. In common with other APNs, the ACNP's scope of practice is broadly set forth in statements by professional nursing organizations. State governments, as regulatory agencies, further delineate the scope of practice in statutes such as nurse practice acts or title-protection statutes. Because ACNPs

frequently provide their services within health care delivery systems such as hospitals, subacute care facilities, nursing homes, and clinics, their scope may be further defined by policies within these institutions, organizations, and health care entities and even by the needs of a clinically specialized patient population. And last, individual ACNPs will further define the scope of their practice based on their own talents, strengths, and attributes. How ACNP practice is configured at each of these levels is described in the following sections.

National (Professional Organizations)

At the national level, the scope of ACNP practice is influenced by the *Domains and Competencies of Nurse Practitioner Practice* (National Organization of Nurse Practitioner Faculties [NONPF], 2006) and the *Acute Care Nurse Practitioner Competencies* (National Panel for Acute Care Nurse Practitioner Competencies, 2004), which describe entry level competencies for graduates of master's and post-master's ACNP educational programs; the *Scope and Standards of Practice of the Acute Care Nurse Practitioner* (American Association of Critical-Care Nurses, 2006), which describes expert ACNP role performance; and the ACNP national certification examinations.

The *Domains and Competencies of Nurse Practitioner Practice* (NONPF, 2006) document has undergone several revisions, and the newest revision (NONPF, 2006) has been broadened to describe general practice competencies at the entry level for all NPs regardless of specialty setting. In 2002, the National Organization of Nurse Practitioner Faculties (NONPF) also convened a National Panel to develop more specific competencies for primary care NP subspecialties in the report *Nurse Practitioner Primary Care Competencies in Specialty Areas: Adult, Family, Gerontological, Pediatric, and Women's Health* (NONPF & American Association of Colleges of Nurses [AACN], 2002). Subsequently, a National Panel for Acute Care Nurse Practitioners was convened in 2003 to develop the *Acute Care Nurse Practitioner Competencies* (National Panel for Acute Care Nurse Practitioner Competencies, 2004). The first phase involved development of specific ACNP competencies within the domains of general NP practice, using information and data from ACNP role delineation studies and other existing literature as the basis. As part of the development phase, a survey was conducted of the 63 existing ACNP educational program directors to assess the extent of ACNP training relative to skills and procedures (see Table 14-3) and served to inform these recommendations (Kleinpell, Hravnak, Werner, & Guzman, 2006). In the next phase a Validation Panel was convened to further develop and refine the competencies to reflect national consensus. The document was then endorsed by nursing organizations and was available in 2004. This document serves to address the scope of ACNP practice in that it identifies entry level knowledge and skills that should be achieved by the student at program completion and at entry to ACNP practice (Box 14-1).

The *Scope and Standards of Practice for the Acute Care Nurse Practitioner,* initially developed jointly by the American Nurses Association and the American Association of Critical-Care Nurses in 1995 and later revised by the American Association of Critical-Care Nurses in 2006 (American Association of Critical-Care Nurses, 2006), further describes the scope of practice and standards of clinical and professional performance of the expert ACNP. This publication, when identifying scope of practice, indicates that the

---

Box 14-1 ACUTE CARE NURSE PRACTITIONER SPECIALTY CENTRAL COMPETENCIES FOR DIRECT CLINICAL PRACTICE: HEALTH PROMOTION, HEALTH PROTECTION, DISEASE PREVENTION, AND TREATMENT (ENTRY LEVEL)

A. ASSESSMENT OF HEALTH STATUS

Assesses the complex acute, critical, and chronically ill patient for urgent and emergent conditions, using both physiologically and technologically derived data, to evaluate for physiological instability and potentially life-threatening conditions.

Obtains and documents a health history for complex acute, critical, and chronically ill patients.

Performs and documents complete, system-focused, or symptom-specific physical examinations on complex acute, critical, and chronically ill patients.

Assesses the need for and performs additional screening, based on initial assessment findings.

Performs evaluations for substance use, violence, neglect and abuse, barriers to learning, and pain.

Distinguishes between normal and abnormal developmental and age-related physiological and behavioral changes in complex acute, critical, and chronic illness.

Assesses for multiple interactive and synergistic effects of pharmacological agents, including over-the-counter (OTC) preparations and alternative and complementary therapies, in patients with complex acute, critical, and chronic illness.

Assesses the impact of an acute, critical, and/or chronic illness or injury on the individuals:
- Health status (physical and mental).
- Functional status, including activity and mobility.
- Growth and development.
- Nutritional status.
- Sleep and rest patterns.
- Quality of life.
- Family, social, and educational relationships.

Provides for the promotion of health and protection from disease by assessing for risks associated with the care of complex acute, critical, and chronic illness, such as the following:
- Physiological risk, including but not limited to immobility, impaired nutrition and immunocompetence, fluid and electrolyte imbalance, invasive interventions, therapeutic modalities, and diagnostic tests.
- Psychological risk, including but not limited to impaired sleep and communication, and crisis related to threat to life, self-image, finances, medication side-effects, home and educational environment, and altered family dynamics.
- Health care system risk associated with care of complex patients, including but not limited to multiple caregivers, continuity of care, coordination of the plan of care, polypharmacy, communication with family or between multiple care providers.

Prioritizes data collection, according to the patient's immediate condition or needs, as a continuous process in acknowledgement of the dynamic nature of complex acute, critical, and chronic illness.

Assesses the needs of families and caregivers of complex acute, critical, and chronically ill patients.

B. DIAGNOSIS OF HEALTH STATUS

Diagnoses acute and chronic conditions that may result in rapid physiological deterioration or life-threatening instability.

Manages diagnostic tests through ordering, interpretation, performance, and supervision in the assessment of complex acute, critical, and chronically ill patients.

Adapted from National Panel for Acute Care Nurse Practitioner Competencies. (2004). *Acute care nurse practitioner competencies.* Washington, DC: National Organization of Nurse Practitioner Faculties.

Continued

Box 14-1 ACUTE CARE NURSE PRACTITIONER SPECIALTY CENTRAL COMPETENCIES FOR DIRECT CLINICAL PRACTICE: HEALTH PROMOTION, HEALTH PROTECTION, DISEASE PREVENTION, AND TREATMENT (ENTRY LEVEL)—CONT'D

B. DIAGNOSIS OF HEALTH STATUS—cont'd

Utilizes specialty-based technical skills in the performance of diagnostic procedures to confirm or rule out health problems.

Synthesizes data from a variety of sources to make clinical judgments and decisions about appropriate recommendations and treatments.

Prioritizes health problems during complex acute, critical, and chronic illness.

Formulates differential diagnoses by priority considering multiple potential mechanisms causing complex acute, critical, and chronic illness states.

Distinguishes complications of complex acute, critical, and chronic illness considering multi-system health problems.

Distinguishes common mental health and substance use or addictive disorder/disease, such as anxiety, depression, and alcohol and drug use, in the presence of complex acute, critical, and chronic illness.

Reformulates diagnoses by priority based on new or additional assessment data and the dynamic nature of complex acute, critical, and chronic illness.

C. PLAN OF CARE AND IMPLEMENTATION OF TREATMENT

Formulates a plan of care to address complex acute, critical, and chronic health care needs:
- Integrates knowledge of rapidly changing pathophysiology of acute and critical illness in the planning of care and implementation of treatment.
- Prescribes appropriate pharmacological and nonpharmacological treatment modalities.
- Utilizes evidence-based practice in planning and implementing care.

Implements interventions to support the patient with a rapidly deteriorating physiological condition, including the application of basic and advanced life support and other invasive interventions or procedures to regain physiological stability.

Manages, through ordering, performance, interpretation, or supervision:
- Interventions that utilize technological devices to monitor and sustain physiological function.
- Diagnostic strategies to monitor and sustain physiological function and ensure patient safety, including but not limited to ECG interpretation, x-ray interpretation, respiratory support, hemodynamic monitoring, and nutritional support.

Performs therapeutic interventions to stabilize acute and critical health problems, such as suturing, wound debridement, tube and line insertion, and lumbar puncture.

Analyzes the indications, contraindications, risk of complications, and cost-benefits of therapeutic interventions.

Manages the plan of care through evaluation, modification, and documentation according to the patient's response to therapy, changes in condition, and to therapeutic interventions to optimize patient's outcomes.

Manages the patient's response to life support strategies.

Manages pain and sedation for patients with complex acute, critical, and chronic illness:
- Prescribes pharmacological and nonpharmacological interventions.
- Monitors patient's response to sedation.
- Evaluates patient's response to therapy, and changes the plan of care accordingly.

Implements palliative and end-of-life care in collaboration with the family, patient (when possible), and other members of the multidisciplinary health care team.

Initiates appropriate referrals, and performs consultations.

Ensures that the plan of care is individualized, recognizing the dynamic nature of the patient's condition, reflecting the patient's and family's needs, and considering cost and quality benefits.

Coordinates interdisciplinary and intradisciplinary teams to develop or revise plans of care focused on patient and/or family concerns.

Incorporates health promotion, health protection, and injury prevention measures into the plan of care within the context of the complex acute, critical, and chronic illness.

Facilitates the patient's transition between and within health care settings, such as admitting, transferring, and discharging patients.

Adapted from National Panel for Acute Care Nurse Practitioner Competencies. (2004). *Acute care nurse practitioner competencies.* Washington, DC: National Organization of Nurse Practitioner Faculties.

purpose of the ACNP is to provide advanced nursing care to meet the specialized physiological and psychological needs of patients with acute, critical, and complex chronic health conditions. The population for which the ACNP provides care includes acutely and critically ill patients experiencing episodic illness, stable and/or progressive chronic illness, acute exacerbation of chronic illness, or terminal illness. The ACNP's focus is the provision of curative, rehabilitative, palliative, and maintenance care. Short-term goals include stabilizing the patient for acute and life-threatening conditions, minimizing or preventing complications, attending to co-morbidities, and promoting physical and psychological well-being. Long-term goals are restoring the patient's maximum health potential or providing palliative and end-of-life care and evaluating risk factors in achieving these outcomes. The practice environment for the ACNP is "any inpatient or outpatient setting in which the patient requires complex monitoring and therapies, high-intensity nursing interventions, or continuous nursing vigilance within the range of high-acuity care" (American Association of Critical-Care Nurses, 2006, p. 12). The "standards of clinical practice" and "standards of professional performance," along with measurement criteria examples for the ACNP as specified in this document, are summarized in Box 14-2. These standards, which are closely aligned with the APN core competencies in Chapter 3, describe a competent level of care and professional performance common to all ACNPs regardless of setting, by which the quality of expert ACNP practice can be judged. Some common themes in the standards of ACNP clinical practice and professional performance that distinguish the practice of ACNPs from other NP specialties are the dynamic nature of the patient's health and illness status, the vulnerability of the patient population, the need for continuous assessment and adjustment of the management plan in the face of rapidly changing patient conditions, and the complexity of the required monitoring and therapeutics. Additional themes include the collaborative nature of the practice and the interactive relationship between the ACNP and the health care system.

And last, a resource that does not define scope of practice but does specify the knowledge necessary to perform within the specialty scope is the ACNP national certification examination. The purpose of national certification is to provide documentation for the public that a licensed professional has demonstrated mastery of knowledge and skills necessary for safe and competent practice (Hravnak & Baldisseri, 1997). APN specialty certification serves as a primary criterion for APN practice (see Chapters 3 and 21). In addition, Medicare regulations stipulate completion of a national certification examination as a requirement for ACNPs to obtain reimbursement. ACNP certification examinations are offered by the American Nurses Credentialing Center (ANCC) and the American Association of Critical-Care Nurses (American Association of Critical-Care Nurses, 1995; American Nurses Credentialing Center [ANCC], 2004). While it is evident that the content of a certification examination should not "drive" educational standards or curriculum development, the topics and content for the ACNP certification examinations have been validated by role delineation studies and are consistent with the other documents delineating ACNP practice scope. As such, they serve to further articulate the scope of ACNP practice.

State (Government)

Each state's government provides the second mechanism whereby the ACNPs professional scope of practice is defined. The nurse practice statute for each state governs nursing practice. NP practice rules and regulations that are intended to define NP practice vary from state to state (Lugo, O'Grady, Hodnicki, & Hanson, 2007; Pearson, 2007).

Licensure, granted by the state, is required to practice a profession, guarantees a safe level of practice, and is generally not specialty-specific (Hravnak & Baldisseri, 1997). In all states, APN regulation for practice is based on basic nursing licensure, but many states have additional rules and regulations that delineate specific requirements and define and limit who can use a specific advanced practice nursing title with protection (see Chapter 21). Many states do not differentiate between NP practice specialties (family, adult, pediatric, acute care), nor do they provide a list of skills, tasks, or procedures permissible within the specialty scope. When there is doubt regarding the interpretation of the nurse practice act for application in a specific employment situation, such as an acute care facility or practice plan, it may be helpful to seek the opinion of the employer's legal counsel for clarification (Hravnak, Rosenzweig, Rust, & Magdic, 1998b). Although at the state level it is relatively easy to define limitations in scope of practice based on the age of the patient population, it is more difficult to determine scope based on patient acuity and practice

Box 14-2   STANDARDS OF CLINICAL PRACTICE AND PROFESSIONAL PERFORMANCE
FOR THE ACUTE CARE NURSE PRACTITIONER (EXPERT LEVEL)

NOTE: All reference to "patient" refers to patients with acute, critical, and complex chronic illness.

STANDARDS OF ACUTE CARE NURSE PRACTITIONER CLINICAL PRACTICE

Standard I: Assessment
The ACNP collects patient data.
Measurement criteria examples:
- Collects data in a continuous process in recognition of the dynamic nature of acute, critical, and complex chronic illness.
- Promotes and protects health by assessing for risks associated with care of acute, critical, and complex illness including physiological, psychological, and health care system risks.

Standard II: Diagnosis
The ACNP analyzes the assessment data in determining diagnoses.
Measurement criteria examples:
- Orders, performs, interprets, and supervises diagnostic tests and procedures that contribute to the formulation of the differential diagnoses, working diagnoses, and subsequent plan of care.
- Prioritizes diagnoses based on the interpretation of available data and the complexity and severity of the patient's condition.

Standard III: Outcome Identification
The ACNP identifies expected outcomes individualized to the patient.
Measurement criteria examples:
- Identifies expected outcomes that incorporate scientific evidence and are achievable through the implementation of evidence-based practices.
- Collaborates with the patient, the family, and the interdisciplinary team in establishing desired restorative, curative, rehabilitative, maintenance, palliative, and end-of-life care outcomes.

Standard IV: Planning
The ACNP develops a plan of care that prescribes interventions to attain expected outcomes.
Measurement criteria examples:
- Is individualized and dynamic and can be applied across the continuum of acute care services.

- Prescribes the diagnostic strategies and therapeutic interventions (both pharmacological and nonpharmacological) needed to achieve expected outcomes.
- Incorporates health promotion, health protection, and injury prevention measures that are specific to acute, critical, and complex chronic illness.

Standard V: Implementation
The ACNP implements the interventions identified in the interdisciplinary plan of care.
Measurement criteria examples:
- Prescribes interventions consistent with the established interdisciplinary plan of care.
- Implements interventions to support the patient with a rapidly deteriorating physiological condition, including application of basic and advanced life support and other invasive interventions or procedures to regain physiological stability.

Standard VI: Evaluation
The ACNP evaluates the patient's progress toward attainment of expected outcomes.
Measurement criteria examples:
- Performs a systematic and ongoing evaluation of each patient to assess the effectiveness and appropriateness of the interventions.
- Incorporates the use of quality indicators, scientific evidence, and the risk/benefit analysis of the treatment process when evaluating the patient's progress toward expected outcomes.
- Consults and makes appropriate referrals as needed, based on the evaluation process.

STANDARDS OF ACUTE CARE NURSE PRACTITIONER PROFESSIONAL PERFORMANCE

Standard I: Professional Practice
The ACNP evaluates his or her clinical practice in relation to institutional guidelines, professional practice standards, and relevant statutes and regulations.
Measurement criteria example:
- Collects and analyzes data regarding the performance of procedures, delivery of care, the incidence and types of individual care complications, and the resulting effect on patients, in order to evaluate and improve practice.

Adapted from American Association of Critical-Care Nurses. (2006). *Scope and standards of practice for the acute care nurse practitioner.* Aliso Viejo, CA: Author.
ACNP, Acute care nurse practitioner.

Box 14-2 STANDARDS OF CLINICAL PRACTICE AND PROFESSIONAL PERFORMANCE FOR THE ACUTE CARE NURSE PRACTITIONER (EXPERT LEVEL)—CONT'D

STANDARDS OF ACUTE CARE NURSE PRACTITIONER PROFESSIONAL PERFORMANCE—cont'd

Standard II: Education

The ACNP acquires and maintains current knowledge in advanced nursing practice.

Measurement criteria example:

- Is accountable for self-engagement in educational activities related to the clinical care of acute, critical, and complex chronically ill individuals, and professional practice.

Standard III: Collaboration

The ACNP collaborates with the patient, family, and other health care providers in patient care.

Measurement criteria example:

- Consults and collaborates with the patient, family, and other health care providers to provide coordinated, interdisciplinary care.

Standard IV: Ethics

The ACNP integrates ethical considerations into all areas of practice.

Measurement criteria example:

- Contributes to individual and system responses in the resolution of ethical dilemmas.

Standard V: Systems Management

The ACNP develops and participates in organizational systems and processes promoting optimal patient outcomes.

Measurement criteria example:

- Analyzes organizational system enhancements and barriers that have an impact on patient care.

Standard VI: Resource Utilization

The ACNP considers factors related to safety, effectiveness, and cost in planning and delivering care.

Measurement criteria example:

- Assists interdisciplinary team members, patients, and families in selecting therapies that integrate perspectives of cost and quality or benefits.

Standard VII: Leadership

The ACNP provides leadership in the practice setting and the profession.

Measurement criteria examples:

- Promotes dissemination of knowledge and advances the profession through writing, publishing, and presenting to professional or lay audiences.
- Demonstrates leadership through teaching, coaching, and supporting others in the advancement of the plan of care for patients with acute, critical, and complex chronic illness.

Standard VIII: Collegiality

The ACNP contributes to the professional development of peers, colleagues, and others.

Measurement criteria examples:

- Identifies and participates in opportunities to share skills, knowledge, and strategies for patient care and system improvement with colleagues and other health care providers.
- Promotes a mutually respectful environment that enables nursing and other health care personnel to make optimal individual contributions, and systems to function most effectively.

Standard IX: Quality of Practice

The ACNP systematically evaluates and enhances the quality and effectiveness of advanced nursing practice and care delivery across the continuum of acute care services.

Measurement criteria examples:

- Participates in formal and informal evaluations of the quality and effectiveness of care delivered to patients with acute, critical, and complex chronic illness.
- Formulates recommendations to improve clinical practice based on data obtained from the work environment, quality-of-care activities, and scientific evidence.

Standard X: Research

The ACNP continually explores scientific knowledge, identifies specific research priorities in practice, and strives to enhance knowledge and skills through participation in research studies and provision of evidence-based practice.

Measurement criteria examples:

- Demonstrates informational literacy through the application of evidence-based practice to support decision making and improve practice.
- Implements diagnostic strategies and treatment interventions substantiated by relevant research.

setting. Regulations relative to acuity and setting are not well defined and vary considerably by state (Percy & Sperhac, 2007).

Institutional

As noted previously, the majority of ACNPs provide patient care within health care institutions. Institutions may further delineate the ACNP's scope of practice within that facility by identifying the patient population the ACNP serves and the process for collaboration with other health care providers in the institution (Magdic, Hravnak, & McCartney, 2005). This further specification of the ACNP's practice scope may be set forth in job descriptions, in hospital policy, or through the health care agency's credentialing and privileging process.

An employer is responsible for the acts an employee performs on the employer's behalf, but the employer is not held responsible if an employee steps beyond the bounds the employer sets forth (Cummings, 1997). Hospitals bear a legal responsibility to protect their clientele and hold some degree of vicarious liability for the actions of both physician and non-physician providers serving their patient population even when they are not employees of the hospital. Employers and hospitals therefore have the right to further delineate a specific health care provider's scope of practice within the employment situation. Documentation of initial training as well as ongoing provider competence in the application of specific skills is needed. This "scope of employment" may not exceed the scope of practice specified by the state's nurse practice act but may be curtailed based on the needs and mission of the employer. The institutional "scope of employment" may take the form of a job description, hospital policy, or both (Cummings, Fraser, & Tarlier, 2003; Hravnak et al., 1998b). In settings in which the ACNP role is being newly introduced, a job description may not exist. In general, the job description should include ACNP performance standards and responsibilities as they relate to patient care, collaborative relationships, professional conduct, and professional development, and these institutional performance standards can provide a template for ACNP performance evaluation.

When providing care within a health care institution, the ACNP will also need to undergo the process of provider credentialing and privileging by the institution, whether the ACNP is an employee of the hospital or an employee of a hospital-affiliated or private practice plan (see Chapter 21). The ACNP is required to provide proof of licensure, certification, educational preparation, (generally) malpractice insurance, and skill performance (training, numbers performed, proof of competency) (Hravnak & Baldisseri, 1997). Institutional credentialing is necessary for the ACNP to provide care to patients within the institution, although the ACNP may or may not hold a medical staff appointment.

Once an individual is credentialed, a determination is made regarding the clinical privileges that may be granted and is the process whereby the institution determines which medical procedures may be performed and which conditions may be treated by both physician and non-physician providers (Magdic, Hravnak, & McCartney, 2005). Although an appropriately educated provider may be permitted by statute to perform certain acts or skills, the hospital is not bound to grant the provider this privilege. The clinical privileges of the ACNP are based partly on the ACNP's professional license, certification, and inherent scope of practice, documented training, experience, competence, and health status. For example, the ACNP who has received educational preparation for performing invasive diagnostic procedures such as insertion of central line catheters and endotracheal intubation may request that these privileges be a part of his or her "institutional" scope of practice if he or she can provide proof of training and competency along with documentation that the skill is required for the job. An ACNP may periodically request new privileges based on evolving mastery of skills, further training, and changes in services needed by the patient population and institution. ACNPs must understand that although they may be qualified to perform certain procedures, privileges to perform these acts may not necessarily be granted or renewed (usually on a biannual basis) if the patient population the ACNP serves does not require these skills or if ongoing application and competency in the skill during the renewal period cannot be documented.

Most ACNPs will be required to participate in institutional credentialing and privileging processes. In a survey of 321 ACNPs, Kleinpell (2005) reported that most were credentialed (81%-86%) and had privileges (79%-84%). The majority reported receiving their credentials and privileges from the medical staff office (69%-83%), whereas the minority received theirs from the department of nursing (8%-12%) or human resources department (2%-4%). Because credentialing and privileging are forms of peer review, it is imperative that APNs participate in the process (Briggs, Heath, & Kelley, 2005).

Service Related

The functions of the ACNP are also adjusted according to the needs of the specialty patient population served or of the care delivery team (i.e., service) in the organization with which the ACNP is affiliated. This service-related scope outlines the clinical functions and tasks that may be administered by the ACNP specific to the service team with which the ACNP works and the needs of the specialty patient population served (Hravnak et al., 1998b). For example, an ACNP working with a cardiology service may initiate treatment for myocardial ischemia or infarction; an ACNP working with an oncology service may perform bone marrow aspirations or order antibiotics for suspected opportunistic infection; an ACNP on a renal medicine service may write orders for hemodialysis and insert central venous dialysis catheters; an ACNP with the cardiovascular surgery service may harvest the vein grafts for coronary artery bypass surgery; and an ACNP in the medical intensive care unit (MICU) may intubate and place arterial and central venous catheters. Therefore service-related scope may vary among ACNPs affiliated with various services or specialties within the same institution and even among those who function under the same generic job description. The service-related scope outlines a more detailed and specific description of the types of activities the ACNP will perform as a member of the practice.

In states in which physician collaboration is a requirement or in cases in which the health care organization has collaborative guidelines, the ACNP's institutional and service-related scope of practice and clinical privileges may be determined collaboratively by the physician and ACNP and set forth in a written agreement. This written agreement for collaborative practice then provides the source document on which the hospital makes privileging decisions. Written agreements, often formatted as a checklist, are frequently helpful because the detail included in a written agreement usually cannot be spelled out in a job description. Job descriptions, by their very nature, tend to be more general to cover ACNPs working in a variety of settings within the institution. In addition to outlining the specific activities that the ACNP performs, the agreement might also specify the level of communication or degree of supervision between the ACNP and the physician that is required before the performance of a specific function (Shapiro & Rosenberg, 2002). An ACNP with novice skills in central line insertion may require direct supervision for a specified period or number of successful attempts, but as the ACNP approaches expert status, the level of supervision may be decreased to minimal or none. Eventually, as the ACNP's expertise continues to advance, he or she may supervise medical trainees or novice ACNPs in these skills. As skills progress, the written agreement, if required, will also need to be modified. In some cases, the written agreement may be used to communicate the ACNP's scope of employment to other members of the health care team, such as staff nurses and pharmacists.

When negotiating the written agreement, both the ACNP and the collaborating physicians need to ensure that no function is in conflict with the individual state's nurse practice act and the policies of the particular institution. Nevertheless, the agreement should not serve as a barrier to practice but, rather, be written as broadly as reasonable to allow for practicality, flexibility, and optimization of practice within the context of experience and safety.

Individual

The final determinant of scope of practice is role individualization by each ACNP. Experience, specialization, interest, motivation, self-esteem, personal ethics, personality traits, and communication style affect the employment opportunities, clinical specialties, skills, practice arrangements, and the degree of autonomy the ACNP will seek out and/or apply in his or her uniquely personal enactment of the role (Hravnak et al., 1998b).

COMPETENCIES OF THE ACUTE CARE NURSE PRACTITIONER ROLE

The central and core competencies for the APN, as explained in Chapter 3, form the foundation of ACNP practice. The central competency for all APNs is direct clinical practice in concert with the other six core competencies of coaching/guidance; consultation; research skills; clinical, professional and systems leadership; collaboration; and ethical decision-making skills. The ways in which ACNPs enact these core competencies are consistent with other APN specialties, as discussed in Chapters 5 through 11. In addition, ACNPs share common entry-level competencies in accordance with the *Domains and Competencies of Nurse Practitioner*

Practice (NONPF, 2006). Although the ACNP may need to use specialty skills and knowledge in the care of acutely and critically ill adults, ACNPs have the following factors in common with the other NP specialties: (1) a generalist nursing foundation, (2) a health promotion basis to their practice, and (3) the development and appreciation of diagnostic reasoning skills. ACNPs prepared at the Doctor of Nursing Practice (DNP) level may have additional knowledge and skills including refined communication, indepth scientific foundations, analytic skills for evaluating and providing evidence-based practice, advanced knowledge of the health care delivery systems and population-based care, the business aspects of practice, and an emphasis on independent and interprofessional practice (AACN, 2005; National Panel for NP Practice Doctorate Competencies, 2006).

Acute Care Nurse Practitioner Specialty Competencies

In addition to the core APN competencies, each of the NP specialties has unique competencies that differentiate practice. As just noted, ACNP entry level competencies are illustrated in *Acute Care Nurse Practitioner Competencies* (National Panel for Acute Care Nurse Practitioner Competencies, 2004) and expert competencies in the *Scope and Standards of Practice for the Acute Care Nurse Practitioner* (American Association of Critical-Care Nurses, 2006). A discussion of how these ACNP competencies are carried out within the framework of the APN core competencies in Chapter 3 follows.

Acute Care Nurse Practitioner Specialty Central Competency: Direct Clinical Practice. Direct clinical practice, the central competency of ACNP practice, is the function that consumes the greatest percentage of ACNP practice time (Kleinpell, 2005; Rosenfeld, McEvoy, & Glassman, 2003). Prior clinical nursing expertise is essential for the ACNP role, since even the novice ACNP cares for acutely and critically ill patients who may precipitously manifest life-threatening conditions that mandate an immediate response. These situations demand a strong clinical practice foundation.

The specialty practice of ACNPs consists of both short-term goals of care (stabilize patients, minimize complications, promote physical and psychological well-being) and long-term goals (restore maximum health potential, evaluate risk factors) (American Association of Critical-Care Nurses, 2006). ACNPs

achieve these specialty practice goals through the performance of cognitive skills common to all APNs, such as patient assessment, critical thinking, diagnostic reasoning, case management, and the prescription of therapeutic interventions. Assessing and intervening in complex, urgent, or emergency situations are key components of ACNP specialty competencies (Kleinpell & Hravnak, 2002; National Panel for Acute Care Nurse Practitioner Competencies, 2004).

The central competencies of direct clinical practice as they apply to ACNP specialty practice can be broadly characterized as those related to (1) diagnosing and managing disease and (2) the promotion and protection of health (see Box 14-1).

Acute Care Nurse Practitioner Central Competency: Direct Clinical Practice— Diagnosing and Managing Disease. For ACNPs to achieve the specialty competencies to diagnose and manage disease in their specialty patient population, they must demonstrate mastery of advanced pathophysiology, completion of a prioritized health history and both comprehensive and focused physical examinations, rapid assessment of unstable and complex health problems, implementation of diagnostic strategies and therapeutic interventions to stabilize health care problems, demonstration of technical competence with procedures, modification of the plan of care based on a client's changing condition and response to interventions, and collaboration with other care providers to facilitate positive outcomes (Kleinpell & Hravnak, 2002; National Panel for Acute Care Nurse Practitioner Competencies, 2004). The varied practice settings of individual ACNPs across the continuum of acute care delivery services result in associated variance in some of the competencies that they perform (Barkley & Rogers, 2001). Most ACNPs practice in acute and critical care settings that include subacute care, emergency care, and intensive care settings. These include but are not limited to acute and critical care neurology (Sarkissian & Wennberg, 1999), pulmonology (Burns & Earven, 2002), transplantation (Martin, 1999; Reel, 1999), presurgical and perioperative care (Fox, Schira, & Wadlund, 2000; Guido, 2004), emergency care (Cole & Kleinpell, 2006), pain management services (Barkley & Whitney, 2001), and cardiac surgery (Meyer & Miers, 2005). A growing number of ACNPs also practice in specialty-based practice settings, such as clinics, medical rehabilitation, home care, long-term care, sports medicine, holistic medicine, occupational medicine, employee health, mental health services, and medical flight programs (Kleinpell, 2005; Kleinpell-Nowell, 2001). Individual elements of the ACNP role differ depending on these varied practice settings and on the specialty patient populations served, but the basic elements necessary to function as a generalist ACNP remain. Kleinpell (2005) reported results of a 5-year longitudinal study of ACNP respondents (certified between 1996 and 1998) (n = 445 in year 1, and n = 321 in year 5). Most respondents were women (95%) and white (95%) with a mean age of 43 years (range 29-63 years). Nearly three quarters of the ACNP respondents reported having at least some of their work responsibilities in tertiary care settings, with up to 26% seeing patients in coronary intensive care units (ICUs), 18% in surgical ICUs, 19% in cardiothoracic ICUs, 16% in medical ICUs, 8% in neurological ICUs, and 4% in transplant ICUs. Other areas of specialty practice included emergency care, oncology, and multi-practice clinics. Respondents to the survey indicated that their principal role responsibility was direct patient care, with 85% to 89% of their time spent in that responsibility (Table 14-1). They also reported being involved, albeit to a lesser degree, in teaching, research, department projects, program development, administrative responsibilities, and quality assurance projects. Rosenfeld and colleagues (2003) corroborated Kleinpell's finding that although ACNPs assume responsibilities beyond their predominant activity of direct patient care, the amount of time spent in other activities is much less.

The performance of patient procedures, some of which are invasive, also constitutes a portion of ACNP's direct clinical practice. Technical procedures most commonly performed by respondents to Kleinpell's survey are listed in Table 14-1. The literature corroborates ACNP technical skill performance, such as endotracheal intubation, central line placement, pulmonary artery line placement, needle thoracotomy, chest tube insertion and removal, and cricothyrotomy for the trauma critical care focus (Keough, Jennrich, Holm, & Marshall, 1996); nerve block, joint needle aspiration, diagnostic peritoneal lavage, needle decompression of the chest, lumbar puncture, chest tube insertion, cricothyrotomy and tracheostomy, suturing of lacerations and wounds, and splinting of injuries for the emergency care focus (Cole & Ramirez, 2000); endotracheal and nasotracheal intubation, chest tube insertion and removal, arterial puncture, and insertion of central

lines for the critical care focus (Kleinpell, Hravnak, Werner, & Guzman, 2006). An imperative understanding is that procedural skill performance is not limited to the task itself but also includes knowledge of the indications, contraindications, complications, and skill in managing complications. When performing a procedural skill to derive physiological data, such as mean arterial pressure, pulmonary artery pressure, or lumbar cerebrospinal fluid pressure, the ACNP must be able to use this information skillfully for patient evaluation. ACNPs are also compelled to collect their individual practice data related to procedure performance, including number and type of complications, and use these data to document ongoing skill competence and facilitate patient safety. The practice of an ACNP in a cardiothoracic surgical ICU, which illustrates the integration of technical skills within the context of diagnosis and management of disease, is provided in Exemplar 14-1.

Acute Care Nurse Practitioner Central Competency: Direct Clinical Practice— Promoting and Protecting Health and Preventing Disease. In addition to disease diagnosis and management, ACNPs also provide services to promote and protect health and prevent disease (American Association of Critical-Care Nurses, 2006; National Panel for Acute Care Nurse Practitioner Competencies, 2004). These services include providing anticipatory guidance and counseling to patients and their families. Inevitably, some of the methods ACNPs use to implement health promotion/protection and disease prevention vary from those used by NPs in the primary care specialties. Variations in application are related to the prioritization of needs during acute and critical illness. In some practice models, the episodic nature of the relationship between the ACNP and the patient/family is limited to a single acute illness event. Hospitalization can provide a critical window of opportunity for ACNPs to address health promotion and disease prevention with patients (Genet Kelley & Daly, 2001).

ACNPs are skilled in a unique form of health promotion/protection and disease prevention: recognizing and modifying health risk factors associated with an inpatient stay. These "system" factors are inherent to patients experiencing an acute critical illness requiring hospitalization and are consequences of the methods and realities of "institutionalized" care (Hravnak, 1998). The ACNP is qualified to identify the additional health problems for which the acutely and

Table 14-1   SURVEY RESULTS FROM 320 ACUTE CARE NURSE PRACTITIONERS REPORTING ACTIVITIES AND PROCEDURES PERFORMED*

Activities		Procedures	
Activity	**% Respondents Performed**	**Procedure**	**% Respondents Performed**
DIRECT PATIENT CARE		Examine and clean wounds	70%
Discuss care issues with patients and family members	96%	Perform defibrillation	52%
Order and interpret routine clinical laboratory tests	96%	Insert nasogastric feeding tubes	47%
Order and interpret radiographs	93%	Apply local anesthetics	47%
Initiate specialty consultation	94%	Pack wounds	47%
Interpret 12-lead electrocardiograms	81%	Perform wound care and debridement	45%
Initiate discharge planning	82%	Perform routine incision and drainage	35%
Initiate and adjust intravenous infusion rates	82%	Perform cardioversion	33%
Initiate blood component therapy	69%	Suture superficial lacerations	29%
Give nursing in-service training	67%	Manipulate pulmonary artery catheter	24%
Initiate and adjust nutritional feedings	52%	Initiate use of central venous catheters	19%
Manage resuscitative efforts	52%	Initiate use of arterial catheters	19%
Initiate and adjust vasoactive drug infusions	51%	Remove intracardiac catheters	18%
Initiate quality improvement/quality assurance study	40%	Initiate use of peripheral venous catheters	18%
Initiate use of muscle relaxants	43%	Perform needle thoracentesis	9%
Manage patients receiving mechanical ventilation	32%	Perform lumbar punctures	9%
Initiate and adjust mechanical ventilation	28%	Perform endotracheal intubations	9%
Adjust temporary pacemaker settings	27%	Insert pulmonary artery catheters	9%
Adjust settings on cardiac assistive devices	13%	Insert chest tubes	7%
Administer chemotherapy	6%		

Adapted from Kleinpell, R.M. (2005). Acute care nurse practitioner practice: Results of a 5-year longitudinal survey. *American Journal of Critical Care, 14,* 211-221.

*As reported by 320 ACNPs certified from 1996 to 1998, participating in the fifth year of a longitudinal survey.

TABLE 14-1   SURVEY RESULTS FROM 320 ACUTE CARE NURSE PRACTITIONERS REPORTING
ACTIVITIES AND PROCEDURES PERFORMED*—CONT'D

Responsibility	% Respondents Performed	Responsibility	% Respondents Performed
INDIRECT PATIENT CARE			
Administrative	26.8%	Research	23.4%
Department projects	21.5%	Program development	15.3%
Teaching	40.8%	Quality assurance	20.2%

 EXEMPLAR 14-1   Acute Care Nurse Practitioner Practice in an Intensive Care Unit

In the CTICU, the ACNP Marie functions collaboratively with the critical care provider team consisting of the ACNP, an attending physician (intensivist), one or two critical care medicine fellows, a clinical pharmacist, and other members of the delivery team including bedside nurses, primary care nurses, and respiratory therapists. The team works in collaboration with the surgeons, surgical fellows, and residents on the cardiac, thoracic, transplant, vascular, and trauma services. As the CTICU ACNP, Marie manages the patient from admission to discharge from the unit.

The day begins with a report from the team members who provided care during the previous night, highlighting changes in patients' conditions and providing information on new patients. Marie participates in dynamic patient-focused rounds during which each patient is examined at the bedside and interviewed when possible. A wealth of other data is reviewed, including vital signs, hemodynamic data (pulmonary artery pressures, central venous pressures, cardiac outputs), ventilator settings, and results of previous weaning trials, chest radiographs and diagnostic testing, laboratory and culture data, and a complete list of medications, continuous infusions, and fluid balances. Based on the clinical examination and review of data and with input from members of the provider and delivery team, a comprehensive plan of care is devised for the patient. Marie assumes varying roles during these patient-focused rounds (e.g., presenting and reviewing data, doing the physical examination, writing orders, calling consultants). During this time, Marie is noting issues to be addressed later, treatment outcomes to follow up, planned procedures, culture and diagnostic test results to review, family conferences, and expected admissions and discharges. Once rounds are complete, Marie will begin to address some of the specific issues on her work list.

Marie begins by seeing the four patients who are to be transferred out of the CTICU care unit that morning. She briefly examines each patient and reviews their data to ensure that the patients' responses to interventions are appropriate. She verifies that these patients have been weaned from their vasoactive medicines and removes their chest tubes. Marie reviews each patient's H&P and restarts home medications that are appropriate to the patients' cardiac conditions and co-morbidities. She writes transfer orders and collaborates with the bedside nurse to ensure that all patient care issues have been addressed in the orders. One patient has a history of active smoking, and Marie discusses with the patient the relationship between smoking and heart disease, as well as smoking cessation strategies. One patient needs to maintain a central intravenous access on the hospital ward. Marie converts the 14-gauge introducer in the patient's right internal jugular vein to a triple-lumen catheter using re-wire technique. One patient has developed an arrhythmia with some hemodynamic instability, and Marie initiates appropriate treatment, cancels the patient's transfer to the floor, and informs the intensivist of the change in condition. One patient is being transferred to a subacute-care facility. Marie collaborates with the unit case manager to finalize transfer plans, speaks

ACNP, Acute care nurse practitioner; *CQI,* continuous quality improvement; *CTICU,* cardiothoracic intensive care unit; *H&P,* history and physical.

Continued

EXEMPLAR 14-1   **Acute Care Nurse Practitioner Practice in an Intensive Care Unit—cont'd**

with the patient's family before discharge, and speaks with the receiving team in the subacute-care facility to ensure continuity of care. During the course of the day, Marie might perform other invasive procedures, such as inserting arterial lines, central venous lines, dialysis catheters, chest tubes, and nasoduodenal feeding tubes and performing thoracentesis, endotracheal intubation, and removal of intra-aortic balloons. Health promotion and protection assessment and intervention are integral to Marie's role but in different areas than one might expect in the primary care setting. For example, in the CTICU, Marie addresses stress ulcer prophylaxis, preventing complications from immobility, promoting skin integrity, and nutritional support.

Marie will continuously monitor the patients on the unit throughout the day and provide problem-focused care in response to changing patient needs and condition. She will be contacted by the nurse providing bedside care for the patient to address patient problems such as hypotension, hypertension, low cardiac output, low urine output, bleeding, low oxygen saturations, fever, difficulty with ventilation or ventilator changes, agitation and delirium, mental status changes, inadequate pain management, arrhythmias, electrolyte abnormalities, and problems with lines or catheters. She will see patients multiple times throughout the day in response to these concerns, each time assessing possible causes, performing directed physical examinations, formulating a treatment plan, and reassessing clinical findings to evaluate response to therapy. Some treatments Marie initiates independently, whereas other more complex situations may require her to consult with the intensivist and/or surgeon to review the management options. Marie will provide consultative services to the cardiologists, who visit their patients daily.

During the day, Marie also participates in the care of patients newly admitted after surgery. As patients arrive from the operating room, Marie receives a brief report from the anesthesiologist and surgical fellow. She reviews the chart, examines the patient, and reviews initial laboratory results, electrocardiograph results, and chest radiograph results. She reviews the plan of care with the critical care nurse and respiratory therapist. She documents a progress note and writes orders and then returns frequently to reassess the patient's status and adjust the plan. One postoperative patient is bleeding severely. Marie alerts the surgeon, orders and reviews a coagulation profile, and ensures that the patient is being rewarmed. She orders blood products to correct the abnormality and monitors the patient to determine whether this therapy is effective or whether the patient will have to return to the operating room for mediastinal exploration.

At the end of the day, the team rounds again, seeing the new patients, evaluating the progress of and plans for other patients, and developing a plan for the next 12-hour period. The dynamic environment of the CTICU and the changing CTICU team members require the ACNP to frequently assess and reassess patient condition, remain flexible and responsive to subtle changes, and carefully organize and manage time.

As a permanent member of the critical care team, Marie provides needed continuity to care. She is available to interact with social services, case managers, physical and occupational therapists, and nutritional consultants. She is able to participate in discharge planning. She is readily available to the nursing staff for questions or problem solving. She participates in the CTICU's CQI activities. She participates in research protocols, screens patients for eligibility criteria, and educates others concerning the research initiatives. Marie plays an important role in communication with patients and families and has a unique opportunity for teaching and reinforcing teaching.

ACNP, Acute care nurse practitioner; *CQI,* continuous quality improvement; *CTICU,* cardiothoracic intensive care unit; *H&P,* history and physical.

critically ill are at risk and to implement strategies to minimize or prevent that risk. This area forms a distinctive health promotion and health protection aspect of ACNP practice. As direct care providers, ACNPs have the ability to activate strategies and systems to implement primary, secondary, or tertiary prevention initiatives related to these unique inpatient risk factors. For example, some of the risk factors imposed by an inpatient stay are physiological in nature: immobility, decreased nutritional intake, fluid and electrolyte imbalance, altered immunocompetence, impairment of self-care ability, existing or developing co-morbid disease states, and risks associated with invasive diagnostic and therapeutic interventions. Other risks have a psychological foundation: psychological consequences of alterations in the patient's physical abilities and alteration of his or her environment, sleep deprivation, communication impairment, alteration of self-image, role reversal, financial challenges, knowledge deficits, and the consequences of medication administration including but not limited to delirium and depression. Families are also influenced by many of these risks and require ACNP services. In addition, risk factors related to hospitalization itself and the multiplicity of caregivers include discontinuity of care, polypharmacy, system inefficiency and redundancy, miscommunication with families, and miscommunication among caregivers (American Association of Critical-Care Nurses, 2006; Hravnak, 1998; National Panel for Acute Care Nurse Practitioner Competencies, 2004). The ACNP is competent to assess patients for these unique risks and implement interventions to prevent their occurrence or minimize their consequences. Although these skills are common to all ACNPs, those prepared at the DNP level are equipped to assume leadership roles in developing, implementing, and evaluating evidence-based interventions to address and improve population health and clinical prevention (AACN, 2005).

ADDITIONAL ADVANCED PRACTICE NURSE CORE COMPETENCIES AS ENACTED BY ACUTE CARE NURSE PRACTITIONERS

In addition to direct clinical practice, the ACNP also performs the APN core competencies described in Chapter 3, with specialization unique to the ACNP role. Providing expert guidance and coaching of patients, families, and other health care providers is a core competency that is an essential part of ACNP care. In the primary care area, the plan of care may be mutually determined and fully implemented between the NP and patient/family dyad. In contrast, the process of assessment and diagnosis, care planning, implementation, and evaluation in the acute care setting, while still centering on the ACNP and patient/family dyad, will likely include a number of other individuals, including but not limited to physicians, other nurses, respiratory therapists, dietitians, pharmacists, physical and occupational therapists, social workers, and clergy. In this complex setting, the ACNP's ability to plan, interpret, and explain the plan of care while educating others about disease processes is a valued aspect of the ACNP role. Often, critical illness can require many complex treatments, and ACNPs are able to provide teaching to families, nursing staff, and other members of the health care team to facilitate knowledge of indicated care. The core competency of coaching and guidance is played out at the highest levels when ACNPs prepare patients for discharge after serious illness or when they assist and prepare family members to care for loved ones who have undergone catastrophic or debilitating health problems (Rhodes & Carlson, 2001). At times, patients (particularly the poor and uninsured) may not have a consistent primary care provider in the outpatient setting. In this case, the ACNP becomes an important source for health information and health promotion/protection interventions during the inpatient encounter (Genet Kelley & Daly, 2001). Some patients may be more receptive to health teaching that occurs in proximity to an acute health event (e.g., diet and exercise information after an acute myocardial infarction). ACNPs also provide coaching for both experienced and inexperienced nurses in complex care settings.

ACNPs often provide consultation; use, promote, and conduct research; and provide clinical, professional, and systems leadership. The consultative activities of the ACNP may take the form of a formal medical consultation. Sometimes consultative services by the ACNP are delivered in more informal exchanges regarding the patient's condition and plan of care with other health care providers. This aspect of the ACNP's practice is invaluable in the teaching hospital setting. In this environment, attending physicians and medical trainees rotate on and off the service and staffing patterns may result in inconsistencies in bedside nursing care. As the consistent member of the health care provider team, the ACNP is able to use consultative skills to keep the team informed of the patient's condition and changing plan of care during the entire length of stay. ACNPs have also demonstrated that their consultative services in evaluating patients after ICU discharge to lower-acuity care settings can decrease ICU readmission rates (Green & Edmonds, 2004). Research competencies may also vary among ACNP providers. All ACNPs use research to deliver evidence-based medical and nursing care, whereas a smaller number of ACNPs may actively participate in or lead research initiatives.

All ACNPs provide some form of professional, clinical, and systems leadership in their provider role: by serving as mentors and role models for staff nurses; by taking on selected administrative responsibilities in the health care agency; and by acting as care facilitators and change agents within the health care system. ACNPs prepared at the DNP level perform these activities at an even higher level of specificity and autonomy. ACNPs coordinate care delivery in the health care system, and several studies have demonstrated that this aspect of ACNP practice reduces inpatient length of stay (Burns & Earven, 2002; Russell, VorderBreugge, & Burns, 2002). Promoting a positive healing environment and espousing assertiveness and conflict negotiation skills are beneficial qualities for ACNPs. ACNPs work to facilitate both individual practice and health care system change through their participation in quality assurance or continuous quality improvement (CQI) initiatives (Kleinpell, 2005; Rosenfeld, McEvoy, & Glassman, 2003, Rundio, 2001a). Participating in the planning and implementation of system-wide cost-containment or cost-effective initiatives is also an aspect of the ACNP role. The range of opportunities to create system change in the ACNP role is infinite. With their other APN colleagues, all ACNPs bear responsibility for providing leadership to advance health care policy that affects not only their practice but also the quality of care for patients and families in the acute and critical care environment (Riley-Bryan & Barkley, 2001).

Collaboration is one of the most frequently practiced core competencies of ACNPs. Collaborative practice in the clinical setting means "cooperatively working together, sharing responsibility for solving problems and making decisions to formulate and carry out plans for patient care" (Baggs & Schmitt, 1988; see also Chapter 10). In the acute care setting, patient care delivery is always a collaborative effort of the multiple members of the multidisciplinary health care team. Therefore the ability to collaborate successfully is one of the critical components of the ACNP role. In a collaborative practice model, the emphasis is on patient outcomes. Each professional should be responsible for providing the care for which he or she is best prepared. A collaborative practice model in acute care focuses on the idea that each patient needs the services of different types of providers simultaneously (King & Baggs, 1998). It has been suggested that the dyad of APN and physician forms the core of collaborative practice in acute care (King & Baggs, 1998; Shapiro & Rosenberg, 2002). The advantage to this model is the ongoing continuity and coordination of care. To formulate a collaborative dyad between the ACNP and physician, each partner must achieve full professional status. This means that each partner has completed basic and postgraduate education, which, in turn, allows him or her to take advantage of and use the full scope of practice of each of the partners. In turn, this assump-

tion refutes the resident replacement model that has been put forth by some as a role for APNs (King & Baggs, 1998).

Although there has been much support for collaborative practice between nurses and physicians, barriers still exist. Unfortunately, these barriers are created between those for whom collaborative practice should be the focus—other nurses and physicians. Incomplete understanding of the ACNP role may lead to concern among both physicians and nurses that, perhaps, ACNPs are inappropriately adopting or selling out to the medical model and trying to practice like "mini-doctors" (King & Baggs, 1998). However, there is growing recognition that the ACNP role promotes a collaborative model of care (Kleinpell, 1999; Kleinpell & Hravnak, 2002).

Electronic communication is another competency that is particularly enacted in the ACNP role. Much if not all of the data retrieval and care documentation that ACNPs perform occurs via electronic clinical information systems within health care institutions. Communication regarding institutional or practice-group–based quality improvement or benchmarking frequently happens electronically. Advances in technology and the use of electronic devices such as personal digital assistants (PDAs) in the clinical setting have impacted patient care in acute and critical care settings and help facilitate coordination of care and the application of treatment protocols. ACNPs may also use electronic devices and programs to track their patient caseload and activities and record procedures—all of which are a necessary part of institutional credentialing and privileging.

The final core competency comprises ethical decision making. ACNPs often find themselves acting as advocates for patients in care dilemmas. The age of the acutely and critically ill patient population (Miller, 2001), the routine application of life-sustaining interventions (Penas & Barkley, 2001), aggressive resuscitation, and a patient pool that often includes victims of violence or abuse (Greenberg, 1996) frequently place ACNPs and their patients in ethical emergencies. Because ACNPs are often involved in planning and implementing end-of-life care, ethical decision-making skills are an essential component of ACNP practice (American Association of Critical-Care Nurses, 2006; Rundio, 2001a). In helping facilitate ethical decision making, ACNPs can be instrumental in resolving moral issues and building ethical practice environments (see Chapter 11).

PROFILES OF THE ACUTE CARE NURSE PRACTITIONER ROLE

Although the majority of ACNPs practice in acute and critical care settings, they have transitioned into a variety of role implementation models in ever-expanding specialty-area practice sites (Kleinpell, 2005). One ACNP role implementation model focuses on episodic management of patients in a single clinical specialty unit, one model involves following a caseload of hospitalized patients throughout their hospitalization, and another focuses on managing patients across the entire continuum of acute care services, from hospitalization to home.

The ACNP model focusing on *episodic care of patients on a specialty clinical inpatient unit* provides the earliest model of ACNP practice (Howie-Esquivel & Fontaine, 2006; Kleinpell & Hravnak, 2005). Under this model, the ACNP, in collaboration with a physician specialist, might manage the care of a patient admitted to a specialty inpatient unit with an acutely unstable medical or surgical condition. Once the patient is stabilized, the patient is transferred to another clinical unit under the care of another provider. Under this model, ACNPs confine their practice to episodic care at a defined level of acute care, permitting them to develop their skill and knowledge about specific conditions in a delineated setting. Exemplar 14-1 provided an example of this model. The limitation of this model is that it does not allow for continuity of care across the continuum.

In another model of role implementation, the ACNP directly manages the *care of a caseload of patients throughout their entire hospitalization,* providing individualized ongoing care with continuity to the patient and family. The goal of this model is to facilitate and coordinate a patient's hospital stay to provide high-quality and cost-effective care (Green & Newcommon, 2006; Kleinpell & Hravnak, 2005; Meyer and Miers, 2005). In this model, the ACNP will, in collaboration with a physician, admit the patient to the hospital, complete the admission history and physical examination, assess the patient's initial clinical status, order and interpret diagnostic and therapeutic tests, perform procedures, evaluate and adjust the plan of care, and prepare the patient for discharge. The ACNP will provide care continuously for patients as they move from high-acuity to lower-acuity inpatient care units, facilitate patients' movement through the acute care system, and plan for and implement discharge. Exemplar 14-2 illustrates this model.

In another model of care, the ACNP delivers *comprehensive specialty care to a group of patients across the entire continuum of care services.* For example, an ACNP member of a heart failure care team may oversee patient management during hospitalization, provide post-discharge clinic follow-up, and ultimately manage home-based infusion therapy. With the growth of specialty-based practices, the number of ACNPs working in this type of model of care is increasing. Exemplar 14-3 illustrates this model with an ACNP in a pulmonary practice who also bills for her services.

Diagnostic reasoning and advanced therapeutic interventions, consultation, and referral to other physicians, nurses, and providers are intrinsic components of this role as described by the ACNP scope of practice (American Association of Critical-Care Nurses, 2006). Although ACNPs might require some variation in skill sets, depending on the model within which their role is implemented, strong commonalties exist. As with other APN roles, all ACNPs are proficient in advanced physical assessment, clinical decision making (diagnostic reasoning), ordering and interpreting laboratory studies and procedures, and collaborating in the development and implementation of a treatment plan that includes prescribing medication. Using diagnostic reasoning, the ACNP diagnoses the origin of a complex medical problem that develops in an acutely or critically ill patient (see Chapter 5). The skills inherent in effective diagnostic reasoning include the fundamental skills of the ACNP role: history taking, physical examination skills, pattern recognition, the ability to analyze and synthesize data, and the ability to generate a working diagnosis. A number of factors affect the quality of diagnostic reasoning when applied to the acutely and critically ill, such as multisystem deterioration, hemodynamic instability, depressed level of consciousness, and unavailability of significant others to supply, corroborate, or supplement patient information. All of these factors challenge the ACNP's ability to accurately and expeditiously diagnose an acutely or critically ill patient's ever-changing physical condition.

Another inherent portion of the ACNP practice profile is the performance of technical skills, as indicated earlier. Patient needs within a specialty practice ultimately influence the type and level of therapeutic and diagnostic psychomotor skills that an individual ACNP performs (Kleinpell & Hravnak, 2002). The ACNP role is one of evidence-based practice, which

EXEMPLAR 14-2   Acute Care Nurse Practitioner Practice in an Inpatient Specialty Service

On the inpatient cardiology service of a large university teaching hospital, patients are assigned to either the ACNP team or the medical resident team (teaching team). The service covers approximately 50 monitored cardiology beds, including general cardiology patients, interventional cardiology patients, heart failure patients, and electrophysiology patients. Approximately two thirds of the patients are assigned to the ACNP team. In addition, the ACNP team is responsible for seeing outpatients for their pre-procedure evaluation in the cardiac catheterization suite. The ACNP team comprises 10 full-time positions and is responsible for providing care 7 days a week from 7 AM until 6 PM, when the service is signed out to night coverage, usually provided by an upper-level cardiology fellow. The day begins when Kate, who is the leader of the four-member ACNP team for the day, receives a sign-out of patients from the cardiology fellow covering the previous night. The fellow reports on the status of the patients on the ACNP team and also adds four new patients to the list who had been admitted overnight. Kate communicates the information to the other three ACNPs on the team and assigns the new patients; she then reviews her nine patients and begins to plan her day. A computer census is generated, and she reviews the daily laboratory results, vital signs, intake and output, weight, and current medication list for each patient.

Kate begins to see her patients starting with the newly admitted patient from the previous night. She reviews this patient's data, reviews the H&P examination findings, and looks at the chest radiograph and ECG. She interviews and examines the patient, validating the H&P findings. This 74-year-old man with a history of hypertension and non-insulin-requiring type 2 diabetes was admitted with chest pain and found to be in atrial fibrillation with a rapid ventricular response. During the night, he was treated with rate-controlling agents and this morning has converted to normal sinus rhythm and does not have chest pain. Kate discusses her plan for ordering an echocardiogram and an exercise stress test with imaging with the attending cardiologist and then returns to the patient to inform him of this plan. She describes the two tests, explaining the reasons for doing the studies. After answering his questions, she communicates the plan of care to the nurse. Next she writes orders for the studies and carefully reviews the medications, adjusting as needed. She writes a progress note and then notifies the patient's primary care physician of the patient's admission and discusses the planned course of action.

Kate next moves on to two patients who are to be discharged. After examining the patients and reviewing the data, she writes discharge orders, completes necessary prescriptions, writes a final progress note, and dictates a discharge summary. In coordination with the nurse, she identifies discharge teaching points and arranges post-discharge follow-up appointments with the cardiologist. One patient will require intravenous antibiotics for a pacemaker wound infection, so home care follow-up is arranged as well.

Over the remainder of the morning, Kate sees the other six patients in similar detail. One patient has chest pain with new ECG changes and is sent for emergency catheterization. The patient receives a coronary stent and is transferred to the CCU. Kate will not continue to follow the patient in the CCU but notifies the CCU resident and provides a verbal sign-out. Kate completes the progress notes on her other patients and follows up on the interventions she has ordered throughout the day.

During the day, Kate has fielded multiple calls regarding new admissions to the service and has assigned them to herself or her colleagues accordingly. An H&P is completed and dictated on each newly admitted patient, admission orders written, and a plan of action coordinated with the attending physician. Kate has collaborated with the other ACNP team member who is stationed in the pre-procedure area of the cardiac catheterization suite to coordinate the admission of patients to the post-procedure area after their coronary interventions.

At the end of the day, each of the four ACNPs completes a sign-out for the night coverage fellow, and a computer-generated census is completed for their reference. The ACNP team updates an electronic database daily that tracks patient volumes, admissions and discharges, and case mix. The ACNPs are also involved in precepting ACNP students, formal lecturing and teaching, and enrolling patients in research protocols.

ACNP, Acute care nurse practitioner; *CCU*, coronary care unit; *EKG*, electrocardiogram; *H&P*, history and physical.

EXEMPLAR 14-3 Acute Care Nurse Practitioner Practice Across the Continuum of Acute Care Services

A community-based pulmonary practice consists of three physicians and Suze, an ACNP. Suze has been with the practice for 4 years. When she was hired, Suze applied for her Medicare PIN/UPIN number. In 2008, she received her Medicare NPI number, which replaced the PIN/UPIN effective May 2007. Suze has assigned her NPI number to the practice. This means that when Suze bills for her services, the bill is submitted under her number but payment comes to the practice. Suze's reimbursement rate is at 85% of the physician fee schedule regardless of whether she bills in the office or in the hospital.

Each member of the practice sees patients both in the office and in the hospital on a rotating basis. During morning conference, Suze participates with the physicians in reviewing the schedule of that day's office appointments and list of inpatients who need to be followed. Suze sees those patients who have specialized needs relative to learning, treatment adherence, smoking cessation, and caregiver burden or unavailability. While each one of them has his or her own daily office schedule of patients, the list of inpatients is divided between Suze and the physician assigned to cover inpatients for the week.

Today, Suze will follow up on 15 inpatients: 3 new overnight admissions and 12 continuing inpatients. On one newly admitted patient, Suze reviews the history and physical examination findings, the chest radiograph, and additional diagnostic results. She interviews the patient to confirm and gain additional historical information. She then conducts a physical examination. This particular patient is a 55-year-old male admitted for exacerbation of his COPD and possible pneumonia. He was treated overnight with broad-spectrum antibiotics, intravenous steroids, oxygen, and nebulizer and is currently less dyspneic. Suze discusses with the pulmonologist her plan to order a chest CT scan because this is the patient's third COPD exacerbation in the past 8 weeks. She is concerned that an underlying condition may be causing the exacerbations. In addition, knowing that he is a current cigarette smoker, she changes the antibiotic to cover organisms more likely to occur in smokers. She discusses smoking cessation with the patient, and they agree to collaborate on developing his smoking cessation strategy at his first office appointment after hospital discharge. Suze and the pulmonologist review the case and treatment plan. He agrees and states that he will also look at the chest radiograph from the office computer but has no need to see the patient that day. Suze writes her progress note and additional orders. At the end of the day, Suze submits her bill for this inpatient under her NPI number to the office manager. Payment will be made to the practice at 85% of the physician fee schedule.

The following day, Suze sees this patient again. She interviews him, performs a physical examination, and reviews the laboratory results and the CT scan. She calls the pulmonologist to tell him that the CT scan is normal. The pulmonologist reviews the CT scan with Suze and visits the patient, asks a few questions related to symptoms, and listens to the patient's lung sounds. He agrees that the chest CT scan is negative, writes a note, which refers to Suze's note and opinion, and documents his H&P examination findings and interpretation of CT scan. Because both Suze and the pulmonologist have seen the patient and performed some part of the service, the total work is combined and Suze submits this day's bill as a shared visit under the physician's number. In this case, the practice will be paid at 100% of the physician fee schedule. Had the pulmonologist not seen the patient and performed and documented a part of the service, the bill would have been submitted only under Suze's NPI number.

The patient is discharged to home on his routine metered-dose inhalers, a steroid taper, and oral antibiotic. He returns in 2 weeks for a follow-up office appointment scheduled with Suze. Suze interviews the patient, who states he is feeling much better; she performs a physical examination. She finds his lung sounds are much improved. They discuss smoking cessation, and the patient agrees to set a stop-smoking date. Suze writes a prescription for a drug to help reduce nicotine cravings and also writes refill prescriptions for his inhalers. She documents the events of the visit and later discusses the plan with the pulmonologist. Suze submits the bill under her own NPI number, and the practice is reimbursed 85% of the physician fee schedule.

ACNP, Acute care nurse practitioner; *COPD,* chronic obstructive pulmonary disease; *CT,* computed tomography; *NPI,* national provider identifier; *PIN/UPIN,* provider identification number/unique provider identification number.

should be evident in clinical decision making and intervention selection.

Additional skills for continued ACNP role development are based on practice doctorate education. As ACNP education transitions to the DNP, emphasis on promoting evidence-based practice for patients with acute, critical, and complex chronic illness and the use of information systems and technology for improving health care will actively bring new opportunities for ACNP practice, as well as leadership opportunities focused on systems change and quality improvement.

Acute Care Nurse Practitioner Differences and Commonalties with Other Advanced Practice Nurse and Physician Assistant Roles

The ACNP role differs from other APN roles with regard to the type of patient care problems encountered, the acuity of the patient's condition, the need for rapid and continuous assessment, the planning and intervention, and the setting in which the care is delivered. For example, the clinical nurse specialist (CNS) enacts the APN role through three spheres of influence: at the patient level, in direct care; at the nurse level, as with staff development; and at the institutional level, providing oversight for care. In comparison, the ACNP uses clinical assessment skills to assess complex and acutely ill patients through health history taking, physical and mental status examination, performing procedures, and risk appraisal for complications. Both the ACNP and CNS roles are targeted to a patient-centered approach to care for patient populations, but the continuous on-unit presence of the ACNP at the bedside of patients often differentiates the role of the ACNP from the CNS role. Staff education and system change responsibilities represent a larger percentage of the CNS's role than of the ACNP's role. Conversely, CNSs are generally not involved in carrying out many of the procedures and interventions that characterize the ACNP role. Institutional variations in role implementation for CNSs and ACNPs sometime lack clear-cut differentiation in role responsibilities. Yet, it is acknowledged that the CNS and NP roles are distinct, with distinct practice foci (Becker, Kaplow, Muenzen, & Hartigan, 2006; Mick & Ackerman, 2002).

Table 14-2 can assist the reader in conceptualizing where the main focus of ACNP practice falls within the health care continuum and where there might be differences or overlap with the primary care NP role.

Within the table are examples of management strategies for common patient health care problems encountered in the traditional primary, secondary, and tertiary health care settings (Hravnak et al., 1995; Kleinpell & Hravnak, 2002). With diabetes care, for example, ACNP practice involves predominantly strategies directed toward management of the patient during an acute exacerbation of his or her diabetes. Because of the severity of symptoms, the patient must be admitted to the hospital, where he or she can be continuously monitored and where management strategies may change from hour to hour (tertiary care). During this same hospitalization, the patient may need to have an infected foot ulcer treated with intravenous antibiotics (secondary care). Once the crisis is over but while the patient is still hospitalized, the ACNP may provide discharge teaching on routine foot care (primary care), as well as diabetic diet and glucose monitoring. At this point, the patient may be referred back to his or her primary care provider for further follow-up and management. In comparison, the primary care NP's practice involves predominantly strategies directed toward management of the patient's diabetes when it is stable (primary care). This would include ongoing surveillance of the patient's self-management of his or her diabetes along with education on diabetic risk factors and assessment of signs of disease progression and complications. The primary care NP may also assess when the patient's diabetes is not well controlled and requires adjustment of insulin or oral hypoglycemic agents (secondary care). At the point when the patient is not responding or becomes acutely ill, the primary care NP will recognize the need for the patient to be referred to a setting where continuous monitoring and management is provided (tertiary care). Using this example helps educators and clinicians understand that there is a natural overlap in some areas of knowledge and practice between acute care and primary care NPs. However, each NP specialty also has its own distinct focus. The knowledge base and practice of the ACNP cannot be limited to only unstable conditions requiring complex technological diagnostic and management strategies for which the acutely or critically ill patient may be admitted to the hospital; the ACNP also needs to be prepared to manage the range of health care problems that accompany the patient. This includes not only the acute illness or exacerbation of chronic illness that requires acute care services but also the patient's co-morbidities, which also must be cared for while in the acute care setting. For

Table 14-2   PATIENT CARE PROBLEMS AND MANAGEMENT INTERVENTIONS TRADITIONALLY
ASSOCIATED WITH HEALTH CARE DELIVERY SETTINGS

| | Health Problem and Interventions | | |
Delivery Setting	Diabetes	Hypertension	Pneumonia
Tertiary care management (ICU setting)	Diabetic ketoacidosis management Fluid replacement Electrolyte titration IV insulin	Continuous vasoactive drugs Arterial pressure monitoring Evaluation/management of possible CVA	Mechanical ventilation and artificial airway Pulmonary toilet Culture assessment Sepsis management Continuous monitoring
Secondary care management (inpatient ward)	Diabetic exacerbation management Sliding scale insulin administration and monitoring Hydration Etiology work-up	Hypertensive crisis management Additional antihypertensives Adjunct therapy as needed	IV antibiotics Oxygen therapy Advanced assessment CXR, arterial blood gases, SpO$_2$
Primary care management (outpatient setting)	Initial Dx or stable management Oral antihyperglycemics or subcutaneous insulin Diet Prevention/assessment associated complications Foot care Risk factor management	Diet Oral agents Lifestyle changes Prevention/assessment of associated complications Risk factor management	Oral or intramuscular antibiotics

Adapted from Hravnak, M., Kobert, S.N., Risco, K.G., Baldisseri, M., Hoffman, L.A., Clochesy, J.M., et al. (1995). Acute care nurse practitioner curriculum: Content and development process. *American Journal of Critical Care, 4,* 179-188.
CVA, Cerebrovascular accident; *CXR,* chest x-ray; *Dx,* diagnosis; *ICU,* intensive care unit; *IV,* intravenous; *SpO$_2$,* peripheral arterial oxygen saturation.

example, the hospitalized diabetic patient previously discussed may also have stable hypertension, stable asthma, osteoarthritis, and an episode of vaginitis. While the patient is hospitalized, the ACNP must also simultaneously attend to these stable co-morbid health conditions to maintain their quiescence.

APNs, including ACNPs, are different from physician assistants (PAs). The PA role is under the jurisdiction of physician licensure, which is supervisory rather than collaborative and does not allow for independent functions. Although some of the care provided by PAs is similar to that provided by ACNPs, the philosophy, education, scope of practice, and patient approach of the APN and PA differ (Daffurn, 1998; Mittman, Cawley, & Fenn, 2002). Some overlap exists between the ACNP and PA in terms of the management of disease; however, the ACNP's direct clinical practice competencies also provide for nursing's holistic perspective, as well as

the promotion and protection of health. Whereas PAs are trained in the medical model to focus on providing illness-based care to patients, ACNPs, with their nursing background and practice, bring expertise in patient and family education, communication, collaboration, and health promotion/disease prevention for individuals and populations. A further differentiation is that ACNP practice also incorporates additional APN core competencies around leadership and coaching.

Acute Care Nurse Practitioners and Physician Hospitalists

The hospitalist is an internal medicine physician who is responsible for managing the care of hospitalized patients in the same manner that a primary care physician is responsible for managing his or her outpatients. Physicians first described this emerging role in 1996 as a consequence of the explosive growth of the primary care and internist role secondary to managed care. Hospitalist specialists have a central role in hospitals in Great Britain and Canada, but until recently, such a specialist has been a scarce commodity in the United States (Wachter, 1999). However, the physician hospitalist role is now being incorporated in many academic teaching centers and community settings, and the ACNP recently has been added as a member of this health care team. Some ACNPs function as members of the hospitalist team and manage patients independently in collaboration with the physician hospitalist. A primary care physician refers the patient to the hospitalist team for management during the acute care admission. The team provides care for the patient during hospitalization and refers the patient back to the primary care provider at the time of discharge. The goal of this service is to provide seamless, cost-effective care. This can be an advantage for a primary care physician with busy office hours who may have limited time to make hospital visits and may not be sufficiently familiar with acute care management. The specific role of the ACNP, as a member of the hospitalist team, is similar to the roles previously described, including obtaining an admission history and physical examination, performing daily physical examinations, making rounds with the physician, developing a treatment plan, reviewing laboratory studies and radiographs, and performing procedures. Furthermore, coordinating patient care management when many consultants are involved in decision making is a significant part of the role, as is consultation with the case managers to effectively facilitate discharge planning (Cowan et al., 2006; Howie & Erickson, 2002; Nyberg, 2006).

Outcome Studies Related to Acute Care Nurse Practitioner Practice

Measuring outcomes of practice (see Chapters 24 and 25) is an acknowledged component of establishing the value of any APN role. Positive outcomes of ACNP care have been demonstrated in subacute transitional and rehabilitation care (Casara & Polycarpe, 2004; Green & Edmonds, 2004), emergency care (Cooper, Lindsey, Kinn, & Swann, 2002), surgical services (Hylka & Beschle, 1995), inpatient medical services (Howie & Erickson, 2002), geriatric inpatient care (Lambing, Adams, Fox, & Divine, 2004), cardiovascular care (Meyer & Miers, 2005), neuroscience care (Green & Newcommon, 2006), respiratory care (Burns & Earven, 2002; Hoffman, Tasota, Scharfenberg, Zullo,

& Donahoe, 2002, 2003), perioperative care (Hylka & Beschle, 1995), intensive care (Hoffman, Miller, Zullo, & Donahoe, 2006; Scharfenberg, Hoffman, Tasota, Happ, & Donahoe, 2003), and as rapid response team leaders (Morse, Warshawsky, Moore, & Pecora, 2006). Research studies have demonstrated the positive impact of ACNP care, including decreased costs, decreased hospital length of stay, decreased use of laboratory tests, lower rates of urinary tract infections and skin breakdown, time savings for house physicians, similar care outcomes compared with physician practices, patient and family satisfaction, and an increased role in discussing patient outcomes with nurses and families, among others.

Although these studies exploring ACNP effectiveness have been conducted in several types of care settings, continued research on the impact of ACNP practice is needed (Kleinpell, 2002). The majority of the studies on utilization and outcomes of ACNPs have focused on comparing ACNP care with physician care, reducing costs, or discussing the impact of ACNP care on a focused area of care. No study has fully evaluated the impact of ACNPs; it would be useful to study a variety of outcomes associated with patient care managed by ACNPs (Howie & Erickson, 2002). If ACNPs are to delineate the impact of their care and justify their existence, it is imperative that their worth be supported by careful research (see Chapters 24 and 25).

ACUTE CARE NURSE PRACTITIONER ROLE IMPLEMENTATION EXAMPLES

Four exemplars have been provided elsewhere in this chapter to describe the ACNP practicing in an intensive care unit (Exemplar 14-1), an inpatient specialty service (Exemplar 14-2), across the continuum of acute care service (Exemplar 14-3), and ACNP role implementation following DNP preparation (Exemplar 14-4 on p. 428). Additional vignettes illustrate the ACNP in other role implementation models.

Role Vignettes in Other Clinical Practice Settings

The ACNP might participate as a member of a specific clinical specialty or consult service practicing within an acute care setting. Examples might include an ACNP working as part of an internal medicine team, trauma service, surgical service, acute stroke team, emergency department, renal medicine team, pulmonary medicine service, electrophysiology service, preadmission surgical service, oncology service, or medical emergency/rapid response team.

Bone Marrow Transplantation Services.
The ACNP working as a member of the bone marrow transplantation service has an autonomous role while functioning as a part of a collaborative practice model; the team comprises a resident, a fellow, an attending physician, and the ACNP. The ACNP provides the continuity of care for the service by being the only consistent member of the academic health care team where physicians rotate between clinical and research activities. The ACNP carries a caseload of patients and follows them through their hospital stay until discharge. Role responsibilities include preliminary rounding daily on each patient, performing physical examinations, interpreting laboratory tests (electrolytes and x-ray studies), performing marrow aspirations, and consulting specialists (e.g., in gastroenterology, infectious disease, pulmonary medicine) to assist in patient management. On the basis of the information gathered, the ACNP collaborates with the other provider team members during daily rounds to develop the daily and long-term treatment plan. In addition, the ACNP teaches the house staff and nursing staff and incorporates health teaching and health promotion/protection (especially risk associated with immunosuppression) activities into his or her practice.

Diagnostic and Interventional Services.
In preadmission surgical services, the major clinical functions of an ACNP include history taking and physical examinations; performing pre-procedure evaluations; providing patient and family education; obtaining and interpreting laboratory, electrocardiographic, and radiological data; identifying at-risk individuals in need of preadmission discharge planning; initiating contacts with social services; and discharge planning and making management recommendations for patients in the surgical holding area. The ACNP consults with the anesthesiologist and surgeon regarding patient health problems that may affect or preclude anesthesia delivery or surgery. ACNPs may provide services similar to those in the cardiac catheterization suite or the gastrointestinal procedure laboratory.

Alternatively, an ACNP may function as part of a team that provides care in continuity across a spectrum of clinical encounters or settings.

Heart Failure Services.
In this example, a team of three ACNPs on the heart failure service in a university medical center collaborate with each other and with physician team members to optimize continuity of care for their patients. Each ACNP has a caseload of patients for whom he or she assumes responsibility in the outpatient area. They see each patient in clinic on a regular basis, examine patients, and adjust the treatment plan. They perform follow-up by phone contact on a weekly basis, helping patients assess their symptoms, follow daily weights, discuss dietary changes, and adjust oral mediations as needed. Based on this discussion, the ACNP may have the patient come to the outpatient clinic for further clinical assessment and treatment (e.g., a dose of intravenous diuretic, adjustment of continuous inotropic medication infusions). When a patient requires admission to the hospital for an acute exacerbation of heart failure, one ACNP (each ACNP team member provides in-hospital coverage on a weekly rotating basis) along with the physician manage the patient in the hospital setting. They are familiar with the patient's problems and treatment plan, can provide continuity, have established a trusting relationship with the patient and the care delivery team, and can readily facilitate discharge planning and follow-up when the patient is ready for discharge to home.

Orthopedic Services.
The role of the ACNP working with patients with orthopedic problems covers a full spectrum of practice settings including coverage for the emergency room, the orthopedic clinic, and the inpatient orthopedic service. The orthopedic ACNP works closely with the attending physicians, staff nurses, and residents to coordinate care from preadmission testing to discharge. Each of the ACNPs carries a caseload of hospitalized patients and outpatients undergoing short procedures. This role may include perioperative management as first-assistant in the operating room.

Rapid Response Team.
A newer role for the ACNP may be as team leader or team member of hospital medical emergency teams or rapid response teams. When hospitalized patients develop sudden physiological instability outside of critical care areas, a mismatch between patient needs and available supportive resources occurs. Rapid response teams have been developed to deploy personnel and other resources to meet patient needs in a crisis in any area of

the hospital (DeVita et al., 2006). These teams consist of multidisciplinary members such as ACNP, physician, critical care nurse, respiratory therapist, and nursing supervisor. The team might be activated to respond to such conditions as hypotension, acute mental status changes, bleeding, respiratory distress, chest pain, or oliguria. The ACNP may be the team leader, coordinating the assessment, triage, and treatment plan, or he or she may participate as a team member enacting problem-focused response protocols, placing peripheral or central venous lines, assisting with airway management, and coordinating transfer to another level of care if necessary (Morse, Warshawsky, Moore, & Pecora, 2006).

PREPARATION OF ACUTE CARE NURSE PRACTITIONERS

At present, ACNPs are registered nurses who are prepared at the master's level of graduate nursing education. The majority of ACNP educational programs also require prior clinical nursing experience, although these requirements vary widely between programs (Kleinpell & Hravnak, 2002). Programs are emerging to prepare ACNPs with additional knowledge and skills in a clinical practice, awarding the title of *Doctor of Nursing Practice (DNP)*. All ACNP programs should provide for program requirements outlined in the *Criteria for Evaluation of Nurse Practitioner Programs* (National Task Force on Quality Nurse Practitioner Education, 2002).

The ACNP curriculum incorporates the graduate core, the advanced practice core, the NP specialty curricula, and the ACNP subspecialty curricula. Programs that prepare ACNPs at the DNP level do not negate the master's core but, rather, build upon it (AACN, 2005). DNP curricula also combine foundational or core competencies for all DNP program graduates, as well as ACNP specialty competencies for the practice doctorate.

A number of publications have addressed ACNP educational preparation and curricular recommendations (Curran & Roberts, 2002; Kleinpell & Hravnak, 2002; Schwertz, Piano, Kleinpell, & Johnson, 1997). The ACNP specialty content should focus on knowledge and skills essential to diagnose and manage the episodic and chronic problems commonly experienced by patients with acute, critical, and complex chronic illness while performing health promotion/protection and disease prevention activities within the context of the continuum of the acute care delivery system (American Association of Critical-Care Nurses,

2006). As illustrated in the conceptual model of care services previously presented in Table 14-2, ACNPs diagnose and manage not only the acute health problems associated with the patient's chief complaint but also quiescent, stable co-morbid health conditions. Because ACNPs must be prepared to manage health problems across the full continuum of acute health care services, their didactic information and clinical experiences should provide for this broad focus. Likewise, the program should provide didactic and clinical preparation in the competencies delineated in both the *Acute Care Nurse Practitioner Competencies* (National Panel for Acute Care Nurse Practitioner Competencies, 2004) and the *Scope and Standards of Practice for the Acute Care Nurse Practitioner* (American Association of Critical-Care Nurses, 2006). Teaching skills in screening and prevention specific to acute care practice are also essential (Heath, Andrews, Thomas, Kelley, & Friedman, 2002). Because ACNP graduates must be competent in critical incident management, clinical simulation is often used in ACNP education (Hravnak, Beach, & Tuite, 2007; Scherer, Bruce, Graves, & Erdley, 2003). Technical skills training is also commonly incorporated into ACNP programs, as indicated in Table 14-3.

More recently, ACNP education is transitioning to DNP preparation, either as entry into ACNP practice or as a post-master's program. These programs prepare ACNPs for the highest levels of leadership in practice and scientific inquiry. Graduates have received additional didactics and experiences to achieve the level of competence indicated in *The Essentials of Doctoral Education for Advanced Practice Nursing* (AACN, 2005). This expansion in direct practice abilities includes advanced communication (interpersonal and technological), utilization of an expanded scientific foundation in providing an evidence basis for practice across settings, advanced participation, collaboration and leadership within the health care delivery system and the business of health care, and a focus on independent practice (NONPF, 2006). An example of the practice skills of an ACNP who has received practice doctorate education is in Exemplar 14-4.

Last, NPs who have been educated in another NP specialty but who are now working in an acute care setting, where additional competencies and skills are required, must ensure that their educational preparation is consistent with the focus of their practice (Kleinpell et al., 2005). Neither certification nor licensure grant

Table 14-3   SKILLS MOST FREQUENTLY
TAUGHT IN ACUTE CARE NURSE
PRACTITIONER EDUCATIONAL
PROGRAM (RESULTS OF A
SURVEY OF 56 ACNP PROGRAMS)

Most Frequently Taught Skills	% of Programs Teaching the Skill
12-lead electrocardiogram interpretation	100%
Chest x-ray interpretation	98%
Hemodynamic monitoring	91%
Suturing	89%
Spirometry and peak flow assessment	78%
Local anesthesia application	70%
Papanicolaou smear	70%
Central venous line insertion	66%
Arterial puncture/cannulation	55%
Intracranial pressure monitoring	55%
Sedation for procedures	52%
Defibrillation/cardioversion	50%
Chest tube insertion	48%
Endotracheal intubation	48%
Wound debridement	48%
Discontinuation of chest tubes	46%
Intra-aortic balloon pump management	45%
Wound packing	41%
Superficial abscess incision and drainage	41%

Kleinpell, R.M., Hravnak, M., Werner, K.E., & Guzman, A. (2006). Skills taught in acute care NP programs: A national survey. *The Nurse Practitioner, 31*, 7-13.

universal practice rights (Smolenski, 2005), and it is important that NP practice is substantiated by the appropriate education. Individuals with master's preparation in another APN specialty may seek a post-master's or DNP ACNP program to ensure that they undergo didactic and supervised clinical practica to adequately prepare for caring for this unique and vulnerable patient population (Kleinpell et al., 2005).

REIMBURSEMENT FOR ACUTE CARE NURSE PRACTITIONERS

It is important that ACNPs become knowledgeable about billing and payment mechanisms for professional services in addition to policy issues that affect ACNP reimbursement (Hravnak, Rosenzweig, Rust, & Magdic, 1998a; Rundio, 2001b). Obtaining reimbursement for services provided by NPs continues to be a universal challenge for every NP specialty, particularly ACNPs. Some of these challenges include securing admission to provider panels, determining whether a service is covered, billing for critical care time, and deciding which billing option—direct, incident to, or shared (see Chapter 19)—to use. The complexities of how federal and state laws apply to specific practice situations can deter groups from fully using ACNPs (Buppert, 2005a; Buppert, 2005b). In addition, how an ACNP demonstrates financial productivity impacts an employer's decision to hire and/or retain ACNP providers.

Although there are many considerations as to which billing option to use, there are compelling reasons why ACNPs should, along with their other APN colleagues, bill directly under their own number. Among these reasons are (1) recognition of the ACNP's financial worth as a result of produced income, and (2) tangible recognition of the ACNP's professional standing, which in turn leads to professional satisfaction and peer recognition (Richmond, Thompson, & Sullivan-Marx , 2000). Direct reimbursement also brings visibility to the quantity and type of care for which an ACNP is compensated. Visibility is accomplished through documentation and monitoring of billed services in the National Claims History File established by the Center for Medicare and Medicaid Services (CMS) (Richmond et al., 2000). Through evaluation of services billed by ACNPs at the national level, an aggregate profile of ACNP practice with respect to billable direct patient care activities can be developed (Richmond et al., 2000).

Almost every encounter between an ACNP and a patient is associated with a payer. The five major categories of payers, each with its own policies and legal structures, are Medicare, Medicaid, indemnity-type insurance, managed care organizations (MCOs), and businesses that contract for certain services (Buppert, 2004). Reimbursement for ACNP services within the Medicare framework is the focus of this chapter. Although Medicare serves as the most common form of reimbursement of NP services, other payers may have their own unique variations. If an ACNP understands Medicare regulations, he or she

EXEMPLAR 14-4   Acute Care Nurse Practitioner Role Implementation Following Doctor
of Nursing Practice Preparation

Joyce is a DNP-prepared ACNP currently working in a nephrology practice. The practice consists of one ACNP and five physicians. The practice is organized such that each provider has his or her own caseload of patients and follows these patients in the office as well as in the hospital. In addition, Joyce is responsible for one of the outpatient dialysis clinics where she sees patients three times per week. This particular dialysis clinic is located in a neighborhood consisting mainly of Hispanics and African-Americans. Every month, members of the practice meet for breakfast to discuss issues related to patient care as well as the logistics of the practice. Her usual schedule consists of daily morning rounds on her hospitalized patients followed by afternoon office hours on Tuesdays and Thursdays and outpatient dialysis clinic patients on Mondays, Wednesdays, and Fridays.

To track her patients, Joyce uses software on her PDA. As she makes her rounds, she enters the patient data and, at the end of the day, uploads the information into her office computer. Having patient data on a PDA allows Joyce to quickly access patient information when, for example, she admits a patient who was seen in the office a week ago, but she herself was not in the office.

Recently, Joyce launched a new set of standard admission orders for patients admitted to the hospital with a diagnosis of chronic renal failure. The standard orders resulted from a series of complications that occurred when new medical residents did not order the appropriate laboratory tests or all the routine medications used to treat renal failure. The result was increased hospital stay and cost. Joyce searched the literature to provide evidence to support orders she believed necessary and then collaborated with the medical staff, the nurses, the nutritionist, the pharmacist, and the manager of the laboratory to develop this order set. Consensus was reached in 6 months, and the orders were approved. Joyce then collaborated with the nursing staff to develop a quality assurance project that looked at whether or not these orders positively influenced patient outcomes.

In addition to seeing clinical patients, every third month Joyce participates on the credentialing and privileging committee at the hospital. She participates in the review of applicants to ensure they are qualified to provide competent, safe patient care. Joyce's unique role is to provide peer review on the applications of NPs.

At the dialysis clinic, Joyce is both the administrator and patient care provider. Physicians from the practice also provide patient care on a rotating basis and are available for consultation. The staff comprises registered nurses, nursing assistants, and secretarial support. To maintain optimal patient care, Joyce has implemented policies and evidence-based procedures. A quality assurance committee, led by Joyce, periodically reviews charts for compliance with selected quality indicators. In addition, Joyce coordinates a bi-monthly journal club for the clinic's staff as one mechanism to ensure that the staff is current in their practice. Because of the clinic's location, Joyce sits on the local neighborhood board. Her goal is for the clinic to be a good "neighbor." Joyce collaborates with the board members to provide culturally appropriate educational opportunities on such topics as hypertension and diabetes in an effort to reduce the incidence of renal failure in that community.

Joyce serves as adjunct faculty at the local university. She lectures to the ACNP students on renal disease and also serves as a clinical preceptor for ACNP students. In addition, she is a member of the ACNP program's local advisory board, which meets annually. The purpose of this board is to provide consultation to the ACNP faculty on ways to recruit and graduate outstanding students who can meet the needs of the community. At the last meeting, Joyce pointed out that students had poor recall on current guidelines related to management of diabetes—a leading cause of renal disease. Joyce suggested ways to integrate this information into the curriculum. She pointed out that current guidelines on diabetes management can be found on diabetes professional organization websites and can be downloaded into a PDA for easy access in the clinical area.

ACNP, Acute care nurse practitioner; *DNP,* Doctor of Nursing Practice; *NPs,* nurse practitioners; *PDA,* personal digital assistant.

is better equipped to navigate the policies of other payers (Buppert, 2005a). Detailed descriptions of third-party payers and related issues are described in Chapters 19 and 22).

At the same time Medicare legislation was enacted in the 1960s, the role of the NP was evolving in the area of pediatrics. Consequently, only limited provisions were made for NPs billing for eldercare services. Medicare regulations specified that NPs could receive direct reimbursement only when they provided care in certain geographical locations such as skilled nursing facilities and federally designated rural medically underserved areas. The 1997 Balanced Budget Act (BBA) removed the geographical restrictions on the direct reimbursement option for NPs. However, complexity still exists, and it is important that ACNPs understand the rules surrounding the direct, incident to, and shared billing options. Any or all of these options may be used by the ACNP in certain situations.

Medicare Reimbursement for Acute Care Nurse Practitioners in the Office/Non-Hospital Clinic Setting

Although ACNPs typically provide services to patients in hospital and hospital-affiliated offices and clinics, a portion of their practice may occur in a non-hospital–affiliated setting, as previously described in the discussion of ACNP role implementation models. In the office setting, an ACNP must decide whether to bill directly or incident to. *Direct billing* means that the ACNP provides the evaluation and management (E/M) service and submits the bill under his or her own provider number. Under this option, Medicare will reimburse at 85% of the physician fee schedule. "Incident to" is the part of Medicare law that provides for coverage of services and supplies furnished incident to the professional services of a physician. The decision of which option to use is often a business decision. For more detailed information regarding "incident to" billing, the reader is referred to the Center for Medicare and Medicaid Services, *Medicare Carriers Manual,* Claim Processing, Part 3, Transmittal 1764 (Center for Medicare and Medicaid Services [CMS], 2003a).

A third option addresses instances in which the ACNP and the physician share the E/M service in the outpatient setting where the ACNP performs a portion of an E/M encounter and the physician completes the E/M service. In this situation, the "incident to" requirements are met and the shared outpatient service should be billed under the physician's number. If the "incident to" requirements are not met, the shared outpatient service must be reported using the ACNP's number (CMS, 2003c). Of note, there is no "incident to" billing option for ACNPs providing services to patients in the hospital, emergency department, and hospital-affiliated clinics (CMS, 2003c).

Medicare Reimbursement for Acute Care Nurse Practitioners in the Hospital Inpatient/Hospital Outpatient/Emergency Department

Hospitals and emergency departments are common practice sites for ACNPs. However, billing for ACNP services in these settings can be challenging (Buppert, 2005b). Whether an ACNP can bill for services delivered in the hospital first depends on whether the ACNP's salary is listed on the hospital's Medicare cost report. If it is, then the ACNP's services are already paid for under Medicare Part A. A transmittal issued by CMS dated January 26, 2007, updated the *Medicare Claims Processing Manual* regarding "Direct Billing and Payment for Non-Physician Practitioner Services Furnished to Hospital Inpatient and Outpatients" (Buppert, 2007; CMS, 2007). According to this transmittal, payments for professional services of the NP (as well as CNS and PA) could be unbundled from the payment to the hospital for "hospital services" billed under the hospital's cost report. However, the hospital still bills the fiscal intermediary for the facility fee associated with NP, CNS, or PA services (Buppert, 2007; CMS, 2007). Direct payment for the ACNP's professional services furnished to hospital inpatients and outpatients must be made to the ACNP at 85% of the physician fee schedule unless the ACNP reassigns payment to the hospital (CMS, 2007).

Shared billing is another option for ACNPs in the hospital inpatient, outpatient, and emergency departments (Magdic, 2006). The high patient acuity in these areas fosters a close collaborative relationship with physician colleagues. It is not uncommon for the ACNP and the physician to both provide services to the hospitalized patient on the same day. On October 25, 2002, CMS issued a Change Request (CR) 2321, which updated *Medicare Carriers Manual* §15501 guidelines for E/M services. These guidelines were further clarified by Transmittal 178 in May, 2004 (CMS, 2003b, 2004) and provide direction for billing and reimbursement of E/M services provided by the physician and the ACNP when they are in the same group practice and provide services on the same day, either at the same or different times. A shared visit under these circumstances means that the physician provides some portion of the E/M service and provides supporting documentation. For shared billing to occur between the ACNP and physician, either the ACNP should be employed by the physician practice or both should be employed by the same entity (CMS, 2003b).

Key issues regarding shared E/M services are as follows:

- If the ACNP provides a medically necessary service and there is no face-to-face encounter between the patient and the physician, the service must be billed under the ACNP's provider number. A physician simply reviewing the chart and creating or adding to a note does not constitute a face-to-face encounter (CMS, 2004).
- If both the ACNP and the physician provide portions of the E/M service on the same day at the same or different times and there is a face-to-face encounter between the patient and the physician, then the physician and ACNP may combine their services and bill for a shared visit under either the physician's or the ACNP's provider number at the level supported by their combined documentation (CMS, 2004).

The preceding discussion also applies to billing for ACNP services provided within hospital outpatient or emergency departments. For more information regarding "incident to" and shared billing, the reader is referred to the *Medicare Carriers Manual* of the Center for Medicare and Medicaid Services, Part 3 Claims Process, Transmittal 1764 and *Medicare Carriers Manual* of the Center for Medicare and Medicaid Services, Chapter 12, Section 30.6.4 (CMS, 2003a, 2003c). An example of billing activities of an ACNP in the inpatient setting is provided in Exemplar 14-3. Exemplar 14-3 illustrates the billing practices of an ACNP in a pulmonary specialty practice who sees patients in the hospital and office.

Critical Care Reimbursement for Acute Care Nurse Practitioners

Critical care involves decision making of high complexity to assess, manipulate, and support vital system function and often requires extensive interpretation of multiple data sources and application of advanced technology (CMS, 2003c). Reimbursement

for critical care services can occur in any location where critical care services are performed, including intensive care units, emergency departments, and general medical-surgical floors (CMS, 2003c; Vachani, DeLong, & Manaker, 2003). Critical care services are billed according to time-based Current Procedural Terminology (CPT) codes (Sample & Dorman, 2006). The first 30 to 74 minutes of critical care services on a given calendar date are billed under one specific CPT code. For each additional 30 minutes, a second code is used. A physician may not tie into an ACNP's note for either code. Either the ACNP or the physician, but only one, may provide the initial 30 minutes of critical care time. For each additional 30 minutes, the service is billed by whoever provided the service (Dorman, Loeb, & Sample, 2006). If the total time spent providing critical care services is less than 30 minutes, then other E/M codes must be used (American Medical Association, 2004).

CHALLENGES SPECIFIC TO THE ACUTE CARE NURSE PRACTITIONER ROLE

The role of the ACNP is continuing to evolve and gain progressive recognition. The increased need for ACNPs to directly manage patient care in an expanding health care arena will continue to provide unique practice opportunities. The practice doctorate will provide additional opportunities to expand and increase the emphasis on promoting evidence-based practice and organizational and systems leadership (National Panel for NP Practice Doctorate Competencies, 2006). Simultaneously, ACNPs will face challenges to practice that will need to be resolved to firmly establish the role. Practicing ACNPs continue to report that physicians and hospital administrators are unfamiliar with the role and the differences between the ACNP and primary care NP specialties. Also, some physicians feel threatened by the role. Misunderstandings about ACNP practice and labeling of the role as a *physician extender* have stemmed from the perception that ACNPs are replacements for house staff and function as "resident replacements." Many of these perceived threats and misperceptions can be addressed through education. ACNPs can use both formal and informal opportunities to educate the professional public about the purpose and practice of ACNPs, providing clear and concrete examples of their utilization and efficacy (Richmond & Becker, 2005). To articulate their role, it is extremely important for ACNPs to frame their practice within the nursing paradigm (Hravnak & Magdic, 1997), one that uses the admitting history and physical examination to develop a plan of care that includes the patient's holistic problems as well as the medical diagnosis; to address these nursing and medical problems throughout the hospital stay; to use interventions that not only diagnose and manage disease but also promote and protect health; to frame the discharge summary so that patients have a continuum of nursing as well as medical care as they return to the community; and to apply all the ACNP role competencies, not only those related to direct clinical care, to their practice.

Exposure to the comprehensive care that ACNPs provide and education of the health care team regarding the role will lead to continued role recognition and role acceptance. Educating administrators and other health care professionals can facilitate acceptance of the role, which will in turn provide an opportunity for independent contracting for ACNP professional services. Awareness of worth in terms of billable revenue and the care that ACNPS are able to provide is imperative for successful contract negotiations and marketing purposes.

In addition to individual efforts, Cummings and colleagues (2003) suggest five specific recommendations to assist with organizational change when implementing ACNPs on a system-wide level:

- Employ a change model to guide the change process and integrate ongoing evaluation for feedback.
- Assign a champion—one or two individuals to support, coordinate, and market the change on both micro and macro levels within the organization.
- Articulate a vision—clarify and communicate a consistent definition and expectations of the role (including an organization-wide job description that is not service-specific and indicates practice boundaries and reporting lines) and anticipated outcomes of role implementation.
- Establish a forum to facilitate open and ongoing communications among all players.
- Attend to cultural and personality transitions.

Whitcomb, Craig, and Welker (2000) further suggest that organization-wide efforts to measure ACNPs' performance and outcomes help demonstrate job justification and organizational impact.

Changing employment trends have also affected ACNP practice (Geier, 2000; Kleinpell & Hravnak,

2002). Originally, ACNPs were hired predominantly into tertiary medical center settings. ACNPs now report increased employment with physician practice groups, MCOs, independent subacute care facilities, and even individual contractual relationships, yet these opportunities also bring the challenges of negotiating legal contracts, multiorganizational credentialing and privileging, group practice and MCO policies, and reimbursement issues (Cummings, Fraser, & Tarlier, 2003; Kleinpell & Hravnak, 2002; see also Chapters 20 and 21).

ACNPs need to continue to develop strong collaborative relationships with physicians and others to provide optimal patient care. The practice doctorate for NPs advocates for advanced interprofessional collaboration for improved health outcomes (AACN, 2005). Working to negotiate a collaborative practice partnership can be a challenge. In working to establish collegial interactions and by sharing successful practice models, ACNPs can promote enhanced collaborative relationships (see Chapter 10).

In the future, ACNPs may practice in multiple settings with individually negotiated contracts. Managing episodes of acute illness or exacerbation of chronic illness in home health care, subacute care, and outpatient settings might be directed by the ACNP, as is already the case in some areas. These areas are natural extensions of acute care services and encompass the scope of ACNP practice—the stabilization of acute and chronic disease. Myriad opportunities relative to acute and chronic therapeutic management exist—for example, the management of renal dialysis or ventilator-dependent patients.

Cost reduction within acute care services will continue. Currently, collaborative teams composed of a physician, resident, and ACNP are popular in many practice settings. In the future, certain patient populations may be managed by teams composed of several ACNPs with one physician, as in the heart failure service vignette described earlier and in other examples in the literature (Figueira, 2003; McMullen, Alexander, Bourgeois, & Goodman, 2001; Shapiro & Rosenberg, 2002).

Monitoring the outcomes of ACNP practice remains essential. Although a growing number of utilization and outcome-based studies of ACNP practice have been conducted and published, the need to demonstrate the impact of ACNP care in a growing number of practice arenas remains. The emphasis on continuous quality improvement will continue to mandate the need for ACNPs to become proactive and involved in measuring the impact of their care.

With all ACNPs holding master's degrees and some holding doctoral degrees, there is an increased potential to apply scientific knowledge to clinical practice and to establish and uphold evidence-based practice. ACNPs are expected to assume leadership roles in evaluating the scientific literature and applying findings to change and improve care (see Chapters 8 and 9).

ACNPs must accept the challenge to continually improve and advance themselves and their profession. Strategies for success in the ACNP role include maintaining competency, networking, demonstrating outcomes of practice, and communicating about the role (Kleinpell & Hravnak, 2005). To provide safe, high-quality, efficient care, the ACNP must persistently pursue ongoing education to be knowledgeable about recent advances in health care and judicious in the application of research findings. ACNPs should not only read the literature but also publish on both clinical and role topics. Sharing their clinical expertise and experiences can benefit their peers as those peers seek to develop and enhance their roles. It is important that ACNPs be involved in their NP professional and clinical specialty organizations so that the issues unique to ACNP practice gain recognition by the leaders of the national organizations and also to ensure that ACNPs have a voice in the legislative and political decision-making process. Collaboration with public policymakers to influence legislation issues related to the ACNP role or, on a larger scale, health policy issues is also an imperative for all ACNPs (American Association of Critical-Care Nurses, 1995; see also Chapters 10 and 22).

CONCLUSION

The ACNP role provides an opportunity for NPs to have a significant impact on patient outcomes at a dynamic time in the history of health care delivery. As the role continues to evolve along with market forces and as health care systems respond to economic change, opportunities to further develop the ACNP role will arise. Future development of the ACNP role should be based on the evaluation of the need for the role, understanding the scope of the role, assessment of the practice or organization, and the service needs of the patient population (Irvine et al., 2000). Because the ACNP role continues to evolve, participation in national organizations to refine consensus regarding role components, program curriculum,

marketing, and role evaluation is necessary. ACNP educators and clinicians must work together to ensure that the preparation and practice of ACNPs is safe, effective, and fully represented as the movement of doctoral APN education evolves. ACNPs must be strong activists in efforts to gain full recognition of the role within their proper scope of practice across acute care settings. In the evolving health care arena, ACNP practice is rapidly expanding and holds unlimited potential.

REFERENCES

American Association of Colleges of Nursing (AACN). (2005). *The essentials of doctoral education for advanced practice nursing.* Washington, DC: Author.

American Association of Critical-Care Nurses. (1995). *Advanced nursing practice: Facts and strategies for regulation, reimbursement and prescriptive authority.* Washington, DC: Author.

American Association of Critical-Care Nurses. (2006). *Scope and standards of practice for the acute care nurse practitioner.* Aliso Viejo, CA: Author.

American Medical Association. (2004). *CPT 2004.* Professional edition. Chicago: AMA Press.

American Nurses Credentialing Center (ANCC). (2004). *A role delineation study of seven nurse practitioner specialties.* Silver Spring, MD: Author.

Baggs, J.G., & Schmitt, M.H. (1988). Collaboration between nurses and physicians. *Image: The Journal of Nursing Scholarship, 20,* 145-149.

Barber, P.M., & Burke, M. (1999). Advanced practice nursing in managed care. In M.D. Mezy & D.O. McGivern (Eds.), *Nurses, nurse practitioners* (pp. 203-218). New York: Springer.

Barkley, T.W., & Rogers, J.E. (2001). Dynamic roles and scope of the acute care nurse practitioner. *Nurse Practitioner Forum, 12,* 115-120.

Barkley, T.W., & Whitney, F. (2001). The acute care nurse practitioner's role in pain and pain management. *Nurse Practitioner Forum, 12,* 166-174.

Becker, D., Kaplow, R., Muenzen, P.M., & Hartigan, C. (2006). Activities performed by acute and critical care advanced practice nurses: American Association of Critical-Care Nurses study of practice. *American Journal of Critical Care, 15,* 130-148.

Briggs, L.A., Heath, J., & Kelley, J. (2005). Peer review for advanced practice nurses: What does it really mean? *AACN Clinical Issues, 16,* 3-15.

Buppert, C. (2004). Reimbursement for nurse practitioners services. In C. Buppert, *Nurse practitioner's business practice and legal guide* (2nd ed., p. 269). Boston MA: Jones & Bartlett.

Buppert, C. (2005a). Billing For nurse practitioner services—Update 2005. Guidelines for NPs, physicians, employers, and insurers. *Medscape* July 22, 2005.

Buppert, C. (2005b). Capturing reimbursement for advanced practice nurse services in acute and critical care: Legal and business considerations. *AACN Clinical Issues, 16,* 23-35.

Buppert, C. (2007). *CMS clarifies payment mechanism for NP professional services furnished to hospital inpatients and outpatients. Annapolis, MD. Law Office of Carolyn Buppert.*

Burns, S.M., & Earven, S. (2002). Improving outcomes for mechanically ventilated medical intensive care unit patients using advanced practice nurses: A 6-year experience. *Critical Care Nursing Clinics of North America, 14,* 231-243.

Casara, M., & Polycarpe, M. (2004). Caring for the chronically critically ill: Establishing a wound-healing program in a respiratory care unit. *American Journal of Surgery, 188*(Suppl. 1A), 18-21.

Center for Medicare and Medicaid Services (CMS). (2003a). *Medicare carriers manual,* Claim Processing, Part 3, Transmittal 1764. Section 2050.0-2050.3. Retrieved February 22, 2007, from www.cms.hhs.gov/ manuals/pm_trans/R1764B3.pdf.

Center for Medicare and Medicaid Services (CMS). (2003b). *Medicare carriers manual,* Claim Processing, Part 3, Transmittal 1776. Section 15501. Retrieved February 22, 2007, from www.cms.hhs.gov/ manuals/pm_trans/R1776B3.pdf.

Center for Medicare and Medicaid Services (CMS). (2003c). *Medicare carriers manual,* Claim Processing, Chapter 12, Section 30.6.4. Retrieved February 22, 2007, from www.cms.hhs.gov/manuals/downloads/clm104c12.pdf.

Center for Medicare and Medicaid Services (CMS). (2004). *Medicare carriers manual,* Claim Processing, Part 3, Transmittal 178. Retrieved February 22, 2007, from www.cms.hhs.gov/transmittals/Downloads/R178CP.pdf.

Center for Medicare and Medicaid Services (CMS). (2007). *Medicare carriers manual,* Claim Processing, Part 3, Transmittal 1168. Retrieved February 22, 2007, from www.cms.hhs.gov/transmittals/downloads/R1168CP.pdf.

Chang, W.C., Mu, P.F., & Tsay, S.L. (2006). The experience of role transition in acute care nurse practitioners in Taiwan under the collaborative practice model. *Journal of Nursing Research, 14,* 83-92.

Clinton, P., & Sperhac, A.M. The acute care pediatric nurse practitioner. (2005). *Journal of Pediatric Health Care, 19,* 117-120.

Cole, F.L., & Kleinpell, R.M. (2006). Expanding acute care nurse practitioner practice: Focus on emergency department practice. *Journal of the American Academy of Nurse Practitioners, 18,* 187-189.

Cole, F.L., & Ramirez, E. (2000). Activities and procedures performed by nurse practitioners in emergency care settings. *Journal of Emergency Nursing, 26,* 455-463.

Cooper, M.A., Lindsey, G.M., Kinn, S., & Swann I.J. (2002). Evaluating emergency nurse practitioner services: A randomized controlled trial. *Journal of Advanced Nursing, 40,* 721-730.

Cowan, M.J., Shapiro, M., Hays, R.D., Afifi, A., Vazirani, S., Ward, C.R., et al. (2006). The effect of a multidisciplinary hospitalist/physician and advanced practice nurse collaboration on hospital costs. *Journal of Nursing Administration, 36,* 79-85.

Cummings, C.M. (1997). Scope of employment vs. scope of practice. *Advance for Nurse Practitioners, 5,* 17.

Cummings, G.G., Fraser, K., & Tarlier, D.S. (2003). Implementing advanced nurse practice roles in acute care: An evaluation of organizational change. *Journal of Nursing Administration, 33,* 139-145.

Curran, C.R., & Roberts, W.D. (2002). Columbia University's competency and evidence-based acute care nurse practitioner program. *Nursing Outlook, 6,* 232-237.

Daffurn, K. (1998). Roles of acute care nurse practitioners, physician assistants, and resident physicians in acute care settings. *American Journal of Critical Care, 7,* 253-254.

Daly, B., & Gent, C. (1997). Influence of the health care environment. In B. Daly (Ed.), *The acute care nurse practitioner* (pp. 29-56). Washington, DC: American Nurses Publishing.

Devita, M.A., Bellomo, R., Hillman, K., Kellum, J., Rotondi, A., Teres, D., et al. (2006). Findings of the first consensus conference on medical emergency teams. *Critical Care Medicine, 34,* 2463-2478.

Dorman, T., Loeb, L., & Sample, G. (2006). Evaluation and management codes: From current procedural terminology through relative update commission to Center for Medicare and Medicaid Services. *Critical Care Medicine, 34*(Suppl. 3), S71-7.

Figueira, M. (2003). ACNP's role in heart failure management. *The Nurse Practitioner, 28,* 57-58.

Fox, V.J., Schira, M., & Wadlund, D. (2000). The pioneer spirit in perioperative advanced practice: Two practice examples. *AORN Journal, 72,* 241-248, 250-253.

Geier, W. (2000). The evolving role of the acute care nurse practitioner. *Nurse Practitioner, 25,* 126-129.

Genet Kelley, C., & Daly, B.J. (2001). Prevention in the inpatient setting. *Journal of the American Academy of Nurse Practitioners, 13,* 354-358.

Goolsby, M.J. (2005). 2004 AANP National Nurse Practitioner Sample Survey, Part II: Nurse practitioner prescribing. *Journal of the American Academy of Nurse Practitioners, 17,* 506-511.

Green, A., & Edmonds, L. (2004). Bridging the gap between the intensive care unit and general wards: The ICU liaison nurse. *Intensive Critical Care Nursing, 20,* 133-143.

Green, T., & Newcommon, N. (2006). Advancing nursing practice: The role of the nurse practitioner in an acute stroke program. *Journal of Neuroscience Nursing, 38*(Suppl. 4), 328-330.

Greenberg, E.M. (1996). Violence and the older adult: The role of the acute care nurse practitioner. *Critical Care Nursing Quarterly, 19,* 76-84.

Guido, B.A. (2004). The role of a nurse practitioner in an ambulatory surgery unit. *AORN Journal, 79,* 606-615.

Heath, J., Andrews, J., Thomas, S.A., Kelley, F.J., & Friedman, E. (2002). Tobacco dependence curricula in acute care nurse practitioner education. *American Journal of Critical Care, 11,* 27-33.

Hoffman, L.A., Miller, T.H., Zullo, T.G., & Donahoe, M.P. (2006). Comparison of two models for managing tracheostomized patients in a subacute medical intensive care unit. *Respiratory Care, 51,* 1230-1236.

Hoffman, L.A., Tasota, F.J., Scharfenberg, C., Zullo, T.G., & Donahoe, M.P. (2002). Management of ventilator-dependent patients: 5-month comparison of acute care nurse practitioner (ACNP) versus physician in training (PIT). *American Journal of Respiratory and Critical Care Medicine, 165,* A388.

Hoffman, L.A., Tasota, F.J., Scharfenberg, C., Zullo, T.G., & Donahoe, M.P. (2003). Management of patients in the intensive care unit: Comparison via work sampling analysis of an acute care nurse practitioner and physicians in training. *American Journal of Critical Care, 12,* 436-443.

Howie, J.N., & Erickson, M. (2002). Acute care nurse practitioners: Creating and implementing a model of care for an inpatient general medical service. *American Journal of Critical Care, 11,* 448-458.

Howie-Esquivel, J., & Fontaine, D. (2006). The evolving role of the acute care nurse practitioner in critical care. *Current Opinion in Critical Care, 12,* 609-613.

Hravnak, M. (1998). Is there a health promotion and protection foundation to the practice of acute care nurse practitioners? *AACN Clinical Issues, 9,* 283-289.

Hravnak, M., & Baldisseri, M. (1997). Credentialing and privileging: Insight into the process for acute care nurse practitioners. *AACN Clinical Issues, 8,* 108-115.

Hravnak, M., Beach, M., & Tuite P. (2007) Simulator technology as a tool for education in cardiac care. *Journal of Cardiovascular Nursing, 22,* 16-24.

Hravnak, M., Kobert, S.N., Risco, K.G., Baldisseri, M., Hoffman, L.A., Clochesy, J.M., et al. (1995). Acute care nurse practitioner curriculum: Content and development process. *American Journal of Critical Care, 4,* 179-188.

Hravnak, M., & Magdic, K. (1997). Marketing the acute care nurse practitioner. *Clinical Excellence for the Nurse Practitioner, 1,* 9-13.

Hravnak, M., Rosenzweig, P., Rust, D., & Magdic, K. (1998a). Reimbursement, liability and insurance. In R. Kleinpell & M. Piano (Eds.), *Practice issues for the acute care nurse practitioner* (pp. 27-40). New York: Springer.

Hravnak, M., Rosenzweig, P., Rust, D., & Magdic, K. (1998b). Scope of practice, credentialing, and privileging. In R. Kleinpell & M. Piano (Eds.), *Practice issues for the acute care nurse practitioner* (pp. 41-46). New York: Springer.

Hylka, S.C., & Beschle, J.C. (1995). Nurse practitioners, cost savings, and improved patient care in the department of surgery. *Nursing Economic$, 13,* 349-354.

Irvine, D., Sidani, S., Porter, H., O'Brien-Pallas, L., Simpson, B., McGillis-Hull, L. (2000). Organizational factors influencing nurse practitioners' role in acute care settings. *Canadian Journal of Nursing Leadership, 12,* 28-35.

Kaan, A., & Dunne, J. (2001). Development of a nurse practitioner role in heart failure management: An Australian experience. *Progress in Cardiovascular Nursing, 16,* 33-34.

Keough, V., Jennrich, J., Holm, K., & Marshall, W. (1996). A collaborative program for advanced practice in trauma/critical care nursing. *Critical Care Nurse, 16,* 120-127.

King, K., & Baggs, J. (1998). Collaboration: The essence of acute care nurse practitioner practice. In R. Kleinpell & M. Piano (Eds.), *Practice issues for the acute care nurse practitioner* (pp. 67-78). New York: Springer.

Kleinpell, R.M. (1999). Evolving role descriptions of the acute care nurse practitioner. *Critical Care Nurse Quarterly, 21,* 9-15.

Kleinpell, R.M (2002). The acute care nurse practitioner: An expanding opportunity for critical care nurses. *Critical Care Nurse, February*(Suppl.), 12-16, 74.

Kleinpell, R.M. (2005). Acute care nurse practitioner practice: Results of a 5-year longitudinal study. *American Journal of Critical Care, 14,* 211-221.

Kleinpell, R.M., & Hravnak, M. (2002). The acute care nurse practitioner. In M.K. Crabtree & R. Pruitt (Eds.), *Advanced nursing practice: Building curriculum for quality nurse practitioner education* (pp. 113-126). Washington, DC: National Organization of Nurse Practitioner Faculties.

Kleinpell, R., & Hravnak, M. (2005). Strategies for success in the acute care nurse practitioner role. *Critical Care Nursing Clinics of North America, 17,* 177-181.

Kleinpell, R.M., Hravnak, M., Werner, K.E., & Guzman, A. (2006). Skills taught in acute care NP programs: A national survey. *The Nurse Practitioner, 31,* 7-13.

Kleinpell, R.M., Perez, D.F., & McLaughlin, R. (2005). Educational options for acute care nurse practitioner practice. *Journal of the American Academy of Nurse Practitioners, 17,* 460-471.

Kleinpell-Nowell, R. (2001). Longitudinal survey of acute care nurse practitioner. *AACN Clinical Issues, 12,* 447-452.

Lambing, A.Y., Adams, D.L., Fox, D.H., & Divine, G. (2004). Nurse practitioners' and physicians' care activities and clinical outcomes with an inpatient geriatric population. *Journal of the American Academy of Nurse Practitioners, 8,* 343-352

Lugo, N.R., O'Grady, E., Hodnicki, D, & Hanson, C. (2007). Ranking state NP regulation: Practice environment and consumer healthcare choice. *American Journal of Nurse Practitioners, 11,* 8-24.

Lundberg, S., Wali, S., Thomas, P., & Cope, D. (2006). Attaining resident duty hours compliance: The acute care nurse practitioner program at Olive View—UCLA Medical Center. *Academic Medicine, 81,* 1021-1025.

Magdic, K.S. (2006). Acute care billing: Shared visits. *The Nurse Practitioner, 31,* 9-10.

Magdic, K.S., Hravnak, M., & McCartney, S. (2005). Credentialing for nurse practitioners: An update. *AACN Clinical Issues, 16,* 16-22.

Martin, R.K. (1999). Organ transplantation: The role of the acute care nurse practitioner across the spectrum of care. *AACN Clinical Issues, 10,* 285-292.

McMullen, M., Alexander, M.K., Bourgeois, A., & Goodman, L. (2001). Evaluating a nurse practitioner service. *Dimensions of Critical Care Nursing, 20,* 30-34.

Meyer, S.C., & Miers, L.J. (2005) Cardiovascular surgeon and acute care nurse practitioner: Collaboration on postoperative outcomes. *AACN Clinical Issues, 16,* 149-158.

Mick, D.J., & Ackerman, M.H. (2002). Deconstructing the myth of the advanced practice blended role: Support for role divergence. *Heart & Lungs 31,* 393-390.

Miller, S.K. (2001). Gerontology and geriatrics: Considerations for the acute care nurse practitioner. *Nurse Practitioner Forum, 12,* 155-160.

Mittman, D.E., Cawley, J.F., & Fenn, W.H. (2002). Physician assistants in the United States. *British Medical Journal, 325,* 485-487.

Morse, K.J., Warshawsky, D., Moore, J.M., & Pecora, D.C. (2006). A new role for the ACNP: The rapid response team leader. *Critical Care Nursing Quarterly, 29,* 137-146.

National Association of Pediatric Nurse Practitioners (NAPNAP). (2004). *Position statement on the acute care nurse practitioner.* Retrieved February 27, 2007, from www.napnap.org.

National Organization of Nurse Practitioner Faculties (NONPF). (2006). *Domains and competencies of nurse practitioner practice.* Washington, DC: Author.

National Organization of Nurse Practitioner Faculties (NONPF) and the American Association of Colleges of Nursing (AACN). (2002). *Nurse practitioner primary care competencies in specialty areas: Adult, family, gerontological, pediatric, and women's health.* Rockville, MD: United States Department of Health & Human Services Health Resources and Services Administration, Bureau of Health Professions, Division of Nursing.

National Panel for Acute Care Nurse Practitioner Competencies. (2004). *Acute care nurse practitioner competencies.* Washington, DC: National Organization of Nurse Practitioner Faculties.

National Panel for NP Practice Doctorate Competencies. (2006). *Practice doctorate nurse practitioner entry-level competencies.* Washington, DC: National Organization of Nurse Practitioner Faculties.

National Task Force on Quality Nurse Practitioner Education. (2002). *Criteria for evaluation of nurse practitioner programs.* Washington, DC: National Organization of Nurse Practitioner Faculties.

Norris, T., & Melby, V. (2006). The acute care nurse practitioner: Challenging existing boundaries of emergency nurses in the United Kingdom. *Journal of Clinical Nursing, 15,* 253-263.

Nyberg, D. (2006). Innovations in the management of hospitalized patients. *Nurse Practitioner, Spring*(Suppl.), 2-3.

Pearson, L. (2007). The Pearson Report: A national overview of nurse practitioner legislation and healthcare issues. *The American Journal for Nurse Practitioners, 11,* 10-101.

Penas, C. D., & Barkley, T.W. (2001). Ethical theory and principles of decision-making for the acute care nurse practitioner. *Nurse Practitioner Forum, 12,* 161-165.

Percy, M.S., & Sperhac, A.M. (2007). State regulations for the pediatric nurse practitioner in acute care. *Journal of Pediatric Health Care, 21,* 29-43.

Reel, V.K. (1999). Utilization of the acute care nurse practice in lung transplantation. *Clinical Excellence for Nurse Practitioners, 3,* 80-83.

Rhodes, R.S., & Carlson, J.H. (2001). Patient teaching tips for the acute care nurse practitioner. *Nurse Practitioner Forum, 12,* 96-91.

Richmond, T.S., & Becker, D. (2005). Creating an advanced practice nurse-friendly culture: A marathon, not a sprint. *AACN Clinical Issues, 16,* 58-66.

Richmond, T.S., Thompson, H.J., & Sullivan-Marx, E.M. (2000). Reimbursement for acute care nurse practitioner services. *American Journal of Critical Care, 9,* 52-61.

Riley-Bryan, K.D., & Barkley, T.W. (2001). Health policy concerns for the acute care nurse practitioner. *Nurse Practitioner Forum, 12,* 98-105.

Rosenfeld, P., McEvoy, M.D., & Glassman, K. (2003). Measuring practice patterns among acute care nurse practitioners. *Journal of Nursing Administration, 33,* 159-163.

Rundio, A. (2001a). Continuous quality improvement and problem solving techniques for the acute care nurse practitioner. *Nurse Practitioner Forum, 12,* 97-92.

Rundio, A. (2001b). Reimbursement hieroglyphics for the acute care nurse practitioner. *Nurse Practitioner Forum, 12,* 138-146.

Russell, D., VorderBruegge, M., & Burns, S. (2002). Effect of an outcomes-managed approach to care of neuroscience patients by acute care nurse practitioners. *American Journal of Critical Care, 11,* 353-362.

Sample, G.A., & Dorman, T. (2006). *Coding and billing for critical care: A practice tool* (2nd ed.). Des Plains, IL: Society of Critical Care Medicine.

Sarkissian, S., & Wennberg, R. (1999). Effects of the acute care nurse practitioner role on epilepsy monitoring outcomes. *Outcomes Management for Nursing Practice, 3,* 161-166.

Scharfenberg, C., Hoffman, L.A., Tasota, F.J., Happ, M.B., & Donahoe, M.P. (2003). Advantages and disadvantages of an acute care nurse practitioner (ACNP) and physicians in training (PIT): Perceptions of ICU clinicians. *American Journal of Respiratory and Critical Care Medicine, 167,* A102.

Scherer, Y.K., Bruce, S.A., Graves, B.T., & Erdley, W.S. (2003). Acute care nurse practitioner education: Enhancing performance through the use of clinical simulation. *AACN Clinical Issues, 14,* 331-341.

Schwertz, D.W., Piano, M.R., Kleinpell, R., & Johnson, J. (1997). Teaching pharmacology to advanced practice nursing students: Issues and strategies. *AACN Clinical Issues, 8,* 132-146.

Shapiro, D., & Rosenberg, N. (2002). Acute care nurse practitioner collaborative practice negotiation. *AACN Clinical Issues, 13,* 470-478.

Silver, H.K., & McAtee, P. (1988). Speaking out: Should nurses substitute for house staff? *American Journal of Nursing, 88,* 1671-1673.

Smolenski, M.C. (2005). Credentialing, certification, and competence: Issues for new and seasoned nurse practitioners.

Journal of the American Academy of Nurse Practitioners, 17, 201-204.

Vachani, A., DeLong, P., & Manaker, S. (2003). Documentation and coding of critical care professional services. *Clinical Pulmonary Medicine, 10,* 85-92.

van Soeren, M.H., & Micevski, V. (2001). Success indicators and barriers to acute care nurse practitioner role implementation in four Ontario hospitals. *AACN Clinical Issues, 12,* 424-437.

Wachter, R.M. (1999). An introduction to the hospitalist model. *Annals of Internal Medicine, 130*(4 Pt 2), 338-342.

Whitcomb, R., Craig, R., & Welker, C. (2000). Measuring how acute care nurse practitioners impact outcomes. *Nurse Manager, 31,* 49-50.

The Blended Role of the Clinical Nurse Specialist and the Nurse Practitioner

Patricia M. Hentz • Ann B. Hamric

INTRODUCTION

Over the past two decades, there have been calls to merge the clinical nurse specialist (CNS) and nurse practitioner (NP) roles into one advanced practice nursing role (Busen & Engleman, 1996; Cooper, 1990; Deane, 1997; Elder & Bullough, 1990; Finke, 2000; Hanson & Martin, 1990; Hockenberry-Eaton & Powell, 1991; Quaal, 1999; Shuren, 1996; Spross & Hamric, 1983; Wright, 1990; Wright, 1997). The need for a new advanced practice nursing role, the blended CNS/NP, has emerged over time as a response to changes in patient populations, the increase in health care costs, access to care issues, changes in the health professions workforce, and shifts in delivery of care within the health care system. In some specialty areas, the NP and CNS roles have converged over the past 10 years. This trend has been witnessed particularly in the area of psychiatric mental health advanced practice nursing (McCabe & Grover, 1999). These trends indicate that there is a need for blending CNS and NP skills into a new role to best meet the health needs of certain populations (Hanson & Hamric, 2003; Shuren, 1996; Skalla, 2006; Skalla, Hamric, & Caron, 2005).

This chapter defines the blended CNS/NP, which we will refer to as the *blended role advanced practice nurse* (APN). The evolution and current profile of this role are described. Although the authors recognize that there are other possible blendings of APN roles (in fact, the most recent National Sample Survey of RNs revealed blending among all four of the major APN roles [Department of Health and Human Services, 2006]), this chapter focuses on the most common blending between specialty CNS and primary care NP practices. In addition, the blended role in psychiatric mental health nursing will be profiled, as it is actively emerging in that specialty. Challenges in role development and implementation are discussed and illustrated by clinical case presentations and role exemplars. Current issues related to development of the blended role APN are addressed, and recommendations for strengthening and sustaining this role are made.

The blended role APN is a graduate of a graduate degree program in nursing that prepares students to fulfill two APN roles—usually those of CNS and primary care NP. The blended role APN is eligible for dual certification as a CNS in a specialty and as an NP. Although prepared to function in either role, the blended role APN is a unique third role (Skalla, 2006; Skalla, Hamric, & Caron, 2005). Blended role APNs demonstrate the core advanced practice nursing competencies through the provision of comprehensive primary and specialty care to a narrowly defined complex patient population. They have practices that cross settings from primary through tertiary care. Blended role practice includes elements of CNS and NP practices, yet the role is distinct from the practice of these other APNs. The blended role preparation discussed here combines the strengths of two traditional roles: the primary health care skills of NPs and the in-depth specialty and systems knowledge of CNSs. Dual preparation and certification expand the repertoire of knowledge and skills that blended role APNs can offer. The benefits of the blended role are seen in the ability of these practitioners to fulfill a variety of functions, their increased marketability, and the flexibility in their practice. Blended role scope of practice includes expert clinical knowledge of a specialty population, knowledge of complex systems, and skills in consultation, collaboration, and providing cost-effective care with a focus on diagnoses, health promotion, and health education (Busen & Engleman, 1996). Blended role APNs are particularly well prepared to provide care across settings that addresses the health care needs of the underserved, those with multiple chronic illnesses, and those with unusual and complex health problems (Sperhac & Strodtbeck, 1997). "These blended APNs are efficient, effective, and deliver care in seamless coordinated models that do not separate inpatient and outpatient care. These expert specialized nurses provide a full range of health-care services within a holistic...framework" (Sperhac & Strodtbeck, p. 126).

CALLS FOR MERGING CLINICAL NURSE SPECIALIST/NURSE PRACTITIONER ROLES: MERGING VERSUS BLENDING

Before the blended role APN is described, the distinction between the terms *blending* and *merging* must be clarified. We see a difference between "blending" CNS and NP roles into a new configuration with a distinct title and "merging" all CNSs and NPs into one homogeneous product (the term *dual role preparation* could refer to either of these types). In the past decade, the pros and cons of merging CNS and NP roles have been actively discussed (Deane, 1997; Finke, 2000; Mick & Ackerman, 2002; Page & Mackowiak, 1997; Redekopp, 1997; Wright, 1997). Some authors believe that the debate is more theoretical and based on minimal research (Fenton & Brykczynski, 1993). Others suggest that the merger of the CNS and NP roles is inevitable and believe that merging the roles would be advantageous for health care organizations, patient care, and graduate nursing education (Cooper, 1990; Elder & Bullough, 1990; McGivern, 1993; Quaal, 1999; Wright, 1990; Wright, 1997). Still others assert that the roles are distinctly different in scope of practice and setting and should be maintained as such (Beecroft, 1994; King & Ackerman, 1995; Lincoln, 2000; Page & Arena, 1994; Page & Mackowiak, 1997; Zimmer et al., 1990). The National Association of Clinical Nurse Specialists (NACNS) does not recommend either blending or merging CNS and NP roles (NACNS, 2004).

The debate on merging CNS and NP roles reflects the lack of consensus within the profession, as well as differing professional perspectives. However, what is notable in many of these articles is the "either-or" tone, asserting that either the roles must merge or they must stay distinct. The contention here is that this is not an "either-or" debate since no one role can "do it all" in advanced practice nursing. Blending CNS and NP roles into a new role that incorporates elements of each into a new configuration is one productive way to move beyond the "either-or" debate. Blended role APNs as well as individual CNS and NP roles are needed to meet the health care needs of diverse populations in diverse settings.

The psychiatric mental health specialty is interesting in regard to the issue of blending versus merging because it seems to be evolving in both directions: some psychiatric mental health programs are merging their CNS and psychiatric NP components into one role preparation that encompasses all elements of both roles. Other articles describing psychiatric mental health APNs describe a blended role practice as will be discussed here, with elements of the psychiatric CNS and family/adult NP roles blended into a new configuration. The reader will see this distinction in examples provided throughout the chapter.

EVOLUTION OF THE BLENDED ROLE

Early Descriptions of the Blended Role

The development of an advanced practice nursing role that blends the practice of the CNS and NP has evolved in response to societal needs. Dunphy, Youngkin, & Smith (2004) noted that "boundaries of practice are always malleable. They are always subject to myriad external forces—political, economic, social and cultural" (p. 25). Historically, the CNS has been viewed as providing specialized nursing care for a specific patient population, staff development, and systems change in secondary and tertiary inpatient care settings. NPs, on the other hand, have been viewed as generalists who provide primary and preventive care and treat illnesses for a broad patient population in outpatient care settings. Both roles emerged in response to public need (see Chapter 1).

In the 1980s, several authors proposed the idea of an APN who possessed the assessment, diagnostic, and treatment skills of NPs and the direct care, staff coaching, and change agent skills of CNSs (Kitzman, 1983, 1989; Spross & Hamric, 1983). Spross and Hamric proposed one possible model describing future CNS practice in which CNSs would acquire and use competencies traditionally associated with NPs. This future APN would be educationally prepared in both CNS and NP roles, and his or her practice would combine the domains of service and scopes of practice of NPs and CNSs. This APN was seen as a practitioner who would be client-based rather than setting-based, providing care in primary, secondary, and tertiary settings to ensure continuity of services to a specialty-based patient population. Through independent and interdependent practice with physicians, the APN would deliver direct care, such as advanced clinical assessment; manage acute and chronic problems associated with a specific patient population; and provide ongoing guidance about potential diagnosis-specific problems as well as generic primary prevention education. The APN would also provide vital indirect patient care through expert clinical consultation, coordination and facilitation of patient services, and support for mproved nursing practice (Spross & Hamric). Their description of this role is consistent with the blended role described in this chapter. Other authors described similar models (Deane, 1997; Gleeson et al., 1990; Hunsberger et al., 1992).

Recent Developments

The evolution of certain advanced practice specialties such as psychiatric nursing and gerontology has created a climate that can be seen as supporting the development of a blended role (Naegle & Krainovich-Miller, 2001; Tappen & Dunphy, 1998; Verger, Trimarchi, & Barnsteiner, 2002). For example, development of the psychiatric CNS/NP role illustrates the challenges in reshaping existing advanced practice nursing roles in response to patient needs and health care trends. In a review of the literature on advanced practice psychiatric nursing and literature on the creation of educational programs to prepare a blended role psychiatric APN, critical factors related to the evolution of blended roles were evident. First, changing population needs became evident as psychiatric care became more outpatient-based. Second, a trend toward primary care practitioners managing psychiatric medications evolved, and patients wanted one-stop service for prescribing and counseling. Finally, a need arose for practitioners to have more skill in differentiating psychiatric illnesses from co-existing medical problems (Scharer, Boyd, Williams, & Head, 2003). Leaders in the specialty recognized that psychiatric CNS practice was changing and responded by developing curricula that offered a blended role (Naegle & Krainovich-Miller; Scharer et al., 2003; Tappen & Dunphy; Verger et al.). The advanced practice roles in psychiatric nursing have a common set of core competencies with educational programs that are very similar (Haber et al., 2003).

HEALTH CARE TRENDS DRIVING EVOLUTION OF THE BLENDED ROLE

Current development of the blended role has been driven by a variety of forces—chiefly, changes in population dynamics and cost-containment initiatives. The rapid pace of change in the health care delivery system continues to require that APNs adapt. Blended role APN practice represents one such adaptation, as these nurses are prepared to meet a wide range of health care needs.

Changing Population Dynamics and Health Care Needs

The demographics of the United States population are changing. Baby boomers are aging, creating the need and demand for affordable primary care and chronic disease management across primary, acute, and long-term care settings (Tappen & Dunphy, 1998). Prosperity and subsequent medical advances have produced better health care, resulting in a population that is living longer with chronic disease. These forces have caused a shift in the focus of care from younger people with more acute care health needs to older people with more chronic disease issues (Porter-O'Grady, 1997). Also, a significant portion of the population have limited access to health care, including the poor, the homeless, and persons from other cultures (Agency for Healthcare Research and Quality [AHRQ], 2005; White, 2000). Clinically, these trends have created the need for a provider who has both primary NP and CNS skills. As increasing numbers of patients of all ages are living with multiple chronic illnesses, they require a provider who can assess, diagnose, and treat illnesses commonly seen in primary care while practicing in the specialty setting and who can assist these patients to navigate a complex care system. The same emphasis on wellness and prevention found in traditional primary care settings needs to be maintained for patients who are living longer with complex chronic illnesses. The dual preparation of the blended role allows the APN to maintain a holistic perspective—seeing patients and their families across settings, assisting in negotiating multiple life stages and transitions, monitoring chronic disease processes and treatments, and helping patients and families cope with the demands of the illness. To manage complex care needs over time and across settings, blended role APNs must also be able to manage and influence the systems within which they function.

Functionally, the blended role APN also requires skills of staff education, consultation, and leadership to improve nurses' and other providers' abilities to care for these patients. It is important to note that not all patients with complex care needs require a blended role APN; they may be better served by a CNS or an acute care NP (ACNP). In addition, some institutions may have need for a particular APN such as a CNS if staff education and support need to be a primary component of the practice. The issue of which provider is appropriate depends on a variety of factors. However, certain patients with complex care needs require a blended role APN to deliver specialty primary care across settings. This point is illustrated in the literature by the account of a CNS who had used CNS-specific skills to initiate and maintain a chronic disease clinic (Paladichuk, Brass-Mynderse, & Kaliangara, 1997). She found she could not practice independently in diagnosis and treatment, so she returned to an NP program to gain those skills.

Health Care Cost Containment and Quality

The rapid pace of change in today's health care system from an illness-driven health care industry to one emphasizing primary health care and prevention means that organizations and individuals must accommodate multiple, simultaneous changes. Cost containment and improving quality continue to be major driving forces in health care. Cost containment through shorter hospital stays and outpatient medical treatments has increased demand for health care providers (Bryant-Lukosius, 2004). The need to keep health care costs down necessitates that chronically ill patients be treated in outpatient rather than inpatient settings. This has resulted in the movement of specialty care to the outpatient setting (Lesser & Ginsberg, 2001, 2003), creating a population of outpatients who are more acutely ill. Given cost pressures, chronically ill patients are being moved through specialty inpatient services more quickly. More attention is being paid to transitions across settings to improve quality and safety as well as to decrease costs (Coleman, Parry, Chalmers, & Min, 2006). At the same time, as noted previously, increasing numbers of individuals being treated for chronic disease still need preventive and primary care.

Cost-effective health care that prevents disease and provides quality care to those who are acutely and chronically ill is the bottom line. Efforts to control costs and to forge a new balance between primary care and illness services are changing the availability and types of positions in health care. In primary care, the patient is viewed as part of the system from birth to death, moving along a continuum of health. At any particular time, health care practitioners are expected to identify where a particular patient's problem fits most appropriately on the health care continuum with respect to both care and cost. Blended role APNs are prepared to "match" patients to the right point on the continuum to maximize appropriate care that is cost-effective.

The blended role can address many of the clinical management challenges raised by cost-containment efforts while demonstrating cost-effectiveness (Brooten et al., 2002). First, patients can get accessible, timely, and appropriate primary care. In addition, it is well recognized that chronic illness care is expensive. These patients require intense follow-up and, in some cases, multiple hospital admissions, as shown by George and colleagues (1999). In general, their experiences in the health care system have made these patients more sophisticated consumers. They have higher expectations of providers and health care systems with respect to continuity of care, access to health care providers, and decision-making power. Familiarity with both inpatient and outpatient systems allows blended role APNs to cross care settings to provide the continuity of care that promotes effective management of chronic illness. The blended role APN also coordinates complex services to ensure continuity of care for patients in need of specialized long-term follow-up. Routine follow-up, chronic illness monitoring, and management of specialty medical problems are done by blended role APNs in collaborative practices with physicians. Blended role practitioners can play a pivotal role in assisting patients to navigate the health care system by providing both direct care and care coordination. The APN's specialty expertise enables him or her to recognize critical turning points in a patient's illness course and prevent unnecessary use of health care resources through early intervention and prevention. For example, a palliative care blended role APN may recognize that an ambulatory patient with cancer who presents with abdominal pain is having narcotic-related constipation and prescribes aggressive bowel management, whereas a primary care provider, without this specialized knowledge, might assume that the patient has a bowel obstruction and admit the patient to the hospital for emergency surgery.

The effectiveness of cost-containment initiatives depends, in large part, on educated consumers. Because APNs have in-depth specialty knowledge and are involved with individual patients across settings, they have credibility with consumers. Research by Litaker and colleagues (2003) demonstrated a high level of patient satisfaction with the care received from blended role APNs. Patients preferred a collaborative NP–physician (MD) team as compared with the usual care group. The NP-MD team spent more time with them. The care included health teaching, written information, referrals as needed, prescription management, and follow-up visits. The APNs provided affordable care. In addition, their interpersonal skills were also rated higher by patients.

Access and Affordability

Access and affordability continue to be difficult issues (Lesser & Ginsberg, 2003). The number of underinsured persons has increased, adding to populations that are underserved such as those in rural areas and those in poor, urban settings. Rural populations, in particular, have difficulty accessing the specialized services of tertiary academic medical centers, and fewer specialists are in these areas, which may mean delays in appointments for referrals and consultations. These patients are treated in a wide variety of settings, including hospitals, freestanding clinics, private offices, public clinics, rural outreach clinics, and other "mobile" settings.

Complex care provided by blended role APNs improves access not only for people in urban and suburban areas but also for rural populations that are currently underserved because of distance and costs. Health care economics cannot support both specialists and primary care medical providers in these areas, but blended role APNs can enhance physician practice or provide a reasonable, cost-effective alternative to help bridge this gap and improve access to quality care.

Increasing Specialty Knowledge Base

An ever-increasing knowledge base is to be mastered within specialties. For example, in advanced practice psychiatric nursing, the specialty content has witnessed a tremendous surge of information (White, 2000). Curricula include psychopathology, psychotherapy, concepts from biological psychiatry, neurobiology, and psychopharmacology. At the same time, the high incidence of co-morbid medical conditions such as heart disease and diabetes means that blended role APNs must have broad advanced physical assessment skills and knowledge of pathophysiology. Blended role APNs in this specialty are often presented with patients who have a chronic psychiatric illness as well as complex physical needs. Combining CNS and NP roles enables holistic care that addresses both the physical and psychological needs of psychiatric patients (Scharer et al., 2003).

Growth in specialty and subspecialty knowledge and practices has helped spur the growth of blended roles. For example, Skalla (2006) noted that the subspecialty of palliative care is well suited for blended role APN practice.

Impact of Physician and Nursing Workforce Shortages

Cost containment continues to drive policymakers to reexamine provider training and workforce needs. There are greater demands for primary care physicians to manage overall patient care and reduce costly specialty care. In the early 1990s, the Council on Graduate Medical Education advocated a decrease in specialty residency programs and a restructuring of medical training to attract more physicians to primary care. The goal was to have a more even distribution of physician expertise, with 50% of physicians being generalists and 50% being specialists (Kindig, Cultice, & Mullen, 1993). This goal has not been realized; more medical school graduates chose a non–primary care specialty than family practice in 2003 (American Academy of Family Physicians, 2003). Tracking of family medicine positions from 1995 through 2007 has demonstrated no notable change in the numbers of medical school graduates choosing family practice (American Academy of Family Physicians, 2007). The need for more primary care providers is even greater, given the growth of the older population and the increase in the number of chronic conditions seen as individuals age (Wolff, Starfield, & Anderson, 2002). High-level specialists who focus on one body system (e.g., the cardiovascular system) may overlook patients' other chronic problems (e.g., chronic urinary tract infections, women's health issues). This situation is one important reason that blended role APNs, with their holistic focus and delivery of primary care in specialized settings, are such a timely innovation in the current health care system.

The other dynamic in relation to the physician workforce is the mandated decrease in residency hours. Since 2003, the Accreditation Council for Graduate Medical Education has required resident hours to be restricted to 80 hours of work per week, averaged over a month (Romano, 2003). This change has dramatically reduced available hospital resident coverage and has already left some institutions in a quandary as to how they will meet patient care needs. This change represents an opportunity for a number of APNs, notably ACNPs, certified registered nurse anesthetists (CRNAs), and blended role APNs. Blended role APNs with specialty expertise can assist with patient management in inpatient settings as well as deliver specialty care in primary care settings.

The current nursing shortage also represents an opportunity for blended role APNs. Compared with NPs for whom the emphasis of the role is on direct clinical practice, blended role APNs have explicit responsibility for developing, educating, and supporting nursing staff to be better able to care for patients with complex specialty care needs. In this capacity, blended role APNs can promote nursing retention and help staff better design unit systems to deal with staff shortages. One institution reported an 8% increase in its nursing retention rate since implementing the blended APN role (Whitcomb et al., 2002). Faculty shortages are receiving attention as more faculty reach retirement age. As Hanson and Hamric (2003) noted, new APN roles that can replenish clinically active nursing faculty ranks need to be encouraged; the blended role APN is such a role.

PROFILE OF THE BLENDED ROLE ADVANCED PRACTICE NURSE

Profiling this role is difficult because many nurses who practice in blended roles do not identify themselves as such. Because the NP role is more familiar to patients, many blended role APNs describe themselves under the single title *NP*. This is borne out by the most recent data from the National Sample Survey of Registered Nurses (RNs) (DHHS, 2006): 66% of the blended CNS/NP responders had *NP* as their position title. Only 6% used the *CNS* title; 18% reported their titles as *instructor/faculty* or *staff nurse*. The other 10% may have had a blended role title, but this was not reported. Given the regulatory recognition and authority granted to the NP title in most states, it is understandable that most blended role APNs would use this title. However, this practice is problematic because it does not clarify whether the APN is functioning in a blended role nor does it clearly show the extent of blended role practice currently in the health care system.

The trend for the number of registered nurses (RNs) educated both as CNSs and NPs demonstrated a dramatic increase from 1996 (the first year data were available) to 2000. The number of RNs with dual preparation increased from 7,802 to 14,643, an 88% increase (DHHS, 2002). However the 2000 to 2004 survey data (DHHS, 2006) indicated that this trend did not continue; the number of RNs with dual preparation showed only a minimal increase from 14,643 to 14,689 (see Chapter 3 for more discussion

of general APN numbers). As noted from the position titles, these numbers do not necessarily indicate that all these nurses are working in blended role positions. Data on blended role positions are more difficult to obtain because most specialty groups do not have a specific designation for a blended role APN in their member database.

Settings

Practice settings for blended role APNs range from hospitals to private practice, from intensive care units to the home setting, and from rural outreach clinics to tertiary care centers. Patient care needs dictate both the settings and the focus of practice. Regardless, crossing settings to provide continuity of care is a key distinguishing characteristic of the blended role APN.

The diversity of settings illustrates the range of practice demands placed on the blended role APN. Despite the challenges, many settings in which the skills of the blended role APN have positively affected patient care have been identified. For example, blended role APNs can be found staffing congestive heart failure clinics in the acute care setting (Paul, 1997), delivering comprehensive care in an outpatient oncology clinic (Jacobs & Kreamer, 1997) and a breastfeeding clinic (Gibbins, Green, Scott, & MacDonell, 2000), managing patients in an organ transplant program (Martin, 1999), managing palliative care needs of oncology patients (Skalla, 2006), managing complex care needs of older adults in a life-care community, functioning in rural oncology outreach settings (Shuren, 1996), or practicing in the subspecialty of gastroenterology (Dudley-Brown, 2006).

Core Competencies: Framework for Practice

A framework for practice remains the biggest challenge facing blended role APNs. Practice has not yet been standardized across practice settings but is currently evolving with the role. It is critical to articulate blended role practice for several reasons. First, blended role APNs have a broad range of skills. Those skills must be identified in collaborative practice to clearly define the scope of practice for the blended role APN. Second, for blended role APNs to properly market themselves, both to potential employers and to the public, a framework for practice must be developed and communicated so that others may understand this role. Third, blended role APNs themselves must be educated to have an understanding of their unique role so they identify themselves as blended role APNs and track outcomes resulting from their practice.

Figure 15-1 provides a conceptualization of the blended role. It is important to understand this role as a distinctive practice with a distinctive title and not as a term for any APN with dual educational preparation as a CNS and NP. It is the regular use of the combined CNS/NP competencies that defines the blended role APN (Hanson & Hamric, 2003). The figure demonstrates that the core competencies common to all advanced practice nursing are at the center of blended role practice. Selected CNS and NP competencies combine with features unique to the blended role to shape this practice. Expert specialty practice with a narrowly defined and complex patient population, crossing settings to deliver care, and dual CNS/NP educational preparation are three distinguishing characteristics of the blended role. This discussion of APN competencies illustrates the

common APN core competencies (see Chapter 3 and Part II) as they are implemented in a blended role. As such, the following sections operationalize Figure 15-1 and illustrate the distinct ways in which blended role APNs practice.

Expert Clinical Practice. Direct care of a narrowly defined population of patients with complex needs is the primary component of blended role practice. Patient care is delivered by the blended role APN as an individual or as a member of a formal team. Clinical responsibilities vary depending on the practice setting and specialty. Expert clinical reasoning and skillful performance are used to provide basic wellness and preventive care, diagnosis and management of illness at the level of a primary care practitioner, and management of the sequela of chronic illnesses within specialty settings.

The blended role APN usually functions within a team to deliver care. Team members range from dyad models of physician–blended role APN in collaborative practice to group practices or hospital services. Team responsibilities may include patient rounds, case presentations at weekly team meetings, cross-coverage, and on-call duties. As integral members of health care teams, blended role APNs must delineate the expanded scope of their practice and negotiate patient coverage during off time in collaboration with peers and physician colleagues.

Criteria should be agreed upon to identify the in-patients and outpatients whose care will be the APN's responsibility. A maximum caseload of patients must be determined to prevent overextension and to enable the APN to provide the range of services that he or she can offer. In addition, time and activities relating to ambulatory patient care should be stipulated. Specifically, the APN should have standard clinic schedule limitations on numbers of patients seen per clinic, guidelines for decision making, and protocols for staff who triage patient phone calls. Human resources and other resources, such as clinical assistants and computers to address clerical functions, need to be negotiated during the hiring process. Ignoring this aspect of providing care may mean that the APN performs these functions by default, compromising productivity, cost-effectiveness, and the role itself. Other personal and political consequences may ensue, such as job dissatisfaction and devaluation of the APN's contributions.

Emphasis on the direct care component of the blended role necessitates that the time required to

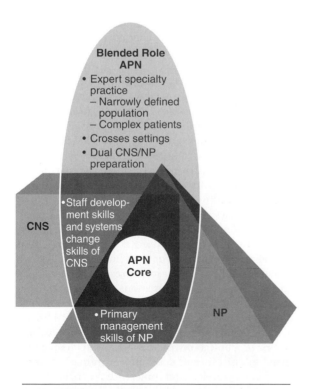

FIGURE **15-1:** Conceptual model of the blended role: framework and competencies. *APN,* Advanced practice nurse; *CNS,* clinical nurse specialist; *NP,* nurse practitioner.

address direct patient care issues be protected. For example, system responsibilities, including staff consultation, form a smaller component of blended role practice than seen in CNS practice. Alternatively, less time is spent on the direct care component for a blended role APN than for an ACNP because of the blended role APN's emphasis on other role components. Within the direct care component, more emphasis is on primary care for a primary care NP than for a blended role APN whose main focus is specialty care and whose secondary focus is primary care.

The holistic approach to direct care is particularly well suited to the skills of blended role APNs as they work with patients and staff. The dual knowledge base of specialty practice and primary care permits the blended role APN to provide comprehensive care for patients. Interviews with recent graduates of psychiatric CNS/NP programs demonstrated that this ability to practice holistically is a major source of job satisfaction (Scharer et al., 2003). The direct care management of blended role practice is illustrated in Exemplar 15-1.

Ethical Decision Making. Ethical decision-making skills (see Chapter 11) are part of the holistic approach to care provided by blended role APNs to assist patients through their illness process. Ethical decision making is necessary to help both patients and staff manage a range of issues, for example, advance directives, durable power of attorney for health care, or sedation at the end of life.

Some of the first author's (PMH) role functions as an APN have involved ethics committee work and education and consultation in actual practice situations (Hentz, 2007). Many nurses have expressed how much easier it is to resolve an ethical dilemma in a case study textbook because they do not know the patient. The ethical dilemmas nurses encounter in practice are "human dilemmas." They are relational in nature and contextually complex. In addition, much of the moral anguish nurses face in ethical situations centers on the awareness of the patient's pain and suffering. By providing a person-centered approach, the relational context becomes critical to the analysis of the ethical dilemma (this is a core tenet of care-based ethics; see Chapter 11). In discussing these cases with an APN skilled in ethical thinking, nurses become more aware that there is no consensus as to which ethical theory is "best" and that it is possible to have conflicting but equally valid moral judgments. In essence, there is no single right answer. Nurses gain an understanding of

the concept *plurality of perspective*—how others view the ethical situation and how they construct meaning and perspective. Because they have the opportunity to see patients across the continuum of care, blended role APNs can bring up end-of-life issues with patients before they are admitted to an acute care facility. They can work with other providers to explain the patient's trajectory and situation outside the hospital setting and clarify the patient's values, which can lead to better ethical decision making. Such a preventive ethics approach (see Chapter 11) can forestall ethical dilemmas before they occur. In addition, providing such information can help other providers to better respect and work with these patients in non-adherence situations.

Expert Guidance and Coaching of Other Care Providers, Patients, and Families. Blended role APNs, like all APNs, must be skilled coaches because they fulfill a variety of educational functions. Patients and families, communities, and professionals all benefit from their guidance and coaching. In addition, blended role APNs have the educational competencies to serve as formal educators for nurses and other care providers (see Chapter 6).

Coaching Nursing Staff, Other Providers, and Students. Because they work across settings and their scope of practice crosses both medicine and nursing, blended role APNs are in a strong position to influence the delivery of health care by educating providers across disciplines. Like other APNs, blended role APNs have opportunities to teach and role model for nurses and other clinicians. What may be unique for the blended role APN is the opportunity to teach and influence staff across settings—in acute, ambulatory, and home care. For example, blended role APNs engage in formal and informal teaching and role modeling of behavior for staff nurses, home care nurses, and ambulatory care nurses. Formal teaching includes classroom presentations and clinical mentoring of both graduate advanced practice nursing students and staff nurses. Blended role APNs may teach in formal educational institutions as guest lecturers or clinical instructors. They are frequently asked to assist in staff development through presentations at in-services and conferences, particularly for issues within their clinical specialty. Informally, education of peers and other providers occurs during consultation for specific patient issues as specialty knowledge is shared.

EXEMPLAR 15-1   **Direct Care Component of Blended Role Practice***

A.B. is a 79-year-old female who has Alzheimer's disease that was initially diagnosed 9 or 10 years ago when she moved into an apartment in a continuing care retirement community. She has been a resident in the health center's Alzheimer's unit for the past 3 years. Her level of dementia is considered to be moderate to severe, with language disturbance, severely impaired memory/recall, and dependence in all activities of daily living. Her days are filled with walking in the halls, singing, and occasional interchange with staff during therapeutic activities.

A.B. has had numerous falls without injury, but after an unwitnessed fall in the evening, she was unwilling to stand and was holding onto her right hip/thigh. The RN present was unable to examine the leg because of A.B.'s agitation. The blended role APN who was on call that evening was contacted, and the situation was described. It seemed very likely from the description of the fall and the limited examination that A.B. had sustained a fracture. She had been lifted into bed and seemed comfortable if she was not moved. Knowing the risk of delirium inherent in sending a patient with dementia to the emergency department for evaluation, the blended role APN concluded that it was preferable to keep A.B. in familiar surroundings.

Consequently, she prescribed oral medications to treat the pain and ordered an x-ray examination of the hip with a mobile x-ray unit in the morning.

The next day, together with A.B.'s brother, the physician, and an orthopedic consult, the blended role APN determined a course of action/plan of care. The x-ray film confirmed a nondisplaced intertrochanteric fracture, and plans were made to admit A.B. to the acute care facility at 6 AM on the second day after the fracture for a multiple pinning procedure, with recovery in the evening and immediate transport back to the extended care facility. The orthopedic surgeon also understood that A.B. would begin physical therapy immediately after surgery so that she would not experience muscular atrophy resulting from immobility and would maintain baseline cognition.

Before admission, the blended role APN communicated with the hospital, providing great detail about A.B., her dementia, and those interventions that could be used to calm her, such as singing if she became agitated while hospitalized. It was clearly communicated that A.B. should not receive psychotropics and should not be restrained. A.B. was readmitted to the long-term care unit at 9 AM the morning after surgery and began touch-down weight-bearing on postoperative day 2. The staff was supported with education regarding the orthopedic procedure done and why she would resume activity so quickly. Her baseline cognition remained unchanged, and within 3 weeks she was walking with assistance and was singing in the halls.

*The authors gratefully acknowledge Brenda Jordan, MS, ARNP, CS, Kendall at Hanover, NH, for her assistance with this exemplar.
APN, Advanced practice nurse; *RN,* registered nurse.

For example, the first author (P.M.H), along with three other blended role psychiatric APNs, worked directly with a nursing staff to develop strategies to help manage agitated and confused older patients. The blended role APNs assessed the staff's patterns of interacting and then identified some of the staff behaviors that were triggering the older patients' aggressive responses. One major difficulty identified was that the staffs' manner and approach were often too abrupt with these patients. An ABC model (antecedents, behavior, consequences) was presented to the staff along with the APNs modeling the behavior with patients (Landreville, Dicaire, Verrault, & Levesque, 2005). In this situation, the blended role APNs were able to share expert knowledge and experience and serve as role models to change practice on the adult psychiatric inpatient unit.

When they are caring for patients with complex needs, it is critical that blended role APNs communicate to the nurses who care for those patients on a daily basis how to provide the best possible nursing care. Conducting similar activities with medical students and residents may fall informally within the scope of practice, but the practitioner must evaluate whether to make it a formal part of his or her practice. Exemplar 15-2 illustrates this competency.

Coaching Patients, Families, and Communities. In contemporary health care, the patient is expected to take an active role in health maintenance, and so patients must be effectively educated in order to be partners in their care. Paradoxically, at a time when patients need more information, providers have less time to provide it because of the

EXEMPLAR 15-2   Expert Coaching and Guidance in Blended Role Practice*

A tertiary care medical center with a well-established oncology program established an outreach site at a community hospital 100 miles away. The physician/blended role APN team model in effect at the cancer center was implemented at the outreach clinic. Shortly after the clinic began treating patients, it became clear that the medical/surgical nursing staff in the community hospital were not comfortable treating patients receiving chemotherapy. Community hospital administrators asked the APN to address the situation and design an educational program to meet the nurses' needs.

Needs assessment, design, and implementation were enhanced by the APN's dual competencies of CNS and NP. The inpatient nursing staff were already familiar with the APN through her clinical visits to oncology inpatients. Using adult education principles and change theory, the APN developed a 4-hour program for the nurses caring for patients who would be receiving or had received chemotherapy in the past 48 hours. In collaboration with one of the clinic oncology nurses, the majority of the medical/surgical and critical care nurses at the community hospital were taught safe handling of antineoplastic drugs, patient assessment around chemotherapy administration, and precautions to observe after the chemotherapy had been administered. Vital components of the program that promoted greater acceptance were the APN's first-hand experience with administering the drugs that were being discussed and her daily experience assessing patients in the process of receiving chemotherapy and managing the accompanying side effects. The program was a success, as measured by the staff's increased comfort and skill in caring for their patients receiving chemotherapy.

*The authors gratefully acknowledge the contribution of Karen Skalla, MSN, ARNP, AOCN, and Paula Caron, MS, ARNP, AOCN, Dartmouth-Hitchcock Medical Center, Lebanon, NH, for this exemplar.
APN, Advanced practice nurse; *CNS,* clinical nurse specialist; *NP,* nurse practitioner.

reimbursement constraints imposed by the health care system. Adding to the burden, medical advances have produced a wealth of knowledge about which patients, as well as providers, need to be informed. Blended role APNs are in an excellent position to offer both individual and programmatic patient education. Knowledge of both primary and specialty care enables them to identify the patient education needs for a defined patient population, critique existing material for applicability, and assist in development of programs and materials.

Although some portion of patient education is billable, funding group educational programs is frequently a challenge. Familiarity with the research process enables blended role APNs to identify and act on potential sources of grant funding for group education, while contacts made in their activities as educators and consultants help them pursue private or corporate sources of funding.

Information seeking on the Internet has become an integral part of patient education today as both providers and patients identify resources, referrals, and educational materials from this source. Much of this information can be overwhelming and misleading to patients. Blended role APNs, in utilizing their research and coaching competencies, can act as resources to filter and validate much of this information while providing the expertise to explain complex information in a way that patients can understand. Blended role APNs can focus on topics that explore how attention to primary care and health promotion in the context of chronic illness improves the quality of life for chronically ill patients. Intensive and ongoing education of this population is critical to successful clinical management. In addition, blended role APNs integrate teaching and coaching activities into the direct clinical time they spend with patients. As pressures mount to see more patients in less time, this critical activity must be safeguarded.

Community or public education is also an important point of practice for blended role APNs. Their visibility across settings and their credibility as nurses make them ideal for educating groups and organizing specialty screening clinics and events. Their expert practice within the specialty gives them the added ability to offer diagnostic/screening services and make referrals to specialists based on the findings of the screening.

Consultation. Blended role APNs may find themselves in the role of consultant, although in blended practice this activity will likely play a smaller part than it would for a CNS (see Chapters 7 and 12). In a review of consultation in nursing, Berragan

(1998) described internal and external consultation. Internal consultation occurs within the context of the practitioner's role. External consultation occurs when the practitioner is an independently practicing consultant. Although prepared to do both, the blended role APN functions primarily as an internal consultant. As practitioners across health care settings, these APNs are consulted on a variety of patient and family issues. Consultation usually focuses on specific patient problems such as symptom management but may address broader issues such as initiating and delivering palliative care. Consultation frequently occurs between blended role APNs and physicians or other nonspecialty providers over specific patient care issues with respect to diagnosis and treatment. In a study of psychiatric CNS/NPs, a process of cross-consultation was identified (Scharer et al., 2003). Not only did the blended role APNs consult with physicians, but physicians and non-psychiatric NPs consulted with the APNs. In primary care settings, physicians asked for help with psychiatric–mental health problems, and in the psychiatric setting, psychiatrists asked for assistance in managing medical problems. This consultation with physicians is in contrast to the role of the CNS, who most frequently consults with nursing staff for nursing care or organizational issues.

Opportunities for external consultation are uncommon but may occur depending on the practitioner. One example of the first author's (PMH) experience as a blended role psychiatric APN was as a consultant to a group of community health nurses who were caring for pregnant and postpartum women. The nurses had questions on how best to screen for depression. In the role of external consultant, an educational session was provided. Nurses were given information on signs and symptoms of depression, on which depression instruments were most reliable and how they could be used, on the best times to screen for depression during pregnancy and postpartum, and on treatment options. Nurses were also able to call with questions, and a follow-up educational session was available as needed. Outcomes of the consultation included increased depression screening during the first trimester of pregnancy and a significant increase in identified cases of depression with resulting referrals to mental health services.

Research. All APNs are prepared by graduate education to utilize research in clinical practice, to collaborate with researchers, and to use evidence-based practice approaches (see Chapter 8). A variety of opportunities exist for integrating research into blended role practice. As an expert clinician and problem solver, the blended role APN is well suited to identify research topics for investigation of complex patient problems and then to follow through in research utilization and dissemination. For example, many nationally developed clinical guidelines provide answers to clinical questions such as how best to manage pain or incontinence, which may take on added complexity when applied to a particular patient group. Blended role APNs promote continuity of care by utilizing and disseminating these guidelines as they manage patients whose chronic problems cross care settings. For example, a blended role APN in oncology used evidence-based clinical guidelines to help the staff develop a pain management plan for a terminally ill patient admitted to the hospital and then followed up with that patient in the ambulatory care setting to modify the plan as the patient's condition changed. In collaboration with staff, the blended role APN can identify areas of practice that are problematic and subsequently model evidence-based practice. When faced with a clinical question, the practitioner can locate current research or collaborate with others to develop an evidence-based approach to answering the question—whether it is a research-based practice guideline as part of a quality improvement project or a pilot study to evaluate the need for a specific practice change (Drenning, 2006). Involvement in professional activities provides a network of colleagues who may be consulted for assistance with applying evidence or identifying potential sources of research funding for projects. Furthermore, the blended role APN may professionally present or publish the findings in order for others to benefit from the experience.

In addition to research utilization and dissemination, the blended role APN may have the opportunity to collaborate in research efforts within institutions and in large multicenter cooperative studies. As frontline providers, blended role APNs are also in an excellent position to recruit patients for participation in studies.

Leadership: Clinical, Professional, and Systems. The variety of activities fulfilled by blended role APNs gives them the broad skills necessary to be credible leaders. Diverse experiences help mold blended role APNs into expert practitioners, change agents, and negotiators who communicate effectively. Leadership activities can be conducted locally or nationally through organizational committees or professional groups. Organizational responsibilities vary, depending on how APNs are utilized within their organization. APNs may be asked to provide staff development programs in their area of specialty or participate in a committee that forms practice guidelines for a particular patient population. In working with a particular population, they identify systematic changes that affect the care of their patients. For example, a palliative care blended role APN may identify an urgent need for designated beds within his or her institution, since the population he or she works with increasingly needs inpatient placement. The APN identifies that this need has arisen because financial concerns have forced family members to work rather than provide care at home. The APN then works at the administrative levels necessary to effect the required changes.

Leadership within the health care delivery system is critical to successful implementation of the blended role. This component develops over time with practice and experience. It includes management of patient care through the health care continuum and so requires the practitioner to manage diverse systems of care in order to treat the patient. Skill at working the system is gained by utilizing familiar activities of the blended role APN: problem solving, negotiation, collaboration, and education. The complexity of the health care delivery system demands creative management approaches to patient problems, whereas the complexity of the modern patient demands expert clinicians.

Utilization of leadership in the political arena enables APNs to be particularly effective in legislative advocacy and lobbying for health care reform. One way to do this is to assist legislators (Hamric, 1998; Milstead, 1997) by developing connections with them, providing fact sheets, statistics, and personal vignettes. As nurses, blended role APNs are innately trusted by the public as patient advocates. As clinicians, they have the specialty expertise to identify problems, particularly related to their respective specialties, and the experience across care settings to identify creative solutions. Considerable impact on health care systems is possible if APNs utilize their leadership skills in policy development and implementation. For example, the blended role perspective can be applied to lobby successfully for such things as increased coverage for specialty medications for Medicare patients.

Collaboration. Interdisciplinary care has received increased attention as a model of delivery in health care systems (Litaker et al., 2003; Zwarenstein & Reeves, 2002). By virtue of working across settings and interacting with a number of providers and staff in different settings, blended role APNs frequently enact the collaboration competency (see Chapter 10). They are in a position to communicate on behalf of patients and their families with their caregivers at different points within the health care system, reducing the burden on patients to re-explain to yet another person their history, needs, and so forth. This competency is integrated into blended role practice on many levels, as demonstrated by the variety of peers and providers with whom blended role APNs interact. Collaborative efforts facilitate continuity of patient care across settings, aid in problem solving, and provide many professional opportunities. Interdisciplinary care environments provide opportunities to develop true collaborative practice with physicians, because patients such as those with chronic mental illness are in need of integrated care from both medicine and nursing. Exemplar 15-3 demonstrates how a blended role APN collaborated with psychiatrists in an inpatient psychiatric facility to enhance quality of care.

Differentiating Blended Role Practice from Other Advanced Practice Nurse Roles

What differentiates blended role practice from other APN roles? As shown in Figure 15-1, three characteristics distinguish the blended role APN. First, blended role APNs are educationally prepared differently from other practitioners—they learn both CNS and NP roles and expectations. Second, because of this preparation, blended role clinical practice differs from that of the CNS and NP—the blended role APN crosses settings while clinically managing a specialty population. These two characteristics have created the third characteristic—blended role APNs care for a more narrowly defined complex patient population than do other APNs. For example, an adult psychiatric mental health blended role APN had a practice focused in a subspecialty area of addictions. Working on an inpatient addictions unit, her role included completing the initial history and physical examination and ordering any relevant laboratory studies or other tests. With a CNS's in-depth specialty knowledge in the area of addictions together with her NP education, she was also able to screen for medical complications that often co-occur with addictions.

EXEMPLAR 15-3   Collaboration in Blended Role Practice

Mrs. J. is an 85-year-old women currently living in an extended care facility. She has a history of COPD and bipolar I disorder. Over the past 3 years, Mrs. J. has been followed by a blended role psychiatric APN who has met with her weekly, has conducted family meetings, and has managed her psychiatric medications. The blended role APN collaborates with a geriatric psychiatrist and carries her own caseload of patients at the extended care facility.

During a routine visit with Mrs. J, the APN detected that Mrs. J. was having some respiratory difficulty. Staff reported that she had not been eating or taking fluids and seemed a bit confused at times. The APN notified the collaborating psychiatrist regarding the patient's change in mental status, initiated a medical consult to Mrs. J.'s attending physician, and ordered a lithium level. The lithium level was elevated (1.4 mEq/L). Mrs. J.'s lithium dose was decreased, and daily lithium levels were ordered. The consulting attending physician recommended starting Mrs. J. on an oral steroid regimen to address the exacerbation of COPD symptoms. The APN shared with the attending physician that there is an increased

risk of precipitating a bipolar manic episode with steroid treatment. Together they weighed the pros and cons and decided that, given the severity of the patient's respiratory symptoms, steroid treatment was necessary. The APN informed the nursing staff of the treatment plan and alerted them to contact her if they detected any manic symptoms. Indeed, the steroids did induce a manic attack, which required Mrs. J. to be admitted into the psychiatric intensive care unit. Because the extended care facility and psychiatric facility were part of the same organization, the APN was able to follow the patient and was able to do the admitting psychiatric evaluation. The APN was able to relay to the inpatient psychiatrist the patient's history and the series of events that led to the manic episode. She was also able to contact the family and set up time to explain Mrs. J.'s condition. The APN worked with the psychiatrists to adjust Mrs. J.'s lithium dose while she was being tapered off of the steroids. Within a week, Mrs. J.'s mood was stable and her respiratory function back to baseline. She was discharged back to the extended care facility, and the APN continued to see her weekly.

APN, Advanced practice nurse; *COPD,* chronic obstructive pulmonary disease.

To enhance the clarification of the blended APN role, Hanson and Hamric (2003) listed practices that are *not* blended CNS/NP practice, stating the following:

> We would submit that the blended CNS/NP role is NOT: a CNS who has returned to school for an NP credential and is practicing as an NP . . . ; a graduate of an educational program that has homogenized the distinctive features of the CNS and NP so that neither role is clearly taught . . . [or] a specialty NP that crosses settings but has a strictly patient-focused practice. (pp. 208-209)

Critical to the blended APN role is that both CNS and NP components of the role are well articulated within the practice and understood by administrators and staff.

The blended role APN's scope of clinical practice differs from the ACNP's scope in the amount of outpatient follow-up that is incorporated into clinical responsibilities, as well as the CNS activities of staff support and systems change. Unlike the ACNP, who is responsible for a variety of acutely or critically ill

patients and for limited ambulatory care activities (if any), the blended role APN is responsible for ongoing follow-up of a particular patient population across settings. The blended role APN has a greater focus on primary care than does the ACNP and a greater opportunity to meet primary care needs as patients present for follow-up in outpatient clinics. For example, the blended role APN may discover that a breast cancer survivor has not had a colonoscopy as recommended by current guidelines for colon cancer screening and would follow up with the appropriate referral. A blended role APN who cares for a woman with chronic obstructive pulmonary disease (COPD) may treat her for a simple urinary tract infection while also seeing her for an exacerbation of COPD. As this practitioner cares for a patient with complex needs, the care delivered is "complete" in that the whole person must be addressed. Although utilizing a holistic perspective, the ACNP is more often treating a specific acute problem and referring primary or non-acute care issues to other providers.

The blended role APN is also distinguished from the CNS who completes a certificate NP program but returns to his or her current position, functioning strictly as a CNS without an expanded focus on direct and primary care. It is challenging to clarify the role differences among NP, CNS, and blended role APN. CNSs and NPs are currently in practice who identify their role as blended but who may not practice in a true blended role. One distinction is that the blended role APN utilizes elements of both the NP and the CNS roles in a specialty setting. As noted earlier, various examples of the blended role in different practice settings are beginning to appear in the literature. The blended role APNs in these settings describe clinical responsibility for their specialty population across settings; the educational role with patients, families, and staff; the research role of evaluating clinical outcomes; and the systems focus in managing system/organizational issues.

EVALUATION OF BLENDED ROLE PRACTICE

In addition to assessing the impact of the blended APN role on patient outcomes, evaluation is necessary for financial justification of the position and future role development. Cost analysis should focus not only on dollars saved or earned by virtue of having a blended role APN but also on clinical outcomes so that value can be demonstrated. Initial research supports the validity of this role (Naylor et al., 1999). Models have been developed to test outcomes specific for advanced practice nursing that support the need for blended role functions (Brooten et al., 2002). Increased ability to use information systems/technology to support and improve patient care systems has been identified as an essential requirement for advanced practice (American Association of Colleges of Nursing [AACN], 2006). APNs must support their practice by aggressive use of computer technology to track data in local and national databases to demonstrate accountability for their outcomes (see Chapter 25).

A lack of specific historical measures upon which to base blended role practice evaluation has slowed research for the blended role; such measures are important to provide validity and illustrate the value of the role to health care institutions. MacDonald, Herbert, and Thibeault (2006) highlighted several studies that have indicated positive outcomes of APN practice in the care of women with breast cancer and the care of frail older adults. However, the APN title broadly included NPs and CNSs and did not indicate whether the effectiveness of these APNs differed or whether any were dually prepared.

The first step is identification or development of valid and reliable tools that can be used in a variety of settings. Many tools exist to standardize health care data collection. Although no evaluation tool currently captures the blended role, many contain useful measures of patient outcomes that could be used to demonstrate the impact of this practice. For example, the Healthcare Effectiveness Data and Information Set (HEDIS), which measures performance, is useful as a tool both to address liability issues and to demonstrate a blended role APN's impact on the quality of care. (These issues are discussed more extensively in Chapter 25.) Blended role practice may have the added value of improving both processes of care and outcomes such as patient satisfaction, adherence to therapy, and improved health maintenance. These outcomes should be studied in settings where blended role APNs practice.

Consultation with outcome managers (Fleschler & Luquire, 1998) in hospital quality improvement departments and outcome management programs or faculty in schools of nursing (Drenning, 2006) can help the blended role APN address such issues as when to measure an outcome, to what level of analysis the research should be taken, and how to achieve appropriate scientific rigor for what is being studied. To conduct complete outcome studies, the issue of admission privileges for blended role APNs must be addressed. For example, tracking admission and readmission rates could be very useful for evaluating a practitioner's ability to manage a patient population clinically across settings and over time. Although great progress has been made in APNs being granted admitting privileges, this is still an issue in some states (Buppert, 2004). When admission rates cannot be accurately determined for an individual blended role APN, it is exceedingly difficult to conduct outcome studies that measure improvement resulting from the continuity of care facilitated by blended role practice.

It is clear that comprehensive practice evaluation must be a priority for all APNs in order to describe their roles and measure their practice. The reader is referred to Chapters 24 and 25 for more discussion of APN outcomes research, evaluation, and performance improvement.

CHALLENGES IN IMPLEMENTATION OF THE BLENDED ROLE

Many issues are raised in blending the CNS and NP roles that, if not addressed, can create confusion both inside and outside the profession. It is critical to focus on blended role APN definition and clarity, not the job title (Hanson & Hamric, 2003; see also Chapter 3), to avoid confusion. The blended role is relatively new, so the degree of clarity that facilitates a consensus as to titling does not yet exist. This lack of clarity is the first hurdle to overcome to strengthen implementation of blended role practices. Blending the CNS and NP roles affects not only individual practitioners but also the disciplines of both medicine and nursing. In addition, as noted earlier, health care consumers have a stake in how this role evolves and, indeed, may affect future role implementation.

Titling

Difficulties with advanced practice nursing titling (Fitzpatrick, 1998) and a summary of efforts to build consensus around the meaning of advanced practice nursing (see Chapter 3) have been described. More recently, a legislative update (Haber et al., 2003) reviewing titling in the specialty area of psychiatric nursing identified 14 different advanced practice titles. Therefore it must be acknowledged that even though the term *advanced practice nurse* is becoming accepted by the profession and policymakers as embracing a variety of advanced practice nursing positions, the issue of titling the blended role APN has remained difficult.

In the past, some authors advocated using the generic title of *APN* for the blended role (Snyder & Mirr, 1995). This stance supports the merging of CNS and NP roles into one advanced practice nursing role. Combining the skills and competencies of the CNS and NP is the focus of this chapter and is an important trend in the continuing evolution of advanced practice nursing. However, the title *APN* is recognized as an umbrella term to describe all advanced practice roles, including CNS, certified nurse-midwife (CNM), CRNA, NP, and ACNP, as well as the blended CNS/NP role (see Chapter 3). Titles should reflect the actual practice and should be unique if the practice is unique.

An alternative title of *CNS/NP* has not been widely explored, nor has it been used often in the literature. This title was seen in one article that used the designation *psychiatric CS/NP*, indicating both the specialty and the blending of CNS (with use of the initials *CS* for clinical specialist) and NP roles (Scharer et al., 2003). This possibility deserves to be considered, because it clarifies the specialty focus of the APN and explicitly denotes both CNS and NP roles merged into one practice. However, this option may be viewed as cumbersome and confusing to consumers. As the blended role is becoming more clearly definable as a distinct advanced practice nursing role, this lack of a consensus title represents a problem in marketing (Bryant-Lukosius et al., 2004). Employers may have some understanding of what role they need but not enough of an understanding to properly advertise and attract the appropriate candidates. As noted, examples of blended role practice were found with authors referring to themselves as *NPs*, or just *APNs* (Paladichuk et al., 1997; Paul, 1997).

Titling has been further complicated by variability in state regulation. For example, in the area of psychiatric nursing, several states designate the title of *APN* to both psychiatric mental health CNSs and NPs without any practice distinctions; that is, they merge the roles. The first author's (PMH) experience with such states is that nurses who hold a single certification as a CNS or NP often see no need to pursue education for the blended role because they can legally practice in either role. As noted, in many states the NP credential is more recognized and versatile. These may be reasons why the statistics for the blended role APN have shown a negligible increase in numbers of blended role APNs but dramatic growth in NPs from 2000 to 2004. However, this trend is problematic because NP scope and characteristics of practice do not reflect blended role practice, with its requirement for CNS educational preparation.

Consequently, the blended role is an APN role that continues to need a clear title to articulate its uniqueness to both professionals and the public.

Balancing Nurse Practitioner and Clinical Nurse Specialist Responsibilities in the Blended Role

Both CNSs and NPs come to blended role practice with special skills and a role identity developed through education, experience, and socialization. Therefore both will need to create a new identity as blended role APNs (Hanson & Hamric, 2003; Skalla, 2006; Wright, 1997). This may present a challenge as the role itself evolves. Role identification and clarification require both a degree of tolerance for ambiguity and the determination to define a new role. In the quest to define this role, blended role APNs must be careful to maintain their nursing focus. Blended role APNs frequently work within a medical model in collaborative practice with physicians. It would be easy to adopt a medical model, but the greatest strength of the role is the nursing focus it brings to health care. As cost-control efforts continue, a real concern is the increasing demands of health care systems for blended role APNs to see more patients in less time, as is currently the case for physicians and NPs. This issue needs to be addressed by NPs and blended role APNs at both the institutional and national levels to advocate that critical nursing functions remain a part of patient care.

Institutions that have converted their CNSs to blended role APNs must also carefully consider the consequences for staff support. Provision of staff support is an important component of blended role practice. However, the blended role APN is unable to provide staff support to the extent that a CNS can. The impact of blending in the inpatient setting has been to create a need for additional CNSs dedicated to staff support, because blended APNs primarily move across settings and are not as available for extended staff support. Because of their greater direct care management responsibilities, blended role providers spend significant time with outpatients and so are limited in the amount of time they have to provide support to staff. It is critical for institutions to recognize this; otherwise, the gains made in improving the care of chronically ill patients by blended role APNs will be offset by patient readmissions caused by a lack of staff education, increased staff turnover, and/or poor nursing care resulting from lack of support by a CNS (Page & Arena, 1994). Therefore the development of the blended role must progress with concurrent support of CNS positions.

Impact on Physicians

The blended CNS/NP role clearly affects physicians. Within primary care, the blended role APN can strengthen what the primary care physician has to offer. APNs prepared in a specialty can expand the ability of a primary care practitioner to manage a wide range of chronic illnesses and the symptoms resulting from those illnesses. Alternatively, blended role APNs can ensure that primary care issues are addressed and appropriately managed in the specialty setting. The beneficial effects of adding a blended role APN into a specialty physician practice can be seen in Exemplar 15-4.

Although this example cites the obvious positive effects the blended role APN can have in practice, many negative perceptions remain within the medical profession. Some physicians have expressed a perceived loss of identity: if blended role APNs can

---

 EXEMPLAR 15-4   Effect of Blended Role Advanced Practice Nurses on Physician Practice

One blended role APN specializing in psychiatric mental health nursing was managing a patient who was being treated for bipolar depression. During the patient's routine visit, the APN noted a fine tremor and increased agitation and restlessness. The APN had been following this patient for 6 months. Although she knew to draw a lithium level, she was also concerned that the presentation of symptoms appeared somewhat different from that seen with high lithium levels. Consequently, she also ordered a thyroid screen. It was discovered that the patient was actually hyperthyroid and her lithium level was within normal limits. This APN carries her own caseload in an outpatient clinic 2 days a week and works collaboratively with two psychiatrists in that setting. The other days she sees patients on an inpatient unit along with two other blended role APNs and the

psychiatrists. Patient satisfaction data have improved significantly with the addition of the APNs, as patients report that they feel they are seen more often and for longer visits. They often ask to see the APN because they know the APN will spend more time with them. The collaborating psychiatrists have commented, "We do not know how we did it without the APNs." The psychiatrists report that they are able to spend the time needed for the most complex cases and rely on the APNs to address the needs of patients who are a good match for their level of knowledge and expertise. It is important to mention that this collaborative relationship has evolved and that the bond of trust took some time. Key ingredients in building collaboration included the proven competence of the blended role APNs along with the openness of the psychiatrists.

APN, Advance practice nurse.

do the tasks of a physician, then what is left for that physician to do? This can lead to the perception of being threatened and can result in conflict over issues related to competition. Clear communication with local primary care physicians should take place in a collaborative fashion to determine how the blended role practitioner can best serve patients within his or her community. The emphasis should be on the value-added complement to medical care that the blended role APN brings to patients and to the practice (see Chapter 3). In addition, the blended role APN's ability to function is often different when the APN is providing primary care versus specialty care. An example is in the oncology specialty in which blended role APNs, licensed to function as primary care NPs, can diagnose and treat primary care problems in the specialty setting but are not licensed to initially diagnose and treat a disease within the specialty. However, this is not the case for all specialty areas, which, of course, adds to the confusion. In addition, practice guidelines vary from state to state. In Exemplar 15-4 cited earlier, practice in the state of Maine permits the psychiatric blended role APN to diagnose within the specialty.

Finally, it is important for blended role APNs to be aware of the role privileges and limitations as dictated by national credentialing bodies and by the privileging system within their own institutions. Both national and institutional credentialing guidelines are important and should be utilized by blended role APNs who may find themselves asked to stretch beyond their scope of practice.

Accountability Issues

By definition, the blended role APN is both CNS and NP. This raises the question, "To whom is the blended role APN organizationally accountable?" Accountability entails both a reporting structure and a philosophical clinical practice alliance. Various possibilities should be considered thoroughly when this role is implemented. Historically, the CNS has been accountable to nursing, and this is a strong reason to implement the blended role position under the direction of nursing. The functions of educator, consultant, and researcher are likely to be most utilized by nursing. However, the clinical component of the position may be more logically aligned with medicine. Collaborative practice models and many NP positions are often structured with accountability to medicine or jointly to medicine and nursing. There is no one correct answer to

this question (see Chapter 23 for more discussion of organizational placement considerations). Each practitioner must assess the practice and strengths and weaknesses of the system and use his or her negotiation skills to establish an appropriate route of accountability for a given position and setting. It is critical, however, for the accountability structure to support a balanced practice so that both CNS and NP components are visible.

PROMOTING SUCCESSFUL ROLE DEVELOPMENT AND IMPLEMENTATION: STRATEGIES AND BARRIERS

The journey to the blended CNS/NP role certainly has its challenges both within and outside of the profession. Discarding or modifying a former role socialization in favor of a new one can be uncomfortable, and making the transition from expert to novice to expert can be unsettling (see Chapter 4). The practitioner faces a variety of issues that need to be addressed for success to be achieved. Recognition of the role's duality is the first issue to address, because it creates the biggest challenge in meeting the demands of diverse role activities in a blended role position. Although diversity is a central component of role success, excellent time management skills are required to balance the demands that this diversity creates. Consensus regarding scheduling and workload, together with role clarity, can help the blended role APN balance multiple demands. This consensus must be negotiated with key stakeholders at the time the APN is hired and should be formally reviewed on a regular basis.

One example of role confusion occurred for a blended role APN who specialized in psychiatric mental health nursing. She was practicing as the first blended role APN to be hired at a psychiatric inpatient facility. She negotiated her job description before starting her position and carefully defined her practice. Within 1 month of her employment, she was asked to take on additional responsibilities, specifically to do Papanicolaou (Pap) tests on the psychiatric patients who needed them. Given her NP preparation, this activity was actually within her scope of practice. However, she viewed doing Pap tests for her psychiatric patients as a boundary problem. She noted to her employer that the psychiatrists were not asked to do Pap tests on their patients. The APN gained support for her stance from the psychiatrists with whom she collaborated.

She also contacted the state board of nursing, who also supported her position not to do Pap tests, and the request was withdrawn. The lesson learned was that she needed to be clear on her role functions in that setting and needed to honor her professional integrity.

Several keys to success in APN development can be applied specifically to the blended role (Brown, 1998). First, as noted earlier, a clear scope of practice mutually agreed upon in a collaborative practice is critical for the blended role APN to function efficiently and avoid turf issues. Second, organizational support for the role must exist. The organization must understand and value the blended role APN and provide support for a balanced role. Effective leadership can facilitate role development and support within the practice setting or institution. An effective leader who can mentor, advocate for academic time, negotiate hours and responsibilities, and encourage research development will ultimately foster development of the successful blended role practitioner. Third, interdisciplinary networks for collaboration, consultation, and referral should be available for the practitioner to be most effective. Developing interdisciplinary and intradisciplinary relationships and lines of support is important to role success. Fourth, one priceless asset in development of the successful blended role is peer support. Peer support is vital to assist in problem solving, provide collegial support, maintain clarity regarding the boundaries of the role, and collaborate in outcomes research. The blended role is among the newest APN roles to be developed. Therefore it is critically important that opportunities for sharing issues regarding development and implementation of the role be provided to facilitate problem solving. A setting without multiple peers is common, but developing a regional peer network through online discussions, formal meetings, and informal consultation should be integral to the practice of any blended role APN.

Exemplar 15-5 articulates these points.

Dealing with Role Strain

An important question to ask given the multiple expectations of blending CNS and NP practice is, "Is the blended role APN trying to be everything to everyone?" It is important to understand the processes that underpin the development of role strain. Simply stated, role strain presents a risk when the demands of a role exceed the actual or perceived

resources to manage the demands. The following are some of the conditions that contribute to this imbalance:

- Situations in which there is a lack of clarity or role confusion
- Pressure to work outside the boundaries of the role
- Lack of support needed to function in the role
- Expectations that exceed the APN's ability in relation to time and resources needed to carry out the role functions
- Conflicts regarding professional standards and role boundaries
- Losing sight of one's own ability to meet the demands and consistently overextending one's self.

APNs who try to be everything to everyone will soon find themselves overloaded with more responsibility than they can handle. They run the risk of doing an inferior job with too broad a scope of practice rather than doing a good job with a limited scope of practice. These risks are analogous to those experienced by CNSs in the 1980s (Hamric, 1989).

One example of how this issue arises is in the performance of medical procedures such as a lumbar puncture, paracentesis, or special surgical techniques. When determining whether to include either a medical task or any other responsibility in blended role practice, the APN must make a decision based on patient need and role clarity. The following are some questions that may be helpful:

- Is the task within the state's nurse practice act, and is it legal?
- Is the task nursing or medical, and is this issue important?
- Will adequate training be provided for the APN to take on this new task or responsibility?
- How much time will be spent doing the task, and how much will it benefit the specific patient population?
- What aspect of practice will the provider have to give up to make room for the added responsibility?
- What is the risk/benefit ratio of the task for the provider and/or the patient?
- What are the political ramifications of accepting or declining the responsibility?

Investigation of these questions can be used to clarify limits on practice that are consistent with meeting the needs of both the patients and the institution.

EXEMPLAR 15-5   Peer Support in Developing Blended Role Practice

Author P.M.H. worked with four other blended role psychiatric APNs in a very progressive psychiatric hospital. Over a period of 4 years, the hospital went from one blended role psychiatric APN to four and was actively recruiting for four new positions. The first APN was truly a pioneer. The psychiatrists were not sure how such an APN could function and what the scope of practice might entail, and they felt a bit threatened. However, after only 1 year, they were pleasantly surprised. They found that the APN was very competent in psychiatric evaluations and was able to follow up with patients throughout their hospitalization. Patients were being seen more often, the APN's assessments were excellent, and appropriate referrals were made to the psychiatrists and the medical staff. The nursing staff also saw benefits. The APN covered several units and was available for consultation. The APN offered educational programs and was available as an expert. The hospital administration soon saw the benefits of the APN in terms of patient satisfaction and cost containment. The second year, three additional blended role APNs were hired. The APNs created a peer group supervision forum and worked together collaboratively. The psychiatrists provided clinical supervision and a high degree of support.

Over the 4 years, the APNs were able to more fully utilize their blended role preparation. Each saw patients in the inpatient setting but also worked 1 to 2 days in another setting including an extended care facility, an outpatient clinic, and a women's health clinic (the blended role APN who worked in the women's health clinic was a certified family NP and had extensive experience in women's health). Because each site was affiliated with the hospital, the APNs were able to refer patients as needed and to follow up with patients who required admission to the psychiatric hospital.

Overall, the APNs enjoyed a high level of job satisfaction. However, a few areas still presented challenges. These challenges revolved around salary and scope of practice. The APNs had proven to be very cost-effective, but the question of fair compensation needed to be addressed. In the fourth year, the APNs negotiated a new model for compensation that factored in the revenue they generated. The psychiatrists had been practicing under this model, and it made sense for the APNs to adopt it. This proved to be a wise decision, because the APNs increased their annual salary by an average of 30%. The second challenge, scope of practice, was ongoing. Because APN practice was cost-effective, administration often had suggestions for additional areas of practice in which to expand blended APN involvement. With strong support from the collaborating psychiatrists, the APNs were able to maintain realistic practice parameters that were in alignment with their scope of practice. This group of APNs also remained well aware of the risks of fragmenting practice and becoming overextended.

APN, Advanced practice nurse; *NP,* nurse practitioner.

As noted, success in the blended role requires balance and time management. Careful reflection and vigilance are needed to maintain balance in practice. Balance in this role may be difficult to achieve, but the balanced practice as described earlier must be maintained. For example, blended role APNs may be asked to participate in multiple educational programs in the settings where they practice. Over time, accepting too many of these commitments can lead to difficulty in managing competing priorities. Skilled negotiation with administrators and colleagues to balance activities such as patient care, research, patient and staff education, and improving system practices is critical. The goal is to avoid excessive emphasis on any one activity, and this presents a challenge, particularly because the clinical component generates revenue. However, a balance must be created in order to successfully fulfill the responsibilities that the blended role requires and to avoid burnout and maintain job satisfaction.

Educational Issues
There are multiple pathways to prepare for a blended role. One common pathway is to begin with CNS preparation and then obtain a post-master's certificate from an NP program. This has been the most common pathway in the psychiatric specialty, as well as most others. CNSs may be motivated to return for NP education because of changes in their clinical populations, reorganization of nursing roles in their settings, changes in state regulations (Quaal, 1999), nursing workforce initiatives (Tappen & Dunphy, 1998), or

other personal or professional goals. NPs may also return to graduate programs to gain CNS skills, but this path seems less common. It is important to note that programs preparing CNSs or NPs alone are not preparing students for blended APN practice.

Many programs have now been developed that offer tracks specifically for the blended role (Scharer et al., 2003; Sperhac & Strodtbeck, 1997; Tappen & Dunphy, 1998; Verger et al., 2002). The increasing interest in preparing blended role APNs is evident in a report of enrollment in graduate education programs (Fang, Wilsey Wisniewski, & Bednash, 2007). As of autumn 2006, 55 programs offering combined NP and CNS preparation enrolled or graduated 1542 students, or 4% of total APN graduates. Sixteen different clinical track titles in combined NP and CNS programs were listed, in addition to an "other" category. While most included primary care NP preparation, the largest number of programs (n = 25) were for adult psychiatric mental health NP/psychiatric mental health CNS-adult. Ten programs offered blended preparation for acute care NP/adult acute and critical care CNS.

As noted, graduate programs that offer a combined CNS/NP blended role curriculum should be longer to ensure sufficient preparation for both roles and may need to incorporate up to a year of extra education for graduates to be eligible to sit for both NP and specialty certifications. This factor may make the DNP degree attractive to nurses wanting blended role APN preparation (see "A Look to the Future," p. 457).

Generic programs that merge content and do not prepare students for the specific CNS and NP competencies needed for blended role practice are doing their students a disservice, and potential students should examine curricula carefully for evidence that both roles are taught. As Scharer and colleagues (2003) said, "as new content and skills are added to accommodate the NP component of the role, it is essential that critical CS content and skills are not lost" (p. 143).

Several criteria should be considered when programs for blended role education are chosen. Clinical practica in blended role programs should be sequenced, beginning with basic competencies of each role and then increasing the complexity with experiences for the blended role APN. Faculty, by necessity, must closely mentor the integration of the roles to ensure that students are adequately prepared and subsequently confident to implement the role. Based on evaluation of graduates of a blended psychiatric CNS/NP program, Scharer and colleagues (2003)

noted the importance of including content on managing complex medical conditions and content and practice experiences related to CNS skills of system negotiation and consultation. In addition, the quality of faculty is critical. As discussed by Sperhac & Strodbeck (1997), faculty need to keep pace with changes in practice. Faculty teaching in blended role programs should have the knowledge and skills related to both roles and have CNS and/or NP experience, preferably in a blended role. The availability of appropriate clinical sites is also critical. A site that already employs blended role APNs is ideal, but the availability of preceptors who have expertise in each of the roles is critical.

CNSs seeking to obtain the NP credential should investigate both the quantity and nature of clinical time necessary to complete the educational program to ensure that clinical hours are sufficient to meet requirements to sit for certification. Some programs have applicants develop a portfolio to identify the applicant's strengths and abilities to fulfill a blended role. The CNS, as an expert in a specialty, may find the transition from expert to novice in an NP program stressful. Lost wages from clinical practice should be considered in factoring educational costs. Negotiation with employers to share the cost and provide time for training can be undertaken by using the value-added aspects of blended role practice as a rationale for funding. There are tremendous benefits from successful blended role education. Students gain a thorough background and subsequently benefit their patients, their clinical sites, and ultimately future employers. This is demonstrated in Exemplar 15-6.

Finding appropriate continuing education can also be a challenge for blended role APNs. The practitioner must take the responsibility to maintain continuing education (CE) in both specialty and primary care practices. For blended role APNs, national meetings of primary care NP and specialty organizations are likely to provide the best opportunities for advanced practice nursing–related CE. APNs also have opportunities to pursue CE on the Internet and through journal subscriptions. Blended role APNs have the challenge of staying informed about both roles.

Certification

Certification issues for blended role practice are complex. In some specialties, such as psychiatric mental health nursing, separate APN examinations exist for CNSs and NPs. In reality, the examination content

EXEMPLAR 15-6 Developing Blended Role Skills in a Graduate Program*

The advanced practice nursing curriculum at Rush University blends PNP and CNS content. The education program and the capstone project, an evidence-based protocol, demonstrate synthesis and application of the blended APN role components that are expected of students near the completion of the program.

One student developed and implemented a comprehensive program to address practice inconsistencies in the treatment of infants with diarrhea in an inner-city, hospital-based ambulatory clinic. During her clinical experiences, the student observed that information given by the pediatricians to parents of infants with diarrhea often differed from that given to them by the PNP. The student surveyed the pediatricians and the PNPs in the group practice about their recommendations to parents of children with diarrhea, compiled the data, conducted a literature search, and obtained the American Academy of Pediatrics guidelines for diarrhea management.

After she disseminated this information to the group for discussion, the group members reached consensus on a uniform approach to treating these infants. The student then developed a practice protocol that was later adopted by the primary care provider group. She also developed and delivered formal in-services for the clinic's professional and ancillary staff on the protocol and developed parent information sheets.

After implementing the practice changes, a formal evaluation was conducted on the education and protocol used in the treatment of children with diarrhea. In a subsequent accreditation visit by TJC, the diarrhea program was highlighted as an example of effective quality improvement.

*The authors gratefully acknowledge the contribution of Arlene Sperhac, PhD, RNC, PNP, Rush University College of Nursing, Chicago, for this exemplar.
APN, Advanced practice nurse; *CNS*, clinical nurse specialist; *PNP*, pediatric nurse practitioner; *TJC*, The Joint Commission.

overlaps, and interesting differences can be seen in the evolution of certification examinations in this specialty. The American Nurses Credentialing Center (ANCC) is currently collaborating with the American Psychiatric Nurses Association (APNA) to move from two examinations to one for advanced practice adult psychiatric mental health nursing. The development of this examination will begin in 2008.

In other specialties and subspecialties, APN examinations for CNSs and NPs do not exist, so practitioners must identify more general areas, such as primary care NP, in which to become certified.

Given these different approaches to certification in the various specialties (see Chapter 21 for updated certification information), one potential trend could be that students graduating from blended role programs may elect for certification in only one role. For example, in the integrated program the first author (PMH) developed, graduates elect to take only the ANCC psychiatric mental health NP examination. They found their practice reflected the blended role and the additional certification did not change the way they practiced. Regardless of the certification path blended role APN students choose, they should be prepared as both a CNS and an NP and thus eligible to sit for two examinations and maintain their certification in both areas.

A LOOK TO THE FUTURE

The Practice Doctorate

One recommendation for APN education with potential opportunity for the blended role is the practice doctorate. A number of authors have advocated expanding education for advanced practice nursing to the doctoral level, in programs geared toward practice rather than the traditional research-oriented PhD (Draye, Acker, & Zimmer, 2006; Fitzpatrick, 2003; Marian et al., 2003; Mundinger et al., 2000). There are a number of reasons the DNP degree may benefit blended role APN education. First, blended role APN educational requirements involve additional courses along with additional clinical hours, which could be accommodated in longer DNP curricula. Second, providing doctoral-level recognition for the blended role APN's additional effort and depth of knowledge and expertise could spur interest in these roles. Third, the DNP prepares graduates for "new dimensions of practice rather than merely 'adding on' courses to a master's degree program" (Draye et al., 2006, p. 125). The DNP program at the University of Washington School of Nursing is an example of a program that builds on the master's-level NP. The APN who is prepared in a practice doctorate gains an increased depth and breadth of knowledge and expertise in practice along with added leadership and clinical research skills. As societal need and the health care system present new challenges, these challenges can become opportunities for nursing. It may be that the blended role APN is part of a natural transition to the DNP.

New Blending Configurations

This chapter has described the blending of primary care NP and CNS roles, but other possibilities for blended roles exist. For example, a blended CNS/neonatal NP role has been described in Canada as a preferred role for a breastfeeding clinic (Gibbins et al., 2000). For the first time, the report of the 2004 National Sample Survey of RNs (DHHS, 2006) listed the numbers of nurses who have various combinations of APN specialties. For example, there are 2892 NP/CNMs and 1365 APNs with other permutations, including CNS/CRNA, CNS/CNM, and NP/CRNA. APNs have always been flexible and proactive in responding to changes in the health care system and changing patient needs. New permutations of APN blending can be seen in this light.

Evolving specialties such as wound, ostomy, and continence nursing and transplant nursing (see Chapter 18) may benefit from proactive development of blended role educational programs to develop the competencies needed to care for their complex patient populations. The challenge as specialties and subspecialties proliferate is to define a cohesive understanding of blended role practice to guide education and role enactment. This chapter has described such an understanding.

A Call for a Cohesive Deliberative Approach

Even while responding to the demands of the health care system, the nursing profession must maintain control and integrity over the development of the blended role. It is critical that the profession be deliberative and cohesive in its approach to this role rather than allow blended role practice to evolve haphazardly or impulsively in ways not consistent with our understanding of advanced practice nursing. The role must be driven by the need for quality patient-centered care delivered by nurses who bring a wide variety of specialized skills to patients across settings. The employment of blended role APNs is one practice alternative to augment the ranks of CNSs and NPs in expanding the profession's ability to deliver advanced nursing care to patients with complex needs.

CONCLUSION

"For APNs who embrace change, there are unlimited opportunities to actively participate in the redefinition of health care, the transformation of practice settings, and the creation of provider roles" (O'Malley & Cummings, 1995, p. 6). New models of education and increased clarity regarding definition and titling will be needed for the blended role APN to develop to its full potential. As mentioned earlier, it may be that a natural transition for the blended APN is toward the DNP degree as the optimal educational level.

On a societal level, patient satisfaction and quality improvement are becoming increasingly important goals in a competitive health care market. As consumers, patients are demanding high-quality care at an affordable price. To thrive, nursing must meet the health care challenges of today while preparing for the challenges that lie ahead. One niche for the blended role may in fact lie with chronic disease management, in which the combined skills of the blended role APN can ensure holistic care and state-of-the-art symptom management for patients facing longer lives with chronic disease. This APN role continues to evolve as an alternative to NP and CNS roles. Blended role APN practice can help meet the needs of specialty populations who require complex coordinated care in a dynamic health care system.

REFERENCES

Agency for Healthcare Research and Quality (AHRQ). (2005). *National healthcare disparities report, 2005.* Rockville, MD: Author. Retrieved July 4, 2007, from www.ahrq.gov/qual/nhdr05/nhdr05.htm.

American Academy of Family Physicians. (March 20, 2003). *Medical student interest in primary care continues to decline.* Retrieved September 1, 2003, from www.aaf.org/x20098.xml.

American Academy of Family Physicians. (March 15, 2007). *Fewer medical students choose primary care, patients may suffer.* Retrieved July 17, 2007, from http://aafp.org.online.en.home.press.aafpnewsreleases/20070301 releases/20070315.

American Association of Colleges of Nursing (AACN). (1996). *Nursing's social policy statement.* Washington, DC: Author.

American Association of Colleges of Nursing (AACN). (2006). *The essentials of doctoral education for advanced nursing practice.* Washington, DC: Author.

Beecroft, P.C. (1994). CNS: Thriving or heading for extinction? *Clinical Nurse Specialist, 8,* 63.

Berragan, L. (1998). Consultancy in nursing: Roles and opportunities. *Journal of Clinical Nursing, 7,* 139-143.

Brooten, D., Naylor, M.D., York, R., Brown, L.P., Munro, B.H., Hollingsworth, A.O., et al. (2002). Lessons learned from testing the quality cost model of advanced practice nursing

(APN) transitional care. *Journal of Nursing Scholarship, 34,* 369-375.

Brown, S.J. (1998). A framework for advanced practice nursing. *Journal of Professional Nursing, 12,* 117-120.

Bryant-Lukosius, D. (2004). Advanced practice nursing roles: Development, implementation and evaluation. *Nursing and Health Care Management and Policy, 48*(5), 519-529.

Buppert, C. (2004). *The nurse practitioner's business practice and legal guide* (2nd ed.). Boston: Jones & Bartlett.

Busen, N., & Engleman, S.G. (1996). The CNS with practitioner preparation: An emerging role in advanced practice nursing. *Clinical Nurse Specialist, 10*(3), 145-150.

Coleman, E.A., Parry, C., Chalmers, S., & Min, S.J. (2006). The care transitions intervention: Results of a randomized controlled trial. *Archives of Internal Medicine, 166,* 1822-1828.

Cooper, D. (1990). Today—assessments and intuitions: Tomorrow—projections. In P.S.A. Sparacino, D.M. Cooper, & P.A. Minarik (Eds.), *The clinical nurse specialist: Implementation and impact* (pp. 285-311). Norwalk, CT: Appleton & Lange.

Deane, K.A. (1997). CNS and NP: Should the roles be merged? *Canadian Nurse, 93,* 24-30.

Department of Health and Human Services (DHHS), Division of Nursing. (2002). *The registered nurse population March 2000: Findings from the National Sample Survey of Registered Nurses.* Washington, DC: Author.

Department of Health and Human Services (DHHS), Division of Nursing: (2006). *The registered nurse population March 2004: Findings from the National Sample Survey of Registered Nurses.* Washington, DC: Author.

Draye, M.A., Acker, M., & Zimmer, P.A. (2006). The practice doctorate in nursing: Approaches to transform nursing practitioner education and practice. *Nursing Outlook, 54*(3), 123-129.

Drenning, C. (2006). Collaboration among nurses, advanced practice nurses, and nurse researchers to achieve evidence-based practice change. *Journal of Nursing Care Quality, 21,* 298-301.

Dudley-Brown, S. (2006). Revisiting the blended role of the advanced practice nurse. *Gastroenterology Nursing, 29*(3), 249-250.

Dunphy, L.M., Youngkin, E.Q., & Smith, K. (2004). Advanced practice nursing: Doing what had to be done; radicals, renegades and rebels. In L.A. Joel (Ed.), *Advanced practice nursing: Essentials for role development* (pp. 3-25). Philadelphia: F.A. Davis.

Elder, R.G., & Bullough, B. (1990). Nurse practitioner and clinical nurse specialists: Are the roles merging? *Clinical Nurse Specialist, 4,* 78-84.

Fang, D., Wilsey Wisniewski, S., & Bednash, G.D. (2007). *2006-2007 Enrollment and graduations in baccalaureate and graduate programs in nursing.* Washington, DC: American Association of Colleges of Nursing.

Fenton, M.V., & Brykczynski, K.A. (1993). Qualitative distinctions and similarities in the practice of clinical nurse specialists and nurse practitioners. *Journal of Professional Nursing, 9,* 313-326.

Finke, D. (2000). Blending CNS and NP roles increases employment opportunities. *Journal of Emergency Nursing, 26,* 98.

Fitzpatrick, E.R. (1990). Analysis and synthesis of the role of the advanced practice nurse. *Clinical Nurse Specialist, 12,* 106-107.

Fitzpatrick, J. (2003). The case for the clinical doctorate in nursing. *Reflections on Nursing Leadership, 29*(1), 8-9, 37, 52.

Fleschler, R., & Luquire, R. (1998). Advanced practice role of the outcomes manager. *Outcomes Management for Nursing Practice, 2,* 54-56.

George, M.R., O'Dowd, L.C., Martin, I., Lindell, K.O., Whitney, F., Jones, M., et al. (1999). A comprehensive educational program improves clinical outcome measures in inner-city patients with asthma. *Archives of Internal Medicine, 159,* 1710-1716.

Gibbins, S.A., Green, P.E., Scott, P.A., & MacDonell, J.W. (2000). The role of the clinical nurse specialist/neonatal nurse practitioner in a breastfeeding clinic: A model of advanced practice. *Clinical Nurse Specialist, 14,* 56-59.

Gleeson, R.M., McIlvain-Simpson, G., Boos, M.L., Sweet, E., Trzcinski, K.M., Solberg, C.A., et al. (1990). Advanced practice nursing: A model of collaborative care. *MCN, The American Journal of Maternal Child Nursing, 15,* 9-12.

Haber, J., Hamera, D., Hillyer, D., Limandri, B., Pagel, S., Staten, R., et al. (2003). Advanced practice psychiatric nurses: 2003 legislative update. *Journal of the American Psychiatric Nurses Association. 9*(6), 205-216.

Hamric, A.B. (1989). History and overview of the CNS role. In A.B. Hamric & J.A. Spross (Eds.), *The clinical nurse specialist in theory and practice* (2nd ed., pp. 2-18). Philadelphia: Saunders.

Hamric, A.B. (1998). Using research to influence the regulatory process. *Advanced Practice Nursing Quarterly, 4,* 44-50.

Hanson, C., & Martin, L.L. (1990). The nurse practitioner and clinical nurse specialist: Should the roles be merged? *Journal of the American Academy of Nurse Practitioners, 2,* 2-9.

Hanson, C.M., & Hamric, A.B. (2003). Reflections on the continuing evolution of advanced practice nursing. *Nursing Outlook, 51,* 203-211.

Hentz, P. (2007). Ethical decision-making: Blending the voice of reason and the voice of compassion. *Pennsylvania Nurse, 62*(1), 14-15.

Hockenberry-Eaton, M., & Powell, M.L. (1991). Merging advanced practice roles: The CNS and NP. *Journal of Pediatric Health Care, 5,* 158-159.

Hunsberger, M., Mitchell, A., Blatz, P., Paes, B., Pinelli, J., Southwell, D., et al. (1992). Definition of an advanced nursing role in the NICU: The clinical nurse specialist/nurse practitioner. *Clinical Nurse Specialist, 6,* 91-96.

Jacobs, L.A., & Kreamer, K.M. (1997). The oncology clinical nurse specialist in a post-master's nurse practitioner program: A personal and professional journey. *Oncology Nursing Forum, 24,* 1387-1392.

Kindig, D., Cultice, J., & Mullen, F. (1993). The elusive generalist physician: Can we reach a 50% goal? *JAMA: The Journal of the American Medical Association, 270*, 1069-1073.

King, K.B., & Ackerman, M.H. (1995). An educational model for the acute care nurse practitioner. *Critical Care Nursing Clinics of North America, 7*, 1-8.

Kitzman, H.J. (1983). The CNS and the nurse practitioner. In A.B. Hamric & J. Spross (Eds.), *The clinical nurse specialist in theory and practice* (pp. 275-290). New York: Grune & Stratton.

Kitzman, H.J. (1989). The CNS and the nurse practitioner. In A.B. Hamric & J.A. Spross (Eds.), *The clinical nurse specialist in theory and practice* (2nd ed., pp. 379-394). Philadelphia: Saunders.

Landreville, P., Dicaire, L., Verrault, R., & Levesque, L. (2005). A training program for managing agitation of residents in long-term care facilities: Description and preliminary findings. *Gerontological Nursing, 31*(3), 34-42.

Lesser, C.S., & Ginsberg, P.B. (2001). Back to the future? New cost and access challenges emerge: Initial findings from HSC's recent site visits. *Issue Brief (Center for Studying Health System Change), 35*, 1-4.

Lesser, C.S., & Ginsberg, P.B. (2003). Health care cost and access problems intensify: Initial findings from HSC's recent site visits. *Issue Brief (Center for Studying Health System Change), 63*, 1-6.

Lincoln, P.E. (2000). Comparing CNS and NP role activities: A replication. *Clinical Nurse Specialist, 14*, 269-277.

Litaker, Mion, L.C., Planavsky, L., Kippes, C., Mehta, N., & Frolkis, J. (2003). Physician-nurse practitioner teams in chronic disease management: The impact on cost, clinical effectiveness, and patients' perception of care. *Journal of Interprofessional Care, 17*(3), 223-237.

MacDonald, J., Herbert, R., & Thibeault, C. (2006). Advanced practice nursing: Unification through a common identity. *Journal of Professional Nursing, 22*(3), 172-179.

Marion, L., Viens, D., O'Sullivan, A., Crabtree, K., Fontana, S., & Price, M. (2003). The practice doctorate in nursing: Future or fringe? *Topics in Advanced Practice Nursing eJournal, 3*, 2. Retrieved May 21, 2003, from www.medscape.com/viewarticle/453247.

Martin, R.K. (1999). The role of the transplant advanced practice nurse: A professional and personal evolution. *Critical Care Nursing Quarterly, 21*, 69-76.

McCabe, S., & Grover, S. (1999). Psychiatric nurse practitioner versus clinical nurse specialist: Moving from debate to action on the future of advanced psychiatric nursing. *Archives of Psychiatric Nursing, 13*, 111-116.

McGivern, D.O. (1993). The evolution to advanced nursing practice. In M.D. Mezey & D.O. McGivern (Eds.), *Nurses, nurse practitioners: Evolution to advanced practice* (pp. 3-30). New York: Springer.

Mick, D.J., & Ackerman, M.H. (2000). Advanced practice nursing role delineation in acute and critical care: Application of the Strong Model of Advanced Practice. *Heart & Lung, 29*, 210-221.

Milstead, J.A. (1997). Using advanced practice to shape public policy: Agenda setting. *Nursing Administration Quarterly, 21*, 12-18.

Mundinger, M.O., Cook, S.S., Lenz, E.R., Piacentini, K., Auerhahn, C., & Smith, J. (2000). Assuring quality and access in advanced practice nursing: A challenge to nurse educators. *Journal of Professional Nursing, 16*, 322-329.

Naegle, M.A., & Krainovich-Miller, B. (2001). Shaping the advanced practice psychiatric-mental health nursing role: A futuristic model. *Issues in Mental Health Nursing, 22*, 461-482.

National Association of Clinical Nurse Specialists (NACNS). (2004). *Statement on clinical nurse specialist practice and education.* Harrisburg, PA: Author.

Naylor, M.D., Brooten, D., Campbell, R., Jacobsen, B.S., Mezey, M.D., Pauly, M.V., et al. (1999). Comprehensive discharge planning and home follow-up of hospitalized elders. *JAMA: The Journal of the American Medical Association, 281*, 613-620.

O'Malley, J., & Cummings, S.H. (1995). Change…more change … and change again. *Advanced Practice Nursing Quarterly, 1*, 1-6.

Page, N.E., & Arena, D.M. (1994). Rethinking the merger of the clinical nurse specialist and the nurse practitioner roles. *Image: The Journal of Nursing Scholarship, 26*, 315-318.

Page, N.E., & Mackowiak, L. (1997). Role play: The clinical nurse specialist and nurse practitioner—Complementary roles. *Journal of the Society of Pediatric Nurses, 2*, 188-190.

Paladichuk, A., Brass-Mynderse, N., & Kaliangara, O. (1997). Chronic disease management: An outpatient approach. *Critical Care Nurse, 17*, 90-95.

Paul, S. (1997). Implementing an outpatient congestive heart failure clinic: The nurse practitioner role. *Heart & Lung, 26*, 486-491.

Porter-O'Grady, T. (1997). Over the horizon: The future and the advanced practice nurse. *Nursing Administration Quarterly, 21*, 1-11.

Quaal, S.J. (1999). Clinical nurse specialist: Role restructuring to advanced practice registered nurse. *Critical Care Nursing Quarterly, 21*, 37-49.

Redekopp, M.A. (1997). Clinical nurse specialist role confusion: The need for identity. *Clinical Nurse Specialist, 11*(2), 87-91.

Romano, M. (2003). Resident restrictions: Most teaching hospitals ready for work-hour rules. *Modern Healthcare, 33*, 10-11.

Scharer, K., Boyd, M., Williams, C.A., & Head, K. (2003). Blending specialist and practitioner roles in psychiatric nursing: Experiences of graduates. *Journal of the American Psychiatric Nurses Association, 9*, 136-144.

Shuren, A. (1996). The blended role of the clinical nurse specialist and nurse practitioner. In A.B. Hamric, J.A. Spross, & C.M. Hanson (Eds.), *Advanced nursing practice: An integrative approach* (pp. 375-394). Philadelphia: Saunders.

Skalla, K. (2006). Blended role advanced practice nursing in palliative care of the oncology patient. *Journal of Hospice and Palliative Nursing, 8*(3), 155-163.

Skalla, K., Hamric, A.B., & Caron, P.A. (2005). The blended role of the clinical nurse specialist and nurse practitioner. In A.B. Hamric, J.A. Spross, & C.M. Hanson (Eds.), *Advanced practice nursing: An integrative approach* (3rd ed., pp.515-550). Philadelphia: Saunders.

Snyder, M., & Mirr, M.P. (Eds.). (1995). *Advanced practice nursing: Guide to professional development*. New York: Springer.

Sperhac, A.M., & Strodtbeck, F. (1997). Advanced practice in pediatric nursing: Blending roles. *Journal of Pediatric Nursing, 16,* 120-126.

Spross, J., & Hamric, A. (1983). A model for future clinical specialist practice. In A.B. Hamric & J. Spross (Eds.), *The clinical nurse specialist in theory and practice*. New York: Grune & Stratton.

Tappen, R.M., & Dunphy, L. (1998). Blended role advanced practice in gerontological nursing. *The Florida Nurse, 46*(8), 21-22.

Verger, J., Trimarchi, T., & Barnsteiner, J.H. (2002). Challenges of advanced practice nursing in pediatric acute and critical care: Education to practice. *Critical Care Clinics of North America, 14,* 315-326.

Whitcomb, R., Wilson, S., Chang-Dawkins, S., Durand, J., Pitcher, D., Lauzon, C., et al. (2002). Advanced practice nursing:

Acute model in progress. *Journal of Nursing Administration, 32*(3), 123-125.

White, J. (2000). Developing a CNS role to meet the mental health needs of the underserved. *Clinical Nurse Specialist, 14*(3), 141-149.

Wolff, J.L., Starfield, B., & Anderson, G. (2002). Prevalence, expenditures, and complications of multiple chronic conditions in the elderly. *Archives of Internal Medicine, 162,* 2269-2276.

Wright, J.E. (1990). Joining forces for the good of our clients. *Clinical Nurse Specialist, 4,* 76-77.

Wright, K.B. (1997). Advanced practice nursing: Merging the clinical nurse specialist and nurse practitioner roles. *Gastroenterology Nursing, 20,* 57-60.

Zimmer, P., Brykczynski, K., Martin, A.C., Newberry, Y.G., Price, M.J., & Warren, B. (April 1990). *Advanced nursing practice: Nurse practitioner curriculum guidelines* (Final Report: NONPF Education Committee). Paper presented at the National Organization of Nurse Practitioner Faculties, Washington, DC.

Zwarenstein, M., & Reeves, S. (2002). Working together but apart: Barriers and routes to nurse-physician collaboration. *The Joint Commission Journal on Quality Improvement, 28.* Retrieved June 23, 2007, from www.jcrinc.com.

16

The Certified Nurse-Midwife*

Cheryl A. Sarton • Maureen A. Kelley

INTRODUCTION

Because midwifery/nurse-midwifery in the United States and around the world represents different levels of preparation, we begin by distinguishing between four different types of midwives in the United States. The common denominator for all midwives is being "with woman" during pregnancy and birth. **Certified nurse-midwives (CNMs)** are individuals educated in the two disciplines of nursing and midwifery who possess evidence of certification according to the requirements of the American College of Nurse-Midwives (ACNM) (American College of Nurse-Midwives [ACNM], 2004b). The educational program must be accredited by the ACNM Accreditation Commission for Midwifery Education (ACME), and the individual must pass a national certification examination administered by the American Midwifery Certification Board (AMCB). **Certified midwives (CM)** are individuals educated in the discipline of midwifery who possess evidence of certification according to the requirements of the ACNM (ACNM, 2004a). According to the Midwives Alliance of North America (MANA), the term *CM* can also be used in certain states as a designation of certification by the state or midwifery organization (Midwives Alliance of North America [MANA], 2007). **A certified professional midwife (CPM)** is an individual who is a knowledgeable, skilled, and professional independent midwifery practitioner who has met the standards of certification set by the North American Registry of Midwives (NARM) and is qualified to provide the Midwifery Model of Care (MANA, 2007). A CPM is certified via an examination administered by the NARM. In addition to CNMs, CMs, and CPMs, there are also **direct entry midwives (DEMs),** lay midwives (also known as *"granny" midwives, traditional midwives, traditional birth attendants, empirical*

midwives, and *independent midwives*), and licensed midwives. Some of these practitioners are legally recognized, some have had formal training, and some have had apprenticeship training. The authors focus on CNMs who are practicing in an advanced practice nursing role. For the purpose of this text, *midwife* and *CNM* are used interchangeably and when issues related to non-nurse midwives are addressed, an attempt is made to make that clear.

Nurse-midwifery in the United States has its roots in nursing and has made many contributions that have paved the way for advanced practice nursing to flourish. These efforts have included the development of standards, core clinical competencies, and successful legislative and regulatory initiatives. Nurse-midwifery activities that have been instrumental in securing prescriptive authority and direct reimbursement by insurers for CNMs have also had a favorable direct or indirect impact on all APNs. The pioneering efforts of CNMs have helped cultivate a clinical and political climate of acceptance not only for themselves but also for clinical nurse specialists (CNSs), certified registered nurse anesthetists (CRNAs), and nurse practitioners (NPs) as legitimate and visible providers of care across all settings.

The ACNM believes that midwifery education should (1) reflect a philosophy that supports women as partners in their health care choices, (2) prepare practitioners whose knowledge and skills reflect current ACNM core competencies for basic midwifery practice, (3) be affiliated with an institution of higher learning that is accredited by an accrediting agency recognized by the United States Department of Education, and (4) be incorporated into a program of professional studies that either requires a baccalaureate degree upon entrance or grants no less than a baccalaureate degree upon completion (ACNM, 2005d). An ACNM position statement on degree requirements for CNM practice states that, as of 2010, completion of a graduate degree will be required for entry into practice (ACNM, 2006b). However, the ACNM has not endorsed the 2004 American Association of Colleges

---

*We wish to acknowledge Margaret W. Dorroh and Sheila F. Norton for their important contributions to the first edition of this text (Dorroh & Norton, 1996) and Margaret W. Dorroh and Maureen A. Kelley for their contributions to the third edition of this text (Dorroh & Kelley, 2005).

of Nursing (AACN) (AACN, 2004b) "Position Statement on the Practice Doctorate in Nursing," emphasizing that the Doctor of Nursing Practice (DNP) "may be one option for some nurse-midwifery programs, but should not be a *requirement* for entry into midwifery practice" (ACNM, 2007d).

The purpose of this chapter is to describe nurse-midwifery practice in the United States so that the reader can appreciate both why it can be seen as an advanced practice nursing role and why there are concerns within midwifery if it is seen *only* as an advanced practice nursing role. As authors, we offer our own perspectives on the issues that prevent full integration of nurse-midwifery into advanced practice nursing. Nurses and CNMs alike have a stake in issues related to this level of professional practice. The reflections in this chapter are meant to foster dialogue, understanding, and wisdom as nurses and CNMs work to accomplish their goals related to practice. It is our hope that all nursing will continue to work productively and collaboratively in activities to promote advanced practice nursing.

HISTORICAL PERSPECTIVE

Midwifery predates nursing and medicine. Throughout time and in all cultures, the midwife has played a recognized and respected role. In Biblical times, the midwife assisted a woman in labor, helped birth the baby, and provided for after-care of mother and infant. Novice midwives acquired knowledge and skill by apprenticing with experienced midwives and through their own observations and experience.

In colonial times, midwives were an integral part of community life and were highly respected members of society. In the early 1900s, a number of developments considerably diminished that respect and led to an ebb in the practice of midwifery. The immigrant population was served by European immigrant midwives, and African-American women from the South were cared for by traditional African-American midwives. These midwives lacked a national organization, methods of communication, access to the health care system, and legal recognition (Burst, 2005). An active campaign was waged to discredit midwives even though data demonstrated good care outcomes for these providers (Dawley, 2003). During this same time frame, physicians took over the role of birth attendant and birth moved into the hospital setting. The medicalization of birth did much to eliminate midwifery and continues to influence and regulate the practice of nurse-midwifery.

Although midwifery remained part of mainstream health care in many European, Asian, and African countries, the renaissance of midwifery in the United States did not occur until the 1940s and 1950s. Strong nursing leaders and the childbirth education movement largely shaped the reappearance of midwifery as a nursing role (Dawley, 2003). Like other forms of advanced practice nursing that emerged later, the resurgence of midwifery and the evolution of nurse-midwifery occurred in response to the need for care by the underserved. By the late 1960s, the contributions of nurse-midwifery were accepted and recognized. Demand for nurse-midwifery services increased, and the profession responded by opening more education programs and more midwifery practices. However, the need was not completely met, and by the 1990s, other practitioners began to practice midwifery skills without adequate education and practice. The ACNM, at the request of state regulatory agencies, developed accreditation and certification for non-nurse midwives, for which graduates would receive the credential *certified midwife (CM)*. The first CM credential was awarded in 1997 (Burst, 2005). A critical component of this decision was the commitment by the ACNM to assert and uphold an equivalent standard among midwives in education, certification, and practice (Fullerton, Schuilling, & Sipe, 2005). As these educational programs evolved, the ACNM proposed changing its name to the *American College of Midwives* in an effort to be more inclusive of non-nurse midwives who achieved ACNM certification. In a demonstration of allegiance to nursing, the ACNM membership voted to retain *Nurse* in the name of the organization (Kraus, 1997). Because the identity of the professional organization continues to be a matter of controversy among some members, this motion was reintroduced in 2007. The membership has not voted on this issue to date. However, in 2000, the official publication of the ACNM, the *Journal of Nurse-Midwifery* changed its name to the *Journal of Midwifery and Women's Health* to reflect the evolution of contemporary midwifery (Shah, 2000).

Table 16-1 presents a timeline of key events that influenced the development of modern nurse-midwifery as described by Varney, Kriebs, & Gegor (2004) (see also Chapter 1).

THE NURSE-MIDWIFERY PROFESSION IN THE UNITED STATES TODAY

As of 2007, 11,021 nurse-midwives have been recognized as CNMs by the ACNM, and 62 have been recognized as CMs (ACNM, 2007a; American Midwife

Table 16-1   THE EVOLUTION OF NURSE-MIDWIFERY: A TIMELINE OF CRITICAL EVENTS

Year	Event	Significance
Colonial times to early 1900s	Midwives traveled to the colonies. They were respected in communities and trained in apprenticeships. Practices were often handed down from mother to daughter.	Midwifery had a strong basis in service to others beyond an occupation—often seen as a "calling." The women who practiced midwifery tended to be rich in life experience if not in formal education.
Early 1900s	Midwifery was co-opted by organized medicine.	Decreased number and experience of practitioners effectively put midwives "in the closet."
1925	Frontier Nursing Service was founded in Hyden, Kentucky.	Imported British-trained midwives utilized the nursing model. Designed to meet the specific needs in an underserved area. Births took place in homes. Low neonatal mortality rate 9.1/1000 births from 1925 to 1951 (not matched by United States at large until 1990s).
1931	The Maternity Center Association in New York City opened the Lobenstine Clinic.	Provided care for immigrant families in upper Manhattan tenements.
1932	The first nurse-midwifery education program was developed at the Lobenstine Clinic.	Offered advanced preparation in midwifery to public health nurses. Acknowledged relationship of nursing and midwifery.
1941	The Tuskegee School of Nurse-Midwifery opened in Alabama.	Access to nurse-midwifery education for minorities.
1943	The Catholic Maternity Institute was founded in Santa Fe, New Mexico.	Many nurse-midwifery leaders came from this program.
Mid-1940s	The National Organization of Public Health Nurses (later absorbed into the American Nurses Association) was established for nurse-midwives.	Recognition of midwifery as having a foundation in nursing.
1955	The American College of Nurse-Midwives was founded.	Began formalizing standards for education, certification, and practice. The basic certificate program was the norm. Also provided a formal voice for nurse-midwives.
Early 1960s	A CNM pilot project was conducted in Madera County, California.	Continues to be used as "gold standard" in assessing nurse-midwifery care.
Late 1960s and 1970s	Nurse-midwifery services and educational programs (mostly certificates) proliferated; autonomous birth centers were developed.	Increased utilization of and demand for CNMs in a variety of settings.
1980s	Malpractice crisis arose.	Closed some practices and threatened closure at some programs until issue resolved.
1980s and 1990s	CNMs moved to graduate-level education.	Majority of programs now prepare students at master's level.
1990s	The milieu for health care practice is changing; CNMs are moving toward primary care of women.	CNMs adapting to environment in which quality, access, and cost must all be addressed.

CNMs, Certified nurse-midwives.

Certification Board [AMCB], 2007). In addition, there are over 7000 active and student members of the ACNM. Of that number, approximately 6200 are in clinical practice. In 2004, the most current year for which data are available, CNMs attended 308,113 births, which constituted 10.7% of all vaginal births in the nation (ACNM, 2005a, 2007a; Declercq, 2007). As of 2007, there were 41 ACNM-accredited nurse-midwifery education programs in the United States. Three of these are post-baccalaureate certificate programs, and 37 are graduate programs. One is a free-standing institution of higher education. Thirty-one of the programs are located in schools of nursing (ACNM, 2007a, 2007c). Overall, 68% of CNMs hold master's degrees and 4% have doctorates. Approximately 1% of CNMs are men (ACNM, 2007a; Kovner & Burkhardt, 2001). Nurse-midwifery practice is legal in all 50 states, and nurse-midwives have prescriptive authority in 48 states and the District of Columbia (ACNM, 2007a).

Education and Accreditation

The ACNM established a national mechanism for the accreditation of nurse-midwifery education programs in 1962. Because the organization wanted to have its process subject to peer review and recognition, it applied to the U.S. Department of Education (DOE) for recognition as an accrediting agency. Since 1982, the ACNM Division of Accreditation (which changed its name effective June 2007 to the *Accreditation Commission for Midwifery Education [ACME]*) has been recognized by the U.S. DOE as a programmatic accrediting agency for certificate, post-baccalaureate, graduate degree, and pre-certification programs in nurse-midwifery/midwifery. In addition, ACME was recently recognized for accrediting educational institutions, such as the Frontier School of Midwifery and Family Nursing (ACNM, 2005d, 2006c). ACNM-accredited programs must receive pre-accreditation status before enrolling students, and once the initial accreditation has been granted, the program must be reviewed at least every 8 years.

The ACNM ACME is responsible for setting and maintaining the standards of midwifery education that reflect the competencies and standards set by the profession. When the ACNM accepted direct entry as a pathway for professional midwifery, ACME delineated the core competencies from the health sciences that can be obtained from prior nursing preparation and that were needed before midwifery education. These skills, knowledge, and behaviors were added as part of the direct entry midwifery curriculum, confirming that existing ACNM core competencies were those of professional midwifery regardless of the point of entry into an education program. This supports ACNM's definition of CNMs as being educated in the two disciplines of nursing and midwifery and CMs as being educated in the discipline of midwifery (ACNM, 2005d). Although ACME supports different educational pathways, it mandates (1) that all ACNM-accredited educational programs either require a baccalaureate degree upon entrance or grant no less than a baccalaureate upon graduation (ACNM, 2005d, 2005e) and (2) that by 2010, a graduate degree will be required for entry into clinical practice (ACNM, 2006b, 2006c; Farley & Camacho, 2003).

As previously mentioned, in 2004, the AACN recommended the requirement of a DNP for entry into clinical practice for advance practice nursing (AACN, 2004a, 2004b). Many CNMs have expressed concerns about what this would mean for midwifery education and clinical practice, given that the majority of education programs are in schools of nursing and the majority of midwifery practice is regulated through state boards of nursing. In 2005, the ACNM ACME released a statement that has subsequently been affirmed by the ACNM Board of Directors as a position statement (ACNM, 2007d). It states that the ACNM continues to support a variety of educational pathways to midwifery education, continues to support and promote the development of independent schools of midwifery, and does not support the DNP as a requirement for midwifery education and clinical practice. They based this statement on 40 years of expertise in setting standards for accreditation for midwifery education programs that have been recognized by the U.S. DOE since 1982. The ACNM ACME has decades of evidence of preparation of successful graduates in all aspects of midwifery, including leadership, political action, and service to women and childbearing families regardless of the terminal degree (ACNM, 2007a). They also recognize the need for midwifery care and the national and global shortage of midwives. And last, the ACNM ACME states that evidence is inadequate to support the advantages of a practice doctorate in the provision of care to women and their families, especially in light of rising health care costs (ACNM, 2005d, 2006c). Despite these expressed concerns, as of Fall 2007, 12 nursing programs in which there are ACNM-accredited nurse-midwifery programs will have initiated DNP options for students (retrieved July 3, 2007, from *www.aacn.nche.edu/DNP/DNPprogramlist.htm*.

The accreditation process rests on two cornerstones. The first is the "Criteria for the Evaluation of Education Programs" (ACNM, 2003a). These criteria specify the elements necessary to develop and maintain a nurse-midwifery program. Because they evaluate the specialty content of midwifery (i.e., content that addresses the hallmarks and components of midwifery, including but not limited to intrapartum care), these criteria apply regardless of the academic "house" in which the program resides (nursing, public health, allied health, medicine, freestanding). In addition, the criteria apply regardless of the level at which the student is being educated (certificate, baccalaureate, master's, or doctoral). This approach to education is not without difficulties. Individual state laws may require a certain level of education to practice or perform certain aspects of practice, such as prescribing medications. In addition, it can affect reimbursement for services from Medicare and Medicaid. The criteria require that a midwifery program be directed by a midwife, that clinical faculty have a minimum of a master's degree and 1 year of clinical nurse-midwifery experience before teaching, and that the faculty remain current in clinical practice. Any clinical faculty without a master's degree must be responsible to a qualified faculty member who has a master's or doctoral degree (ACNM, 2006a). The ACNM criteria are revised every 5 years to maintain currency and are due for revision in 2008.

The second cornerstone of the accreditation process is the "Core Competencies for Basic Midwifery Practice," which is revised every 5 years, with the most recent revision occurring in 2007 (ACNM, 2007b). This document represents the delineation of the fundamental knowledge, skills, and behaviors expected of a new practitioner. It is divided into six sections:

- Hallmarks, which speak to the art and science of midwifery
- Professional responsibilities, which delineate the non-clinical requirements of the professional midwife
- The midwifery management process, which is the clinical decision-making framework for practice
- The fundamentals of midwifery care
- The primary health care of women
- The care of the childbearing family

This document ensures equivalent preparation for all graduates of midwifery education programs accredited by the ACNM ACME. It likewise helps inform the blueprint for the certification examination for CNMs (ACNM, 2002a).

Certification/Certification Maintenance

A national certification examination for entry into practice was instituted in 1971. At that time, certification rested within the ACNM. In 1991, certification was separated from the professional organization. The AMCB, formerly the ACNM Certification Council (ACC), was incorporated as a distinct organization charged with developing and administering the examination for nurse-midwives and midwives. Within the AMCB, there are committees charged with keeping the examination content current and appropriate. The Examination Committee works closely with test consultants and annually reviews examination specifications and content outline. The Research Committee conducts a survey of the "face validity" of the national certification examination known as the *Task Analysis of Midwifery Practice*. The Task Analysis is done every 5 years (AMCB, 2007).

As of January 1, 1996, the certification became time-limited, valid for 8 years from the date of issue. Mechanisms for certification maintenance, administered by the Certification Maintenance Program (CMP), include options such as certification maintenance modules, continuing education units, and retaking the certification examination. The CMP is sponsored by the AMCB. At this juncture, the time-limited certificate does not apply to midwives certified before 1996, and therefore the CMP is optional for this group. Instead, the continuing competency assessment mechanism, developed in 1987, may be used. Individual state regulations may affect which method of maintenance a nurse-midwife must follow.

Continuing Competency Assessment

In 1986, the ACNM developed a Continuing Competency Assessment (CCA) mechanism for its members in clinical practice. Its purpose is to demonstrate that clinicians continue to maintain contemporary knowledge and demonstrate competency in the provision of health care to women, newborns, and their families. This 5-year cycle requires that practicing midwives either acquire 50 contact hours of continuing education appropriate to midwifery practice or retake the certification examination. The ACNM Continuing Education Committee grants continuing education units for programs that meet the guidelines of the International Association of Continuing Education and Training.

The ACNM initially "mandated" competency assessment but modified this position in 1995, placing the decision to mandate participation in the hands of state regulators or employers. The ACNM still sets the standard that all CNMs must demonstrate continuing competency, and a number of states and employers have adopted ACNM's continuing competency mechanism as evidence for meeting the requirement for licensure or employment (ACNM, 2005c).

Re-entry to Practice

The ACNM has developed a flexible, individualized pilot program designed to provide a framework for midwives who are not currently engaged in clinical practice and wish to re-enter clinical practice. The program contains two components: continuing education and a clinical refresher course based on individual needs. The program can also be structured to meet the needs of midwives who have been practicing a limited scope and wish to return to full scope of practice (i.e., have been providing women's health care but now wish to include labor and birth) (ACNM, 2007e). The Re-entry Program is in an active pilot stage, and the committee working on revisions is discussing issues such as the following:

- How long a hiatus from clinical practice would require a refresher course and/or being precepted by a qualified practicing midwife?
- If no midwife is available to precept a returning midwife, can a physician be a preceptor?
- At what point must the certification examination be retaken?
- If a refresher course is required, is it available and at what cost?

Regulation, Credentialing, and Reimbursement

As with all health care providers in the United States, CNM practice is regulated on a state-by-state basis. CNMs must comply with the legal requirements for the practice of nurse-midwifery in the jurisdiction in which they practice (District of Columbia, the Virgin Islands, and Puerto Rico, as well as the 50 states). The practice of nurse-midwifery differs in the various jurisdictions because of legal, regulatory, and other influences. Such influences include statutes, rules and regulations, opinions of the state attorney general, court decisions, licensure, registration, and certification. This variability results in differences in regulatory parameters such as which state agency regulates midwifery practice, whether midwives have prescriptive privileges, what educational degrees are required for practice, and what types of employers and practice arrangements are permitted.

States may also have regulations about private insurance reimbursement and are required to set the Medicaid reimbursement schedule for CNMs (ACNM, 2006e, 2006f, 2006h). The effect that this variation in state law and regulation has on midwifery practice was examined by Declercq, Paine, Dejoseph, and Simmes (1998). They found that, when compared with states with low regulatory support for nurse-midwifery practice, states with high regulatory support had a nurse-midwifery workforce three times larger than other states, three times the number of midwifery-attended births, and two times as many midwife-patient contacts.

The political climate affects nurse-midwifery practice and can promote or restrain the practice of CNMs. For example, the relative power of constituencies such as medical and nursing organizations and consumer groups and the relationships among them can shape legislation and patterns of referral to CNMs. Laws and other ordinances that regulate CNM practice should ensure that all practitioners are qualified to practice nurse-midwifery. In 36 states, nurse-midwifery is regulated by boards of nursing, in three states by a board of nursing and another regulatory body, in nine states by non-nursing boards, and in two states by boards of nurse-midwifery.

The ACNM recently reaffirmed the autonomy with which the CNM practices. The ACNM's official clinical practice statement on independent midwifery practice is presented in Box 16-1.

In addition to state regulation, hospitals and health plans have established credentialing requirements for health care professionals. These credentialing standards determine who may have hospital admitting privileges, who may be employed by health care systems, and who may be listed on managed care provider panels. An optimum system would create a mechanism that is consistent with the profession's standards, recognize midwifery as distinct from other health care professions, and recognize processes that permit CNMs to build upon entry-level competencies within their statutory scope of practice.

The American College of Nurse-Midwives

During the 1940s, the National Organization of Public Health Nurses (NOPHN) established a section for nurse-midwives. During the reorganization of national nursing organizations, the NOPHN was absorbed into

Box 16-1 CLINICAL PRACTICE STATEMENT ON INDEPENDENT MIDWIFERY PRACTICE

It is the position of the American College of Nurse-Midwives (ACNM) that midwifery practice is the independent management of women's health care, focusing particularly on women, pregnancy, childbirth, the postpartum period, and care of the newborn. The practice occurs within a health care system that provides for consultation, collaborative management, or referral as indicated by the health status of the client.

Independent midwifery enables certified nurse-midwives (CNMs) and certified midwives (CMs) to utilize knowledge, skills, judgment, and authority in the provision of primary women's health services while maintaining accountability for the management of patient care in accordance with ACNM Standards for the Practice of Midwifery.

Independent practice is not defined by the place of employment, the employee-employer relationship, requirements for physician co-signature, or the method of reimbursement for services. Nor should independent be interpreted to mean alone, as there are clinical situations when any prudent practitioner would seek the assistance of another qualified practitioner.

Collaboration is the process whereby health care professionals jointly manage care. The goal of collaboration is to share authority while providing quality care within each individual's professional scope of practice. Successful collaboration is a way of thinking and relating that requires knowledge, open communication, mutual respect, a commitment to providing quality care, trust and the ability to share responsibility.

From the American College of Nurse-Midwives. (2004b). Position Statement: *Independent midwifery practice.* Washington, DC: Author.

the American Nurses Association (ANA) and the National League for Nursing (NLN). These two organizations did not include a recognizable entity for nurse-midwives. Midwives at the 1954 ANA convention formed The Committee on Organization. This committee approved the definition of a nurse-midwife and a statement of purposes of a midwifery organization. For various reasons, the NLN and the ANA could not find a home for the nurse-midwives. The Committee on Organization voted at their May 1955 meeting to form a separate nurse-midwifery organization—The American College of Nurse-Midwifery (Dawley, 2005; Dawley & Burst, 2005; Varney, Kriebs, & Gegor, 2004).

The growth and development of American nurse-midwifery was fostered by the ACNM, founded in 1955 as the professional organization for certified nurse-midwives and later certified midwives. The mission of the ACNM is to promote the health and well-being of women and infants within their families and communities through the development and support of professional midwifery. The organization establishes clinical standards, creates liaisons with state and federal agencies and members of Congress, administers and promotes continuing education programs, supports midwifery-relevant research and practice, and supports the accreditation mechanism.

The ACNM Philosophy (ACNM, 2004a) (Box 16-2) and Code of Ethics (ACNM, 2005b) (Box 16-3) embody the spirit of the profession. The ACNM has professional moral obligations. The code identifies the

obligations that guide the CNM in the practice of nurse-midwifery and clarifies what consumers, the public, other professionals, and prospective practitioners can expect of the profession. Nurse-midwifery exists for the good of women and their families; this good is safeguarded by practice that is consistent with the ACNM Philosophy (ACNM, 2004a) and ACNM Standards for the Practice of Midwifery (ACNM, 2003b). The belief that pregnancy and childbirth are normal life processes is at the heart of nurse-midwifery practice. The CNM learns to be "with woman" (the original meaning of midwife) without having to "manage" pregnancy, labor, or delivery.

The Code of Ethics further describes expectations regarding practice competence, CNM-patient relationships, ethical responsibilities, collegial practice, and nondiscrimination. Responsibilities for conducting research in nurse-midwifery and for supporting community and political activities that promote access to health care are also delineated. CNMs take responsibility for implementing the Health Insurance Portability and Accountability Act (HIPAA) regulations in an understandable and usable format in their individual practices. Other essential documents, position papers, and fact sheets about ACNM can be found on its Internet website. The website can be accessed at either *www.acnm.org* or *www.midwife.org.* The site is also rich in information for consumers and the second web address makes it accessible to the lay public.

Box 16-2 American College of Nurse-Midwives Philosophy

We, the midwives of the American College of Nurse-midwives, affirm the power and strength of women and the importance of their health in the well-being of families, communities, and nations. We believe in the basic human rights of all persons, recognizing that women often incur an undue burden or risk when these rights are violated.

We believe every person has a right to:

- Equitable, ethical, accessible quality health care that promotes healing and health
- Health care that respects human dignity, individuality, and diversity among groups
- Complete and accurate information to make informed health care decisions
- Self-determination and active participation in health care decisions
- Involvement of a woman's designated family members, to the extent desired, in all health care experiences

We believe the best model of health care for a woman and her family:

- Promotes a continuous and compassionate partnership
- Acknowledges a person's life experiences and knowledge

- Includes individualized methods of care and healing guided by the best evidence available
- Involves therapeutic use of human presence and skillful communication

We honor the normalcy of women's lifecycle events. We believe in:

- Watchful waiting and non-intervention in normal processes
- Appropriate use of interventions and technology for current or potential health problems
- Consultation, collaboration, and referral with other members of the health care team as needed to provide optimal health care

We affirm that midwifery care incorporates these qualities and that women's health care needs are well-served through midwifery care.

Finally, we value formal education, lifelong individual learning, and the development and application of research to guide ethical and competent midwifery practice. These beliefs and values provide the foundation for commitment to individual and collective leadership at the community, state, national, and international level to improve the health of women and their families worldwide.

From the American College of Nurse-Midwives. (2004). *Philosophy of the American College of Nurse-Midwives.* Washington, DC: Author.

IMPLEMENTING ADVANCED PRACTICE NURSING COMPETENCIES

Overview of Advanced Practice Nurse and Certified Nurse-Midwife Competencies

Nurse-midwifery is constantly evolving and has a broader scope of practice now than it did 75 years ago (Barger, 2005). Nurse-midwifery has six core competencies that are similar to the APN competencies (see Chapter 3). As with Hamric's model, the direct care role is integral to CNM practice and is well substantiated in both exemplars included later in this chapter. Consistent with the expanded scope of advanced practice nursing, nurse-midwives assume responsibility and accountability for their practice as primary health care providers (ACNM, 1997a, 2002a, 2002b, 2004b, 2006g). Patient-centered assessment and management are hallmarks of all aspects of CNM care. CNMs have, in common with

all APNs, the characteristics of using a holistic, evidence-based perspective. CNMs use research methodologies and ethical decision making to support a caring, low-technology approach to childbirth. ACNM has well-defined position statements on consultation and collaboration in midwifery practice (ACNM, 1997a) that have helped inform APN practice (see Chapters 7 and 10). CNMs have demonstrated leadership in the development of freestanding birth centers and in efforts to remove legislative barriers restraining midwifery practice. It is informative to take a closer look at the competencies related to advocacy and patient education to further understand midwifery practice. The ACNM-defined competencies in advocacy and patient education parallel the advanced practice core competencies of ethical decision making and coaching and guidance. CNMs enact the seven competencies of advanced practice nursing as described in the following discussion.

Box 16-3   AMERICAN COLLEGE OF NURSE-MIDWIVES CODE OF ETHICS

Certified nurse-midwives and certified midwives have three ethical mandates in achieving the mission of midwifery to promote the health and well-being of women and newborns within their families and communities. The first mandate is directed toward the individual women and their families for whom midwives provide care, the second mandate is to a broader audience for the "public good" for the benefit of all women and their families, and the third mandate is to the profession of midwifery to assure its integrity and in turn its ability to fulfill the mission of midwifery.

Midwives in all aspects of professional relationships will:

- Respect basic human rights and the dignity of all persons
- Respect their own self worth, dignity, and professional integrity

Midwives in all aspects of professional practice will:

- Develop a partnership with the woman, in which each shares relevant information that leads to informed decision-making, consent to an evolving plan of care, and acceptance or responsibility for the outcome of their choices

- Act without discrimination based on factors such as age, gender, race, ethnicity, religion, lifestyle, sexual orientation, socioeconomic status, disability, or nature of the health problem
- Provide an environment where privacy is protected and in which all pertinent information is shared without bias, coercion, or deception
- Maintain confidentiality except where disclosure is mandated by law
- Protect women, their families, and colleagues from harmful, unethical, and incompetent practices by taking appropriate action that may include reporting as mandated by law

Midwives as members of a profession will:

- Promote, advocate for, and strive to protect the rights, health, and well-being of women, families, and communities
- Promote just distribution of resources and equity in access to quality health services
- Promote and support the education of midwifery students and peers, standards of practice, research, and policies that enhance the health of women, families, and communities

From the American College of Nurse-Midwives. (2005c). *Code of ethics of the American College of Nurse-Midwives.* Washington, DC: Author.

Direct Clinical Practice

CNMs manifest a high level of expertise in the assessment, diagnosis, and treatment of the complex responses of women with regard to pregnancy, labor, birth, postpartum, and women's health issues. CNMs perform many of the same interventions used in nursing but have a greater depth and breadth of knowledge, ability to synthesize data, and ability to intervene in complex situations.

Nurse-midwives form partnerships with the women they care for, empowering them to be active participants in their own health care. They provide information and support to clients, enabling them to make informed decisions and assume responsibility for their health. Nurse-midwives incorporate scientific evidence into clinical practice, are familiar with complementary and alternative therapies, exercise expert clinical thinking and skillful performance, and demonstrate a holistic approach in the care they provide.

The ACNM position statement on CNMs as primary care providers/case managers (ACNM, 1997c)

states that CNMs are providers of primary health care for women and newborns. In direct clinical practice, CNMs evaluate, assess, treat, and refer as required. They provide preconception counseling, care during pregnancy and childbirth, gynecological and contraceptive services, and care for the perimenopausal and postmenopausal woman (ACNM, 2003b, 2007b, 2007f).

Expert Guidance and Coaching of Patients, Families, and Other Care Providers

Expert guidance and coaching are functions of advanced practice nurses that assist patients through life transitions such as illness, childbearing, and bereavement (see Chapter 6). Nurse-midwives offer skillful communication, guidance, and counseling throughout the nurse-midwifery management process (ACNM, 2007b). Client education is a cornerstone of nurse-midwifery practice. Evidence that nurse-midwives invest time in patient education is supported by Paine (2000), who reported that nurse-midwives spent more time during office visits providing patient education and counseling than physicians spent. For example, when a nurse-midwife counsels a pregnant woman regarding fetal testing, she not only educates the patient about how the test is done but also advises the woman as to what the results might indicate, what further testing would then be offered, and what decisions the woman and her partner may need to make and offers to provide additional coaching as the process unfolds. In the instance of the quadruple screen, a blood test offered between 15 and 19 weeks' gestation, the woman would learn that it is a blood test conducted on the mother that screens for neural tube defects or Down's syndrome in the fetus. She is informed that it is not diagnostic and that a positive screen means there is increased risk for the problem, not that the fetus has the problem. A positive result would mean that she would then have to decide whether to have further testing, such as an amniocentesis or a high-level ultrasound. The procedures, risks, and benefits of these tests would then be presented. If the woman opts for further testing and the results are diagnostic for a complication, she would then need to decide whether to continue the pregnancy or have a medical termination. This level of coaching patients requires time and commitment.

As mentioned by Spross in Chapter 6, coaching is an interaction between an expert (the nurse-midwife) and the learner (the patient) that enables the learner to develop knowledge and skills within an area of the coach's expertise. Nurse-midwives are expected to apply their knowledge to guide women with regard to pregnancy, birth, breastfeeding, parenthood, changes in family constellation, family planning, and women's health-related issues.

Consultation

Consultation is discussed in detail in Chapter 7. Nurse-midwives use consultation in their practice, both as the consultant and as the consultee. Patients consult with midwives regarding health care and health promotion. For example, a patient may see a nurse-midwife regarding the desire to quit smoking. She wants to know what is available to help her be successful. The nurse-midwife would then discuss her options, help her devise a plan for cessation, and provide guidance and medication if she so chooses. The patient is free to adopt these recommendations or not. Nurse-midwives often provide consultation in

the hospital setting. During a labor and birth, nurses and nurse-midwives may consult each other regarding a fetal monitor heart tracing. Nurse-midwives sit on hospital committees to improve quality of care, where they can advocate for evidence-based policies. Physicians may consult nurse-midwives regarding complementary therapies, breastfeeding, or alternative birthing options.

Nurse-midwives also consult other professionals. There are many instances in which a nurse-midwife would make use of another's expertise to provide the best care for his or her patients. For example, a midwife caring for a pregnant woman with a low platelet count might consult with the midwife's collaborating physician or with a hematologist to decide on the appropriate care and provider for this woman and her fetus. Nurse-midwives frequently consult with lactation consultants to assist women who are having breastfeeding difficulties or with physical therapists to advise on mobility and discomfort problems. Nurse-midwives also consult with other nurse-midwives when seeking the best course of action for their patients.

Collaboration

The ACNM has a position statement on collaborative management in midwifery practice for medical, gynecological, and obstetrical conditions (ACNM, 1997a, 2006g) (Box 16-4). In the 1997 statement, a focus is on midwifery management as independent, primarily intended for healthy women; however, in the event of complications, collaborative management or co-management allows for consultation, collaboration, or referral. The 2002 statement also recognizes the need for nurse-midwives and physicians to collaborate but stresses the working relationship, respect for each other's abilities and knowledge, and professional responsibility and accountability.

When a complication occurs, the nurse-midwife can continue to be instrumental in the woman's care while benefiting from collaboration with an obstetrician-gynecologist. This involves the nurse-midwife and the physician jointly managing the care of a woman whose case has become medically, gynecologically, or obstetrically complicated. The collaborating physician and the nurse-midwife mutually agree on the scope of care each will provide. If the physician needs to assume the main role in the woman's care, the nurse-midwife will still participate to some degree in the physical care and to a large degree in counseling, guidance, teaching, and support.

Box 16-4   COLLABORATIVE MANAGEMENT IN MIDWIFERY PRACTICE FOR MEDICAL, GYNECOLOGICAL, AND OBSTETRICAL CONDITIONS

The American College of Obstetricians and Gynecologists (ACOG) and the American College of Nurse-Midwives (ACNM) recognize that in those circumstances in which obstetricians-gynecologists and certified nurse-midwives/certified midwives collaborate in the care of women, the quality of those practices is enhanced by a working relationship characterized by mutual respect and trust as well as professional responsibility and accountability. When obstetricians-gynecologists and certified nurse-midwives/certified midwives collaborate, they should concur on a clear mechanism for consultation, collaboration, and referral based on the individual needs of each patient.

Recognizing the high level of responsibility that obstetricians-gynecologists and certified nurse-midwives/certified midwives assume when providing care to women, ACOG and ACNM affirm their commitment to promote appropriate standards for the education and certification of their respective members, to support appropriate practice guidelines, and to facilitate communication and collegial relationships between obstetricians-gynecologists and certified nurse-midwives/certified midwives.

From the American College of Nurse-Midwives and American College of Obstetricians-Gynecologists. (2002b). *Joint statement of practice relations between obstetricians-gynecologists and certified nurse-midwives/certified midwives.* Washington, DC: American College of Nurse-Midwives.

For example, a nurse-midwife caring for a pregnant woman identifies that inadequate fetal growth may be an issue. The nurse-midwife then consults with the collaborating physician and together they decide on what further testing and care is required under these circumstances. In this instance, the testing does show inadequate growth; therefore the woman will alternate her prenatal visits between the physician and the nurse-midwife so that together they can provide frequent fetal surveillance and the best possible outcome for mother and baby. Effective communication is essential in ongoing collaborative management to maintain an effective working relationship and to provide comprehensive care to the individuals under the collaborators' care.

In addition to obstetrician-gynecologists, nurse-midwives collaborate with other providers. During labor, nurse-midwives often collaborate with doulas (labor support providers) to provide the laboring woman with the best birth experience possible and to meet the goals of her individual birth plan. Nurse-midwives collaborate with nurses and maternity unit managers to develop nursing policies. Nurse-midwives collaborate with other nurse-midwives, labor and delivery nurses, and physician colleagues to develop practice standards and guidelines. These are just a few examples of the myriad ways in which nurse-midwives collaborate.

Research

The advanced practice of nursing core competency of research involves interpretation and use of research in practice, evaluation of one's own practice and nursing practice, and participation in research (Chapter 8). In nurse-midwifery, the research component is enacted throughout the core competencies. Nurse-midwives are charged with incorporating scientific evidence into clinical practice to evaluate, apply, interpret, and collaborate in research (ACNM, 2006d). The ACNM recognizes the importance of research to the profession. One of the missions of the ACNM Division of Research (DOR) is to contribute to knowledge about the health of women, infants, and families and to advance the practice of midwifery. The DOR promotes the development, conduction, and dissemination of midwifery research (ACNM, 2007f). The ACNM through the DOR is developing a research agenda that will foster research that makes a difference to women and the midwifery profession (Kennedy, Schuiling, & Murphy, 2007). The agenda is promoting research that focuses on policy, evidence-based practice, education, collaboration, visibility/message, and organizational/leadership development (ACNM, 2007f; Kennedy et al., 2007). Nurse-midwifery has its own journal, the *Journal of Midwifery & Women's Health*, a peer-reviewed, clinically focused publication that publishes research pertinent to maternal-child, well-woman gynecology, family planning, primary care of women, and health care policy.

Since the early days of our country, midwives have contributed to knowledge regarding women and infants. Martha Ballard's diary from 1785 to 1812 details the care she gave to women and their families in her rural community. Her diary demonstrates skills, knowledge, outcomes, and political forces that began to control the practice of midwifery by physicians

(Ulrich, 1990). Midwifery research has grown significantly since Martha Ballard's time.

Cheryl Beck has conducted extensive qualitative and quantitative research on postpartum depression. Besides advancing our knowledge about this timely and important topic, her research has provided a list of predictors for postpartum depression (Beck, 1998, 2001, 2002, 2006) and given us the Postpartum Depression Screening Scale (Beck & Gable, 2000, 2001a, 2001b, 2002). This scale is unique in that it not only screens postpartum women for depression but also gives a picture of their symptomatology, enabling providers to tailor their treatment to the symptoms.

The majority of nurse-midwifery education is conducted in institutions of higher learning (37 of the 41 midwifery educational programs). By promoting advanced degrees, the ACNM is providing for a research-knowledgeable cohort that will continue to build and support evidence-based practice in the field of women's health and midwifery.

Clinical and Professional Leadership

Leadership skills are professional responsibilities that are core competencies for nurse-midwives. Not only are nurse-midwives knowledgeable regarding national and international issues and trends in women's health and maternal/infant care but also they are expected to be leaders in bringing those issues to the forefront. Nurse-midwives are expected to exercise leadership for the benefit of women, infants, and families; the profession of midwifery; and the ACNM. To this end, the ACNM sponsors leadership seminars four times a year in various locations throughout the United States.

The mission of the ACNM Division of Women's Health Policy and Leadership (DWHP&L) is to improve the health of women at the community level through the development, implementation, and promotion of public policy and public information initiatives (ACNM, 2005f). The goals and objectives of the DWHP&L include the following:

- Assisting in the development of policies and making recommendations regarding policy issues to the ACNM Board of Directors
- Evaluating policies that impact women's health
- Identifying advocacy needs, and developing advocacy groups
- Being a source of information for lobbying activities
- Enhancing the capacity of CNMs/CMs and the ACNM to acquire positions of authority

- Facilitating networking among the ACNM and women's health organizations
- Creating a culture of recognizing and valuing the work of CNMs/CMs in policy arenas that are not practice-focused

Ethical Decision Making

"The goal of midwifery practice is to promote the health and well-being of women and childbearing families, wherever they reside, raising cultural, value, and ethical concerns that need to be respected and understood before making a final decision on a plan of care or action in the political arena" (Ament, 2007, pp. 280-281). The goal of ethical midwifery practice is to do the right thing for the right reason.

Codes of ethics guide moral behavior and are considered to be part of the criteria that make a practice a profession (Thompson, 2002). The latest edition of *The Code of Ethics* approved by the ACNM Board in 2005 has three mandates (see Box 16-3). The first is directed toward the individual woman and her family. The second is for the benefit of all women and their families. The third is to the profession of midwifery. These mandates are reflected in the "Core Competencies for Basic Midwifery Practice," the philosophy of the ACNM (see Box 16-2), and the "Standards for the Practice of Midwifery" (Box 16-5).

Nurse-midwives are faced with ethical decisions in their daily practice, especially as concerns technology, informed consent, and health as a basic right for all (Ament, 2007). Whether and when to use electronic fetal monitoring is an excellent example. It has become "standard of care" to monitor the fetal heart rate (FHR) in labor with electronic fetal monitoring. Most places of birth (mainly hospitals) have protocols and guidelines concerning this practice. Many nurse-midwives care for women in hospital settings where they are confronted with these guidelines. They are expected to monitor the FHR even though the monitor may be intrusive to the woman and not part of her birth plan. In addition, there is no supporting evidence that electronic FHR monitoring when the woman is low-risk improves outcomes. In fact, it is well known that overuse of the fetal monitor has increased the cesarean section rate without improving the health and well-being of mothers or infants (Ament, 2007). At this time, no informed consent accompanies the use of fetal monitoring that addresses any of these issues.

Box 16-5   STANDARDS FOR THE PRACTICE OF MIDWIFERY

STANDARD I
Midwifery care is provided by qualified practitioners.

STANDARD II
Midwifery care occurs in a safe environment within the context of the family, community, and a system of health care.

STANDARD III
Midwifery care supports individual rights and self-determination within the boundaries of safety.

STANDARD IV
Midwifery care is comprised of knowledge, skills, and judgments that foster the delivery of safe, satisfying, and culturally competent care.

STANDARD V
Midwifery care is based on knowledge, skills, and judgments which are reflected in written practice guidelines.

STANDARD VI
Midwifery care is documented in a format that is accessible and complete.

STANDARD VII
Midwifery care is evaluated according to an established program for quality management that includes a plan to identify and resolve problems.

STANDARD VIII
Midwifery practice may be expanded beyond the ACNM Core Competencies to incorporate new procedures that improve care for women and their families.

From the American College of Nurse-Midwives (ACNM). (2003b). *ACNM standards for the practice of midwifery.* Washington, DC: Author.

Traditional biomedical ethics developed after the atrocities of World War II and the increase of scientific research. Biomedical ethics is a discipline focused on moral philosophy, normative theory, abstract universal principles, and objective problem solving in dilemmas (Thompson, 2002, 2003). The medicalization of health care has directed the education and practice of nursing and midwifery, and bioethics has guided their codes of ethics. The essence of ethical midwifery practice occurs through human engagement, relationships, and the flow of power within those relationships. In addition, Thompson (2003) proposes that the ethics of engagement fosters ethical midwifery practice by encouraging practitioners to focus on "being with" the woman through human engagement.

Advocacy

Advocacy, which can be considered part of the ethical decision-making competency as described in the APN model in Chapter 3, is a competency that is central to nurse-midwifery practice. Client education and support of clients' rights and self-determination inform every aspect of nurse-midwifery care. These values have been challenged by the burgeoning growth of medical technology over the past two decades and the incursion of managed care in the 1990s. The availability of highly technical interventions for many

aspects of childbearing—such as infertility, monitoring pregnancies and birth—conflicts with the traditionally low-tech, low-interventionist approach of nurse-midwives. This presents nurse-midwives with several challenges (ACNM, 2003c):

- To evaluate technologies to determine whether and how they can be incorporated into their practice
- To incorporate such therapies into practice in ways that are consistent with nurse-midwifery's values
- To explain technology in a way that empowers women to make informed decisions
- To provide equal access to the technology

The ACNM launched a public awareness campaign in 2005 to raise awareness about women's health concerns. The intent was to draw attention to the myriad major issues in women's health care, such as the rise in unnecessary and elective cesarean sections and the "gap" in access to care between women of color and white women. The website *www.WithWomen.org* provides information about the most pressing issues in women's health and connects visitors to key organizations combating these issues.

The advent of cost-containment strategies in health care has often restricted the choices that women can make for their personal health care. The ACNM is strongly supportive of legislation ensuring that consumers have access to the full spectrum of qualified health care providers. To that end, women should be able to designate a nurse-midwife as their primary care provider (ACNM, 1998, 2004b, 2004d).

THE CURRENT PRACTICE OF NURSE-MIDWIFERY

Scope of Practice
Originally, midwifery practice was limited to prenatal, intrapartum, postpartum, and newborn care. Nurse-midwifery care today has expanded to include the primary care of women, as well as preconception, gynecological, contraceptive, and infertility care. Nurse-midwives provide care for teenage women, women in their childbearing years, women in midlife, and older women. This expansion is largely the result of consumer demand and the need for greater access to these services. Of interest, in many other countries midwifery practice continues to be somewhat restricted to care related to childbirth only.

A general discussion of the scope of advanced practice nursing can be found in Chapter 21. *Scope of practice* (ACNM, 2007e) refers to what nurse-midwives are actually doing in practice, based on the "Core Competencies for Basic Midwifery Practice" (ACNM, 2007b) and "Standards for the Practice of Midwifery" (ACNM, 2003b). The ACNM provides a guide for the evaluation and addition of other skills and procedures to nurse-midwifery practice (1997b). Thus procedures such as circumcision, vacuum extraction delivery, endometrial biopsy, colposcopy, and elective termination of pregnancy can be included in some nurse-midwives' practice. The term *scope of practice* is also used to differentiate nurse-midwifery practice that is office-based, in which no labor and delivery care is provided, from full-scope practice, which includes labor and delivery care (ACNM, 2007e). Both types of practice may or may not include the additional procedures previously mentioned.

The ACNM core competencies (ACNM, 2007b) codify knowledge and practice expectations of the graduate nurse-midwife/midwife, serve as a guide for education programs, and represent basic nurse-midwifery/midwifery practice to other organizations, health care professionals, and practice settings (Roberts & Huser, 2002). Nurse-midwifery practice incorporates knowledge of the following: normal human physical and psychological development, anatomy and physiology, physiological and psychological deviations from

normal, embryology and genetics, reproduction, sexuality, and pharmacology. Nurse-midwives recognize indicators of developmental changes throughout women's life cycles and can counsel women regarding health promotion measures specific to these changes. They recognize indicators of problems with sexuality and can counsel or initiate consultation or referral for problems outside the scope of nurse-midwifery practice.

Like all advanced practice nurses (APNs), nurse-midwives are familiar with deviations from normal risk factors, appropriate preventive measures, and interventions for selected pathology. Whatever a woman's developmental stage or health care concern, nurse-midwives are expected to teach and counsel patients regarding self-care practices, health promotion, nutritional issues, emotional concerns, and sexuality. Nurse-midwifery practice includes well-defined processes for interacting with physicians and other colleagues to ensure high-quality care (ACNM, 1997a, 2002b, 2006g; American Medical Association [AMA], 1995). The ACNM core competencies, practice guidelines, and an agency's standards of care together with state regulations (ACNM, 1997d, 2006i) determine the scope of practice for a particular agency or practice setting.

Nurse-Midwifery Management Processes
Regardless of the practice setting, nurse-midwifery care encompasses four aspects of management: independent management, consultation, co-management (collaborative management), and referral (ACNM, 1997a, 2002b, 2006g). Implicit in these processes are timely action and documentation of the three aspects other than independent management. The key differences among these aspects of management relate to accountability (see Chapter 7).

Independent Management. Nurse-midwives are responsible and accountable for the management decisions they make in caring for patients. Nurse-midwives provide independent management when they systematically obtain or update a complete and relevant database for assessment of the patient's health status. This includes the history, the physical examination results, and laboratory data. On the basis and interpretation of these findings, nurse-midwives accurately identify problems and diagnoses and implement a plan of action. They delineate health care goals and formulate and communicate a complete needs/problem list in collaboration with the woman and her significant other. Nurse-midwives know when consultation, co-management, or referral is needed and initiate these interactions in a timely manner.

Consultation. When nurse-midwives identify problems or complications, they seek advice from another member of the health care team—often a physician but not always an obstetrician. When they retain independent management responsibility for the patient while seeking advice, this is called *consultation* (ACNM, 1997c, 2004b). A consultation may center on an ongoing health problem (e.g., hypothyroidism), a non-obstetrical, time-limited problem that arises during pregnancy (e.g., bronchitis or food poisoning), or an obstetrical complication (e.g., size-date discrepancy). After consultation, the nurse-midwife and the woman discuss the recommendations, if any, and modify the plan of care accordingly. In the process of consultation, nurse-midwives retain responsibility for decisions. If there is concern with the plan of care, another consultant can be approached. Thus the process of consultation used by nurse-midwives is consistent with the consultation process described in Chapter 7. It is fair to say that novice nurse-midwives are likely to consult often and to use most of the recommendations they receive until they acquire more experience. Consulting is one way of continuing to learn. The experienced nurse-midwife is likely to have a tentative plan in mind when he or she consults with another health care provider and to use consultation to verify the approach or to seek alternatives. It is important to emphasize that nurse-midwives assume direct responsibility for implementing the plan of care in light of their independent management role.

Co-Management or Collaborative Care. One outcome of consultation may be the decision to shift to co-management or collaborative care. This usually occurs if part of the woman's care is related to an ongoing medical, gynecological, or obstetrical complication beyond the scope of the nurse-midwife's practice. In this situation, the nurse-midwife and physician collaboratively treat the patient, with the nurse-midwife defining and retaining accountability for nurse-midwifery aspects of care (ACNM, 1997a, 1997c, 2002b). (See Chapters 7 and 10 for further discussions of consultation and collaboration, respectively.)

Referral. When nurse-midwives identify the need for comprehensive management and care that are outside the scope of nurse-midwifery practice,

they direct the patient to a physician or another professional for treatment of the particular problem (ACNM, 1997c, 2007e). Referral involves the transfer of some or all of the care and some or all accountability to another provider. This management aspect is usually temporary, and once the patient's condition returns to that which is within the nurse-midwife's scope of practice, the nurse-midwife resumes independent management or co-management. For example, the nurse-midwife would refer a woman to an internist for hospitalization for pneumonia, to a surgeon for appendicitis, or to an obstetrician for a cesarean delivery. Once the woman regains her health or recovers from surgery, she could return to the care of the nurse-midwife. The details of these aspects of management are developed by individual nurse-midwives in concert with obstetrical consultants/backups and the practice settings in which the nurse-midwife practices. In addition to providing these aspects of care, nurse-midwives also serve as consultants to or co-managers with other providers, including physicians, advanced practice nursing colleagues, registered nurses, physical therapists, mental health colleagues, or other nurse-midwives.

Practice Settings

There are many different practice styles in nurse-midwifery, from full-scope practice to prenatal only to only women's health. Nurse-midwives practice in urban, suburban, and rural areas. Their practice settings can include private practice (midwife-owned or physician-owned), hospitals, freestanding birth centers, clinics, or homes. Nurse-midwifery practice can be part of a group practice (with any combination of physicians, nurse-practitioners, physician assistants, or other health care providers) or solo practice. The nurse-midwife's actual practice depends on the needs of the population he or she is serving, his or her willingness to undertake a variety of functions, the availability of educational resources for the many different clinical practices a nurse-midwife performs in a specific setting, the particular requests of patients, the availability of physicians and nurse-midwife colleagues for backup and coverage, and finally, personal and philosophical beliefs of the individual midwife (Ament, 2007).

Nurse-midwifery–assisted birth can take place in homes, freestanding birth centers, birth centers within hospitals, or traditional hospital settings (community, regional, or tertiary). For nurse-midwives and the women for whom they provide care, the choice of setting may be a matter of philosophy, comfort, convenience, degree of medical risk, or a combination of these factors. Each setting has unique advantages and disadvantages.

Home births are very family-centered. Risks of iatrogenic and nosocomial infections are minimized. After the birth, the woman can rest or sleep in her own bed, nurse her infant at will, and enjoy the attention and support of her family and friends. The major disadvantage of home birth is the distance from emergency services should the need arise.

The freestanding birth center has a home-like environment with some select emergency equipment. Nurse-midwives and patients are in one location, making it possible to care for more than one woman at a time should the need arise, and generally a second birth attendant is in attendance to assist when needed. Disadvantages are similar to those of a home birth in that emergency transport to a hospital may be necessary if conditions exceed the birth center's capabilities. In addition, the mother and baby do need to make the trip home within a few hours of birth.

Birth centers within the hospital may at first glance appear ideal. They do try to have a home-like environment but do not have the same ambiance as home or freestanding birth centers. Emergency equipment and personnel are immediately available but so are other technologies and medicines that tend to interfere with low-risk labors.

The traditional hospital labor, delivery, and maternity unit are designed to care for several women at a time, making the units easier for staff to function in but not necessarily conducive to the normal labor process. The tendency is to use available technology despite birth plans or evidence-based recommendations. They are suitable for high-risk women and infants who need special care nurseries.

Differences in Practice Between Nurse-Midwives and Other Providers

The most significant difference between nurse-midwives, obstetrical-gynecological nurse practitioners, family practice nurse practitioners, women's health nurse practitioners, and clinical nurse specialists is the management of labor and birth. Other APNs do not provide independent care or co-management care during labor and birth.

As mentioned in the introduction of this chapter, not all midwives are nurse-midwives (ACNM, 2004c; MANA, 2007). Their definition and scope of practice are determined by their educational background, certification, and/or licensure in the state in which they practice. Non-nurse midwives include certified midwives (CMs), licensed midwives (LMs), certified professional midwives (CPMs), direct entry midwives (DEMs), and traditional birth attendants (TBAs). They are most likely to practice in their communities, providing care to pregnant women and attending home births. Their practices are determined partly by the degree to which a particular jurisdiction regulates midwifery and partly by the prevailing consumer demand and level of medical support for this type of care (ACNM, 2007a). Non-nurse midwives do not provide primary care or gynecological care to women.

Nurse-midwives and obstetricians differ most prominently in the processes they use in providing care, which can be explained by the differing values of medicine and nursing. Nurse-midwives approach the care of women, particularly during pregnancy, with the expectation that all will be normal until proven otherwise. They are educated in the normal but able to recognize the abnormal. During midwifery education, it is not uncommon to be told "when you hear hoof beats, don't look for zebras." Obstetricians are educated to diagnose and treat the abnormal. They approach health care with the expectation that problems are likely to occur and that a normal birth is a diagnosis after delivery.

Certified Nurse-Midwife Practice Summary

Nurse-midwives, through care provided, scope of practice, management processes, and practice settings, have many opportunities to influence women's health care. Nurse-midwifery care is woman-focused, independent, and collaborative. It offers a woman the opportunity to obtain, throughout her life as well as during her reproductive years, accessible, understandable, high-quality care that is safe, satisfying, and individualized to her and her families needs.

EXEMPLARS OF NURSE-MIDWIFERY PRACTICE

The day-to-day practice of midwifery is similar in all settings. In this section, an author in an earlier edition of this text (MWD) describes the practice she established in an autonomous nurse-midwife–owned freestanding birthing center (Exemplar 16-1); one of the authors of this chapter (CAS) describes her private hospital-based practice (Exemplar 16-2). These exemplars illustrate how the components of nurse-midwifery care are enacted in different settings.

EXEMPLAR 16-1 **Nurse-Midwifery Practice in a Birth Center Setting**

Our patient education process begins before a patient is accepted into the practice. Orientation sessions are held to provide prospective patients with information to assist them in determining whether they want to have their baby in a birth center. These sessions, conducted by the CNM, are designed to provide both information and a tour of the physical facility. Prospective patients can see firsthand the comfort measures (e.g., the whirlpool tub) and the equipment on hand to handle normal deliveries and emergencies. Finances are discussed. The cost of care in the birth center is approximately half of that for obstetrical care in a hospital setting with a physician. Many insurers, Medicaid, and Medicare provide reimbursement.

In an autonomous setting such as this, clinical documentation must be meticulous, and an individualized health record ensures that accurate, consistent, and complete information is obtained. Thorough health and family histories are taken. The questions elicit information about the woman's physical health and her psychological well-being. How does she feel about being pregnant? What kind of support system does she have in place? What resources might she have that are not currently being called upon? Was the pregnancy planned or a surprise? What are her family circumstances? Is there a stable relationship? Are there other children? It is important to document both positive and negative influences that can have an impact on the patient's health and the health of her baby. Once the assessment is complete, risk factors that would prevent us from being able to accept a patient are reviewed; if we cannot accept a patient, we make a referral. If no risk factors are identified, we schedule the patient's first visit.

When patients are accepted into the practice, they are told that they are equal partners in their care. It is the goal of patient education to bring this to reality. To be active participants in their care, patients are taught to weigh themselves and do their own urine dipstick tests. They participate in charting the information, thus noting the progress of their pregnancy firsthand. The program of care for pregnant patients at our birth center includes 10 to 15 prenatal visits, childbirth classes, labor and delivery in the birth center, a home visit within 72 hours of birth, and two office follow-up visits for mother and baby—one at 1 week and the other at 6 weeks after birth.

Clinical hours are held daily. The CNMs in the practice share in doing patient visits, teaching classes, and on-call time. Other responsibilities include administration and facility maintenance. We see pregnant patients, postpartum patients with their babies, and gynecological patients. The amount of time scheduled for a visit is based on need. A first visit for a pregnant patient is 1 hour long. An established gynecological patient who is coming for her contraceptive medication requires only a few minutes, long enough to establish that she is having no problems.

A pregnant patient is given the CNM pager number and instructions on how and when to use it. When a patient is in active labor or her membranes have ruptured, she calls the CNM on duty. She is met at the birth center and examined. Most often when the woman arrives, she is in active labor. We attribute this largely to the educational process that has taken place. On the rare occasion of false labor or very early labor, we are able to individualize care. If a patient lives far away, we may elect to observe progress for a number of hours. If the woman is sleep-deprived, she and her labor may benefit from some sedation. We remain with our patients in the birth center during labor. An RN is on call for every delivery. If the CNM attending the patient is tiring from having been up for a long labor, or several labors, the RN can be called to come in early to care for the patient while the CNM rests. Sometimes, the RN is not needed until close to time for the birth.

The mother-to-be helps us accommodate her wishes by preparing a birth plan. As her due date nears, one of her tasks (along with packing a bag to bring to the birth center and readying her home for a baby) is to write a birth plan, which will become a part of her record. This form allows her to tell us who she wants with her during labor, what she imagines labor will be like, what she hopes labor will be like, and what comfort measures would assist her during labor. We use this tool in several ways. We evaluate the effectiveness of our teaching by reading what the woman thinks labor will be like. Mention of fears not previously revealed gives us an opportunity to resolve any emotional factors that could hinder a successful labor. Knowing the person(s) the patient wants with her during labor informs us about her support system. The people present during labor are an important factor in enhancing the woman's experience of labor.

The list of comfort measures is mainly a reminder to us, although it is a key contribution from the patient. In the midst of labor, a woman may

CNM, Certified nurse-midwife; *RN,* registered nurse.

EXEMPLAR 16-1   Nurse-Midwifery Practice in a Birth Center Setting—cont'd

forget that she was looking forward to the whirl-pool tub for relaxation and pain relief. A glance at the birth plan helps us try the things the patient has already identified as potentially helpful to her. The birth plan helps emphasize to the patient that this is her labor, with its inherent responsibilities and rights. Her dignity and worth as a human being are underscored. We try to nourish the woman's self-esteem and strengths that help in labor, life, and motherhood. The stronger the woman is in every way, the better her outcome is going to be.

Patients are given ample written material to help with their recall of information covered in classes. (If a patient is unable to read, extra time is spent providing information verbally and making sure the patient understands it.) To help the patient assume responsibility for herself and her labor, she is expected to bring with her to the birth center food and beverages that she would like to have available during labor and certain supplies, such as perineal pads, bed pads, and diapers. Patients take their babies home dressed in their own clothes and wrapped in their own blankets. They take with them an instructional booklet that they were given in the postpartum class. The booklet describes mother and baby care for the first few days in detail. Because mothers and babies are discharged early, often in 4 to 6 hours, it is imperative that the mother be prepared to check the baby's temperature and respirations, to check her own uterus, and to be able to recognize signs of complications that require attention. These are all enumerated in the instructions, and there is room for notes and questions. Having a reference helps new moms feel more secure. If something needs attention, they can always call the nurse-midwife, but they usually find what they need to know in the booklet. It often confirms what they sensed—either that everything was okay or that they need to get in touch with the nurse-midwife. Thus new mothers start out having faith in their own perceptions regarding their infants reinforced.

Empowering our patients, enhancing their decision-making abilities, reinforcing the mind-body connection, and enhancing family life by helping women find their personal power are goals of CNM care at the birth center. When I think of the enormous effects of empowerment, two new moms come to mind.

M.L.'s case is proof positive of the benefits of teaching new mothers to trust their feelings and make decisions based on them. On the third or fourth day after delivery, M.L.'s baby ceased nursing well. He had been nursing vigorously and now was not. Nursing poorly is one of the signs listed in our booklet as requiring professional help. M.L. insisted to her husband that they had to go to the emergency room immediately. They lived a long distance from the birth center, and it had been decided earlier that, if there should be a problem that seemed serious, she should go to a nearby emergency room rather than try to get to the CNM. Initially, doctors could find nothing wrong, but M.L. insisted they keep looking. As it turned out, the baby had a congenital heart defect that does not show up on clinical examination until 3 or 4 days after birth. M.L. said she was glad she had been given the information at the birth center; it gave her the confidence to trust her feelings that something was seriously wrong. The baby had heart surgery and is doing well.

A woman with confidence and trust in herself can do almost anything, as the case of S.J. shows. S.J. was 26 years old and came to the birth center soon after it opened to have her fourth child. She had a high school education and was home with her children, all of whom were younger than 5 years. Her self-esteem was negligible. Her husband came to a few of the prenatal classes but was sullen and unsupportive. S.J. seemed to droop, but she was an excellent mother and was an attentive and fast learner at everything to do with childbirth, childrearing, and health in general. Her interest and enthusiasm grew as we reinforced her abilities and strengths. By the time she gave birth to her son, she seemed a different person from the withdrawn, self-effacing young woman we had met 7 months earlier. Two years after this baby's birth, S.J. visited the birth center. "I just wanted to thank you," she said. "Before I came here, I never felt I was any good at anything. You told me I was a good mother, you noticed how well cared for my children were, and you encouraged me to learn all about birth and even let me borrow books and tapes. Well, I learned I was good—at a lot of things! You all showed me that. And I wanted you to know I'm in nursing school now because I want to be able to do what you do—not just take care of people physically, but help people grow."

EXEMPLAR 16-2   Nurse-Midwifery Practice in a Hospital Setting

At the first prenatal visit, a complete family and health history is taken, a complete physical examination is done, a risk assessment is completed, an outline of midwifery care for the pregnancy is presented, laboratory work and other tests are explained, and the client is provided with education to make informed decisions regarding the care. The woman is asked how she feels about being pregnant, what her support system is, what the relationship with her partner is like, and if there are any issues she would like to discuss. The woman is made aware that if at any time she develops risk factors that are beyond the scope of midwifery care, the nurse-midwife will consult, collaborate, co-manage, or transfer her care to a physician. The woman is encouraged to be a partner in her care and is provided with the knowledge to make informed choices.

The woman is made aware of the office set-up, such as office hours and who all the health care providers are. She is given numbers to call if she has any questions, concerns, or problems. She is made aware of the call schedule and is also made aware that a physician is always available if the need arises but is not routinely present for births. It is also explained that on occasion her appointment may be canceled because the nurse-midwife she was to see is at the hospital with a laboring woman. Even though the women are going to be giving birth in a hospital in which there are obstetrical nurses, the nurse-midwife attends the laboring woman, providing the support the woman and her family desire. A laboring woman can expect to have a nurse-midwife with her for her labor, birth, and the first 2 hours after birth. She can then anticipate daily visits and sometimes more than once a day if there are any concerns, such as breastfeeding difficulties.

Throughout her prenatal care, all tests and options are explained and she is asked how she is feeling, what questions she may have, and any issues she wishes to discuss. She is encouraged to develop a flexible birthing plan. The majority of each visit is based on the individual needs and requests of the client. From the first visit until the last, the birthing process is discussed. The woman is offered a wide range of classes on birthing, breastfeeding, and parenting that she may attend in preparation for the birthing experience and parenting.

The woman is encouraged to visit both hospitals before deciding where she would prefer to give birth. After choosing the hospital, her prenatal records are sent there so that when she is admitted,

a complete record of her pregnancy will be available for review. Accurate record keeping during the pregnancy, labor, and birth is very important for providing continuity of care that is competent and complete.

The day the woman is discharged from the hospital, the midwife provides her with discharge instructions reiterating many of the issues that have been discussed throughout the pregnancy. These include physical and emotional issues, comfort measures, diet, rest, exercise, need for birth control, sexuality, when to return for follow-up visits, symptoms she should call the office about, a reminder that she can call for any questions, and reassurance that she has the ability to care for herself and her infant.

Mrs. S.H.'s prenatal care is an excellent demonstration of nurse-midwifery care. After deciding she would like nurse-midwifery care for her pregnancy, Mrs. S.H. was scheduled for her first prenatal visit at 8 weeks' gestation. At her initial visit, her health history was taken and a complete physical examination including a pelvic examination and vaginal cultures was performed. Midwifery care was discussed with her, as well as options regarding hospital of choice and prenatal testing. Mrs. S.H. was given an order for routine prenatal laboratory tests, to which she had agreed, and was scheduled to return in 4 weeks unless she had any concerns before then. She was given information regarding diet, activity, fetal development, and prenatal classes. Mrs. S.H.'s care remained routine until her 28-weeks' prenatal visit when she tested positive for gestational diabetes. The midwife referred her to the diabetic clinic for diet counseling and instruction in daily glucose testing. Mrs. S.H. was also scheduled to see the consulting physician after 1 week of daily glucose testing and an 1800-calorie diet. This consultation with the collaborating physician was part of the practice guidelines that the nurse-midwife and the physician had established. Gestational diabetes does increase the risk for potential problems with the pregnancy and with the birth. Because her glucose levels were stable on her 1800-calorie diet, it was decided that she could continue with nurse-midwifery care with monitoring of her glucose levels, weight, and fetal growth and fetal surveillance.

Mrs. S.H.'s pregnancy continued without further difficulties, her blood glucose remained within normal levels, and fetal growth appeared to be appropriate. Nonstress tests the last 4 weeks of the pregnancy and a biophysical profile the last week

EXEMPLAR 16-2   Nurse-Midwifery Practice in a Hospital Setting—cont'd

of the pregnancy provided reassurance of fetal well-being. Mrs. S.H. felt that she was able to contribute to the well-being of herself and her infant by being knowledgeable regarding gestational diabetes and taking appropriate care of herself. She understood the need for extra fetal surveillance at the end of the pregnancy because of increase risk for fetal macrosomia (large for gestational age) and other potential complications of gestational diabetes. When Mrs. S.H. was in labor, a physician was readily available in case of difficulties with the birth because of fetal size. All went well, and after a 12-hour labor, she gave birth to a 9-pound male in good health. Afterwards, Mrs. S.H. commented on how important it was to her to be involved in her plan of care and that it gave her confidence to labor and give birth without unnecessary medical interventions.

The ability to have such a positive impact on others is very satisfying. However, it is clear that being a CNM does not entail "doing it all" for our patients. It is far more important, and healthier for all concerned, to teach patients so that they are empowered to provide themselves and their families with the best possible care for every situation. We cannot be there for every health difficulty our patients may have, but we can give them the confidence to know when something is wrong and the knowledge of what to do in various situations. Nurse-midwives give from the core of their being. They listen, which is one of the crucial skills nurse-midwives bring to their practice. Listening is more than an auditory experience. Nurse-midwives listen observantly to hear clearly. They communicate confidence in the care of their patients in everyday matters. They hear clearly, and their patients respond.

The rewards of nurse-midwifery practice are many, but we have faced some challenges, too. On the rare occasions that things go wrong, we are scrutinized intensely. Vacation coverage is difficult to find. Other challenges include complying with regulations and legislation, finding appropriate resources for medical consultation and referral, and dealing with misperceptions of our practice within the larger health care system. These issues are not unique to our practice, as the following section demonstrates.

PROFESSIONAL ISSUES

Image

Although there is universal recognition of the term *midwife*, the word also conjures up a variety of images—some positive and others negative. Rather recently, the term *midwife* has come into common usage as a metaphor for positive experiences of guidance, compassion, strength, or peace (Paine, 2000). After their first encounter with a nurse-midwife, many people comment that they are surprised at how "normal" or how "professional" or how "knowledgeable" he or she was, but most are unable to say just what they expected. Stereotypes that have been voiced about midwives include "old, stooped, with stringy gray hair," "someone shuffling around in jeans and Birkenstocks," a "hippie," "someone practicing illegally," and "backward." These images are damaging and misleading. In contrast, actual experiences with nurse-midwives are judged overwhelmingly positive. A commonly heard refrain from patients of nurse-midwives is that every woman should have the privilege of being cared for by a nurse-midwife.

Part of the confusion about the image of the midwife stems from the different types of midwives in the United States—CNMs, CMs, CPMs, DEMs, LMs, and TBAs. In addition to the variety of midwives, there is also variety among nurse-midwives. Some nurse-midwives have certificates in midwifery, some have baccalaureate degrees, some have master's degrees, and a few have doctorates. An unfortunate result of this lack of standardization has been marked variation among practitioners and thus difficulty in characterizing this practice as professional.

In addition to confusion over who is a midwife and what is their educational background, the variety in scope of practice of nurse-midwives is somewhat surprising. Some nurse-midwives practice full-scope midwifery, which includes birth; some provide only prenatal care; and others provide only gynecological and women's health care.

From this discussion, it is no wonder that the public image of the nurse-midwife is unclear. In addition to consumer confusion, there has been a fair amount of professional resistance to nurse-midwives from the medical community. This is not unlike their response to other APNs. Despite both the confusion and resistance, the ACNM is committed to ensuring that a positive image of the professional CNM/CM emerges and seeks media opportunities to educate consumers about the role of the CNM/CM. Even with these efforts, each CNM in clinical practice also spends a portion of the day explaining who he or she is and striving to both educate and improve the image of the midwife—one patient at a time.

Credentialing Non-Nurses (Direct-Entry Midwives)

In 1994, the ACNM made the difficult decision to develop a mechanism to accredit midwifery education programs that do not require a nursing credential (ACNM, 1999, 2005d). The ultimate reason for the ACNM's decision was to advance a single standard for professional midwifery in this country. Although a discussion of the process and outcomes of this decision is beyond the scope of this chapter, the decision is relevant to discussions about credentialing APNs.[1]

This decision by the ACNM has been met with mixed reactions. Some believe that these initiatives further obscure advanced practice nursing and make it even more difficult for APNs to attain some of the regulatory and legislative support they seek. However, the ACNM may be at the cutting edge of developing a transdisciplinary workforce—a legion of people with different backgrounds but the same core set of midwifery competencies. It is difficult to predict where such practitioners will fit into the current and future health care system. Part of their ability to succeed will rest on the state regulatory agencies. In 16 states, midwifery without a registered nursing credential is regulated by a state agency. In 13 other states, the practice of midwifery by non-nurses is legal but unregulated (ACNM, 2006b, 2006c). If the demand for this type of practitioner grows and states use the ACNM national standards, which demonstrate equivalent preparation, the public will be assured of well-qualified providers.

The ACNM continues to support multiple pathways to midwifery education, non-nurse midwives as members of the College, and research that demonstrates the safety of midwife deliveries.

---

[1]Text from prior editions has been moved to the Evolve website for faculty use.

Credentialing Nurse-Midwives

Multiple levels of credentialing must be met by CNMs in order to practice. To meet professional standards, nurse-midwives must pass the ACNM certification examination that the AMCB administers. To meet regulatory requirements, they then need to be licensed in the state in which they are going to practice. Each state and U.S. jurisdiction has its own set of requirements that must be met for licensing. Included in those requirements are certification, education, graduation from an accredited program, and a current RN license (ACNM, 1997d, 2006h, 2006i). If the state grants prescriptive privileges, a specific number of hours of pharmacology course work usually is required. If the nurse-midwife's practice includes attending labors and births, then, in addition to meeting state requirements, he or she must become credentialed and privileged at the hospital or freestanding birth center with which he or she will be associated. Midwives must be cognizant of state laws and regulations that affect midwifery practice. It is important that legislators, regulatory boards, and hospital bylaws committees avoid the use of "direction and supervision" with regard to midwives, because these terms can have a negative impact on the practice of midwifery. Licensed independent practitioners (LIPs) are by definition "without direction or supervision," and midwives need to maintain that status to practice independently (Ament, 2007). ACNM publishes *Nurse-Midwifery Today: A Handbook of State Laws and Regulations* to help nurse-midwives understand regulation as it relates to nurse-midwifery.

To help nurse-midwives meet the various credentialing requirements, a number of resources are available. The resources discussed here are particularly useful for helping CNMs navigate the process of credentialing within a hospital or birth center. The ACNM publishes a handbook—*Clinical Privileges and Credentialing*—that provides an in-depth look, checklists, and practical advice for midwives who are applying for privileges to practice in a health care facility. The information in this handbook enables the nurse-midwife to approach the credentialing process with the correct information to proceed appropriately. In addition, The Joint Commission (TJC) has adopted medical staff standards that recognize that the medical staff may include licensed individuals that are not physicians and dentists, such as nurse-midwives. These standards usually guide agency credentialing committee reviews of an individual's credentials before privileges to practice in their facility are granted. Nurse-midwives usually need to obtain clinical privileges to provide care to women, their families, and the community in hospitals, birthing centers, and other clinical settings. The credentialing committee obtains, verifies, and assesses the qualifications of an applicant to provide patient care, treatment, and services in or for a health care organization (Ament, 2007). After credentials have been evaluated, the committee submits a written recommendation to the governing board that describes specific practice privileges granted to the individual and establishes an ongoing method for monitoring the care he or she provides. Nurse-midwives must go through this process to provide care for women at a health care facility or organization.

Congruence/Incongruence of Midwifery Practice with Advanced Practice Nursing

The fact that the ACNM includes non-nurse midwives in its pool could be seen as a divergence from the vision that nurse-midwives are APNs. Several observations can be made, however, that suggest that the mainstreaming of nurse-midwifery within advanced practice nursing may still occur.

Despite the fact that inconsistencies exist regarding the nurse-midwifery role within advanced practice nursing, nurse-midwives are developing in ways congruent with the vision that is bringing together CNSs, CRNAs, NPs, and other APNs (National Council of State Boards of Nursing [NCSBN], 2006). The core competencies defined by the ACNM and their implementation are consistent with the core competencies of advanced practice described in Chapter 3. Thirty-seven of the 41 accredited midwifery educational programs are in schools of nursing or colleges of nursing. As of 2010, completion of a graduate degree will be required for entry into clinical midwifery practice (ACNM, 2006b, 2006c). Clinical and regulatory issues such as access to and availability of services, as well as second licensure for APNs, are likely to engage nurse-midwives in collaborative efforts to promote the values and vision driving advanced practice. Twenty-three states already require a master's degree for licensing as an APN (including nurse-midwives) and/or for prescriptive authority; others have established a date by which a master's degree will be required. These precedents could well affect federal funding for nurse-midwifery education.

It is unlikely that nurse-midwives will risk the legal privileges for which they fought so hard by resisting efforts to ensure a common definition of advanced practice nursing across state and federal laws and regulations. In the current climate, however, it is difficult to anticipate how nurse-midwifery will address the regulatory complexity that is likely to result from the entry of non-nurses into midwifery. Whether the regulatory climate will be more or less open to innovative programs such as those contemplated by the ACNM is not clear.

These are the driving forces that may carry nurse-midwives and nurse-midwifery along in their wake as APN roles are defined and regulated at federal and state levels. Failure to be involved or opposition to the changes may undermine nurse-midwifery's efforts to secure accessible health care for individuals and may well undo its historical legislative achievements, which have enabled nurse-midwives to practice autonomously.

It is interesting to note a recent editorial debate in the *International Journal of Nursing Studies* (Thompson, Watson, & Stewart, 2007), in which international nursing authors recommend that nursing and midwifery agree to an amicable divorce, based on the prevailing view of midwifery as a separate entity from nursing. An American nurse-midwifery respondent remarked that midwifery is a separate discipline from nursing despite the fact that one half of the world's midwives are nurses. She asserted that these nurses are practicing midwifery when they care for women and childbearing families—not nursing and not obstetrics. However, she also emphasizes that collaboration and partnership are the keys to making a difference in health care and that this discussion does little to accomplish this aim (Thompson et al., 2007). It seems unfortunate and ill-timed to spend time or energy on the question of "divorce" on either the national or international level. The ACNM defines a CNM as an "individual educated in the two disciplines of nursing and midwifery" and a CM as an "individual educated in the discipline of midwifery." Currently, fewer than 0.5% of ever-certified CNM/CMs are CMs. U.S. midwifery has placed itself in a difficult position by combining both nurses and non-nurses in its profession, given the educational, political, and regulatory environment in which we function. Continuing to work with the nursing and advanced practice community is an important facet of our continued development as a profession. This does not preclude working with other groups to achieve our goals, including consumers and other women's health advocates.

Congruence with Physicians

Professional relationships between obstetrician-gynecologists and nurse-midwives are addressed in a joint statement agreed upon by the American College of Obstetricians and Gynecologists and the ACNM (Shah, 2002) (see Box 16-4). Nurse-midwives educate, attend women in birth, assist women with reproductive health issues, work with women across the lifespan, and involve their families and significant others in the process. Physicians diagnose and treat injury and disease. Midwifery and medicine have different but complementary purposes (Ament, 2007).

Individual nurse-midwives and individual physicians often develop the kind of mature, collaborative relationships described in Chapter 10. However, the current health care environment, in which organizations and providers are scrambling to cut costs and services, is not conducive to building the kind of CNM-physician rapport that has made so many CNM-run practices successful.

Barriers to effective working relationships between nurse-midwives and physicians can arise within organizations. Organizations themselves often spend time and money on efforts to restrict nurse-midwives ability to practice autonomously. These efforts include lobbying against federal and state laws and regulations that are favorable to nurse-midwives and other APNs. Chapter 20 describes the American Medical Association's public relations campaign to convince the public that APNs and other non-physician providers are incompetent. Nurse-midwives who enjoy excellent collaborative relationships with individual physicians should be alert to the activities of organized medical groups, both nationally and within their jurisdictions, so that they can protect their rights to practice nurse-midwifery and encourage their physician colleagues to speak out against limitations on nurse-midwifery practice.

Physicians sit on the boards and credentialing committees of hospitals. They have the power and authority to grant or not grant institution privileges to nurse-midwives and other APNs. Whether they need clinical privileges or not, CNMs must have physician consultation and medical backup. This requirement may be incorporated into a state practice act, but even if it is not, clinical practice and ACNM standards demand it.

PRACTICE ISSUES

Legislative, Regulatory, and Financial Barriers

Unfortunately, midwifery practice is inherently political. Laws affecting women's health care and midwifery practice are commonplace, ever changing, and differ among states (Ament, 2007). Restrictions to practice nurse-midwifery/midwifery can be found at the local, state, and federal levels. Physician control remains apparent at all levels of regulation for nurse-midwives and advanced practice nurses, from hospital privileges to malpractice insurance availability.

If interpersonal, marketing, and public relations efforts fail to secure admitting and clinical privileges for nurse-midwives, legislation that ensures nurse-midwives and other APNs access to these privileges will be needed (ACNM, 2006e, 2006f). Inequitable reimbursement for services remains a problem for nurse-midwives in many states. Nurse-midwifery care should be an option in managed care systems, but it may not be if APNs and consumers do not make their voices heard. Nurse-midwives must have nationwide prescriptive authority. Greater uniformity and consistency of regulations at the federal and state levels for prescribing and dispensing medications are needed. Nurse-midwives must be assured of a continuing source of professional liability insurance and at a cost they can afford. Allocations for nurse-midwifery education from federal and state funding agencies are at risk in the current political climate, in which many politicians are seeking to minimize government initiatives that promote health and education. Medicare and Medicaid must ensure facility fee payment for freestanding birth centers.

Workload

For nurse-midwives, who are in a full-scope midwifery practice, the stress and commitment of on-call time in addition to regular office hours can be overwhelming. If the practice has several nurse-midwives and the call is shared (e.g., one or two nights of call a week for each midwife), then it is manageable. For many nurse-midwives, especially those in solo or independent practices, however, the schedule can be daunting. To give their best to their patients and to stay healthy, nurse-midwives with a heavy on-call schedule need to develop self-care strategies that enable them to balance work with personal responsibilities and relationships.

Some nurse-midwives choose between full-scope practice and partial practice to deal with everyday living. Other nurse-midwives are employed by hospitals covering the labor and delivery unit in 12-hour shifts. Finding other nurse-midwives who can cover for vacation and sick time can become a crisis. A recent survey of Connecticut nurse-midwives (Holland & Holland, 2007) described state-specific data about practice environments. As reported in the article, these CNMs worked an average of 77 hours per week, taking two 24-hour calls and working 3 office days per week. Seventy-five percent of respondents provided full-scope antepartum, intrapartum, and gynecological care. Expanded scope of practice was also reported by respondents, including but not limited to endometrial biopsies, surgical assist at cesarean birth, water birth, and ultrasound. Salaries were slightly higher than the national average for nurse-practitioners, possibly taking into account the expanded work week.

The physical and emotional demands of birthing babies, the long hours and periods of sleep deprivation, and the liability concerns mean that nurse-midwifery is not for everyone. For those who love it, the satisfaction of providing care to a pregnant woman, following her through her pregnancy, assisting her through the physical and mental demands of labor and birth, anticipating the unpredictability of birth, and the joy of a family greeting their newborn make nurse-midwifery fascinating, exciting, and personally worth the physical and emotional investment of self that may be required. It is a privilege to be with families who are experiencing pregnancy and birth. In making this investment, however, midwives struggle to achieve a work-life balance that maintains personal well-being.

Malpractice

As mentioned earlier, physicians sit on hospital credentialing committees, their national and state organizations lobby against pro-midwifery and advanced practice legislation, and even their malpractice insurance companies have control over the ability of nurse-midwives to obtain malpractice insurance (Ament, 2007; Summers, 2005). In general, nurse-midwifery malpractice insurance rates are higher than for other APNs, which reflects the malpractice climate of obstetrical care. These rates have been cited as reasons for some midwifery practices to be discontinued. Therefore the professional organization and individual nurse-midwives seek to stay abreast of legislative and practice changes that may help reframe the litigious environment in which health care occurs, especially for practitioners of midwifery and obstetrics.

Quality and Safety

Quality and safety issues have become of paramount concern to nurse-midwives. As reported by Clancy (2006), two thirds of serious injuries and deaths in the delivery room are the result of human error and the median award for "medical negligence in childbirth" is $2.3 million (ACOG, 2003). The professional organization has increased the activity of the Division of Standards and Practice, which includes committees on clinical practice, quality improvement, and professional liability. A recent ACNM position statement "Creating a Culture of Safety in Midwifery Care" (2006aa) outlines the importance of evidence-based practice, interdisciplinary team communication, active involvement of patients in their care, and participation in quality management programs. ACNM also maintains a current website entitled "Quality Improvement and Patient Safety in Women's Health," which directs midwives to resources including organizational links of importance to quality and safety for practitioners. Nurse-midwives are participating in the Institute for Healthcare Improvement's Learning and Innovation Community on Improving Perinatal Care (*www.ihi.org/IHI/Results/WhitePapers/IdealizedDesignofPerinatalCareWhitePaper/htm*). They are also eligible to participate in the Tax Relief and Health Care Act of 2006 and the CMS Pay-for-Performance Initiative and have a representative on the CMS taskforce for non-physician providers. In as many ways as possible, midwives are striving to raise their awareness and become partners in improving care to women and infants.

CONCLUSION

The demand and need for CNMs' unique services are growing. CNMs focus on women, their families, and their communities. They have been thinking globally and acting locally long before it became trendy to do so. They are called to do what they do. As long as there are pregnant women who wish to give birth in an informed and caring fashion, CNMs will be needed. Indeed, there are those in the profession who feel that midwifery holds the key to contemporary obstetrical problems (Baldwin, 1999; Rooks, 1998).

Nurse-midwifery, advanced practice nursing, and the profession of nursing in general are at a critical juncture. Although nurse-midwifery is standing somewhat apart from advanced practice efforts, it seems clear that a need exists to recognize the interdependence of advanced practice nursing and nurse-midwifery. By examining the separate yet related courses being charted by the nursing profession (related to advanced practice nursing) and by CNMs (to meet demands for midwifery services), one can see that potential for divisiveness is great at a time in our history when we need to be unified.

CNMs have often led the nursing profession into the future, and many of the initiatives mentioned in this chapter indicate that the profession continues to move forward. It may now be time for CNMs to join forces with the nursing profession, which is investing its energy and resources in preserving and expanding the climate for autonomous nursing practice that CNMs helped create.

REFERENCES

Ament, L.A. (2007). *Professional issues in midwifery*. Sudbury, MA: Jones & Bartlett.

American Association of Colleges of Nursing (AACN). (2004a). *The essentials of doctoral education for advanced nursing practice*. Washington, DC: Author.

American Association of Colleges of Nursing (AACN). (2004b). *AACN position statement on the practice doctorate in nursing*. Washington, DC: Author.

American College of Nurse-Midwives (ACNM). (1997a). *Collaborative management in midwifery practice for medical, gynecological and obstetrical conditions*. Silver Spring, MD: Author.

American College of Nurse-Midwives (ACNM). (1997b). *Expansion of midwifery practice and skills beyond basic core competencies*. Silver Spring, MD: Author.

American College of Nurse-Midwives (ACNM). (1997c). Position Statement: *Certified nurse- midwives/certified midwives as primary care providers/case managers*. Silver Spring, MD: Author.

American College of Nurse-Midwives (ACNM). (1997d). *State practice acts and regulations*. Silver Spring, MD: Author.

American College of Nurse-Midwives (ACNM). (1998). *Healthcare/managed care reform*. Silver Spring, MD: Author.

American College of Nurse-Midwives (ACNM). (1999). *Direct entry midwifery: A summary of state laws and regulations*. Silver Spring, MD: Author.

American College of Nurse-Midwives (ACNM). (2002a). *Core competencies for basic midwifery practice*. Silver Spring, MD: Author.

American College of Nurse-Midwives (ACNM). (2002b). *Joint statement of practice relations between obstetricians, gynecologists and certified nurse-midwives/certified midwives*. Silver Spring, MD: Author.

American College of Nurse-Midwives (ACNM). (2003a). *Criteria for the evaluation of education programs*. Silver Spring, MD: Author.

American College of Nurse-Midwives (ACNM). (2003b). *Standards for the practice of midwifery*. Silver Spring, MD: Author.

American College of Nurse-Midwives (ACNM). (2003c). Position Statement: *Appropriate use of technology in childbirth*. Silver Spring, MD: Author.

American College of Nurse-Midwives (ACNM). (2004a). *Philosophy of the American College of Nurse-Midwives*. Silver Spring, MD: Author.

American College of Nurse-Midwives (ACNM). (2004b). Position Statement: *Independent midwifery practice*. Silver Spring, MD: Author.

American College of Nurse-Midwives (ACNM). (2004c). Position Statement: *Definition of midwifery practice, certified nurse-midwives and certified midwives*. Silver Spring, MD: Author.

American College of Nurse-Midwives (ACNM). (2004d). Position Statement: *Health care for all women and families*. Silver Spring, MD: Author.

American College of Nurse-Midwives (ACNM). (2005a). *CNM-attended births continue to rise*. Silver Spring, MD: Author.

American College of Nurse-Midwives (ACNM). (2005b). *Code of ethics*. Silver Spring, MD: Author.

American College of Nurse-Midwives (ACNM). (2005c). *Continuing competency assessment*. Silver Spring, MD: Author.

American College of Nurse-Midwives (ACNM), Division of Accreditation. (2005d). *Statement on midwifery education*. Silver Spring, MD: Author.

American College of Nurse-Midwives (ACNM). (2005e). *Midwifery education*. Silver Spring, MD: Author.

American College of Nurse-Midwives (ACNM). (2005f). *Division of Women's Health Policy & Leadership: Goals and objectives*. Silver Spring, MD: Author.

American College of Nurse-Midwives (ACNM). (2006aa). Position Statement: *Creating a culture of safety in midwifery care*. Silver Spring, MD: Author.

American College of Nurse-Midwives (ACNM). (2006a). Position Statement: *Faculty degree requirements*. Silver Spring, MD: Author.

American College of Nurse-Midwives (ACNM). (2006b). Position Statement: *Mandatory degree requirements for entry into midwifery practice*. Silver Spring, MD: Author.

American College of Nurse-Midwives (ACNM). (2006c). Position Statement: *Midwifery education*. Silver Spring, MD: Author.

American College of Nurse-Midwives (ACNM). (2006d). *Nurse-midwifery in 2006. Evidence-based practice*. Silver Spring, MD: Author.

American College of Nurse-Midwives (ACNM). (2006e). *Principles for licensing and regulating midwifery and other maternal-child health providers*. Silver Spring, MD: Author.

American College of Nurse-Midwives (ACNM). (2006f). *Principles of credentialing and privileging certified nurse-midwives and certified midwives*. Silver Spring, MD: Author.

American College of Nurse-Midwives (ACNM). (2006g). *Requirements for signed collaborative agreements between physicians and certified nurse-midwives/certified midwives*. Silver Spring, MD: Author.

American College of Nurse-Midwives (ACNM). (2006h). *States that require master's degree for nurse-midwifery practice*. Silver Spring, MD: Author.

American College of Nurse-Midwives (ACNM). (2006i). *State fact sheets*. Silver Spring, MD: Author.

American College of Nurse-Midwives (ACNM). (2007a). *A comparison of certified nurse-midwives/certified midwives and certified professional midwives*. Silver Spring, MD: Author.

American College of Nurse-Midwives (ACNM). (2007b). *Core competencies for basic midwifery practice.* Washington, DC: Author.

American College of Nurse-Midwives (ACNM), Division of Accreditation. (2007c). *ACNM overview.* Silver Spring, MD: Author.

American College of Nurse-Midwives (ACNM). (2007d). Quick Info: *Reentry to midwifery practice.* Silver Spring, MD: Author.

American College of Nurse-Midwives (ACNM). (2007e). Quick Info: *Scope of practice.* Silver Spring, MD: Author.

American College of Nurse-Midwives (ACNM), Division of Research. (2007f). *Mission and activities.* Silver Spring, MD: Author.

American College of Obstetricians and Gynecologists (ACOG). (2003). Survey on professional liability. Washington, DC: Author.

American Medical Association (AMA) Board of Trustees. (1995). Model guidelines for physician and nurse practitioner integrated practice. *Journal of Nurse-Midwifery, 37,* 150-154.

American Midwifery Certification Board (AMCB). (2007). *Policies and procedure manual.* Linthicum, MD: Author.

Baldwin, K.A. (1999). The midwifery solution to contemporary problems in American obstetrics. *Journal of Nurse-Midwifery, 44*(1), 75-79.

Barger, M.K. (2005). The history of nurse-midwifery/midwifery practice. *Journal of Midwifery and Women's Health, 50*(2), 87-90.

Beck, C.T. (1998). A checklist to identify women at risk for developing postpartum depression. *Journal of Obstetric, Gynecologic, and Neonatal Nursing: JOGNN, 27*(1), 39-46.

Beck, C.T. (2001). Predictors of postpartum depression: An update. *Nursing Research, 50*(5), 275-285.

Beck, C.T. (2002). Revision of the postpartum predictors inventory. *Journal of Obstetric, Gynecologic, and Neonatal Nursing: JOGNN, 31*(4), 394-402.

Beck, C.T. (2006). Further development of the postpartum depression predictors inventory—revised. *Journal of Obstetric, Gynecologic, and Neonatal Nursing: JOGNN, 35*(6), 735-745.

Beck, C.T., & Gable, R.K. (2000). Postpartum depression screening scale: Development and psychometric testing. *Nursing Research, 49*(5), 272-282.

Beck, C.T., & Gable, R.K. (2001a). Further validation of the postpartum depression screening scale. *Nursing Research, 50*(3), 155-164.

Beck, C.T., & Gable, R.K. (2001b). Comparative analysis of the performance of the postpartum depression screening scale with two other depression instruments. *Nursing Research, 50*(4), 242-250.

Beck, C.T., & Gable, R.K. (2002). *Postpartum depression screening scale.* Los Angeles, CA: Western Psychological Services.

Burst, H.V. (2005). The history of nurse-midwifery/midwifery education. *Journal of Midwifery & Women's Health, 50*(2), 124-137.

Clancy, C. (2006). The culture of safety. Speech presented at the Nurse Alliance of Service Employees International Union (SEIU) Networking Conference on Quality. St. Louis, MO, September 25, 2006. Agency for Healthcare Research and Quality, Rockville, MD. Retrieved September 1, 2007, from http://www.ahrq.org/news/sp092506.htm.

Dawley, K. (2003). Origins of nurse-midwifery in the United States and its expansion in the 1940s. *Journal of Midwifery and Women's Health, 48*(2), 86-95.

Dawley, K. (2005). Doubling back over roads once traveled: Creating a national organization for nurse-midwifery. *Journal of Midwifery and Women's Health, 50*(2), 71-82.

Dawley, K., & Burst, H.V. (2005). The American College of Nurse-Midwives and its antecedents: A historic time line. *Journal of Midwifery and Women's Health, 50*(1), 16-22.

Declercq, E. (2007). Trends in CNM-attended births, 1990-2004. *Journal of Midwifery and Women's Health, 52*(1), 87-88.

Declercq, E., Paine, L.L., Dejoseph, J.F., & Simmes, D. (1998). State regulation, payment policies, and nurse-midwife services. *Health Affairs, 17,* 190-200.

Dorroh, M.W., & Kelley, M.A. (2005). The certified nurse-midwife. In A.B. Hamric, J.A. Spross, & C.M. Hanson (Eds.), *Advanced practice nursing: An integrative approach* (pp. 551-581). Philadelphia: Saunders.

Dorroh, M.W., & Norton, S.F. (1996). The certified nurse-midwife. In A.B. Hamric, J.A. Spross, & C.M. Hanson (Eds.), *Advanced nursing practice: An integrative approach* (pp. 395-429). Philadelphia: Saunders.

Farley, C., & Camacho, K.C. (2003). New directions in midwifery education: The master's of science in midwifery degree. *Journal of Midwifery & Women's Health, 48*(2), 133-137.

Fullerton, J., Schuiling, K.D, & Sipe, T.A. (2005). Presidential priorities: 50 years of wisdom as the basis of action agenda for the next half century. *Journal of Midwifery & Women's Health, 50*(2), 91-101.

Holland, M.L., & Holland, E.S. (2007). Survey of Connecticut nurse-midwives. *Journal of Midwifery & Women's Health, 52*(2), 106-115.

Kennedy, H.P., Schuiling, K.D., & Murphy, P.A. (2007). Developing midwifery knowledge: Setting a research agenda. *Journal of Midwifery and Women's Health, 52*(2), 95-97.

Kovner, C.T., & Burkhardt, P. (2001). Findings from the American College of Nurse-Midwives annual membership survey, 1995-1997. *Journal of Midwifery & Women's Health, 46,* 24-29.

Kraus, N. (1997). What's in a name: Defining the professions of midwifery. *Journal of Nurse-Midwifery, 42*(2), 69-70.

Midwives Alliance of North America (MANA). (2007). *Definitions.* Washington, DC: Author.

National Council of State Boards of Nursing (NCSBN). (2006). *Vision paper: The future regulation of advanced practice nursing* (Draft). Chicago, IL: Author.

Paine, L.L. (2000). Midwife is a metaphor (Editorial). *Journal of Midwifery & Women's Health, 45*(5), 367.

Roberts, J., & Huser, S. (2002). The evolution of midwifery as reflected in the 2002 revisions of the ACNM's core competencies. *Journal of Midwifery & Women's Health, 47*(5), 301-302.

Rooks, J.P. (1998). Unity in midwifery: Realities and alternative. *Journal of Nurse-Midwifery, 43*(5), 315-319.

Shah, M.A. (2000). The Journal of Midwifery & Women's Health: Celebrating its heritage—forging its future (Editorial). *Journal of Midwifery & Women's Health, 45*(1), 1-2.

Shah, M.A. (May 27, 2002). *Professional visions...contemporary realities*. Presidential address delivered at the 47th annual meeting of the American College of Nurse-Midwives, Atlanta, GA.

Summers, L. (2005). Liability concerns: A view from the American College of Nurse-Midwives. *Journal of Midwifery & Women's Health, 50*(6), 531-535.

Thompson, D.R., Watson, R., & Stewart, S. (2007). Nursing and midwifery: Time for an amicable divorce? *International Journal of Nursing Studies, 44*(4), 523-524.

Thompson, F.E. (2002). Moving from codes of ethics to ethical relationships for midwifery practice. *Nursing Ethics, 9*(5), 522-536.

Thompson, F.E. (2003). The practice setting: Site of ethical conflict for some mothers and midwives. *Nursing Ethics, 10*(6), 588-601.

Ulrich, L.T. (1990). *A midwife's tale: The life of Martha Ballard, based on her diary, 1785-1812*. New York: Knopf/Random House.

Varney, H., Kriebs, J.M., & Gegor, C.L. (2004). *Varney's midwifery* (4th ed.). Sudbury, MA: Jones & Bartlett.

CHAPTER 17

The Certified Registered Nurse Anesthetist

Margaret Faut-Callahan • Michael J. Kremer

INTRODUCTION

As noted in Chapter 1, nurse anesthesia is the oldest organized specialty in nursing. Standardized postgraduate education, credentialing, and continuing education are all areas pioneered by certified registered nurse anesthetists (CRNAs). CRNAs were the first nurse specialists to receive direct reimbursement for their services. This chapter discusses professional definitions of nurse anesthesia practice and issues important to the specialty. A profile of current CRNA practice is described, and challenges and future trends are proposed. The American Association of Nurse Anesthetists (AANA) is described, and the model of professional competence for CRNAs is presented.

Brief History of Certified Registered Nurse Anesthetist Education and Practice

The first organized program in nurse anesthesia education was offered in 1909, although nurses have provided anesthesia for over 125 years. There are currently 105 accredited nurse anesthesia programs with over 1500 clinical sites in the United States and Puerto Rico. These programs are affiliated with or operated by schools of nursing, allied health, or other academic entities.

In 2006, over 2000 nurse anesthesia students graduated and took their certification examinations. CRNAs must be recertified every 2 years, which includes meeting practice requirements and obtaining a minimum of 40 continuing education credits. Nurse anesthetists were among the first advanced practice nurses to require continuing education.

The AANA implemented a certification program in 1945 and instituted mandatory recertification in 1978. In 1952, the AANA established a mechanism for accreditation of nurse anesthesia educational programs that has been recognized by the U.S. Department of Education since 1955. The CRNA credential came into existence in 1956.

In 1990, the U.S. Department of Health and Human Services (USDHHS) published findings indicating a growing need for additional nurse anesthetists.

Despite a current workforce of some 36,000 CRNAs, the 12% vacancy rate continues to be a concern as demands for CRNA services grow. For example, the *2004 National Hospital Discharge Survey* (Centers for Disease Control and Prevention [CDC], 2005) indicated that 45 million inpatient procedures were performed in that year and CRNAs administered 65% (over 29 million) of the involved anesthetics for those procedures. CRNAs are the primary anesthesia providers in rural America, enabling health care facilities in these medically underserved areas to offer obstetrical, surgical, and trauma stabilization services. In some states, CRNAs are the sole anesthesia providers in nearly 100% of rural hospitals.

According to a 1999 report from the Institute of Medicine (IOM), anesthesia care today is nearly 50 times safer than it was 20 years ago. Outcomes studies have demonstrated that there is no difference in the quality of care provided by CRNAs and their physician counterparts (Jordan, Kremer, & Crawforth, 2001; Pine, Holt, & Lou, 2003; Simonson, Ahern, & Hendryx, 2007).

Nurse anesthetists have been the main providers of anesthesia care to U.S. military men and women on the front lines since World War I. Nurses first provided anesthesia to wounded soldiers during the Civil War. During Operation Iraqi Freedom, data released from the U.S. Department of Defense revealed that a total of 364 CRNAs and 77 anesthesiologists were deployed to provide anesthesia care (Bettin, 2004).

Across the country, nurse anesthesia professional liability premiums are 34% lower than 18 years ago. When adjusted for inflation, the decrease in coverage costs is 42%. Legislation passed by Congress in 1986 provided direct billing for CRNAs under Medicare Part B. As of 2007, 14 states have opted out of the requirement for physician supervision as a condition of reimbursement for Medicare Part A when CRNAs provide anesthesia services. No harmful effects as a result of opt-outs have been reported in any of the opt-out states. Physicians and CRNAs continue to work cooperatively in states where opt-outs have been enacted.

Males have historically been more represented in nurse anesthesia compared with nursing as a whole. Approximately 46% of the nation's 36,000 nurse anesthetists and student nurse anesthetists are men, compared with about 8% in the nursing profession as a whole. When all employed CRNAs are examined, 44.5% are male and 55.5% are female. The gender balance shifts significantly with part-time employees: 85.1% of part-time CRNAs are women, whereas 14.9% are men. Currently, more than 90% of U.S. nurse anesthetists are members of the AANA (American Association of Nurse Anesthetists [AANA], 2006).

Role Differentiation Between Certified Registered Nurse Anesthetists and Anesthesiologists

CRNAs provide anesthesia services in collaboration with surgeons, anesthesiologists, dentists, podiatrists, and other qualified health care professionals. When anesthesia is administered by a nurse anesthetist, it is recognized as the practice of nursing; when administered by an anesthesiologist, it is recognized as the practice of medicine. Regardless of their educational backgrounds, all anesthesia providers adhere to the same standards of care. Nurse anesthetists practice in every setting in which anesthesia is delivered: traditional hospital surgical suites and obstetrical delivery rooms; critical access hospitals; ambulatory surgical centers; the offices of dentists, podiatrists, ophthalmologists, plastic surgeons, and pain management specialists; and U.S. military, Public Health Services, and Department of Veterans Affairs health care facilities.

PROFILE OF THE CERTIFIED REGISTERED NURSE ANESTHETIST

A CRNA is a registered nurse (RN) who is educationally prepared at the graduate level and certified as competent to engage in practice as a nurse anesthetist, rendering patients insensible to pain with anesthetic agents and related drugs and procedures. Anesthesia services are delivered by anesthesia providers upon request, assignment, or referral by the operating physician or other health care providers authorized by law to facilitate diagnostic, therapeutic, or surgical procedures. In addition to general or regional anesthesia techniques, as well as monitored anesthesia care, a referral or request for consultation or assistance may be initiated for provision of obstetrical anesthesia services, ventilator management, or treatment of acute or chronic pain through performance of selected diagnostic or therapeutic blocks or other forms of pain management (AANA, 2002b).

CRNAs are responsible and accountable for their individual professional practices and are capable of exercising independent judgment within the scope of their education (credentials), demonstrated competence (privileges), and licensure. CRNAs are recognized in all 50 states by state regulatory bodies, primarily boards of registered nursing. Nurse anesthesia is a recognized nursing specialty role and is not a medically delegated act.

Certified Registered Nurse Anesthetist Scope and Standards of Practice

The "Scope and Standards of Nurse Anesthesia Practice," as set forth by the AANA, is comprehensive and includes all aspects of anesthesia care (AANA, 2002a). Regardless of the settings in which CRNAs practice, their role includes meeting individual anesthesia care needs of patients in the perioperative period including the following:

- Performing a physical assessment
- Participating in preoperative teaching
- Preparing for anesthetic management
- Administering anesthesia to keep the patient pain-free
- Maintaining intraoperative anesthesia
- Overseeing recovery from anesthesia
- Following the postoperative course of the patient from recovery room to patient care unit

The scope of practice of the CRNA encompasses the professional functions, privileges, and responsibilities associated with nurse anesthesia practice. These activities are performed in collaboration with qualified and legally authorized professional health care providers. CRNAs are prepared to recognize situations in which health care requirements are beyond their individual competencies and to seek consultation or referral when such situations arise (AANA, 2002a).

Anesthesia care is provided by CRNAs in four general categories: (1) preanesthetic evaluation and preparation; (2) anesthesia induction, maintenance, and emergence; (3) postanesthesia care; and (4) perianesthetic and clinical support functions. Parallels between nursing and nurse anesthesia can be seen. CRNAs perform preanesthetic assessments, plan appropriate anesthetic interventions, implement planned anesthetic care, and evaluate patients postoperatively to determine the efficacy of their interventions. CRNAs working alone routinely perform all of these aspects of clinical practice. When CRNAs and anesthesiologists work together in "team" anesthesia, a variety of factors, such as local anesthesia practice patterns, determine to what extent each practitioner is involved in specific anesthesia care areas.

Preoperative evaluation has become more complex with the increasing acuity of surgical patients. Thorough preanesthetic assessments, combined with specialty consultation as needed, are essential activities at which nurse anesthetists must be proficient. Other aspects of preanesthetic patient preparation are requesting diagnostic studies; selecting, obtaining, ordering, or administering preanesthetic medications and fluids; and obtaining informed consent for anesthesia (AANA, 2002a).

Developing and implementing an anesthetic care plan is another aspect of CRNA practice. This care plan is formulated with input from the patient, the surgeon, and, in team anesthesia settings, the collaborating anesthesiologist. Similarly, the choice of administering regional or general anesthesia is not solely the province of any one of the aforementioned participants. Input from the patient, the surgeon, and the anesthetist is relevant in the important decision about which type of anesthetic to administer in a given situation. Compromise and flexibility may be necessary to achieve the goals of surgery and anesthesia to maximize safety and minimize risks during the procedure and post-procedure period.

The scope of practice for CRNAs varies depending on institutional credentialing. Whereas the majority of CRNAs provide general anesthesia and monitored anesthesia care, survey data show a noticeable decrease in the frequency with which regional anesthesia is performed relative to general anesthesia. Placement of invasive monitoring lines and pain management techniques are less commonly performed by nurse anesthetists. Practice restrictions may not always be explicitly documented; some clinicians choose not to perform certain types of procedures.

Certified Registered Nurse Anesthetist Credentialing Requirements

To become a CRNA, one must meet the following requirements:

- Complete a bachelor of science degree in nursing or other appropriate baccalaureate degree.
- Hold current licensure as an RN.
- Practice at least 1 year as an RN in an acute care setting.

- Graduate from a nurse anesthesia program accredited by the Council on Accreditation of Nurse Anesthesia Educational Programs (COA) or its predecessor.
- Successfully complete the certification examination administered by the Council on Certification of Nurse Anesthetists or its predecessor.
- Comply with criteria for biennial recertification as defined by the Council on Recertification of Nurse Anesthetists. These criteria include evidence of (1) current licensure as an RN; (2) active practice as a CRNA; (3) appropriate continuing education; and (4) verification of the absence of mental, physical, and other problems that could interfere with the practice of anesthesia.

Certified Registered Nurse Anesthetist Certification

Nurse anesthesia was the first nursing specialty to have mandatory certification. The Council on Certification, like other AANA councils, is administratively independent of the AANA. The mission of the certification council is to certify nurse anesthesia graduates by examination, thus protecting and assuring the public regarding CRNA competency. The Council on Certification utilizes psychometricians, an academy of test item writers, and computer adaptive testing to assess beginning-level competence in nurse anesthesia graduates.

Another AANA council, the Council on Recertification, was developed in the late 1970s. The impetus for its development was the need to document for the public continued professional excellence for practicing CRNAs. The certification period for CRNAs is every 2 years and is renewable. Documentation of anesthesia practice and continuing education activities are required for recertification. Continuing education programs must be approved by the council to meet requirements for recertification (AANA, 2002b).

These two councils, plus the Council for Public Interest in Anesthesia, endeavor to assure the public that the education and practice of CRNAs is more than adequate for the demands of the specialty.

Institutional Credentialing of Certified Registered Nurse Anesthetists

CRNAs practice according to their expertise, state statutes or regulations, and local institutional policy. Institutional credentialing procedures may require additional evidence of clinical and didactic education in areas such as cardiothoracic or regional anesthesia. State nurse practice acts and practice patterns in the anesthesia community contribute to variability in the scope of nurse anesthesia practice in different settings.

Competence can be partially assured through institutional credentialing processes. A hospital may delineate procedures that the CRNA is authorized to perform by the authority of the governing board. Guidelines for granting CRNAs clinical privileges are found in the "Scopes and Standards for Nurse Anesthesia Practice" (AANA, 2002a). Recommended clinical privileges for CRNAs are in the areas of preanesthetic preparation and evaluation; anesthesia induction, maintenance, and emergence; postanesthetic care; and perianesthetic and clinical support functions.

American Association of Nurse Anesthetists Data Supporting Certified Registered Nurse Anesthetist Practice Profiles

The average student nurse anesthetist works at least 1694 clinical hours and administers more than 790 anesthetics.

Data that comprise CRNA practice profiles are derived from annual practice surveys completed by CRNAs when they pay their AANA dues. The response rate to these surveys has been as high as 72%, providing a reasonable degree of generalizability despite the limitations of self-reported data. The AANA member database, 2005 Practice Profile Survey, and demographic surveys distributed by AANA show over 35,000 members (Rivera, 2006). These data demonstrate an additional 10,000 CRNA members between 1996 and 2006. This 28% growth rate bodes well for the future of nurse anesthesia, along with the continued availability of high-quality, cost-effective anesthesia services, especially to rural and medically underserved citizens. This growth rate reflects the effective work of the National Commission on Nurse Anesthesia Education (American Association of Nurse Anesthetists, 1990), which provided the profession with workforce data projections and related strategies to ensure that the market demand for nurse anesthetists would be met. The marked growth in numbers of nurse anesthesia programs, clinical sites, and graduates since 1990 is significant, with a greater than 300% increase in the number of program graduates over that time.

This growth is attributed to the advocacy of AANA, through the National Commission on Nurse Anesthesia Education, for the development of new educational programs to meet increasing needs for anesthesia services (Mastropietro, Horton, Oullette, & Faut-Callahan, 2001).

Similar to the nursing workforce, demographic data on practicing nurse anesthetists indicate an average age of 48 years. Although it is clear that many people continue to work beyond the traditional retirement age range, the profession has been proactive in expanding the number of nurse anesthesia educational programs to ensure a ready supply of CRNAs. Furthermore, with life expectancy increasing, it is clear that population growth in older adults will contribute to additional surgical and diagnostic procedures that require anesthesia.

Years of practice as a CRNA also reflect the aging nurse anesthesia workforce. Forty percent of CRNAs have practiced for more than 20 years, and 22% have been in practice for 11 to 20 years (Figure 17-1). Overall employment patterns demonstrate that 81% of AANA members work full-time; 14% are part-time employees; 4% are retired, and 1% of survey respondents are unemployed.

At one time, CRNAs were primarily hospital-employed. With cost shifting that has occurred more recently, 37% of CRNAs report that they are employees of practice groups; 34% are hospital employees; 15% are independent contractors; 6% are employees in other settings; 5% are owners or partners in professional groups; and 3% of CRNAs currently are military, government, or Veterans Administration employees. CRNAs provide 90% of the anesthesia care in U.S. military combat zones globally (Bettin, 2004) (Figure 17-2).

The majority (97%) of nurse anesthetists are practicing clinicians. Departmental management and administration are listed as primary employment positions by 1.8% of CRNA survey respondents, and 1.3% of nurse anesthetists are educators. This paucity of educators with an increase in the number of nurse anesthesia educational programs has prompted concerted efforts to recruit and retain nurse anesthesia faculty (Starnes-Ott & Kremer, 2007).

Most practicing CRNAs report that they are clinical generalists (83%). Areas of specialty for practicing CRNAs include obstetrics (3.8%), cardiovascular surgery (1.9%), plastic surgery (1.6%), pediatrics (1.6%), and ophthalmology (1.3%).

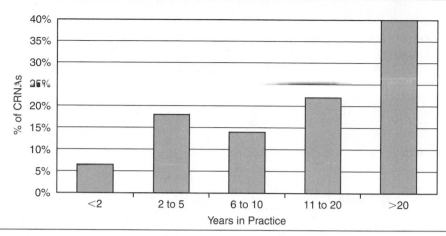

FIGURE **17-1:** Years in practice as a CRNA.

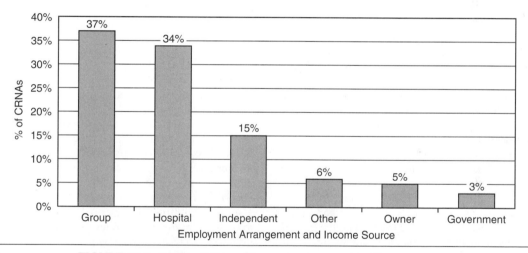

FIGURE **17-2:** Primary CRNA employment arrangement and income source.

Hospitals are the most common primary CRNA practice setting, with 82% of survey respondents reporting that they practice in these settings. Ambulatory surgical centers (ASCs) are the employment setting for almost 10% of nurse anesthetists, followed by university hospitals (6.3%), office-based surgery (1.7%), and all other practice settings (0.5%).

Compensation along with the role-related autonomy and responsibility continues to attract qualified applicants to this advanced practice nursing specialty. The most recent data for full-time CRNAs, excluding those who are self-employed, show a mean salary of $140,013. Medicare payment decreases of over 7% were imposed in 2007, with significant reimbursement implications for all anesthesia providers given the prevalence of Medicare in most payer mixes. Further cuts in Medicare payments are anticipated over time (AANA, 2007a).

Although these reimbursement decreases are a concern, the number of surgical and diagnostic procedures performed annually continues to increase. It seems reasonable to project that demand for CRNAs will remain high with the associated compensation growing at a slower rate than in the past (Figure 17-3).

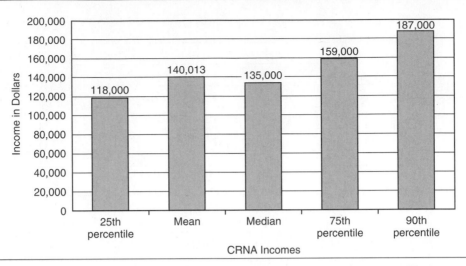

FIGURE **17-3:** Calendar-Year 2004 total compensation for non–self-employed CRNAs.

Given the average CRNA age, it is not surprising that slightly more than half of nurse anesthetists possess graduate degrees. The COA imposed the requirement for a master's degree that became effective in 1998. Most nurse anesthesia programs voluntarily moved to the master's level in the 1980s. The progression from certificate to baccalaureate to master's exit degrees for nurse anesthesia occurred in a relatively short time frame, from the 1970s through the 1990s.

The CRNA practice profile is influenced by the work of the AANA Practice Committee and professional Practice Affairs Department. The Practice Affairs Department participates in safety and quality issues. AANA is represented at the National Patient Safety Foundation and involved with the Ambulatory Surgery and Office Surgery Safety Initiative. AANA is a major stakeholder and participant in the National Quality Forum, addressing patient safety issues, and has been involved in a summit that addressed wrong-sided surgery.

AANA works with accrediting bodies to review standards revisions. CRNAs are represented on The Joint Commission (TJC) Professional Technical Advisory Committees. TJC has announced more specific credentialing requirements for all categories of allied health providers, a development that AANA is monitoring closely. CRNAs are surveyors for the Accreditation Association for Ambulatory Health Care (AAAHC).

Employment Factors

Shortage Predictions. A recent study determined the current trends in supply, demand, and equilibrium in the market for CRNAs. The researchers also forecast future needs for CRNAs given varying scenarios. The impact of the current availability of CRNAs, projected retirements, and changes in the demand for surgeries were considered relative to future needs for CRNAs. The study used data from many sources to estimate models associated with the supply and demand for CRNAs and the relationship to relevant community and policy characteristics such as per capita income of the community and managed care. These models were used to forecast changes in surgeries and the supply of CRNAs in the future. The study showed an overall CRNA vacancy rate of 12% (Merwin, Stern, & Jordan, 2005).

Although the supply of CRNAs has increased in recent years, stimulated by workforce shortages, the increases have not offset the number of retiring CRNAs to maintain a constant age in the CRNA population. The average CRNA age will continue to increase for the near term, despite increases in the numbers of CRNAs trained. The supply of CRNAs related to the number of surgeries is expected to increase in the near future (Merwin et al., 2005).

Recent research related to nurse anesthesia faculty workforce revealed that there was no difference in the expected years to retirement for faculty versus non-faculty CRNAs: 36% of both groups plan to retire by 2014; 64% expect to retire after 2014. The expected increase in demand for nurse anesthesia faculty in the future is significant given the significant growth in the number of nurse anesthesia programs and graduates. The salary differential between clinical and academic settings was the biggest barrier to recruitment of academic faculty. Other identified barriers in this study were academic credential, benefits, workload, and loss of clinical time. Program directors earn a median $10,000 more per year than other CRNAs but work an average of 10 hours per week more (Merwin, Stern, & Jordan, 2007).

Of those CRNA faculty members without a doctorate or not currently pursuing doctoral studies, 20% indicated that they would stop teaching if a doctorate was required to continue teaching. Age and being a clinical faculty member were the only predictors of an individual's plan to stop teaching if doctoral degrees were required for faculty. Major hurdles perceived by CRNA faculty research subjects to obtaining a doctoral degree included time, finances, availability of programs, value, their age, desire, and workloads (Merwin et al., 2007). A requirement for doctoral education is an ongoing concern, given an increasing emphasis on the desirability of earned doctoral degrees in the academic community.

The faculty workforce study found that 66% of programs had no CRNA faculty vacancies. The mean vacancy rate per program was 0.5 full-time equivalent (FTE). There were 52 reported CRNA faculty vacancies nationally at the time these data were collected (Merwin et al., 2007). High reliance on volunteer faculty makes some nurse anesthesia programs depend on goodwill and reciprocal benefits. Should the economic or political climate change, hospitals may be less willing in the future to support clinical faculty participation in the education of nurse anesthesia students (e.g., providing release time from clinical responsibilities) (Merwin et al., 2007). The profession will continue to address faculty workforce issues proactively, because faculty resources are essential to maintain the needed number of graduates for the anesthesia workforce. Websites such as *www.gaswork.com* feature clinical CRNA employment opportunities. At the time of this writing, 2426 CRNA positions were posted on this website (GasWork.com, 2008). Given the existing vacancy rate and projected retirements, a high demand for nurse anesthetists should continue.

External funding, such as federal traineeships, has helped to offset expenses for nurse anesthesia students and to meet CRNA workforce needs. The AANA closely monitors each proposed federal budget for potential changes in Title VIII funding. In testimony before the House Appropriations Subcommittee in 2005, Louise Hershkowitz, CRNA, MSHA, requested $210,000,000 for fiscal-year 2006 to effect nursing shortage relief through Title VIII. The goal of this testimony was to secure $3,000,000 for nurse anesthesia education, $85,000,000 for advanced practice nursing education, and $210,000,000 for nursing education (Oklahoma Association of Nurse Anesthetists [OANA], 2005). In 2007, significant cuts to Title VIII funding were proposed by the Bush administration.

Regarding the anesthesia workforce needs in academic medical centers, a 2006 survey of 128 academic anesthesiology departments yielded a 73% response rate. These research findings demonstrate the integral role CRNAs play in academic settings, along with significant CRNA vacancy rates in these settings. Significant reported findings from this study are as follows:

- The average department employed 45 faculty members, and 81% of those departments had an average of 3.3 open positions.
- 91% of the departments employed CRNAs, with an average of 25 CRNAs per department. Of those departments, 73% had an average of 4.2 open CRNA positions.
- The average department received $3,787,835 or $97,621 per CRNA faculty in institutional support. This was an increase over the 2003 amount of $85,607 per CRNA faculty. In 36.6% of departments, a portion of these support dollars ($1,888,111) was provided to support CRNA salaries.

The investigators concluded that an ongoing shortage of anesthesiology faculty existed and that continued institutional support was needed to keep anesthesiology residency programs viable (Tremper, Shanks, & Morris, 2006).

The continued high demand for nurse anesthetists in clinical and academic settings is not expected to change. The safety, cost-effectiveness, and high quality of nurse anesthesia care coupled with the advocacy provided by members through the AANA keep nurse anesthesia at the forefront of the health care workforce.

CERTIFIED REGISTERED NURSE ANESTHETIST SETTINGS FOR PRACTICE

CRNAs provide services in conjunction with other health care professionals such as surgeons, dentists, podiatrists, and anesthesiologists in diverse clinical settings. Nurse anesthetists provide anesthesia services on a solo basis, in groups, and collaboratively. Some CRNAs have independent contracting arrangements with physicians or hospitals (AANA, 2007d).

Today, most surgery is performed on an ambulatory basis, a paradigm shift related to the vigorous efforts to decrease average length of hospital stay over the past 25 years. In 1980, outpatient surgery made up 16% of all surgeries performed. By 2002, outpatient surgeries accounted for 63% of all surgeries performed in hospitals nationally (Agency for Healthcare Research and Quality [AHRQ], 2003), with many additional surgeries performed on a same-day admissions basis. Anesthesia practices have adjusted to accommodate this change in delivery of surgical services. Multiple mechanisms, ranging from preoperative telephone interviews to preanesthesia clinics, are used to conduct preanesthesia assessment and to allow anesthesia providers a venue to discuss care options, procedures, and risks with patients. However, detailed physical assessment and establishing rapport between the anesthesia provider and patient often still occur on the day of surgery.

Anesthesia services can facilitate diagnosis, as in the case of the "curare test" for myasthenia gravis. Anesthesia as a therapeutic modality is seen in the treatment of acute and chronic pain; it is also used in psychiatry for conducting interviews under the influence of ultra-short-acting intravenous barbiturates, and for accelerated detoxification of opioid-dependent patients. However, the most common use of anesthesia resources is for the administration of surgical anesthesia. Anesthesia services are frequently used in obstetrics, for providing analgesia and anesthesia to women in labor. Regional anesthesia and applied pharmacology have greatly advanced obstetrical anesthesia, which in the past relied on systemic drugs that could cause neonatal depression. Epidural analgesia has become increasingly common for vaginal and cesarean section delivery, often obviating the need for general anesthesia and its attendant risks. In addition to using regional anesthesia in obstetrical and postpartum settings, CRNAs have long worked collaboratively with other clinicians in these areas to manage intrapartum and postpartum pain with a variety of pharmacological and nonpharmacological modalities (Faut-Callahan & Paice, 1990).

Access to Care

Access to health care remains an ongoing concern across the country with geographical maldistribution being a major factor. U.S. manpower trends in anesthesia have been studied (Kaye, Scibetta, & Grogono, 1999). The authors suggest that because of changes in graduate medical education (GME) funding, fewer physicians are pursuing anesthesia residencies. An increased need for nurse anesthetists in academic medical centers (Miller, Rampil, & Cohen, 1999) and community and rural hospitals in the United States has been noted (Fallacaro, 1998). Some argue that inefficiencies in the allocation of labor in United States anesthesia departments have lead to serious concerns. Nurse anesthetists are acknowledged by physician health care policy analysts to make significant contributions to health care in rural and medically underserved areas, within and beyond the United States (Cromwell & Rosenbach, 1988). The optimal use of nurse anesthetists and physician anesthesiologists may garner a 1% reduction in commercial health costs (Klein, 1997).

CRNAs provide 27 million anesthetics annually in the United States. In some rural settings, 100% of the anesthesia, trauma stabilization, and obstetric anesthesia services are provided by nurse anesthetists. Without the services of CRNAs in rural and underserved communities, many small hospitals would close, leaving few alternatives for health care. Some rural CRNAs have completed additional training in the management of acute and chronic pain and offer services such as pain clinics so that patients do not have to travel to distant centers for pain treatment. Academic medical centers and government-operated facilities heavily rely on nurse anesthetists. Many CRNAs practice in the Veterans Administration hospital system, dealing with high acuity patients undergoing complex surgical procedures. The military relies heavily on and actively recruits nurse anesthetists. A CRNA may be the only anesthesia provider on a Navy vessel. This essential access to anesthesia care for military men and women is part of nurse anesthesia history, dating back to the American Civil War. In such a situation, knowledge of regional anesthesia and the ability to practice autonomously enable the CRNA to capably respond to mass casualty situations in which many trauma victims simultaneously require anesthesia.

A recent study described the correlation between anesthesia providers by type (e.g., CRNA or anesthesiologist) and their respective rural or urban practice settings across America. Analyses were based on county-level data contained in several distinct databases with the assumption that most providers practice and reside in the same rural or urban designation category. Research findings demonstrated that 91.6% of active, practicing anesthesiologists resided in metropolitan counties and that 8.4% lived in non-metropolitan counties. Regarding CRNAs, 81.4% resided in metropolitan counties versus 18.6% in non-metropolitan counties. Overall analyses showed that out of 3140 counties, there were 843 counties in which neither anesthesiologists nor CRNAs resided. Of these counties, 97% are non-metropolitan (Fallacaro & Ruiz-Law, 2004). It is clear that a higher proportion of nurse anesthetists reside in non-metropolitan counties, and these providers are responsible for delivering the majority of anesthesia care in these population centers, providing key access for patients.

CRNAs continue to provide essential health care access to citizens in rural and medically underserved areas. The increasing number of surgical and diagnostic services across practice settings requires safe, cost-effective CRNA providers to ensure that access to appropriate health care services for all citizens is maintained.

International Practice Opportunities

The International Federation of Nurse Anesthetists (IFNA) was founded in 1989 by 11 countries in which nurse anesthetists were educated and practiced. IFNA now has 34 member countries. The IFNA mission (IFNA, 2007)

> …is dedicated to the precept that its members are committed to the advancement of educational standards and practices which will advance the art and science of anesthesiology and thereby support and enhance quality anesthesia care worldwide. The IFNA establishes and maintains effective cooperation with institutions that have a professional interest in nurse anesthesia. [The IFNA vision is to be] …the authoritative voice for nurse anesthetists and nurse anesthesia, supporting and enhancing quality anesthesia care worldwide… [IFNA seeks to] … serve as the authoritative voice of nurse anesthesia internationally; to provide a means of communication among nurse anesthetists throughout the world; to promote the independence of the nurse anesthetist as a professional specialist in nursing.

IFNA describes these organizational objectives (IFNA, 2007):

> To promote cooperation between nurse anesthetists internationally
>
> To develop and promote educational standards in the field of nurse anesthesia
>
> To develop and promote standards of practice in the field of nurse anesthesia
>
> To provide opportunities for continuing education in anesthesia
>
> To assist nurse anesthesia associations to improve the standards of nurse anesthesia and the competence of nurse anesthetists
>
> To promote the recognition of nurse anesthesia
>
> To establish and maintain effective cooperation between nurse anesthetists, anesthesiologists and other members of the medical profession, the nursing profession, hospitals and agencies representing a community of interest in nurse anesthesia

IFNA member countries include 19 European countries, 9 African countries, and 4 Asian countries. Since its inception in 1989, IFNA has developed Standards of Education, Standards of Practice, and a Code of Ethics for Nurse Anesthetists. Model international nurse anesthesia curricula have been developed. IFNA was initially recognized as a Professional Resource Group by the International Council of Nurses (ICN). Currently, IFNA is an affiliate member of the ICN. Research findings have shown that nurse anesthetists participate in 80% of the anesthetics administered worldwide and are sole providers in 60% of the anesthetics (Henry & McAuliffe, 1999).

CERTIFIED REGISTERED NURSE ANESTHETIST ROLE DEVELOPMENT AND MEASURES OF CLINICAL COMPETENCE

Nurse Anesthesia as a Subculture of Advanced Practice Nursing

Horton (1998) conducted a comprehensive study of the views of CRNAs to determine implicit and explicit ideas about the culture of nurse anesthetists. Dominant rules of behavior were identified (Box 17-1).

Foundational to nurse anesthesia practice, CRNAs identified two major domains of professional activity: (1) to remain active and vigilant in defending and

Box 17-1   DOMINANT RULES OF BEHAVIOR OF NURSE ANESTHETISTS IN THE UNITED STATES

- Able to control and manage stressful clinical situations
- Able to make independent judgments quickly
- Accepts a high degree of responsibility
- Belongs to a professional organization (AANA)
- Committed to life-long learning of scientific facts
- Demonstrates self-confidence
- Effective in using assertiveness to facilitate role as patient advocate
- Engages in political activities

- Enjoys short-term patient care
- Functions effectively and calmly in life and death situations
- Ability to be organized with meticulous attention to detail
- Possesses intelligence and current knowledge
- Technically skilled, efficient, and clinically competent
- Upholds patient care values
- Willing to work hard and dedicate long hours to the job

Horton, B. (1998). Nurse anesthesia as a subculture of nursing in the United States. Doctoral dissertation, Rush University. *Dissertation Abstracts International, 9912475.*
AANA, American Association of Nurse Anesthetists.

maintaining practice rights, and (2) to demonstrate dedication to patient care. Inherent to their dedication to patient care, CRNAs note the following as key elements of protective patient care: individualized care, technology, touch, surveillance, vigilance, and honesty. Horton (1998) found that CRNA dominant values include autonomy, education, continuing education, achievement, group cohesiveness, identity as a CRNA, membership in the AANA, political activism, and technology.

The role of the nurse anesthetist encompasses many facets. Callahan (1994) described a competency-based model for nurse anesthesia practice that demonstrated areas in which nurse anesthetists must strive to achieve competence (Figure 17-4). The unifying themes of caring, collaboration, communication, and technology are defined in Box 17-2. Many of the characteristics of advanced practice nursing described in Chapter 3 are found in this model. Although the model is in its infancy and further research with its use is in progress, it depicts the many facets of the CRNA role. Munguia-Biddle, Maree, Klein, Callahan, and Gilles (1990) defined components of the model and suggested that the nurse anesthesia process is a problem-solving model that utilizes assessment, analysis, planning, implementation, and evaluation in the complex decision making and actions that exemplify CRNA practice within the health care environment. They further define lifelong learning as a part of the nurse anesthesia process. This essential process function is in concert with the changing characteristics of nurse anesthesia practice.

Additional clarification of the components of the model is found in Box 17-3. The nurse anesthesia process parallels the nursing process and emphasizes the importance of this approach to comprehensive anesthesia care following the model and its components; CRNA practice is based on the advanced practice nurse (APN) competencies found in Chapter 3. Some of these competencies are discussed here and in the three exemplars that describe CRNA practice.

Direct Patient Care

CRNAs select, obtain, or administer the anesthetics, adjuvant drugs, accessory drugs, and fluids necessary to manage the anesthesia, to maintain physiological homeostasis, and to correct abnormal responses to anesthesia or surgery (AANA, 2002b). When CRNAs perform these activities, they are recognized legally to be providing anesthesia services on request, not to be prescribing as defined by federal law. With the advent of legislated prescriptive authority for CRNAs and other APNs, these providers can prescribe legend and in some cases Schedules II through V controlled substances. However this authority varies from state to state and is an ongoing tension between medicine and APN nursing.

Monitoring is another vital area in which CRNAs participate. Nurse anesthetists select, apply, and insert appropriate noninvasive and invasive monitoring modalities for collecting and interpreting physiological data. These activities are all recognized components of anesthesia services performed on request by CRNAs and are not prescriptive. Criteria for the use of invasive monitors and who places them vary by institution and geographical region. At times, professional fees associated with the placement of devices such as pulmonary artery catheters leads to conflict

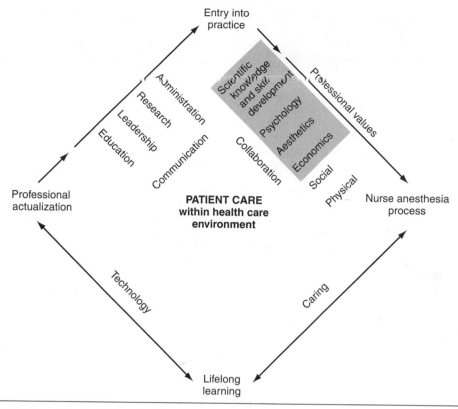

FIGURE **17-4:** **Nurse Anesthesia Practice Model.** (From Munguia-Biddle, F., Maree, S., Klein, E., Callahan, L., & Gilles, B. [1990]. *Nurse anesthesiology competence evaluation: Mechanism for accountability.* Unpublished document, American Association of Nurse Anesthetists, Park Ridge, IL.)

Box 17-2   Nurse Anesthesia Practice Model

The advanced practice of nursing in the specialty of nurse anesthesia has special attributes that speak to the strength and uniqueness of the CRNA role in the provision of anesthesia care in the health environment.

Caring for the patient as a holistic being is an important tenet of CRNA professional behavior. CRNAs strive to be altruistic human beings, believing that caring is essential to one's personal development.

Collaboration between the nurse anesthetist and other members of the health care team takes place in separate and joined activities and responsibilities that are directed at attaining mutual goals of excellence in patient care.

Communication is sharing information to achieve mutual understanding. Communication skills are a cornerstone of patient interviews, imparting information to other health professionals, documentation of practice, and participation as a contributory member in meeting society's health needs.

Technology denotes an area rich in technological advances and scientific content that requires strengthening and updating through the professional life. Practitioners have the ability to apply the nursing process to complex problems at a high level of competence.

From Munguia-Biddle, F., Maree, S., Klein, E., Callahan, L., & Gilles, B. (1990). *Nurse anesthesiology competence evaluation: Mechanism for accountability.* Unpublished document, American Association of Nurse Anesthetists, Park Ridge, IL.
CRNA, Certified registered nurse anesthetist.

Box 17-3 DEFINITION OF NURSE ANESTHESIA PRACTICE MODEL COMPONENTS

PROFESSIONAL ACTUALIZATION

Professional actualization is a dynamic, ongoing endeavor to realize maximum development of professional potential.

- **Education** provides an environment that allows for exploration and application of strategies to facilitate the preparation of future practitioners, thereby assuring continuance.
- **Leadership** demonstrates the ability to define reality, set goals, communicate a vision, and influence the willing participation of others in purposeful action that is directed to goal achievement.
- **Research** encourages active involvement in scientific inquiry as a consumer, participant, or contributor. It is the driving force of actualization that validates our role in the provision of anesthesia services, enhances growth for the nurse anesthetist and the profession, and leads to new knowledge and improved safety in patient care.
- **Administration** provides the interface between people, groups, departments, organizations, professions, and society that enhances individual and collective professional growth.

PROFESSIONAL VALUES

A **profession** may be defined in terms of the domains of human endeavor valued by the members of the profession. Such are the following domains within the profession of nurse anesthesia practice.

- **Intellectual.** Integral concepts within this domain are based on advanced knowledge in the fields of anatomy, physiology, pathophysiology, technology, and pharmacology as applied to anesthetic practice. The continued development of technical expertise and competence in practice are inherent in this area of concern.
- **Psychological.** The professional nurse anesthetist is concerned with enhancement of the patient's coping skills in a time of possible

physical and emotional disruption produced by the perioperative experience. Recognition of the needs of the practitioner are expressed as concern with issues such as communication, autonomy, counseling, and impairment or incompetence practice within the workplace and the profession as a whole.

- **Aesthetics.** Spiritual growth and religious preferences are recognized and respected as inherent to full development of human potential within the patient and the nurse anesthetist. Ethical development and involvement within the political realm encompassing the nurse anesthetist as a member of society are held to be continual and necessary growth processes.
- **Economics.** CRNAs place great value on the historical role of the nurse anesthesia profession in providing continuity of anesthesia care that supports an economically viable health care industry. The exploration of strategies leading to resolution of liability issues as well as mechanisms to increase feelings of potential job security are recognized as valuable to continued professional and personal growth and well-being.
- **Social.** Valued concepts within this domain include enhancement and preservation of the professional role of nurse anesthetists in the societal health care delivery system, legal and legislative responsibility for competent patient care, constant development of improved standards of care, patient education, and continued liaison with other health care providers.
- **Physical.** Patient safety and the interface between technology and humankind or machines and the patient are of paramount concern. The appropriateness of physical work that considers the impact of schedules, stress, fatigue, and vigilance must be demonstrated in the clinical setting as important factors in securing the patient care environment.

From Munguia-Biddle, F., Maree, S., Klein, E., Callahan, L., & Gilles, B. (1990). *Nurse anesthesiology competence evaluation: Mechanism for accountability.* Unpublished document, American Association of Nurse Anesthetists, Park Ridge, IL.
CRNA, Certified registered nurse anesthetist.

over which practitioner (e.g., anesthetist or surgeon) will place invasive monitors and receive the associated reimbursement.

Nurse anesthesia practice also includes airway management using endotracheal intubation, mechanical ventilation, and pharmacological support both within

and outside the operating room. In some settings, CRNAs are the sole providers of this service. A combination of technical skills required for airway management using a variety of instruments and knowledge of respiratory anatomy and physiology and pharmacology is important. For example, clinicians continue to

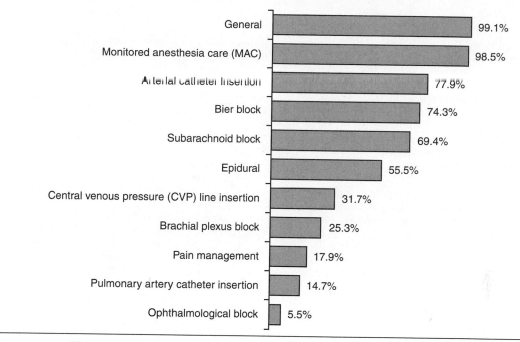

FIGURE 17-5: Techniques performed by CRNAs in clinical practice (Rivera, 2006).

develop efficacious approaches to sedation and analgesia for ventilator-dependent patients. Opportunities exist for collaborative research in this area (Weinert & Calvin, 2007). CRNAs need to remind clinicians caring for ventilator-dependent patients that sedative/amnesic drugs and analgesics need to be included when critically ill patients are mechanically ventilated. As well, the role of the CRNA in helping patients and families understand these procedures is important (Figure 17-5).

Nurse anesthetists manage emergence and recovery from anesthesia by selecting, obtaining, ordering, or administering medications, fluids, or ventilatory support to maintain homeostasis, to provide relief from pain and anesthesia side effects, and/or to prevent or manage complications (AANA, 2002b). These activities also fall within the scope of providing anesthesia services and are not prescriptive in the traditional sense (e.g., where a CRNA would write a prescription that a pharmacist would fill). The CRNA can release or discharge patients from a postanesthesia care area. Providing postanesthesia follow-up evaluation and care related to anesthetic side effects or complications is another CRNA function.

Regional anesthesia is used by many CRNAs in the management of surgical anesthesia, labor pain, and postoperative pain. CRNAs are increasingly involved with pain management services. The use of epidural analgesic infusions and patient-controlled analgesia has greatly contributed to the effective treatment of preventable pain. Nurse anesthetists should have a role in the formulation of protocols and staff education when acute pain protocols are introduced.

Nurse anesthetists respond to emergency situations by providing airway management skills and by implementing basic and advanced life support techniques. CRNAs can provide leadership in these settings, away from the operating room, reinforcing the need for nationally promulgated standards of anesthesia care. One of these standards of care, for example is the measurement of end-tidal carbon dioxide to rule out esophageal intubation (AANA, 2002a). Nurse anesthetists are bound by the standards of practice adopted by the profession as shown in Box 17-4.

Collaboration

As with other advanced practice nursing roles, nurse anesthesia practice is based in a collaborative model. Collaboration, one of the seven APN competencies described in Chapter 3, is defined as a dynamic process

Box 17-4   STANDARDS FOR NURSE ANESTHESIA PRACTICE

INTRODUCTION

These standards are intended to:

- Assist the profession in evaluating the quality of care provided by its practitioners.
- Provide a common base for practitioners to use in their development of a quality practice.
- Assist the public in understanding what to expect from the practitioner.
- Support and preserve the basic rights of the patient.

These standards apply to all anesthetizing locations. While the standards are intended to encourage high quality patient care, they cannot assure specific outcomes.

STANDARD I

Perform a thorough and complete preanesthesia assessment.

Interpretation: The responsibility for the care of the patient begins with the preanesthetic assessment. Except in emergency situations, the CRNA has an obligation to complete a thorough evaluation and determine that relevant tests have been obtained and reviewed.

STANDARD II

Obtain informed consent for the planned anesthetic intervention from the patient or legal guardian.

Interpretation: The CRNA shall obtain or verify that an informed consent has been obtained by a qualified provider. Discuss anesthetic options and risks with the patient and/or legal guardian in language the patient and/or legal guardian can understand. Document in the patient's medical record that informed consent was obtained.

STANDARD III

Formulate a patient-specific plan for anesthesia care.

Interpretation: The plan of care developed by the CRNA is based upon comprehensive patient assessment, problem analysis, anticipated surgical or therapeutic procedure, patient and surgeon preferences, and current anesthesia principles.

STANDARD IV

Implement and adjust the anesthesia care plan based on the patient's physiological response.

Interpretation: The CRNA shall induce and maintain anesthesia at required levels. The CRNA shall continuously assess the patient's response to the anesthetic and/or surgical intervention and intervene as required to maintain the patient in a satisfactory physiologic condition.

STANDARD V

Monitor the patient's physiologic condition as appropriate for the type of anesthesia and specific patient needs.

- **Monitor ventilation continuously.** Verify intubation of the trachea by auscultation, chest excursion, and confirmation of carbon dioxide in the expired gas. Continuously monitor end-tidal carbon dioxide during controlled or assisted ventilation. Use spirometry and ventilatory pressure monitors.
- **Monitor oxygenation continuously** by clinical observation, pulse oximetry, and if indicated, arterial blood gas analysis.
- **Monitor cardiovascular status continuously** via electrocardiogram and heart sounds. Record blood pressure and heart rate at least every 5 minutes.
- **Monitor body temperature continuously** on all pediatric patients receiving general anesthesia and when indicated on all other patients.
- **Monitor neuromuscular function and status** when neuromuscular blocking agents are administered.
- **Monitor and assess the patient's positioning** and protective measures.

Interpretation: Continuous clinical observation and vigilance are the basis of safe anesthesia care. The standard applies to all patients receiving anesthesia care and may be exceeded at any time at the discretion of the CRNA. Unless otherwise stipulated in the standards, a means to monitor and evaluate the patient's status shall be immediately available for all patients. As new patient safety technologies evolve, integration into the current anesthesia practice shall be considered. The omission of any monitoring standards shall be documented and the reason stated on the patient's anesthesia record. The CRNA shall be in constant attendance of the patient until the responsibility for care has been accepted by another qualified health care provider.

From the American Association of Nurse Anesthetists. (2002). *Scope and standards for nurse anesthesia practice.* Park Ridge, IL: Author.
CRNA, Certified registered nurse anesthetist.

Box 17-4   Standards for Nurse Anesthesia Practice—cont'd

STANDARD VI
There shall be complete, accurate, and timely documentation of pertinent information on the patient's medical record.
Interpretation: Document all anesthetic interventions and patient responses. Accurate documentation facilitates comprehensive patient care, provides information for retrospective review and research data, and establishes a medical-legal record.

STANDARD VII
Transfer the responsibility for care of the patient to other qualified providers in a manner which assures continuity of care and patient safety.
Interpretation: The CRNA shall assess the patient's status and determine when it is safe to transfer the responsibility of care to other qualified providers. The CRNA shall accurately report the patient's condition and all essential information to the provider assuming responsibility for the patient.

STANDARD VIII
Adhere to appropriate safety precautions, as established within the institution, to minimize the risks of fire, explosion, electrical shock, and equipment malfunction. Document on the patient's medical record that the anesthesia machine and equipment were checked.
Interpretation: Prior to use, the CRNA shall inspect the anesthesia machine and monitors according to established guidelines. The CRNA shall check the readiness, availability, cleanliness, and working condition of all equipment to be utilized in the administration of the anesthesia care. When the patient is ventilated by an automatic mechanical ventilator, monitor the integrity of the breathing system with a device capable of detecting a disconnection by emitting an audible alarm. Monitor oxygen concentration continuously with an oxygen supply failure alarm system.

STANDARD IX
Precautions shall be taken to minimize the risk of infection to the patient, the CRNA, and other health care providers.
Interpretation: Written policies and procedures in infection control shall be developed for personnel and equipment.

STANDARD X
Anesthesia care shall be assessed to assure its quality and contribution to positive patient outcomes.
Interpretation: The CRNA shall participate in the ongoing review and evaluation of the quality and appropriateness of anesthesia care. Evaluation shall be performed based upon appropriate outcome criteria and reviewed on an ongoing basis. The CRNA shall participate in a continual process of self evaluation and strive to incorporate new techniques and knowledge into practice.

STANDARD XI
The CRNA shall respect and maintain the basic rights of patients.
Interpretation: The CRNA shall support and preserve the rights of patients to personal dignity and ethical norms of practice.

---

in which individuals interact with the genuine intent to inform each other and problem solve to achieve outcomes (Hanson & Spross, 2005). Partnerships are formed to provide the best care to patients (Hanson and Spross, 2005; Kyle, 1995) (see Chapter 10). Baggs (1994) identified six critical elements in physician-nurse collaborative practice: cooperation, assertiveness, shared decision making, communication, planning together, and coordination. Research on the impact of collaborative care has consistently found an association between care and improved patient outcomes and enhanced quality of care (Kyle, 1995).

Nurse anesthetists first formed collaborative relationships with surgeons dating back to the late nineteenth century. At the request of surgeons, nurses were called upon to administer anesthesia because of high surgical mortality. Today, approximately 80% of nurse anesthetists collaborate with physician/consultant anesthesiologists in daily practice. No statutory requirements exist for the supervision of nurse anesthetists by attending anesthesiologists. Therefore CRNAs also legally collaborate with surgeons, podiatrists, and dentists. Surgeons who collaborate with CRNAs have no increased legal liability, since CRNAs are responsible for their own actions (Blumenreich, 2007).

Howie (2007) described an effective use of collaboration in a unique CRNA-surgeon team providing care in the field. General anesthesia and sedation are sometimes required in environments that are uncommon. The nurse anesthetist and surgeon provided definitive operative services to patients injured in the field. This occurred when the patient could not be transported to a medical facility. CRNAs collaborate with other physicians by sharing their assessment and plan of care for anesthesia. At the same time, collaboration occurs with the patient so a mutually agreeable anesthetic plan can be developed; procedures, risks, and benefits associated with the anesthetic are discussed. Nurse anesthesia services are always provided in collaboration with the operating physician, dentist, podiatrist, or consultant anesthesiologist, and this has proved to be a beneficial collaborative practice model.

Evidence-Based Practice and Leadership

Research is a core APN competency that is valued by CRNAs. CRNAs have long advocated the use of evidence in their daily practice but have not accumulated a large body of research-based literature to date. The AANA publishes evidence-based position statements that address practice issues (Box 17-5). Further, CRNAs are the authors of seminal texts that provide the foundation for practice (Foster & Faut-Callahan, 2001; Naglehout & Zaglaczyncy, 2005). The *AANA Journal* routinely publishes evidence-based continuing education courses on key topics of importance to the overall mission to promote patient safety. Most important are the contributions that CRNAs make to the literature through case study and research publications. Emphasis on continued competency, patient safety, and the development of scholarship is consistent with the values described by Horton (1998).

The influx of CRNAs with graduate degrees into the profession, combined with expectations of consumers, legislators, and regulators, provides opportunities to objectively assess clinical practices in terms of safety and economy. In this era of rapidly shifting resources and changing models of care, CRNAs must demonstrate quality and cost-effective patient care. Historically, quality of anesthesia care has been studied measuring variables such as mortality, morbidity, length of stay, readmission, and cost. Methods have not been readily available to define quality in terms of the effect of care delivery on the health of patients. Combined administrative and health-related databases are essential, albeit limited, in elucidating the outcomes associated with nurse anesthesia practice. Development of methodologically sound research will require the preparation of more scholars in the specialty who have expertise in research design and measurement (Kremer & Faut-Callahan, 2000). Some recent publications describe trends in nurse anesthesia research.

Box 17-5   SELECTED AANA EVIDENCE-BASED PRACTICE POSITION PAPERS

- Certified Registered Nurse Anesthetists' Utilization of Invasive Monitoring Techniques
- Considerations for Policy Guidelines for Registered Nurses Engaged in the Administration of Sedation and Analgesia
- Guidelines for the Management of the Obstetrical Patient for the Certified Registered Nurse Anesthetist
- Infection Control Guide
- Informed Consent
- Informed Consent Form (English and Spanish version)
- AANA-ASA Joint Statement Regarding Propofol Administration
- AANA Latex Protocol
- Needle & Syringe Reuse = Infection Risk
- Patient Safety and CRNAs on Drug Therapy Regimens for Pain Management
- Postanesthesia Care Standards for the CRNA

- Quality of Care in Anesthesia
- Standards for Office-Based Anesthesia Practice
- Minimum Elements for Providing Anesthesia Services
- Anesthesia Equipment & Supplies Checklist
- Preparedness for Treatment of Malignant Hyperthermia
- Pain Management
- Unintended Awareness Under General Anesthesia
- Qualified Providers of Sedation and Analgesia
- The Separation of Operator/Anesthesia Provider Responsibilities
- Provision of Pain Relief by Medication Administered via Continuous Epidural, Intrathecal, Intrapleural, Peripheral Nerve Catheters, or Other Pain Relief Devices
- Removal of Epidural Catheters

AANA, American Association of Nurse Anesthetists; *ASA*, American Society of Anesthetists; *CRNA*, certified registered nurse anesthetist.

One study compared research reported in the *AANA Journal* in 1995-1996 (n = 38 studies); 1985-1986 (n = 18); and 1975-1976 (n = 14). The amount of research published in the *AANA Journal* has increased steadily, with a stable focus on clinical practice. In addition, an increase in educational and safety-related research has been reported. Another 28 articles authored by CRNAs were found in other medical and nursing journals for the 1995-1996 period (Connelly, Schretenthaler, & Taunton, 2002).

By the 1990s, all studies contained at least one indicator of theoretical orientation. Convenience samples of hospitalized patients were the most frequently represented sampling technique. Reporting on reliability and validity of data and the psychometric evaluation of research tools was minimal. The authors recommended increased emphasis on methodological studies, multisite studies, programs of research, collaboration among CRNAs, nurses in other specialties, and practitioners from other disciplines (Connelly et al., 2002).

Kremer and Blair (2006) described the rare condition of Ludwig angina. This is a critical disease because loss of airway control can result in catastrophic events. The authors found that clinicians must be aware of the etiology of this rare disease because of the imperative that this condition be rapidly recognized and treatment options implemented immediately to diminish risk to the patient.

Simonson and colleagues (2007) demonstrated that no differences exist when anesthesia for cesarean section is administered by a CRNA and by an anesthesiologist. Using data from the Comprehensive Abstract and Reporting database, they studied 134,806 patients and found care delivered by CRNAs alone and anesthesiologists alone was comparable. Some of the other interesting findings were that (1) in CRNA-staffed hospitals, more Medicaid patients were treated; (2) teaching and rural hospitals were in a greater proportion; and (3) very young patients (younger than 17 years) were cared for. The anesthesiologists-only hospitals had more emergency admissions and cared for more older mothers (older than 35 years). Simonson and colleagues (2007) noted, "The study results clearly demonstrate that OB anesthesia complications are not different between the CRNA-only and anesthesiologist-only staffing models" (p. 6).

Forrester, Benfield, Matern, Kelly, and Pellegrini (2007) demonstrated that the use of meclizine in combination with standard drug therapies improved the management of postoperative nausea and vomiting (PONV) in high-risk patients. Subjects (n = 77) were randomized and screened using a PONV risk assessment. The use of prophylactic meclizine lowered PONV. The results of this study provide evidence to support practice changes with the intended result being to increase patient comfort and satisfaction and reduce health care costs.

These papers demonstrate CRNA-authored research with tangible practice implications. These are valuable additions to the anesthesia literature and contain useful, data-based practice recommendations. Websites that are useful to CRNA practice are found in Box 17-6.

With the challenges described, the future of nurse anesthesia is promising. More CRNAs hold graduate degrees, and there is potential for additional CRNA-conducted basic and applied research. Additional graduate education in nursing, the basic sciences, and business will better enable CRNAs to collaborate with other investigators in the arenas of clinical and bench research; practice, legislation, and policy formulation will also be enhanced by this additional educational preparation. A greater nurse anesthesia voice in policy formulation has already been felt, with CRNA members securing places on state boards of nursing and other governmental positions.

The tradition of strong leadership meeting challenges directly continues. Former AANA Executive Director John Garde, CRNA, MS, FAAN, asserts (Garde, 1998):

> The profession has an optimistic future. I point out with pride the commitment that AANA members have toward [the future of their profession]—a commitment that encompasses being outstanding anesthesia practitioners who belong to their Association. I am reminded, too, what each of you brings every day to your patients. Dick Davidson, president of the American Hospital Association, said when asked about what will remain in health care 100 years from now, 'There will always be personal contact and caring. We will always have hands touching patients. Everything we do is about human need. That's the constant over time.' And, that is the legacy of the nurse anesthesia profession. (p. 15)

Accountability and Ethics

CRNAs are legally liable for the quality of the services they render (Blumenreich, 2007). They make independent judgments and decisions as to the appropriateness of their professional services and the probable effects of those services on the patient. A CRNA who believes that the anesthesia care plan for a particular

Box 17-6   POPULAR ANESTHESIA WEBSITES

American Association of Nurse Anesthetists	www.aana.com
Anesthesiology—The Journal of the American Society of Anesthesiologists, Inc.	www.anesthesiology.org
Anesthesia & Analgesia	www.anesthesia-analgesia.org
Anesthesia & Intensive Care	www.aaic.net.au/home.html
Anesthesia Online	www.priory.co.uk/anes.html
Internet Journal of Anesthesiology	www.ispub.com/journals/ija.htm
Journal of Clinical Anesthesia	www.sciencedirect.com/science/journal/ 09528180
Journal of Cardiothoracic and Vascular Anesthesia	www.jcardioanesthesia.com
Pain (the journal of the International Association for the Study of Pain)	www.sciencedirect.com/pain
Survey of Anesthesiology	www.gasnet.mail.yale.edu/periodicals/sa
International Trauma Anesthesia and Critical Care Society	www.trauma.itaccs.com/news.html
GASNets—anesthesiology discussion list archives	www.gasnet.med.yale.edu/

patient is inappropriate should seek consultation for more appropriate direction. CRNAs should be patient advocates and always seek resolution to these and other ethical issues. If reasonable doubt continues, it is the responsibility of the CRNA to consider withdrawal from rendering the service, provided that the well-being of the patient is not jeopardized. Expected professional responsibilities of the APN ethics competency for the CRNA are explicitly stated in the "Code of Ethics for the Certified Registered Nurse Anesthetist" (Box 17-7).

EXEMPLARS

Exemplars 17-1, 17-2, and 17-3 explain how CRNAs use the APN competencies to enact their APN role. The direct care competency is central to CRNA practice, and the exemplars show the importance of the other six supporting competencies for successful implementation of the CRNA APN role.

Many of the observations in Chapter 16 about the role of the certified nurse-midwife (CNM) pertain to the CRNAs depicted in these exemplars. Many rewards are associated with their practice, but there are also challenges. Surgical or anesthetic morbidity and mortality understandably result in close internal and some external scrutiny. CRNAs must be able to defend their actions in terms of congruence with standards of care and existing hospital policies. Vacation coverage can be difficult to find and expensive, given the current undersupply of CRNAs. As with CNMs, CRNAs find that

complying with regulations (e.g., Medicare/Medicaid) and other health policy legislation can be challenging. Fortunately, state and national professional associations are available for consultation on these issues. Like CNMs, CRNAs deal with "misperceptions of our practice from within the larger health-care system" (Dorroh & Norton, 1996, p. 214). The ongoing challenges for CRNAs and other APNs are to have effective public relations and government relations strategies in place to minimize these misperceptions.

J.R. (Exemplar 17-1), F.M. (Exemplar 17-2), and D.S. and P.R. (Exemplar 17-3) demonstrate qualities shared by many of their professional predecessors. They are practice-setting leaders, teachers, and risk-takers. Their willingness to push conventional practice limits ultimately advances the profession. These exemplars exemplify the implementation of all of the APN competencies described in Chapter 3 and Part II.

NURSE ANESTHESIA EDUCATION

Nurse anesthesia education occurs in diverse settings. Diversity is demonstrated by the many academic units that house nurse anesthesia educational programs such as nursing, allied health sciences, and medicine. However, the relative value of this diversity has never been quantified in terms of an academic power base or educational credibility. This diversity exists because the nurse anesthesia educational community values various undergraduate degrees for entrance into nurse anesthesia programs and because of the initial difficulty nurse

PREAMBLE

Certified Registered Nurse Anesthetists practice nursing by providing anesthesia and anesthesia related services. They accept the responsibility conferred upon them by the state, the profession, and society. The American Association of Nurse Anesthetists has adopted this Code of Ethics to guide its members in fulfilling their obligation as professionals. Each member of the American Association of Nurse Anesthetists has a personal responsibility to uphold and adhere to these ethical standards.

1. RESPONSIBILITY TO PATIENTS

Certified Registered Nurse Anesthetists (CRNAs) preserve human dignity, respect the moral and legal rights of health consumers, and support the safety and well being of the patient under their care.

1.1 The CRNA renders quality anesthesia care regardless of the patient's race, religion, age, sex, nationality, disability, social or economic status.

1.2 The CRNA protects the patient from harm and is an advocate for the patient's welfare.

1.3 The CRNA verifies that a valid anesthesia informed consent has been obtained from the patient or legal guardian as required by federal or state laws or institutional policy prior to rendering a service.

1.4 The CRNA avoids conflicts between his or her personal integrity and the patient's rights. In situations where the CRNA's personal convictions prohibit participation in a particular procedure, the CRNA refuses to participate or withdraws from the case provided that such refusal or withdrawal does not harm the patient or constitute a breach of duty.

1.5 The CRNA takes appropriate action to protect patients from healthcare providers who are incompetent, impaired, or engage in illegal or unethical practice.

1.6 The CRNA maintains confidentiality of patient information except in those rare events where accepted nursing practice demands otherwise.

1.7 The CRNA does not knowingly engage in deception in any form.

1.8 The CRNA does not exploit nor abuse his or her relationship of trust and confidence with the patient or the patient's dependence on the CRNA.

2. COMPETENCE

The scope of practice engaged in by the Certified Registered Nurse Anesthetist is within the individual competence of the CRNA. Each CRNA has the responsibility to maintain competency in practice.

4. RESPONSIBILITY TO SOCIETY

4.1 Certified Registered Nurse Anesthetists work in collaboration with the healthcare community of interest to promote highly competent, safe, quality patient care.

4.2 Certified Registered Nurse Anesthetists collaborate with members of the health professions and other citizens in promoting community and national efforts to meet the health needs of the public.

5. ENDORSEMENT OF PRODUCTS AND SERVICES

Certified Registered Nurse Anesthetists endorse products and services only when personally satisfied with the products or service's safety, effectiveness and quality. CRNAs do not state that the AANA has endorsed any product or service unless the Board of Directors of the American Association of Nurse Anesthetists has done so.

5.1 Any endorsement is truthful and based on factual evidence of efficacy.

5.2 A CRNA does not exploit his or her professional title and credentials for products or services which are unrelated to his or her professional practice or expertise.

6. RESEARCH

Certified Registered Nurse Anesthetists protect the integrity of the research process and the reporting and publication of findings.

6.1 The CRNA evaluates research findings and incorporates them into practice as appropriate.

6.2 The CRNA conducts research projects according to accepted ethical research and reporting standards established by public law, institutional procedures, and the health professions.

6.3 The CRNA protects the rights and well being of people and animals that serve as subjects in research.

6.4 The CRNA participates in research activities to improve practice, education, and public policy relative to health needs of diverse populations, the health workforce, the organization and administration of health systems, and healthcare delivery.

7. BUSINESS PRACTICES

Certified Registered Nurse Anesthetists, regardless of practice arrangements or practice settings, maintain ethical business practices in dealing with patients, colleagues, institutions, and corporations.

7.1 The contractual obligations of a CRNA are consistent with the professional standards of practice and the laws and regulations pertaining to nurse anesthesia practice.

7.2 The CRNA will not participate in deceptive or fraudulent business practices.

Adapted from American Association of Nurse Anesthetists. (2008). *Code of Ethics for the Certified Registered Nurse Anesthetists.* Retrieved March 25, 2008, from www.aana.com/resources.

EXEMPLAR 17-1   The Certified Registered Nurse Anesthetist Role in Pain Management

J.R. has been a practicing CRNA for 12 years. The strongest influences in her professional development are "believing in our profession, my knowledge, skills and competencies, while seizing any and all opportunities for professional advancement that crossed my path."

Her interest in nurse anesthesia was stimulated by early exposure to the CRNA role. Her father was an otolaryngologist who practiced in a Midwestern city with a population of 60,000. At the hospital where he practiced, three anesthesiologists and a CRNA were on staff. At that time, the surgeons were allowed to post their cases to the surgery schedule and choose the anesthesia provider. J.R.'s father usually chose the CRNA to provide anesthesia care for his patients. He stated she had excellent skills and was wonderful with pediatric patients.

J.R. has practiced as a staff CRNA in a large physician-owned anesthesia group with 11 physicians and 26 CRNAs in the Midwest. She has also been a hospital-employed chief CRNA for an obstetrical anesthesia practice involving three network hospitals in another Midwestern city. Most recently, her practice has moved into the realm of interventional pain management for a neurosurgical group. Her time currently is divided between direct patient care (80%); teaching (10%); administration (5%); and professional activities (5%). J.R. acknowledges that working as an employee of a large neurosurgical group in an office-based interventional pain practice is unique. AANA member survey data show that a significant number of respondents are involved in pain management, and CRNA involvement in this specialty area has been contested by other providers.

J.R.'s current practice developed after an initial contact by another APN who was employed by the neurosurgical group. She was asked to meet with the group to discuss a practice opportunity. The group was interested in hiring a CRNA to reopen an interventional pain clinic that had been closed for over a year. J.R. was contacted because of her experience in regional anesthesia as well as her leadership activities within her state nurse anesthesia association. After she met with the physician who championed this effort, she was interested in accepting the challenge. The position "gave me an incredible opportunity for clinical growth and I strongly felt this was a perfect example of how CRNAs are beneficial in an area outside the traditional operating room setting."

A typical day in J.R.'s practice begins with a quick review of her schedule and a safety check of equipment and medications. Her day usually consists of a mixture of diagnostic and therapeutic interventional procedures such as epidural steroid injections, nerve root blocks, joint blocks, trigger point injections, and lumbar diskography.

"In our pain clinic, a patient checks in at the front desk and an escort assesses his or her vital signs, and brings them to an exam room. A nurse will interview the patient, answer questions, and obtain informed consent." During that time, J.R. "reviews the chart, imaging studies, assessment forms, and the order for treatment." She also interviews the patient before the procedure to answer questions or obtain additional information pertinent to the treatment plan before deciding on the type and targeted site of injection.

The patient is then taken to the fluoroscopic suite, where he or she is prepped and draped under sterile technique. J.R. then performs a diagnostic or therapeutic injection under fluoroscopic guidance. The patient is assessed immediately after the injection and returns to the examination room for 30 minutes. Before discharge, the patient is reassessed and information is recorded concerning the type and amount of pain relief provided by the injection. The patient is educated concerning onset and duration of the injected medications and possible complications of the medication/injection and is given discharge and follow-up information.

J.R. describes the greatest challenges in her practice as "initially...obtaining the necessary knowledge, skills, and competencies to perform the procedures requested by the group that oversees me as there was no other employment situation identical to this practice. Overall, it is dealing with the political environment as there are physicians who feel a CRNA should not be providing pain management care."

J.R.'s story demonstrates the value of professional collaboration, mentoring, networking, and organizational involvement. Her willingness to take risks and improve care elevates the profession.

AANA, American Association of Nurse Anesthetists; *APN*, advanced practice nurse; *CRNA*, certified registered nurse anesthetist.

EXEMPLAR 17-2   Certified Registered Nurse Anesthetist Role: Leadership and Autonomy

F.M. has been a CRNA for 12 years. His initial interest in the profession was engendered by a family friend who was a CRNA and encouraged F.M. to pursue a career as a nurse anesthetist. The factors that have most influenced F.M. in his professional development are his interests in multiple areas including complex pathophysiology; matching anesthesia techniques to complex patient presentations, pharmacology, and the desire for autonomous practice. F.M. notes, "I get paid to do anesthesia!" This enthusiasm for his specialty is typical of many practicing CRNAs.

F.M. was an active duty military CRNA and practiced at several armed services medical centers. As a civilian CRNA, he has moved into a group practice based at a rural critical access hospital in the Midwest. He currently spends 90% of his time in direct patient care. Some of that time he is with a student rotating through his facility, since he remains with the student and patient at all times. The balance of F.M.'s time is spent "in "the business of anesthesia," related to being part-owner of his practice.

A typical day in F.M.'s practice includes meeting in the group's office with colleagues for coffee at 6 AM. After that, he prepares the anesthetics he will administer that day. He then meets with patients, conducts preanesthesia interviews and physical assessments, plans their anesthetic care, and implements the planned anesthetic for the first and subsequent cases of the day, until the cases are done. If he is on call, he spends the afternoon in the preoperative clinic performing preoperative assessments and interventions for complex patients who will be coming to the OR in the future.

Some of the unique aspects of F.M.'s practice include autonomy and the use of regional anesthesia techniques. He enjoys the challenges of caring for high-acuity patients undergoing complex surgical procedures in a small community hospital. This practice is proactive in the use of regional anesthesia techniques, such as ultrasound-guided continuous peripheral nerve blocks, for postoperative analgesia. This technique avoids the potential risk of epidural hematomas associated with enoxaparin (Lovenox) therapy (Chan & Bailin, 2004).

F.M. describes the greatest challenges in his practice as "autonomy—having to make decisions while caring for very sick/complicated patients with no input from other anesthesia providers; the complexity of the patients and the procedures we are performing on them." He also notes that managing a very busy private practice anesthesia group is challenging—"ensuring that we cover all the surgeons/hospitals but at the same time protecting our staff from overwork..."

The practice in which F.M. is a partner evolved from a small hospital-employed group of one anesthesiologist and two CRNAs. As the workload grew and more surgeons were added, the group grew larger. "We eventually ended up with three anesthesiologists and six CRNAs. Unfortunately, several members decided to move closer to family. At this point we decided to take advantage of the turmoil and go independent. We formed our own private practice group (a service corporation). We have been functioning like this for the last 4 years."

F.M.'s military background provided knowledge about infrastructure and resources for personal and professional development that have carried over into his later career. His practice partners are all former military CRNAs, and their principal clinical site is a clinical affiliation site for military and civilian nurse anesthesia programs. F.M. has had extensive involvement with his state and national professional organizations and presents to these groups on clinical and non-clinical topics.

CRNA, Certified registered nurse anesthetist; *OR,* operating room.

anesthesia educators met when trying to move certificate nurse anesthesia programs into schools of nursing. Since 1998, all nurse anesthesia programs have been at the graduate level. However, this requirement does not dictate the movement of programs into one academic discipline. A reason for this factor may stem from those programs that in the 1970s established relationships with whichever academic unit was open to affiliating with a nurse anesthesia program. Programs that pioneered nurse anesthesia education at the graduate level established relationships with those departments in colleges and universities that were willing to take risks with the small numbers of students in nurse anesthesia programs. This diversified model of nurse anesthesia education has proliferated in the past 15 years, and many of these long-established programs would find it difficult to change their academic affiliations.

In the mid-1970s, over 170 nurse anesthesia educational programs existed. Currently, 106 CRNA educational programs operate in the United States

EXEMPLAR 17-3   **Implementation of Advanced Practice Nurse Competencies**

D.S. and P.R. are hospital-employed CRNAs at a community hospital in central Illinois. D.S. has practiced as a CRNA for 20 years and P.R. for 22 years. Their practice includes a physician anesthesiologist, who is also hospital-employed. The hospital has four operating rooms and an active obstetrics department, where labor epidurals are provided by the CRNAs and the anesthesiologist. All three anesthesia providers rotate taking call. They act as backups for each other if additional help is needed, such as caring for a multiple-trauma patient.

The nurse anesthetists have deep ties with the community in which they practice. Because it is a town of 30,000, many people know each other. D.S. and P.R. are active in church and community groups. They are very cognizant of the perceptions of their professional and personal lives. They work with the same surgeons and obstetricians routinely. Competence, caring, and dependability are qualities that D.S. and P.R. convey; these attributes help solidify their roles as trusted APNs in the community.

Because the majority of their surgical cases are performed on an outpatient basis, preanesthetic assessment takes place on the outpatient unit, one floor below surgery. The CRNAs or the anesthesiologist conduct a preoperative interview in a private room with the patient. This time is crucial for establishing the rapport necessary between the patient and his or her anesthesia provider. The health history is obtained, and patients are prompted for additional information as necessary. Anesthetic options are explained using easily understood language. The risks and benefits associated with each anesthetic option are described. Sometimes, surgeons indicate preferences for particular anesthetic techniques; however, the anesthesia provider ensures that patients are comfortable with the proposed anesthetic, its benefits, and potential risks.

On a typical day, several elective surgical cases are scheduled. Emergency cases may be scheduled at any time later in the day. Other clinical activities for D.S. and P.R. include the placement and management of labor epidurals, helping with venous access, emergency airway management, and acting as team leaders during cardiac arrests. The CRNAs are consulted on pain and ventilator management. They serve on the pharmacy and therapeutics committee because perioperatively administered medications constitute a large part of the hospital formulary. They are also members of the operating room committee. This committee has representation from operating room nursing, surgery, and anesthesia. Time and resource allocation are two of the priority areas for this committee.

This exemplar clearly demonstrates the core APN competencies:

1. **Expert direct clinical practice**: The CRNAs have to be highly competent because the other anesthesia providers are frequently busy when they are performing their duties. When taking call, the CRNAs, collaborating with the staff physicians and nurses, are responsible for expert anesthetic assessment, crisis management, decision making, implementation, and evaluation skills.

2. **Expert guidance and coaching of patients, families, and other care providers**: This core competency is evident in both the perioperative and obstetrical arenas. In the obstetrical area, the CRNAs provide expert guidance and coaching to patients and their families regarding labor analgesia that they provide with labor epidurals. The guidelines used for implementation and management of labor epidurals were collectively developed by the anesthesia department, the staff obstetricians, and the labor and delivery unit nurses.

3. **Consultation**: The CRNAs are consulted for pain management; treatment of postoperative/post-procedure nausea and vomiting; ventilator management; acquisition of new equipment for the operating room and intensive care units; oral intake guidelines for surgery and other diagnostic and therapeutic procedures; and their expertise with sedation techniques.

4. **Research skills**: The CRNAs read anesthesia journals and visit anesthesia websites (e.g., *www.aana.com;* www.anesthesia-analgesia.org; http://gasnet.med.yale.edu) regularly. See also Box 17-6. The rapid development of new technology and pharmacology in anesthesia mandates an ability to critique and utilize these developments to ensure evidence-based practice. CRNAs also collaborate in clinical research about anesthesia and pain management.

5. **Clinical and professional leadership**: This core competency is evident on multiple levels. The CRNAs are regarded as clinical leaders in the operating room. Their counsel on positioning, monitoring, and fluid management is important to surgeons and operating room nurses. Professional leadership opportunities exist both in the hospital and through local forums, as well as in state and national organizations. D.S. and P.R. have served on committees for their state professional organization and stay actively involved in developments

APN, Advanced practice nurse; *CRNA,* certified registered nurse anesthetist.

EXEMPLAR 17-3   Implementation of Advanced Practice Nurse Competencies—cont'd

affecting their national organization (e.g., influencing legislators, chairing committees).

6. **Collaboration:** Collaboration is key to nurse anesthesia practice. The CRNAs collaborate with surgeons, dentists, podiatrists, nurses, and the anesthesiologist in their department. There is significant mutual respect between the CRNAs and these clinicians. The long record of clinical competence, dependability, and affability that D.S. and P.R. exhibit helps maintain their position as valued collaborators in their practice setting.

7. **Systems leadership:** The CRNAs bring their knowledge, skills, and abilities in perioperative monitoring, pain management, and airway management to their colleagues. One example of how D.S. and P.R. brought about change was to advise the hospital to purchase two anesthesia machines with computerized record-keeping capabilities. Rather than having to keep an anesthetic record by hand, this technology requires the anesthetist to enter only patient demographics, drugs and fluids administered, and other information deemed

necessary for the case. A laser-printed anesthetic record is printed at the end of each case. The information entered into the computer can also be used for billing and continuous quality improvement.

8. **Ethics:** These CRNAs experience a variety of ethical situations in the perioperative setting. A variety of decision-making models and resources are available to assist the CRNA with the resolution of these ethical situations. Bosek (2001) notes that each ethical situation needs to be evaluated with respect to values, customs, policies, and other nuances that affect the decision to be made.

On a typical day, P.R. or D.S. may deal with cases as diverse as an elective cesarean section, a hip pinning in an older patient, a closed reduction of a Colles' fracture in a 10-year-old, and placement of labor epidurals. The labor epidurals require monitoring for adequate analgesia as well as potential side effects. Each patient has unique requirements for anesthesia management; often, family members will have questions for the anesthesia providers.

and Puerto Rico (Council on Accreditation of Nurse Anesthesia Educational Programs, 2007). Several new CRNA educational programs are on the horizon. A rapid decline in the numbers of nurse anesthesia programs occurred in the 1980s. This change was of great concern to the specialty. The closures were attributed variously to physician pressure, declining support, the inability of hospitals to continue support of small programs, and lack of a geographically accessible university with which a nurse anesthesia program could affiliate (Faut-Callahan, 1991). Those who argued that nurse anesthesia programs closed solely because of the graduate degree mandate offered little evidence to support that claim. One can surmise that if the requirement for graduate education were the only reason for program closures, those programs would have remained open until 1998, when the master's degree was required (Figure 17-6).

Despite the decline in the overall numbers of nurse anesthesia programs, many of which were certificate programs that had enrollments of fewer than five students, the level of educational programs changed dramatically. After an initial decline in graduates, the newer graduate programs increased

their admissions. The overall number of CRNA graduates has continued to rise. The period between 1996 and 2006 demonstrated a significant increase in the number of students enrolled in nurse anesthesia educational programs. In 1995, about 1800 students were enrolled in nurse anesthesia programs. By 2005, almost 5000 students were studying to become CRNAs. To accomplish this, programs had to increase the numbers of clinical training sites. The result has been a strengthened educational system, deeply entrenched in an academic model. The anticipated number of nurse anesthesia graduates in 2007 is greater than 2000. Today there are over 1550 clinical training sites.

Colleges of nursing are more frequently becoming the sites for nurse anesthesia programs as nurse anesthesia and other APN groups increasingly collaborate on legislative, policy, and educational matters. Agatha Hodgins' expressed desire for a separate professional organization and education process for nurse anesthesia has been partially supplanted by the rapprochement between nursing and nurse anesthesia (Mungia-Biddle et al., 1990). Coalitions of APNs have been effectively working together on the state and federal levels with health care reform issues.

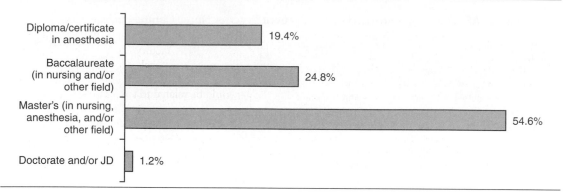

FIGURE **17-6:** Highest level of education completed by CRNA respondents in 2005.

Program of Study

Nurse anesthesia educational curricula include time requirements for both didactic and clinical activities that reflect minimum standards for entry into practice. Academic content areas are crucial to the preparation of practitioners for beginning-level competence in a highly demanding, rapidly changing specialty. Various colleges and schools that administratively house nurse anesthesia programs may have additional academic requirements. Nurse anesthesia programs in colleges of nursing include core graduate-level courses taken by all graduate-level nursing students. These courses include graduate-level nursing theory, nursing research, advanced physical assessment, and pharmacology. The following are the mandated content areas for nurse anesthesia programs (Council on Accreditation, 2006):

- Pharmacology of anesthetic agents and adjuvant drugs, including concepts in chemistry and biochemistry, 105 hours
- Anatomy, physiology, and pathophysiology, 135 hours
- Professional aspects of nurse anesthesia practice, 45 hours
- Basic and advanced principles of anesthesia practice including physics, equipment, technology, and pain management, 105 hours
- Research, 30 hours
- Clinical correlation conferences, 45 hours

The clinical component requires that the student administer a minimum of 550 anesthetics. An external agency, the Council on Certification of Nurse Anesthetists, requires that students complete given numbers of surgical procedures and anesthetic techniques. For example, all students must administer at least 25 general anesthetics using a mask airway (versus endotracheal intubation), and must care for patients across the life span. Similarly, required numbers of specific clinical experiences, such as endotracheal intubations or thoracic surgical cases, must be met for nurse anesthesia graduates to be eligible to take the national certification examination. Most programs exceed these minimum requirements. The average student nurse anesthetist works at least 1694 clinical hours and administers more than 790 anesthetics. In addition, many require study in methods of scientific inquiry and statistics, as well as active participation in student-generated and faculty-sponsored research.

The Council on Accreditation (COA) of Nurse Anesthesia Educational Programs accredits nurse anesthesia educational programs. Council members include nurse anesthesia educators and practitioners, nurse anesthesia students, health care administrators, university representatives, and the public. The COA conducts mandatory, on-site program reviews with a maximum accreditation period of 10 years. Nurse anesthesia educators and the COA have found that retaining a prescriptive curriculum in terms of hours and types of clinical experiences has helped the survival of educational programs. That is, when documented deviations from established standards for nurse anesthesia educational programs occur (e.g., physicians restricting clinical access), program directors can cite COA standards mandating these experiences.

Doctor of Nursing Practice

In the educational arena, debate continues about the preparation of CRNAs. Currently, the minimum length of nurse anesthesia programs is 24 months.

However, because of the combination of didactic and clinical time requirements, many programs are 27 to 36 months long. Nurse anesthesia curricular requirements can overload the typical master's curriculum. Because of the time commitment and academic rigor necessary for this specialty area, there is increasing interest in a clinical doctoral degree as the exit degree in nurse anesthesia. The vision of nursing leader Dr. Luther Christman that nurses be prepared with advanced degrees both in their discipline and in a basic science reflects the trend to propose preparation beyond the master's degree for entry into this and other advanced practice specialty areas (Christman, 1977). Doctoral programs in nurse anesthesia are being developed. Currently, approximately 1% of practicing nurse anesthetists possess doctoral degrees in disciplines including education, nursing, physiology, and pharmacology.

The COA of Nurse Anesthesia Educational Programs has mandated doctoral preparation for nurse anesthesia program directors by 2014. Currently, 40 of the 106 program directors (38%) listed in the *COA List of Recognized Educational Programs* (2007) have doctoral degrees. CRNAs continue to seek doctoral education, but the incentives for pursuing this type of education are quite different from those for a practice-oriented master's degree. In the wake of the Doctor of Nursing Practice (DNP) initiative (AACN, 2004), an AANA task force conducted a study to investigate the feasibility of a doctoral degree for nurse anesthetists. Results of the involved survey showed that 65% of the respondents did not support a doctoral degree for entry into practice; 60% of nurse anesthesia education programs stated it was not feasible to offer doctoral degrees at their institutions because of insufficient faculty resources (Jordan & Shott, 1998). There was no statistically significant relationship between year of graduation from an anesthesia program and doctorate entry support for all respondents. A significant association was found between planned retirement year and doctorate entry support for female respondents. Respondents who believed that the AANA should promote doctoral programs tended to be more recent graduates (median graduation year, 1982) than those who did not agree with this concept (median graduation year, 1980) ($P = 0.044$) (Jordan & Shott, 1998).

The themes that emerged for faculty related to doctoral education were in three major areas. Adequate time for doctoral studies was an impediment for almost half the respondents (44%). Inadequate finances for doctoral education was identified as an area of difficulty by 27% of respondents, and 25% of responding CRNA faculty members had no interest in obtaining a doctoral degree (Jordan & Shott, 1998). The lack of interest in pursuing a doctoral degree could be related to time demands on program directors.

AMERICAN ASSOCIATION OF NURSE ANESTHETISTS

Organization and Structure
The AANA was among the first nursing specialty organizations. At a 1931 regional nurse anesthesia meeting, Agatha Hodgins, founder of AANA, described her vision for the essentials for a national organization of nurse anesthetists (Thatcher, 1953):

> Improvement of the present situation is in the hands of the nurse anesthetists themselves. If the work is to be properly safeguarded and hoped-for progress attained, it is necessary that remedies to be applied to certain conditions now acknowledgedly exist. It would seem that the first step should be the awakening of deeper interest and the development of constructive leadership. Following in logical order would be: self-organization as a special division of hospital service…educational standards, post-graduate schools of anesthesia…required to conform to an accepted criteria of education; state registration, putting right the nurse anesthetist to practice her vocation beyond criticism; constant effort toward improving the quality of work by means of study and research, thus affording still greater protection to the patient; [and] dissemination of information gained through proper channels. (p. 183)

Early efforts of nurse anesthetists to affiliate with the American Nurses Association (ANA) did not occur because each organization had different ideas of what such an affiliation would entail (Gunn, 1990; Thatcher, 1953). With time, the breach between nursing and nurse anesthesia has narrowed considerably. Since its inception as the National Association of Nurse Anesthetists (NANA) in 1931, the AANA has placed its responsibilities to the public above or at the same level as its responsibilities to its membership. The association has produced education and practice standards, implemented a certification examination for nurse anesthetists in 1945, and developed an accreditation process that was implemented in 1952. The AANA has been a leader in the formation of a multidisciplinary council with public representation to fulfill the autonomous credentialing functions of the profession, including accreditation, certification, and recertification.

When AANA founder Agatha Hodgins became ill, Gertrude Fife, who provided anesthesia for pioneering heart surgeon Claude Beck, assumed the role of developing NANA in its early days (Thatcher, 1953). The name of the association was changed to the American Association of Nurse Anesthetists in 1939. Helen Lamb, who served two terms as AANA president (1940-1942) provided anesthesia exclusively for Dr. Evarts Graham, one of the first modern thoracic surgeons (Bankert, 1989). The first anesthesia administered for correction of tetralogy of Fallot was given by a nurse anesthetist, Olive Berger, at Johns Hopkins Hospital. Early nurse anesthesia leaders were involved in complex practice settings with surgeons who were also influential in their fields. In addition to development of a professional identity for nurse anesthesia, early nurse anesthetist leaders developed curricular standards for nurse anesthesia educational programs. These standards initially included a minimum program length of 6 months with subsequent institution of mandatory certification and recertification policies.

The board of directors oversees and governs the association in its efforts "to be the pre-eminent association of anesthesia providers by putting patients first and taking a leadership role in policy making, nurse anesthesia education, and research to ensure high quality, safe anesthesia practice...." (AANA, 2007b). Seven AANA committees support the work of the association. Several committees have student representatives.

Mission and Vision

The AANA mission statement is "advancing patient safety and excellence in anesthesia." The accompanying vision statement reads, "recognized leaders in anesthesia care." The core values of the profession are integrity, professionalism, advocacy, and quality. The association seeks to support its members and protect patients. Current areas of activity for AANA are safety and quality, compliance issues, employment issues, and responsiveness to other trends identified through ongoing environmental scanning.

SAFETY AND QUALITY ISSUES

Regarding safety and quality, specific areas addressed by the AANA include outpatient anesthesia practice and work with the National Patient Safety Foundation in that area. Scope of practice issues are monitored

and addressed by AANA staff and committee members. The AANA has been a participant in Medicare "pay for performance" initiatives, which are intended to encourage improved quality of care in all health care settings in which Medicare beneficiaries receive their health care services (Purcell, 2007).

Non-governmental regulation of nurse anesthesia practice is closely monitored by the AANA related to the activities of TJC, the Accreditation Association for Ambulatory Health Care, and other agencies whose policies may impact nurse anesthesia practice.

Reimbursement issues related to Medicare, Medicaid, and other payers are closely monitored by the AANA, since changes in reimbursement can have a major impact on earnings. The AANA office also provides members with resources on how to start a business, contracts, reimbursement, practice models, management and staffing, pain management, and disability.

Practice trends monitored by the AANA include pain management and scope of practice issues. Provision of sedation and analgesia by non-anesthesia providers is closely monitored by the AANA. Other areas in which the association provides support to its members include strategies to address workplace harassment, expert witness identification, and development of skills and resources for mass casualty and bioterrorism situations.

An AANA subsidiary, AANA Insurance Services (*www.aana.com/insurance*), provides malpractice coverage for many nurse anesthetists. Trends monitored by this agency include the decreasing number of insurers covering CRNAs and all health care providers. The remaining insurers are being more selective about whom they cover. Consequently, malpractice liability insurance premiums are increasing. The St. Paul Fire and Marine Casualty Company withdrew from providing malpractice coverage to CRNAs in 2001. After that decision, the TIG Insurance Company announced its withdrawal from the malpractice insurance market in 2002. The principal insurer for CRNAs who need to obtain coverage, as opposed to those who work for self-insured entities, is now CNA Insurance. Applicants must meet underwriting guidelines and criteria (AANA, 2007f).

The AANA closely monitors trends in patient safety and malpractice litigation. There are numerous continuing education meetings across the country with patient safety topics, which is integral to the association's mission. Reinforcing the 11 standards of care (e.g., performing preanesthesia assessments, routine use of pulse oximetry, end-tidal carbon dioxide monitoring) described in the "Scope and Standards for Nurse Anesthesia Practice" (AANA, 2002a) is central to these presentations.

The Council for Public Interest in Anesthesia, a multidisciplinary body concerned with monitoring issues involving safe anesthesia care, oversees the AANA Wellness Program. The goals of the Wellness Program are to promote wellness and healthy lifestyles for professionals and to coordinate peer assistance activities. The Wellness Program was established by the AANA Board of Directors in 2004 in response to several wellness concerns, including the growing problem of substance abuse (Kremer & Litwin, 2006). Built upon recommendations from an expert panel, the program incorporates a website *(www.aana.com/resources),* peer assistance activities, a wellness assessment, and resources for areas of improvement for personal well-being. Wellness and patient safety are interrelated—as professionals working in high-risk, high-stress environments, nurse anesthetists and student nurse anesthetists are vulnerable to events that can impact physical and mental health. The Wellness Program provides resources for AANA members to become better educated and more aware of how to manage these stressors (AANA, 2007e).

CONTINUED CHALLENGES

Reimbursement for Nurse Anesthesia Clinical Services

From the inception of this specialty through the 1950s, CRNAs were often paid as employees of either the surgeon or the hospital that employed them. In rural areas, CRNAs often contracted with hospitals to provide services based on fee-for-service structures—that is, a set amount of compensation per case as opposed to a straight salary for hours worked (Simonson & Garde, 1994). The advent of private payers such as Blue Cross/Blue Shield led to the compensation of only physicians and hospitals through these plans. Other health care providers, such as nurse anesthetists, psychologists, and physical therapists, would submit charges to the hospital or treating physician. The hospital or physician would then obtain reimbursement for these services as "incident to" their own and pass the money on to the non-reimbursed provider (Simonson & Garde, 1994).

Escalating health care costs in the late twentieth century caused Medicare to institute a prospective payment system (PPS) in 1983. This legislation ini-

tially affected only Medicare Part A (hospital costs) and subsequently also impacted Medicare Part B (physician and non-physician) costs. PPS legislation mandated a fixed payment rate for all hospital care, covering Part A services paid to hospitals based on the diagnosis-related group (DRG) classification of the patient. This fixed rate was to cover all costs associated with hospital admission, including services provided by non-physician health care providers. CRNAs were in great jeopardy under this system. In their cost-cutting efforts, hospitals had no incentive to hire CRNAs, since the related employment costs would come directly from the hospital DRG payment. Congress inadvertently created reimbursement disincentives for the use of CRNAs while bolstering incentives for the use of anesthesiologists. The AANA lobbying efforts caused the Health Care Financing Administration (HCFA)—now the Centers for Medicare & Medicaid Services (CMS)—to rewrite portions of this legislation, enabling all CRNAs to obtain Medicare reimbursement or to sign over their billing rights to their employer (Broadston, 2001; Simonson & Garde, 1994).

Historically, anesthesia charges have been based on direct time involvement, either as a charge for simple time or as a charge based on a combination of time and the complexity of the anesthetic. The resource-based relative value scale (RBRVS), developed in the 1960s, is used to determine anesthesia charges based on the complexity of a surgical procedure. The result is charges for "base units," or surgical procedures described by anatomical or functional units. Additional "modifier units" can be added to base units for factors such as emergency procedures, extremes of age, or anesthetic risk. After adding base and modifier units, time units are calculated at one unit per 15 minutes. The value of time units is determined by the payer (e.g., Medicare or Blue Cross/Blue Shield) and the market. One unit of anesthesia time may be billed at from $15 to over $70. The total of base, modifier, and time units determines the professional fee for administration of anesthesia. Many third-party payers, such as Medicare and some Blue Cross insurers, completely ignore the charges of the practitioner and determine payments from their own fee schedules. These payments are often determined by what providers charge "on average" for their services (Broadston, 2001; Simonson & Garde, 1994).

CRNAs can evaluate their clinical and financial outcomes through data collected, often by billing services, over specified time periods (e.g., monthly, quarterly, or annually). The total number of anesthetics administered during the specified timeframe needs to be determined. Then, the total number of relative value units generated is calculated. This is accomplished through multiplication of the total number of anesthetics administered by the average number of relative value units per case, which might be 10.5 units. The surgical case mix and payer mix breakdowns need to be determined (e.g., 15% commercial, 35% Medicare, 10% Medicaid). Finally, the specific reimbursement rates per relative value unit per section of the case mix/payer mix are calculated. If the specific unit rate is not available, the usual unit conversion factors are used (e.g., Medicare, $15 per unit; health maintenance organization [HMO], $30 per unit; private, $40 per unit) (Broadston, 2001). Payer mix will vary with practice settings, and this information is helpful as part of the assessment of a potential new practice setting (see Chapter 19).

Attempts to control spiraling health care costs and improve access to care resulted in the development of managed care contracts and resurgent interest in HMOs with capitated payment schemes. Fee-for-service reimbursement structures may become less common because of the imposition of additional cost-containment measures by payers and the national economy. Cost containment in health care does not ensure client access to APNs based on cost-effectiveness. Transitional mechanisms in vertical integration strategies, such as combining payers, providers, and a wide spectrum of network services, still focus on physicians and hospitals as the principal health care resources.

There are ongoing efforts by the CMS to reduce reimbursement to providers under Medicare. Initial results in anesthesia led to a slight increase for a few procedures, but the majority of procedures were assigned lower values (Lester, 2003). In 2006, Congress proposed a 13.7% decrease in Medicare anesthesia reimbursement, which was reduced by 5.1% through lobbying efforts (AANA, 2007c). Health care providers received additional payment incentives in exchange for reporting quality measures to Medicare. Providers who report specified quality measures to Medicare will be able to obtain an additional 1.5% incentive payment. Therefore the original proposed CRNA Medicare payment cut for 2007 of −13.7% was reduced to −8.6% and −7.1% for those reporting quality measures. These quality measures include maintenance of perioperative normothermia, appropriate timing of prophylactic preoperative antibiotics, and pain management planning (AANA, 2007c).

The AANA estimated that the mean national anesthesia conversion factor would decline from $17.76 in 2006 to $16.23 in 2007 under the provisions of the legislation adopted by Congress. Without congressional intervention, the CMS would have decreased the 2007 anesthesia conversion factor to $15.33, lower than the 1992 level of $15.75 (AANA, 2007c). Continued cost-containment efforts from all payers are likely, given the increasing portion of the gross domestic product allocated to health care costs.

The AANA was asked by the American Society of Anesthesiologists (ASA) to join them in an effort to seek congressional help to reverse the CMS proposal and seek increases for all surgical procedures. Paradoxically, the ASA actively opposed an AANA effort to change Medicare Part A supervisions requirements and was not supportive of efforts to obtain reimbursement for medically directed CRNAs working with nurse anesthesia students (Lester, 2003). These experiences demonstrate the ongoing efforts to decrease anesthesia reimbursement and that complex policy initiatives are difficult to achieve unilaterally.

The AANA continues to work for the creation of teaching rules under Medicare that would allow reimbursement for teaching CRNA students. The AANA and CRNAs have advocated that congress should include in the Medicare package reform of teaching rules to capture the services of CRNAs and anesthesiologists. However, at this writing, no changes have been made by congress to the Medicare anesthesia payment teaching rules, including changes proposed by the ASA that would have benefitted anesthesiologists only. Federal fiscal constraints contributed to congressional disinclination to adopt multiple payment reforms sought by health care advocates, including teaching rules reforms sought by anesthesia providers in 2006 (AANA, 2007c).

Nurse Anesthesia Educational Funding

At the time of this writing, serious concerns exist related to the Federal Advanced Education Nurse (AEN) Training and the Nurse Anesthesia Traineeship (NAT) programs. AEN funding provides critical support for nurse anesthesia students during their first year of education. The administration has proposed to eliminate the $57 million in funding in fiscal year 2008 for this program, which will dramatically affect the supply of nursing faculty and APNs, including CRNAs. These cuts come at a time when there is a documented faculty shortage and growing numbers of older adults requiring services (AANA,

2007g). NAT funding supports nurse anesthesia students during the second year of studies. This is a time when all nurse anesthesia students are required to be full-time students and are not able to work because of the rigor of the program, often requiring more than 60 hours of clinical education per week.

Medicare Anesthesia Payment Teaching Rules

The Medicare Academic Anesthesiology and CRNA Payment Improvement Act proposes to eliminate the inequity in how anesthesia services are reimbursed when a nurse anesthesia student participates in the care of a Medicare beneficiary. Today, "Medicare cuts its anesthesia fee by 50% in certain educational settings involving nurse anesthetists and anesthesiologists, if one case involving a teacher's student overlaps for even a minute with a second case involving another student of the same teacher" (AANA, 2007h). This proposed act differs from other approaches suggested by the American Society of Anesthesiologists, which seek to solve the problem for situations involving anesthesiology residents only. Should such an approach continue, the disincentive for an organization to support nurse anesthesia education will continue. "It is vital that the Medicare anesthesia payment rules treat both CRNAs and anesthesiologists the same" (AANA, 2007h).

SUMMARY

Nurse anesthesia, the earliest nursing specialty, was also the first nursing specialty to have standardized educational programs, a certification process, mandatory continuing education, and recertification. Nurse anesthetists have been involved in the development of anesthetic techniques along with physicians and engineers. Nurse anesthetists have been nursing leaders in obtaining third-party reimbursement for professional services and in coping with challenges such as the prospective payment system, managed care, and physician supervision.

Nurse anesthetists provide surgical and nonsurgical anesthesia services in a variety of settings, both in the United States and in other parts of the world. CRNAs work in collaboration with physicians as do other APNs and are capable of providing the full spectrum of anesthesia services.

Activism in the state and federal legislative and regulatory arenas is a recognized CRNA activity. Increasing coalition building between nurse anesthetists, other APNs, and nursing educators is congruent with a shared nursing vision. This vision values health care for all Americans provided in a safe and cost-effective manner by APNs collaborating with other health care professionals.

REFERENCES

Agency for Healthcare Research and Quality (AHRQ). (2003). *Ambulatory surgery in U.S. hospitals, 2003.* Retrieved April 8, 2007, from www.ahrq.gov/data/hcup/factbk9/factbk9a.htm.

American Association of Colleges of Nursing (AACN). (2004). *Position statement on the practice doctorate in nursing.* Washington, D.C.: Author.

American Association of Nurse Anesthetists. (1990). *Report of the National Commission on Nurse Anesthesia Education.* Park Ridge, IL: Author.

American Association of Nurse Anesthetists (AANA). (2002a). *Scope and standards for nurse anesthesia practice.* Retrieved April 8, 2007, from www.aana.com/resources.

American Association of Nurse Anesthetists (AANA). (2002b). *Qualifications and capabilities of the CRNA.* Retrieved April 8, 2007, from www.aana.com/resources.

American Association of Nurse Anesthetists (AANA). (2006). *2006 report practice profile and demographic surveys.* Park Ridge, IL: Author.

American Association of Nurse Anesthetists (AANA). (2007a). *Following AANA and CRNAs' actions, Congress OKs some Medicare cuts relief for CRNAs, but leaves teaching rules alone.* Retrieved April 3, 2007, from www.aana.com/advocacy.

American Association of Nurse Anesthetists (AANA). (2007b). *About AANA.* Retrieved April 3, 2007, from www.aana.com/aboutaana.

American Association of Nurse Anesthetists (AANA). (2007c). *Advocacy.* Retrieved April 5, 2007, from www.aana.com/advocacy.

American Association of Nurse Anesthetists (AANA). (2007d). *Becoming a CRNA.* Retrieved April 5, 2007, from www.aana.com/becomingcrna.

American Association of Nurse Anesthetists (AANA). (2007e). *Resources.* Retrieved April 10, 2007, from www.aana.com/resources.

American Association of Nurse Anesthetists (AANA). (2007f). *Insurance.* Retrieved April 10, 2007, from www.aana.com/insurance.

American Association of Nurse Anesthetists (AANA). (2007g). *Reverse nurse anesthesia education budget cuts.* Retrieved April 3, 2007, from www.aana.com/resources.

American Association of Nurse Anesthetists (AANA). (2007h). *Fix Medicare anesthesia payment teaching rules for CRNAs and anesthesiologists equally.* Retrieved April 3, 2007, from www.aana.com/resources.

Baggs J. (1994). Development of an instrument to measure collaboration and satisfaction about care decisions. *Journal of Advanced Nursing, 20,* 176-182.

Bankert, M. (1989). *Watchful care: A history of America's nurse anesthetists.* New York: Continuum.

Bettin, C. (2004). *Certified registered nurse anesthetists play pivotal role in U.S. efforts to combat worldwide terrorism.*

Retrieved April 4, 2007, from www.canainc.org/news/2004archive/pdfs/011304-CRNAs.pdf.

Blumenreich, G. (2007). Another article on the surgeon's liability and anesthesia negligence. *AANA Journal, 75,* 89-93.

Bosek, M. (2001). Ethical decision making in anesthesia. In S. Foster & M. Faut-Callahan (Eds.). *A professional study and resource guide for the CRNA.* Park Ridge, IL: AANA Publishing.

Broadston, L. (2001). Reimbursement for anesthesia services. In S. Foster & M. Faut-Callahan (Eds.). *A professional study and resource guide for the CRNA.* Park Ridge, IL: AANA Publishing.

Callahan, L. (1994). Establishing measures of competence. In S. Foster and L. Jordan (Eds.), *Professional aspects of nurse anesthesia practice* (pp. 275-290). Philadelphia: Davis.

Centers for Disease Control and Prevention (CDC). (2005). *2004 National hospital discharge survey.* Retrieved April 2, 2007, from www.cdc.gov/nchs/fastats/insurg.htm.

Chan, L., & Bailin, M. (2004). Spinal epidural hematoma following central neuraxial blockade and subcutaneous enoxaparin: A case report. *Journal of Clinical Anesthesia, 16*(5), 382-385.

Christman, L. (1977). Doctoral education: A shot in the arm for the nursing profession. *Health Services Manager, 10*(5), 6, 7.

Connelly, L., Schretenthaler, J., & Taunton, R. (2002). Nurse anesthesia research: A follow-up study. *AANA Journal, 70,* 463-469.

Council on Accreditation of Nurse Anesthesia Educational Programs. (2006). *Standards for accreditation of nurse anesthesia educational programs.* Author.

Council on Accreditation of Nurse Anesthesia Educational Programs. (2007). *List of recognized educational programs.* Author.

Cromwell, J., Rosenbach, M.. (1988). The economics of anesthesia delivery, *Health Affairs,* 118-131.

Dorrah, M., & Norton, S. (1996). The certified nurse-midwife. In A.B. Hamric, J.A. Spross, & C.M. Hanson (Eds.), *Advanced nursing practice: An integrative approach* (pp. 395-420). Philadelphia: Saunders.

Fallacaro M. (1998). An inefficient mix: A comparative analysis of nurse and physician anesthesia providers across New York State. *Journal of New York State Nurses' Association, 29*(2), 4-8.

Fallacaro, M., & Ruiz-Law, T. (2004). Distribution of U.S. anesthesia providers and services. *AANA Journal, 72,* 9-14.

Faut-Callahan, M. (1991). Graduate education for nurse anesthetists: Master's versus a clinical doctorate. In *National Commission on Nurse Anesthesia Education Report* (pp. 110–115). Park Ridge, IL: AANA Publishing.

Faut-Callahan, M., & Paice, J. (1990). Post-operative pain control for the parturient. *Journal of Perinatal and Neonatal Nursing, 4*(1), 27-41.

Forrester, C., Benfield, D., Matern, C., Kelly, J., & Pellegrini, J. (2007). Meclizine in combination with ondansetron for prevention of postoperative nausea and vomiting in a high risk population. *AANA Journal, 75*(1), 27-33.

Foster, S., & Faut-Callahan, M. (2001). *A professional practice guide for the CRNA.* Park Ridge, IL: AANA Publishing.

Garde, J. (1998). Annual report of the executive director. *AANA News Bulletin,* p. 14-16.

GasWork.com. *CRNA job listings.* Retrieved January 8, 2008, from www.gaswork.com.

Gunn, I. (1990). The history of nurse anesthesia education: Highlights and influences. In *National Commission on Nurse Anesthesia Education report* (pp. 33-41). Park Ridge, IL: AANA Publishing.

Hanson, C.M., & Spross, J.A. (2005). Collaboration. In A.B. Hamric, J.A. Spross, & C.M. Hanson (Eds.). *Advanced practice nursing: An integrative approach* (3rd ed., pp. 341-378). Philadelphia: Saunders.

Henry, B., & McAuliffe, M. (1999). Practice and education of nurse anesthetists. *Bulletin of the World Health Organization, 77*(3), 267-270.

Horton, B. (1998). Nurse anesthesia as a subculture of nursing in the United States. Doctoral dissertation, Rush University. *Dissertation Abstracts International,* 9912475.

Howie, W. (2007). Anesthesia "Go team" for trauma patients: Field-based anesthesia. *AANA Journal, 75*(2): 107-110.

International Federation of Nurse Anesthetists (IFNA). (2007). *Overview of the International Federation of Nurse Anesthetists.* Retrieved April 8, 2007, from http://ifna-int.org/ifna/page.php?16.

Jordan, L., & Shott, S. (1998). Feasibility of a doctoral degree for nurse anesthetists. *AANA Journal, 66,* 287-298.

Jordan, L., Kremer, M., & Crawforth, K. (2001). Data-driven practice improvement: The AANA Foundation Closed Malpractice Claims Study. *AANA Journal, 69*(4), 301-316.

Kaye D., Scibetta W., & Grogono, A. (1999). Anesthesia manpower and recruitment 1998. An update. *Advances in Anesthesia 9*(16), 1-27.

Klein, J.D. (1997). When will managed care come to anesthesia? *Journal of Health Care Finance, 23,* 62-86.

Kremer, M., & Blair, T. (2006). Ludwig angina: Forewarned is forearmed. *AANA Journal, 74*(6), 445-451.

Kremer, M., & Faut-Callahan, M. (2000). Outcomes assessment in nurse anesthesia. In R. Kleinpell. (Ed.). *Outcomes assessment in advanced practice nursing* (pp. 227-260). New York, Springer.

Kremer, M., & Litwin, L. (2006). Stop medication diversion in its tracks. *Men in Nursing, 1*(6), 42-50.

Kyle, M. (1995). Collaboration. In M. Snyder & M. Mirr (Eds.), *Advanced practice nursing: A guide to professional development* (pp. 169-182). New York: Springer.

Lester, R. (2003). President's message. *AANA NewsBulletin,* 57(4), 2.

Mastropietro, C., Horton, B., Oullette, S., & Faut-Callahan, M. (2001). The National Commission on Nurse Anesthesia: Ten years later, Part 1. *AANA Journal, 69*(5), 379-385.

Merwin, E., Stern, S., & Jordan, L. (2005). Supply, demand, and equilibrium in the market for CRNAs. *AANA Journal, 74,* 287-293.

Merwin, E., Stern, S., & Jordan, L. (2007). *Executive summary of AANA Foundation faculty workforce study.* Park Ridge, IL: AANA Foundation.

Miller, R.D., Rampil, L., & Cohen, N. (1999). Fewer residents: Financial, educational, and practical implications. *Anesthesia and Analgesia, 88,* 964-965.

Munguia-Biddle, F., Maree, S., Klein, E., Callahan, L., & Gilles, B. (1990). *Nurse anesthesiology competence evaluation: Mechanism for accountability.* Unpublished document, American Association of Nurse Anesthetists, Park Ridge, IL.

Nagelhout, J., & Zaglaniczny, K. (2005). *Nurse anesthesia* (3rd ed.). Philadelphia: Saunders.

Oklahoma Association of Nurse Anesthetists (OANA). (2005). *AANA Federal Government Affairs.* Retrieved April 3, 2007, from www.oana.org/news/2005/04222005.htm.

Pine, M., Holt, K., & Lou, Y. (2003). Surgical mortality and type of anesthesia provider. *AANA Journal, 71,* 109-116.

Purcell, F. (2007). Pay for performance boosts quality at hospitals. *AANA Federal government affairs hotline, 8* (4), 1.

Rivera, L. (2006). *2005 Practice profile and demographic surveys.* Personal communication: AANA Senior Director of Executive Affairs.

Simonson, D., Ahern, N., & Hendryx, M. (2007). Anesthesia staffing and anesthetic complications during cesarean delivery: A retrospective analysis. *Nursing Research, 56* (1), 9-17.

Simonson, D., & Garde, J. (1994). Reimbursement for clinical services. In G. Foster & L. Jordan (Eds.), *Professional aspects of nurse anesthesia practice* (pp. 129-142). Philadelphia: F.A. Davis.

Starnes-Ott, K., & Kremer, M. (2007). Recruitment and retention of nurse anesthesia faculty: Issues and strategies. *AANA Journal, 75,* 13-16.

Tremper, K., Shanks, A., & Morris, M. (2006). Trends in the financial status of United States anesthesiology training programs. *Anesthesia and Analgesia, 102*(2), 517-523.

Thatcher, V. (1953). *History of anesthesia with emphasis on the nurse specialist.* Philadelphia: Lippincott.

Weinert, C., & Calvin, R. (2007). Epidemiology of sedation and sedation adequacy for mechanically ventilated patients in a medical and surgical intensive care unit. *Critical Care Medicine, 35*(2), 635-637.

CHAPTER 18

Evolving and Innovative Opportunities for Advanced Practice Nursing

Jeanne Salyer • Ann B. Hamric

INTRODUCTION

Technological advances and economic and sociocultural conditions have sustained a climate of change in the health care environment, and opportunities for advanced practice nursing continue to emerge in the wake of these changes. As specialties have emerged, many new roles have evolved from specialty nursing practice and have expanded to incorporate some or all of the core attributes of advanced practice nursing (see Chapters 1 and 3). Some of these roles have clearly evolved as advanced practice roles, whereas others are in various stages of evolution. Not all specialties, however, will evolve into advanced practice roles, for a variety of reasons. For example, some specialties evolve away from the core definition of advanced practice nursing, which encompasses direct clinical practice and clinical expertise as essential ingredients (see Chapter 3). Some of these specialties, such as informatics and nursing administration, arise as specialties and remain specialties because direct clinical practice is not a requisite role component.

The purpose of this chapter is to examine some currently evolving specialties and characterize stages in their continuing evolution from specialty nursing practice to advanced practice nursing. Some of these specialties have not yet fully evolved to an advanced level; however, movement within the specialty toward advanced practice may be accelerated as Doctor of Nursing Practice (DNP) programs target these specialties for development. The focus of the discussion, however, is on the various specialties—not on particular advanced practice nursing roles, such as clinical nurse specialist (CNS), nurse practitioner (NP), certified nurse-midwife (CNM), or certified registered nurse anesthetist (CRNA). Specialties selected for inclusion in this discussion were chosen for one or more of the following reasons:

- The specialty has the potential to transition to the DNP.
- The specialty has the potential to evolve to advanced practice nursing given the complexity of care required by the patient population,

and direct care is likely to be a defining characteristic.
- The specialty has arisen as a result of scientific and/or technological advances and the influence of these advances on the delivery of health care.
- The specialty is growing because of the rising incidence of health problems in the population.
- The specialty's patient population needs sophisticated care across settings in the complex health care environment.

Opportunities in these evolving specialties for advanced practice nurses (APNs) are discussed, and a framework for evaluating progress toward advanced practice status is illustrated. Exemplars provided by APNs in the specialty were deliberately chosen to illuminate the *added value* of advanced practice competencies to these evolving specialties

PATTERNS IN THE EVOLUTION OF SPECIALTY TO ADVANCED PRACTICE NURSING

Before discussing the evolution of specialty nursing practice into advanced practice nursing, it is important to make a distinction between the two, as well as to clarify the use of the term *subspecialty* in this chapter. *Specialization* reflects a concentration in a selected clinical area in nursing. Specialties can be further characterized as "nursing practice that intersects with another body of knowledge, has a direct impact on nursing practice, and is supportive of the direct care rendered to patients by other registered nurses" (American Nurses Association [ANA], 2003). As the profession of nursing has responded to changes in health care, the need for specialty knowledge has increased. For example, in the wake of the National Cancer Act of 1971, which was enacted as a consequence of the increasing incidence of cancer in the population and the need to advance national efforts in prevention and treatment, the oncology specialty became more widely recognized (Oncology Nursing Society [ONS], 2007). The ONS traces its origin to the first National Cancer Nursing Research Conference, supported by both the ANA and the American Cancer Society, in 1973, after which a small group met to discuss the need for a national organization to support their professional development. From these early efforts, this organization, which was incorporated in 1975, has become a leader in cancer care—both in the United States and around the world (ONS, 2007).

The classic specialties in nursing have been pediatric, psychiatric/mental health, obstetrics (now termed *women's health*), community/public health, and medical-surgical nursing (now termed *adult health*). Newer specialties that have emerged include, for example, concentrations in acute and critical care, neonatal, and geriatric nursing. As a given specialty coalesces, nurses often form specialty nursing organizations out of clinicians' needs to share practice experiences and specialty knowledge. Some examples include the American Association of Critical-Care Nurses, the Oncology Nursing Society, and the Association of Women's Health, Obstetric, and Neonatal Nurses (AWHONN). Scope and standards of practice statements legitimize specialty designation and prompt efforts to provide opportunities for specialty education and certification. The efforts of the International Transplant Nurses Society (ITNS) to develop and approve of a scope of practice statement, a core curriculum, and specialty certification for registered nurses is but one recent example (ITNS, 2007).

Advanced practice nursing *includes specialization* but goes beyond it—involving expansion, which legitimizes role autonomy, and advancement that is characterized by the integration of a broad range of theoretical, research-based, and practical knowledge (ANA, 2003; see also Chapter 3). Thus advanced practice nursing reflects concentrated knowledge in a specialty that offers the opportunity for expanded and autonomous practice based on a broader practical and theoretical knowledge base.

The term *specialty* suggests that the focus of practice is limited to parts of the whole (ANA, 1995). For example, family NPs, who classically see themselves as generalists, have in fact specialized in one of the many facets of health care, namely primary care. *Subspecialization* further delineates the focus of practice. In subspecialty practice, knowledge and skill in a delimited clinical area is expanded further. With this expanded knowledge and skill, there is potentially further advancement of theoretical, evidence-based, and practical knowledge in caring for a specific patient population base. Examples of subspecialty

practices within the specialty of adult health nursing include diabetes, transplant nursing, and palliative care nursing. Examples of subspecialty practice within the specialty of psychiatric/mental health nursing include substance abuse/addiction and geriatric psychiatry. Notably, most of the practice opportunities chosen for discussion in this chapter are subspecialty practices. This distinction between specialty and subspecialty is important, particularly for certification and regulatory reasons. The National Council of State Boards of Nursing (NCSBN) is proposing the regulation of advanced practice nursing in terms of certification requirements at the broad "population foci" level, with subspecialty certification being voluntary (NCSBN, 2007). Regulatory considerations aside, the expansion of advanced practice nursing is increasingly occurring in subspecialty practice. Indeed, expanding the boundaries of specialty nursing practice into subspecialties places APNs on the cutting edge of clinical care delivery in a complex, ever-changing, health care environment. However, for the sake of brevity in the remainder of the chapter, we refer to both *specialty* and *subspecialty practices* as *specialties*.

The evolution of specialty nursing practice to advanced practice nursing follows a trajectory that has been described by several authors (Beitz, 2000; Bigbee & Amidii-Nouri, 2000; Hamric, 2000; Lewis, 2000; see also Chapter 1). Hanson and Hamric (2003) synthesized these observations and characterized this evolution as having four distinct stages (Table 18-1). Initially, the specialty develops in response to changing patient needs—needs that are usually a result of new technology, new medical specialties, and/or changes in the health care workforce. For example, a lack of pediatric residents created an opportunity for development of the neonatal NP role (DeNicola, Klied, & Brink, 1994).

A second phase of development is characterized by progress to the point that organized "training" in the specialty begins. This training is often institution-specific, on-the-job training that develops experts in the specialty. Some of these institution-specific programs develop into certificate programs; however, the content may not be standardized, and the quality of these programs may vary. Examples include early transplant coordination roles in major transplant centers (see "Clinical Transplant Coordination" section) and, more recently, clinical research coordination.

In the third phase, the knowledge base required for specialty practice becomes more extensive and the

Table **18-1**   Four Stages in the Evolution of Advanced Practice Nursing

Stage	Characteristics
Stage I* Specialty Begins	Specialty develops in practice settings Development driven by increasing complexity in care demands, new technology, changing workforce opportunities On-the-job training and expansion of practice Not exclusively nursing
Stage II* Specialty Organizes	Organized training for specialty practice begins Institution-specific training develops Initially uses apprenticeship model Progresses to certificate training Specialty organization forms Certification examination develops but may not be nursing-specific Writings appear on role of nurse in specialty
Stage III* Pressures Mount for Standardization	Knowledge base grows; pressures mount for standardization and graduate education Knowledge base keeps growing, and scope of practice expands for practitioners in the specialty Expanded practice leads to expanded regulatory oversight Leaders call for transition to graduate education and differentiated practice to standardize practice in the specialty APNs migrate to specialty, or specialty nurses return to school Articles appear differentiating APN role in the specialty
Stage IV Maturity and Growing Interdisciplinarity	APN practice in the specialty is well articulated and recognized by other providers APNs practice collaboratively with other practitioners in the specialty APNS are experts in the specialty or subspecialty Shared knowledge base with other health care professionals is recognized Interdisciplinary certification examinations are developed

*Adapted from Hanson, C.M., & Hamric, A.B. (2003). Reflections on the continuing evolution of advanced practice nursing, *Nursing Outlook, 51*, 204.
APN, Advanced practice nurse.

scope of practice of the nurse with specialty training expands. There is growing recognition of the additional knowledge and skill needed for increasingly complex practice in the specialty. It is not unusual at this stage to see APNs in other specialties migrate into an evolving specialty and further expand the specialty by infusing it with advanced practice core competencies, making the specialty resemble advanced practice and creating new calls for evolution to this higher level. This transition is clearly evident in wound, ostomy, and continence nursing (see "Wound, Ostomy, and Continence Nursing" section), as well as in palliative care nursing. Over time, pressure for standardization of education and skills involved in the specialty arise from clinicians, the profession, and regulators. Certificate-level training programs move into graduate schools that assume responsibility for preparing nurses for these evolving

specialties—improving standardization, elevating the status of the specialty, and fostering its emergence as an advanced practice role. In this third stage of the trajectory, graduate education becomes an expected level of preparation (Hanson & Hamric, 2003).

Stage four is characterized by mature and recognized APN practice in the specialty, along with an emerging understanding of a shared interdisciplinary component. Nurse practitioners in human immunodeficiency virus (HIV) medicine who have attained certification as an HIV specialist, awarded by the American Academy of HIV Medicine, are an example of mature, expert practitioners who share an interdisciplinary clinical knowledge base with physicians in this specialty.

It is important to note that these stages are dynamic and not mutually exclusive. It is not unusual for specialties to show characteristics of more than

Box 18-1   Issues in the Evolution of Specialty to Advanced Practice Nursing

- Defining the attributes of advanced practice in the specialty
- Delineating the core competencies of the specialty as encompassing the core competencies of advanced practice
- Delineating a vision of advanced practice that may step outside of nursing's traditional vision of what constitutes an advanced practice role and gaining support within nursing and the health care community for the role

- Standardizing curricula for achieving competency at the advanced practice level
- Clarifying certification and credentialing requirements
- Overcoming legal and regulatory issues that are barriers to patient and/or consumer access to APNs
- Promoting recognition of APNs and nursing as a profession
- Clarifying APN role titles to be consistent and decrease confusion

Adapted from Hanson, C.M., & Hamric, A.B. (2003). Reflections on the continuing evolution of advanced practice nursing, *Nursing Outlook, 51,* 205. *APN,* Advanced practice nurse.

one stage simultaneously (e.g., graduate programs began to develop at the same time that most practitioners in the specialty were prepared in certificate programs). In addition, the duration of each stage may significantly vary by specialty. We contend that the evolution from specialty to advanced practice nursing can represent a natural maturation that should result from deliberate, logical planning to strengthen the education and broaden the scope of practice of specialty nurses. Some of these roles evolve to fulfill needs of specific patient populations or the needs of organizations. In some cases, changes in the legal recognition and regulation of practice also influence the movement toward advanced practice nursing. Complex and often controversial issues must be addressed both before and during this process (Box 18-1). In the following sections, the evolution of particular specialties to advanced practice nursing is described and these issues are discussed. Some specialties are struggling to evolve, and change is haphazard. Others are following a planned course of action and have emerged (or will soon do so) at the advanced practice level. Two challenges all evolving specialties share are the need to gain support both within and external to nursing for these roles and the need to clearly delineate their potential contributions in the health care environment.

INNOVATIVE PRACTICE OPPORTUNITIES: STAGE I

The initial stage of the evolution from specialty practice to advanced practice is characterized by the development of a specialty focus. Numerous examples are apparent in the history of nursing, which is replete with accounts of nursing's response to unmet patient needs. As a consequence, definable specialties emerge as nurses expand their practice to include the knowledge and skills necessary to meet the needs of patients requiring specialty care. Examples from our history include the specialty of enterostomal therapy (ET) nursing, now known as *wound, ostomy, continence (WOC) nursing,* and forensic nursing, which encompasses the care provision in correctional facilities, psychiatric settings, and emergency departments as nurse examiners care for sexual assault and child abuse victims (Burgess, Berger, & Boersma, 2004; Doyle, 2001; Hutson, 2002; Maeve & Vaughn, 2001; McCrone & Shelton, 2001). As specialties begin to coalesce, the practice may not be viewed as a nursing role. For example, early enterostomal therapists were lay persons with ostomies. However, as the specialty evolves, the valuable contributions of nurses begin to distinguish them from other care providers.

Several evolving roles in nursing are characterized as being "innovative." Some of these roles do not reflect the core competencies of advanced practice nursing, and the role components differ significantly, in some cases, from those of an APN. For example, if the focus of practice in forensic nursing had remained on the gathering of legal evidence, not sustained clinical practice using advanced practice core competency elements, the role would not be evolving to an advanced practice level. Regardless, nurses functioning in these specialties, some of whom are APNs, make unique contributions to the health of specific populations of patients. One such role to be explored as a stage I specialty is that of the acute care nurse practitioner (ACNP) hospitalist.

Acute Care Nurse Practitioner Hospitalist Practice

The ACNP emerged in the early 1990s as an advanced practice role that originated, in part, from the need for oversight of patients with acute and critical conditions. Since then, ACNP practice has evolved to incorporate a variety of practice settings and specialty-based care (Cole & Kleinpell, 2006). One of the earliest practice settings to benefit from the ability of these APNs to manage more complex patients was the emergency care setting. In this setting, essential aspects of practice, as proposed in the Emergency Nurses Association (ENA) scope-of-practice statement for NPs, included advanced assessment skills; the ability to triage and prioritize, resuscitate, and stabilize; and the ability to intervene in crisis situations as essential aspects of practice (Cole, Ramirez, & Luna-Gonzales, 1999). More recently, an opportunity to practice in a relatively new, innovative specialty has evolved out of the physician hospitalist model of care (Nyberg, 2006); see Exemplar 18-1.

The development of the hospitalist movement over the past 10 years represents a break in the tradition of primary care physicians (PCPs) managing patients in both inpatient and outpatient settings. In this model, inpatients are cared for by a *hospitalist physician*—a term coined by Wachter and Goldman (1996)—whose primary professional focus is the general medical care of hospitalized patients (Coffman & Rundall, 2005). Inpatient management is voluntarily transferred by the PCP to the hospitalist during the hospital admission, and upon discharge, care is resumed by the PCP.

The Society of Hospital Medicine (SHM), with over 6000 members, is a multidisciplinary organization (physicians, physician assistants [PAs], NPs) with the following goals (Society of Hospital Medicine, 2007):
- Promote high quality care for all hospitalized patients.
- Promote education and research in hospital medicine.
- Promote teamwork to achieve the best possible care for hospitalized patients.
- Advocate a career path that will attract and retain the highest quality hospitalists.
- Define the competencies, activities, and needs of the hospitalist community.
- Support, propose, and promote changes to the health care system that lead to higher quality and more efficient care for all hospitalized patients.

This organization recognizes the contributions of non-physician providers and has established a committee within the organizational structure to develop initiatives and programs to promote and define the role of NPs and PAs in hospital medicine (SHM, 2006). Depending on the outcomes of these endeavors, there are three distinct possibilities with respect to hospitalist providers: (1) the hospitalist model will remain a physician-only model; (2) the practice will become interdisciplinary; or (3) a transfer of technology will occur, and ACNPs and PAs will be the majority providers. The first and last options seem least likely in light of the efforts of the SHM to include non-physician providers in organizational decision making—implying an interest in and willingness to support a collaborative practice model. What seems most likely to occur is the development of non-physician (PA, ACNP)–physician teams to provide differentiated levels of care in the inpatient setting.

Commentary: Stage I

Hospitalist practice is a quickly emerging specialty within medicine. Although NPs, particularly ACNPs, are beginning to practice in this medical specialty, we see this as a stage I specialty for two reasons: (1) the specialty is not a nursing specialty, and describing unique distinctions between an ACNP hospitalist and a physician hospitalist have not yet been attempted; and (2) ACNP preparation for hospitalist practice is on-the-job because programs preparing ACNPs for this role do not exist. One challenge for this stage I specialty is to clearly articulate the unique contributions that ACNPs can bring to the care of hospitalized patients that may decrease fragmentation of care and improve interdisciplinary collaboration. In addition, to transition away from an on-the-job training model, graduate nursing programs offering ACNP education can ensure that hospital practice, based on the identified competencies in hospital medicine (Dressler, Pistoria, Budnitz, McKean, & Amin, 2006), is incorporated in required clinical practica. The challenge to any APN moving into this specialty is to maintain APN competencies and avoid a practice that is *strictly* an extension of medical practice.

SPECIALTIES IN TRANSITION: STAGE II

Stage II roles are characterized by progress in the evolution of the specialty to the point that organized training in the specialty begins. This training is often institution-specific, on-the-job training that develops

The Hospital Medicine Nurse Practitioner Service at Strong Memorial Hospital/University of Rochester Medical Center was started in 1995 as an initiative to reduce length of stay. Four nurse practitioners (NPs) were hired along with a hospitalist to start a short-stay unit. Patients included those with myocardial infarction rule-outs, new-onset atrial fibrillation, and simple cellulitis, as well as those needing observation after procedures. The NPs covered the unit 10 hours per day, 5 days per week, with fellows and other housestaff covering the remaining hours (Mary Alice Terboss, personal communication, October 26, 2007).

Since its inception, the service has grown exponentially, primarily in response to the reduced number of medical resident positions and tighter restrictions on resident work hours by the Accreditation Council on Graduate Medical Education (ACGME). In addition, the team's census grew along with the hospital census when two hospitals in the city closed. Other changes include an increase in patients, the addition of physician assistants (PAs) to the team, and orthopedic surgery patients attended to by the Hospital Medicine Service. The service has expanded to cover patients on 15 patient care units, 24 hours per day, 7 days per week, including holidays.

The specialty of hospital medicine is relatively new, and therefore the role of the acute care nurse practitioner (ACNP) varies from hospital to hospital. At Strong Memorial, ACNPs have a variety of roles and responsibilities. They collaborate with the Hospital Medicine Division physicians and community-based primary care providers and share responsibility for examinations, note and order writing, and discharge planning. The ACNPs also follow patients admitted to subspecialty services such as gastroenterology, nephrology, cardiology, and infectious diseases. Whereas the subspecialist attending physician or fellow may focus on the organ of interest, the ACNP independently manages co-morbidities, updates families, and coordinates care, all of which provide a more holistic perspective to the patient's hospital stay.

Concrete, defined tasks include admitting histories, physical examinations, orders, discharge instructions and summaries, and a daily visit with a progress note. ACNPs order and interpret diagnostic and laboratory tests, participate in multidisciplinary unit rounds, and update an electronic sign-out system for safer handoffs. Procedures such as line placement are usually provided by residents as part of their educational experience.

Many of the ACNP's responsibilities are less easily defined or measured. However, in these functions the ACNP adds value to the care provided by the Hospital Medicine Service. These functions include coordination of care among the variety of consultants, other health professionals (e.g., physical therapists, nutritionists, social workers), and unit management. In addition, ACNPs update patients and families to maintain open communication and keep them informed of the care plan. They also orient new ACNPs to their role and mentor ACNP students. Most importantly, ACNPs collaborate with the bedside nurses and unit staff. Communication of updates, orders, and plans is essential to ensuring safe, timely, and quality care. The accessibility of the ACNP promotes collaboration and many opportunities for informal teaching. As advanced practice nurses, ACNPs are often the most knowledgeable about medication information, technology management, or even basic nursing care and can serve as resources for newer, less experienced nurses. Teaching and mentoring are important to ensure staff development and retention as well as safe patient care. The importance of these activities has been difficult to quantify. It has been and continues to be a challenge to the Hospital Medicine Service to measure these contributions and illustrate their value.

The future for ACNPs on Hospital Medicine teams is promising. The specialty is growing along with the acuity of inpatients and the complexities of discharge planning—both of which ACNPs are well-suited to manage. ACNP programs are incorporating hospital medicine into their curricula and into clinical rotations. The ACNPs on the Hospital Medicine Service have precepted many of these students—some of whom have gone on to join our team. Many challenges are ahead, including finding ways to quantify our contribution in terms of quality of care, length of stay, and patient and staff satisfaction. Orienting new ACNPs to handle the complexity of these inpatients and recruiting for 24-hour, 7-days-per-week positions is also a challenge.

I find my role as an ACNP on the Hospital Medicine Service to be highly satisfying because I care for patients with a wide variety of health problems. I also have the opportunity every day to teach, learn, and make a difference for a patient or another nurse. Finally, it is very rewarding to work on a *team* of APNs who are so dedicated to hospital medicine, providing excellent patient care, and supporting and helping each other. I am proud to be an ACNP in hospitalist practice.

*We gratefully acknowledge Elizabeth Palermo, MS, RN, APRN-BC, Rochester, NY, for her assistance with this exemplar.

experts in the specialty. The two roles that are discussed as demonstrating predominantly stage II characteristics but may exhibit some characteristics of stage III are those of the clinical transplant coordinator (CTC) and the forensic nurse. The CTC role is clearly subspecialty practice, whereas the forensic nursing role can best be characterized as a specialty having several subspecialty opportunities.

Clinical Transplant Coordination

There is mounting evidence that the role of the CTC is evolving to the level of advanced practice nursing in response to patient care requirements in the referral and evaluation phase for patients, their families and living donors, and in the pre- and post-transplant management phases of candidates and recipients. One issue for this evolving specialty is that not all CTCs are nurses—individuals with widely differing preparation assume these roles. Organized training in the specialty in the form of an introductory course (for new clinical and procurement transplant coordinators) and continuing education (for those with more experience) is offered by the North American Transplant Coordinators Organization (NATCO), but institution-specific, on-the-job education and experience are widely embraced. Continuing education opportunities are also offered by specialty organizations such as ITNS and specialty scientific societies.

Unlike the efforts to move specialty education into graduate nursing programs described by WOC nurses (Gray, Ratliff, & Mawyer, 2000), health care providers in diabetes care (Melkus & Fain, 1995), and other established advanced practice roles (Bjorklund, 2003; Lynch, Cope, & Murphy-Ende, 2001; Murphy-Ende, 2002; Naegle & Krainovich-Miller, 2001), expertise in transplantation nursing is gained in clinical practice and through continuing education (McNatt & Easom, 2000). However, ITNS recently published a core curriculum for the specialty (Ohler & Cupples, 2007), and a newly developed scope and standards of practice statement, developed in conjunction with the ANA, is available on the organization's website (ITNS, 2007). This document clearly addresses the scope of practice for generalist transplant nurses, clinical and procurement transplant coordinators, and advanced practice transplant nurses—both NPs and CNSs. Building on the practice of the registered nurse generalist and transplant nurse coordinator by demonstrating a greater depth and breadth of knowledge, greater synthesis of data and interventions, and

significant role autonomy that may include medical diagnosis and prescriptive authority, APNs working in transplant centers integrate and apply a broad range of theoretical and evidence-based knowledge using both specialized and expanded knowledge and skills (ITNS, 2007).

CTCs are essential for the continuity of care provided to transplant recipients. Most transplant centers employ coordinators; however, in some centers the role does not require that coordinators possess skills that reflect the core competencies of an APN (Reel, 1999). Specialty nurses with expertise in transplant nursing recognize the complex needs of their patients. Many obtain graduate education to better prepare them to deal with the realities of transplant nursing. To the benefit of their patients, these coordinators have expanded the specialty by incorporating advanced practice core competencies.

It can be argued that the complex needs of patients with end-stage organ disease require higher levels of clinical reasoning and analytical skills, such as those possessed by APNs; however, to advance the CTC role (not just individuals in the role) to this higher level, attention to several issues is necessary. First and foremost, leaders in the specialty must systematically determine whether advanced practice core competencies (see Chapter 3 and Part 2) are required to fully enact the role or whether two levels of differentiated practice—generalist professional and APN—should be defined for the specialty. Second, the specialty's leadership must agree that the role is a nursing role. Making these decisions may disenfranchise many committed and experienced transplant professionals who are essential care providers. Similar to the levels of certification proposed for diabetes educators (Daly, Kulkarni, & Boucher, 2001; Hentzen, 1994), some similar method of differentiation, which would recognize the added value that advanced practice knowledge and skill brings to the CTC role, might serve to acknowledge the contributions of both APNs and other transplant professionals. Both the ITNS and NATCO seem to be moving in this direction by (1) delineating the core competencies required for clinical and procurement transplant coordinators (North American Transplant Coordinators Organization [NATCO], 2004), (2) development of a core curriculum for transplant nursing at the generalist level (Ohler & Cupples, 2007), and as of 2004, (3) initiating a certification examination for the clinical transplant nurse (certified clinical transplant nurse [CCTN]) (in addition to certification as a transplant coordinator) (American Board for Transplant Certification [ABTC], 2007).

Certification as a transplant coordinator is conferred by the ABTC by written examination. Advanced education is not required for certification. Because this organization credentials all categories of transplant professionals, licensure as a registered nurse (RN) is also not a requirement. Recertification is achieved through continuing education. The issue of specialty versus subspecialty certification is an issue for all evolving advanced practice nursing specialties. We consider the case of transplantation in some detail to illustrate the complex issues surrounding the certification process for any evolving role.

A model proposed by McNatt and Easom (2000) addressed the credentialing and certification of APNs in nephrology nursing and renal transplantation, as an example. Currently, nephrology nurses are certified through the American Nephrology Nursing Association (ANNA), a subspecialty certification that does not require specific educational preparation. McNatt and Easom suggest that nephrology APNs should have a graduate nursing degree in a defined clinical specialty, should have national specialty certification in their area of advanced practice (e.g., as NPs or CNSs), and should be board-eligible for or certified in nephrology nursing. Transplant coordinator certification (certified clinical transplant coordinator [CCTC]) would be an additional certification for APNs. They would be differentiated from other transplant professionals who hold the same certification by their expanded scope of practice as well as their credentials as CNSs or NPs. McNatt and Easom's model essentially depicts a modular certification configuration for nephrology and renal transplantation nurses that may have utility for other transplant specialties (e.g., cardiac, lung, liver).

This conceptualization is similar to an option proposed by Lyon (2002) regarding specialty versus subspecialty certification for CNSs, in which she described an examination process to test for core competencies (for legal recognition) and a subspecialty certification to test advanced clinical knowledge. Hanson and Hamric (2003) suggest expanding on this idea, with different modules being developed to evaluate advanced practice core competencies as well as knowledge required for functioning in various advanced practice roles (e.g., CNS, ACNP, CNM). Because some advanced practice nursing is subspecialty practice (e.g., organ transplantation, diabetes), a model that incorporates subspecialty certification, in addition to a credentialing process that evaluates core competencies and knowledge required for a particular APN role, should be considered as long as the process is not unnecessarily restrictive. McNatt and Easom's model addresses this modular certification approach, as well as the need for standardization of education and skills involved in the specialty. It can facilitate role and scope of practice differentiation among renal transplantation professionals and may have utility for other evolving subspecialties beyond the transplantation arena.

Educational institutions that prepare APNs must consider the certification options available and address methods of preparing students for certification beyond currently available credentialing requirements. They must also ensure that their graduates are eligible to sit for APN certification examinations approved for legal recognition of an APN role.

The CTC role in organ transplantation is evolving from a traditional model focusing on coordination of services to one incorporating the knowledge and skill of an advanced practice nurse (Martin, 1999; Morse, 2001; Reel, 1999). This evolution has been haphazard as a result of inattention to several issues. Most notably, the lack of recognition that the role requires advanced practice competencies and the lack of opportunities for subspecialty certification may impede expansion into advanced practice nursing as an expectation of coordinator roles. The issue of subspecialty certification (at the generalist level) has been addressed, but no plans for advanced practice certification have been proposed. Also, some disagree about the preferred advanced practice role for the specialty, with some authors advocating the CNS and others the blended CNS/NP or ACNP (Martin, 1999; Morse, 2001; Reel, 1999). The scope of practice document recently developed by the ITNS clearly embraces both CNS and NP roles, so this disagreement may become moot in the future. Clearly, there is a commitment to advanced practice nursing in transplantation, and given that commitment, more attention to these issues will be necessary for the CTC role to evolve to stage III.

Exemplar 18-2 demonstrates the complexity of care required for transplant candidates, recipients, and their families. In addition to expertise in advanced practice core competencies, the exemplar also highlights the skill of the CNS in dealing with systems issues and staff education, both of which are important components of providing care to this challenging

EXEMPLAR 18-2   Heart Transplant Coordinator*

Given the complexity of care associated with solid organ transplant patients, most transplant programs have multidisciplinary teams that care for candidates and recipients (Donaldson, 2003). The clinical transplant coordinator's role is to facilitate the care of the patient, in collaboration with the multidisciplinary team, throughout the transplant process—a process that begins with the patient's initial referral to the transplant program and often continues for the rest of the patient's life.

As a CNS, my clinical transplant coordinator position affords me the opportunity to incorporate the core competencies of advanced practice nursing. My clinical practice role includes both direct and indirect care activities. For example, key direct care activities involve coordinating detailed discharge planning, seeing patients in transplant clinic, and triaging telephone calls from candidates, recipients, and family members. Indirect care activities include participating in interdisciplinary clinical rounds (e.g., transfer conferences as patients transition from the intensive care unit to the intermediate care unit), developing protocols and patient education materials, participating in performance evaluation and improvement activities, initiating referrals to other health care specialists, and facilitating staff support groups. One example of staff support involved a transplant candidate with biventricular mechanical support who remained hospitalized for over 12 months until a suitable donor organ became available. Over the course of this prolonged hospitalization, the nursing staff encountered several challenging problems. Many of the patient-staff conflicts revolved around the patient's desire for autonomy and the staff's need to provide care in a timely manner (e.g., dressing changes, physical therapy). Consultative sessions with the transplant team's neuropsychologist and social worker were held biweekly. The neuropsychologist enhanced the staff's understanding of the patient's cognitive status, and the social worker helped the staff articulate their frustrations. Over time, in concert with the patient, mutually acceptable strategies were devised and implemented. For example, staff members negotiated with the patient in developing a daily schedule that permitted him to "sleep in" on weekends when the census was typically low and the staff had more flexibility in providing care. In turn, the patient agreed to follow a more rigid schedule on weekdays.

My role affords many opportunities for staff and patient education. Staff education is both formal (e.g., teaching in the critical care nurse internship program) and informal (e.g., answering staff nurses' questions during rounds). Patient education involves extensive teaching sessions with prospective transplant candidates and their family members. The purpose of these sessions is to provide patients with information so they can make informed decisions about whether they wish to proceed with transplantation. Once a patient decides to proceed and is placed on the waiting list, additional education is provided during monthly support group meetings. After the transplant procedure, recipients and family members attend comprehensive discharge education sessions. Post-discharge education is provided through newsletters, support group meetings, and individual counseling sessions during clinic visits.

One example of my role as collaborator is my participation with the interdisciplinary team that discusses, plans, implements, and evaluates the ongoing care of transplant candidates and recipients. One of our major responsibilities is to determine whether a particular patient meets the heart transplant program's physiological and psychosocial eligibility criteria for placement on the waiting list. A second example concerns technology transfer, more specifically, the transfer of scientific advances of mechanical assist device technology into clinical practice. When the heart transplant team was about to discharge our first patient with an LVAD, I collaborated with the heart transplant research nurse, social worker, NP, physicians, hospital administrators, MedStar flight crew members, and community resource providers (e.g., the local power company) in facilitating this process. The purpose of this collaborative effort was to establish physiological and psychosocial criteria for discharge and to develop policies and procedures regarding emergent and routine follow-up care.

Last, I have had the opportunity to collaborate with an international, multidisciplinary task force in reviewing the literature pertaining to the biopsychosocial outcomes of cardiothoracic transplantation, evaluating the strength of the evidence, and developing specific recommendations for future research designed to improve psychosocial and clinical outcomes.

*We gratefully acknowledge Sandra A. Cupples, DNSc, RN, Washington, DC, for assistance with this exemplar.
CNS, Clinical nurse specialist; *LVAD*, left ventricular assist device; *NP*, nurse practitioner.

patient population. It is our view that the knowledge and expertise of advanced practice nurses could fully enable the potential of the CTC position.

Forensic Nursing

Forensic nursing has emerged as a specialty as a result of the severity of the national public health problems associated with violence. Recognition of the severity of the problem was first addressed in 1985 at the Surgeon General's Workshop on Violence and Public Health. In opening remarks, C. Everett Koop, MD, championed a multidisciplinary approach that addressed both prevention of violence and providing better care for victims of violence. The severity of the problem was again addressed by the World Health Organization (WHO) in the World Report on Violence and Health (World Health Organization [WHO], 2002). As the first comprehensive summary on the global impact of violence, it stated that more than 1.6 million people die from violence every year and more are injured and suffer mental health consequences.

In 1991, the ANA published a position statement on violence as a nursing practice issue, and in 1995, at the request of the International Association of Forensic Nurses (IAFN), they officially recognized forensic nursing as a specialty. In the wake of the ANA position statement, the American College of Nurse Midwives (in 1995) and the Emergency Nurses Association (in 1996) issued similar statements (Burgess et al., 2004). The scope and standards of forensic nursing practice was published in 1997 (ANA, 1997).

Since the 1970s, nurses have been formally recognized providers of health care services to victims of violence. Nurses have volunteered at rape-crisis centers and by the mid-1980s were widely acknowledged for the expertise they had developed. In addition, nurses were also being recognized for their research competence. This combination of factors opened doors for nurses to collaborate with other care providers, initiate courses and programs of research on victimology and traumatology, influence legislation and health care policy, and ultimately create a new specialty (Burgess et al., 2004). Exemplar 18-3 depicts APN competencies in the forensic specialty.

Forensic nursing practice is, according to the IAFN (2007), the application of nursing science to public or legal proceedings and often involves work with perpetrators and victims of interpersonal violence (sexual assault, abuse, domestic violence), death investigation, legal and ethical issues. Forensic nurses interact with forensic psychiatric nurses, correctional nurses, emergency nurses, and trauma nurses. Forensic nurses may work for specialized hospital units, in medical examiners' offices, or for law enforcement and social services agencies (IAFN).

Like most stage II specialties, forensic nursing has traditionally been taught outside of formal educational programs. Some of the earliest programs were institution-based programs preparing nurses as sexual assault nurse examiners (SANEs). Certification is obtained through the Forensic Nursing Certification Board (FNCB), established in 2002 to promote the highest standards of forensic nursing practice. The FNCB offers the sexual assault nurse examiner–adult/adolescent (SANE-A) certification, as well as a sexual assault nurse examiner–pediatric (SANE-P) certification. Newer educational programs, such as those that prepare sexual assault forensic examiners (SAFEs) or forensic nurse examiners (FNEs), have begun to replace SANE programs and will expand the scope of forensic nursing practice to include not only sexual assault incidents but also the gathering of forensic evidence in cases of domestic abuse or vehicular accidents (Burgess et al., 2004). The IAFN believes that the attainment of a common knowledge base, utilization of the nursing process, and a high level of skill in the practice setting are required for the specialty practice of forensic nursing.

The trend of educating forensic nurses in certificate programs is changing as graduate nursing programs are established; thus forensic nursing is a specialty in transition. Similar to the efforts to move WOC nursing into graduate nursing education programs (Gray et al., 2000), forensic nursing has been taught at the graduate level in a few institutions for several years. Although certificate programs are often the route to preparation (and certification), recently some of these programs have transitioned to offer a DNP in forensic nursing.

Commentary: Stage II

Forensic nursing provides a different perspective on evolving specialties and is used here to illustrate a stage II specialty practice that may become an advanced practice role integrating multiple specialties. In stage II, the specialty becomes more organized and visible. Formal training programs develop, specialty organizations form, and certification moves beyond individual institution-based certificates for completion of training to national certification examinations. All of these developments lend strength

EXEMPLAR 18-3 Forensic Nurse Examiner*

Prevention and prosecution of violent crimes has become a priority in today's society. Because many of the victims of violence seek medical care in addition to justice services, many disciplines provide services. The role of the forensic nurse examiner (FNE), as part of a team of care providers, is to initiate medical care, collect evidence, collaborate with law enforcement, and testify as an expert witness.

As both a team member and the director of the FNE team, I demonstrate the core competencies of an APN. My practice includes patient care, participation on a community-based multidisciplinary team, ethical decision making, clinically focused research, and staff education. Even though most of my practice is related to the care of sexual assault victims, I also provide direct care and consultative services for victims of physical assaults (e.g., gunshot wounds, stabbings).

Clinical practice is at the core of my role as an APN and includes both direct patient care and other APN competencies. Examples of direct care include initiation of necessary medical treatments such as pregnancy and sexually transmitted infection prophylaxis, immediate crisis intervention, discharge care standards, and follow-up with victims. By standardizing the care of sexual assault and child abuse victims, they receive comprehensive care with an introduction to available resources in the community. Examples of other competencies include consultation in the development of protocols for evidence collection and clinical and systems leadership in the implementation of systems to assure confidentiality related to photographs, especially after a sexual assault. Other examples include collaborative participation in the development of sexual assault resource teams and local child advocacy centers. The sexual assault resource teams include health care professionals (forensic nurses and physicians), law enforcement officers, prosecutors, individuals who provide victim and child and adult protective services, and forensic interviewers. These teams bring together all available community resources to strengthen the response to violent crimes. In addition, team members have the opportunity to voice concerns regarding services that might not put victims' needs first. A team approach that involves direct care providers who act as advocates creates the opportunity for a FNE to help meet the immediate needs of victims without compromising the police investigation. Although this may seem to limit

what the FNE provides, this collaborative approach to managing a complex situation allows for evidence collection and referral to other health care providers and victims' services.

In dealing with victims of violence, ethical decision making is embedded in the practice of all the FNE team members. Issues to be confronted include personal feelings about the victim's appearance, behavior, and demeanor; confidentiality; and maintaining the integrity of the evidence. As an APN, I role model ethical behaviors related to these issues for other FNE team members in order to guide and develop their practice. I often have opportunities to coach team members through situations that may reflect ethical dilemmas or those that create moral distress related to dealing with victims of violence or abuse and providing victim's services.

Research is a strong component of my practice. Recent challenges to expert witness testimony regarding injuries following a sexual assault compared with injuries following consensual intercourse brought to light the lack of scientific evidence in two sexual assault cases: Commonwealth of Virginia *v.* Johnston and Commonwealth of Virginia *v.* Velasquez (Canaff, 2004). Both cases challenged the limits of medical expert testimony in situations in which the issue of consent to intercourse was being questioned. Because of these questions, I initiated a program of research to examine some of these issues. With the assistance of other experts in the field, my research examines differences between microscopic genital injuries after sexual assault and consensual intercourse to determine differences in the types, number, and location of the injuries. Information obtained from my research is still preliminary and needs to be replicated; the findings are, however, being used in court testimony.

Developing a Sexual Assault Nurse Examiner (SANE) training program is an example of staff guidance and coaching that is a major focus of my role. When the SANE program was started at the University of Virginia, nurses were trained primarily to collect evidence for adult sexual assault victims. As the nurses have continued developing in this role, SANE team members have expanded their forensic nursing expertise and the types of services they can offer by attending numerous training programs. Additional training in forensic photography, death investigation, child sexual and physical abuse, and expert witness testimony has

*We gratefully acknowledge Sarah Anderson PhD, RN, Charlottesville, VA, for assistance with this exemplar.
IAFN, International Association of Forensic Nurses.

EXEMPLAR 18-3   Forensic Nurse Examiner*—cont'd

allowed the team to expand the types of services offered, enhanced the quality of photographic and written documentation of evidentiary findings, and expanded the realm of expert court testimony.

At this point in the development of the forensic nursing specialty, formal graduate education is not required and is not locally available. To help our program expand, I began a forensic nursing training program that develops new team members by using the expertise of experienced team members. By developing the program of study, which includes educational content based on the standards set by the IAFN, I was able to incorporate the most recent research into the curriculum, promote retention of current team members, recruit new team

members, and provide research and teaching opportunities for interested nurses. For example, current team members who have developed proficiency in specific areas incorporated in the curriculum are mentored to develop their ability to teach. By providing coaching and guidance, I help them develop their abilities to plan and deliver information on topics that reflect their areas of clinical expertise.

As an APN in forensic nursing, my role incorporates expert clinical practice, consultation, collaboration, leadership, guidance and coaching, ethical decision making, and research for an important but underserved population—victims of violent crimes.

and credibility to the specialty and its practitioners. Although many forensic nurses are prepared in certificate programs, being a specialty in transition to advanced practice nursing presents some opportunities for this particular specialty to evolve. Some of the graduate forensic nursing programs, which have existed as master's and post-master's programs, are transitioning to DNP programs and, as a consequence of these efforts, may be able to hasten their progress.

One of the major challenges in stage II is demonstrating that the specialty is a nursing specialty. There are a number of evolving specialties, such as clinical research coordinators and clinical transplant coordinators, whose practitioners include non-nurses as well as nurses. Clearly, these roles cannot emerge as advanced practice nursing roles without clear distinctions being drawn between non-nursing practice and nursing practice in the specialty. Specialty organizations with members who are non–health care providers, such as the NATCO, must face this challenge. In the case of transplantation, for example, recognition of an APN level of practice or a sanctioning of practice at the APN level for all specialty providers may be evolving. For CTCs or other advanced practice nurses working with transplant candidates or recipients, a mechanism for certifying advanced practice transplant nurses (e.g., through the ITNS) is necessary to recognize nursing's essential role in transplantation without diminishing the contributions of others who also provide essential care and services.

EMERGING ADVANCED PRACTICE NURSING ROLES: STAGE III

In the third stage of evolution to advanced practice, a specialty's knowledge base is growing and the scope of practice of nurses with specialty education is expanding. There is growing recognition of the additional knowledge and skills needed for increasingly complex practice in the specialty (Hamric, 2000). Pressures for standardization of education and skills required for specialty practice create incentives to move certificate-level training programs into graduate-level educational settings, both to increase standardization and to raise the status of the specialty to an advanced practice level (Hanson & Hamric, 2003). According to Hanson and Hamric (2003), antecedents to legitimizing advanced practice roles must be addressed for a given specialty to evolve to advanced levels of practice (see Box 18-1). Two organizations that are addressing the issues necessary to legitimize advanced practice roles in their specialties are the Wound, Ostomy and Continence Nurses Society (WOCNS) and the International Society of Nurses in Genetics (ISONG). Although these organizations have adopted differing approaches to advancing practice in their respective specialties, the process, in each case, was unified and proactive and depicts a framework that can guide other specialty organizations as they chart a course to advanced levels of practice.

Wound, Ostomy, and Continence Nursing

Wound, ostomy, and continence (WOC) nursing, a specialty that developed in response to unmet patient needs after fecal or urinary diversion surgery, has evolved significantly since its inception in the 1960s. Historically, lay persons developed the specialty, dedicated exclusively to the care of ostomy patients (Wound, Ostomy and Continence Nurses Society [WOCNS], 1998). As health care changed and new patient needs arose, the original ET role evolved into a nursing specialty whose scope of practice expanded to include wound, skin, and continence care in addition to ostomy care. These WOC nurses became increasingly valued team members in acute care, outpatient settings, extended care facilities, and home care (Doughty, 2000).

The educational preparation for WOC nurses, which began as clinical training programs based heavily on experiential knowledge about ostomy management, has been provided within post-baccalaureate educational programs. Some of these programs have begun to offer graduate-level course work in the specialty. Thus the content has been integrated into graduate curricula of some universities throughout the United States (Gray et al., 2000). Growing expectations for research (Bryant, 1995; Gray, 1998; Palmer, 2000) and evidence-based practice (Roe & Moore, 2001) require research skills best taught in graduate nursing programs. Thus the WOCNS and the Wound Ostomy Continence Nursing Certification Board (WOCNCB) now differentiate entry-level from advanced practice certification.

To be eligible for entry-level nursing certification, *one* of the following requirements must be met by RNs seeking this credential: (1) graduation from an accredited WOC educational program requiring 120 didactic hours and 120 clinical hours; (2) completion of 1500 hours of clinical practice and 50 continuing education units (directly related to the specialty for which the certification is being pursued) within the past 5 years (for each specialty for which certification is being pursued; and (3) completion of a graduate-level program in nursing with documentation of clinical coursework equivalent to two semester hours in WOC nursing content. Advanced practice in WOC nursing as either a CNS or NP requires (1) a master's or doctoral degree in a related specialty area of nursing, (2) being clinically active in the WOC nursing specialty, and (3) advanced knowledge of the WOC nursing specialty via a valid and reliable measure of competency in the specialty (e.g., certification examination or professional portfolio) (WOCNS, 2007).

Recent decisions by the WOCNCB to differentiate certification based on education clearly represent progress in addressing the added value of APNs in this specialty. This is a critical decision point for this stage III specialty. Similar to the work done by the International Society of Nurses in Genetics (ISONG), who established levels of genetics knowledge, practice, and certification, WOC nursing has advocated for APNs as having unique characteristics and contributions to make. These contributions reflect advanced practice core competencies obtained in graduate nursing education in addition to competencies attained in a specialty program aimed at preparing WOC nurses. The advanced practice certification seems to build on the entry-level certification and offers an incentive to entry-level WOC nurses to complete graduate nursing education as an APN; it also further legitimizes the advanced practice of WOC nursing.

APNs in the specialty may also want to pursue additional recognition for advanced practice competency. Some nurses with graduate education in wound, ostomy, and/or continence nursing may seek certification as a wound management specialist (certified wound specialist [CWS]) awarded to qualified clinicians by the American Academy of Wound Management, a multidisciplinary organization, or as a urological specialist, for CNSs or NPs, by the certification board of the Society of Urologic Nurses and Associates. In particular, the CWS certification recognizes a shared clinical knowledge base among professionals providing care to patients with complex wounds and may foster collaborative relationships that would further advance this specialty.

Genetics Advanced Practice Nursing

Mapping of the human genome and the relevance of the Human Genome Project to health and disease are revolutionizing the provision of genetics services (specifically) and health care (generally). New genetic discoveries have made available an increasing number of genetic technologies for carrier, prenatal, diagnostic, and presymptomatic testing for genetic conditions. These discoveries are creating changes in the delivery of genetic services, the most immediate being the integration of genetics into the prevention and treatment of, for example, cardiovascular disease (Arnett et al., 2007), obesity (Yang, Kelly, & He, 2007), and cancer (Balmain, Gray, & Ponder, 2003). Although brought to the forefront of public awareness by the mapping of the human genome, genetics services initially emerged out of a need for professionals who could provide genetic information, education, and support to patients and families with current and future genetic health concerns. Genetics specialists in academic medical, public health, and community-based settings have traditionally provided these services. In each setting, genetics professionals, including medical geneticists, genetics counselors, and genetics APNs, provide genetics services to patients and families. Working with other team members, genetics specialists obtain and interpret complex family history information, evaluate and diagnose genetic conditions, interpret and discuss complicated genetic test results, support patients throughout the genetics counseling process, and offer resources for additional individual and family support. Over time, through interaction with these specialists, patients and family members come to learn and understand relevant aspects of genetics to make informed health decisions and receive support in integrating personal and family genetics information into their daily lives (Lea, Jenkins, & Francomano, 1998).

According to the ISONG, the scope of genetics nursing practice is both basic and advanced. At the basic level, genetics nurses are prepared to perform assessments to identify risk factors, plan care, provide interventions such as information, and evaluate for referral to genetic services. At the advanced level, master's-prepared nurses provide genetics counseling, case management, consultation, and evaluation of patients, families, resources, or programs (ANA/International Society of Nurses in Genetics [ISONG], 2007). Nurses in genetics clinical practice are certified by the Genetic Nursing Credentialing Commission (GNCC), established in 2001 in cooperation with the ISONG. Two levels of practice and recognition, which correspond to the scope of genetics nursing practice, currently exist: the genetics clinical nurse (GCN) and the APN in genetics (APNG). The credentials conferred by the GNCC mandate that specific educational, practice, and professional service requirements are met. The process is accomplished using a portfolio review. Noteworthy is the fact that the GNCC, in collaboration with the American Nurses Credentialing Center (ANCC) on this process, developed the portfolio with the intent that it become a benchmark for the profession (Monsen, 2005). Eligibility for the APNG credential requires a minimum of 3 years of experience as a clinical genetics nurse, completion of 300 hours of genetics practicum experiences (supervised by graduate nursing faculty with research or clinical emphasis in genetics, an APN in a genetics health care setting, board-certified health care professionals, or other clinicians who have a genetics

research or clinical background in their specialty area), and extensive documentation of patient care experiences reflecting the ISONG standards of clinical genetics nursing practice (ANA/ISONG, 2007).

The National Coalition for Health Professional Education in Genetics (NCHPEG), established in 1996 in cooperation with the ANA, the American Medical Association, and the National Human Genome Research Institute at the National Institutes of Health, has provided leadership in bringing advances in genetics to health care providers. The NCHPEG is a coalition of more than 100 professional organizations collaborating to promote professional education about advances in genetics. An interdisciplinary working group has developed recommendations for core competencies and curricula guidelines in genetics essential for nurses regardless of education, role, or clinical specialty (Jenkins & Calzone, 2007; Lewis, Calzone, & Jenkins, 2006).

Very few programs offer graduate-level genetics programs for nurses. Currently, educational preparation for APNs occurs in master's programs in nursing; genetics content is usually obtained later within post-baccalaureate educational programs or through continuing education courses. Course content must reflect information in human genetics; molecular and biochemical genetics; ethical, legal, and social issues in genetics; genetic variations in populations; and clinical application of genetics, including genetics counseling to meet requirements for certification. Growing expectations for evidence-based practice, which has the potential to transform health care because of integration of genetics knowledge, requires the knowledge and skill acquired in graduate nursing programs. In addition, the ethical decision-making skills of APNs are important to this specialty (see Chapter 11). Thus the ISONG may soon be faced with the choice of recommending advanced practice nursing education as minimum preparation for all nurses practicing in this specialty. This seems a particularly pressing issue because graduate nursing educational preparation, required for the APNG credential, will place these nurses at the same level as other genetics services providers and has the potential to foster professional diversity and interdisciplinary collaboration.

The American Board of Genetics Counselors (ABGC) certifies some nurses; however, this avenue is not open to nurses unless they complete graduate education and clinical practice requirements in genetics medicine, human genetics, and/or genetic counseling. Those nurses who wish to pursue graduate education in nursing are not eligible for this certification. Because the scope of practice for the APNG is much broader than that of a genetics counselor, differentiation based on credentials is appropriate. Collaboration among these professionals is necessary for appropriate genetics services delivery. Toward this end, the National Society of Genetics Counselors and the ISONG have jointly developed a position statement advocating a multidisciplinary and collaborative approach to enhance the quality of genetic services and care (ISONG, 2006). These efforts by the ISONG position the specialty to transition to a stage IV specialty as a result of collaborative efforts with genetics counselors.

Commentary: Stage III

The specialties discussed here that are in stage III are characterized by a growing knowledge base and an expanded scope of practice that is differentiated from basic professional practice in the specialty. Changes in the law and regulation of practice, particularly those expanding the scope of practice for APNs, have also affected this stage. As shown in Exemplar 18-4, the commitment of leaders in the specialty organizations has been the driving force behind the evolution of these roles to the advanced practice level. In each instance, the advancement efforts have been unified and proactive. However, attention to several issues is still necessary for the roles to fully emerge at the advanced level (Box 18-2). For example, WOC nurses have identified levels of WOC nursing practice to differentiate advanced practice from basic professional practice and now further differentiate entry level and advanced practice nursing through their credentialing process. The ISONG has made tremendous progress in defining various roles for health care providers, fostering a collaborative relationship with genetic counselors, and differentiating levels of practice within multidisciplinary teams. These efforts provide an excellent example to other organizations that are considering advanced practice opportunities in their specialties.

ESTABLISHED ADVANCED PRACTICE NURSING ROLES: STAGE IV

The fourth stage in the evolution of specialty practice to advanced practice is characterized by specialties that are mature. APNs practicing in those specialties are experts in the specialty or subspecialty, secure in understanding the unique contributions that they make in the direct care of patients. Yet they embrace the notion that aspects of their practice are shared by experts from other disciplines essential to the care of their patients. Because of its origins in interdisciplinary practice, the advanced diabetes manager best characterizes an established APN role.

Advanced Diabetes Manager

The rising incidence of diabetes mellitus (DM) has created new opportunities for APNs. Advances in the science and technology of diabetes care and findings from two clinical research trials have redefined the roles of health care providers in diabetes care. Two classic studies, the Diabetes Control and Complications Trial (DCCT) (1993) and the United Kingdom Prospective Diabetes Study (UKPDS) (1998), demonstrated the value of multidisciplinary teams consisting of dietitians, nurses, and pharmacists in the clinical management of individuals with DM. Before the results of these clinical trials were released, however, the American Association of Diabetes Educators (AADE) (1992) published multidisciplinary scope and standards of practice guidelines, which were revised as recently as 2005 (Martin, Daly, McWhorter, Shwide-Slavin, & Kushion, 2005). An advanced practice task force was established in 1993, and the dialogue among the three major disciplines constituting the membership of the association (nurses, dietitians, pharmacists) and their credentialing bodies was begun (Hentzen, 1994; Tobin, 2000). These collaborative efforts resulted in a definition of advanced practice in diabetes as the highest of various levels of practice utilized along the full continuum of diabetes care (Hentzen; Tobin). These levels are identified as the certified diabetes educator (CDE), and the board-certified advanced diabetes manager (BC-ADM) (Martin et al.).

The CDE is a health care provider who meets educational and practice requirements, successfully completes the certification examination for diabetes educators, and is credentialed by the National Certification Board for Diabetes Educators (NCBDE). The CDE can provide case management; diabetes education program development, coordination, and implementation; and referral to advanced practitioners, other health care team members, or community resources.

The BC-ADM (which was launched in 2000 as a result of unprecedented multiorganizational collaboration) is credentialed by the ANCC. This advanced practice credential focuses on *management of diabetes*, including prescribing medications, rather than on *diabetes education*. Thus this credential distinguishes

EXEMPLAR 18-4 Insights from Leaders in the Specialty*

In 1976, the Genetic Diseases Act was passed by Congress, and the Genetic Diseases Services Branch of the Office of Maternal Child Health, Health Services Administration, Department of Health and Human Services, was established. At that time, a small and academically diverse group of nurses were working with genetics programs in tertiary health care settings. They tended to come from practice backgrounds in pediatrics or obstetrics, which made sense because genetic services at that time were centered primarily on the delivery of prenatal diagnostic procedures and evaluation of the dysmorphic child or the child with developmental delays. A relatively small number of master's-prepared genetics counselors also were working in settings similar to those of the nurses. In the 1980s, however, medical geneticists started to employ nurses rather than counselors for a variety of reasons, including the limited number of counselors available and the broader scope of practice of nurses.

Differing perspectives emerged regarding basic requirements for certification and the appropriate credentialing body for awarding certification. Genetics counselors required a degree from an approved master of science in genetics counseling program and were credentialed through the ABMG. In contrast, nurses advocated for a professional nursing organization as an appropriate credentialing body and graduate education in nursing as an acceptable educational route.

The number of genetics counselors increased faster than the number of genetics nurses in the 1980s. This led to the educational meetings of the NSGC becoming focused on the learning needs of genetics counselors—not consistently and sufficiently addressing the issues that confronted genetics nurses. After the initial NSGC educational meetings, a bond was formed among those nurses working in genetics, and monies were found to form the Genetics Nurse Network. In 1987, there was significant discussion among the members of the network regarding the benefits of establishing a formal professional organization for genetics nurses. The lack of a professional "home" and the inability to obtain certification that would be recognized by the nursing profession led to the development of the ISONG. Membership in the organization has continued to grow since 1987; however, the issue of certification remained unresolved. Nurses working in genetics had academic preparation ranging from diplomas to doctoral degrees. Some were already certified as genetics counselors, and others were certified as nurse practitioners in their specialty area. After significant discussion among the membership of the ISONG, it was thought that the core knowledge required by genetics nurses was broader, but there was also the issue of recognition of a credential provided by a non-nursing organization being accepted by the nursing community. In addition, it was understood that at that time there were not enough nurses to sit for a written examination to provide for test item validation. Therefore the GNCC was established to investigate alternatives that would address these issues. After extensive work, the GNCC announced the establishment of the APNG credential and awarded the first credentials in 2001.

As genetics knowledge continues to develop, genetics will become an integral part of the clinical practice of all nurses. The ISONG has worked with the NCHPEG to develop competencies for health care professionals at both the generalist and specialty levels and has collaborated with the ANA to publish competencies specific to nurses. The ISONG continues to grow and develop to meet the needs of nurses who are anywhere on the novice-expert continuum and who focus on clinical practice, professional or consumer education, or research.

*We gratefully acknowledge Shirley Jones, PhD, RN, Louisville, KY, and Judith Lewis, PhD, RN, Richmond, VA, for their assistance with this exemplar. *ABMG*, American Board of Medical Genetics; *ANA*, American Nurses Association; *APNG*, Advanced Practice Nurse in Genetics; *GNCC*, Genetic Nursing Credentialing Commission; *ISONG*, International Society of Nurses in Genetics; *NCHPEG*, National Coalition for Health Professionals Education in Genetics; *NSGC*, National Society of Genetics Counselors.

between two sets of skills (Daly et al., 2001; Valentine, Kulkarni & Hinnen, 2003). This level of credentialing is designed for licensed health care professionals, including registered dietitians, registered nurses, and registered pharmacists, who hold graduate degrees and have recent clinical diabetes management experiences after they have been licensed. Credentialing as a CDE is not required to take the advanced management examination.

Notably, the BC-ADM designation is unique. Although each discipline eligible for credentialing takes a different examination (Valentine et al., 2003), it is

Box 18-2   QUESTIONS FOR LEADERS TO ADDRESS IN CHARTING THE COURSE OF SPECIALTY EVOLUTION

- Are advanced practice nursing competencies required to fully enact specialty practice, or are they an added value?
- What are the distinct advanced practice nursing roles within the specialty?
- How can the organization best recognize and value existing providers while moving to new expectations?
- How should certification and educational expectations be structured, especially if differentiated practice between non-APNs and APNs continues within the specialty?
- How should subspecialty certification within the context of advanced practice nursing regulation be addressed?
- How can the centrality of direct clinical practice be maintained?

APN, Advanced practice nurse.

the first multidisciplinary approach to certifying nurses, dietitians, and pharmacists ever developed by the ANCC (Daly et al., 2001; Valentine et al., 2003). The fact that the ANCC supported the AADE's request to support the advanced-level examination for disciplines other than nursing, to promote team collaboration and improve quality of care for individuals with diabetes, represents the emergence of a *new model of collaboration* among practitioners who, in the past, may have competed for recognition by patient/consumer groups. The potential benefits of multidisciplinary certification include increased credibility (with colleagues, patients/consumers, employers, and other health care professionals) as a result of a shared knowledge base; differentiation of these providers as having advanced-level expertise in diabetes management; greater autonomy in the delivery of care and services; and improved reimbursement (Daly et al., 2001). In this multidisciplinary model, APNs fill a niche in the care of these patients. Nurses constitute the largest group of health care professionals who deliver care to individuals with DM across the life span and in a variety of settings; therefore graduate-level preparation for APNs in diabetes management (consistent with American Diabetes Association standards) would fulfill the need for care providers in both acute and primary care settings.

Commentary: Stage IV

Caring for persons with diabetes has become complex, requiring the expertise and efforts of interdisciplinary teams. Because the nature of caring for patients with diabetes has historically required interdisciplinary collaboration, health care providers from these disciplines are secure in understanding the unique contributions they make in the management of patients. They are experts—secure in both their individual and shared clinical knowledge base—and embrace the challenges and opportunities inherent in multidisciplinary collaboration. This model of collaboration is somewhat unique and has been expertly developed by leaders in the AADE. The trajectory of change that was initiated in the early 1990s is exemplary of the natural maturation of the specialty resulting from deliberate, logical planning to strengthen the education and broaden the scope of practice of practitioners in the specialty.

The following are the requirements for other specialties to evolve to this advanced stage of development:

- Attention (at a minimum) to defining and clarifying the attributes of advanced practice in the specialty
- Delineating the core competencies of the specialty as encompassing the core competencies of advanced practice nursing
- Delineating a vision of advanced practice that may step outside of nursing's traditional vision of what constitutes an advanced practice role
- Gaining support within nursing and the health care community for the role as part of an interdisciplinary team
- Standardizing curricula across disciplines

These activities allow APN specialties at the stage IV level to achieve competency in advanced practice nursing and to recognize unique and shared clinical knowledge.

SUMMARY AND CONCLUSIONS

As can be seen from Chapter 1, the evolution of specialties in nursing has a long and rich history that continues in the present. Many specialties are evolving toward advanced practice nursing along a trajectory that for some has been haphazard, whereas others have evolved as a consequence of a cohesive vision communicated by leaders in the specialty. The progress made by members of specialty organizations that have evolved their specialties to advanced levels of practice (stages III and IV) can serve as examples for others that are struggling to evolve (stage II) or are newly emerging (stage I).

In this chapter we have examined each of these stages in the context of selected specialty groups and the evolving and innovative roles that characterize progression toward advanced practice nursing. Clearly, the ability to be deliberate in efforts to evolve the specialty speeds progress, as demonstrated by organizations such as the WOCNS, AADE, and ISONG. Some specialties have haphazardly evolved. Others may not evolve into advanced practice nursing; without commitment from the nursing community and attention to the issues noted in Boxes 18-1 and 18-2, the move toward advanced practice nursing may be an unrealistic goal. It is important to recognize that progression to advanced levels of practice is neither inevitable nor necessary. For example, staff development educators are a respected specialty group within the nursing profession, yet their competencies are not consistent with advanced practice nursing (Hanson & Hamric, 2003). As specialties move through the stages described here, one important question for the specialty's leadership is whether the specialty is best advanced by deliberate evolution to the advanced level of practice, development of differentiated levels of practice with distinct expectations and certifications, or continued development as a specialty (see Box 18-2). In these decisions, it is critically important to affirm the roles and value of ALL providers in the specialty, even as differentiation occurs for advancement and strengthening of specialty roles.

Concern over whether a role is a nursing role (versus *exclusively* a nursing role) is an issue that will need to be examined in particular specialties. In the history of nursing, some roles were characterized as sharing attributes with other types of health care providers. For example, some psychiatric CNSs attained the credentials to practice as licensed professional counselors. Other health care providers (e.g., counselors, psychologists) also receive this same credential, despite educational differences. Failure to acknowledge the value of multidisciplinary teams, shared knowledge, and overlapping expertise may limit opportunities for APNs in the current health care environment and impede advancement of specialties within the discipline. As a profession, nursing must embrace the notion that some roles are not exclusively nursing and endorse differentiated practice models.

At the same time, the profession must define the advanced level of practice within the interdisciplinary model. This is critical for regulatory purposes, for standardization of APN competencies in the practice, and for recognition by the public and insurers. In addition to the AADE, other multidisciplinary specialty organizations (Table 18-2) certify health care providers who share a common knowledge base. These organizations are models of collaboration that communicate to consumers, other providers, third-party payers, and other stakeholders that there are national standards in the specialty that are upheld by these specialty care providers. These multidisciplinary collaborative models represent a trend in health care that has given rise to a fourth stage in the evolution of advanced practice nursing—a stage characterized by APNs who are mature, expert practitioners in a specialty or subspecialty, secure in understanding the unique contributions that they make in the direct care of patients, yet embracing the notion that some aspects of their practice are shared by experts from other disciplines essential to the care of their patients.

The proliferation of role titles seen in evolving specialties requires special attention as APNs begin practicing in the specialty. For example, within the transplant specialty, role titles such as *clinical transplant coordinator, transplant coordinator, transplant nurse, transplant NP,* and *transplant CNS* have been used in practice settings. The advanced practice role titles of *CNS, NP,* and *CNM* need to be consistently applied to APNs who are practicing in particular specialties to decrease role confusion. In addition, such consistency is important for promoting the recognition of advanced practice nursing within evolving specialties and the profession as a whole. For specialties that develop both nonadvanced and advanced levels of practice, consistent titles are necessary to avoid confusion among providers and patients.

This is an extraordinarily interesting time in the history of the nursing profession. Opportunities and

Table 18-2 SPECIALTY ORGANIZATIONS OFFERING ADVANCED-LEVEL CERTIFICATION

Specialty Organization	Credentialing Organization/Credential Awarded	Graduate Nursing Education Required?
American Academy of HIV Medicine*	American Academy of HIV Medicine/HIV Specialist	Implied (must be licensed as an NP)
American Academy of Wound Management*	American Academy of Wound Management/CWS	Yes (for diplomate or fellow status)
American Association of Critical-Care Nurses	AACN Certification Corporation/CCNS	Yes
American Association of Diabetes Educators*	American Nurses Credentialing Commission/BC-ADM	No (master's in nursing or related field)
Association of Nurses in AIDS Care	HIV/AIDS Nursing Certification Board/AACRN	Yes
Hospice and Palliative Care Nurses Association	National Board for Certification of Hospice & Palliative Care Nurses/APRN, BC-PCM	Yes
International Society of Nurses in Genetics	Genetic Nursing Credentialing Commission/APNG	Yes
International Nurses Society on Addictions	Addictions Nursing Certification Board/CARN-AP	No (master's in nursing or related field)
Oncology Nursing Society	Oncology Nursing Certification Corporation/AOCNS, AOCNP	Yes
Wound, Ostomy and Continence Nursing Society	Wound Ostomy Continence Nursing Certification Board/CWOCN, CWN, COCN, or CCCN	Yes
Society of Urologic Nurses & Associates*	Certification Board of Urologic Nurses & Associates/CUNP or CUCNS	Yes (must already be NP or CNS)

*Multidisciplinary membership.
CNS, Clinical nurse specialist; *NP,* nurse practitioner.

challenges for advanced practice nursing abound. What will the history books say about this period in the evolution and expansion of the nursing profession? As the second author (ABH) wrote in addressing the WOC specialty group (Hamric, 2000):

> [Our] hope is that they will say [we] clearly saw patients' needs and developed [our] skills to meet those needs; that [we] grasped the role opportunities that were possible and created new ones; and, most importantly, that [we] moved forward together. (p. 47)

REFERENCES

American Association of Diabetes Educators (AADE). (1992). The scope of practice for diabetes educators and the standards of practice for diabetes educators. *The Diabetes Educator, 18,* 52-56.

American Board for Transplant Certification (ABTC). (2007). *Candidate handbook: Clinical transplant coordinators, procurement transplant coordinators, clinical transplant nurses.* Lanexa, KS: Author.

American Nurses Association (ANA). (1995). *Nursing's social policy statement.* Washington, DC: Author.

American Nurses Association (ANA). (1997). *Scope and standards of forensic nursing practice.* Washington, DC: Author.

American Nurses Association (ANA). (2003). *Nursing: Scope and standards of practice,* Washington, DC: Author.

American Nurses Association (ANA)/International Society of Nurses in Genetics (ISONG). (2007). *Genetics/genomics nursing: Scope and standards of practice.* Washington, DC: Author.

Arnet, D.K., Baird, A.K., Barkley, R.A., Basson, C.T., Boerwinkle, E., Ganesh, S.K., et al. (2007). Relevance of genetics and genomics for prevention and treatment of cardiovascular disease: A scientific statement from the American Heart Association Council of Epidemiology and Prevention, the Stroke Council, and the Functional Genomics and Translational Biology Interdisciplinary Working Group. *Circulation, 155,* 2878-2901.

Balamin, A., Gray, J., & Ponder, B. (2003). The genetics and genomics of cancer. *Nature Genetics, 33*(Suppl.), 238-244.

Beitz, J.M. (2000). Specialty practice, advanced practice, and WOC nursing: Current professional issues and future opportunities. *Journal of Wound, Ostomy, and Continence Nursing, 27*, 55-64.

Bigbee, J.L., & Amidii-Nouri, A. (2000). History and evolution of advanced nursing practice. In A.B. Hamric, J.A. Spross, & C.M. Hanson (Eds.), *Advanced nursing practice: An integrated approach* (2nd ed., pp. 3-32). Philadelphia: Saunders.

Bjorklund, P. (2003). The certified psychiatric nurse practitioner: Advanced practice psychiatric nursing reclaimed. *Archives of Psychiatric Nursing, 17*, 77-87.

Bryant, R. (1995). Establishing a WOCN research program. *Journal of Wound, Ostomy, and Continence Nursing, 22*, 1-3.

Burgess, A.W., Berger, A.D., & Boersma, R.R. (2004). Forensic nursing: Investigating the career potential in this emerging graduate specialty. *American Journal of Nursing, 104*(3), 58-64.

Canaff, R.A. (2004). Limits and lessons: The expert medical opinion in adolescent sexual abuse cases. *American Prosecutors Research Institute, 17*(3), 1-4.

Coffman, J., & Rundall, T.G. (2005). The impact of hospitalists on cost and quality of inpatient care in the United States: A research synthesis. *Medical Care Research Review, 62*, 379-406.

Cole, F.L., & Kleinpell, R. (2006). Expanding acute care nurse practitioner practice: Focus on emergency department practice. *Journal of the American Academy of Nurse Practitioners, 18*, 187-189.

Cole, F.L., Ramirez, E., & Luna-Gonzales, H. (1999). *Scope of practice of nurse practitioners in emergency care* (p. 4). Des Plaines, IL: Emergency Nurses Association.

Daly, A., Kulkarni, K., & Boucher, J. (2001). The new credential: Advanced diabetes management. *Journal of the American Dietetic Association, 101*, 940-943.

DeNicola, L., Klied, D., & Brink, L. (1994). Use of pediatric physician extenders in pediatric and neonatal intensive care units. *Critical Care Medicine, 22*, 105-106.

Diabetes Control and Complications Trial (DCCT) Research Group. (1993). The effect of intensive treatment of diabetes on the development and progression of long-term complications in insulin-dependent diabetes mellitus. *New England Journal of Medicine, 329*, 977-988.

Donaldson, T.A. (2003). The role of the transplant coordinator. In S.A. Cupples & L. Ohler (Eds.), *Transplantation nursing secrets* (pp. 17-26). Philadelphia: Hanley & Belfus.

Doughty, D. (2000). Integrating advanced practice and WOC nursing education. *Journal of Wound, Ostomy, and Continence Nursing, 27*, 65-68.

Doyle, J. (2001). Forensic nursing: A review of the literature. *Australian Journal of Advanced Nursing, 18*, 32-39.

Dressler, D.B., Pistoria, M.J., Budnitz, T.L., McKean, S.C.W., & Amin, A.N. (2006). Core competencies in hospital medicine: Development and methodology. *Journal of Hospital Medicine, 1*(1), 48-56.

Gray, M. (1998). Continence research in the JWOCN: A report card. *Journal of Wound, Ostomy, and Continence Nursing, 25*, 61-62.

Gray, M., Ratliff, C., & Mawyer, R. (2000). A brief history of advanced practice nursing and its implications for WOC advanced nursing practice. *Journal of Wound, Ostomy, and Continence Nursing, 27*, 48-54.

Hamric, A.B. (2000). WOC nursing and the evolution to advanced practice nursing. *Journal of Wound, Ostomy, and Continence Nursing, 27*, 46-47.

Hanson, C.M., & Hamric, A.B. (2003). Reflections on the continuing evolution of advanced practice nursing. *Nursing Outlook, 51*, 203-211.

Hentzen, D. (1994). AADE moves to advanced practice model for diabetes education and care. *The Diabetes Educator, 20*, 190.

Hutson, L.A. (2002). Development of sexual assault nurse examiner programs. *Nursing Clinics of North America, 37*, 79-88.

International Association of Forensic Nurses (IAFN). (2007). *IAFN mission.* Retrieved July 9, 2007, from www.iafn.org/about/aboutHome.cfm.

International Society of Nurses in Genetics (ISONG). (2006). *Provision of quality genetic services and care: Building a multidisciplinary, collaborative approach among genetic nurses and genetic counselors.* Retrieved July 7, 2007, from www.isong.org/aboutus/ps_multidisciplinarygeneticcare.cjm.

International Transplant Nursing Society (ITNS). (2007). *Scope and standards of transplant nursing.* Retrieved July 9, 2007, from http://itns.org/scope-and-standards-of-transplant-nursing.

Jenkins, J., & Calzone, K.A. (2007). Establishing the essential nursing competencies for genetics and genomics. *Journal of Nursing Scholarship, 39*(1), 10-16.

Lea, D.H., Jenkins, J., & Francomano, C.A. (1998). *Genetics in clinical practice: New directions for nursing and health care.* Sudbury, MA: Jones & Bartlett.

Lewis, J.A. (2000). Advanced practice in maternal/child nursing: History, current status, and thoughts about the future. *Maternal Child Nursing, 25*, 327-330.

Lewis, J.A., Calzone, K.M., & Jenkins, J. (2006). Essential nursing competencies and curricula guidelines for genetics and genomics. *MCN: American Journal of Maternal Child Nursing, 31*(3), 146-153.

Lynch, M.P., Cope, D.G., & Murphy-Ende, K. (2001). Advanced practice issues: Results from the ONS Advanced Practice Nursing Survey. *Oncology Nursing Forum, 28*, 1521-1530.

Lyon, B.L. (2002). The regulation of clinical nurse specialist practice: Issues and current developments. *Clinical Nurse Specialist, 16*, 239-241.

Maeve, M.K., & Vaughn, M.S. (2001). Nursing with prisoners: The practice of caring, forensic nursing or penal harm? *Advances in Nursing Science, 24*, 47-64.

Martin, C., Daly, A., McWhorter, L.S., Shwide-Slavin, C., & Kushion, W. for the 2004-2005 American Association of Diabetes Educators Professional Practices Committee. (2005). The scope of practice, standards of practice, and standards of professional performance for diabetes educators. *The Diabetes Educator, 31*, 487-512.

Martin, R.K. (1999). The role of the transplant advanced practice nurse: A professional and personal evolution. *Critical Care Nursing Quarterly, 21,* 69-76.

McCrone, S., & Shelton, D. (2001). An overview of forensic psychiatric care of the adolescent. *Issues in Mental Health Nursing, 22,* 125-135.

McNatt, G.E., & Easom, A. (2000). The role of the advanced practice nurse in the care of organ transplant recipients. *Advances in Renal Replacement Therapy, 7,* 172-176.

Melkus, G.D., & Fain, J.A. (1995). Diabetes care concentration: A program of study for advanced practice nurses. *Clinical Nurse Specialist,* 9, 313-316.

Monsen, R.B. (2005). *Genetics nursing portfolio: A new model for the profession.* Washington, DC: American Nurses Association.

Morse, C.J. (2001). Advance practice nursing in heart transplantation. *Progress in Cardiovascular Nursing, 16,* 21-24, 38.

Murphy-Ende, K. (2002). Advanced practice nursing: Reflections on the past, issues for the future. *Oncology Nursing Forum, 29,* 106-112.

Naegle, M.A., & Krainovich-Miller, B. (2001). Shaping the advanced practice psychiatric–mental health nursing role: A futuristic model. *Issues in Mental Health Nursing, 22,* 461-482.

National Council of State Boards of Nursing (NCSBN) Advanced Practice Registered Nurse Joint Dialog Group. (2007). *Consensus statement on advanced practice registered nursing: Report of the APRN Consensus Work Group* (Draft). Chicago, IL: Author.

North American Transplant Coordinators Organization (NATCO). (2004). *Core competencies for the clinical transplant coordinator and the procurement transplant coordinator.* Lanexa, KS: Author.

Nyberg, D. (2006). Innovations in the management of hospitalized patients. *Nurse Practitioner, Spring*(Suppl.), 2-3.

Ohler, L., & Cupples, S. (Eds.). (2007). *Core curriculum for transplant nurses,* St. Louis: Mosby.

Oncology Nursing Society (ONS). (2007). *About ONS.* Retrieved August 31, 2007, from www.ons.org/about/.

Palmer, M.H. (2000). The RU-3 project: Research utilization and practice. *Journal of Wound, Ostomy, and Continence Nursing, 27,* 98-99.

Reel, V.K. (1999). Utilization of the acute care nurse practitioner in lung transplantation. *Clinical Excellence for Nurse Practitioners, 3,* 80-83.

Roe, B., & Moore, K.N. (2001). Utilization of continence clinical practice guidelines. *Journal of Wound, Ostomy, and Continence Nursing, 28,* 297-304.

Society of Hospital Medicine (SHM). (2006). *Non-physician provider committee.* Retrieved July 9, 2007, from www.hospitalmedicine.org/AM/Template.cfn?Section=Committees&TEMPLATE=/CM/ContentDisplay.cfm&contentid=10360.

Society of Hospital Medicine (SHM). (2007). *Mission statement and goals.* Retrieved July 9, 2007, from www.hospitalmedicine.org/Content/NavigationMenu/AboutSHM/MissionStatementGoals/Mission_Statement_Go.htm.

Terboss, M.A. (October 26, 2007). Personal communication.

Tobin, C.T. (2000). A rainbow of opportunities: Advanced practice. *The Diabetes Educator, 26,* 216, 326-327.

United Kingdom Prospective Diabetes Study (UKPDS) Group. (1998). Intensive blood glucose control with sulfonylurea or insulin compared with conventional treatment and risk of complications in patients with type 2 diabetes. *Lancet, 352,* 837-853.

Valentine, V., Kulkarni K., & Hinnen, J. (2003). Evolving roles: Diabetes educator to advanced diabetes manager. *The Diabetes Educator, 29,* 598-610.

Wachter, R.M., & Goldman, L. (1996). The emerging role of "hospitalists" in the American health care system. *New England Journal of Medicine, 335,* 514-517.

World Health Organization (WHO). (2002). *World report on violence and health: summary.* Geneva: Author.

Wound, Ostomy and Continence Nurses Society (WOCNS). (1998). *Commemorative program for opening session: 30th Anniversary Conference.* Laguna Beach, CA: Author.

Wound, Ostomy and Continence Nurses Society (WOCNS). (2007). *Candidate handbook.* Retrieved January 2, 2008, from www.wocncb.org/pdf/examhandbook2007updated.pdf.

Yang, W., Kelly, T., & He, J. (2007). Genetic epidemiology of obesity. *Epidemiologic reviews advance access.* Retrieved July 7, 2007, from http://epirev.oxfordjournals.org/cgi/content/abstract/mxm004v1.

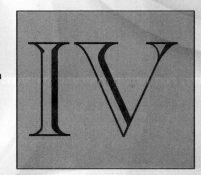

PART IV

Critical Elements in Managing Advanced Practice Nursing Environments

Business Planning and Reimbursement Mechanisms

Charlene M. Hanson • Sally D. Bennett

INTRODUCTION

In today's complex health care environment, communities and families need and demand health services beyond those that have been traditionally available. From the patient's perspective, services must be accessible and affordable. From the payer's perspective, they must be cost-effective. Both groups desire and demand high-quality services. In sum, the work of the health care system and subsequently the advanced practice nurses (APNs) practicing in it is to give the right care, to the right person, at the right time, and to do this within an increasingly demanding environment. Many different processes contribute to this system, most of which may be classified either as those related to direct patient care (with a clinical focus) or as those that support the patient care process indirectly (with an administrative focus). Successful APNs develop, implement, and continuously analyze the direct and indirect processes of care used to meet patient outcomes while being cognizant of the other critical environmental elements that affect their practice. Success is measured by the ability of the APN using these existing processes to attain desired patient outcomes within the constraints of available resources and reimbursement.

The current health care environment provides significant tension for change. Through the political leadership of national organizations and the active participation of nurses in the political process, nurses have the ability to influence the direction of that change (see Chapter 9). By virtue of their expanded knowledge and skill set, APNs are uniquely poised as effective alternatives to the traditional physician provider. Factors providing support for additional providers for patients include the acceptance of the need for change by health care organizations, the commitment of APNs to nursing's professional ethics, and the covenant nurses hold with society. Doctoral education will assist APNs in achieving both the direct and indirect goals of care by enhancing their ability to design and deliver effective care to patients (American Association of Colleges of Nursing [AACN], 2006). Enhanced leadership, policy

making, and collaboration skills will augment their ability to make positive change at both the system and practice setting level.

One particular innovation in patient care settings that has been successful over time is the conceptualization and organization of the direct and indirect processes of patient care within the context of systems thinking (Reel & Abraham, 2007; Solberg, Kottke, Brekke, & Magnan, 2000). Simply put, any system represents the flow of resources through a process that results in the desired outcomes (Figure 19-1). The size and complexity of the developed system depends on the number and complexity of processes being used to attain the desired outcome. Evaluation of any system includes assessment and evaluation of the resources used, the processes used, and the outcomes attained. This chapter focuses on the process of APN business planning from a systems approach. Although the emphasis is on an APN-managed practice, all APNs, whether they are employers or employees, need to be aware that patient care delivery is conceptualized as comprising the direct and indirect care processes that ensure that available resources are allocated in a manner that meets desired patient outcomes. Business planning is itself a process that focuses primarily on the development, implementation, and evaluation of those indirect processes that support patient care. It stands in contrast to a business plan, which is a document used by legal and financial advisors to evaluate the success potential of a particular business venture, such as an individual APN practice. The business plan may be conceptualized as an outcome or product of the business planning process. Reimbursement, as part of overall business planning, is another indirect process supporting patient care and is one of the critical elements affecting APN success. Examples are provided to illustrate these important concepts. It is important to note that much of the information discussed throughout this chapter changes from year to year. Federal, state, and professional websites contain the most current information and should be consulted for the latest changes.

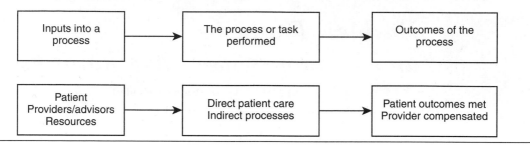

FIGURE **19-1:** Flowcharts of processes.

Table **19-1**   EXAMPLES OF DIRECT AND INDIRECT PROCESSES AND SKILLS

Clinical/Direct Processes and Skills	Administrative/Indirect Processes and Skills
Disease management	Risk management and assessment
Wound management	Support staff supervision
Childbirth education	Presentation/teaching/precepting
Lactation consultation	experience
Suturing	Grant-writing capabilities
Intrauterine contraceptive device	Computer literacy
insertion	Budget development
Pain management	Medical billing
Intubation	Word processing/desktop publishing
Counseling	Compliance monitoring
Minor procedures	Quality/safety monitoring

BUSINESS PLANNING: PRINCIPLES OF PRACTICE MANAGEMENT

Designing and Delivering Care to Patients

Success in and satisfaction with one's APN role revolve around the right match between APNs and the work they do and the ability to be flexible and innovative within the scope of that role. As noted, APNs participate in both direct and indirect care processes as they enact their roles. Examples of indirect processes are the steps taken to register a patient and collect demographics, the process of third-party billing, and the identification of medical and office supplies vendors. Table 19-1 lists examples of clinical and administrative processes and skills. Both direct and indirect processes are essential to the successful management of any health care system, whether it be a small, self-contained APN or physician practice or a large, multihospital network.

Over an APN's career, the balance between direct and indirect process involvement and the size of the system in which these processes occur may vary. At any given time, such shifts in balance and size of the system may require that APNs adopt an entrepreneurial approach, an intrapreneurial approach, or a mixture of both (Dayhoff & Moore, 2005). Both entrepreneurs and intrapreneurs are individuals who continually search for and who are receptive to opportunities and innovation. Innovation comes through the creation of a new process (whether direct, indirect, or both) or through radical changes to an existing process so that it seems "like new." An *entrepreneur* plans, organizes, finances, operates, and participates in a new health care delivery organization. Entrepreneurs have control over and responsibility for an increased proportion of indirect processes of care in their roles as compared with intrapreneurs. An *intrapreneur* is generally an employee of an existing health care system, in which many of the indirect processes of the care delivery system may be controlled and managed by other employees or departments. The intrapreneur improves, redesigns, or augments an employer's current direct care processes, with a lesser role in day-to-day business administrative functions. Entrepreneurs function within the context of the larger, societal health care system. Intrapreneurs function within an institutional health care system—a microcosm of the larger arena. Both entrepreneurs and intrapreneurs are risk takers. Entrepreneurs are likely to take bigger risks and have a higher tolerance for the accompanying uncertainty.

When embarking on program or practice oversight, the APN needs to understand the balance between direct and indirect processes as well as the size the business will have over time. A large portion of time is dedicated to clinical visits and must be financially productive, so there must be a realistic balance between direct and indirect care. The decision about the proportion of one's role to devote to direct care versus indirect processes is based on the professional and personal values and goals of the APN and the needs and demands of the practice.

A self-assessment may assist the APN in clarifying professional and personal values. Types of questions to consider include the following and are intended to be illustrative only and are not assumed to be exhaustive:

- *Theoretical basis for practice.* What model of nursing practice or approach to care delivery best describes how I perceive my own nursing practice? Do the options before me favor this model or some other approach? If they favor another approach, how compatible is it with my own beliefs? (See Chapter 2.)
- *Preference for intrapreneurial or entrepreneurial approach.* Do I thrive on risk taking, like some risk, or prefer situations with a conservative level of risk involved? How is a "loss" or being "unsuccessful" defined? If I like taking risks, how much of a loss can I afford to take—both professionally and personally—if my venture proves to be unsuccessful? (The more risk one is willing to take, the more entrepreneurial one is likely to be.) Do I prefer being a part of a team or being on my own? If I like being on a team, what other team members would I like to be included on this team? How big a team am I most comfortable with? If I prefer working on my own, how will I interact with my colleagues? (See Chapters 7, 9, and 10.)

Inventory of Skills

A skills inventory can serve as a springboard for the clarification of the APN's professional goals. The extent to which the APN balances the clinical role with administrative demands depends on the APN's skills and preferences and begins with an inventory of those clinical skills and administrative talents that the APN would like to bring, or acquire, in an ideal advanced practice role. Box 19-1 lists some questions that may refine one's ideal inventory.

The questions in Box 19-1 are among the many questions to be answered by APNs before deciding how extensive their role will be in the management of their program or practice. Fortunately, several resources help clinicians better understand the indirect processes, or "business," of clinical practice. The reader is referred to Buppert (2004; 2008) for an in-depth discussion of nurse practitioner (NP) business and legal concerns. The American Medical Association (AMA) (1996, 1999, 2002a, 2002b, 2002c), in collaboration with the Coker Group, has published a series regarding independent practice management that is useful for any APN role. *Entrepreneur* and other business magazines provide useful information related to business management and administration. The Small Business Administration *(www.sba.gov)* provides general and specific information regarding business management and referral to local supports, including the local office of the Service Corps of Retired Executives (SCORE *[www.score.org/business_toolbox.html]*). There are many online resources related to business management. Specific websites that may be useful to the development of small businesses include the following:

- *www.americanexpress.com* (American Express Company, 2003): Go to "small business network" to find advice about business start-up and community networking.
- *www.smallbizsearch.com:* This website offers information about a wide variety of issues around financing, technology, and business opportunities.
- *www.dol.gov/osbp:* The Department of Labor, Office of Small Business Programs, offers good information about minority- and women-owned businesses.
- *www.pftweb.org:* In the "Building Your Practice" section of the Partnerships for Training website (George Washington University Medical Center/Faculty Resources, 2006) is an excellent resource that has in-depth coverage of all of the concerns just mentioned. This interactive, interdisciplinary Web resource offers a wealth of resources, information, and pearls of wisdom for clinicians who wish to develop a practice.

Box 19-1   INVENTORY OF SKILLS

DIRECT CARE PROCESSES

Can I clearly articulate my existing area of clinical expertise?

Do I have well-developed advanced clinical skills? If so, what are they?

What tasks do I particularly enjoy, feel neutral about, and particularly dislike?

Of those that I dislike but that need to be performed, do mechanisms exist for those tasks to be performed by someone else?

What processes would I like to do more of or learn more about?

Does the current situation provide opportunities for me to do them?

COLLABORATION STYLE

Do I get along with peers if a partnership were to form?

How well do I collaborate?

Am I comfortable with sharing business decision making and financial loss or gain?

INDIRECT CARE PROCESSES

Internal and External Loci of Support

Do I have the unflagging support of those closest to me, both personally (e.g., significant other, children, friends) and professionally (e.g., physician collaborators, APN colleagues, financial and legal advisors)?

Basic Management Skills

Do I have well-honed organizational skills?

Do I enjoy paying attention to details?

Am I comfortable in a leadership position?

Financial Management Skills

Am I familiar with or willing to learn the budgeting cycle and processes of my employer?

Have I participated in budget preparation and resource allocation in the past?

Am I comfortable developing a budget for my own practice?

External Regulatory Guidelines Affecting Practice

Do I know where to locate copies of the applicable regulations affecting my practice?

Do I understand or do I have access to advisors who understand the specific ramifications of state and federal laws applicable to this program such as those pertaining to the Clinical Laboratory Improvement Amendments (CMS, 2006b)?

Are there any institutional rules and regulations that may limit my ability to practice within the full scope of my role?

What are the procedures for obtaining approval of the various institutional committees that may be involved?

FINANCIAL RESOURCES

Where will funding for the program (capital for start-up expenses) come from?

Do I have the financial ability to live without a steady income for at least 1 year while the practice is growing or if the grant is not refunded?

HUMAN RESOURCES SKILLS AND SYSTEMS

Am I willing to be responsible for the work of others? What does that entail?

Are administrative systems in place for hiring, evaluating, and terminating staff for the duration of the program/practice?

APN, Advanced practice nurse.

DIRECT PROCESSES OF CARE

Direct Patient Care

Direct care of patients and families is the central competency for APNs (see Chapters 3 and 5). The direct process of care for a given practice or practice population is defined as those patients who will receive direct clinical care by the APN within a practice environment. High-quality care and patient satisfaction sustain any level or configuration of practice over time. The patient population served, components of care and procedures based on APN role, scope of practice, and mission must be carefully considered before implementing care. Ongoing evaluation with regard to patient outcomes and patient satisfaction is an important tool to maintain high-quality, safe direct care over time. The therapeutic relationships that are the trademark of APN direct practice provide opportunities for innovative business opportunities (Thomas, Finch, Schoenhofer, & Green, 2004).

One way to think about practice environments is that they represent small health care systems based on a patient population with identified needs. This patient population is identified through a variety of means, including individual APN expertise and preference based on the role and scope of practice of the individual APN. For certified nurse-midwives (CNMs) and certified registered nurse anesthetists (CRNAs), the patient population is essentially defined by their roles with childbearing women and their families and with patients undergoing surgical anesthesia, respectively. NPs and clinical nurse specialists (CNSs) have a broader population base (e.g., family NP, psychiatric CNS; see Part III). Sometimes APNs identify patient populations through other modifiers, such as age, health promotion specialty, or disease state specialty (e.g., CNMs who care for adolescent mothers-to-be, CRNAs who specialize in providing anesthesia in pain management centers, and adult NPs or CNSs who specialize in management of asthma or diabetes). In other instances, it is the geographical location or organizational setting that differentiates one's patient population of interest. Examples of these populations are the rural underserved populations cared for by National Health Service Corps providers, veterans cared for by the Veterans Affairs Medical Centers, and participants in Kaiser Permanente's health maintenance organization (HMO) who are cared for by their own staff of providers. APNs must be able to clearly and succinctly define the patient populations being served by their clinical practice.

Mission, Vision, and Values

After the patient population has been identified and the patient care processes have been outlined, the APN will need to formalize this information in a mission and vision statement. The mission and the vision statement describe to patients and prospective funding agencies the APN practice's reason for existence and future direction; the brief statement serves to remind the APN entrepreneur about where the program or practice's priorities should lie. Professional values include those tenets of nursing practice that provide significance and meaning to the APN's practice of nursing (American Nurses Association [ANA], 2001). The mission and goal statements of national APN organizations clearly portray these values as well (see Chapter 11). One's professional and personal values influence one's comfort with risk taking and one's preference as to the arena in which care is delivered. The written summary of program or practice values may be combined with the mission and the vision statement into one document, such as a brochure or program information sheet. This summary is available for review by any interested party and should be given to every patient at the time of the first practice encounter.

The mission states the goal of the direct processes of care in one sentence. For example, "comprehensive primary care and wellness care for pediatric and adult individuals and families." The vision statement describes the "ideal" 5-year goal, that is, what the APN envisions the clinical care to be 5 years from inception. The mission and vision statements should enhance transparency and interdisciplinary collaboration as APNs clearly articulate their values, goals, and vision of patient care to existing and potential colleagues, consultants, and third-party payers. If the APN is functioning through an intrapreneurial approach, the organization's mission and vision should be examined to ensure that the practice or program fits into the overall goals of the organization and into the APN's personal goals. If the program's mission conflicts with that of the organization, problems may take the form of delays in funding, changes to the program's direct or indirect processes of care, barriers to program implementation, and outright denial of program development. If other providers, individuals, or groups have a stake in the program, the mission and vision statement should be determined through consensus of the group. See SCORE at *www.score.org/business_toolbox.html*.

The values of a practice or program describe the focus, preferences, and ethical precepts that underlie relationships among the provider, the practice, the patients, and external groups. They may be related to direct or indirect care processes. Professional ethics are discussed in Chapters 11 and 21. Ethical precepts pertaining to patient-focused values are described briefly here.

Informed Consent. Informed consent is both an ethical and legal mandate that requires providers to obtain a competent patient's fully informed and voluntary consent before any medical or nursing treatment. The APN must describe the general nature of the treatment and any consequences involved, the normal risks and hazards inherent to the treatment, any known side effects or complications that may occur, and any alternative treatments available to the patient. Final informed consent comprises the patient's understanding of this information and the agreement to proceed with treatment. Both the APN's information and the patient's agreement within the informed consent discussion must be documented as part of the patient's medical record.

Compliance with Health Insurance Portability Accountability Act.

Privacy and confidentiality are important ethical issues that require careful consideration. The balance between the patient's right to privacy and society's need to be protected is important. State laws clearly explicate those patient issues, such as sexually transmitted diseases, abuse, or tuberculosis, that are reportable by law. Patient confidentiality is critical to the provider-patient relationship. Other than legal reporting obligations, it is the patient's right to decide what information the APN and all other members of the health care team may share with others. The federal Health Insurance Portability and Accountability Act (HIPAA) became law in 1996. Mandatory compliance with federal regulations began in 2003. HIPAA mandates the proper use and disclosure of personal health information. Providers must have policies and trained personnel in place to implement privacy standards (Buppert, 2003; see also Chapter 22). An APN employee must be knowledgeable about office policy and all HIPAA compliance regulations. HIPAA guidelines are detailed on the Centers for Medicare & Medicaid Services [CMS] website at *www.cms.hhs.gov/hipaa.* This site provides a good overview of the Privacy Rule, as well as answers to frequently asked questions about implementation.

In addition to the right to confidentiality regarding their health information, patients are entitled to a degree of personal privacy within the clinical encounter. Courtesy demands that the patient's dignity be maintained, including providing the patient with well-fitting patient gowns and cover sheets during the physical examination. Privacy includes careful attention to cross-cultural issues that may be unfamiliar to American APNs. Attention should be paid to the physical layout of the patient encounter area, ensuring that conversations cannot be overheard and that the room is secure from line of gaze through open doors and/or windows.

Safety and Security.

The APN must advocate for measures that improve safety and security within the office environment. There must be a sense of well-being for staff, patients, and their families. Policies should clearly articulate how to maintain patient, provider, and staff safety, including provisions for securing a patient's valuables during procedures and for managing hostile persons in the area (including a policy for managing violent and armed persons). The waiting room door should be locked to the patient care area. Adequate lighting, railings, and paved walkways are necessary, as well as adequate parking close to the facility. The level of security needed depends on the APN's practice environment, knowledge of staff about patients' conditions and potential safety issues, and available resources within the facility.

Patient Communication.

Ethical clinical practice demands honesty and integrity in all patient interactions. Under the best circumstances, communication lines will be open and both the APN and the patient will understand each other and feel as if they have been understood. When misunderstandings occur, the APN should manage the issue as if it were a patient complaint—seeking to address the concerns in an objective and timely manner. Risk management policies and protocols must be enacted to ensure that timely and thorough communication is delivered to the patient regarding all visit outcomes, plans of care, and diagnostic test results. This is of vital importance to the legal and ethical success and safety of the APN practice. Samples of risk management guidelines may be acquired through the malpractice insurance carriers or as described by Buppert (2004, 2006). Dealing with difficult and nonadherent patients requires experience and understanding. Over time, many issues can be resolved between the patient and the caregiver. Should termination of the provider-patient relationship be necessary, this may be accomplished in many ways. It is important to provide alternatives for another provider so that the patient does not feel abandoned. *Finally,* whatever rules the APN practice has set as grounds for termination of this relationship must be in writing, well documented, and sent to the patient as a certified, return-receipt letter.

Resolution of Complaints.

Resolving complaints is not usually an ethical issue; however, it is good business practice to monitor patient satisfaction with the clinical experience from the time the patient enters the waiting room through the time the final bill for services is paid. Many valid, reliable patient satisfaction tools are available to health care providers to measure patients' responses to the way care is delivered (Kleinpell, 2001; see also *www.qualitymeasures.ahrq.gov/*). Despite one's best efforts, however, patients may be dissatisfied with some aspect of their experience at some point during an APN's career. It is important that any patient complaint or sign of dissatisfaction be addressed immediately, preferably at the time of the complaint (Buppert, 2004). A formal policy related to the management of patient complaints includes how patient complaints are recorded, who investigates and responds to the patient's concerns, and how quickly the complaint is addressed. Specific guidelines for managing patient complaints may be supplemented by risk management information provided by the APN's malpractice carrier.

Clinical Relationships with Other Staff and Providers

Although the APN is assumed to be the primary provider in this discussion, attention must be paid to the development of clinical relationships with other APNs, physicians, pharmacists, and allied health colleagues. (In-depth discussions related to clinical mentorship, consultation, and collaboration are found in Part II.) To be successful, the APN must maintain a collegial relationship with other health care providers (Almost & Laschinger, 2002; Horns et al., 2007; Lindeke, 2005). An important legal consideration is defining the parameters of the association with a collaborating physician through the development of a collaborative practice or contracting agreement (see Appendixes A and B). Many state statutes for APNs require some form of medical collaboration. Even without state statute, strong collegial relationships that provide support and coverage for time off are essential to the success of APN practice. As well, in APN-owned practices, impediments to care can occur when referring to out-of-area facilities for diagnostic testing. Most facilities want a Doctor of Medicine (MD) as referring provider to be identified on patient orders and correspondence. If APNs' names are not accepted as the primary provider, patient test results may be sent to the collaborating MD, who is off-site and unable to prescribe or otherwise care for patients. APNs must be able to track these results to provide adequate, safe care for patients.

APNs need to find consultants and referral sources for patients whose medical problems require additional expertise from a specialist. Locating referrals for indigent or uninsured patients who need specialized medical care or hospitalization may be difficult because of the lack of services or reimbursement for these populations. A list of consultants and referral sources should be generated that outlines the services they offer and their willingness to accept referrals for indigent patients, as well as their participation in third-party payer plans. Consultants are identified through word-of-mouth recommendations from clinical mentors and colleagues, through the recommendation of lay public support groups who have worked with certain specialty groups, and through direct provider interviews. Over time, the APN develops a referral and consultation base and develops strong relationships with those providers who are able to assist the APN in meeting patients' needs. Once relationships are established, acknowledging a consultant's assistance and support is equally important. This acknowledgment may be as simple as learning from the consulting registration staff what demographic information they need in order to schedule the patient, providing the most recent office notes to the consultant in time for the patient's appointment, and sending seasonal cards thanking them for their support.

The numbers and variety of APN providers that are available in local communities is growing (see Part III). APN colleagues who can serve as peer consultants or serve as potential partners are an added strength that can be fully utilized to build practice relationships.

APNs must also carefully decide about the support staff that will assist with the direct care of patients. Staff positions include nurses, certified nurse aides, office manager, and clerical staff. Other staff such as respiratory and physical therapists, pharmacists, and nutritionists may be on site on a daily basis. All permanent and part-time staff need to be oriented to the organization and the goals of care with clear role delineation. Staff should be clearly identified so that the consumer is aware of their roles in the provision of care; in particular, non-nursing personnel should not be identified as nurses.

INDIRECT PROCESSES OF CARE

Indirect processes support patient care and include administrative and operational structures and functions. Although they require a different set of advisors, staff, and equipment, indirect processes are equally important to successful APN practice. Business relationships and business structures are necessary to define the context and framework under which clinical practice is performed. Knowledge of the external regulatory bodies that have an impact on APN practice is essential in today's complex and rapidly changing health care arena. This discussion presents an overview of these issues but in no way is intended to be comprehensive. The APN is referred to business consultants for up-to-date information reflective of the laws and guidelines within a particular state and practice setting.

Business Relationships

Separate from but as important as the clinical advisors and resources described earlier are the administrative advisors and resources required to develop and maintain smooth indirect processes to support patient care. An independent practice will need to contract or consult with an accountant, attorney, banker, and insurance agent for specific services (Buppert, 2004). In addition, the services of a practice management consultant with medical billing expertise should be enlisted (George Washington University Medical Center/Faculty Resources, 2006; Reel 2007). The accountant should assist the APN in setting up an accounting system, establishing internal controls, and preparing an operating budget. The accountant should set up the practice to ensure that the best tax advantages and flexibility are obtained (Buppert, 2004). Attorneys with expertise in health care law should establish the legal structure of the practice and provide advice on an as-needed basis for special purposes. The attorney and accountant should have a working relationship so that the legal structure selected provides the best legal, financial, and tax advantages for the providers involved. The banking relationship serves to establish a line of credit or business loan (if needed) and to meet business banking needs (AMA, 1996; George Washington University Medical Center/Faculty Resources, 2006). A business insurance agent provides expertise in the areas of health, liability, and Workers' Compensation insurance programs. The practice management consultant serves to develop policies and procedures manuals, billing procedures and fee schedules, and job descriptions for an entrepreneurial enterprise (Buppert, 2006; Letz, 2002). A medical billing expert provides guidance in both the efficient completion and processing of billing forms in order to receive third-party reimbursement or capitation payment for the provider's services and the thorough and accurate completion of any third-party payer's contracting paperwork required for the APN's participation in selected contracts. The APN needs to carefully decide which of these functions can be done by the APN/APN practice staff and which need to be purchased as externally contracted services. It is important for the APN entrepreneur to ask the following: Is this an area of strength and interest, or is this an area that I do not want to attend to? Is this an indirect process of care to which I want to devote time and energy? More important, is up-front capital sufficient to sustain the practice until it can generate its own income—usually at least 6 months to 1 year.

The organization of day-to-day administrative support staff services (separate from the services of business advisors) revolves around the processes of care being delivered and the environment in which services are delivered. Once the APN knows what the direct patient care processes will include and has identified those indirect processes that will support the patient encounter, additional ancillary personnel may be needed. The APN maintains ultimate responsibility for all operations if he or she owns the clinic. APN employees must be aware of their specific responsibilities and understand which belong to them and which belong to the owner. In a community-based primary care setting, the practice may require someone to assist in patient registration and scheduling (the first process box in Figure 19-1), someone to assist the clinician in certain elements of patient care (the second box), and someone to collect or process patient fees (the third box). Any additional administrative roles support these primary roles and may include someone to manage patient medical records, someone to triage acutely ill patients by telephone, and someone to perform office cleaning functions. The individuals who fill these roles should have skills and qualifications that are complementary to those of the APN and should be able to meet practice goals for patient care. In hospital-based settings, CRNAs, CNSs, and CNMs often collaborate with the nurse managers of the area in which they practice to obtain the assistance of the unit's support staff and ancillary personnel. An organizational chart and job descriptions of the roles required should be developed, placed in a common personnel manual, and shared among staff members so that everyone is aware of his or her role within the successful functioning of the system. An example of an organizational chart is presented in Figure 19-2. Some payers require a copy of the organizational chart before enrolling the provider, as Medicaid does for APNs providing children's services. The experience, education, and other qualifications of the APN, other professionals providing services, and support staff should be described briefly and made available to interested parties.

Program and Business Structure

The structure that a particular intrapreneurial program takes depends on the organization's overall guidelines for program development. For example, a hospital may wish to open a satellite primary care or oncology clinic staffed partially by APNs. The structure of the new clinic would fall under the business

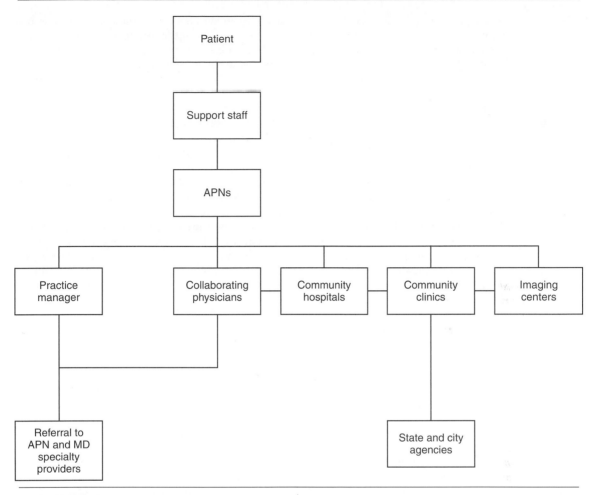

FIGURE **19-2:** Example of an organizational chart. *APN,* Advanced practice nurse; *MD,* Doctor of Medicine.

structure and plan of the hospital. An entrepreneurial program structure is often dictated by the requirements of whichever funding agency has provided the start-up and operating capital. The APN developing a program that depends on the guidelines of other organizations is referred to the particular organization participating in program sponsorship. Many grant-funding agencies have criteria for funding and program guidelines available on the World Wide Web.

APNs may adopt one of several business structures, depending on the organizational context in which the practice is set. Practices may be hospital-based or community-based. Hospital-based practices may be inpatient or ambulatory in nature. Community-based practices are usually primary care

settings, freestanding health centers, birthing centers, or convenient care clinics. They may also be a part of a managed care organization (MCO) or other payer-based primary care site. Practices may be established on a for-profit or not-for-profit basis. APNs should consult with business advisors to determine the best business structure to match their values and goals.

The three basic ways to structure the practice are a sole proprietorship, a partnership, or a corporation (Buppert, 2004). The primary differences among these structures lie in differing tax restrictions and liability. The simplest form of business organization is a *sole proprietorship*, which involves one owner. It is relatively straightforward and inexpensive to establish, and control remains with the sole owner. For tax purposes, the business income is taxed at the personal tax rate. The major disadvantage of the sole proprietorship is the unlimited liability that accompanies the structure. The owner assumes all liability, including that for any negligent acts of employees. Most medical practices are *for-profit partnerships*. A general partnership may be advantageous for the APN because partnering with another professional may attract venture capital. The unlimited liability for each individual partner remains, as does the personal tax rate on business income. A disadvantage of this structure is the possibility of personality conflicts and disagreements arising between the partners over control and decision making. As mentioned previously, the legality of relationships between different professionals is often dictated by state law. For example, CRNAs can join business arrangements as consultants to hospitals and anesthesia groups.

A *corporation* is a separate legal entity for both tax and liability purposes. Incorporation protects the owners from some, though not all, liability because a corporation's liability is limited. Consequently, because the medical professional owners retain a portion of any liability incurred, it is strongly advised that APNs and other providers have an individual liability policy. A professional corporation can elect a small business (Subchapter S) status, which allows owners to retain the benefit of taxation at the personal rate or, as is sometimes said, to avoid double taxation—first on corporate income and second on shareholder dividends. Other advantages of a corporation include the ability to start pension and profit-sharing plans and the possibility of attracting venture capital investors. The main disadvantage for a corporation not electing small business status is the higher tax rate incurred by corporations. A corporation may also be more expensive to establish and operate.

Most APN practices are eponymous (named after the owner). However, selecting a name for the practice may be an option worth considering in certain situations. For example, a specific practice name may assist in describing the services offered and reflect the business focus (e.g., *Coastal Cardiac Rehabilitation* suggests a geographical location and a type of service). Many professionals use their own name to connote a more personalized service, as well as to promote themselves. Most individual states regulate the selection and registration of business names as part of the registration of the business structure process. The process entails registering the business name, conducting a formal state agency search to ensure that the name is not being used by another business, paying a registration fee, and awaiting the receipt of a formal document confirming assignment of the business name to the APN *(www.bizfilings.com/)*. Further, you may want to protect your business name with a federal service mark or trademark *(www.legalzoom.com)*.

External Regulatory Bodies

An interwoven fabric of regulations and guidelines serves as the basis upon which APN professional practice is built and developed (see Chapters 21 and 22 and the individual APN chapters in Part III for an in-depth discussion of APN credentialing and regulation). Federal and state regulations, policies of private insurance companies, and, in some instances, local politics determine in which business structures and practice environments an APN may work and obtain reimbursement and whether this practice is independent or collaborative. Although APN students routinely learn about the importance of the rules and regulations established by many different stakeholders within health care systems, the impact on daily practice may not be appreciated until the student becomes a practicing clinician. The major external regulatory vehicles affecting APN practice include the following:

- Those state and federal statutes pertaining to regulation and credentialing requirements for advanced practice nursing *(www.ncsbn.org* or *www.ncqa.org/)*
- Guidelines for health care organizations regarding multiple facets of the management, environment, and delivery of health care established by The Joint Commission (TJC) *(www.jointcommission.org)*
- Occupational Safety & Health Administration (OSHA) regulations related to safe working conditions for employees *(www.osha.gov)*
- Clinical Laboratory Improvement Amendments (CLIA) regulations pertaining to laboratory services *(www.cms.hhs.gov/clia)*
- Additional Centers for Medicare & Medicaid Services regulations pertaining to Medicare reimbursement processes *(www.cms.hhs.gov/ medicare)*

TJC (The Joint Commission [TJC], 2007) evaluates a health care organization's system performance in both patient-focused (direct care) and organizational (indirect care) areas to improve the quality of care provided to the public. Patient-focused functions include patient rights and organizational ethics, assessment of patients, care of patients, education, and continuum of care. Organizational functions include improving organization performance, leadership, management of the environment of care, management of human resources, management of information, and surveillance, prevention, and control of infection. In addition, TJC examines an organization's governance, management, and functions related to medical and nursing staff. Surveys are performed every 3 years by TJC-employed provider and nonprovider survey teams. An overall score is determined along with any recommendations for improving scoring deficiencies. Accreditation is based on the organization's compliance with TJC guidelines and implementation of any recommendations to resolve deficiencies (The Joint Commission [TJC], 2007; see also *www.jointcommission.org*).

As a result of being expert clinicians, APNs are often involved in patient-focused processes of interest to TJC. Their level of involvement in organizational processes depends on the degree of individual APN responsibility for indirect care processes. Regardless of how many standards directly relate to an individual APN's practice, all APNs should be aware of the guidelines upon which their organization is being evaluated. On an individual level, many of the APN competencies discussed in Part II are touched on by some or many of TJC standards. TJC standards may also assist APNs in the development of their own standards of patient care and professional performance. In this manner, TJC serves as a valuable resource to augment professional nursing standards and guidelines related to the delivery of clinically excellent patient care in caring, compassionate, high-quality health care organizations.

Health care safety management and hazard control are proven processes that produce results by preventing accidents, reducing injury rates, and increasing organizational efficiency *(www.osha.gov)*. Areas include emergency planning and fire safety, general and physical plant safety, managing hazardous materials, managing biological waste, safety in patient care areas, and health care support area safety *(www.osha.gov)*. In terms of external regulators, safety management is carefully scrutinized by both TJC and OSHA. APNs functioning as entrepreneurs or employers must be well-versed in the rules, regulations, and implementation of safety programs governing these areas of safety management and hazard control, especially with respect to the management of biological waste and OSHA guidelines regarding blood-borne pathogens.

Created as part of the Department of Labor, OSHA was charged by the Occupational Safety and Health Act of 1970 to ensure safe and healthful working conditions for American workers. In 2002, Congress amended OSHA to expand research on the "health and safety of workers who are at risk for bioterrorist threats or attacks in the workplace" *(www.osha.gov.)*

Diagnostic Services

Any provider or laboratory service planning to collect, prepare, and analyze patient specimens is bound by CLIA rules and regulations (Centers for Medicare & Medicaid Services [CMS], 2006b). Enacted to safeguard the public, the CLIA established minimum acceptable standards for all categories of laboratory testing in the United States. Providers offering laboratory services must meet the criteria and apply for the appropriate level of CLIA certification. Fees for the certificates are based on the test complexity, the number of specimens being processed, and the cost of surveyor inspection. Four categories of laboratory testing are defined by the CLIA: waived tests, provider-performed microscopy (PPM), moderate-complexity procedures, and high-complexity procedures. If laboratory specimens are going to be performed by the APN, the first two categories of CLIA testing apply to the usual level of procedures performed. Moderate- and high-complexity procedures are generally performed by independent or hospital-based laboratories.

Waived tests are simple laboratory examinations and procedures cleared by the U.S. Food and Drug Administration (FDA) for home use. They are simple and accurate (making the likelihood of error minimal) and pose no significant harm to the patient. Examples of CLIA-waived tests include fecal occult blood, non-automated dipstick or tablet urinalysis, urine pregnancy visual color comparison tests, and all qualitative color comparison pH testing of body fluids. The laboratory would apply and pay for a CLIA Certificate of Waiver, allowing the laboratory to perform only waived tests. The certificate is valid for 2 years. PPM is a subcategory of the moderate-complexity level of testing. These examinations may be performed by clinicians during the patient visit on a specimen obtained from the provider's patient or a patient of the group practice (American Academy of Family Physicians, 2004). Other key criteria related to PPM stipulate (1) that the primary instrument for the test be the microscope; (2) that the specimen must be labile, or a delay in the testing could compromise test accuracy; and (3) that limited specimen handling is required. Examples of PPM procedures include wet mounts, including preparation of vaginal, cervical, or skin specimens; all potassium hydroxide (KOH) preparations; pinworm examinations; and nasal smears for eosinophils. The certificate for this level of laboratory service, the Certificate for Provider-Performed Microscopy Procedures, allows the provider to perform waived tests as well.

With the new structure at CMS, quality and personnel rules for clinical laboratories have been streamlined and simplified. CLIA information may be obtained at the following sites: *www.cms.hhs.gov/clia* and *www.aafp.org/pt*.

If the APN does not intend to perform laboratory testing within the practice setting, he or she will need to identify providers of diagnostic testing services with appropriate CLIA certification who will accept requisitions for diagnostic tests. In the absence of an in-house laboratory, external laboratory services basically include specimen collection, specimen processing, and reporting of results. Some APN practices choose to collect specimens themselves and then send them to the laboratory for processing and reporting. The APN would set up all business agreements and arrangements with the receiving laboratory for complete processing and reporting of the specimens including billing and payment practices. For those practices choosing to collect and process their own specimens, additional equipment and supplies will be needed depending on the nature of the tests being performed.

Recent revisions in Medicare regulations have resulted in the heightened enforcement of the policy of medical necessity with respect to diagnostic services. In an attempt to decrease costs related to inappropriate diagnostic testing, certain laboratory and radiological services have been identified as requiring proof of medical necessity for them to be covered by Medicare, Medicaid, and other carriers. The determination of medical necessity is made by CMS and codified in the International Classification of Diseases (ICD) (discussed in the "ICD-9-CM Codes" section of the "Medical Classification Systems" section) (AMA, 2007), a list of diagnoses and symptoms that will justify the diagnostic service requested. For example, to have thyroid-stimulating hormone (TSH) testing paid for by Medicare, the patient must have an ICD-9-CM (International Classification of Diseases, Ninth Revision, Clinical Modification) diagnosis that is on the list of diagnoses for TSH testing, such as goiter (ICD-9-CM codes 240.0–240.9) or acquired hypothyroidism (ICD-9-CM codes 244.0–244.9).

ICD-9 codes need to be quite specific, adding a fifth digit when possible. Those diagnostic tests for which medical necessity has been determined in specific locales of the United States are listed in local Medicare medical policies found either through the laboratory service or directly from the local Medicare intermediary newsletter (see *www.cms.hhs.gov*). Most other carriers follow the Medicare medically necessary requirements. It is important to note that CMS uses private companies, termed *fiscal intermediaries,* that contract with Medicare to pay Medicare Part A and some Part B bills. These fiscal intermediaries influence what procedures and tests are covered at the local level.

If the patient's diagnosis does not comply with CMS guidelines but testing is determined to be necessary by the provider, the patient must be notified, in advance, that the cost of this testing may become the responsibility of the patient. This notification is formalized in the completion of an Advanced Beneficiary Notice (ABN), detailing the test requested, the symptoms or disease state necessitating the testing, and that the patient has been advised that the testing may not meet the guidelines for Medicare reimbursement. The patient signs the ABN, and the signature is witnessed by another staff person. Although on the surface this process may seem to limit provider discretion, it serves to deepen the provider's knowledge of appropriate utilization of diagnostic testing and recognition that diagnostic testing is an expensive and limited resource with significant financial impact on the health care system. This process also holds true for certain procedures that may be considered cosmetic, such as some lesion removals. The current ABN has been expanded to include any procedure and injection not covered by Medicare *(www.cahabagba.com).*

PROCESS RESOURCES

Facility, Equipment, and Supplies
Using the paradigm of systems thinking, the processes of care to be delivered and the setting in which these processes occur will determine the tools needed to deliver that care. Choice of facility and office space depends on capital resources and is beyond the scope of this chapter. Equipment and supplies will vary depending on the population served and the type of facility used. The most effective way to determine what is needed for a program or practice is to visit a site already in full operation and/or use business planning resources listed in Box 19-2. Inventory lists

Box 19-2   Useful Business Planning Resources for Advanced Practice Nurses

Centers for Medicare and Medicaid Services
7500 Security Blvd
Baltimore, MD 21244-1850
1-800-MEDICARE
1-800-633-4227
www.cms.hhs.gov

Drug Enforcement Administration (DEA)
2401 Jefferson Davis Highway
Alexandria, VA 22301
1-800-882-9539
www.usdoj.gov/dea

Medi-Scripts
500 Rt. 17 South, Suite 308
Hasbrouck Heights, NJ 07604
1-800-283-0140
201-727-1555
www.medipromotions.com

Counselors to America's Small Business (SCORE)
www.score.org

The Joint Commission
One Renaissance Blvd.
Oakbrook Terrace, IL 60181
630-792-5000
www.jointcommission.org

Pharmaceutical Research/Manufacturers of America (PhARMA)
950 F. Street NW
Washington, DC 20004
202-835-3400
fax 202-835-3414
www.phrma.org

Robert Wood Johnson Foundation
www.rwjf.org

Fast Company Business Planner
www.fastcompany.com

Business Statistics
www.bizstat.com

will need to be made for direct and indirect processes of care, including prices. This approach is the basis for cost-based analysis, which examines the actual costs of the supplies, equipment, and personnel needed to perform a particular process of care. Additional expenditures related to overhead such as air conditioning and billing are calculated into the final cost, which is then used to determine the charge to the patient for that process of care. The actual charge for each service should be based on the Medicare relative value unit times a conversion factor amount that not only is necessary for the practice but also is consistent with other services in the area (Reel & Abraham, 2007). By using this system, APNs will be assured that they will not be overcharging or undercharging for clinical services. The charge profile should be reviewed annually.

Additional methods available for identifying needed equipment and supplies include the following:

- Relying on clinical expertise of the APN and his or her familiarity with the items needed to deliver the particular service
- Referring to a clinical procedures manual that lists the equipment needed
- Consulting with the collaborating physician

- Interviewing other providers who are performing the same or similar services
- Interviewing support staff to determine what they require to perform their roles
- Referring to standardized equipment listings

After determining the program/practice needs, lists or inventories are generated. Equipment and supply inventories enable the APN to establish an initial budget and time line for business-planning purposes and provide information related to budgetary requests required by lenders and grantors. (These inventories may be included in any business plan, grant application, or office procedure manual, thus eliminating the need to rewrite them for each application.) Inventories also assist the APN to create an initial ordering list, record business assets, establish minimum par levels for an inventory of disposable supplies, and identify the locations where items are kept in the office to facilitate inventory management.

The initial inventories for medical and office equipment and supplies follow the same template and could be set up as separate spreadsheets such as durable equipment, reusable equipment/supplies, and disposable supplies within any commercial office software package. One advantage to this separation is that it enables the program administrator/practice manager to quickly assess how much money is needed to set up the program/practice, as opposed to how much will be needed on an ongoing basis for replenishment of supplies. Durable equipment includes desks, chairs, file cabinets, examination tables, autoclave, electrocardiograph, and computers, purchased as a one-time expense. Reusable equipment includes items such as otoscopes, stethoscopes, computer software, and trash containers. Disposable supplies can be separated into two lists: one for office supplies (e.g., pens, paper, staples) and one for medical supplies (e.g., syringes, bandages).

For accounting and budgeting purposes, request professional advice to separate these items into capital and noncapital expenses. Each list includes the specific name of the equipment or supply needed and the number of units required. Quotes from potential vendors for disposables should be sought on a yearly basis. Once a vendor is identified, the price per unit (unit cost) and a total price for that item (total cost) are added to the inventory template. It is possible to obtain some disposable supplies free of charge from other sources. For example, in primary care, often the laboratory analyzing the blood specimens drawn at the practice will provide alcohol swabs, small gauze pads, Band-Aids, and other supplies used during venipuncture or other specimen collection as part of its service to the practice. Many pharmaceutical representatives are often willing to provide pens, note pads, and clipboards for free, although these items will have the names of the pharmaceutical company's products on them as part of its marketing plan.

Decisions related to which processes will be performed in house, as opposed to being contracted externally, will affect the types of equipment and supplies needed. Examples of other indirect processes of care that need to be budgeted include the following:

- *Creating a patient database.* Several medical office computerized systems of varying complexity and cost are available for the management of patient information. Some of the processes supported by these programs are appointment scheduling, generation of patient encounter forms (superbills), and electronic claims filing. Electronic claims filing is essential to any practice as a way to keep the accounts receivable under control and should be HIPAA compliant (Buppert, 2003).
- *Transcription services.* For intrapreneurial APNs, transcription services may be available through the larger organization's facilities. For independent APNs, the decision to contract for transcription services should include a review of the available voice-to-text computer software programs that allow the APN to directly dictate the patient's progress note (or other printed material) into a commercially available word processing or desktop publishing program. Several voice-to-text programs are available with different degrees of complexity and adaptability and varying sizes of medical vocabulary lexicons. The prices for these programs range from $150 for a basic voice-to-text program to more than $4000 for a complex system that may be used by several providers at once.
- *Ensuring staff safety.* One staff member should be designated an OSHA officer to maintain OSHA compliance and training for all staff. Medical assistants or other clinical support personnel can be good OSHA officers. All staff must attend OSHA training, which can be done off-site, by the OSHA officer, or through a program subscription purchased online.
- *HIPAA compliance.* HIPAA training must take place annually. Delegate the office manager to train and maintain staff in HIPAA compliance. Off-site training and online training are available, usually at a higher cost. HIPAA materials for patients need to be posted and readable with available copies.
- *Patient education materials.* Patient education materials are available in a variety of formats, including videotape, interactive computer software, and written brochures or pamphlets. The APN should review the direct patient care processes for which educational materials can be anticipated. Part of the initial planning process includes reviewing available materials that can be incorporated into the APN's practice. Educational material should be evaluated for quality, readability/literacy level, availability in different languages, and cost. Oral presentations to individuals or groups are also an important component of patient education.

Managing Prescriptive Authority and Sample Medications

One process of care that requires particular attention is the use of pharmaceutical agents in direct patient care by APNs with prescriptive privileges. Prescriptive authority involves nonpharmacological as well as pharmacological interventions, but the focus here is on pharmacological interventions.

- *Writing the physical prescription.* APNs need to follow the regulating board's rules for prescribing in each state. Prescription pads should include the APN's name and credentials, the name of the APN's practice setting and, in several states, the name of the collaborating physician.
- *Receiving drug samples.* A system to track lot numbers, expiration dates, and the patients to whom the drugs were dispensed needs to be developed to address the issue of lot number recalls and to meet certain states' requirements for oversight.
- *Prescribing controlled substances.* In states where APNs can prescribe controlled substances, the APN must obtain an individual Drug Enforcement Administration (DEA) number. A completed DEA registration form will be required, with the registration fees paid, before the APN can prescribe controlled substances allowed by statute. The DEA registration is renewable every 3 years. Forms may be requested on the Internet (see Box 19-2). In addition to a DEA number, a locked, secure location for storage needs to be established and a procedure for access must be determined before acceptance of a supply if the APN dispenses controlled substances from the office.

Free prescription pads are available through Medi-Scripts, a prescription printing service funded by a collaboration of pharmaceutical companies. Box 19-2 provides further information. Prescription pads should never be left where they may become accessible to patients, family, or unauthorized staff.

The use of medications, herbals, or homeopathy within a program or practice depends on the nature of the services to be delivered but is also constrained by the scope of practice granted by individual state nurse practice acts. When decisions regarding the use of pharmaceutical agents have been made, a listing of anticipated pharmacy supplies, along with cost, vendor, and drug comparison information, may be generated from the same software spreadsheet as the other inventories. When a pharmaceutical inventory is prepared, those practices that provide children's services will find enrollment in the state immunization program extremely useful. States provide immunizations free to children who fall within certain eligibility guidelines (e.g., Medicaid recipients, uninsured patients, participants in a federally funded health center). These programs involve practice enrollment, a monthly vaccine utilization report, and some record keeping regarding recipient eligibility. Some state programs have established a web-based system, allowing practices to report monthly usage and to reorder vaccine online. The maximum benefit of the web-based system is that it allows confirmation of childhood vaccinations to other enrolled practices within a secure and confidential network environment.

When writing prescriptions, the APN must be aware of the patient's financial resources and constraints and know the requirements and procedures for prescribing from insurance companies' formularies or for obtaining prior approval for non-formulary items when indicated. The uninsured and those with low income may have access to prescription assistance from the pharmaceutical company, available on their websites. In addition, a number of foundations assist underinsured patients to meet their co-pay expenses.

It is important to note that certain third-party payers, government agencies, and mail-order prescription drug companies will not accept prescriptions from APNs. The primary reason for this exclusion is that the state to which the prescription and enrollment forms are sent does not permit APNs to write prescriptions. The second reason for this exclusion is that the parent company is unaware of revisions to state practice acts that allow APNs to write prescriptions in particular states. The solution to the first issue is the development of a prescribing policy whereby the APN's collaborating physician writes the prescription for that patient's medications. The solution to the second issue is continued efforts on the part of APNs to educate and collaborate with pharmaceutical companies to ensure that accurate, timely information about current state regulation is being shared. Patients who obtain their prescriptions through the Internet or those patients whose insurance prescription plan requires a written prescription may also experience the inconvenience of being told that the APN cannot write their prescriptions.

THE BUSINESS PLAN SUMMARY

Once the process of business or program planning has been accomplished, the APN should summarize in one document the mission, vision, values, and processes of care and required resources to meet the patient's needs. Traditionally, this summary has taken the form of a business plan (see Chapter 20), which was then distributed to potential sources of financial backing. Even if the program is not seeking external funding, a summary is needed to describe the available services to others. One way of writing this summary is to modify the traditional business plan so that it reflects a systems-thinking approach to patient care. Box 19-3 provides an outline of a program/practice summary. The reader is referred to Reel and Abraham (2007), Buppert (2004), the AMA (2002c), Letz, (2002), the Small Business Administration *(www.sba.gov)*, and local business advisors for additional information and advice.

Consideration must be given to the audience for whom the summary is being prepared. As discussed earlier, funding agencies have specific guidelines for the compilation of the program's operational documentation. If the summary is written for the community of patients being served, issues related to literacy, language, and emphasis need to be addressed. If the summary is written for potential investors or potential physician colleagues, issues related to capital expenditures, numbers of patients to be served, services to be delivered, and expected revenue need to be emphasized. Consequently, the first step in preparing the summary is to identify the anticipated audience.

A successful business plan describes what the business does, how it does it, and how it evaluates the outcomes achieved (Kleinpell, 2001). A successful APN develops, implements, and evaluates both patient care and indirect processes that support outcomes by organizing these tasks as a system. Today's health care consumers demand that patient

---

Box 19-3   OUTLINE OF A PROGRAM/PRACTICE SUMMARY

I. Introductory Elements
  A. Cover page
  B. Overview/summary
    1. Mission and vision statements
    2. Overarching program/practice values
    3. Other required elements
  C. Table of contents
II. Description
  A. Background information
  B. Direct processes of care to be delivered
  C. Key factors in the delivery of patient care
III. Market
  A. Description of the patient population to be served
    1. Patient demographics
  B. Analysis of the market
  C. Marketing strategy
    1. Initial
    2. Ongoing
  D. Competition
  E. Advertising and promotion
IV. Program/Practice Structure
  A. Structure/ownership
  B. Management
  C. Clinical advisors and services offered (includes APN)
  D. Business advisors and services offered
  E. Support staff and services offered
V. Resources
  A. Budget

    1. Projected income
      a. Start-up capital: business loans, grants
      b. Ongoing capital: patient revenues, other funding
    2. Projected expenses
      a. Office space and overhead
      b. Durable equipment
      c. Reusable equipment
      d. Disposable items
      e. Provider and staff compensation
      f . Compliance budget
      g. Technology updates
        i. Software for databases,
        ii. Subscriptions
        iii. Classification updates
VI. Compliance
  A. Federal and/or state regulations
    1. TJC
    2. OSHA
    3. CMS
  B. Other agency regulations
  C. Provider-specific licensing, credentialing, privileging
  D. HIPAA
  E. Risk Management
VII. Outcome Evaluation
  A. APN performance measures
  B. System performance measures
  C. Internal review parameters and timeline
  D. External review parameters and timeline

APN, Advanced practice nurse; *CMS,* Centers for Medicare and Medicaid Services; *HIPAA,* Health Insurance Portability and Accountability Act; *OSHA,* Occupational Safety & Health Administration; *TJC,* The Joint Commission.

care delivery be individualized, compassionate, effective, and resource-efficient. A sound knowledge of the system in which care is delivered enables APNs to meet the demands of today's complex environment and the patients they serve.

Choosing the type of practice to engage in as an APN is a difficult and challenging task, one that the APN will have to live with on a daily basis. Decisions around practice type require careful planning, research, and discussions with other APNs who have entered into various types of practice arrangements. Exemplar 19-1 describes a practice arrangement and illustrates how one APN was able to purchase a "turn key" family practice business in a very short time and eventually employ a second APN.

PAYMENT MECHANISMS FOR ADVANCED PRACTICE NURSES

The process of reimbursement is perhaps the most important and complex indirect process supporting patient care. Figure 19-3 provides an overview of reimbursement. All APNs are involved in the completion of the patient's clinical encounter, the documentation of the encounter in the patient's medical

---

 EXEMPLAR 19-1   The Entrepreneurial Advanced Practice Nurse

Sally is a family NP who was employed by an OB/GYN physician to offer family practice services at his busy private practice. This was her first job as an NP. Her experience included 20 years as a critical care RN, with 7 of those years as an internal medicine office manager in a private practice setting. After 1 year of employment as an NP, her employer decided to move out of the area, offering her first refusal on purchasing the practice. This practice would become a family practice business only. Because his move would take place almost immediately, decisions had to be made quickly. Sally had never really thought about owning her own practice; however, this idea was certainly attractive. A quick feasibility study was necessary.

Sally solicited advice from family and peers, who were supportive. She developed a collaborative practice agreement with a local physician to provide back-up and referral. Sally's collaborating physician had his own practice at another site and believed strongly that this was a great opportunity for her. She received assistance from her employer in writing a business plan and then reviewed the business plan with a local business owner and her accountant friend for advice. Was this a good, sound business investment or not? After receiving positive feedback on her business plan, Sally met with a local banker to discuss financing. A small business loan for women was compared with a conventional bank loan. The small business loan was possible but very restrictive and required frequent reporting. The conventional bank loan was actually a better idea with a more beneficial interest rate. The president of the bank reviewed Sally and her husband's assets and agreed to the loan, with a line of credit for any start-up expense

needed. Sally used the bank's attorney for all legal advice. He advised her to establish a subchapter S–type corporation, set this up for her, and prepared the closing papers and all documents necessary to complete the transaction. Sally's accountant friend agreed to be the business accountant and set up all computer programs for her. He also became her business advisor and a most valuable asset to the success of her practice.

From the time Sally was approached by her employer in May of 2000, the entire process was completed in 8 weeks. Although this went from start to finish quickly, several things were in place to make this happen. Because this was a "turn key" business, all staff, equipment, supplies, medical software, vendor accounts, payroll services, medical records, patients, and accounts receivable were already established. All direct and indirect processes of care were established, with the cost and budget known at time of purchase. Because she was already credentialed with insurance companies under his name, a change of business name and new tax identification number for reimbursement were all that were required. There was no interruption in service to the patients being served by the practice. After 4 years of business success, Sally was able to employ another family NP. Beverly was hired as an employee the first year and then was able to become incorporated and work as an independent contractor to Sally's business in the second year of her employment. Today Sally and Beverly operate one of the most successful practices in the region. Sally attributes much of her success to the attention that the practice pays to each patient and the focus on open lines of communication among staff, patients, and families.

NP, Nurse practitioner; *OB/GYN*, obstetrical/gynecological; *RN*, registered nurse.

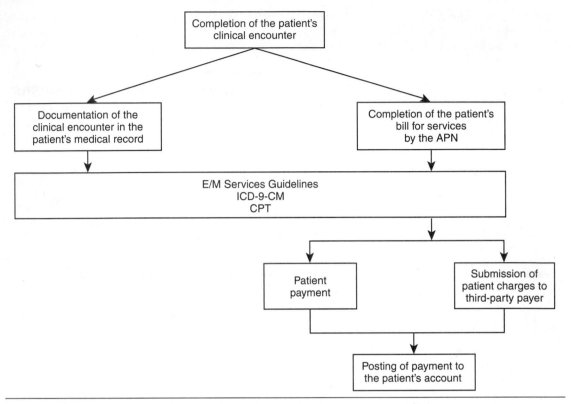

FIGURE **19-3:** An overview of reimbursement. *APN,* Advanced practice nurse; *CPT,* current procedural terminology; *E/M,* evaluation and management; *ICD-9-CM,* International Classification of Diseases, Ninth Revision, Clinical Modification.

record, and, frequently, the completion of the patient's bill for services. APNs must be involved in the subsequent steps in the reimbursement process: the actual payment collection, either from the patient or from the third-party payer; and the posting of the payment to the patient's account in the provider's office. They should be cognizant of the major concepts and issues related to third-party reimbursement and to APN compensation. To ensure profitability, APNs need to check regularly that the reimbursement is consistent with the most recent contracted fee schedules and that monies are collected in a timely manner. As illustrated in Figure 19-3, reimbursement links payment of the APN with the clinical encounter, the patient's medical record, the patient's bill for services, the claim submitted to the appropriate third-party payer (if any), and the payment of the APN for services delivered. In this section, an overview of documentation is presented, along with a description of the major third-party payment schemes and the

patient's financial responsibility for self-pay. Examples are used to illustrate steps in the reimbursement process.

Documentation of Services

Documenting the care given to each patient and maintaining and managing patient records are high-priority tasks for APNs in any type of practice arrangement. Coordinating care across time and various settings and providing continuity for patients with chronic illnesses and multiple co-morbidities require a well–thought-out process, attention to detail, and appropriate documentation for reimbursement purposes. The following discussion provides several approaches to documenting care. Several manuals and classification systems are used to bill for services including these widely accepted medical classification systems: the International Classification of Diseases, Ninth Revision, Clinical Modification (ICD-9-CM) and Current Procedural Terminology

(CPT) codes. The ICD-9 code is developed by the World Health Organization (WHO) in Geneva, Switzerland, and the ICD-9-CM is the American version of ICD-9. ICD-9-CM is continuously updated and contains one more level (decimal) than the original ICD *(www.cdc.gov)*. The evaluation and management (E/M) services guidelines (CMS, 2006a) were developed to compensate providers for clinical and cognitive effort rather than time expended.

Medical Classification Systems

ICD-9-CM Codes. The ICD-9-CM codes are diagnostic codes that identify the diagnosis, symptom, or condition to be treated. Their purpose is to aid in standardizing coding practices across the United States (AMA, 2007) as directed by the CMS. The CMS has prepared guidelines for use of the ICD-9-CM codes in the area of medical billing. These guidelines are available online at the CMS website *(www.cms.hhs.gov)* and from Medicare's local fiscal intermediaries. The codes are published each year in two volumes that are combined into one spiral-bound text for ease of use. Volume 1 contains the Tabular List of Diseases, based on the ICD-9-CM code attached to the diagnosis, symptom, or condition of concern. Volume 2 contains the Alphabetic Index to Diseases, published by Practice Management Information Corporation. To identify the appropriate code for a particular symptom, a clinician would begin the search in Volume 2 under the alphabetical listing. Once the code is obtained from Volume 2, the clinician then turns to the tabular listing of the code itself to determine any additional modifiers necessary to clarify the entity being coded. For example, if an NP diagnoses otitis media, Volume 2 indicates that "Otitis" is coded as 382.9. Volume 2 also indicates that additional information is needed to determine which code best matches the type of otitis media the patient has: acute (382.9), with effusion (381.00), allergic (381.04), serous (381.01), with spontaneous rupture of ear drum (382.01), and so on. A listing of common ICD-9-CM codes used in family practice may be found on the American Academy of Family Practice website *(www.aafp.org)*.

The primary function of the ICD-9-CM is to facilitate medical billing. Therefore it is sometimes used at the point of care to classify the patient's diagnosis (or diagnoses) on the patient's billing form, or superbill. The *superbill* is so named because all subsequent forms generated for that encounter are based on this first bill completed at the time of service. The

superbill may have a listing of frequently seen diagnoses or symptoms accompanied by the appropriate ICD-9-CM code for the provider to check off. This practice is discouraged by CMS because of a concern that diagnostic bias may be introduced by the presence of preprinted diagnoses. The CMS would prefer that the provider write the diagnosis or symptom independently, without the possible influence of the preprinted list. The billing coder for the medical practice then transcribes this code onto a uniform billing form (CMS-1500 claim form) that is submitted for reimbursement, preferably by electronic means. If the provider does not know the code assigned to his or her assessment findings, the coder assigns the code based on the diagnosis (or diagnoses), sign(s), or symptom(s) written on the patient's superbill. In addition, each service or procedure performed for a client must be represented by a diagnosis that would substantiate those particular services or procedures. In other words, the procedure performed must match the diagnosis coded. For example, if a urine dipstick was performed in the office, the superbill should show diagnoses related to urinary tract infection, polyuria, dysuria, and the like. This practice has received particular attention in the realm of diagnostic testing through the use of ABNs (see previous discussion in the "Diagnostic Services" section) for those services that may not fall within Medicare or any other insurer's guidelines for medical necessity.

In addition to its role in reimbursement, the ICD-9-CM serves as a guide to the practicing clinician for the classifications of diseases and symptoms. It is a useful tool in the evaluation of morbidity data for indexing medical records, medical care review, ambulatory and other medical care programs, and basic health statistics (see example in Box 19-4). This tool can be used also for evaluation of outcomes as part of quality improvement initiatives. Supplemental coding information is located in the ICD-9-CM to capture those patient encounters with the health care system that may not entail a disease or injury classified elsewhere in the manual. There are three main types of encounters that fall into this category and receive a "V code":

- When a well person encounters the health care system for some specific purpose (e.g., organ or tissue donation [V42.0 for kidney recipient], prophylactic vaccination [V04.8 for influenza vaccination]).

Box 19-4 ANALYSIS OF ICD-9-CM CODES TO DETERMINE PRACTICE PRIORITIES

An adult NP wants to know which symptoms or diagnoses are most common in her practice. Collaborating with the medical billings administrator in her practice, the APN defines a sort of the administrative billing database by ICD-9-CM code. The sort tallies the numbers of patient encounters associated with each code. The resulting list captures the most frequent diagnoses seen in her practice. Among the top five ICD-9-CM codes represented, hypertension, unspecified (401.9) and type 2 diabetes mellitus, uncontrolled (250.22) rank numbers 1 and 2. Based on this information, the NP commits to implementing the Seventh Report of the Joint National Committee on Prevention, Detection, Evaluation, and Treatment of High

Blood Pressure guidelines (U.S. Department of Health and Human Services, 2003) for the management of hypertension, and the American Diabetes Association (2003) guidelines for the management of diabetes. Flow sheets for blood pressure readings, urinalysis results, glycosylated hemoglobin testing, and scheduled referrals to specialists and routine follow-ups are developed. The following year, the NP commits to evaluating what percentage of patients with hypertension are reaching the goal of systolic blood pressure less than 140 mm Hg and diastolic blood pressure less than 90 mm Hg and what percentage of patients with diabetes are reaching the goal of a glycosylated hemoglobin below 7 gm/dL.

APN, Advanced practice nurse; *ICD-9-CM*, International Classification of Diseases, Ninth Revision, Clinical Modification; *NP*, nurse practitioner.

- When a person with a known disease or illness encounters the system for a specific treatment related to that disease or illness (e.g., chemotherapy [V58.1]).
- When some circumstance exists that influences the person's health status but is not in itself a current illness or injury (e.g., inadequate housing [V60.1], no other household member able to render care [V60.4]).

Environmental events, circumstances, and conditions that are the cause of injury (motor vehicle accidents), poisoning, fire, and/or other adverse effects are assigned "E codes."

Current Procedural Terminology Codes.
CPT codes are those listed in the Current Procedural Terminology manual published annually by the AMA (2008). This text is a listing of the descriptive terms and identifying codes for reporting medical services and procedures (AMA, 2008). As with the ICD-9-CM, the CPT manual serves to provide a uniform language that accurately describes medical, surgical, and diagnostic services. The CPT codes for reimbursement should accurately reflect the services or procedures performed for those ICD-9-CM codes assigned to the patient's diagnosis (or diagnoses) or symptom(s). All services or procedures are assigned a five-digit code and represent procedures consistent with contemporary medical practice and performance by many providers in multiple locations. The CPT manual is divided into several sections: Evaluation and Management (see previous discussion), Anesthesiology, Surgery, Radiology,

Pathology and Laboratory, and Medicine. Medicare and state Medicaid carriers are required by law to use CPT codes for the payment of health insurance claims; all insurance carriers recognize and use CPT codes. Although a CPT code may describe a current medical procedure, a particular insurance carrier may deny reimbursement for that specific procedure.

Occasionally, modifiers are used to indicate that a service or procedure has been performed and not changed in its description or code but altered by some specific or extenuating circumstance. The use of modifiers attached to the end of CPT codes eliminates the need for separate procedure codes in these instances. Understanding the proper use of modifiers substantially affects insurance claim reimbursement. The reader is referred to the CPT manual for an in-depth explanation of the use of modifier codes. CPT codes are also available in paper, disk, and CD-ROM formats from the AMA.

E/M Services Guidelines. The E/M services guidelines (CMS, 2006a) are available online at the CMS website (*www.cms.hhs.gov*) or through the local Medicare intermediary. There are seven components of E/M services, with the first four bearing the most weight:
- *Nature of the presenting problem:* The reason or need for the client's office visit.
- *History:* The client's chief concern, a brief history of the present issue or illness, and a related systems review. A family and/or social history is included.

- *Physical examination:* May be *focused*, addressing only the affected body area or organ system, or *comprehensive*, addressing a complete examination of a single system of concern, or a multiple system physical examination.
- *Medical decision making:* Refers to the complexity in establishing a diagnosis and selecting a certain management strategy. It includes the differential diagnoses and management options, an analysis of medical records, all diagnostic tests, and other information analyzed to make a competent decision.
- *Counseling:* Includes discussions or meetings with client, family, caregivers, and nursing staff (as in long-term care). Counseling can include discussions about disease process, results of diagnostic tests, prognosis, education and instructions on management, and treatment options.
- *Coordination of care:* Refers to time spent working with other health care providers and agencies to direct care. This process must be well documented in the client's medical record if it is intended to denote the type of service or care delivered because other providers may be billing for direct care of the patient.
- *Time:* In the case of encounters that predominantly consist of counseling or coordination of care, time is the key component used to determine the level of E/M services provided. Time is defined as "face-to-face" time in the office; time spent reviewing records and tests and arranging further services; or time spent with staff, such as in the nursing home. Time should be averaged in minutes and recorded in the client's medical record. Time is considered only when coordination, chart review, and counseling services represent more than 50% of the visit.

As noted, the major elements used to determine the level of service provided under the E/M system are the patient history, the physical examination, and the complexity of medical decision making required to manage the patient. Elements of at least these three components must have been performed and consequently documented in the patient's medical record. The documentation guidelines provide minimum assessment data points within each component that will support a particular level of E/M service. Each level of service is assigned a separate five-digit CPT code. The codes vary for new patients and established

patients even if the same level of service has been provided (Box 19-5).

Nursing Classification Systems. Clinically excellent, holistic patient care delivered by APNs includes both nursing and medical diagnoses, interventions, and outcomes. Nursing diagnoses provide the basis for the selection of nursing interventions that achieve the identified patient outcomes for which the nurse is accountable (McCloskey & Bulechek, 2000; NANDA-I, 2007). Thus documentation by an APN on the patient record would reasonably include a combination of both nursing and medical diagnoses, interventions, and outcomes languages. APNs, such as CNSs, work in settings in which documentation standards are based on a nursing taxonomy such as NANDA. However, in many settings, third-party reimbursement requires that medically oriented information be recorded in chronological order in the patient record. Such information includes reason for the visit, health history (including past and present illnesses), physical examination findings, test results, treatments, and outcomes (CNS, 2006a). Therefore APN students precepted by APNs in such settings are not routinely prepared to continue the use of the nursing-sensitive language they learned in their undergraduate nursing education. One likely reason may be economically driven since reimbursement policies are based on medical language. In general, APNs are unable to bill third-party payers or be reimbursed for nursing diagnoses or interventions unless the diagnosis or intervention is also recognized as a medical one. In the future, direct financial compensation may be paid for nursing diagnoses and interventions that are independent of a medical model counterpart, but they have not gained a foothold to date.

NANDA International (NANDA-I) has worked toward the establishment and implementation of a classification system for nursing diagnoses that provides a taxonomy of clinical judgments about individual, family, or community responses to actual or potential health problems/life processes (NANDA-I, 2007). The current strategic goals of NANDA-I 2004-2010, including plans to incorporate NANDA-I diagnoses in standardized language systems and health care databases and research, can be found at *www. nanda.org*. The Iowa Interventions Project developed an evolving codified taxonomy of nursing interventions, the Nursing Interventions Classification (NIC), to list the treatments that nurses perform, to assist practitioners in documenting their care, and to facilitate the evaluation of nurse-sensitive patient outcomes (McCloskey & Bulechek, 2000). The Nursing

Box 19-5   Example of Implementing Documentation Guidelines: Subjective, Objective, Assessment, Plan, Evaluation

S:
R.M. is a 6-year-old boy brought to the office by his mother. He is an existing patient. She reports that R.M. has had a 24-hour history of severe sore throat, headache, and fever to 102° F. He is unable to swallow solids because of throat pain but is taking fluids well. R.M. reports that his best friend has also been ill with similar symptoms. Denies ear pain, nasal congestion, nausea, vomiting, or diarrhea. Mom has been treating his symptoms at home with over-the-counter medications for fever management, salt water gargles, rest, and increased amounts of fluids, with fair symptom relief.
R.M. has been a healthy child, with no prior episodes of acute illness, injury, or hospitalization. He has no known drug or environmental allergies. His only medication is a children's multivitamin. He takes no prescription medications or alternative modality supplements.

O:
GEN: Alert, well-developed, well-nourished, flushed child in mild distress. VS: T, 101.9° F oral; HR, 115; RR, 20; Wt, 35 kg. HEAD: NC. No frontal or maxillary tenderness with palpation or percussion. ENT: Bilateral external auditory canals clear. Bilateral tympanic membranes pink, translucent, neutral, and freely mobile. Bony landmarks clearly visible. Nasal mucosa pink, moist, mildly edematous. Nasal passages partially obstructed by swollen turbinates. Clear rhinorrhea in the vaults. Buccal mucosa pink and moist. Tonsillar pillars, tonsils, and posterior pharynx beefy, swollen, and covered with white purulent exudate. NECK: Supple with

significant tonsillar and anterior cervical adenopathy. QUICK STREP TEST: positive (CPT 87430 Rapid antigen strep testing).

A/P:
Strep pharyngitis (ICD-9-CM 034.0 Streptococcus, unspecified)
Fever (ICD-9-CM 780.6 Fever)
Throat swab for culture and sensitivity (CPT 87070)
Antibiotic regimen based upon weight
Supportive measures including symptomatic management of fever and throat pain with over-the-counter medications (NIC 3900 Temperature regulation)
Anticipatory guidance provided to mother and child regarding streptococcal infection, anticipated course of illness, and treatment implementation (NIC 5602 Teaching: Disease process; NIC 5616 Teaching: Prescribed medication; NIC 7040 Caregiver support)
Risk for infection transmission
Anticipatory guidance provided to mother and child regarding meticulous handwashing and other activities that decrease the spread of infection (NIC 7040 Caregiver support; NIC 5618 Teaching: Procedure/treatment)

E:
Mother to be notified of throat culture results and any need to alter antibiotic therapy based upon sensitivities. If child does not improve or worsens in next 48 hours, he is to return to clinic for reevaluation. R.M. due for next well-child check in 7 months.

E/M:
99213 Expanded services, existing patient.

S, subjective; *O*, objective; *A*, assessment; *P*, plan; *E*, evaluation; *E/M*, evaluation and management.
CPT, Current procedural terminology; *ENT*, ears, nose, and throat; *GEN*, general; *HR*, heart rate; *ICD-9-CM*, International Classification of Diseases, Ninth Revision, Clinical Modification; *NC*, non-contributory; *NIC*, Nursing Interventions Classification; *RR*, respiratory rate; *STREP*, streptococcus; *T*, temperature; *VS*, vital signs; *Wt*, weight.

Outcomes Classification (NOC) exists to codify a standardized language of nursing-sensitive patient outcomes (Iowa Intervention Project, 1997). Familiarity with these standardized languages that capture the nursing care provided by APNs, as well as their consistent use in clinical practice and documentation, provides APNs with valuable tools in support of APN practice now and in the future.

Summary of Documentation

Familiarity with the guidelines and external regulations that govern reimbursement programs for medical care enables the APN to obtain health care reimbursement through existing reimbursement classification structures and demonstrates to third-party payers that the APN is a knowledgeable participant in health care. This degree of professional accountability may reduce barriers to full APN participation as providers of record in their own right and expand the inclusion of nursing care within the realm of reimbursed elements of patient care. The foundation of the reimbursement process is proper patient medical record documentation of medical necessity. Payers require the following information to determine medical necessity: (1) knowledge of the emergent nature or severity of the patient's condition and (2) the signs, symptoms, complaints, or background facts describing the reasons for care. This information must be substantiated by the patient's medical record, and it must be available to payers upon request with a signed patient authorization (AMA, 2002b; see also *www.cms.hhs.gov/*). Failure to document services rendered translates into the nonperformance of the service, which may leave the APN open not only to questions regarding the medical necessity of the encounter but also to potential liability issues.

All services submitted for reimbursement must be supported by appropriate documentation in the patient's medical record. Explanation of unusual services or extenuating circumstances must be clear and unambiguous; there should be no room for misinterpretation or assumption. From a financial standpoint, insurance carriers will frequently limit or deny reimbursement for services because of insufficient documentation. In addition, they may request refunds from the provider if audited medical records do not substantiate the reported services. APNs who are precepting students must also be aware of current CMS regulations concerning reimbursement that may prevent documentation in patient records by certain categories of students *(www.cms.hhs.gov)*.

To bill for services, many insurance carriers require the use of specific medical documentation guidelines, classifications, reimbursement codes, and ongoing evidence of APN credentials. Documentation guidelines provide standardization and structure for the clinical encounter record. The various classifications available provide a standard language, used by both insurance carriers and health care providers, to provide a uniform interpretation of medical conditions and to identify the billable services of the provider. Three main systems are used to record and classify care delivered: (1) the evaluation and management (E/M) services guidelines (CMS, 2006a), (2) the ICD-9-CM codes (ICD-9-CM 2007 Physician Volume 1&2, AMA), and (3) the CPT codes (AMA 2007 Professional Edition; *www.ama.assn.org*) discussed earlier.

Reimbursement for Advanced Practice Nurses

At the conclusion of the patient encounter, two parallel processes occur (see Figure 19-3). The APN documents the clinical encounter in the patient's record and completes the patient's superbill. Ideally, the medical record should provide data in support of the level of service selected, the ICD-9-CM diagnoses used, and the CPT codes used. As discussed previously, it is anticipated that the record will also document nursing diagnoses and interventions appropriate to the clinical scenario. Both medical and nursing outcomes and plans for evaluating the efficacy of the plan of care are expected to be included. Viewed through the lens of process improvement and innovation, the implementation of these external resources allows APNs to improve the existing processes of care while establishing baseline information for reimbursement. Improvement may be obtained through the use of guidelines both to support the appropriate level of third-party reimbursement and to include key elements of patient care. The key to improvement in the quality of care is for APNs to capture the full range of nursing as well as medical interventions. In this way, APNs can be reimbursed for the full range of interventions that they provide. Guidelines can be adapted by individual APNs to create encounter forms incorporating the anticipated elements of the patient's history, physical examination, and diagnostic testing for any particular APN practice. Today's health care economic landscape presents several obstacles to the inclusion of APNs in reimbursement strategies, from the barriers related to scope of practice (see Chapter 21) to the lack of recognition of nursing diagnoses and interventions for monetary compensation. From a systems-thinking approach, APNs must continue efforts to rectify these inequities through an understanding of, active participation in, and knowledge-based improvement of the current processes of reimbursement. An overview of direct patient payer and third-party payer reimbursement strategies is presented here. The reader is referred to the individual programs described for the most recent legislation and information affecting APN participation or enrollment.

Fostering Patient Responsibility. Patients need to assume some level of self-care and financial responsibility for their health care. Self-care measures include active participation in the development and implementation of the plan of care for wellness maintenance and/or illness management. Financial responsibility includes recognition of the valuable services provided by the APN and subsequent compensation of the APN for those services. Patients should be familiar with their insurance programs, particularly with regard to understanding that many programs do not provide the "blanket insurance" elements that were common in the past. Patients without insurance should expect to pay for the services rendered at the time of their delivery unless prior arrangements have been made with the APN.

Financial Responsibility Statement. The billing process includes the development of clear and concise written procedures and policies that will enhance the efficiency of the practice, allow review of individual patient bills to ensure accuracy, and clearly communicate to clients where their responsibilities for payment lie (AMA, 2002b). A clearly written patient financial responsibility statement, specifically describing payment expectations, should be provided to and signed by each client upon entry into the APN's practice. These expectations not only include what is expected from the patient but also describe what the patient may expect from the APN's billing procedures and staff. It would be advantageous to include a signed statement allowing the assignment of insurance benefits directly to the APN as part of the financial responsibility statement. This release expedites the processing of insurance claims when the patient's signature is required and should be renewed annually. Annual renewal of financial responsibility not only complies with most insurance payers but also acts as a reminder to the patient of his or her responsibility. It is extremely important to check the patient's insurance card at every visit, because one release form does not carry to another company. Payment guidelines should be posted in the patient waiting room stating, for example, "Co-pay required at time of service" and "You must have a valid insurance card to be seen."

Installment Plans. In the event that the uninsured or self-pay client is unable to pay for services at the time they are rendered, offering alternative payment plans provides financial flexibility while supporting the patient's financial responsibility to pay for the care delivered. These alternatives should be negotiated and documented before the patient's appointment. The agreed-upon payment should then be collected at the time of service. Based upon systems developed by consumer lenders, installment payment plans enable patients to pay their bills in regularly scheduled partial payments. These plans are negotiated between the APN's practice and the patient on a case-by-case basis, according to predetermined policies established by the practice. Interest is not added to the installment payment because the payment is not considered a financial loan per se; however, a service charge may be added.

Sliding Fee Scales. Sliding fee scale programs set up by the business using state and federal guidelines may be offered to eligible applicants who have been denied Medicaid because they exceed that program's income guidelines. Practices offering sliding fee scales require that the patient apply for and be refused other forms of medical financial aid before applying for the practice's program. From a patient's perspective, the information needed to complete the application for sliding fee scale is often identical to that used for a state Medicaid application. Consequently, it is possible for the patient to have to compile the mandatory financial information only once while applying to two different funding programs.

Failure to Pay. Consequences for failure to meet the agreed-upon payments under practice-based aid programs may result in collection services being initiated against the patient and/or the decision by the provider to not offer services to the patient any longer. As discussed earlier, issues related to denial of care must be clearly documented before the provider takes any action and must include providing the patient with an opportunity to secure the services of another provider.

Payment Mechanisms. There are as many different payment mechanisms as there are different health insurance companies. Each company has its own process for becoming a recognized provider and providing reimbursement for care delivered to its beneficiaries. The unstable health care environment means that the information for each plan can change quickly from month to month and varies from state to state. However, the need for uniformity is ever-present as health care reimbursement becomes more difficult and costly to obtain. The basic process involved in reimbursement, as an independent provider, is illustrated in Figure 19-4. APNs should be familiar with and participate in the major programs that are the mainstay of American health care.

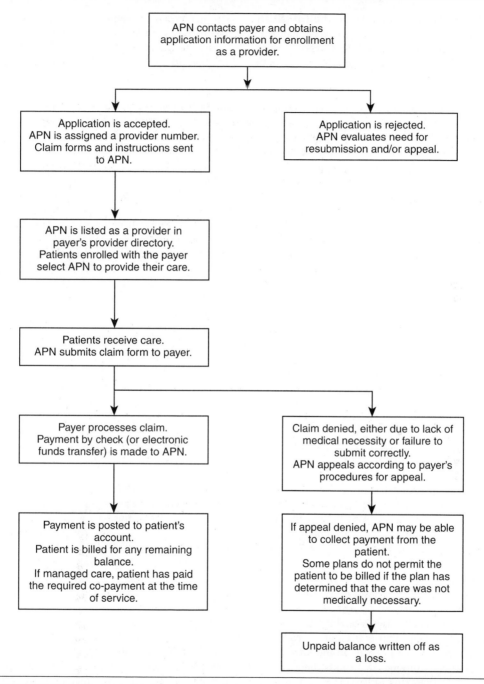

FIGURE **19-4:** The basic third-party payer reimbursement process. *APN,* Advanced practice nurse.

Medicare. Since its authorization by Title XVIII of the Social Security Act in 1965, Medicare has provided access to care to individuals 65 years of age and older. In 1972, Medicare coverage was extended to include those individuals younger than 65 years with long-term disabilities (of at least 2 years' duration and eligible for Social Security Disability Insurance) and those with end-stage renal disease. In 1982, the Tax Equity and Fiscal Responsibility Act introduced a risk-based option, facilitating the involvement of health maintenance organizations (HMOs). In 1983, the inpatient hospital prospective payment system (PPS) was adopted. This system replaced cost-based payments with a plan in which a predetermined rate was paid based on patients' diagnoses. The Balanced Budget Act of 1997 included the most extensive legislative changes for Medicare since its inception. Among these changes are the expansion of covered preventive benefits and the establishment of Part C (Medicare Choice), which creates new managed care and other health plan choices for beneficiaries (*www.cms.hhs.gov/medicare*). In 1997, Medicare opened up to private company HMOs to provide beneficiaries with additional benefits at a proposed lower cost (Northeast Health Care Quality Foundation, 1999). Some of these private HMOs have already left the Medicare program because of the negative impact on their business and financial viability. (See Chapter 22 for further discussion of the Medicare program.)

Medicare coverage consists of two parts. Hospital insurance (Part A) covers inpatient hospital services, short-term care in skilled nursing facilities, post-institutional home health care, and hospice care. Those individuals eligible for Social Security are automatically enrolled in Part A. Other qualified beneficiaries need to initiate the enrollment process. Supplementary medical insurance (Part B) covers physician services, outpatient hospital services, home health care not covered by Part A, and other medical services such as diagnostic testing, durable medical equipment, and ambulance costs. Enrollment in Part B is voluntary to beneficiaries receiving Part A. Medicare Part A is funded primarily through payroll taxes, although beneficiary cost sharing in the form of deductibles and co-insurance also funds the program. Beneficiaries participating in Part B pay into the system through monthly premiums that are established yearly based upon system expenses as well as through deductibles and co-insurance programs for various services. Medicare Choice (Part C) benefits are available through participation in coordinated care or private fee-for-service plans and medical savings accounts (*www.cms.hhs.gov/medicare*).

Beginning January 1, 2006, Medicare Part D prescription drug coverage became available to all people with Medicare. As of June 2006, over 32 million beneficiaries had enrolled in the program (*www.cms.hhs.gov/prescriptiondrug*). Providers are not required to participate in Medicare. For participating providers, the Medicare fee schedule for physicians' professional services, services and supplies provided incident to physicians' professional services (e.g., certain medications and biological agents), and patient physical and occupational therapy services, diagnostic tests, and radiology services is 5% higher than for non-participants (National Heritage Insurance Company [NHIC], 2004). At present, NPs, CNSs, CNMs, and CRNAs in some settings are permitted to bill Medicare as individual providers. Payments are set at 85% of the physician's fee schedule. Visit *www.cms.hhs.gov/provider/* for the current year physician fee schedule.

APNs who are Medicare providers must be participating providers, which means they will accept "assignment," the allowable charge determined by Medicare. As of May 2007, APNs need the following qualifications to be a Medicare provider:

- A state registered nurse (RN) and advanced practice registered nurse (APRN) license
- National certification in an advanced nursing specialty
- A master's degree in nursing
- A National Provider Identifier (NPI) number

The unique provider identification number (UPIN) and all former legacy numbers used to identify APNs with Medicare were replaced by the new NPI number. On May 23, 2007, the NPI became the only means Medicare recognizes to identify APNs in all standard transactions. The NPI also replaced the numbers APNs use in communicating with other payers as well. NPI information can be found at *https://nppes.cms.hhs.gov/* (see Chapter 21).

Medicaid. Medicaid provides health insurance benefits as well as other assistance for eligible low-income individuals and families. Medicaid is a jointly funded state-federal insurance program. Coverage varies by state according to federal requirements that stipulate eligibility and basic services covered. Payment is usually lower than is available through other insurance groups. Privatization has occurred in some states as they have contracted with private HMO companies to administer previously state-funded

Medicaid plans. In 1989, Congress mandated that state Medicaid agencies provide direct reimbursement to family NPs, pediatric NPs, and CNMs. Some states cover the services of other APNs; however, the resulting inconsistencies have caused significant confusion. The Medicaid site at *www.cms.hhs.gov/medicaid* offers links to individual states and their Medicaid rules and regulations. A recent change in Title XXI of the Social Security Act offers services for children through the State Children's Health Insurance Program (SCHIP). (See Chapter 22 and *visit www.cms.hhs.gov/schip* for detailed information about this payment mechanism for APN services.)

A new service offered through CMS is especially helpful to APNs. Regularly scheduled "Open Door Forums" are accessible by phone, on the World Wide Web, or on site, in which APN participants may discuss current issues and concerns about Medicare, Medicaid, and other federal reimbursement programs. To access this resource, go to *www.cms.hhs.gov,* click on "Open Door Forums," and then proceed to the nursing and allied health section to schedule admission to the forum or to read current and recent minutes.

Federal Employee Health Benefit Program (FEHBP). The Federal Employee Health Benefit Program (FEHBP) is the health insurance plan for the approximately 10 million federal employees and their dependents. This is a voluntary, contributory program open to all employees of the federal government. Contracts are held with private health insurance carriers to offer health insurance plans to federal employees. Public Law 101-509, enacted in 1990, allows federal employees enrolled in the FEHBP direct access to NPs, CNSs, and CNMs, thus enabling direct reimbursement for APN services. Under this provision, insurance carriers for federal plans must make payment directly to these APNs if their services are covered under the plan. Collaboration with or supervision by a physician or any other health care provider is not needed. The payment level is determined by the individual health insurance plan. Additional information is available at the Office of Personnel Management website under Federal Employee Insurance Programs *(www.opm.gov/insure/).*

Private Health Insurance—Fee-for-Service Plans. Private health insurance plans include carriers such as Blue Cross/Blue Shield, Aetna, Prudential, and Metropolitan. Many of these carriers are merging into larger entities as the move to managed care demands system-wide changes and efficiencies. These traditional fee-for-service plans reimburse providers for patient charges according to the usual and customary charges for that local area. An insurance policy does not explicitly need to include the coverage of nursing services for APNs to be reimbursed for their services. APNs' direct reimbursement by private insurance carriers varies from state to state (Pearson, 2007). When considering application for third-party reimbursement, the nurse needs to be familiar with the state's nurse practice act, state insurance laws and codes (including reimbursement amendments), judicial decisions, and opinions by the attorney general. State health insurance laws do not necessarily prohibit third-party reimbursement to nurses. In Florida and Maine, for instance, direct third-party reimbursement is essentially a 1:1 process. The individual APN applies to the third-party insurer and requests provider status. If reimbursement is rejected, familiarity with the state's nursing practice act and the state's health insurance laws can assist the nurse in appealing the decision. Some third-party payers reimburse under the APN's collaborating physician's name. APNs should contact each insurance company directly for credentialing and reimbursement protocols. When choosing to become a participating provider with a third-party insurance company, reimbursement is from a negotiated fee schedule. The APN or practice manager has the ability to negotiate for the best fee possible.

Capitated Payment. Capitated payment or managed care denotes a spectrum of arrangements that entail some connection between financing and delivery of care, usually with cost containment (Bodenheimer & Grumbach, 2005). In managed care, the financial risk associated with health care delivery is shared between the payers, the contracted providers, and the enrolled beneficiaries. Risk is lessened for payers by the exclusive enrollment of beneficiaries with a particular health status profile. Risk is lessened for any one provider by the addition of providers to a pool of providers sharing the care for a particular population of patients. Risk is lessened for the beneficiaries through the utilization of providers who are within the contracted pool, or "network," of providers. The distribution of financial risk has received increased media coverage recently as some managed care companies face financial difficulties. Such turmoil is evidenced by the alteration of key components of typical managed care contracts. Examples include changes in patient population (e.g., the disenrollment of Medicare beneficiaries), pharmaceutical coverage

(e.g., the increased practice of allowing a decreased supply of chronic medications to be dispensed at one time to increase collection of co-payments), and departure of companies from a particular catchment location. Managed care entities will usually either discount a clinician's fee for services or require that a predetermined fee be charged. However, the majority of managed care companies pay providers a "capitated fee" (the provider cares for a client population for a prearranged fee per client). Capitation amounts typically vary by age, gender, and risk status and are negotiable. The capitated fee is paid to the provider monthly, based on the number of plan enrollees who have selected that provider as their primary care provider. MCOs encompass any variety of prepaid group practice arrangements. These programs usually offer health care services to members enrolled in the plan for a predetermined, prepaid, or discounted fee. *Prepaid* means that the organization receives a fixed payment or premium to care for members of a certain population and that the organization bears the financial risk for the care that members receive. Participating providers are required to provide services for contracted reimbursement amounts. This reimbursement can range from a discounted fee for service to a lump sum for all services required.

There are four main types of HMOs:

- *Staff-model HMOs* employ clinicians who work in the HMOs' own clinics.
- *Group-model HMOs* contract with a large multispecialty group practice.
- *Individual practice association (IPA) model HMOs* contract with individual clinicians or affiliations of independent physicians.
- *Network HMO models* are similar to IPAs except that they contract with several larger clinical groups.

Some models are mixed combinations of group, staff, network, or IPA models. A preferred provider organization (PPO) is a network of providers, usually physicians and hospitals, that have discounted their fees for an increased volume of patients (Bodenheimer & Grumbach, 2005).

Some MCOs make extensive use of APNs, particularly primary care NPs, to increase the cost-effectiveness of primary care. As discussed earlier, APNs must provide the data needed by states to demonstrate cost-efficiency and must work together at the policymaking level to eliminate these financial restraints to trade where they exist in these various reimbursement systems (Safriet, 1998; see also Chapter 22).

Cash and Credit Card. A minority of patients pay cash for the care they receive or pay a co-payment out of pocket. Cash payment requires that the practice site have the ability to make change for patients who pay cash or who meet sliding scale requirements on a cash basis. The APN provider may choose to honor major credit cards to facilitate payment. Lastly, a practice owner needs to decide whether to extend credit options with the additional billing procedures to their customers.

Reimbursement Summary

Reimbursement is an indirect process supporting patient care that provides a vehicle for APN compensation for the services rendered to patients. The process begins with the appointment for the patient's clinical encounter and ends with the posting of the patient's payment, either through patient payment or through third-party reimbursement. The involvement of APNs in the reimbursement process depends on whether the APN is allowed by the applicable state and federal regulations to practice and bill independently and is able to obtain direct reimbursement for those independently delivered services. The level to which the APN is involved in a practice setting's administrative procedures depends on whether the APN has chosen to practice in an entrepreneurial or intrapreneurial manner. Usually, the process of reimbursement is and should be delegated to an individual familiar with medical billing who can dedicate the time and effort required to become expert in this level of practice management. If the APN decides to become directly involved in reimbursement procedures, it is strongly urged that a professional billing advisor be contracted or hired; this is just as important as consulting with an attorney and accountant during business planning. This advisor serves to provide the APN with the latest and most accurate information regarding this vital process to ensure the APN's financial viability.

Some authors report that reimbursement should equal 90% of the patient's billable charges (Buppert, 2004). The reality of health care economics is that this number varies considerably over time depending on the payer mix (specifically, on the percentage of Medicare, Medicaid, other payments to be received) and the amounts charged to patients. The average expectation is 50% to 55% of billable charges. Medicaid usually pays a lower proportion of billed charges than Medicare pays, based on the local Medicare fee structure. Capitated contracts can result in financial losses if enrolled beneficiaries use the health care system more frequently than the anticipated risk calculation had allocated.

During the business planning phase, the APN should become intimately familiar with the reimbursement rates in the local area, the anticipated mix of the patient population to be served, and the available resources and personnel to design and implement a reimbursement process that meets the APN's financial expectations. APNs should never allow one payer to dominate their practices and should set goals based on the percent of each payer for their practice. As with any system, the reimbursement process should undergo periodical evaluation to determine where improvements may be made, including electronic claim submission, tighter internal audit controls, and efficient cross-training of staff to ensure consistency during staff absences.

Pay for Performance. In the future, entrepreneur and intrapreneur APNs may find themselves being reimbursed under a pay-for-performance (P4P) plan (see Chapter 25). It is clear that payment will be linked to measures of performance. Although care delivered by APNs is included in P4P reimbursement models that are being initiated through the Agency for Healthcare Research and Quality (AHRQ) and sponsored by public and private purchasers of health care services, the question remains as to whether APNs will be included as direct clinical providers in these models. APNs are not present at the table as federal and private programs such as P4P are being developed to link quality improvement to payment. NPs must be in on the ground floor to include nursing measures in the variety of methods used to reward providers financially for achieving targets. P4P plans assess not only clinical performance but also the APN's practice efficiency and use of information technology to report outcomes (Endsley, Baker, Kershner, & Curtin, 2006; Johnson, Harper, Hanson, & Dawson, 2007; see also *www.aafp.org/; www.ahrq. gov/qual/p4pguide.pdf*).

USING INFORMATION SYSTEMS AND TELEHEALTH TO ENHANCE PATIENT CARE AND PRODUCTIVITY

Information technology (IT) is an APN responsibility that is steadily increasing in importance. Proficiency in the evaluation and use of IT is essential for APNs to achieve direct care, leadership, and research (evidence-based practice) competencies. From a business point of view, there are a number of ways that information systems drive the success of APN practice whether the APN owns and manages the business, is an employee, or is in a contract service arrangement (Crosson, Stroebel, Scott, Stello, & Crabtree, 2005). In a health care system in which patients see several providers and have many comorbidities, *electronic documentation on interoperable systems* is essential to facilitate prompt and efficient communication. New interactive systems make it possible for providers to share important information and findings across settings and from home (McBride, 2005). *Electronic budgeting* assists APNs in planning and managing cost and running a business from day to day. The ability to understand budget constraints is accommodated if APNs who work for others can access budget information in order to use resources wisely.

Electronic billing and coding is a most useful application of IT. The ability to track reimbursement and to interface with payers electronically is exceedingly time-advantageous and cost-effective (Miniclier, 2000). From a patient care standpoint, the capacity to develop and access *web-based patient and staff education* is important to APNs in all types of business and practice arrangements. Exciting new models of interactive education targeted to individual patients make it possible for the APN to implement care that is personal and time efficient. In addition, electronic logs and monitoring devices that track patient data such as blood pressure and hemoglobin A_{1C} levels over time make it much easier for the APN to obtain data to evaluate outcomes (Milhailidis, Krones, & Boger, 2006). Also, the opportunity to join with other colleagues to develop, implement, and publish *research initiatives* is greatly enhanced by electronic communication.

APN competencies identified for the Doctor of Nursing Practice (DNP) place a high priority on the need for IT skills at the highest level of expertise (AACN, 2006). Health care services will increasingly depend on electronic systems to manage both the business and patient care aspects of practice. It is incumbent on APNs to be able to appropriately select vendors for clinical, administrative, and database software products that are useful to their practice settings. APN providers will need to continually augment their IT competencies and strive to learn new measures to enhance their ability to communicate and share data electronically. Telehealth or remote monitoring technology is a way for APNs to monitor their community-based patients and reduce visits to the office or house calls without reducing patient contact. With newer technologies that make it possible to connect disparate systems, telehealth is a promising information technology for consultation that offers opportunities for improving quality of care while controlling costs (Waldo, 2003; see also Chapter 7).

NEW BUSINESS OPPORTUNITIES FOR ADVANCED PRACTICE NURSES

Business opportunities abound, and in health care practice businesses continue to flourish as APNs respond to the needs of patients and communities in a complex and mobile society. Nurses have led the way in innovations that make care more accessible to individuals who have busy lifestyles. Both entrepreneur and intrapreneur APNs can take advantage of new arenas to carve out rewarding businesses such as the ones described below.

Convenient Care Clinics

The trend toward APN-delivered health care that is offered in retail locations is growing rapidly because of the need for accessible, affordable, convenient care. As these clinics are appearing faster than they can be regulated, it is extremely important for APNs to provide high-quality, safe care that will set the standard for this type of patient encounter. Retail giants like CVS Pharmacies and Target Stores are opening primary care clinics staffed by NPs who, in addition to providing affordable, episodic care in a convenient, community-based environment, are providing important entrée to other health-related services (Klein, 2006; Lugo, Giorgianni, & Zimmer, 2006). Corporations who are entering the market have little experience with NP care and offer expanding opportunities for APNs to be at the groundbreaking level to set up a new model of APN focused care.

Traveler Health Services

An exciting opportunity for APNs exists in the area of international travel health. Individuals and families travel globally for both business and pleasure with increasing frequency. Although prevention and planning can avert travel-related health problems and protect both the traveler and society in general, little has been done to incorporate travel-related services into routine health care (Lugo, 2007). New models of traveler health services offer business opportunities for knowledgeable NPs, CNMs, and CNSs to offer

their patients education about infectious disease, immunizations, and counseling about co-morbidities both before traveling and after they return.

Pain Management Clinics

Pain management clinics are not a new phenomenon. However, because pain continues to be undertreated and remains a major public health problem *(www. painfoundation.org/),* numerous business opportunities exist for APNs, especially CRNAs and CNSs. Community-based, freestanding pain clinics are rapidly expanding, and APNs' skill in assessing and managing pain is a sought-after commodity. CRNA entrepreneurs are expanding their practices in this area with good success.

Hospitalist Services

APNs are entering the market as important collaborators in hospitalist care. Physician/APN teams are achieving positive results with patients (e.g., fewer readmissions) and have reduced costs. APN competencies in bridging the gap between hospital and community-based care offer an excellent niche for practice that is worth exploring (Cowan et al., 2006; Kleinpell, 2006; see Chapter 18). A hospitalist is an employee of the hospital or part of a contracted group to the hospital. Two models of reimbursement are (1) contract billing with the group and hospital at a flat rate with incentive pay for positive outcomes and (2) split billing—the hospital and group bill separately for services.

These examples are just a few of the many business ventures open to APNs who may want to explore setting up their own practices, contracting their services, or expanding their existing practices. All require careful exploration of needs for services, funding/capitalization in the short term, and the potential for professional satisfaction, financial remuneration, and return on investment over the long term.

CONCLUSION

Through the development of innovative programs and practices grounded in a systems-thinking approach, APNs define, demonstrate, document, and thereby claim their contributions to patient care. Business planning establishes a clear picture of how the APN will function on a daily basis, as well as how midrange and long-term goals are to be met. Knowledge of the processes involved in care delivery increases the sharing of information between APNs and their patients, other health care providers, and colleagues. Reimbursement is identified as the major indirect process of care that has a direct impact on the success of the APN's business planning efforts. Equally important to success is the APN's candid self-evaluation and determination of whether an entrepreneurial or intrapreneurial approach is the most appropriate model under which to deliver patient care. The emergence of clinically focused doctoral education for APNs enhances their ability to recognize and implement new practice models and innovate within existing organizations. The recognition that others, such as other APNs, physicians, attorneys, and practice managers, in the greater health care system have skills and expertise to offer provides the APN with a "safety net" of advisors who can play an active role in the actualization of advanced practice nursing. Above all, the success of the APN is grounded in the professional recognition of and active participation in the larger system to ensure that the needs of patients are met through the delivery of clinically excellent, holistic health care.

REFERENCES

Almost, J., & Laschinger, H.K. (2002). Workplace empowerment, collaborative work relationships, and job strain in nurse practitioners. *Journal of the American Academy of Nurse Practitioners, 14,* 408-420.

American Academy of Family Physicians. (2004). *CLIA and other regulatory information.* Retrieved March 14, 2004, from www.aafp.org.

American Association of Colleges of Nursing (AACN). (2006). *Essentials of doctoral education for advanced practice nurses.* Washington, DC: Author.

American Diabetes Association. (2003). *Clinical practice recommendations.* Retrieved May 26, 2004, from www.diabetes.org.

American Express Company. (2003). *Small business exchange: Creating an effective business plan.* Retrieved May 27, 2004, from www.americanexpress.com/smallbusiness/resources/starting/bizplan.

American Medical Association (AMA). (1996). *Integration strategies for the medical practice: The physician's handbook to integration alternatives.* Norcross, GA: Coker Publishing.

American Medical Association (AMA). (1999). *Automating the medical record.* Norcross, GA: Coker Publishing.

American Medical Association (AMA). (2002a). *Financial management of the medical practice: The physician's handbook for successful budgeting, forecasting and cost accounting* (2nd ed.). Norcross, GA: Coker Publishing.

American Medical Association (AMA). (2002b). *Managing the medical practice: The physician's handbook for successful practice administration* (2nd ed.). Norcross, GA: Coker Publishing.

American Medical Association (AMA). (2002c). *Starting a medical practice: The physician's handbook for successful practice start-up* (2nd ed.). Norcross, GA: Coker Publishing.

American Medical Association (AMA). (2007). *International Classification of Diseases, 9th Revision, Clinical Modification (ICD-9-CM 2008)* (Vols. 1 and 2). Chicago, IL: Author.

American Medical Association (AMA). (2008). *CPT2008.* Chicago, IL: Author.

American Nurses Association (ANA). (2001). *Code of ethics for nurses with interpretive statements.* Washington, DC: Author.

Bodenheimer T., & Grumbach, K. (2005). *Understanding health policy: A clinical approach.* New York: Lange/McGraw/Hill.

Buppert, C. (2002). *Avoiding malpractice: 10 rules, 5 systems, 20 cases.* Annapolis, MD: Law offices of Carolyn Buppert.

Buppert, C. (2003). HIPAA patient privacy. *The American Journal for Nurse Practitioners, 7,* 17-22.

Buppert C. (2004). *Nurse practitioner's business practice and legal guide* (2nd ed.). Boston: Jones & Bartlett.

Buppert, C. (2006). *The top 10 to-dos for billing NP services.* Retrieved June 20, 2007, from www.buppert.com/articles/top-10.php.

Buppert, C. (2008). *Nurse practitioner's business practice and legal guide* (3rd ed.). Boston: Jones & Bartlett.

Centers for Medicare and Medicaid Services (CMS). (2006a). *Evaluation and management documentation guidelines.* Retrieved March 15, 2004, from www.cms.hhs.gov.

Centers for Medicare and Medicaid Services (CMS). (2006b). *CLIA: General program description.* Retrieved May 28, 2004, from www.cms.hhs.gov/clia.

Cowan, M.J., Shapiro, M., Hays, RD., Afifi, A., Vazirani, S., Ward, C.R., et al. (2006). The effect of a multidisciplinary hospitalist/physician and advanced practice nurse collaboration on hospital costs. *Journal of Nursing Administration, 36*(2), 79-85.

Crosson, J., Stroebel, C., Scott, J., Stello, B., & Crabtree, B. (2005). Implementing an electronic medical record in a family medicine practice: Communication, decision making and conflict. *Annals of Family Medicine, 3*(4), 307-311.

Dayhoff, N.E., & Moore, P.S. (2005). CNS entrepreneurs: Innovators in patient care. *The Nurse Practitioner, 30*(Suppl. 1), 6-8.

Endsley, S., Baker, G., Kershner, B., & Curtin, K. (July/August 2006). *Family practice management: What family physicians need to know about pay for performance.* American Academy of Family Physicians. Retrieved March 21, 2008, from www.aafp.org/fpm/20060700/69what.html.

George Washington University Medical Center/Faculty Resources. (2006). *Building a practice in your home community.* Retrieved May 15, 2007, from www.gwumc.edu/healthsci/faculty_resources/health_science_learning_objects.cfm.

Horns, P.N., Czaplijski, T.J., Endelke, M.K., Marshburn, D., McAullife, M., & Baker, S. (2007). Leading through collaboration: A regional academic/service partnership that works. *Nursing Outlook, 55*(2), 74-78.

Iowa Intervention Project, Johnson, M., & Maas, M., Editors. (1997). *Nursing outcomes classification.* St. Louis: Mosby.

Johnson, J., Harper, D., Hanson, C., & Dawson, E. (2007). Forging a quality agenda. *American Journal for Nurse Practitioners, 11*(10), 10-19.

The Joint Commission (TJC). (2007). Joint Commission requirements. Retrieved June 10, 2007, from www.jointcommission.org.

Klein, T.A., (2006). Working in a retail clinic: What nurse practitioners need to ask. *Topics in Advanced Practice Nursing eJournal,* posted 09/20/06.

Kleinpell, R.M. (2001). *Outcome assessment in advanced practice nursing.* New York: Springer.

Kleinpell, R.M. (2006). Expanding opportunities in ACPN practice. *The Nurse Practitioner, Spring*(Suppl.), 8-9.

Letz, K. (2002). *Business essentials for nurse practitioners: Essential knowledge for building your practice.* Fort Wayne, IN: Previcare Inc. Publishing.

Lindeke, L.L., (2005). Nurse-physician workplace collaboration. *Online Journal Issues in Nursing, 10*(1), 1-7. Retrieved March 31, 2007, from http://198.65.150.241/ojin/.

Lugo, N.R, (2007). International traveler health: A national prevention opportunity: A white paper by the Nurse Practitioner Healthcare Foundation. *American Journal for Nurse Practitioners, 11*(3), 51-56.

Lugo, N.R., Giorgianni, S.J., & Zimmer, P.A. (2006). Nurse practitioner services in retail locations: A white paper by the Nurse Practitioner Healthcare Foundation. *American Journal for Nurse Practitioners, 10*(6), 36-40.

McBride, A.B. (2005). Nursing and the informatics revolution. *Nursing Outlook, 53*(4), 183-191.

McCloskey, J.C., & Bulechek, G.M. (Eds.). (2000). *Nursing interventions classification* (3rd ed.). St. Louis: Mosby.

Milhailidis, A., Krones, L., & Boger, J. (2006). Assistive computing devices: A pilot study to explore nurses' preferences and needs. *Computers, Informatics, Nursing: CIN, 24*(6), 328-336.

Miniclier, P. (2000). *Credentialing, reimbursement, and billing for nurse practitioners.* Retrieved April 4, 2007, from www.medscape.com/viewarticle/425419.

NANDA-I. (2007). NANDA International Taxonomy II. Retrieved June 8, 2007, from www.nanda.org.

National Heritage Insurance Company. (2004). *Second update to Medicare physical fee schedule database.* Retrieved May 27, 2004, from www.medicarenhic.com.

Northeast Health Care Quality Foundation. (1999). *Health matters for Medicare consumers* (Vol. 3). Dover, NH: Author.

Pearson, L. (2007). The Pearson report: A national overview of nurse practitioner legislation and health care issues. *The American Journal for Nurse Practitioners, 9*(1), 9-135.

Reel , S.J., & Abraham, I.L. (2007). *Business and legal essentials for nurse practitioners: From negotiating your first job through owning a practice* (Chapter 19). St Louis: Mosby.

Safriet, B. (1998). Still spending dollars, still searching for sense: Advanced practice nursing in an era of regulatory and economic turmoil. *Advanced Practice Nursing Quarterly, 4*(3), 24-33.

Solberg, L.I., Kottke, T.E., Brekke, M.L., & Magnan, S. (May, June 2000). Improving prevention is difficult. *Effective Clinical Practice.* Retrieved June 11, 2007, from www.acponline.org/journals/ecp/mayjune2000/solberg_2.htm.

Thomas, J.D., Finch, L.P., Schoenhofer, S., & Green, A. (2004). *The caring relationship created by nurse practitioners and the ones nursed: Implications for practice.* Retrieved April 4, 2007, from www.medscape.com/viewarticle/496420.

U.S. Department of Health and Human Services. (May 2003). *The seventh report of the Joint National Committee on Prevention, Detection, Evaluation, and Treatment of High Blood Pressure.* Washington, DC: Author.

Waldo, B. (2003). Telehealth and the electronic medical record. *Nursing Economic$, 21*(5), 245-246.

Marketing and Contracting Considerations*

Donna R. Hodnicki

HEALTH CARE AS A BUSINESS: A CALL TO ACTION FOR ADVANCED PRACTICE NURSES

As the health care system and health care needs become more complex and demanding, there is an increased necessity for advanced practice nurses (APNs) to address issues related to health care transformation and health care outcomes. The November 1999 Institute of Medicine (IOM) (1999) report on medication errors supports the need to fix the health care system (see Chapter 22). The IOM reports focused on the fragmented nature of the system and the context in which health care is purchased as being major contributors to the high and inexcusable error rate that compromises patient safety. Changing demographics in our country, including the increase in the numbers of older adults and development of new services and technologies, have contributed to increasing costs (IOM, 2001). One recommendation in the report calls for all health care organizations and professional groups to promote health care that is safe, effective, client-centered, timely, efficient, and equitable (p. 6). In a follow-up report (IOM, 2003), the IOM Committee on the Health Professions Education stated that "all health professionals should be educated to deliver patient-centered care as members of an interdisciplinary team, emphasizing evidence-based practice, quality improvement approaches, and informatics" (p. 3). APNs are part of the solution to improve quality, safety, and efficacy, and to take on this important role, an understanding of marketing is essential.

With more than 8% of the registered nurse (RN) population prepared for advanced practice (Health Resources and Services Administration [HRSA], 2004), the educational preparation of APNs has advanced from certificate and baccalaureate preparation to a graduate degree. Although the preponderance of APNs are currently prepared at the master's level, the balance will begin to shift as the Doctor of Nursing Practice

(DNP) becomes the future norm. With this educational shift, a renewed emphasis on marketing is essential to educate the public, industry, and other professionals of this expanding role development to the DNP in addition to the continuing marketing of the master's-prepared APN. Those prepared as DNP APNs will take on the added responsibility of assessing health care system structures and outcomes to influence policy, provide leadership, and improve outcomes within the health care environment. Continuing and expanded marketing of the APN role is essential to bring about the needed changes in health care delivery and outcomes in this country.

The focus of this chapter is marketing strategies for all APNs. Classic marketing concepts are reviewed, and their application to advanced practice nursing is described. Specific marketing issues such as promotion and APN-specific marketing strategies and contracts are also discussed. For development of a business plan, refer to Chapter 19.

The Influence of Doctor of Nursing Practice Education on Advanced Practice Nursing Marketing

The DNP curriculum is built around eight Essentials as articulated in the American Association of Colleges of Nursing (AACN) *Essentials of Doctoral Education for Advanced Nursing Practice* (AACN, 2006). Some of the DNP *Essentials* (see Chapters 2 and 3) are particularly relevant to marketing the APN role. For example, enhanced leadership and health policy advocacy skills can help APNs gain visibility in the health care marketplace and will require accelerated marketing strategies to increase understanding of the role of the DNP-prepared APN in the complex health care system. With the increased emphasis on collaboration, interdisciplinary efforts, leadership, and use of technology to improve health care outcomes, education and marketing about the expanded role of the APN will be necessary.

With the emerging DNP role, marketing-related issues arise. The current nursing shortage and the diverse strategies to alleviate it make it even more

*The authors and editors express their gratitude to Susan E.D. Doughty, RNC, MSN, WHNP, and Jennifer M. Kellis, RN, MSN, for their contributions to this chapter in previous editions.

important for all APNs to continue to market themselves. Marketing efforts should be directed to their own profession as well as to others, informing them of patient services they are qualified to provide and of their availability for patient care referrals. One area of marketing to be addressed is promotion of reimbursement for improved health care outcomes and the cost savings of APN care. The Centers for Medicare and Medicaid Services (CMS) has a Premier Hospital Quality Incentive Demonstration (HQID) in which 270 hospitals are participating over a 3-year period (Hagland, 2006). Hospitals that have performance levels for inpatient quality care in the top 10% will receive a 2% bonus on their base Medicare diagnosis-related group (DRG) payments for the relevant conditions. Those hospitals that perform poorly in quality areas receive penalties. Bonuses totaling over $8.5 million were awarded the first year of the demonstration project. Hospitals and physician practices are encouraged to use this pay-for-performance (P4P) reimbursement model, and APNs must fit into this context of improved quality of inpatient care.

Whitehead (2000) reported that nursing was doing very little to use the mass media to enhance health promotion. With the advances in technology with iPods, Internet blogs, e-mail, and diverse access to the Internet, the utilization of the mass media to market the role of nursing and APN services is an opportunity yet to be fully utilized. Improved use of the mass media for these last two examples are areas of marketing needs to be addressed by the APN.

The Influence of the Marketplace on Advanced Practice Nursing Marketing

In spite of the increased number of APNs and increased educational preparation, knowledge is still lacking among health care colleagues and consumers about who APNs are and how they can positively impact the health care system. APNs must market themselves to the public, industry, and other health care professionals, especially in light of the changes that the DNP-prepared APNs are expected to bring to the health care arena. Many persons still remain unaware that the term *advanced practice nurse* refers to four groups of nurses: certified nurse-midwife (CNM), clinical nurse specialist (CNS), certified registered nurse anesthetist (CRNA), and nurse practitioner (NP). In the twentieth century, CNMs answered a call for safe birthing practices while CNSs responded to a need for expert practitioners at the nurse-patient interface. The practice realm of the

CRNAs was established to provide anesthesia services *long* before the medical specialty of anesthesiology was developed (see Chapters 1 and 17). The establishment of NP educational programs in the mid-1960s was the result of a cooperative effort of nurse and physician leaders to address the health care crisis of the time, when increased numbers of health care providers were needed to provide patient care services. As the role and scope of practice of APNs have changed over the years, new challenges and growth in services offered provide APNs with diverse health care opportunities to market skills to the public, industry, and other professionals.

Currently, market forces drive health and illness care. In spite of the overall wealth and technological excellence in the United States as a whole, a serious problem still remains in that many Americans cannot obtain or afford even minimal health services. APNs have helped to alleviate some of this health care disparity, but expanded use of APNs is needed to effect significant improvement in health care outcomes. APNs prepared at the DNP level will increase the need for targeted marketing to promote this new role, to assist the profession to comprehend and support the transition to the broader competencies, and to explain a new set of initials in the current "alphabet soup" of credentials.

For the public to be informed about the wide variety of services APNs can provide, it is necessary to market both the role and the services. To effectively market themselves, APNs must understand marketing concepts and utilize marketing strategies. APNs who cannot get beyond an aversion toward marketing themselves will be left behind, both as a group and as individuals.

WHAT IS MARKETING?

Marketing is anything and everything APNs do to promote their roles, practices, and services. It is about meeting the needs of the consumer and positioning services and businesses in the marketplace. Nurses have the respect of the public. For years nursing has been identified as one of the most trusted professions, held in the highest esteem. It is imperative that this trust and high esteem not become eroded. Continued efforts are needed to further enhance the public's trust through education and marketing strategies that communicate the role of the APN in the provision of health care and the services that APNs render. APNs provide quality care similar to that offered by physicians, and they are cost-effective providers (Office of

Technology Assessment [OTA], 1986; Safriet, 1992; see also Chapter 24). Government and national studies indicate that patient satisfaction with APN care has remained high over the years (Druss, Marcus, Olfson, Tanielian, & Pincus, 2003; Hayes, 2007; Mundinger et al., 2000; OTA).

Classic Marketing Categories and Implementation Concepts

The four classic concepts of marketing that need to be addressed are product, price, place, and promotion (Chang, Pfoutz, & Price, 2001; Letz, 2002). Each of these categories provides opportunities to expand APN practice in diverse arenas. A fifth concept, partnering, has become important in contemporary marketing efforts.

Product. A *product* is that entity that is offered to the market. An APN offers health care services that may be specialized and serve a market niche. As APNs become affiliated with institutions/practices, patients are deliberately choosing APNs as care providers. A study by Druss and colleagues (2003) reported that "between 1987 and 1997 the proportion of patients who saw a nonphysician clinician rose from 30.6 to 36.1 percent" (p. 130). More recently, patient care is being offered in covenient care (retail) clinics exclusively by APNs (Klein, 2006). With increasing numbers of individuals seeking care from non-physician providers, it is important that patients are aware of APN roles and the types of care that specific APNs provide and that care is based on a health promotion model that supports prevention strategies. The administrative and clinical staff can have a positive impact on a patient's perception of APN care. In the primary care setting, one strategy that fosters this perception occurs when staff members offer the services of the APN if a patient's preferred provider is unavailable or a walk-in appointment is requested. In an acute care setting, staff nurses can be sure that APNs are consulted promptly to address clinical issues. In any case, the staff with whom APNs work can help APNs educate the public about the benefits of APN care; they can explain that the quality is the same from all providers but that some of the APNs' services are unique or add value, given the patient's needs. It is important that the public understand the similarities between APNs and other providers and that quality and safety are equivalent to that of other providers and that, in some cases, APN care is better.

Disseminating information about APNs to the public is essential. Master's-prepared and doctorally prepared APNs have built their knowledge and skills on a strong nursing foundation. The foundation of any APN role is the holistic consideration of the physical, psychological, spiritual, sociocultural, functional, and environmental aspects of the individual—aspects that emerge in assessment, interventions, and overall health care. Health and wellness are major components of the holistic perspective; however, other assessment and intervention components add to the APN's ability to perceive the wholeness of the situation. Information about APN products and services should emphasize the uniqueness of advanced practice nursing—that is, using a holistic approach, promoting health, identifying health risks, preventing illness, and improving health care systems and outcomes, in addition to diagnosing and managing disease and issues of concern. An individual who is being seen by an APN not only receives a broader range of services relative to maintaining and restoring health but also begins to understand how APN practice differs from that of other providers.

Price. *Price* is the amount of money that the individual will be asked to pay for the product. Price will be strongly influenced by many factors such as office overhead, staff costs, updated equipment costs, and supplies. The expectations of APNs regarding financial rewards from the practice may vary because of locale and the differences in salaries across the United States. Although good statistics on nationwide salaries are difficult to obtain, APNs need to be familiar with regional and local salaries, compensation, and benefits to be competitive in the market (Hayes, Allen, Gruen, Wilson, & Kalmakis, 2001). The quality of care given by APNs has been shown to be cost-effective (see Chapter 24). In some areas, APNs are in demand because they have proven to be cost-effective to the patients and the practice, generating proportionately more revenue compared with that of internists and family physicians. Potential employers and APNs seeking positions need to make sure that salary, benefits, and working conditions are competitive (Lowes, 2007; Weiss, 2007). If the cost of care by APNs is lower than that of competitors in the area, providing price information may be a useful marketing strategy. If lower costs are part of the overall marketing strategy, APNs can inform health care consumers that health promotion, disease prevention, early intervention, and chronic illness management services may prevent more costly diagnostic tests and interventions in the future.

Place. *Place* refers to accessibility and the various tasks that are necessary to make the product more available to the market (Chang et al., 2001). A needed product at a good price must be accessible to be marketed successfully. Historically, APNs have been in the forefront of providing care to vulnerable populations and remain willing to provide care to these groups. Positioning the APN clinic in an area of need, where care is lacking, is one strategy. Selecting a location that is safe, has parking, and is near public transportation will support the establishment of an accessible and user-friendly practice site. Locating convenient office space and developing an aesthetic environment are important considerations (Letz, 2002).

Place extends beyond a physical location. Multiple health care resources are available on the Internet offering detailed information. Helping patients find reliable Internet health care information can be used as a marketing strategy by providing patients a printed tool to identify and evaluate reliable websites. This activity not only supports patients' independence but also markets your support and services when your name, office hours, contact data, and website are on the form. A clinic website with links to reliable information resources provides added value and acts as a marketing strategy. The increased use of technology to extend diagnostic and therapeutic services to populations in need expands the concept of place to far-reaching venues in neighboring counties, states, or even countries.

Promotion. *Promotion* encompasses those activities that communicate the value of the product to the market (Chang et al., 2001). Promotion depends on making the consumer aware of the availability of APN services. A lack of recognition of the availability of a product or the provider by consumers is a barrier to APN practice that can be removed (Lindeke, Bly, & Wilcon, 2001). Nurse practitioners and CNSs have identified the lack of public knowledge about their advanced practice roles and limitations of practice climate as barriers to practice. CNSs also note resistance from physicians and psychiatrists (Chevalier, Steinberg, & Lindeke, 2006; Powers, 2001; Washington Consulting Group, 1994). APN promotional activities that address such barriers include the following:

- Changing a hospital or health care company's promotional materials to ensure that APNs are explicitly mentioned. When you look for Doctors of Medicine (MDs) on a hospital's website, it is easy to find MD names; however, it is more difficult to find APN names. Magnet status hospitals are changing this lack of acknowledgment. (See *www.massgeneral.org/pcs/CCPD/cpd_Professional_Cert.asp;* a directory of APNs is under "Resources"; unfortunately, however, outsiders cannot access it.)
- Prominently displaying the APN name in visible signage along with all other providers in the office.
- Adding a description of APN services in a patient education booklet that provides common management approaches to health care problems (e.g., fever, diarrhea) or posting the same information on the agency website.
- Asking clients on the first visit how they were informed about available APN services.
- Distributing a business card to all patients seen by the APN.
- Having provider business cards available at the checkout counter.
- Encouraging word-of-mouth referrals from patients.
- Sending a thank-you note to the individual who provided a referral.
- Joining local and state APNs groups to network and to remain current on issues.
- Becoming a member of the local business groups.

Another important endorsement for the nursing profession that promotes APN practice is for APNs to use APNs for their personal and family care. Miller (2000) noted that successful promotion depends on APNs getting out into their target communities and being visible. To market one's practice, APNs will need to invest time, money, or both to increase chances of success.

Although advertising or promotion is a small but important part of marketing, advertising has a bad reputation for being focused on materialism. Almost no one believes advertising's claims, yet advertising thrives because it works! Health care professionals may be uncomfortable with the notion of self-promotion, but consumer demands and constantly changing reimbursement mechanisms for health care providers necessitate marketing to both clients and payers (Kendig, 2002). In today's health care market, which is becoming more diversified and competitive, it is important that APNs understand and utilize multiple marketing strategies, including advertising.

Partnering. While the four P's of marketing are classic, consideration of a fifth P, *partnering*, has been proposed as useful in the current, complex health care industry (Liberman & Rotarius, 2001). Partnering or collaboration can be with health care colleagues or groups (see Chapter 10). Nickitas and Valentino (2003), academician and clinician APNs, were asked to consult on a project. Their collaborative consulting with a newly formed for-profit organization provided an opportunity to develop a peer-to-peer partnership that has developed into a successful business venture. A partnering of a health care customer group consists of patient, insurance organizations, and employers with one goal being directed toward keeping health care costs to a minimum. When establishing partnering groups, marketing strategies should include showcasing how one partner group (A,B,C) would be differentiated from another partner group (A,B,D) in terms of the ability to provide selected services and contain costs.

Another approach to partnering in health care is the use of a *consumer-centric approach* (in business circles called *reverse marketing*), which gives patients/consumers control of their own health care and empowers them to obtain what they want from the sellers (health care systems or providers) (MacStravic, 2006). In many instances, a consumer agent intervenes for the consumer to negotiate and organize the care received. This service can be offered through employers as a benefit of employment. It would behoove APNs to make themselves known to consumer agents, since APN care fits the consumer-centric model (see also the discussion of patient navigators in Chapter 6).

The use of a *care transitions coach* is another approach to partnership. Patients who receive care across diverse health care settings are at risk for serious problems with care resulting from a lack of knowledge about how to deal with the management of illness and obtaining services within the complex health care system. A randomized, controlled study of persons older than 65 years determined that coaching chronically ill older patients and their caregivers to ascertain that all of their health care needs were met during care transitions may decrease the number of subsequent rehospitalizations (Coleman, Parry, Chalmers, & Min, 2006). An APN with expertise in geriatrics could market services to health care systems to provide care transition interventions that help the patient and caregiver become more active in self-management, leading to fewer rehospitalizations and reduced health care costs.

A group of self-employed APNs (NPs and CNSs) who were RN first-assistants developed a multidisciplinary surgical-assisting partnership (DeCarlo, 2005). The partnership allowed the group to provide a variety of services that were attractive to their consumer surgeons as the APNs brought diverse expertise and background to the group. The use of *peer consultation groups*, a partnering strategy, supported psychiatric mental health CNSs who had separate practices (Barry, 2006). The peer consultation groups used face-to-face meetings and phone conferences to provide support and discuss complex situations to learn new strategies and approaches to meet patient needs. Characteristics to look for in a partner are listed in Box 20-1.

APPLYING KEY MARKETING CONCEPTS TO ADVANCED PRACTICE NURSING PRACTICE

Utilizing the concepts of price, product, place, promotion, and partnering, the goal of marketing is focused on satisfying the needs and desires of consumers. In order to know the consumer needs, data

---

Box 20-1   CHARACTERISTICS TO LOOK FOR IN A PARTNER

- Conceptual and clinical nursing wisdom
- Excellent interpersonal skills
- Ability to prioritize and organize
- Resourceful and motivated
- Perseverance and tenacity
- Critical thinking capacity
- Time-honored judgment
- Self-confident and self-directed
- Insightful and perceptive
- Strategic and innovative
- Energetic and enthusiastic
- Flexible and curious
- Resiliency
- Steadfastness
- Compassion for self and others

Adapted from Nickitas, D.M., & Valentino, L.M. (2003). Evolving a nursing collegial relationship into a successful consulting business. *Nursing Economic$, 21*(4), 181-187.

are gathered to target marketing strategies. One important marketing strategy organizes information about client needs through the use of a *marketing survey*. The survey assesses two components—service differentiation (product), which is identifying aspects of a service valued by clients yet unmatched by competitors, and market segmentation (place), which divides clients into groups according to factors that influence selection and use of services (Pakis, 1997). Determining service differentiation for an APN practice or service includes gathering data from a group of people about their preferences for a preferred location, hours of service, or availability of follow-up care. Market segmentation data include individual and group characteristics such as age, gender, socioeconomic status, population density, and the benefits or services being sought to define a specific market or market segment being considered (Gershon, 2003).

Good marketing is designed to educate persons and systems about APNs' expertise and to sell a service from a position of strength (Kendig, 2002). It is important for APNs to take a position regarding marketing as it relates to the provision of health care today. APNs cannot afford to be passive. Nursing values and information that is oriented toward the well-being and goals of the consumer can support ethical marketing. Marketing strategies to compete for finite health care resources include health care marketing seminars, hiring of health care marketing consultants by agencies, and the development of marketing jobs in most health care organizations. Until recently, nursing's values have not embraced marketing. However, developing marketing skills and markets for advanced practice nursing could literally determine the survival of APNs.

Corporate marketing strategies aimed at promoting a service or product can work for APNs (Shaw, 2002). The slogans "Finger lickin' good" and "Reach out and touch someone" are well-known branding strategies used by Kentucky Fried Chicken and AT&T. The slogan "Nurses care" has been incorporated by nursing organizations in a variety of ways to market nursing. The slogan has been placed on carry-all bags, pins, and bumper stickers to communicate the fact that the essence of nursing is caring and that the individual person matters to the nurse. The Oncology Nursing Society has used the slogan, "All heart, All mind, No limits," to promote its specialty (J. Spross, personal communication, May 24, 2004). APNs can use similar promotional strategies

to position themselves as unique providers of certain service niches so that consumers automatically think of the APN when they seek that particular service. Examples of marketing service niches for APNs can be found in Box 20-2.

Strategies to market APN services are integrated throughout the chapter; the more common ones include community public speaking, placing ads in community performance programs and church bulletins, giving interviews, legislative lobbying, distributing fact sheets and business cards, and networking with colleagues to educate other professionals and the public about the role of the APN in providing quality health care. In all interactions with patients and consumers, it is essential to identify oneself as an APN and to answer questions as they arise about advanced practice nursing roles.

Based on the overview of marketing just presented, key marketing goals for APNs include the following:

- Educating consumers and colleagues about advanced practice nursing
- Generating income, and obtaining reimbursement for services
- Developing broad-based, interdisciplinary support for advanced practice nursing
- Meeting existing, but unmet, client needs
- Increasing visibility of health care problems that benefit from APN services
- Creating new job opportunities and stable niches in changing delivery systems
- Understanding how to work with a variety of health care practice configurations
- Supporting the use of language that promotes the APN role

Areas of growth in nursing are to be found at the edges of traditional practice (e.g., convenient care clinics, bioterrorism preparation, complementary therapies). The continuing evolution of health care provides APNs areas of expansion. Activities aimed at promotion should educate the public to understand, accept, and request care from an APN. APNs should be seen as necessary providers of acute, primary, and chronic illness care depending on APN role and specialty—not as peripheral providers who exist only on the edge but, rather, as premier providers of health care services. Expanding knowledge and technologies provide opportunities for innovation and marketing to the public.

APNs must broaden their knowledge base to include becoming familiar with economic, political, business, and marketing literature outside of nursing

Box 20-2 Examples of Advanced Practice Nursing Marketing Niches or Services

- Adolescent gynecology specialist
- Architectural consultant
- Bioterrorism preparation
- Birthing center
- Brokering services (e.g., for specific populations)
- Chronic illness management
- Convenient care clinic
- Correctional health care
- Daycare consultant
- Diabetes management
- Disaster preparation
- Older adult care
- Employee programs for health care cost containment
- Fitness/exercise consultant
- First-assistant surgery services
- Genetics
- Health policy consultant
- Health/wellness promotion
- HIV/AIDS care
- Homeless shelters
- Lactation consultant and equipment rental
- Lifestyle change
- Mammography, breast health counseling
- Medical, nursing, health care writing
- Menopause center

- Mobile health services (e.g., mammography van)
- Multidisciplinary clinical practice
- Nurse case manager
- Occupational health/workers' compensation consultant
- Pacemaker center
- Palliative care
- Pain management
- Patient navigator
- Product development (e.g., pharmaceutical, toys, personal care, therapeutic devices, population-focused programs of care [e.g., heart failure clinic])
- Psychiatric counseling
- Radio/television/media consultant
- Retirement center
- Risk management consultant
- Same-day surgery center
- School/college health
- Special populations (e.g., lesbian/gay health, Latino health, immigrant health)
- Stress management consultant
- Transition coach (for health care issues)
- Women's health
- YMCA/YWCA and Boys'/Girls' clubs (for health promotion activities)

AIDS, Acquired immunodeficiency syndrome; *HIV,* human immunodeficiency virus.

to learn about issues that affect care and to become familiar with strategies that improve the context and care of the service provided (see Box 20-3 for website resources). The business concept of *cooperative competition,* or "co-opetition" (Brandenburger & Nalebuff, 1996; Friedman, 2002) offers a way for today's competitors to find new common ground for business collaboration tomorrow. "When competitors reach a standoff in market advantage, they can switch to cooperation to increase their mutual strengths and benefits" (Coile, 1999, p. 5). Creating shared business alliances using co-opetition is one of many concepts APNs can borrow from the corporate world. Integrating business principles with caring practices enhances one's ability to market APN services. To expand services and improve existing care, many health care providers are adopting the use of *customer relationship management* (CRM) and *patient relationship management* (PRM) strategies (Benz & Paddison, 2004). Both CRM and PRM are data-driven approaches to strate-

gic planning and consumer relationship building and strengthening. PRM is directed toward consumers, and CRM encompasses the entire market with a goal of optimizing revenues by identifying consumer and prospective consumer needs and preferences.

Leadership has been an expected competency of APNs. The enhanced leadership strengths of the APN prepared with a DNP will broaden APNs' access to corporate venues previously closed to most APNs. APNs educated as DNPs may actually change the face of marketing. The APN DNP will bring new competencies in the areas of leadership, systems management, and health policy development to the practice arena (AACN, 2006). These competencies prepare APNs who have strong leadership skills, are able to integrate nursing and scientific knowledge that improves evaluation and creates new practice approaches, and are motivated to disseminate information to a broader audience that enhances health care outcomes. A role that encompasses these broader competencies

Box 20-3   INTERNET RESOURCES RELATED TO BUSINESS PLANNING AND MARKETING

www.medscape.com/resource/apn/rc-apn3	Latest on business and legal topics for both new and experienced advance practice nurses
www.buppert.com/trainingmodules	Site describes training modules for purchase to start a business in the health care field
www.sba.gov and www.sba.gov/starting_business/	Help from the government to start your business
www.startupjournal.com	Information from the *Wall Street Journal* on how to start a business
www.business.com	Leading business search engine and business directory designed to help users find the information needed to make business decisions
www.businessknowhow.com	Much pithy advice on real problems faced in starting and early stages of a business
www.FASTcompany.com	Website with multiple marketing and business links including technology and leadership
www.adslogans.co.uk/pages/hall_of_fame.html	Website of best slogans for branding companies
www.cms.hhs.gov	Centers for Medicare and Medicaid Services for reimbursement information
www.score.org	Courses and one-on-one mentoring by retired business experts
www.nawbo.org	National Association of Women Business Owners

invigorates the development of new avenues for impacting health care practice, delivery, and policy.

MARKETABLE PROPERTIES OF ADVANCED PRACTICE NURSES

Realistic self-appraisal of marketable skills is essential, not just for new APN graduates and APNs who change jobs or move to a new area but for *all* APNs in the current health care environment. The ability to market oneself is necessary whether one is (or wishes to be) an employee or an entrepreneur. Much of what we understand about marketing advanced practice nursing is based on the experiences and writings of nurse entrepreneurs (see Chapter 19).

APNs cannot develop markets and sell themselves if they do not clearly recognize their unique skills and how these skills can meet client needs. Such an appraisal helps APNs determine what areas of practice need to be developed to better position themselves for the marketplace. Many NPs are tempted to skip this step because they do not have the time or interest; they may think that the exercise is not valuable (Fitzgerald, 1999). APN entrepreneurs have invested tremendous energy and resources in their careers and

owe it to themselves to perform a self-appraisal, a key step in determining one's marketability. Questions that can help APNs inventory their skills and identify opportunities for applying these unique skills include the following:

1. What motivates me in my practice?
2. What are my strengths?
3. What do I do best in my practice?
4. Where do I get the most satisfaction in my practice?
5. What am I most proud of about my practice?
6. Do I have a skill a consumer or organization would pay for?
7. How might I attract a consumer or organization to pay for my skills?
8. What services can I provide to fill a niche need?

In his book *What Color Is Your Parachute?*, Richard Bolles (2002) aptly described how individuals can determine their best fit in a career and how they can market themselves to attain that goal. Readers are instructed to formulate a picture of their ideal job by identifying the specific wants and needs that allow them to flourish. By applying these strategies, the APN can identify strengths, such as favorite transferable skills, favorite tasks, favorite people with whom

EXEMPLAR 20-1   CNS-Led Clinic Influences System-wide Policy Change

A DNP-prepared CNS employed in a health system found a great deal of satisfaction establishing a nurse-managed center for patients with cardiovascular diseases to improve patient outcomes and to decrease rehospitalizations. The establishment of the clinic was feasible only after researching and discovering that the number of patients who were being rehospitalized for the same cardiovascular problems was increasing. After analyzing the evidence-based literature, she believed that a clinic would promote patient self-care and improve understanding of how lifestyle behaviors would enhance quality of life. She convinced the system administrators that such a clinic in which patients' status would be monitored regularly using technology (e.g., e-mail, phone contacts, video cameras) would eventually decrease system costs because of decreased readmissions. The CNS marketed the concept to the hospital administrators and implemented the clinic. The clinic became an excellent revenue source as well as a marketing tool for the hospital. The clinic was marketed through community brochures and speaking opportunities and by distributing flyers to local physicians and clinics. The DNP CNS was able to change system-wide policy with the development of the first APN-directed clinic for the system.

CNS, Certified nurse specialist; *DNP*, Doctor of Nursing Practice.

 EXEMPLAR 20-2   Advanced Practice Nurses as Practice Owners/Employers*

This exemplar describes two family nurse practitioners, K.B. and S.B., who are graduates of the author's Master of Science in Nursing FNP program. K.B. began the graduate program with the goal to establish a health care clinic in her hometown, because the closest physician practice for the rural community was 30 miles away. The only other provider in the town was her dentist-husband. Together they purchased a building and refurbished it into a combined clinic, with his dentist office on one side and her primary care clinic office on the other side. The entrance foyer, waiting room, receptionist area, and kitchen are shared. To open the clinic, K.B. negotiated with the regional hospital to set up and fund the clinic. She established a collaborative practice agreement with one of the area physicians as required by the Georgia Board of Nursing state practice act for APNs. In addition, she successfully led the effort to have her small town of 1200 persons redesignated as an HPSA. Almost 15 years later, the clinic is thriving and K.B. has purchased the clinic from the hospital. She became an FNP because she saw a need. She developed a plan, marketed her clinic, and established a very successful health care center.

S.B. was employed by a physician for several years. When the physician decided to make changes in his life, she purchased the primary care practice from him and is now the owner/employer and has hired several physicians to provide care to the underserved population of coastal Georgia. S.B. advertises her practice as offering health care and wellness throughout the life span. Working in multiple roles, she is the business administrator and a clinician in this nurse-owned primary care practice. Over time, these two FNP entrepreneurs have worked and supported each other professionally in their practices. Their example shows how APNs can be successful entrepreneurs and demonstrates that a sound marketing plan helps produce positive outcomes. (See Chapter 19 for further description of S.B.'s practice.)

*We gratefully acknowledge Kim Baird, MSN, ARNP, BC, Woodbine, GA, and Sally Bennett, MSN, ARNP, BC, Kingsland, GA, for their contribution to this exemplar.
APN, Advanced practice nurse; FNP, family nurse practitioner; HPSA, health professional shortage area.

to work, and favorite kinds of information with which to work; then the APN can identify the unique services that he or she has to offer. Many APNs have successfully developed unique practices that meet a vital need. Exemplars 20-1 and 20-2 describe APNs' self-appraisals of marketable knowledge and skills.

External and Internal Marketing

Two facets of marketing that are useful to clarify the APN roles in every setting are external marketing and internal marketing (Reel & Abraham, 2007). *External marketing* refers to techniques that APNs can use to promote themselves or their practices to their consumers or the public at large. Suggestions include speaking at community meetings, writing a column in the newspaper, and sending out fliers or brochures about the practice. In addition, using the positive opinions of respected persons to support practice outcomes about using APNs is beneficial. Considering the perceptions of the population targeted for APN services is important. Those persons who have used APN services in the past and high school graduates were noted to have a more positive attitude toward nurse practitioners (Phillips, Palmer, Wettig, & Fenwick, 2000). Telephone surveys to identify the perception of patients toward APN services and knowledge about APNs were used to indicate the receptivity of insured or affluent persons to use the services of APNs in New York City. (Garfield, 2000). The finding that only 23% of the survey participants were familiar with the term *advanced practice nurses* whereas 76% had heard of *nurse practitioners* emphasizes the need to use external marketing strategies to increase the public's familiarity with the term *APNs* for marketing purposes.

Marketing the practice using an external strategy could include mailing a patient education newsletter to existing patients that reminds them about your services. This may help recruit new patients if it goes out to the entire community, including physicians (Anonymous, 2006). Recommendations to increase the success of the newsletter include publishing regularly, assuming the patient's viewpoint, and distinguishing the newsletter from junk mail. It should have a professional presentation and include educational information, and it should not look like a blatant marketing tool. Retention of the existing consumer base while attracting new consumers of the service is an important consideration (Sturm, 2005).

Internal marketing involves differentiating the unique capabilities of APNs in their practice. APNs offer care that is often of higher quality, more complex, more accessible, or less expensive than other clinicians' care (Brunk, 1992). Hallums (1994) considered internal marketing a holistic management process that is important work undertaken by an organization to motivate and train its "internal customers" (employees) to work as a unified group to deliver customer service and satisfaction. Utilizing relationship marketing in the health care clinic helps develop, enhance, and maintain long-term relationships (Bansal, 2004). The emphasis of service quality that influences consumer perceptions is described by these five dimensions: tangibility, reliability, responsiveness, assurance, and empathy. *Relationship marketing* encompasses the three processes of

interaction, dialogue, and value (Gronroos, 1997). Interaction is the core of relationship marketing—the interaction between the consumer and the service supplier (e.g., office personnel, APN). To enhance the interaction, a two-way dialogue needs to be established. The value process demonstrates how the consumer perceives the worth of services over a period of time. Everyone in the organization from the receptionist to the health care provider is important to the establishment of excellent relationships. The utilization of relationship marketing as an internal strategy can enhance and ensure a high-quality experience for the consumer. Grasping the importance of internal marketing is crucial for APNs. Internal marketing strategies are often central to establishing credibility and developing collaborative, interdisciplinary relationships.

Creativity is the hallmark of both external and internal APN marketing. Tapping into one's creativity often gets overlooked when performing routine care and managing patient problems. In Exemplar 20-3, Keller (Doughty & Keller, 2000) used a unique, creative internal marketing strategy that was successful.

PUBLIC RELATIONS, THE MEDIA, AND TECHNOLOGY

Effective promotion of one's product depends on a sound understanding of the relationships among product, promotion, and public relations. Public relations and promotion are closely linked in that promotion incorporates a variety of public relations strategies. The following public relations barriers need to be addressed for the marketing of APN services to be successful:

- Invisibility of APNs and a general lack of knowledge about advanced practice nursing
- Effects of negative publicity in advertising and popular media, which includes inaccurate portrayals of nurses in general and APNs in particular, or adverse publicity, as when a nurse is arrested for deliberately harming a patient or making a medication error
- Traditional images of nurses in the media that portray them as tyrants, sex symbols, ditsy females, or physicians' handmaidens

Invisibility of Advanced Practice Nurses

Although the American Nurses Association (ANA) and other APN role-specific groups speak for APNs at the national level, APNs have the responsibility to market themselves at the state and local levels by educating legislators, physicians, and consumers about what services APNs are educationally prepared to

EXEMPLAR 20-3   **Internal Marketing Strategies to Promote Advanced Practice Nurse Roles***

While working in a multispecialty group practice in the Southwest several years ago, NP and PA colleagues met regularly to discuss practice issues. The group decided that it was necessary to educate physicians, administrators, and clinical and clerical support staff about the role of NPs and PAs in the organization. A presentation was developed titled "A Day in the Life of an NP and a PA." With a total of 85 physicians and 13 NPs and PAs in the practice, the group thought that it was very important for the entire medical staff and top administrators to attend. It was determined that the best forum for the presentation was during the health center's monthly medical and administrative staff meeting. Because this presentation would be a first within the organization, two things were certain: (1) this might be the only chance to capture the attention of physician and administrative colleagues; and (2) the presentation had to be extremely well-prepared to enhance the credibility of the NP/PA group.

After much brainstorming, a creative, humorous, and informative presentation was developed. A listing of the most memorable questions that had been asked of the group was developed. Examples of the questions included, "What do all those letters after your name mean?" "When are you going to become a doctor?" "Do I have to pay the full $5 co-pay to see you instead of a doctor?" "I am so confused . . . what is the difference between an NP and a PA?" "As an NP, are you the one who stands in the room with the doctor when he does a Pap smear?"

The group then enlisted the help of collaborative physicians to serve as "plants" in the audience. Each collaborating physician was provided with the question that was to be addressed by the NP or PA in his or her dyad. *Dyad* was the term that had been mutually agreed upon with the medical director to define the relationship between each NP or PA provider and his or her collaborating physician in the practice. It was thought that the dyad recognition in the presentation was important because some of the physicians had historically been uncomfortable referring patients to NPs and PAs if they were not aware of the dyad arrangement. The overall mood during the presentations was humorous and informal. On cue during the program, each physician "plant" stood up and asked the question assigned to him or her. The corresponding NP or PA then answered the question with factual information illustrating the role of the NP or PA. For example, in response to the question "When are you going to become a doctor?," an NP replied with enthusiasm about positive reasons for choosing to be an APN instead of a physician. In response to the question "As an NP, are you the one who stands in the room with the doctor when he does a Pap smear?," an NP addressed the need for consumer education and widespread external and internal marketing of APNs. Other issues that were addressed in the question-and-answer format were the educational requirements for NPs and PAs, quality-of-service issues, and the role of NPs and PAs as primary care providers.

Before the start of the program, the NPs and PAs were seated in front of the audience with large nametags and were given the opportunity to introduce themselves individually in a brief biographical format (e.g., name, department, site, collaborating physician name, education, related work/volunteer background, and special interests clinically and personally). Many of the staff members had never met each other, so this provided the opportunity for recognition and networking. The feedback the group received was tremendous. Many physicians, administrators, and human resources representatives made a special point to thank the group for a most informative and interesting program. The outcome of the presentation was an overall increase in the numbers of internal referrals to NPs and PAs. As a result of this success, further marketing projects were launched.

A presentation for receptionists and medical assistants about the role of NPs and PAs in health care was provided. The result of this effort was more appropriately scheduled appointments and no more receptionists being overheard to say, "You can't see the doctor today, just the NP or PA. Sorry!" One of the most important outcomes of this overall marketing effort by the NP/PA group was the appointment of the first NP on the medical center's new board of directors. In this setting, it was determined that an aggressive internal marketing strategy was necessary before branching out to external strategies. In this exemplar, thoughtful assessment of the practice situation, group discussions, and strategic planning for the best possible implementation resulted in positive outcomes. One caveat to remember is that it is important never to assume that all of the administrators or physician colleagues have a clear understanding of the role of an APN in a practice setting. Internal and external marketing strategies can help improve the practice milieu and thus have a positive impact on APN job satisfaction.

*We gratefully acknowledge Jennifer M. Keller , RN, MSN, and Susan E.D. Doughty, RNC, MSN, WHNP, for their contribution to this exemplar. *APN*, Advanced practice nurse; *NP*, nurse practitioner; *PA*, physician assistant.

provide. The reality is that APN invisibility is a pervasive problem not only among consumers but also among health care professionals. In an interview, Robert J. Blendon, director of the Harvard Opinion Research Program, stated that national polls regularly do not include questions on nursing and, as a result, more is known about the public's opinion of physicians than nurses (Buerhaus, 2000). In spite of the negative perspective on advanced practice nursing by organized medicine and the lack of information regarding public opinion of advanced practice nursing, the health care community is becoming more aware of APNs, particularly NPs, in part because of new federal guidelines that include their services (Diamond, 2000). Language can be a powerful influence on the visibility or invisibility of particular APN providers. For example, organizations and public media regularly refer to APNs as *physician extenders* or *mid-levels*. These terms denigrate the role of the APN to a lower level of care and imply that APNs are not capable of providing care without physician oversight—both inferences have been proven false. When one says the word *doctor,* everyone knows who is being identified. The terms *nurse-midwife* and *nurse anesthetist* are also clear. However, when one says *advanced practice nurse, nurse practitioner,* or *clinical nurse specialist,* some consumers not only are unfamiliar with these terms but also are often uncomfortable using them. For example, a young administrator (Marie) was describing her child's health care provider to a nurse researcher who had previously practiced as an APN. During the conversation, Marie said "the doctor" did this and that. At the end of Marie's description of her child's visit to the provider, the nurse researcher said, "Marie, the person you are describing sounds a lot like a nurse practitioner." Marie said with some embarrassment, "Well … she is a nurse practitioner." When asked, Marie said that her only reason for using the term *doctor* was that it was easier to say. A teachable moment had arisen, and the nurse researcher had a collegial discussion with Marie about the power of language and its role in concealing nursing's contributions to health care. As a result of the conversation, Marie realized the negative impact (invisibility, unintentional invalidation) that is perpetuated when the appropriate identity of the APN is not used in conversations with others. It is equally important to present oneself as a *nurse practitioner,* a *clinical specialist,* a *nurse-midwife,* a *nurse anesthetist,* or an *APN* instead of a *mid-level provider* or *physician-extender*

because these terms continue to promote APN invisibility. Continued efforts to eliminate the use of these terms and promote a more politically correct term like *advanced practice nurse provider* are needed!

The lack of consistent terminology in nursing for APNs contributes to the invisibility of nursing and confusion within the profession as well as the public. For instance, the titling for nurse practitioner in the 50 states includes *certified registered nurse practitioner (CRNP), advanced practice registered nurse (APRN), advanced practice nurse (APN),* and *certified nurse practitioner (CNP)* (Pearson, 2007). When NPs (and other APNs) have such varied legal titles, how can the public be expected to know what to call APNs? This conundrum may worsen as new roles evolve, as education levels change to DNP, and as the nursing profession deals with advanced practice credentialing and licensing (see Chapter 21).

Effects of Negative Publicity

Physician dominance in the health care market and efforts by organized medicine to discredit APN practice can be obstacles to APN marketing. Fear of encroachment and a lack of understanding about the services APNs are educationally prepared to provide to patients have caused some physicians and organized physician groups to attempt to block legislation that would allow for the full scope of APN practice activities. Since 1995, and modified in 2003, the American Medical Association (AMA) has a policy to assist state and local medical societies in identifying and lobbying against laws that allow APNs to provide medical care without the supervision of a physician (H-160.947) (AMA, Policy [a], 2003). In 2006, the AMA executive summary on convenient care clinics (AMA, 2006) references a policy on limiting the scope of practice of allied health professionals: "With respect to scope of practice issues, the AMA has established a Scope of Practice Partnership with members of the Federation as a means of using legislative, regulatory, and judicial advocacy to restrain the expansion of scope of practice laws for allied health professionals that threaten the health and safety of patients" (p. 5). Attempts by anesthesiologists to require supervision of CRNAs is an ongoing conflict. The continuing full-press effort by organized medicine to limit and control APN practice proceeds despite contrary evidence that shows APN care is safe and cost-effective. Organized medicine continues to attempt to thwart APN practice; a more positive approach of developing partnering relationships between nursing and medicine to provide care to more of the underinsured would be much more beneficial, especially in light of the predicted physician shortage in 2020 (AMA, 2007). The relative invisibility of advanced practice nursing and the public's lack of understanding of the APN role may indirectly support the actions of the AMA.

In many states, state laws that established barriers to APN practice have been challenged and changed to extend APN scopes of practices. In some states (Georgia, Illinois, Maine, Mississippi, Ohio, Oklahoma, Oregon) restrictions are placed on use of the term *doctor* in the clinical setting by doctorally prepared APNs (Pearson, 2007; Rudner, O'Grady, Hodnicki, & Hanson, 2007). This issue needs to be addressed as more doctorally prepared APNs enter practice. Some states allow the term *doctor* to be used as long as the individual is clearly identified by profession on the identification name tag. Patient confusion can be easily alleviated with proper introductions, "Hello, I am Dr. Ima Groundswell. I am an advanced practice nurse (or nurse practitioner, nurse midwife…), and I will be seeing you today." Multidisciplinary teams of "doctors" exist in health care facilities. When one profession limits use of the term *doctor,* this action denies the identity of other professionals and does not allow the patient to know the caliber of the person providing services. These legislative restrictions, occurring within the context of a complex health care market, have led to rising tensions between advanced practice nursing and medicine. The medical profession has become more vocal and has initiated specific activities aimed at limiting APN scope of practice. As a result of these actions, the American public has been exposed to "negative marketing" campaigns directed against APNs.

Organized medicine continues to attempt to create barriers to APN practice (see previous discussion of AMA activities). From a public relations standpoint, it is crucial that APNs support medical colleagues who do value and understand the role of APNs and who refuse to participate in organized medicine's attempts to discredit APNs. It is important to delineate major differences in the practice scopes and the range of services that APNs and physicians are prepared to provide (Moody, Smith, & Glenn, 1999). Those who write health care policy must be clear about how APNs can help meet the health care needs of the country, and APNs must be proactive in contacting state and federal representatives to help them understand the role of APNs as health care providers. It is hoped that positive policy and legislative changes that promote APN practice will increase with the advent of more DNP-prepared APNs assuming leadership positions in health care systems.

Traditional Images of Nurses and Advanced Practice Nurses

Traditional images of nurses in the media indicate that improved, widespread strategic promotion is a particularly important marketing concept for APNs to grasp. Kalisch and Kalisch's (1981) classic work on nurses and the media recommended that nursing specialties work with the media to improve their image, that the public be informed that the primary role of the nurse is to promote health and not serve as handmaiden to the physician, and that nurses are knowledgeable and accountable, as well as sympathetic, caregivers. This advice, given over 26 years ago, is still accurate today. The media continue to present the traditional nurse-physician relationship in a stereotypical fashion (Corser, 2000). In spite of efforts to correct these portrayals, inaccurate perceptions of nursing still exist in many arenas. Suzanne Gordon, a journalist, has written several books portraying the profession of nursing, the contexts in which nurses work, and the resulting exodus of nurses from the profession. Her latest book describes in detail the trials of nurses on the front line of care, the lack of recognition for their work, and the constant confrontation with physicians in order to provide quality care for patients (Gordon, 2006).

In response to the nursing shortage, seven graduate students at Johns Hopkins University School of Nursing came together in April 2001 to form the Center for Nursing Advocacy to address the negative portrayal of nursing by the media. The mission of the Center is to increase public understanding of the central, front-line role nurses play in modern health care (Center for Nursing Advocacy, 2007).

The media are not solely to blame for the traditional negative or stereotypical images of nursing or the current paucity of coverage of nursing issues in the media. APNs and nurses must bear some responsibility for these misperceptions. To be successful in the evolving health care industry, APNs must be more proactive in marketing the profession as a whole in a positive way and in continuing to inform and confront the mass media when inaccurate perceptions are presented.

Americans use the media as their primary source of information about health. "This finding is enormously important to nursing. It means that nursing cannot ignore or underestimate the power of the media to influence nursing's public credibility and prestige both now and well into the twenty-first century" (Buresh, 1998, p. 69). The public needs to be constantly oriented toward several functions that nurses serve in many settings; nurses promote health, teach disease-prevention strategies, and diagnose and treat common illnesses. In addition, some APNs are specially educated to deliver anesthesia and pain management; to provide safe prenatal, intrapartum, and postpartum care; and to broker services for older adults or the chronically ill. To change the public's perceptions of nursing, APNs must make themselves available to consult with entities such as health policy writers, health care journalists, and health planning boards to establish more pro-APN health policies and to increase the number of APN-directed health care centers.

A study on the care provided by NPs from 1995 to 1997 indicated, among other findings, that after the initial appointment (p = .88), overall satisfaction ratings did not differ between the care provided by the NPs and that provided by the physicians (Mundinger et al., 2000). These findings are consistent with observations from those outside the profession. In a *Harvard Business Review* article, the authors suggested that NPs could take on more complex roles than they are doing. Nurse practitioners are capable of treating many ailments that in the past were within the realm of physicians' care (Christianson, Bohmer, & Kenagy, 2000). Widespread reporting of outcomes of APN care, including the public's level of satisfaction with the care provided by NPs, can influence the development of a more positive image of advanced practice nursing.

The public's lack of understanding about nurses contributes to an inaccurate image of nursing and a lack of persons interested in the profession. In 2002, Johnson & Johnson began a national multiyear, multilevel media effort, The Campaign for Nursing's Future, to promote interest in nursing careers and a positive image of nursing. A phone survey conducted by Penn, Shoen, and Berland Associates in December 2001 of 1005 adults older than 18 years in the United States found that only 53% knew that an RN must have a bachelor's degree or an associate's degree. Fewer than half knew that an NP must have a master's degree, and over two thirds did not know that NPs could prescribe medications (Johnson & Johnson, 2002). The data suggest that the lack of information about nurses is associated with the public's lack of understanding regarding the role that nurses and APNs have in health care decision making.

The nursing community has undertaken a national effort to improve the image of nursing. Nursing's Agenda for the Future (American Nurses Association [ANA], 2001), a national plan developed by a steering committee comprising 19 national nursing organizations, is designed to provide guidance for improving nursing's future and the public's right to high-quality health care. The plan is designed around 10 domains. One of the domains is communication, and a primary objective is improving communication with the public about the role nurses play in health care (ANA). These national efforts are, in part, aimed at improving nursing's image and disseminating accurate information to the public about nurses in a media context that continues negative portrayals. As the public's understanding of APN practice, quality of care, and positive care outcomes increases, existing barriers to practice can eventually be removed. However, as health care evolves and comes under continued intense scrutiny, more barriers to effective marketing for APNs can also arise. To counteract current and future barriers, APNs must be willing to go beyond conventional thinking and to perceive barriers as opportunities.

One strategy to improve the public image of nursing is to disseminate the positive and cost-effective outcomes of care provided by APNs in consumer publications as well as to professional journals. A secondary analysis of seven clinical studies (conducted over 22 years) of care provided by APNs indicated that APN interventions consistently resulted in improved patient outcomes and reduced health care costs across the groups studied (Brooten et al., 2002;. see also Chapter 24). Economic outcomes such as these and other studies related to APN practice (Mundinger et al., 2000) can be used effectively to market the APN as a cost-effective, quality health care provider. In light of rapidly escalating health care costs, these types of information must be shared with the public in a way that is readily understood. APNs, whether in private practice or employed in institutions, need to distribute (or help prepare) press releases on innovative and effective clinical programs, as well as important research findings, to the popular press. This strategy can interest journalists in nursing and generate interviews and other media activities that will elicit public interest in and commitment to APNs. These actions need to be ongoing, because not all efforts result in information being picked up by the popular press. Numerous opportunities exist for APNs to improve the public's perception of the image of nursing, the role of APNs, and the variety of ways that nurses improve health care services. Box 20-4 provides media and public relations strategies for marketing APN services.

MARKETING STRATEGIES FOR ADVANCED PRACTICE NURSES

Transition Considerations for New Graduates

Marketing oneself as a new graduate is one of the most challenging tasks for APNs. The transition period from student to APN provides many exciting new opportunities, but it can also be the source of much anxiety. Helping students develop skills to make the transition to new graduate APNs is essential to the success of future marketing strategies. Brown and Olshansky's (1998) research-based model identifies the "Limbo to Legitimacy" transition stages that take into account the experiences of the new NP during the first year in primary care practice. Stage 1 of this developmental, nonlinear model is relevant to all APNs in the first year of practice and raises important marketing considerations. This stage is characterized by a period of recovering from school, seeking employment, negotiating bureaucracies, and worrying about meeting role expectations. Maintaining positive self-esteem is key to a successful completion of this role transition (see Chapter 4). The change from APN student to graduate APN is an added challenging transition. Transition periods can be disconcerting because of leaving the protective context of the academic setting, feeling uncertain about the future, seeking employment, and putting on the APN role for real. Bolles (2002) suggested teaching new graduates five approaches to sustaining a positive outlook during transition periods:

- Keep physically fit by developing an action plan that makes time for positive self-care.
- Deal with emotions by building an effective support network.
- Monitor mental stamina, and focus on positive views.
- Utilize spirituality for support in difficult times.
- Keep active by using time and talents within the community.

Although the new APN may have an ideal position in mind, in reality the position may not exist; therefore flexibility is a characteristic to be desired in all graduates. According to Payne (1997), the role of executives, recruiters, and faculty is to help new graduates stay open to alternative employment options in health care. Key elements include helping them to remain enthusiastic, to market their unique skills, and to understand the need for flexibility. Strategies include encouraging new graduates to view a part-time position as a potential bridge to full-time employment, to perceive cross-training as a challenge, and to consider new or unusual job opportunities as pathways to a rewarding professional nursing career.

Strategies for the Nurse Entrepreneur

An APN nurse entrepreneur *identifies* a need, develops an approach to respond to the need in an effective way, formulates a plan of action, and then executes the plan (Dayhoff & Moore, 2003; see also Chapter 19). APNs as entrepreneurs are creative forces within an organization to increase the quality of patient care (Ieong, 2005). Nurse entrepreneurs are visionary, decision makers, risk takers, problem solvers, self-confident, committed, creative, flexible, and responsible clinicians (Dayhoff & Moore; Palmer, 1996; Price, 2004). Entrepreneurship is a concept that APN programs need to incorporate in business and practice management discussions (Ieong). Friedman (2002) discussed the

---

Box 20-4   MEDIA AND PUBLIC RELATIONS STRATEGIES

- Network with health journalists.
- Gain television news show exposure.
- Write magazine and journal articles.
- Send out press releases.
- Produce public service announcements.
- Publish research reports.
- Write for daily newspapers and news magazines.
- Participate in radio/television news interviews.
- Establish a site on the Internet/World Wide Web.
- Volunteer to give community presentations.
- Volunteer to work in a free clinic and/or provide free services (e.g., homeless shelter).
- Join community organizations.
- Get involved with politics (e.g., run for public office, work on a campaign).
- Publish a patient newsletter for your practice.

EXEMPLAR 20-4   Marketing a Holistic Women's Health Practice*

S.D., an APN in a holistic OB-GYN practice, recognized a need in the community for women in midlife to have access to information about whether to take hormones or herbs, how to improve quality of life, and how to prevent problems of aging that start in midlife. Certain obstacles prevented universal access in that practice. The idea was to create an interdisciplinary holistic center on a bus line, a center with handicapped accessibility and a fund for indigent women. The foundation would be a concept of circle leadership among the disciplines without a medical hierarchy, consistent with the work of Christina Baldwin (1998). According to Baldwin, "The circle is an organizational structure that locates leadership along the rim and provides an inclusive means for consultation. Circling is a useful structure for learning, governance, creating community, providing services, envisioning in starting long-range goals and observing ritual" (p. 38).

After a year of planning with a nurse massage therapist and a highly skilled medical receptionist, the APN completed the business plan and went to the bank. She hoped to get partial funding as a business loan and to secure a personal loan for the remainder of the start-up costs. The bank officials were so impressed with the marketing projections and data in the business plan that they funded the entire start-up costs.

Critical to the success of the women's center was the agreement of a close friend and colleague, another experienced women's health NP with a background in business and a master's degree in business administration, to buy in as a partner. Many of the business decisions that had to be made in the infancy of the practice were tempered with expertise and practical orientation. The new partner believed in the vision, and both practitioners remained connected to the constant question, "How will this decision affect the women who want our services?"

Initially, the other disciplines included massage, mental health, movement, and nutrition. A physical therapist and a gynecologist were recruited. The team sat in "circle" weekly to discuss how the center was doing and how they were doing with the center. They held retreats quarterly to bond as a team. A naturopath also joined the group. Their marketing efforts are detailed in Box 20-5.

Obstacles to third-party reimbursement for APN autonomous practice in Maine precipitated legislation to ensure reimbursement. The state NP group hired a lobbyist who helped them forge this legislation. S.D.'s business partner was extremely active in this effort, gathering data and testimonials. Prior data that had been generated on cost and efficacy influenced the banking and insurance committee, who first heard the bills. Patient testimonials were what convinced all involved that APNs made a difference and needed to have separate identification numbers and reimbursement. A unanimous vote supporting eligibility for reimbursement for certified NPs and CNMs went from the committee to both houses, where it passed without debate.

*We gratefully acknowledge Jennifer M. Keller, RN, MSN, and Susan E.D. Doughty, RNC, MSN, WHNP, for their contribution to this exemplar. *APN,* Advanced practice nurse; *CNM,* certified nurse-midwife; *GYN,* gynecological; *NP,* nurse practitioner; *OB,* obstetrical.

opportunities for hospital growth that exist amid niche facilities. Many of the strategies suggested can also be applied to APNs carving out niches in the health care field by pursuing joint ventures with other providers, using common ground to mutual benefit, and redesigning the business as needed (Friedman).

Nurse entrepreneurs have made changes in the health care service arena using marketing strategies. One strategy is to establish or increase a consumer base for APN practice by creating a practice name that provides as much information as possible (Dirubbo, 2005). For example, the practice name *Effingham Family Nursing and Health Care Center* provides the practice location and the fact that both nursing and health

care services are provided. Other strategies include joining the local chamber of commerce and being listed in the business directory, attending local networking get-togethers, writing an article for the chamber newsletter, sending letters to local service groups offering to be an event speaker, distributing business brochures and cards at all opportunities, participating in local health fairs, and providing "Tell a Friend" 3×5-inch practice information cards to patients to give to friends. These successful and effective marketing tools increased one nurse entrepreneur's patient base by over 23% of her practice plan goal for the year (Dirubbo). The strategies used by an APN's holistic obstetrical-gynecological (OB-GYN) practice are described in Exemplar 20-4 and in Box 20-5.

Box 20-5   MARKETING EFFORTS FOR HOLISTIC OB-GYN PRACTICE

MARKETING THE CONCEPT TO THE BANK FOR START-UP COSTS

The business plan included detailed data based on experience as well as income projections.

MARKETING TO THE COMMUNITY

1. Other providers
   - Contracts with three gynecologists to provide backup care on an urgent basis
   - Community letters and meetings with internists and gynecologists about the niche our service provided to help women with complex midlife needs or hormone therapy that was not working
   - Meetings with a community breast surgeon, oncologist, and nurse practitioners about complex menopausal symptom relief for women who could not take estrogen
2. Potential women clients
   - Open houses highlighting the services of the center
   - Day-long workshops presented by the team about midlife issues. Topics included the following:
        Osteoporosis: Reframing Your Frame
        Heart Disease: Finding Your Heart's Desire

        Mental Clarity: Mysteries of the Menopausal Mind
        The Joy of Soy: Cooking with Soy Made Easy
   - Free monthly menopause support group supported by the American Menopause Foundation, which helped market to area media
   - Multiple community education workshops and lectures to YWCA, women in business, insurance executives
   - Lunch meetings and tours through center
   - Newspaper stories featuring third-party reimbursement hassles for an APN practice
   - Newspaper columns about women's health
   - Newspaper advertisement
   - Promotional fact sheet about center
3. Other APNs who wanted to start similar practices
   - Reprints about the practice
   - Panel discussions with slide show at state APN meetings
   - Meetings, tours, and opportunities for shadowing in the practice (professional fee charged for time spent with us)
   - Lectures to the university NP programs in the city
   - Preceptor to one APN graduate student each semester

Adapted from Doughty, S., & Keller, J.M. (2000). Marketing and contracting considerations. In A.B. Hamric, J.A. Spross, & C.M. Hanson (Eds.), *Advanced nursing practice: An integrative approach* (2nd ed., pp. 655-677). Philadelphia: Saunders.
APN, Advanced practice nurse; *GYN,* gynecological; *NP,* nurse practitioner; *OB,* obstetrical.

Avoiding Marketing Missteps

Economic limitations necessitate the best usage of marketing principles to be successful in disseminating information. Gandolf and Hirsh (2006) list the seven deadly sins of private practice marketing:

- *Deadly Sin 1: Spaghetti Marketing.* This is a scattered and ineffective approach that throws strategies out to see what sticks. It is more effective to have an organized marketing plan that uses marketing professionals working within your budget.
- *Deadly Sin 2: Analysis Paralysis.* No marketing strategy is forever; it can be changed, so do not take forever to make a marketing decision. Consider what you want to do, and do it.
- *Deadly Sin 3: Marketing Decisions by Committee.* Consensus decisions can take forever. Get opinions, but act on what you want to do.
- *Deadly Sin 4: Inadequate Training.* If the frontline staff members do not understand

your service or product, it represents a lost opportunity. Prepare the office staff to handle a variety of questions (frequently asked questions [FAQs]) from potential consumers.
- *Deadly Sin 5: Treating Marketing as a Cost Center.* Marketing is a revenue builder and needs a sufficient budget. Evaluate strategies, and reinvent or revise components when necessary.
- *Deadly Sin 6: Insufficient Delegation.* One person cannot do everything. Use a team approach to handle the marketing components.
- *Deadly Sin 7: Inconsistency.* Keep the message consistent at all times, and make sure that you deliver what consumers were led to expect.

Developing a marketing plan is necessary. To reach your practice goals using marketing strategies, do not hesitate to ask for assistance in order to avoid the pitfalls that will waste time and money. Marketing strategies will need to be tailored to the practice goals to be successful.

Strategies for Seeking Employment

Seeking employment is a primary task for new graduates. During the course of graduate education, strategies for seeking an APN position should be discussed. Specific elements include developing a professional portfolio, a résumé, a curriculum vitae (CV), and query and cover letters. Strategies for interview preparation and negotiating or accepting a position are needed. These issues are briefly covered here.

Professional Portfolio. An accurate self-assessment of individual strengths and a clear conceptualization of one's desired practice arena are essential first steps in developing a personal marketing plan. Developing a professional marketing portfolio is a useful strategy to aid in this process (Burgess & Misener, 1997). A professional portfolio is defined as a representative sample of documents about who you are as a professional and what you have to offer the employer (Letz, 2002). A nursing portfolio provides an accessible resource that can be used to enter a job market, to make a career change, and to enhance professional opportunities (Meister, Heath, Andrews, & Tingen, 2002). A portfolio differs from a résumé or CV in that, in addition to containing a list of all previous positions and educational background, the portfolio contains examples of one's work. Students' and experienced APNs' portfolios are similar with some additions to the latter in terms of mentorship, patient satisfaction, performance evaluations, and employer committee involvement (Meister et al.). Professional portfolios contain a description of skills and provide a profile of the applicant's major accomplishments and contributions (Box 20-6). When a specific employment opportunity arises that an APN desires, the APN chooses from the portfolio only those materials that best relate to the desired position, such as a résumé listing previous positions and responsibilities, a CV listing academic experience and achievements, authored publications, project results, letters of recommendation from former employers, client and colleague recommendations, honors, and awards. Restifo (1999) recommends using the portfolio for communicating personal strengths in situations such as performance appraisals, job and return-to-school interviews, presentations, job fairs, and networking sessions. In addition, an APN who precepts or mentors students or graduate APNs can use

---

Box 20-6 COMPONENTS OF A PROFESSIONAL PORTFOLIO FOR ADVANCED PRACTICE NURSES

Select the components appropriate to the position desired.

PROFESSIONAL BACKGROUND
Résumé or CV
Letters of recommendation
List of professional references
Nursing documents such as license (with COPY written over it and not in color), professional certificates, certification, malpractice insurance information, diplomas, transcripts, continuing-education contact-hour certificates or course information (course descriptions, outlines)
Identification such as a driver's license, Social Security number, passport, and work visa
Health information such as PPD or chest x-ray results, immunization record and immunity titers
Items showing special recognition you have received, such as honors and awards, newspaper clippings, and photos
Statement of professional goals
Personal webpage citation

CLINICAL ACCOMPLISHMENTS
Evidence of your teaching, including programs, presentations, evaluations, lesson plans, and handouts
Performance appraisals or promotion letters
Preceptor performance appraisals
Project/program reports
List of procedures performed
Total clinical log of patients seen, age, diagnosis
Sample of clinical documentation
Patient education materials

SCHOLARSHIP/RESEARCH
Professional activities, including articles or a list of publications and photos (e.g., of posters, exhibits)
Project/research summary reports

SERVICE
Listing of community activities
Copies of thank-you letters recognizing service activities
Professional organization membership (list elected offices, volunteer work)

CV, Curriculum vitae; *PPD,* purified protein derivative (tuberculin skin test).

the personal professional portfolio as an exemplar of how a career develops over time, presenting activities and choices made and providing anticipatory guidance to the novice.

An APN might find it useful to include information in the portfolio that helps differentiate what physicians do from the services that APNs provide. Also helpful are studies that describe the role differentiation between physicians and APNs and how primary care, for example, differs when provided by an APN (Kassirer, 1994; Mundinger et al., 2000; Safriet, 1992). Fact sheets and brochures from professional organizations that describe the advantages of working with particular APNs might also be included in one's portfolio. Thus the portfolio serves as a data bank from which the APN can construct a position-specific marketing tool.

Résumé and Curriculum Vitae. A résumé or CV should be prepared before seeking employment. Résumés are generally one or two pages long and cover relevant experience and responsibilities appropriate to the position sought; they also cover educational background (give expected graduation date if educational program is not completed). Résumés may begin with a brief profile of the applicant and a goal statement. Relevant experience is usually organized chronologically with most recent experience first. It is not sufficient to list places and dates of employment; bulleted phrases under each position describing key responsibilities and accomplishments are necessary (e.g., "was responsible for developing and implementing an oncology certification review course; 20% of staff RNs [n = 10] became certified in oncology nursing within 18 months of program initiation," or "supervised 20 RNs and 10 CNAs"). Do not include salary requirements or other expectations about benefits. Because of concerns about identity theft, the résumé should not have your Social Security number or RN license number. It is sufficient to say that you are licensed (or have applied for a license) in a particular state or states. The résumé is your introduction to a prospective employer and should be visually interesting and brief but substantive. To maximize the possibility that a résumé will be considered, it is advisable to tailor the résumé to highlight the relevance of the applicant's experience to a particular position.

CVs are more comprehensive—they are usually representative of one's entire career, and APN graduates who seek a joint appointment as a clinician and a faculty member may need to have both a résumé and a CV. Although most APN graduates are unlikely to need a CV immediately upon graduation, those APNs who envision teaching at some point in the future may want to create one and update it annually. It is difficult to recreate a comprehensive CV 10 years after graduation if one has not developed some system for keeping track of the professional experiences and activities that are included in a CV.

For both résumés and CVs, accurate contact information must be included (e.g., address, telephone, fax numbers, e-mail addresses, and website if available). Resources such as *www.resume.com* or job search resources such as *www.Monster.com* can be accessed for additional information on résumé preparation. Many job sites have advice on résumé and CV preparation for those seeking positions in health care. Résumés and CVs should be carefully proofread. New graduates are advised to have a colleague or faculty member look at the résumé (and the position advertisement or description, if available) before sending it out to prospective employers.

Query and Cover Letters. APNs who are seeking employment can expand the opportunities for obtaining desirable positions by crafting a well-thought-out letter. Query letters are used to determine whether possibilities for employment exist, especially when no positions have been advertised, and/or to request an informational interview. The first sentence or two must engage the reader—for example, indicate your familiarity with the setting and/or the staff, its vision, or mission; identify the person who referred you to the organization; or state why you want to work there. A query letter should conclude positively and assertively—"I look forward to speaking with you"—and include accurate contact information. If you receive no response within a week of sending a query letter, it is acceptable to follow up with a telephone call or e-mail message.

Cover letters are usually written in response to an advertisement or job board posting about a specific position. Before preparing a cover letter, it is advisable to consult the organization's website and/or marketing material to help you tailor the letter. The cover letter should be brief and, as with the query letter, should engage the reader in the first sentence or two. As with a query letter, indicate why you are interested in the position and highlight the specific strengths you bring to the position. The letter is an opportunity to add additional, relevant information that a prospective employee would find useful. For example, your résumé may indicate that you have experience in teaching, specialty practice, or setting up a practice. If you are applying for a job at a comprehensive cancer center, you can indicate in the letter additional knowledge and skills that may be specific to an oncology setting—those acquired in the medical-surgical setting as well as any additional skills acquired during graduate education. One variation on the cover letter that some human resources staff have recommended is a "T-letter," in which the applicant, after the first two "engaging" sentences, creates a brief table (N. Solomons, personal communication, May 21, 2004). In the left-hand column, list, in bulleted phrases, the job requirements; in the right-hand column, list bulleted substantive phrases of your related experience. Such a letter highlights your relevant knowledge and skills as they relate to the specific requirements of the position. (See query letter example, Appendix C.)

Interview Preparation. Before an interview, homework must be completed. As with the cover letter, it is advisable to be familiar with an organization's public "face"—website, brochures, and other marketing materials—as well as the position description. Using this information, you can prepare questions that will help you better understand the setting and the position expectations. Determine whether you are meeting with more than one person. Sometimes a human resources staff member does an initial interview by phone or in person to verify that a candidate should proceed with an interview with other providers. Other points to attend to are dressing appropriately, scouting the location (if the interview is being held in an unfamiliar location, do a dry run to estimate time), and arriving a few minutes early. If an interview does not result in being selected for the position, ask for some feedback that will help you improve your future interviewing style/skills.

Negotiating/Accepting a Position. Although it is not appropriate to discuss salary in résumés or initial interviews, it is wise to be aware of salary ranges for the type of position you are seeking in the local area. When an offer is made, this knowledge can help in the negotiation of a mutually acceptable salary and benefits package. Other elements to consider when negotiating, once an offer has been made, are reporting relationships (to whom you will report), productivity expectations, available administrative and staff support, on-call

responsibilities, and orientation plan. Seek data so that, once the position is offered, an informed decision can be made for accepting the position.

CONTRACT CONSIDERATIONS
Obtaining a working knowledge of negotiation skills is the foundation for handling contract considerations. Negotiating and advocating for patients is much easier than negotiating a new contract, salary, and/or benefits package. Historically, nurses have been inexperienced with establishing contractual and legal relationships, which are common in the business world. However, a political and economic reality of the current health care environment is that there is still some resistance to recognizing APNs as legitimate providers of care. As members of a largely female profession, nurses may be less comfortable with self-promotion. Keller advised nurses to avoid the "burnt toast" syndrome—a term she coined to describe the self-effacing behavior demonstrated by mothers who make toast for breakfast and keep the burnt piece for themselves while giving the nicely toasted pieces to family members. Nurses can no longer afford to eat "burnt toast" (Doughty & Keller, 2000).

Negotiating a Contract
Robbins' (1998) Negotiation Framework outlines five steps that can help APNs become more comfortable with negotiating:
- Step 1: Prepare and plan
- Step 2: Define the ground rules
- Step 3: Clarify and justify
- Step 4: Bargain and problem-solve
- Step 5: Close and implement

By learning to be a strong negotiator, the APN can increase the probability of achieving desired outcomes. Negotiating a contract is an important marketing skill. As APNs share the market place with other health care providers, they have to acquire new skills, especially in the area of business and leadership (Munden, 2001). The most common contracts or agreements that APNs are likely to encounter are employment contracts, managed care contracts, collaborative practice agreements, and service contracts.

Employment Contracts
An employment contract helps the APN clarify all parameters of a new position, including a section that outlines the requirements for ending the professional relationship. The value of an employment contract is

still being debated, but at the least, some type of written agreement should be obtained. APNs should avoid agreeing to unreasonable restrictive covenants (Buppert, 2001, 2004). Noncompete and gag clauses are restrictive covenants that may be included in a contract. A noncompete clause provides a barrier to future practice in the employer's service area for a period after the professional relationship between the employer and the APN has been terminated. Noncompete clauses refer to areas such as geographical location, patient referrals, and employment opportunities (Zaumeyer, 2003). Depending on applicable state laws, a noncompete clause may be governed by a state statute and is still considered by some to be a restraint of trade (Herman & Zeil, 1999).

APNs must also be alert to gag clauses that constrain clinical practice or interactions with patients during employment and after severance of the professional relationship with the employer. Gag clauses can limit the ability of the provider to provide information to a patient as to why, for example, tests are not covered under a carrier or about other providers outside of the health care organization. The AMA has strongly opposed gag clauses in health maintenance organization (HMO) contracts, which limited the physician's ability to provide needed information to patients (AMA, 1996). In light of the current environment, APNs must read the contract carefully to ascertain that all essential areas are covered and that unreasonable restrictions are not included. All areas of a contract are negotiable, including restrictive clauses. Consider such clauses carefully before signing the contract (Buppert, 2004). In addition, it would be prudent to have a lawyer review any contract before signing it. Box 20-7 lists elements of an employment contract, and a sample employment agreement can be found in Appendix A.

When negotiating an employment contract/agreement, the APN should know in advance what is desired and needed. Although this might seem obvious, nurses often do not anticipate or negotiate for important personal and professional benefits. The essence of a contract will vary according to the nature of individual APN practices, but the goal of negotiating a contract is always to protect the APN by including expectations, objectives, and the nature of the relationships with those with whom the contract is being formed. In addition, APNs must always attend to the certification, licensing, and authorization requirements in states where they will practice (see Chapter 21).

In terms of vacation benefits, APNs should aim for the physician standard in the setting/practice. For continuing education time, they should aim for at least 4 to 5 paid days per year and a minimum of $1000 for continuing education expenses (Fitzgerald, 1999). Buppert (2004) notes additional items that may be desirable to address in an employment contract:

- Extent of support service to be provided to APN
- Expectation as to the number of patients to be seen daily
- Administrative work to be expected
- Listing of APN's name on outside clinic sign, doors, directories, and advertisements
- Use of APN's name when phone is answered
- Release to the APN of the APN's quality performance as measured by health plan auditors
- Release to the APN of the amount of profit brought into the practice by the APN

Managed Care Contracts

Contracts are required by insurers and fall into two categories—managed care and indemnity insurers (Buppert, 2004). Box 20-8 lists the key components of a managed care contract. The goal of managed care is to decrease overall health care costs and to provide more services for less reimbursement through a contract on a capitated or fee-for-service basis. A contract is essential to clarify the responsibilities of a position when participating in managed care; it should provide the details of the services that will be provided and a description of the arrangement between the APN and the managed care organization (MCO) (Buppert, 2004). A practice must be recognized in the MCO provider panel in order to participate. Managed care contracts with providers include an agreement for the APN to provide certain kinds of services for a company, such as pre-employment histories and physical examinations. Provision of health education to employees of a company may or may not include the employee's family members, and this should be clarified by the contract. It is important to make sure that contracts with the MCO specify the APN as a legitimate provider of care to protect APNs from being eliminated from provider panels. While indemnity insurers pay provider fees, unlike an MCO, they have no relationship with the provider other than to pay the bill for the care received by the covered patient (Buppert, 2007). Not all

Box 20-7 ELEMENTS OF AN EMPLOYMENT CONTRACT

Your contract should include the following:

1. Official relationship with physician partnership, medical group, or corporation
2. Terms of employment
   - Start date
   - Probation period
   - Criteria for probationary review
   - Duration of contract
   - Annual review
   - Salary increases
3. Clinical responsibilities and supervision
   - Supervising/consulting MD responsibilities
   - Job description or expected duties
   - Work hours
   - Call hours and responsibilities
   - PA/NP cross-coverage
   - Work sites
4. Compensation
   - Salary and method of calculation
   - Bonuses and/or incentives, profit sharing
5. Benefits
   - Insurance
     Medical
     Dental
     Vision
     Disability (short-term and long-term)
     Life
     Automobile
   - Medical malpractice coverage
   - Retirement plan
6. Business expenses
   - State licensure and supervisory fees
   - Certification fees
   - Hospital medical staff fees

- Automobile costs and insurance
- Association dues
- Books and professional journals
- Equipment
7. Vacation and sick time
   - Vacation conditions
   - Holiday time
   - Sick leave and limits
   - Maternity leave
8. Continuing education
   - Conditions and amounts
   - Listed separately from vacation
9. Contract renewals and terminations
   - Paid leave
   - Option to review
   - Clinician evaluation criteria
   - Termination "for cause" specifics
   - Termination "without cause"
     Notice period
     Compensation/benefit buyout
10. Other standard clauses
    - Contract is total agreement (no verbal agreements accepted—neither contract negotiations nor contract changes)
    - Contract modifications must be signed by both parties
    - Conduct differing from the contract does not waive the right to uphold all contract clauses
    - Other clauses (evaluate impact on practice and/or future employment)
      Gag clause
      Non-compete clause
11. Proper signatures with names and title typed below
12. Date of signing

Adapted from Woomer, S. (1994). Negotiating an employment contract. *The Clinician's Reference Guide 1994* (a supplement to *Clinician Reviews*), pp. 21-28.
MD, Doctor of Medicine; *NP*, nurse practitioner; *PA*, physician assistant.

insurers cover care provided by APNs, and a contract with the insurer may need to be negotiated for coverage of services. Newer legislation is continuing to open doors for APNs to ensure that they are included in the primary care medical provider panels and that they will be reimbursed.

Collaborative Practice Agreements
Depending on the regulatory requirements of particular states (see Chapter 21), APNs may need to make formal arrangements with physicians to ensure that

medical backup is available for patients' concerns that are out of the APN's scope of practice. Typically, such agreements address the nature of the collaborative relationship, parameters for consultation, and physician availability for consultation and emergency care. Such agreements may refer to interdisciplinary guidelines, medical references, and particular standards of care that are to be followed. The agreement should meet the state regulatory requirements and be signed by all involved parties. A sample collaborative practice agreement is found in Appendix B.

Box 20-8   Key Components of a Managed Care Contract

Negotiating a contract with an MCO will demand the assistance of an attorney experienced in negotiating these contracts, because the contract will cover much more than just compensation.

- What is included? What is excluded?
- Requirements for the following:
    Utilization management
    Quality assurance
    Credentialing
    Member grievance
    Record-keeping
    Claims submission
    Hours of operation
    Appointment response times
    On-call coverage
    Employing other providers
    Arranging backup with other groups
    Maximum/minimum number of patients
    Anti-disparagement
    Business confidentiality
- Fee (capitation) schedule
- Special needs programs (carve outs): criteria, process for transfer of care for those eligible
- Stop-loss provisions
- Referral pools

- Withholds
- Level of distribution from withhold/referral pools over prior 5 years
- Bonus system
- Provisions for closing the practice to additional practice from the MCO
- Claims processing: in-house or contracted out?
- Who does laboratory work?
- Renewal of contract: based upon? Renewal rate with provider
- MCO's review of office practices
- Directory listing: How will it read?
- Any prohibition on joining other MCOs?
- Definitions of "experimental emergency" and "preexisting condition"
- Who bears the brunt of a mistake in eligibility or coverage determination?
- Can preadmission or referral approval be rescinded retroactively?
- Formulary contents
- System for verifying member eligibility
- Routine for notification of members selecting practice
- Provisions for dispute resolution
- Marketing provided
- Who owns the records/data?

Adapted from Buppert, C. (2004). *Nurse practitioner's practice and legal guide.* Boston: Jones & Bartlett.
MCO, Managed care organization.

Service Agreements

Service agreements that outline services to be provided over a specified period are often negotiated between APNs and other parties. For example, an oncology clinical nurse specialist employed in a comprehensive cancer center may negotiate with a consortium of rural hospitals in his or her state to provide two chemotherapy certification workshops annually. The service agreement would outline the responsibilities of each party, contingencies for insufficient registration, a budget or specified dollar amount to cover honoraria and expenses (overhead expenses would be included if the contract were negotiated with the APN's agency as opposed to the APN as an independent contractor), and other relevant details. In this example, the APN would meet with his or her department head and the financial officer for the APN's agency to discuss the contract and identify the appropriate agency person to sign the contract. The APN would estimate the number

of days needed to prepare and deliver the programs, the human and material resources needed, and travel expenses. He or she would anticipate factors that might require cancellation/rescheduling (e.g., weather, insufficient registration). Also, the APN would indicate the dates (agreed to by the APN and the consortium representatives) on which the program is to be delivered and identify "in-kind" resources that would not require financial support (e.g., the consortium would be responsible for copying and collating the training manuals). Together, the APN and a financial officer would determine the appropriate activities and budget to discuss with the consortium before signing an agreement. Other examples of a service agreement are a nurse researcher contracting with an NP to provide certain services for research subjects or a CRNA contracting with a rural hospital to administer anesthesia. Similar details would need to be considered for these types of service agreement.

Professional Development Plan

A final and important aspect of professional development is to make an informal contract with oneself to reevaluate short-term and long-term goals. It is to the APN's advantage to review objectives at least quarterly to be able to determine if progress is being made along the anticipated career path and to recommit to the most important employment components to attain personal satisfaction in a position. A critical part of this personal contract includes balancing the physical, intellectual, emotional, and spiritual dimensions of the individual. Reviewing the position to determine whether it is consuming an unbalanced amount of energy is essential to ensure that the interests of the APN, patients, and the organization are being served. Balancing personal and professional lifestyle is imperative to successful practice.

MARKETING A SERVICE

To be successful, a business must be well-planned and the owners must be prepared to offer and market a service that others need and value. Before one can market a service, it is important to prepare a business plan (see Chapter 19).

Approaches to Marketing a Service

It is helpful for the APN to remember that people usually will not appreciate what a professional does unless they are educated to the facts. People want to know more about unique services, yet potential customers (employers, patients, physicians, other providers) may have no concept of the expertise APNs could bring to their businesses or practices and, therefore, would never advertise for one (Weill et al., 1989). In fact, those who have worked with APNs or contracted for APN services often wonder how they ever got along without them. APNs have many strengths that increase their marketability, and these strengths are rooted in basic nursing practice.

Marketing is a social and managerial process by which individuals and groups obtain what they need and want through creating, offering, and exchanging products of value with others (Chang et al., 2001). The keys to marketing a service are variety and reinforcement. According to Stern (1997), using multiple marketing techniques is not an outdated practice because people seek information from multiple sources including traditional, Internet, other media sources, and word of mouth. The basics of marketing are staying focused and not varying the presentation of the image widely (e.g., using one logo on all marketing materials [e.g., the AFLAC duck]), selecting the media format carefully to reach the intended population, tracking marketing results, and remaining flexible in order to change to more effective strategies when necessary.

Differentiation (i.e., how a proposed service differs from that provided by others) is important. Differentiating factors may include such things as higher quality, more accessibility, or different hours of service. Services targeted toward specific, data-based market segments (e.g., retirement centers, hospital staff, individuals living with chronic pain, new mothers needing breastfeeding counseling) help the APN tailor marketing plans for success based on client needs.

Establishing, growing, and improving a business take a sophisticated mix of entrepreneurial vision, business management know-how, and specialized knowledge. Through free small business counseling and support services, the Service Corps of Retired Executives (SCORE) volunteers provide marketing advice and financial and business plan development assistance that could benefit the APN just forming a business or implementing the marketing of a service (see www.score.org). Exemplar 20-4 provides an example of how one APN developed and marketed a unique service to a defined population with health care needs. This exemplar emphasizes how marketing a service effectively depends on making others aware of its unique features. It is helpful to gather data on how clients discovered a service so that future energy and resources can be channeled into what is known to be successful. Brochures, newspaper articles, newsletters, letterhead stationery, business cards, flyers, personal interviews with the media, and group community classes all help promote a unique service. Yellow Pages advertising is expensive, so it is wise to routinely audit how often clients use the publication to initiate contact. Groups such as Rotary, American Association of Retired Persons, American Association of University Women, Junior League, and Kiwanis often invite speakers to address health topics. These opportunities allow the APN not only to promote a service but also to dispel misinformation about APNs and clarify their role. Joining professional and civic organizations is an important part of marketing a service as well, and the opportunity to sit on a board of directors or a health-related committee does much to enhance one's professional reputation (Box 20-9).

To help APN students think about marketing their services, some faculty have students develop a personal website that can be used for creative

Box 20-9   STRATEGIES FOR MARKETING ADVANCED PRACTICE NURSE SERVICES

- Advertise in local phone book.
- Direct mail to specific groups (e.g., teens, housing complex for older adults).
- Distribute flyers with services provided, philosophy, and credentials.
- Mail patient birthday cards.
- Mail reminder cards for heath promotion examinations, or call ahead.
- Distribute useful materials with your name or practice's name and contact numbers.
- Provide free Papanicolaou (Pap) smears on occasion for an underserved population.
- Offer to teach sex education classes for community or local schools.
- Ask your patients to refer family and friends.

- Establish collaborative relationships with other health care providers in the area.
- Establish relationships with pharmaceutical representatives who can provide support in many ways.
- Establish hours that meet patient needs, such as evenings and weekends.
- Distribute business cards and practice brochures generously in the community (e.g., grocery store, fitness club, alternative health care businesses)
- Donate a day for specialty consultation in areas that are hard to manage in primary care.
- Send a generalized brochure about your practice by bulk mail to a targeted zip code.
- Network with local businesses and banks; join the local chamber of commerce.

marketing, employment searching, and patient education purposes (C. Hanson, personal communication, September 2006). The APN must ensure that all marketing complies with the Health Insurance Portability and Accountability Act (HIPAA). For example, if mothers who have given birth are sent invitations to attend a parent education session on caring for the toddler, the APN must make sure that only those mothers who have given consent are contacted. If a patient gave birth and was keeping it secret, an invitation opened by a family member would violate both her privacy and HIPAA rules (Advisory Publications, 2002).

Marketing to Physicians, Consumers, and Others

Presenting oneself to the medical community is an important marketing strategy in promoting a service. During the process of business plan development, an APN has opportunities to meet with physician colleagues and begin building relationships that can lead to referrals. Having confidence about one's skills, knowing one's particular areas of expertise and limitations, and having a collaborative approach are important. Establishing credibility with regard to one's competency and abilities is essential. Successful APN-physician collaboration, including those interactions that lead to positive patient outcomes, helps alleviate such fears (see Chapter 10). When one is outlining possible benefits to physicians for including an APN in their referral network, it is important to stress the

APN's unique areas of expertise: prevention, counseling, education, and the ability to see patients with special, time-consuming needs.

The office staff has a role in helping APNs in this process by having a thorough understanding of the APN's uniqueness and skills in order to share this knowledge with the public. APNs and staff should be able to describe the aspects of APN care that are different from and complementary to other providers' services.

APNs should educate pharmaceutical representatives about the differences between what an APN does and what a physician does. Representatives should be asked to have APNs included as providers in their patient-oriented product brochures. To constantly see the word "doctor," such as "see your doctor with any questions," sends a distinct message to potential clients, health policy decision makers, and legislators (Smithing & Wiley, 1990). Finally, using an APN provider for personal as well as for family care is a strong endorsement for nursing.

A Delphi study of the influences and experiences of becoming nurse entrepreneurs (Wilson, Averis, & Walsh, 2003) found that to be successful, nurses needed recognition from both the public and private systems as well as from nursing bodies. In addition, it was noted that a customer service focus was needed. One can assume that the needs of different businesses are not the same (e.g., academic vs. private practice) and that the marketing strategies would need to correspond to the target populations.

Keeping Up with Population, Clinical, and Business Trends

Knowing the population base is important. Johnson (2006) describes how one size does not fit all in the current "boomer" market. The baby boomers make up about 26% of the consumer segment and are a diverse group, described as *single boomers, new family frontiers,* and *late-blooming boomers.* This diverse group, now turning 60 years of age, will be focusing on health issues and increasing health care service consumption. Knowing the target segment helps APNs use more-focused marketing strategies.

Building relationships is important to maintaining a consumer base. In a relationship management approach, data are gathered to focus on current and prospective patient needs (Benz & Paddison, 2004). Marketing strategies in this approach include interviewing executives to determine growth areas and needs, assessing the market and analyzing the database, identifying individual needs of the population, creating ways to reach the target with appropriate information, and tracking and analyzing the strategy results. Dividing the patient population by age, gender, or high-risk categories and then communicating appropriate information to them by e-mail or postal service (e.g., postcards, letters) will keep the APN services in their sights. These activities could be conducted near patient birthdays. Strategies such as these increased patient visits by 14% in one community health clinic (Benz & Paddison).

The market trend projection for health care is consumer-driven. It is important to meet a consumer need, provide a service that fills a niche, and be competitive. According to a *HealthLeaders Media* publication (2007), retail health care and consumer-driven care will be significant forces now and into the near future. Health care restructuring is taking place as evidenced by the expanding market for in-store convenient care clinics and telehealth care. Important trends in strategic marketing include consumerism, transparency, and competition. Consumers desire convenience, and health plans and convenient care clinics are tapping into this desire. Publicly available reports of statistics about pricing, quality, health care outcomes, surgical outcomes, and other indicators are evidence of the increasing transparency in health care. Competition for the health care consumer is in full swing, with hospitals and retailers marketing to the same populations while trying to develop specialty services desirable to the public.

According to Griffin and Lowenstein (2001), a company has a 60% to 70% chance of selling back to an existing customer. Keeping current patients satisfied should be at the top of any marketing strategy. How many times have you gone to a new store or new restaurant, never to return again because of how you were treated or how you perceived the service? The same can be said of APN services. Efforts must be taken to satisfy the consumer while maintaining the integrity, quality, and standard of care in the services being provided.

Building a corporate memory or data mining is an approach that can be used to increase or maintain relationships with consumers in your care (Sturm, 2004). Electronic data can be analyzed to both improve the practice services and increase the number of consumers served. Data mining can be accomplished with office practice software that can determine which persons use your services frequently, how they learned of your services, and how satisfied they are with the services. Once groups are identified, the APN can determine if services for this group could be added at minimal cost (e.g., updating immunizations, special hours for sports physicals, performing annual Papanicolaou [Pap] smears). With the use of current technology, the ability to keep communication avenues open is at one's fingertips. APNs need to keep their practice on the consumers' minds by sending an e-mail to thank them for using their services, asking if they would like other services offered, sending a birthday congratulatory note, and reminding them of upcoming scheduled visits or the need to make an appointment for an annual examination. Benz and Paddison (2004) described the use of data mining to deliver preventive services to patients based on age, gender, and health need. They developed 137 different versions of a direct mailing and sent personalized reminders for important checkups and screenings to patients ages 3 months to 75 years; the mailings resulted in a 14% increase in visits.

Small is the New Big provides a humorous look at over 100 ideas that can be turned into marketing strategies individualized to each APN's practice (Godin, 2006). One idea is "zooming," which is defined as stretching your limits without creating any threat to what you have already established as your foundation. Zooming is about using new ideas, opportunities, and challenges to improve. "Zooming is about doing the same things as usual, only different" (p. 25). For instance, in health care it is necessary to be time-efficient *and* it is important for patients to understand directions regarding their care. If you usually handwrite directions for patients, use the zoom approach and create an education sheet, give it a title or number, and document in the chart by number that it was provided. This zoom approach will save valuable time while ensuring that consistent education is provided. Another zooming strategy is to develop a progress sheet that can be used on every visit to document history, physical and laboratory results, and education topics for patients with common diagnoses such as diabetes or hypertension. This documentation sheet will provide data over time to analyze patient outcomes, save time, and allow more time for interaction with the patient.

There is an increasing trend to move from a transaction-oriented approach to a relationship marketing view. In this shift, the person is no longer the patient but, rather, a consumer. With a consumer perspective, the emphasis is on maintaining the current consumer, not just continually trying to increase numbers. In this relationship approach, customer satisfaction is essential with a goal of developing mutually satisfying long-term relationships with consumers (Bansal, 2004).

In 1989, Weill and colleagues predicted that the biggest obstacle to future viability of the APN's role was lack of consumer awareness and minimal demand for preventive services as a result of inadequate marketing by APNs. Although we are experiencing a greater demand for preventive services, a lack of consumer awareness about the APN role still remains. An understanding of this notion, a strong belief in oneself and in the APN role, and a strong understanding of one's own APN philosophy are necessary to reverse this trend and enhance the return on the time and energy invested in marketing. When marketing a service, APNs should strive to avoid the common marketing mistakes noted by Abraham (1994) by doing the following on a regular basis:

- Audit clients and others to find which particular strategies provide the best return.
- Continuously ascertain needs for unique services, and develop them.
- Differentiate APN practice from that offered by the competition.
- Always give clients a reason to return for repeat services.
- Address clients' needs as a priority.
- Educate and inform clients about any changes made in the practice, such as in prices, office hours, or services offered.
- Maintain enjoyment in providing the service to avoid burnout.

APNs can learn from other professionals' experiences with marketing missteps. A casebook of scenarios of marketing mistakes, successes, analyses, and practical tips are presented in a book by Hartely (2000).

CONCLUSION

Buppert (2007) summarizes the general principles of marketing a practice that APNs need to consider. To educate consumers about APNs and engage their interest in APN services, APNs must do the following:

- Repeat the marketing message over and over in order to be heard.
- Create in clients a sense of affiliation with the practice.
- Create an image of the practice and a marketing message.
- Strive to exceed the expectations of clients (they not only will stay with the practice but also will share their perceptions with others and encourage them to seek APN services).
- Remember that a new patient is worth the price of the visit, whereas a patient who values and stays with the practice is likely to generate more revenue.

Marketing oneself and one's services is critical to the survival of APNs and might well influence the future of the nursing profession itself. As the health care environment changes, clients are becoming sophisticated about what they want, as well as about what they need. APNs must become familiar enough with marketing concepts and be flexible enough so that they can position themselves to meet client needs. As a result of successful marketing strategies, clients will specifically request APNs and they will demand their services, recognizing the value they provide in the ever-expanding and complex world of health care.

Advanced practice nurses are prepared to address the issues documented in the IOM reports of 1999, 2001, and 2003 relative to patient safety, providing quality care, and collaborating within an interdisciplinary context. Active marketing of APN services and ongoing dialogue between nursing and other health care disciplines will continue to improve health care outcomes in this country, as well as to expand service sites (Lowes, 2007). It is vital that APNs be vocal, proactive, visible, cost-effective, astute to current issues, and involved at all levels of the health care system. Effective marketing of the image and role of the APN to the public and other disciplines is essential to effect positive outcomes for the future of our APN profession and the persons we serve.

REFERENCES

Abraham, J. (1994). *The Abraham experience.* Rolling Hills Estates, CA: Citation Publishing Group.

Advisory Publications. (2002). Make sure your marketing is HIPAA compliant. *Financial Management Strategies, 1,* 5-6. Retrieved May 29, 2003, from www.medscape.com/viewarticle/446400.

American Association of Colleges of Nursing (AACN). (2006). *The essentials of doctoral education for advanced nursing practice.* Washington, DC: Author.

American Medical Association (AMA), Policy (a). (2003). H-160.947. *Physician assistants and nurse practitioners.* Retrieved July 2007 from http://search.ama-assn.org/Search/query.html?qc=public+amnews+pubs&qt=H-160.947.

American Medical Association (AMA). (January 17, 1996). *Statement on ethical concerns regarding managed care physician gag* (AMA press release). Retrieved May 28, 2003, from www.ebglaw.com/article_330.html.

American Medical Association (AMA). (June 2006). *Report 7 of the Council on Medical Services (A-06) Store-Based Health Clinics* (Reference Committee G). Retrieved June 2007 from www.ama-assn.org/ama1/pub/upload/mm/372/a-06cmsreport7.pdf.

American Medical Association (AMA). (May 2007). H-2000.954. *U.S. physician shortage.* Retrieved July 12, 2007, from www.ama-assn.org/apps/pf_new/pf_online?f_n=browse&doc=policyfiles/HnE/H-200.954.HTN.

American Nurses Association (ANA). (2001). *Nursing's agenda for the future.* Retrieved May 26, 2004, from http://nursingworld.org/naf/.

Anonymous. (2006). Market your practice by mailing a patient newsletter. *Health Care Strategic Management, 24*(12), 13-14. Retrieved May 2007 from ABI/INFORM Complete.

Baldwin, C. (1998). *Calling the circle.* New York: Bantam Books.

Bansal, M. (2004). Optimizing value and quality in general practice with primary health care. *International Journal of Health Care Quality Assurance, 17*(4), 180-188. Retrieved March 6, 2007, from ABI/INFORM Complete.

Barry, P. (2006). Perspectives on private practice. *Perspectives in Psychiatric Care, 42*(1), 63-65.

Benz, G., & Paddison, N.V. (2004). Developing patient-based marketing strategies. *Healthcare Executive, 19,* 5. Retrieved March 6, 2007, from ABI/INFORM Complete.

Bolles, R.N. (2002). *What color is your parachute?* Walnut Creek, CA: Ten Speed Press.

Brandenburger, A.M., & Nalebuff, B.J. (1996). *Co-Opetition.* New York: Doubleday.

Brooten, D., Naylor, M.D., York, R., Brown, L.P., Munro, B.H., Hollingsworth, A.O., et al. (2002). Lessons learned from testing the Quality Cost Model of advanced practice nursing (APN) transitional care. *Journal of Nursing Scholarship, 34,* 369-375.

Brown, M., & Olshansky, E. (1998). Becoming a primary care nurse practitioner: Challenges of the initial year of practice. *Nurse Practitioner, 23,* 46, 52-66.

Brunk, Q. (1992). The clinical nurse specialist as an external consultant: A framework for practice. *Clinical Nurse Specialist, 6,* 2-4.

Buerhaus, P.I. (2000). A conversation with Robert Blendon about public opinion and health care, nursing and the 2000 presidential election. *Nursing Outlook, 48,* 203-210.

Buppert, C. (2001). Agreeing not to compete. *The Green Sheet, 3*(7). Retrieved May 29, 2003, from www.medscape.com/viewarticle/407075.

Buppert, C. (2004). *Nurse practitioner's business practice & legal guide.* Gaithersburg, MD: Aspen Publishers.

Buppert, C. (2007). Challenges for NPs thinking about opening their own business. *Nurse Practitioner World News, 12*(2), 1, 8.

Buresh B. (Spring 1998). Healthcare forms new media partnership: Nursing must participate. *Revolution: The Journal of Nurse Empowerment, 8,* 68-75.

Burgess, S.E., & Misener, T.R. (1997). The professional portfolio: An advanced practice nurse job search marketing tool. *Clinical Excellence for Nurse Practitioners, 1,* 468-471.

Center for Nursing Advocacy (CNA). Retrieved February 10, 2007, from www.nursingadvocacy.org/about_us/mission_statement.html.

Chang, C.F., Pfoutz, S.K., & Price, S.A. (2001). *Economics and nursing: Critical professional issues.* Philadelphia: F.A. Davis.

Chevalier, C., Steinberg, S., & Lindeke, L. (2006). Perceptions of barriers to psychiatric mental-health CNS practice. *Issues in Mental Health Nursing, 27,* 753-763.

Christianson, C.M., Bohmer, R., & Kenagy, J. (September-October 2000). Will disruptive innovations cure health care? *Harvard Business Review, 78,* 103-111.

Coile, R.C. (1999). The three C's: Consumerism, cyberhealth, and co-opetition. In R. Gilkey (Ed.), *The 21st century health care leader* (pp. 3-21). San Francisco: Jossey-Bass.

Coleman, E., Parry, C., Chalmers, S., & Min, S. (2006) The care transitions intervention. *Archives of Internal Medicine, 166,* 1822-1828.

Corser, W.D. (2000). The contemporary nurse-physician relationship: Insights from scholars outside the two professions. *Nursing Outlook, 48,* 263-268.

Dayhoff, N.E., & Moore, P.S. (2003). Entrepreneurship: Start-up questions. *Clinical Nurse Specialist, 17,* 86-87.

DeCarlo, L. (2005). Advanced practice nurse entrepreneurs in a multidisciplinary surgical-assisting partnership. *AORN Journal, 82*(3), 418-426.

Diamond, F. (August 2000). Nurse practitioners inch onto the field. *Managed Care, 9,* 24-30.

Dirubbo, N. (2005). Marketing 101: Setting your practice apart. *The Nurse Practitioner, 30*(9), 18.

Doughty, S., & Keller, J.M. (2000). Marketing and contracting considerations. In A.B. Hamric, J.A. Spross, & C.M. Hanson (Eds.), *Advanced nursing practice: An integrative approach* (2nd ed., pp. 655-677). Philadelphia: Saunders.

Druss, B.G., Marcus, S.C., Olfson, M., Tanielian, T., & Pincus, H.A. (2003). Trends in care by nonphysician clinicians in the United States. *New England Journal of Medicine, 348,* 130-137.

Fitzgerald, M.A. (1999). Negotiating your future: Employment, contract and practice issues for the nurse practitioner. *The Clinical Letter for Nurse Practitioners, 3,* 1-11.

Friedman, S. (2002). Opportunities for growth amid niche facilities. *Health Care Strategic Management, 20*(11), 17-18. Retrieved June 2007 from ABI/INFOTM Complete.

Gandolf, S., & Hirsch, L. (2006). 7 deadly sins of private practice marketing. *Healthcare Success Strategies.* Retrieved Feb 26, 2007, from www.healthcaresuccess.com/articles/.

Garfield, R. (2000). The marketability of nurse practitioners in New York City. *Nursing Economic$, 18*(1), 20-22, 31.

Gershon, H.J. (2003). Marketing management: A concept worth exploring. *Journal of Healthcare Management, 48*(6).

Godin, S. (2006). *Small is the new big.* New York: Penguin Group.

Gordon, S. (2006). *Nursing against the odds: How health care cost cutting, media stereotypes, and medical hubris undermine nurses and patient care.* Ithaca, NY: Cornell University Press.

Griffin, J., & Lowenstein, M.N. (2001). *Customer winback: How to recapture lost customers—and keep them loyal.* San Francisco: Jossey-Bass.

Gronroos, C, (1997). Value driven relational marketing: From products to resources and competencies. *Journal of Marketing Management, 13,* 407-419.

Hagland, M. (2006). Pay-for-performance programs show results, spur development. *Health Care Strategies Management, 24*(2), 1-4. Retrieved June 2007 from ABI/INFORM Complete.

Hallums, A. (1994). Internal marketing within a health care organization: Developing an implementation plan. *Journal of Nursing Management, 2,* 135-142.

Hartely, R.F. (2000). *Marketing mistakes and successes.* Indianapolis, IN: Wiley Publishing.

Hayes, E. (2007). Nurse practitioners and managed care: Patient satisfaction and intention to adhere to nurse practitioner plan of care. *American Journal of Nurse Practitioners, 19*(8), 418-426.

Hayes, E., Allen, J., Gruen, S., Wilson, J., & Kalmakis, K. (2001). Nurse practitioner practice patterns, compensation, and professional participation: Western Massachusetts. *Clinical Excellence for Nurse Practitioners, 5,* 52-60.

Health Resources and Services Administration (HRSA.) (March 2004). *National sample of registered nurse population.* USDHHS, HESA, BHP. Retrieved June 19, 2007, from ftp://ftp.hrsa.gov/bhpr/workforce/0306rnss.pdf.

HealthLeaders Media. (2007). Competition, consumerism impact market strategy. *Health Care Strategic Management, 25*(2), 3.

Herman, R., & Zeil, S. (1999). Collaborative practice agreements for advanced practice nurses: What you should know. *AACN Clinical Issues: Advanced Practice in Acute and Critical Care, 10,* 337-342.

Ieong, S.L. (2005). Clinical nurse specialist entrepreneurship. *Internet Journal of Advanced Nursing Practice, 7*(1). Retrieved June 2007 from EBSCOhost.

Institute of Medicine (IOM). (1999). *To err is human: Building a safer health system.* Washington, DC: National Academies Press.

Institute of Medicine (IOM). (2001). *Crossing the quality chasm: A new health system for the 21ˢᵗ century.* Washington, DC: National Academies Press.

Institute of Medicine (IOM). (2003). *Health professions education: A bridge to quality.* Washington, DC: National Academies Press.

Johnson & Johnson. (2002). *Knowledge gap about opportunities for nurses contributing to escalating nursing shortage.* Retrieved May 18, 2003, from www.jnj.com/news/jnj_news/20020506_0949.htm.

Johnson, M. (2006). One size definitely does not fit boomer marketing. *Drug Store News, 28*(8), 101-102. Retrieved February 10, 2007, from ABI/INFORM Complete.

Kalisch, P.A., & Kalisch, B.J. (1981). Communicating clinical nursing issues through the newspaper. *Nursing Research, 30,* 132-138.

Kassirer, J.P. (1994). What role for nurse practitioners in primary care? *New England Journal of Medicine, 330,* 204-205.

Kendig, S.M. (2002). Every woman deserves an NP: Getting your message across. *Women's Health Care, 1,* 29-32.

Klein, T.A. (2006). Working in a retail clinic: What nurse practitioners need to ask. *Topics in Advanced Practice Nursing ejournal, 6*(3). Retrieved September 2, 2006, from http://www.medscape.com/viewarticle/544422.

Letz, K.K. (2002). *Business essentials for nurse practitioners.* Fort Wayne, IN: PreviCare, Inc.

Liberman, A., & Rotarius, T.M. (2001). Marketing in today's health care environment. *The Health Care Manager, 19*(4), 23-28.

Lindeke, L.L., Bly, T.R., & Wilcon, R.A. (2001). Perceived barriers to rural nurse practitioner practice. *Clinical Excellence for Nurse Practitioners, 5,* 218-221.

Lowes, R. (2007). *Medical economics.* Retrieved March 2007 from www.memag.com/memag/content/contentDetail.jsp?if=394848.

MacStravic, S. (2006). Marketing model puts customer in charge. *Health Care Strategic Management, 24*(6), 1, 13-16.

Meister, L, Heath, J., Andrews, J, & Tingen, M. (2002). Professional nursing portfolios: A global perspective. *Medsurg Nursing, 11*(4), 177-182.

Miller, S.K. (2000). Marketing your practice. *Patient Care for the Nurse Practitioner, 3,* 52-53.

Moody, N.B., Smith, P.L., & Glenn, L.L. (1999). Client characteristics and practice patterns of nurse practitioners and physicians. *Nurse Practitioner, 24,* 94-103.

Munden, J. (Ed.). (2001). *Nurse practitioner's legal reference.* Springhouse, PA: Springhouse.

Mundinger, M., Kane, R.L., Lenz, E.R., Totten, A., Tsai, W., Cleary, P.D., et al. (2000). Primary care outcomes in patients treated by nurse practitioners or physicians. *Journal of the American Medical Association, 283,* 59-69.

Nickitas, D.M., & Valentino, L.M. (2003). Evolving a nursing collegial relationship into a successful consulting business. *Nursing Economic$, 21*(4), 181-187.

Office of Technology Assessment (OTA). (1986). *Health technology case study 37: Nurse practitioners, physician assistants, and certified nurse midwives—A policy analysis* (Publication No. OTA-HCS-37). Washington, DC: Government Printing Office.

Pakis, S. (1997). Managing the marketing function for advanced nurse practitioners in a managed care environment. *Seminars for Nurse Managers, 5,* 149-153.

Palmer, J.W. (1996). Thoughts on becoming a nurse entrepreneur. *Emergency Nursing, 22,* 534-535.

Payne, M.E. (July/August 1997). Counseling new graduates to find jobs. *Recruitment, Retention & Restructuring Report, 10,* 4-7.

Pearson, L.J. (2007). The Pearson report. A national review of nurse practitioner legislation and health care issues. *American Journal for Nurse Practitioners, 11*(2), 10-101.

Phillips, C.Y., Palmer, V.V., Wettig, V.S., & Fenwick, J.W. (2000). Attitudes toward nurse practitioners: Influence of gender, age, ethnicity, education and income. *Journal of the American Academy of Nurse Practitioners, 12*(70), 255-259.

Powers, P. (2001). The image of nursing in hospital promotional materials: A discourse analysis. *Scholarly Inquiry for Nursing Practice, 15*(2), 91-107.

Price, R.W. (2004). *Roadmap to entrepreneurial success: Powerful strategies for building a high-profit business.* New York: American Management Association.

Reel, S.J., & Abraham, I.L. (2007). Understanding strategies to build an NP practice. In S.J. Reel & I.L. Abraham (Eds.), *Business and legal essentials for nurse practitioners: From negotiating your first job through owning a practice* (pp. 137-147). St. Louis: Mosby.

Restifo, V. (1999). Your professional portfolio. *Nursing Spectrum, 3,* 17.

Robbins, S. (1998). *Organizational behavior* (8th ed.). Englewood Cliffs, NJ: Prentice-Hall.

Rudner, N., O'Grady, E., Hodnicki, D., & Hanson, C. (2007). Ranking state NP regulation: Practice environment and consumer healthcare choice. *American Journal for Nurse Practitioners, 11*(4), 8-27.

Safriet, B.J. (1992). Health care dollars and regulatory sense: The role of advanced practice nursing. *Yale Journal on Regulation, 9,* 417-487.

Shaw, C. (2002). What can you learn from Coca-Cola? *Nursing Spectrum, 11,* 12.

Smithing, R.T., & Wiley, M.D. (1990). Marketing and management. See your physician. *Journal of the American Academy of Nurse Practitioners, 2,* 38.

Stern, M. (1997). *Marketing for small business.* Retrieved May 26, 2004, from www.digitalstore.com/marketing/mstern/trad_mktg.html.

Sturm, A.C. (2004). Looking for revenue? Try tapping your keyboard. *Healthcare Financial Management, 58*(3), 100. Retrieved March 6, 2007, from ABI/INFORM Complete.

Sturm, A.C. (2005). Misplaced expectations make for marketing missteps. *Healthcare Financial Management, 59*(1), 88-91. Retrieved May 2007 from ABI/INFORM Complete.

Washington Consulting Group. (1994). *Survey of certified nurse practitioners and clinical nurse specialists: December 1992.* Rockville, MD: Division of Nursing, Health Resources and Services Administration.

Weill, J.A., Love, M.G., Pron, A.L., Tesoro, T.A., Grey, M., Hickel, M., et al. (1989). Future potential, phase I: Nurse practitioners look at themselves. *Journal of Pediatric Health Care, 3,* 76-82.

Weiss, G.G. (2007). PAs and NPs: How to bill for their services. *Medical Economics, 84*(4), 32, 35, 39. Retrieved March 2007 from www.memag.com/memag/content/contentDetail.jsp?id=403836.

Whitehead, D. (2000). Using mass media within health-promoting practice: A nursing perspective. *Journal of Advanced Nursing, 32*(4), 807-816.

Wilson, A.W., Averis, A., & Walsh, K. (2003). The influences on and experiences of becoming nurse entrepreneurs: A Delphi study. *International Journal of Nursing Practice, 9,* 236-245.

Zaumeyer, C.R. (2003). *How to start an independent practice.* Philadelphia: F.A. Davis.

CHAPTER 21

Understanding Regulatory, Legal, and Credentialing Requirements

Charlene M. Hanson

INTRODUCTION

At both federal and state levels, this is a time of shifting priorities and changing models for nursing practice in all settings. Advanced practice nurses (APNs) are meeting regularly in national forums to discuss evolving roles and to conceptualize new dimensions for practice (American Association of Colleges of Nursing [AACN], 2007b; National Council of State Boards of Nursing [NCSBN], 2007; see also Chapter 18). It is an environment in which any discussion of regulatory issues is, by definition, fluid, dynamic, and subject to rapid change. APNs must influence health policy at both national and grassroots levels to ensure regulatory configurations that allow for successful advanced practice nursing and reimbursement. This activity may be as simple as interpreting health policy decisions to patients and co-workers locally or as complex as negotiating equitable regulatory decisions about reimbursement with the Centers for Medicare & Medicaid Services (CMS) in Washington, DC (see Chapter 22).

Issues involving education, scope of practice, specialty practice, reimbursement, and prescriptive authority are all embedded in regulatory language. Legal and regulatory issues are governed by multiple federal, state, educational, and professional entities whose work occurs in different venues, and these differences complicate efforts to collaborate (Hanson, 1998). The complexity of regulatory issues and the multiplicity of stakeholders are the bases for the 1998 recommendations by the Pew Health Professions Commission that national policy initiatives are urgently needed to research, develop, and publish national scopes of practice and continuing competency standards for state legislatures to implement (O'Neil & the Pew Health Professions Commission, 1998). This work continues to be vitally important and requires regular and careful input from APNs.

The issues surrounding the titling and credentialing of APNs have been difficult since the inception of the roles. At the state regulatory level, the preference is to use the title *advanced practice registered nurse (APRN)*. APN practices have evolved in differing ways

with multiple titles that confuse policy makers, patients, and the profession. *Credentialing* refers to the process by which APNs are certified, recognized, licensed, and privileged at both the state and local practice level. Dialogue is ongoing between national certifying bodies and state regulators, as well as among agencies that accredit educational programs, to standardize the multiple APN specialties. Certified registered nurses anesthetist (CRNA) and certified nurse-midwife (CNM) certification and credentialing are the most clearly uniform and standardized based on their longevity, singleness of purpose, and specialty. The credentialing and oversight of nurse practitioners (NPs) and clinical nurse specialists (CNSs) is less clear because of the multiplicity of programs and specialties and the continuing need to develop certification examinations in some areas (see Chapters 12 and 13). As new APN roles evolve, the problems around credentialing become increasingly acute.

This chapter describes basic national and state regulatory and credentialing realities and provides a discussion of the critical elements of regulation and credentialing that currently affect APNs. For specific questions about up-to-the-minute, current APN rules and regulations—especially those that pertain to specific state statutes regarding licensing of APNs, prescriptive authority, and reimbursement—the reader should refer to individual local and state regulatory bodies for practice requirements.

The skills required for successful policy activism and advocacy, which are crucial to negotiating regulatory mechanisms, are part of the APN core competency of clinical, professional, and systems leadership. The concepts and skills outlined in Chapters 9 and 10 are crucial to the role APNs play in setting credentialing and regulatory policy mechanisms and should be considered as this chapter is read.

DEFINITIONS

It is important for APNs to understand the language and terms used to describe the credentialing process. Credentialing involves several steps before completion and full authority to practice as an APN. To complicate matters, the credentialing procedures and requirements vary somewhat from state to state and from practice setting to practice setting. Definitions for the major components of APN credentialing are found in Box 21-1.

STATE LICENSURE/RECOGNITION

Individual state nurse practice acts define the practice of nursing for registered nurses (RNs) throughout the 50 states. State laws overseeing advanced practice nursing are divided into two forms: (1) statutes as defined by the nurse practice act are enacted by the state legislature; and (2) rules and regulations are explicated by state agencies under the jurisdiction of the executive branch of state government. Licensure is delegated to the individual states by the Federal Constitution, which provides standards to ensure basic levels of public safety. In 23 states, the board of nursing has sole authority over advanced practice nursing; in others, there is joint authority with the board of medicine, the board of pharmacy, or both (Lugo, O'Grady, Hodnicki, & Hanson, 2007). The states require that all APNs carry current licensure as RNs. Authority to practice is tied to scope of practice and varies from state to state, depending on the degree of practice autonomy the APN is granted. The current status of advanced practice nursing licensure and scope of practice and application information in a particular state can be easily obtained by accessing the National Council of State Boards of Nursing (NCSBN) website *(www.ncsbn.org),* which has a link to each individual state board of nursing.

Some states require a temporary permit for a new graduate to practice as an APN while awaiting national certification results (Pearson, 2007). New graduates should contact the board of nursing and submit the required application for a temporary advanced practice nursing permit if the state allows such practice. With the advent of electronic testing, the time lapse between testing and obtaining results for licensure is minimal and markedly reduces the need for a temporary permit.

Prescriptive Authority

Credentialing and licensure for prescriptive authority also occur at the state level. Pharmacology requirements vary from state to state although, currently, most states require a core advanced pharmacotherapeutics course during the graduate APN educational program and yearly continuing education (CE) credits thereafter to maintain prescriptive privileges. Prescriptive authority may be regulated solely by the board of nursing, as it is in several states; jointly by

---

Box 21-1   ADVANCED PRACTICE NURSE CREDENTIALING DEFINITIONS

Credentialing (state level) The requirements that a state uses to assess minimum standards of competency for APNs to be authorized to practice in an APN role. The purpose of credentialing is to protect the health and safety of the public.

Credentialing (institutional level) The process an individual institution uses to permit an APN to practice in an APN position within the institution. Generally, APNs submit particular documentation to an institutional credentialing committee, who reviews and authorizes the APN's practice.

Legal authority The authority assigned to a state or agency with administrative powers to enforce laws, rules, policies.

Regulations The rules and policies that operationalize the laws and policies that recognize APNs and credential them for practice in an APN role.

Licensure The process by which an agency of state government grants authorization to an individual to engage in a given profession. For nursing, licensure is usually based on two criteria: the applicant attaining the essential education and degree of competency necessary to perform a unique scope of practice; and passing a national examination. APNs are licensed first as RNs and second as APNs.

Certification A formal process (usually an examination, but may be a portfolio) used by a certifying agency to validate, based on predetermined standards, an individual's knowledge, skills, and abilities. Certification provides validation of the APN's knowledge in a particular specialty. It is used by most states as one component of second licensure for APN practice.

Accreditation The voluntary process by which schools of nursing are reviewed by external nursing educational agencies for the purpose of determining the quality of a nursing and/or APN program.

APN, Advanced practice nurse; RN, registered nurse.

the board of nursing and the board of pharmacy, as it is in several others; or by a triad of boards of nursing, medicine, and pharmacy. It is incumbent upon the APN to clearly understand the mechanism of prescriptive authority regulation in his or her state and to understand whether ongoing continuing education is required.

As prescriptive authority has evolved over the past several years, certain basic requirements have become fairly standard for APN prescribers (Box 21-2). These requirements vary from state to state but provide a core regulatory process for prescriptive authority (Buppert, 2004; Pearson, 2007).

As noted, state boards of nursing should clearly document the numbers of hours of pharmacology required for an APN to receive and maintain prescriptive privileges in terms of both the APN educational program and annual CE. APN programs that previously integrated pharmacological content within clinical management courses are required to have a stand-alone advanced pharmacotherapeutics course in order to comply with state requirements and accreditation standards (*www.aacn.nche.edu/Accreditation*). Pharmacology content should be taught by faculty pharmacists or a nurse-pharmacist faculty team who have an in-depth knowledge of therapeutic prescribing. Some states are requiring that APN nursing programs verify specific course and content hours that can be used in a board of nursing application for prescriptive authority. Furthermore, several states require

Box 21-2   Requirements for Advanced Practice Nurse Prescribers

- Graduation from an approved master's- or doctoral-level APN program
- Licensure/recognition in good standing as an APN
- National certification in an APN specialty
- Recent pharmacotherapeutics course of at least 3 credit hours (45 contact hours)
- Evidence of a collaborative practice arrangement (in some states)
- Ongoing CE hours in pharmacotherapeutics to maintain prescribing status
- State prescribing and national DEA numbers in some instances

APN, Advanced practice nurse; *CE,* continuing education; *DEA,* Drug Enforcement Administration.

documentation of the number of hours of CE for pharmacology per year or per cycle. The direction is clearly to require APNs to attend ongoing CE in pharmacology to maintain prescriptive privileges although APNs should update their knowledge in this changing area whether or not their state requires it. Timely CE offerings and distance learning modalities (e.g., podcasts and Web-based offerings) are available to meet the needs of busy clinicians. Over time, the states will probably move in the direction of interdisciplinary pharmacology education for both nurses and physicians. New innovations, including handheld personal digital assistants (PDAs) that offer clinicians on-site information about prescribing modalities and state-of-the-art drug information, are a positive response to the increasing evidence of medication prescribing errors (Huffstutler, Wyatt, & Wright, 2002).

Drug Enforcement Administration Number

In addition to prescriptive authority, APNs who plan to prescribe or dispense controlled substances will need to apply for a Drug Enforcement Administration (DEA) number as required by both federal and state policy. DEA numbers are site-specific; therefore APNs practicing at more than one site will need to obtain additional DEA numbers at a current cost of $390 per site (Klein, 2006; Reel & Abraham, 2007).

SCOPE OF PRACTICE FOR ADVANCED PRACTICE NURSES

By definition, *scope of practice* describes practice limits and sets the parameters within which nurses in the various advanced practice nursing specialties may legally practice. Scope statements define what APNs can do for and with patients, what they can delegate, and when collaboration with others is required. Scope-of-practice statements tell APNs de facto what is beyond the limits of their nursing practice (Cady, 2003). The scope of practice for each APN specialty group differs and is explicated in Chapters 12 through 17. Scope-of-practice statements are key to the debate about how the U.S. health care system employs APNs as health care providers; scope is inextricably linked with barriers to advanced practice nursing. CRNAs, who administer general anesthesia, have a scope of practice markedly different from that of the primary care NP, for example, although both have their roots in basic nursing. In addition, it is important to understand that scope of practice differs from state to state and is based on state laws promulgated by the various state nurse practice acts and the rules and regulations for APNs (Lugo et al., 2007; Pearson, 2007). On the Internet, scope-of-practice statements can be found by searching state government Web pages in the areas of licensing boards, nursing, and advanced practice nursing rules and regulations or by visiting the NCSBN site *(www.ncsbn.org).*

Accountability becomes a crucial factor as APNs move toward increasing authority over their own practices. First, it is important that scope-of-practice statements identify the legal parameters of each APN role. Furthermore, it is crucial that scope-of-practice statements presented by national certifying entities are carried through in language in state statutes. Our society is highly mobile, and APNs must recognize that their scope of practice will vary from state to state; in a worst-case scenario, one can be an APN in one state but not meet the criteria in another state. This factor is discussed more fully in the "Telehealth and Telepractice" section later in this chapter.

APNs owe Barbara Safriet, former Associate Dean at Yale Law School, a debt of gratitude for her vision and clarity in helping APNs understand and think strategically about scope-of-practice and regulatory issues. In her landmark 1992 monograph, Safriet noted that APNs are unique in that there is a multiprofessional approach to their regulation based on ignorance and the fallacy that medicine is all-knowing, particularly about advanced practice nursing. Safriet (1992) reports that:

> States have used a variety of approaches to extend the scope of practice of nursing. Some have revised their nurse practice acts (NPAs) to delete the absolute prohibition on diagnosis and treatment or to add "nursing diagnosis." Some have added an "additional acts" clause to the NPA, authorizing some specially trained nurses to "perform acts of medical diagnosis and treatment" as specified by rules of the state nursing and/or medical boards or as "agreed upon by the professions of nursing and medicine." Some have added a generic category, or specific categories, of APNs and either have defined their scope of practice or have authorized state nursing and/or medical boards to promulgate rules that do so. Some have revised their medical practice acts (MPAs) to authorize physicians to delegate diagnosis and treatment tasks to nurses who have the necessary additional training. (pp. 445-446)

As Safriet's quote implies, restraints on advanced practice result from ignorance about APNs' abilities, rigid notions about professional roles, and turf protection. Safriet (2002) cited reforms in scope-of-practice laws in Colorado that encouraged solutions to long-time tensions over control of practice between organized medicine and nursing. Their new provision defines *practice authority* in terms of ability and thus redirects the regulatory focus from providers' status to the APN's training and skills. This example and the work being done by leadership groups at the NCSBN and the Consensus Group at the American Association of Colleges of Nursing (AACN) offer hope that, in the future, policies can be formulated that will close the gap between what APNs are able to do and what they are allowed to do by scope-of-practice statutes. Scope of practice is hampered in many states where APN practice is carved out of the medical practice act as a "medically delegated" act that precludes reasonable autonomy for the APN (NCSBN, 2007). The ability to diagnose disease and treat patients that is inherent to the role of the APN is fluid and evolving and is, in many instances, tied to the collaborative relationships that APNs have with physician colleagues.

Benchmarks of Advanced Practice Nursing and Education

Three components of APN education and practice are related to scope of practice and provide additional important benchmarks. These benchmarks form the foundation upon which Boards of Nursing develop APN statutes.

Advanced Practice Nurse Competencies.

Underpinning scope-of-practice statements are the *APN competencies,* which are carefully outlined in Part II of this text. They form the core that distinguishes APN practice. Scope is directly linked to the APN competencies of direct clinical practice and coaching and guidance. These two interact with other core competencies to make up the quality care spectrum that APN providers offer to their patients.

Professional Specialty Competencies. In

addition, the professional specialty organizations such as the National Organization of Nurse Practitioner Faculties (NONPF), the National Association of Clinical Nurse Specialists (NACNS), the American Colleges of Nurse-Midwives (ACNM), and the American Association of Nurse Anesthetists (AANA) support each role and specialty with their own set of *specialty competencies.* These more specific competencies provide benchmarks particular to the specialty (see Chapters 12 to 18 for examples and sources for specialty competencies).

Master's and Doctor of Nursing Practice Essentials. Educational groups have promulgated the *Essentials* of master's and the *Essentials* of doctoral education for advanced practice nursing (AACN 1995, 2006a). These documents support scope of practice for APNs by providing the requirements for advanced physical assessment and diagnosis, pathophysiology, and pharmacotherapeutics in addition to existing APN competencies (National Organization of Nurse Practitioner Faculties [NONPF], 2003). At the new Doctor of Nursing Practice (DNP) level, a stronger foundation in population-based care, organizational leadership, collaboration, and information systems enhances APN roles (AACN, 2006a).

Although there has been considerable progress toward a better professional understanding of APN practice and more evidence to support standardization of education and practice, to date this progress has not yet fully translated into standardized regulation. Continued collaborative efforts among practice, education, and regulatory groups are required to bring about needed change in the regulatory environment. Encouraging evidence of progress in this area is presented on pp. 623-624.

Standards of Practice and Standards of Care for Advanced Practice Nurses

Standards of practice for nursing are defined by the profession nationally and help further explicate and delineate scope of practice. Standards are overarching, authoritative statements that the nursing profession uses to describe the responsibilities for which its members are accountable (American Nurses Association, 1996, 2003). As such, they complement and enable the APN core and specialty competencies. APNs are held both to the standards of practice promulgated by the nursing profession and to standards of the various APN specialties. At both levels, standards of practice describe the basic competency levels for safe and competent practice (e.g., see Chapters 16 and 17 for the standards of practice for CNMs and CRNAs, respectively). Professional standards of practice match closely with the core competencies for APNs, outlined in Chapter 3, which undergird advanced practice nursing.

Standards of care differ from the standards of practice set forth by the nursing profession described previously. These standards are often termed *practice guidelines*. Practice guidelines provide a foundation by which health care providers administer care to patients. These guidelines crosscut the health professions' disciplines and provide the framework by which basic safety and competent care are measured. For APNs, this means that the standard used to evaluate advanced practice is often the same as the standard used to review medical practice. Standards of care are derived from evidence-based practice and are continuously evolving. At the federal policy level, the Agency for Healthcare Research and Quality (AHRQ) has responsibility for conducting the research needed to evaluate clinical practice guidelines that define a standard of appropriate care in specific areas (Agency for Healthcare Research and Quality [AHRQ], 2007; Buppert, 2004). The Centers for Disease Control and Prevention (CDC) and many professional medical and nursing specialty organizations also promulgate guidelines for practice. It is very important that APNs be part of interdisciplinary teams that develop and test practice guidelines for care. The ability of APNs to download cutting-edge practice guidelines onto handheld PDAs for use in clinical settings is a major step toward competent and safe practice.

LEGAL CONCERNS SURROUNDING ADVANCED PRACTICE NURSE TITLING

The definition of an APN requires that the role be clinically focused and that the APN give direct clinical care to patients (ANA, 1996; Hamric, 2005). The definition developed in this text goes beyond this requirement and is further explicated in Chapter 3. Currently, four established advanced practice nursing roles are generally recognized: NPs in primary and acute care, CNMs, CRNAs, and CNSs. In addition, some emerging advanced practice nursing roles can be included in these groups (see Chapters 15 and 18). From a legal and regulatory perspective, inclusion in the designation of what constitutes an APN is driven primarily by three factors: the diagnosis and management of patients at an advanced level of nursing expertise, the ability of APNs to be directly reimbursed, and the degree to which nurses desire to hold prescriptive and hospital admitting privileges. Although this may seem restrictive to some, there must be a well-defined and efficacious way for state boards, insurers, prescribing entities, and the like to monitor the scope-of-practice, prescribing, and reimbursement patterns of APNs. These groups need clear criteria that can be validated to ensure patient safety and to monitor proper certification and credentialing.

There are several reasons that the multiplicity of titles and roles for APNs is a problem from a policy viewpoint. The foremost reason is that it is confusing to policymakers and regulators, especially at agencies such as the CMS, where major designations for Medicare and Medicaid reimbursement set the standard for all reimbursement of APNs across the country. In addition, discrepancies in advanced practice nursing definition and licensing criteria among states make mobility difficult for APNs in terms of prescriptive authority and reimbursement. APNs are responsible primarily to and are disciplined by individual state boards of nursing. One of the licensing and credentialing difficulties faced by APNs is the variance in board regulations from state to state. In some states, advanced practice nursing is governed only by the board of nursing; in others, it is jointly administered by the boards of nursing and medicine; and in still others, it is governed by the boards of nursing and pharmacy. In many states, CNMs are answerable to nurse-midwifery boards that are attached to boards of medicine. Although restrictive statements delegating only medical acts approved by the board of medicine and co-signed by a physician preceptor are not as prevalent as they were in the 1980s, they are still the norm in some states, predominantly in the South (Lugo et al., 2007; Pearson, 2007). Currently, states that have delegated medical authority for APNs often require *collaborative agreements* for APNs who diagnose diseases, manage treatment, and prescribe medications for patients. As implied, collaborative agreements provide a written description of the professional relationship between an APN and a collaborating physician that defines the parameters by which the APN can perform delegated medical acts (see further discussion of collaborative practice arrangements later in this chapter; Appendix B at the end of the book contains a sample collaborative practice agreement).

COMPONENTS OF ADVANCED PRACTICE NURSE CREDENTIALING AND REGULATION

Credentialing of APNs to ensure that they meet competency and safety standards that will protect the public has developed rather haphazardly. To try to impose some uniformity on credentialing and licensure of APNs, professional nursing organizations and the NCSBN are moving toward a new model of regulation that embraces all credentialing stakeholders and may include second licensure. *Second licensure* means that an APN must meet certain criteria established by a state board of nursing to receive an additional license or recognition to be authorized to practice at an advanced level of nursing practice. The notion of second licensure is unprecedented among the health professions and is onerous to some nurses, but given the various routes of entry into the nursing profession, it seems the only way to ensure a minimum set of competencies or requirements. The issue of titling and second licensure is a "bread and butter" issue for all APNs and one that individual APNs must pay attention to in order to protect their ability to practice, prescribe, and be reimbursed for their services.

Elements of Regulation for Advanced Practice Nursing

Several important steps lead the way to state licensure as an APN. The regulatory process begins when a student is admitted to a university-based accredited APN program and proceeds through national certification by a specialty organization and then to second licensure and prescriptive authority. Box 21-3 lists the elements of regulation for APNs.

Several definitions and concepts are central to a discussion of credentialing and regulation of APNs in the United States. As APNs become more mobile across state and international boundaries and as communications allow for increased interaction, it is important that credentialing and regulatory parameters be well understood.

Credentialing

Credentialing is an umbrella term that refers to the regulatory mechanisms that can be applied to individuals, programs, or organizations (Styles, 1998). Credentialing can be defined as "getting your ducks in a row" for the purpose of meeting standards, protecting the public, and improving quality. For the purposes of this text, credentialing (as it relates to APNs) is defined as follows: Credentialing is furnishing the

---

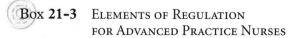

Box 21-3   Elements of Regulation for Advanced Practice Nurses

Education
  • Master's
  • Post-master's
  • Doctoral
Accreditation of APN programs
National Certification
  • Recertification
Licensure
  • Prescriptive Authority (see Box 21-2)

documentation necessary to be authorized by a regulatory body or institution to engage in certain activities and to use a certain title. Credentialing can be at a state level in terms of applying for a second license as an APN. The term can also apply to a local institutional process that requires certain documentation from an APN before the individual is allowed to practice and use an APN title. Credentialing in health care is used to assure the public that the individual meets proposed standards and is prepared to perform the duties implied by the credential. National certification is only one part of credentialing and is used by many states as one vehicle to ensure a basic level of competence to practice; education is the other one. Certification alone does not provide a credential to practice as an APN. Regulatory groups commonly request evidence of the primary criteria of graduate education, national certification, and patient- focused practice (see Chapter 3).

Credentialing may be mandatory, as in state second licensure, or voluntary, as with some states that only register APN providers in the state. In some instances, bodies that regulate APNs to ensure public safety may recognize voluntary credentialing bodies, such as national nursing certification organizations, as a part of their mandatory state credentialing mechanism.

APN program accreditation and approval, scope of practice, standards of practice, practice guidelines, and collaborative practice agreements all have important implications for APNs in terms of proper credentialing and interactions with the court system. The documents specified in Box 21-4 create the standard

by which advanced practice nursing is monitored and regulated and deemed safe or unsafe and by which APNs are disciplined from state to state. The components of advanced practice nursing education and practice are described in the following sections.

Advanced Practice Nurse Master's and Doctoral Education

The first criterion that any new APN must meet is successful graduation from an approved APN program. Over time, most educational programs have moved their curricula to the graduate nursing level, and within the decade, many programs will move from master's to doctoral level education for APNs. The recommendation by the AACN is that at least until 2015, the master's will be the level at which APNs are credentialed (AACN, 2006b). In most states, both eligibility to sit for national certification and the ability to obtain advanced practice nursing licensure or recognition by the state require a transcript showing successful completion of a master's degree from an accredited university in the designated nursing specialty (Buppert, 2004). This is rapidly becoming the norm for APN licensure or recognition in all states, with the current exception of credentialing for midwifery. However, as of 2010, all nurse-midwives will be required to obtain a graduate degree before being credentialed into midwifery practice (American College of Nurse-Midwives [ACNM], 2006).

Advanced Practice Nurse Program Accreditation. For a graduate nursing program (either master's or doctorate) preparing APNs, credentialing has a somewhat different meaning. Program credentialing may include accreditation by the Commission on Collegiate Nursing Education (CCNE) or the National League for Nursing Accreditation Center (NLNAC); regional and state university boards and commissions; or groups such as the ACNM or the AANA (AANA, 2007; Summers & Williams, 2003). For an institution (hospital, clinic), credentialing may include adhering to The Joint Commission (TJC) and Occupational Safety and Health Administration (OSHA) guidelines.

Graduate programs in nursing and related fields that prepare APNs must be accredited as educationally sound, with appropriate content for the specialty and adequate clinical hours of supervised experience. As noted, the NLNAC and CCNE accredit graduate programs in the nursing major (Commission on Collegiate Nursing Education [CCNE], 1998). Accreditation

---

Box 21-4 OVERVIEW OF ADVANCED PRACTICE NURSE CREDENTIALING

- Graduation from an accredited graduate-level nursing program
- Attainment of national APN-level certification
- State licensure/recognition as an RN and APN
- Collaborative practice agreement with a physician if required in the state
- Approval for prescriptive authority
- Medicare/Medicaid provider numbers
- NPI number
- DEA number to prescribe controlled substances
- Approval of hospital privileges

APN, Advanced practice nurse; *DEA,* Drug Enforcement Administration; *NPI,* National Provider Identifier; *RN,* registered nurse.

procedures for the practice doctorate are being developed. The accreditation process provides an overall evaluation of the graduate program but currently does not deal with the specifics of approval of specialty advanced practice nursing content. Oversight of specialty education for APNs occurs with the use of several different models. The clearest models are those administered by the ACNM and the AANA, which oversee and review CNM and CRNA educational programs. These bodies provide a process to review and regulate CRNA and CNM programs across the country that is separate from the overall graduate nursing accreditation processes of the CCNE and the NLNAC. Furthermore, certifying agencies such as the ANCC and the AANP review programs, to some degree, to sanction eligibility for APN graduates to sit for national APN certification examinations. Many educators feel that this process comes too late. There is a need for educators, certifiers, and regulators to be proactive and oversee program appropriateness and strength before students graduate and are ready for credentialing. Given the increased numbers of advanced practice nursing programs in a variety of nursing specialties, more work needs to be done to standardize education for APNs.

A new change, based on the work of the NCSBN and consensus groups, that was suggested by Hanson and Hamric (2002) is the planned introduction of pre-accreditation procedures before the start of new programs. Pre-accreditation will ensure that all new programs are well developed and lead to graduates who can be licensed as APNs. The use of grandfathering mechanisms to protect APNs during transition periods of standardization provides leeway for positive change to occur (NCSBN, 2007). For example, students who are in educational programs that are phasing out or phasing into new configurations will be allowed to graduate, sit for certification, and be credentialed until the transition period is complete.

The review and monitoring of NP education at the specialty level is much more complex because of the multiplicity of specialties. The NONPF, the National Certification Board of Pediatric Nurse Practitioners and Nurses (NCBPNP/N), the NACNS, and other like bodies provide curriculum guidelines, program standards, and competencies to assist APN programs with curriculum planning. The most clearly established review processes for NP programs are those administered by the NCBPNP/N, which approves pediatric NP programs, and the National Association of Women's Health, which accredits women's health programs (Association of Women's Health, Obstetric, Neonatal Nurses; and the National Association of Nurse Practitioners in Reproductive Health). In 2002, the National Task Force on Quality Nurse Practitioner Education established national criteria by which to monitor and evaluate NP programs according to broad-based criteria in six overarching areas (Box 21-5). In 2007 the National Task Force Guidelines for Quality NP Education were updated and revised, and these guidelines are scheduled for ongoing revision every 5 years (*www.nonpf.com*). The National Task Force on Quality Nurse Practitioner Education (1997, 2002) were developed and endorsed by a consortium of NP education and practice associations, NP regulators, and NP national certifiers and accreditors. The AACN's *Essentials of Master's Education for Advanced Practice Nursing* (1995) and *Essentials of Doctoral Education for Advanced Nursing Practice* (2006a) define graduate nursing core and advanced practice nursing core (advanced pathophysiology, physical assessment, and pharmacology) curriculum requirements. These three documents provide needed structure and guidance for NP nursing education.

Box 21-5   NATIONAL TASK FORCE CRITERIA FOR NURSE PRACTITIONER PROGRAM EVALUATION

Criterion I—Organization and administration	Institutional support of nurse practitioner programs
Criterion II—Students	Student admission and progression
Criterion III—Curriculum	Content areas, competencies, basic course work
Criterion IV—Resources, facilities, and services	Physical resources, clinical site, preceptorship resources
Criterion V—Faculty and faculty organization	Faculty preparation, credentialing, clinical practice
Criterion VI—Evaluation	Program, students, faculty, clinical sites

Data from the National Task Force on Quality Nurse Practitioner Education. (2002). *Criteria for evaluation of nurse practitioner programs*. Washington, DC: Author.

The CNS community is working toward clear structure and progression of CNS specialty education to ensure compliance with credentialing and regulation as APN providers (National Association of Clinical Nurse Specialists [NACNS], 2004). Currently, momentum is strong among nursing accreditors, APN certifiers, and APN specialty organizations such as the NONPF and NACNS to better align the overarching accreditation process (AACN, 2007b; NCSBN, 2007).

Postgraduate Education. The number of postgraduate APN programs targeted to students who have already attained a graduate degree in nursing but who wish to become APNs or want to work in a different APN role markedly increased in the late 1990s but has leveled off more recently. The new educational initiative is the development of post-master's programs that offer the practice doctorate (AACN, 2006b; Fang, Wisniewski, & Bednash, 2007; NONPF, 2006). Post-master's APN education is often tailored to meet the individual needs of post-master's students. Currently, post-master's education does not fall within the purview of formal graduate nursing accreditation. New accreditation criteria for post-master's and practice doctorate programs are recommended in the vision statements by the NCSBN and the AACN (2007b) and are under development. It is important that master's-prepared nurses who aspire to do postgraduate work to acquire a new or additional APN credential identify programs that offer curricula that meet the standards of eligibility for national certification and state licensure for the particular APN role they seek to attain.

Dual and Blended Role Education. New configurations of programs and tracks for specialty APNs that are dual or blended (see Chapters 3 and 15 for clarification of these roles) are widespread (Fang et al., 2007). These programs require careful consideration of content and meaningful clinical experiences to ensure mastery of basic advanced practice nursing competencies and clinical experiences in both specialty areas. Dual and blended advanced practice nursing programs are, by necessity, longer and require more clinical experiences. Many APNs are dually prepared and thus must sit for more than one national certification. Today's complex health care system makes this a viable option for many APNs who are functioning in diverse settings. The practice doctorate offers a new educational path that allows practicing APNs to attain new knowledge and skills that can lead to additional APN certification.

National Advanced Practice Nurse Specialty Certification

National certification for APNs is the other primary vehicle used by state boards of nursing to ensure regulatory sufficiency. Advanced practice nursing certification is national in scope, and it is a mandatory requirement for APNs to obtain and maintain credentialing in most states (Pearson, 2007). Multiple stakeholders for certification such as the American Nurses Association (ANA), faculty groups (e.g., NONPF), specialty organizations (e.g., AANP, AANA, Oncology Nursing Society [ONS]), and many others have worked to accomplish the multifaceted tasks needed for successful advanced practice nursing certification. These efforts have resulted in a broad range of certification and credentialing requirements. Typically, certification mechanisms develop when a role delineation study is undertaken to define the competencies that provide the framework for appropriate testing within the APN specialty. More and more state regulatory bodies are currently including national certification examinations as a component of their advanced practice nursing credentialing mechanism. CRNAs are credited with the first national certification in 1945, with other APN specialties following suit, although few standards for certification were in place early on (Hodnicki, 1998). A perceived weakness of APN certification is the multiplicity of certification configurations for advanced practice nursing.

Much work is being done to enhance transparency among the NCSBN, individual state boards of nursing, and APN certifiers. The groups are striving for a way to regulate all APNs who diagnose, prescribe, and are reimbursed for services. The situation creates challenges for graduate programs as they develop and revise curricula to prepare students to be eligible for particular advanced practice nursing certifying examinations. Visit the specialty certification websites listed in Box 21-6 to see criteria for eligibility, test outlines, and recertification and practice requirements.

Recertification. Overall, APNs must fulfill CE and practice requirements to successfully maintain their national certification, although requirements differ from specialty to specialty. Each advanced practice nursing certification entity clearly lays out the requirements and time frame for recertification.

Box 21-6   INTERNET ADDRESSES TO NATIONAL ADVANCED PRACTICE NURSING
ACCREDITATION, REGULATION, AND CERTIFICATION WEBSITES

American Academy of Nurse Practitioners (AANP)	www.aanp.org
American Association of Colleges of Nurses (AACN) and Commission on Collegiate Nursing Education (CCNE)	www.aacn.nche.edu (links to CCNE)
American Association of Nurse Anesthetists (AANA)	www.nursecredentialing.org
American College of Nurse-Midwives (ACNM)	www.acnm.org
American Nurses Credentialing Center (ANCC)	www.nursecredential.org
Pediatric Nursing Certification Board (PNCB)	www.pncb.org
National Certification Corporation (NCC) for obstetrical, gynecological, and neonatal nursing specialties	www.nccnet.org
National Council of State Boards of Nursing (NCSBN)	www.ncsbn.org
National League for Nursing (NLN) and National League for Nursing Accreditation Corporation (NLNAC)	www.nln.org/nlnac
National Association of Nurse Practitioners in Women's Health (NPWH)	www.npwh.org

Generally, national certification for most specialties lasts from 5 to 8 years and requires that the candidate retest unless the established parameters are met.

Mandatory Continuing Education Requirements. CE requirements differ from specialty to specialty as to the type and amount of CE needed to maintain current national certification. Individual advanced practice nursing specialties determine the number of hours required for successful recertification. Instruction should be in the area of the APN specialty, although it may be interdisciplinary. For example, CRNAs may choose to attend a conference with collaborating anesthesiologists, or family NPs may attend a conference with family practice physicians. It is encouraging to note that more and more conferences are offering interdisciplinary speakers and panels at specialty-specific conferences. APN expert clinicians are serving as conference faculty for medical CE and vice versa. Ongoing CE hours can be met by attending CE courses and workshops; working toward degree requirements; completing journal CE offerings; writing for publication; and completing online offerings, simulations, audiotape, and CD-ROM materials. Many nursing and medical journals offer CE credit to subscribers. The move to interdisciplinary offerings has broadened the scope of information available.

Mandatory Practice Requirements. Most APN specialties have built in specific requirements for an adequate number of clinical practice hours between the years of recertification to ensure that APNs are remaining clinically current and competent through regular practice. Each certification process clearly spells out the clinical hour practice requirement for the specialty. Some advanced practice nursing specialties accept clinical teaching and other modalities as part of the practice requirement. This is problematic because such graduate-level teaching may not involve providing APN-level direct clinical care to patients or require regular use of other APN core competencies. If individuals are not maintaining an APN practice, they should not represent themselves as APNs (see Chapter 3). APNs who do not meet stipulated CE and practice requirements must retake the national certifying examination to continue to practice. One concern is that standardization of quality will be lost in the face of multiple advanced practice nursing specialties and specialty certifications. Certification is one way to ensure that competent APNs provide needed health care to patients and families. Therefore standardization of APN certification and recertification processes is critical to ensure the credibility of advanced practice nursing specialties (Hodnicki, 1998; NCSBN, 2007).

Institutional Credentialing
The need for hospital privileges for APNs varies according to the nurse's practice. For example, CNMs and many rural NPs cannot properly care for patients without the ability to admit patients to the hospital should the need arise. Conversely, many CNSs are

employed by hospitals and have no need for admitting privileges. CRNAs and some NPs have not needed to admit patients to the hospital independently in order to give comprehensive care, but they may need to see patients in the emergency room.

The rules for practice as part of the hospital staff are even more specific and variable than those for state regulation and are bound to the local hospital or medical facility and the medical staff of the granting institution. Unfortunately, most of the criteria and guidelines are written exclusively for medical practitioners and therefore are not compatible with the APN's education and supporting credentials. In many hospitals, professional privileges are granted by a committee made up of physicians and administrators. More and more committees are adding APN members to privileging committees as APNs gain stature in hospital settings.

The first step for APNs seeking hospital privileges is to ask the top-level nurse administrator how the credentials committee is organized, who makes up the membership, and what support there is for non-physician applicants. Is there a process for nurses or others to petition for privileges? Nursing administrators are often members of these committees, and the APN should meet with nurse colleagues for advice and support before the application process. A second step is to obtain the application package and begin to collect the necessary documents, which include, for example, licenses and certifications, transcripts, letters of support, and provider numbers. Support from collaborating physicians is key; in some committee structures, a collaborating physician may serve as the petitioner for a nurse colleague. Dialogue between the hospital administration, physician staff, and other stakeholders such as APN colleagues and other team members is necessary if admitting privileges are required for the desired practice role. Alliances with consumers often add support to the application. Some hospitals have specific guides and protocols for all non-physician providers; others do not.

The determination of the specific privileges desired is critical to the process. For example, is it necessary to be able to admit or discharge patients, write orders, perform particular procedures, visit in-hospital patients, or take an emergency room call? Many hospitals have different levels of hospital privileges, ranging from "full" privileges to modified privileges for specific functions. Asking for full privileges may not be prudent or useful in a particular setting. A good rule is to ask for what is needed, establish a solid track record, and expand privileges later as the need arises. In today's market, professional turf issues are losing ground and opportunities for hospital privileges are opening the door for new APN practice alternatives.

ISSUES THAT AFFECT ADVANCED PRACTICE NURSE CREDENTIALING AND REGULATION

Collaborative Practice Arrangements

The general term *practice guidelines* can be confusing to the APN in that it is used in several different contexts. First, as defined earlier, it is an evidence-based standard of care. Practice guidelines are used by health care clinicians and provide interdisciplinary support for state-of-the-art practice. However, the term may sometimes be used to refer to a collegial agreement between an APN and physician to define parameters of practice for the APN. Many states require this as part of APN licensure (Lugo et al., 2007). A collaborative agreement or arrangement may take many forms, from a one-page written agreement defining consultation and referral patterns to a more specific prescribed "protocol" for specific functions based on state statutes for advanced practice nursing. Collaborative agreements need to be written as broadly as possible to allow for practice variations and new innovations.

The term *protocol* in relation to advanced practice nursing was common several years ago as a physician-directed, specified guideline for the medical aspects of practice that defined each patient problem and the treatment approach. Some states used this "cookbook" approach to NP practice as a way to oversee prescriptive and other treatment modalities. For the most part, specific protocols for care are no longer used in most settings because it is difficult to update them and tailor them to the individual needs of patients and practices. More important, advanced practice nursing has evolved. As APNs have proven their ability to provide competent care with positive outcomes, protocols have been replaced by evidence-based practice guidelines and collaborative practice agreements. However, it is important to note that the specificity of the collaborative arrangement is usually based on trust and respect between the collaborating APN and physician colleague. For example, a newly graduated APN might have a more tightly drawn collaborative agreement than a more experienced one in a new practice arrangement. APNs must often "earn their stripes" as competent health care providers in the medical world before they are granted more autonomous practice. Although it should not be this way, physicians are, de facto, assumed to be competent in the workplace whereas APNs need to prove their worth.

The norm today in APN regulation is shifting toward loosely configured collaborative relationships that offer support to all parties and protect the safety of patients. In any case, to achieve compliance with state regulations for practice, the collaborative agreement, if required in a given state, must be updated annually, must have a current signature, and must provide relevant and up-to-date information. Collaborative relationships vary widely from advanced practice nursing specialty to specialty. APNs who expand their scope in a practice (e.g., from pediatric to family NP) must update their collaborative practice agreement accordingly. The chapters in Part III of this text help explain the differences in collaborative structures for APNs. Appendix B offers an example of a collaborative practice agreement.

National Provider Identifier Number
In addition to prescriber and DEA registration, APNs will need to apply for a National Provider Identifier (NPI) number. The Administrative Simplification provisions of the Health Insurance Portability and Accountability Act (HIPAA) of 1996 mandated the adoption of a standard unique identifier for health care providers. The National Plan and Provider Enumeration System (NPPES) collects identifying information on health care providers and assigns each a unique NPI. Every APN should go to *https://nppes. cms.hhs.gov* for further information or to apply for an NPI enumerator. NPI numbers are important for APN prescribers because many drugs are on insurance company formularies and prescriptions are billed via the NPPES system *(https://nppes.cms.hhs. gov/NPPES)*.

Medicare/Medicaid Provider Numbers.
The new NPI number for APNs will replace Medicare billing numbers, but currently APNs still need to register with the state for a Medicaid provider and a State Children's Health Insurance Plan (SCHIP) number. Visit *www.cms.org/Medicaid* and individual state Medicaid websites for instructions.

Reimbursement
On a par with the need to be able to prescribe medications for patients is the need to be appropriately reimbursed for care. Clearly, APNs should be paid for services rendered for health care whether they work independently, share a joint practice with a physician colleague, or are employed within an institution or provider network. Although the insurance industry is regulated by the individual states, many of the private-pay insurance standards that are used to set payment mechanisms are modeled after federal Medicare and Medicaid policy (see *www.cms.gov*). Federal mandates that encourage direct payment of non-physician health care providers are often blocked at the state level by discriminating rules and regulations. The terms *non-physician provider* and *mid-level provider* both denote caregivers who are not prepared as medical doctors. This category includes NPs, CNSs, CNMs, CRNAs, physician assistants (PAs), psychologists, and other reimbursable providers of care. Most third-party reimbursers, including some major insurance companies, are now reimbursing APNs and other non-physician providers directly; others are not. As states move more directly into reimbursement models for APNs, in both the private and public sectors, and into large purchasing groups in which APNs are providing care as part of interdisciplinary teams, reimbursement is becoming more readily available. However, tensions persist with regard to provider status and membership on patient panels. From a credentialing standpoint, attention to CMS rules, Medicare and Medicaid provider numbers, Clinical Laboratory Improvement Act (CLIA) *(www. cms.hhs.gov/clia/)* regulations, and provider requirements is extremely important to ensure that APNs are reimbursed. How APNs fit into reimbursement systems is a critical issue for nurses. It is important for APNs to know how to contract for their services at the individual level as they negotiate employment packages, but even more important, they need to be present at the negotiating table as members of management teams who are setting the policies for provider services where the rules for payment are made. Exemplar 21-1 describes the many credentialing requirements needed to begin practice as an APN.

Payment for advanced practice nursing services has long been controversial. Issues surrounding substitutive care offered by non-physician providers versus value-added care by APNs that enhances medical care are complex and profoundly affect direct and indirect reimbursement. It is important that APNs differentiate and clearly articulate the differences between their practices and those of physician extenders. The argument continues about whether nurses should be paid the same fee for service as a physician or be

EXEMPLAR 21-1 **Meeting the Requirements for Credentialing and Regulation**

Jeni is in the final semester of her master's FNP program at a state university. She is in the process of negotiating a contract with a provider network of physicians and APNs in a satellite HMO practice. Jeni knows that she must begin the process of acquiring the necessary credentials to be able to practice in her state. When she applied to her FNP program, she made sure that the university and graduate program were accredited in good standing. Now that she is ready to leave, she must prepare for a new and challenging professional life.

In her seminar class, Jeni received the application to sit for national certification the month after she graduates and has sent the application forward to register the date for her examination. Her next step is to access the Internet and download the advanced practice nursing rules and regulations for her state as well as the application for a temporary permit to practice as an APN for the interim between graduation and the time that she gets the results from her national certifying examination. Jeni reviews both of these documents carefully so that she fully understands the application process and the materials and fee that she will need to submit.

Jeni carefully notes in the advanced practice nursing rules and regulations that, to be able to prescribe in her state, she must show proof that she has completed a 45-contact-hour, approved course in pharmacotherapeutics and that she must complete 6 hours of CE in pharmacotherapeutics

each year to maintain her status as a prescriber. She makes a note to request the transcript for her pharmacotherapeutics course to attach to her application for her advanced practice nursing license.

The HMO in which Jeni plans to practice has sent her several documents that she must complete to be able to practice. First, upon signing her contract, she will need to negotiate a written collaborative arrangement with the precepting physician colleague, who will see the patients who are beyond her scope of practice. Second, she needs a Medicaid provider number in order to see children in the Medicaid program and a Medicare number in order to see older adults. She will need to apply for her NPI and DEA numbers. In addition, this managed care system requires that Jeni apply to the local hospital and nursing home privileging committees so that she can see patients on rounds, do admitting and discharge planning, and follow nursing home patients on a regular basis.

As part of her "package," Jeni has negotiated for the employer to pay the premium on her malpractice insurance as an APN. She needs to call her insurance carrier to discuss the transfer of her student policy to a full policy to cover her as a certified APN with the appropriate scope of practice that she will need in her new position. Jeni uses the support of her colleagues and mentors as she works through this important process of preparing her credentials to practice as an APN.

APN, Advanced practice nurse; *CE,* continuing education; *DEA,* Drug Enforcement Administration; *FNP,* family nurse practitioner; *HMO,* health maintenance organization; *NPI,* national provider identifier.

paid only a percentage of the physician payment. Should APNs demand equal pay for equal service, or should they cast themselves as more cost-effective providers to patients? This is always a negotiable issue, and there is disagreement within medicine and nursing alike. Payment by private insurers is contract-specific and varies with each state's insurance commission. The current climate of large-scale mergers between major private insurance companies to accommodate complex managed care structures has important relevance for reimbursement for APNs. It is critical that APNs position themselves to sit on policymaking boards for private enterprise. To accomplish this, APNs must have visibility with local, state, and national entities that make the important decisions for health care. Both the ACNM and the AANA vigilantly monitor reimbursement to stay on the cutting edge of payment schemes for APNs.

Another key issue exists regarding reimbursement for APNs. In capitated contracts, the level of reimbursement is immaterial. APNs and all other providers must deliver care at a fixed, preset price; this can be an advantage if APNs are less costly to employ. Thus it becomes critical for APNs to fully understand how much it costs them to provide care for patients who present with a variety of preventive, acute, episodic, and chronic health problems and to be able to articulate to contractors that they are competitive in the marketplace. Research data demonstrating the cost-effectiveness of APNs (see Chapter 24) are mounting and can strengthen an APN's case.

Policy issues surrounding the reimbursement of APNs require careful reflection before strategies to remove constraints to payment are undertaken. For all health care providers, outcomes of care will take precedence in reimbursement over all other issues, so attention to quality of care is a paramount consideration. Several other important questions should be considered when policy is being shaped. For example, for what services do APNs want to be paid? Are they different from physician services or the same? Are there specific nursing services that need to be reimbursed? Is direct payment the issue, or does it matter who gets the payment? Will the payment level be the same as or lower than what physicians receive for equivalent service? These are important questions because, in most states, APNs historically have been reimbursed indirectly, "incident to" physicians and at a considerably lower rate (Buppert, 2004; Reel & Abraham, 2007).

As mentioned earlier, "incident to" billing is a difficult issue. An APN can charge the full physician rate if billing is "incident to," but only 85% if billing is done directly by the APN, an unfortunate disincentive for doctors to let APNs bill independently. Most physicians desire to bill under their own Medicare number to receive the highest rate of reimbursement. On the other hand, APNs want and need to bill independently to be viewed as the caregivers of record. Many rules are associated with "incident to" billing, including the need for the physician to be on the premises. The CMS is currently studying "incident to" billing to better understand the prevalence of APN care and the cost to the system for billing APN services through the physician for a higher fee for service. It is advantageous for APNs who are planning to practice clinically, no matter what the setting or physician relationship, to seek counsel about the reimbursement realities in their state and in their particular practice setting(s) before beginning to care for patients. In particular, it is important to identify the third-party payers of the majority of patients the APN will be caring for and to learn their requirements for reimbursement of APNs. Only then are APNs in an appropriate position to seek status as reimbursable providers with Medicare, Medicaid, and the many private payers (see Chapter 19).

There are several areas in which reimbursement schemes directly affect the regulation of advanced practice nursing. Medicare and Medicaid, commercial insurers, and managed care organizations (MCOs) (health maintenance organizations [HMOs] and preferred provider organizations [PPOs]) cover most health care cost in today's market. These entities build networks of providers by hiring, purchasing services from, or contracting with physicians and APNs, hospitals, and others to provide health care services to patients. Often, these systems are capitated; that is, providers are prepaid a fixed amount to care for a population of patients. When APNs join a provider network, they must meet all of the requirements, regulations, and standards of care established by the plan. For example, a primary care NP applying for a position in an HMO would need to meet all of the criteria listed in Box 21-2 and obtain appropriate Medicare and Medicaid provider status, as well as malpractice history and coverage. It is incumbent upon the APN to have all credentials and regulatory documentation in good and accessible order when preparing to practice, because third-party payers are often located in and governed by reimbursement administrators in a distant state.

Risk Management, Malpractice, and Negligence

Although malpractice suits involving APNs are rare, malpractice issues are ever present for all providers of health care, regardless of credential or setting. In an unstable health care environment, patients look to the tort system to ease their apprehension and anxiety about the care they receive. Patients are more likely to seek redress if they mistrust their provider or believe they have been harmed by the system. First and foremost, APNs need to clearly understand what constitutes negligent practice and grounds for malpractice and to put safeguards in place so that they do not have to confront the legal system.

By definition, negligence is the failure to act in a reasonable way as a health care clinician. Negligence may lead to malpractice and legal action. The following four factors must exist for a malpractice suit to be valid (Buppert, 2004):

- A duty of care must be owed to the injured party, either through direct office or hospital care OR through phone or e-mail advice, and a patient-nurse relationship must be established.
- The accepted standard of care must be breached.
- The patient must have sustained an injury.
- There must be causation demonstrated—that is, the patient suffered an injury that was caused by the APN clinician. (Often there are multiple causation implications based on care by several caregivers over time.)

Within the court system, care is evaluated by preset criteria in the form of medical and advanced practice nursing standards. National professional organizations set the standards for appropriate care. APNs are often held to the medical standard of care as advanced practice nursing standards continue to be developed. There is much blurring between medical and nursing standards, leading toward a need for truly interdisciplinary standards of care that will hold care providers to the same standards as their peers (Buppert; Letz, 2002). There are several ways that legal standards of care are established in a particular case. By far the most common is through expert testimony offered by a person who is qualified by education, experience, knowledge, and skill level to judge the actions of the providers in the case. Other mechanisms include review of professional literature, manufacturers' package inserts, and documented professional standards of care. Letz suggested four ways to prevent malpractice events: establish a good rapport with patients over time; follow an established standard of care to ensure competence; document accurately and completely; and take a course in risk management.

Many risk management resources to assist APNs are available through professional advanced practice nursing organizations and though public and private entities. Visit the professional websites suggested throughout this text to find comprehensive risk management tools and a current discussion of legal questions confronting APNs. Box 21-7 provides a list of 10 rules compiled by Buppert (2002) to help APNs avoid malpractice.

Liability Insurance. APNs need a thorough understanding of liability insurance coverage, types of policies, and extent of coverage required. It is important to understand the difference between the two most common types of professional liability insurance plans—"claims-made" and "occurrence." A "claims-made" insurance policy covers claims made against the APN only while the policy is in effect. Coverage must be continued indefinitely to ensure coverage for claims filed in the future for actions that occurred in the past. On the other hand, with an "occurrence" policy, the APN is covered for alleged acts of negligence that occurred during the time when the policy was in effect. The benefit of occurrence coverage is that even if the policy is cancelled at some future date, coverage for events that occurred while the policy was in effect will be honored. For more information about advanced practice nursing liability insurance, visit the websites for the major malpractice insurance carriers. It is also important to understand the extent of coverage per incident and how personal legal costs are covered in your policy.

It is important that APNs carry their own individual liability coverage even if they are covered by an employer group practice. Employer-based insurance contracts are geared to protect the institution or practice as a whole and are not targeted to the individual APN. The comfort of having your own council during litigation far outweighs the cost of individual liability insurance. Conferences, workshops, and Internet offerings are available to assist APNs in choosing the appropriate insurance carrier and plan (Reel & Abraham, 2007).

As APNs move in and out of what is considered the domain of medicine, serious thought must be given to the standard by which APNs will be judged

---

Box 21-7   Rules to Avoid Malpractice

- Know the "red flag" complaints and conditions for your specialty.
- Rule out the worst thing first.
- Know the risk factors that call for screening tests.
- For diagnostic tests or referrals ordered, be able to answer "yes" to these three questions: Was it done? Are results on record? If abnormal, was the condition, symptoms, or finding followed up to a definitive diagnosis or rule-out?
- Revisit an unresolved problem until it is resolved.

- With every prescription, go through a script analysis: Side effects; Contraindications; Right patient, right drug, right dose, frequency, duration, and route; Interactions; Precautions; Transmittal legible.
- Have office systems and policies in place for ensuring follow-up.
- Audit charts for mistakes or omissions.
- Treat every medical opinion you give as if it were rendered during an office visit.
- If the patient doesn't really need something, don't order it.

Adapted with permission from Buppert, C. (2002). *Avoiding malpractice: 10 rules, 5 systems, 20 cases.* Annapolis, MD: Law Offices of Carolyn Buppert. (*www.buppert.com*)

if they are deemed to have made an error. Although not many documented cases cite APNs who have injured patients by wrongful actions, the question about whether APNs should be tried by the courts according to medical or nursing standards is important and needs to be clarified. It is incumbent upon APNs to set clear standards for practice that are based on clinical competency.

Privacy Issues

Health Insurance Portability and Accountability Act. The federal HIPAA became law in 1996. Legal requirements were finalized by the U.S. Department of Health and Human Services in 2002, and mandatory compliance with federal regulations was required by April 14, 2003. Visit *www.hhs.gov* to view the ruling and its latest amendments and documentation.

HIPAA mandates implementation of uniform minimum patient privacy standards within the states. The main goal of HIPAA is to protect the privacy of a patient's identifiable health information that is maintained or transmitted by health care providers and insurers. This information includes any information that would identify the patient, the patient's problem, the plan of care, or the way that care is paid for. The regulations for privacy established by HIPAA place a new level of legal responsibility on health providers including APNs. If APNs accept third-party reimbursement or transmit any health information in any form, they are required to comply with HIPAA regulations.

Providers and facilities need to adhere to several operating standards to comply with HIPAA regulation.

The rules state that providers are required to train all of their staff members regarding HIPAA rules and on-site procedures. Facilities and providers can design their own policies and procedures to meet the needs and scope of their practice, but the policies must adhere to all of the standards that are included in the operating standards of HIPAA (Buppert, 2003). Penalties are severe and include civil monetary fines and, in some cases, felony criminal penalties (*www.hhs.gov/ocr/hipaa/privacy.html* or *www.buppert.com*).

Telehealth and Telepractice

Federal and state legislation change daily as new and better ways to connect through virtual innovations emerge. Regulatory issues surrounding the changes in the way health care providers practice based on electronic capabilities will continue to challenge policymakers and APNs well into the twenty-first century. A model described as mutual recognition allows an APN licensed in a home state to be recognized as licensed in another state. The mutual recognition model would hold the APN accountable for the laws and regulations in the state where the APN provides the health care but would rely on the licensure from the home state (NCSBN, 2002b, 2007). Exemplar 21-2 illustrates an interstate practice.

It is interesting to note that new technologies and a system of "virtual practice," as described in Exemplar 21-2, focus attention on pervasive barriers that have plagued APNs for many years (Safriet, 1998). Although implementation of a mutual recognition system is well underway for RNs, the same type of recognition is lagging behind for APNs because of the lack of stability and standardization of

 EXEMPLAR 21-2 **Interstate Practice**

As a pediatric NP in an HMO practice, Alice has been co-managing, with Dr. Pete Johnson, the health care of 4-year-old David in North Carolina. Alice and Dr. Johnson have taken care of David since he was born. David has insulin-dependent diabetes mellitus. The child and his mother have grown to trust and depend on Alice's care for David over time. While on vacation at Disneyland in Florida, David develops diarrhea and vomiting. His mom chooses to e-mail Alice for advice rather than take David to an unfamiliar emergency room and provider. Alice responds back to the mother with directions about management of the gastroenteritis and potential changes in David's insulin dosage if needed. In providing this guidance, Alice has cared for David in a state other than the one in which she is licensed and recognized as an APN. A system of mutual regulatory recognition between Florida and North Carolina would allow for Alice to care for David using her North Carolina advanced practice nursing credentials. Without a system of mutual recognition between states, Alice would be practicing in Florida without a license.

APN, Advanced practice nurse; *HMO,* health maintenance organization; *NP,* nurse practitioner.

regulatory schemes from state to state with regard to scope of practice, prescriptive authority, and reimbursement. Although the dysfunctional aspects of this current regulatory climate for APN providers are problematic, they may provide a basis for positive change. Based on the Comprehensive Telehealth Act of 1997 and new legislation currently under consideration, physicians and other health care providers, including nurses, fall within the boundaries of electronic practice and all require regulation (see Chapter 7). Telehealth legislation could provide the catalyst needed to ensure that all states recognize and authorize key elements of scopes of practice for APNs (e.g., prescriptive authority).

A national strategy and the work of the NCSBN APRN Advisory Committee are underway to advance this issue. It will be important for APNs to carefully monitor the development of practice across state boundaries and work closely with advanced practice nursing associations to effect regulatory change that removes barriers and augments practice.

From a legal and regulatory standpoint, clear statutes are needed that offer broad practice standards to allow for mobility across state lines. This change will require national standards of practice as well as certification and credentialing requirements that can satisfy many different jurisdictions and advanced practice nursing specialty groups—not an easy task! These standards will require diligent collaboration among educators, state boards of nursing, the specialty professional associations, and all practicing APNs (AACN, 2007b; NCSBN, 2007). Part of the professional agenda that APNs must address is the need for accountability and responsibility for competence in practice. As a professional group, APNs must build strong national standards of practice, scope, and skills.

Safety and Cost-Containment Initiatives

Although more work is needed on the outcomes of advanced nursing, research has shown that APNs are safe and cost-effective alternatives to physician-based health care (see Chapter 25). This increased visibility makes it imperative that APNs monitor the competencies of their own practices and clearly understand the costs of providing care to patients.

Acts of Congress since the events of 9/11 and the current war in Iraq have cut federal programs for the poor. These factors plus the increase in older adults with chronic illness will augment the need for APNs even while funds to pay for this care are reduced, causing increased stress on underserved populations with health problems. Bodenheimer and Grumbach (2005) suggest several alternatives to painful cost controls that APNs can implement. Certainly, initiating simple policies such as the judicious use of supplies and prudent choice of diagnostic tests and procedures is a first step. Physician groups have moved quickly to fill the quality gap because they recognize the potential relationship of quality to payment issues, which is now a fact of practice through pay-for-performance programs. APNs need to understand the broad scope of pay-for-performance projects as a way to ensure both the quality and cost-effectiveness of their practice (Johnson, Harper, Hanson, & Dawson, 2007).

The Institute of Medicine's (IOM's) reports such as "To Err is Human" (1999) and "Crossing the Quality Chasm" (2001) focused on human factors that influence patient safety. In addition to a healing environment for patients, initiatives that enhance patient safety such as enlarging the safety knowledge base of caregivers and providing technological assistance in the form of PDAs, cell phones, and bedside Internet capabilities are receiving much attention. Funding opportunities are increasing for research, demonstration projects, and other activities to improve safety outcomes and decrease errors (Seifert & Hickman, 2005).

INFLUENCING THE REGULATORY PROCESS

APNs can directly influence the regulatory process in several ways, including using political strategies. At all levels, regulators are keen to find practicing APNs and advanced practice nursing educators who will take an active role in assisting them to develop and implement sound regulatory policies and procedures. The information explosion has brought the ability to communicate and connect with others at a moment's notice and makes it easier for APNs to directly influence the system. Chapters 9 and 22 provide in-depth discussions of skills needed for leadership and political advocacy. Following are some additional ways that novice and expert APNs can actively engage in any regulatory process that affects their practice.

For Novice or Any Advanced Practice Nurses

Participate in professional organizations, and get involved in regulatory activities such as educating lawmakers on APN issues, writing letters, and being part of campaign activities.

- Monitor current APN legislation and legislation that affects patients.

- Offer to participate on the test-writing committees for national certification examinations as item writers and/or reviewers.
- Respond to offers to review/edit/provide feedback on circulated draft regulatory policies that directly affect advanced practice nursing education and practice.

For Experienced or Expert Advanced Practice Nurses

- Seek out a gubernatorial appointment to the board of nursing or to the advanced practice committee that advises the board of nursing in your state.
- Seek membership as the APN or consumer member of the advisory council for either the state medical board or the state board of pharmacy.
- Seek appointment to CMS panels where Medicare and Medicaid provider issues are decided.
- Seek appointment to hospital privileging committees, and ensure that privileging materials are appropriate for APNs.
- Seek appointment on advisory committees and task forces that are advising the NCSBN and other regulatory and credentialing bodies.
- Offer testimony at state and national hearings at which proposed regulatory changes in advanced practice nursing regulation, prescriptive authority, and reimbursement schemes will be aired.

To accomplish these activities, APNs need to use research data—a powerful tool for shaping health policy (Hamric, 1998). By actively participating in the regulatory process, APNs ensure themselves of a strong voice in regulatory and credentialing processes. At the very least, it is incumbent upon the practicing APN to carefully monitor the process through websites and newsletters to stay informed.

CURRENT PRACTICE CLIMATE FOR ADVANCED PRACTICE NURSES

The current practice environment is a positive one for APNs in all venues. Population growth, new technologies and modes of delivery of services, and growing APN collaborative and autonomous practice are creating new opportunities for exploration. Change is noted in media awareness as APNs are finally approaching a juncture where their roles are visible and part of the health care agenda. However, the differences in education, certification, and individual scope-of-practice regulations from one advanced nursing specialty to another complicate issues for policymakers and regulators (Hanson & Hamric, 2002).

The climate within nursing practice is greatly affected by what is happening in other health care disciplines. For example, the move toward group practice rather than solo medical practice has implications for APNs (Deighton, 2003; Rentmeester & Kindig, 1994). The continued preference of physicians for specialty practice and away from primary care practice is important for APNs to consider. Within the nursing profession, although nursing school enrollments are increasing, serious shortages in nursing faculty have profound implications for advanced practice nursing education and practice over time (AACN, 2007a). Currently, the combined health care needs of an aging population and a period of economic retrenchment in health care have fostered mixed trends for advanced practice nursing. Community-based health care systems that rely on interdisciplinary health care team approaches have positively benefited from APN specialties but in some instances have heightened tensions between the disciplines of medicine and nursing. In addition, recent issues around physician malpractice and tort reform directly affect APNs and require constant vigilance (Deighton). Health policy issues surround APN practice parameters, reimbursement, and patients' abilities to choose APN providers. All of these environmental phenomena have an impact, either directly or indirectly, on the credentialing and regulatory policies that govern advanced practice nursing.

Nursing's earliest efforts to establish professional identity for APNs focused on advancing APN education as well as gaining independent authority for nursing practice and autonomy from the medical community. These efforts were critical to the evolution of advanced practice in nursing, and great strides have been made over the years (see Chapter 1). At the same time, complex health care systems and patient population needs that require a multifaceted approach to multiple problems demand effective interdisciplinary team-building. "Parallel play," or working side by side, is not enough; a true blending of nursing and medical models to offer a comprehensive health care approach is needed. Larger teams of health care providers must collaborate fully to provide comprehensive care to families and whole communities. To be able to move forward as full-fledged team members in cooperation with other interdisciplinary health care providers, APNs need to shift their practice ideal from one of complete autonomy to a truly collegial interdisciplinary paradigm. This change in practice stance is necessary and long overdue. Does any health care professional, including the most renowned vascular surgeon, practice with full independence? Or does this surgeon call upon the internist, the CNS, and the physical therapist to assist with providing competent and expert care? Will APNs do themselves a disservice if they maintain an isolationist stance based on barriers and professional turf issues? Have APNs reached a point in their evolution at which they can feel comfortable as peers and colleagues with providers in other disciplines? These are all questions that APNs struggle to answer.

It is important to understand that when APNs seek to change statutes and regulations, it is not because they see themselves as needing to practice in a vacuum of independence apart from the rest of the health care team. It is a hard fact that APNs must have authority over their own practices and the decisions they make about patient care. They must be able to defend their actions within the legal system based on nursing-driven standards and regulation. Only in this way can an APN move out of the darkness of being a shadow provider (Wilcox, 1995). Issues related to being a shadow provider are best exemplified by "incident to" billing by NPs using the physician's Medicare number. Advanced practice nursing care is invisible to regulators and reimbursers with this type of billing procedure. This is one example of the challenges for APNs across the nation who are working to clarify statutory policies within state boards of nursing. It may be that APNs will feel comfortable only when their position within the health care community is fully secure in all states, and this will require focused and coordinated political and legislative work related to credentialing and regulatory issues.

VISIONING FOR ADVANCED PRACTICE

Impressive strides have been made over time in the areas of credentialing and regulation of APNs. The health care provided by APNs has had far-reaching effects on members of society, and thus the evolution of advanced practice nursing in the United States is a source of pride to nurses. However, with success comes ever higher accountability and the need for more standardized ways to credential, certify, regulate, and sanction competent practice for a growing number of APNs. Forces within health care as well as needs within the regulatory and educational milieu

of advanced practice nursing have set the stage for a climate of progressive change. The movement toward the practice doctorate in nursing has implications for education, practice, and regulation. Advancing technologies, enhanced mobility of APNs across state lines, and diversity among state regulatory mechanisms have brought together APN leaders and stakeholders to craft a new vision for the future of APN education and practice.

The Doctor of Nursing Practice

Since the early 1960s, master's-level education for APNs has been an espoused standard for the preparation of APNs. The movement toward clinically based doctoral education for APNs will unfold over the next several years. It is clear that APNs will continue to be credentialed at the master's level during this intermediate period, so the move to the practice doctorate will not change credentialing in the foreseeable future. Although master's-level education for APNs will continue to be the standard for education and practice currently, new opportunities for doctoral education are designed to strengthen the research and systems leadership base of clinically prepared clinicians.

The National Council of State Boards of Nursing Vision for a New Regulatory Model for Advanced Practice Nurses

Over the past 4 years, the NCSBN has been working to craft a model for regulation that will be synchronized with other regulatory stakeholders such as accreditors, certifiers, and educators. Vast differences exist regarding rules and regulations and the credentialing process among states. State rankings analyzed by Lugo and colleagues (2007) using the 2006 Pearson Report data (Pearson, 2007) demonstrated wide variations, which indicates that in many states APNs are not able to reach their full potential to practice. This same study analyzed the data from the perspective of patient access to NPs and NP services, again finding wide variation from state to state (Lugo et al., Pearson).

The NCSBN's vision is to implement one national regulatory scheme that is most beneficial to patients and that allows APNs to be innovative and to meet patient needs (NCSBN, 2007). The NCSBN vision speaks to the recommendations of the Quality Chasm report (IOM, 2001) that suggested that various regulatory bodies need to develop forms of regulation that are most beneficial to patients. Several recommendations in this important report heightened the need for collaboration, transparency, evidence-based decision making, and information exchange, all of which support doctoral education for APNs (O'Sullivan, Carter, Marion, Pohl, & Werner, 2005).

Although there is consensus within the APN community that regulation for practice is needed for public safety and protection and that the public has a right to rely on the credentials of health care providers in making choices and decisions regarding health care (NCSBN, 2002a, 2002b), tension exists among stakeholders about how the process plays out for specific advanced practice nursing roles. The NCSBN and others believe that advanced practice nursing licensure should be designated in relatively broad categories of practice and not at the subspecialty level in order to ensure baseline competency and experience with common health care problems (NCSBN, 2007). On the other hand, APN specialty organizations are developing subspecialty examinations in areas such as oncology to deal with the burgeoning knowledge bases required for advanced-level subspecialty practice.

The Consensus Group Vision for Education and Practice

At about the same time that the NCSBN began its work (March 2004), stakeholders including leaders from the AACN (AACN, 2006c, 2007b), the NONPF, the NACNS, the AANA, the ACNM, and several APN certifying bodies, accreditors, and regulators began meeting to establish a process that would result in a consensus statement on the credentialing of APNs. The strength of this group and the NCSBN Vision Group is that both are coming close to reaching consensus about a regulatory model that will establish a collaborative model of education, certification accreditation, and licensure to strengthen and standardize the public and private regulatory processes that govern APN education and practice. The collaborative efforts of both of these groups confirm the importance of the APN leadership competency. Bold steps are being taken to meet current regulatory guidelines as well as to allow for the growth of future APN roles and specialties. Most important, this work paves the way for interstate mobility and telehealth conformations of the future.

FUTURE REGULATORY CHALLENGES FACING ADVANCED PRACTICE NURSES

Health professions reports disseminated over the past decade continue to recommend the need for generic benchmarks and standards for health care education and practice for all of the health professions (AACN, 2006b; Gelmon, O'Neil, Kimmey, & the Task Force on Accreditation of Health Professions Education, 1999; IOM, 2001; Johnson et al., 2007; NCSBN, 2007; O'Neil & the Pew Health Professions Commission, 1998). The Pew Commission recommended interdisciplinary competence for all health care professionals. More specifically, advanced practice nursing leaders were charged to "develop standard guidelines for advanced nursing practice and reinforce them with curriculum guidelines, examination requirements, and accreditation regulations" (O'Neil & the Pew Health Professions Commission).

The future requires that APNs promulgate clear, competency-based standards for both education and practice that will allow for growth and movement across state lines. It is important that APNs accomplish this work in preparation for the next phase—interdisciplinary credentialing and regulation based on defined patient outcomes—because this phenomenon is becoming a reality in some specialties such as advanced diabetes management (see Chapter 18). The wave of the future is to move to interdisciplinary regulation whereby, for example, family practice physicians, family NPs, and CNMs caring for menopausal women would all be held to a like standard of education and practice. Burroughs, Dmytrow, and Lewis (2007) and Safriet (2002) suggest that regulation for the health professions will require a new approach that dispels notions of exclusivity, exclusion, or independence from other disciplines. This move toward overarching regulation for the health professions, when and if it comes to pass, will require much higher levels of collaboration among the disciplines and specialties than now exist (see Chapter 10) and, most important, broad-based standards and regulations for advanced practice nursing. New models of regulation will require strong leadership and enhanced involvement by practicing APNs, as exemplified in the competencies put forth by the DNP *Essentials* (AACN, 2006a).

CONCLUSION

At no time has it been more important for APNs to understand and value the important relationships among groups that control the complex processes and systems that regulate practice. New models of health care and varying configurations of how APNs practice in interdisciplinary teams escalate the importance of regulatory considerations. The growth of telehealth and telepractice modalities makes the picture even more complex. APNs will need to provide leadership and clear direction to policymakers to ensure the development of broad-based practice standards that will satisfy state statutes and "fit" all of the advanced practice nursing specialties. The current work toward a new APN regulatory model that is reaching fruition places APNs in an excellent position of leadership for the future.

REFERENCES

Agency for Healthcare Research and Quality (AHRQ). (2007). *Clinical guidelines index.* Retrieved March 14, 2007, from www.ahrq.gov.

American Association of Colleges of Nursing (AACN). (1995). *Essentials of master's education for advanced practice nursing.* Washington, DC: Author.

American Association of Colleges of Nursing (AACN). (October 2006a). *The essentials of doctoral education for advanced nursing practice.* Washington, DC: Author. Retrieved March 14, 2007, from www.aacn.nche.edu/pdf/essentials.

American Association of Colleges of Nursing (AACN). (July 2006b). *DNP roadmap Task Force Report* (Draft). Washington, DC: Author.

American Association of Colleges of Nursing (AACN). (December 2006c). *Consensus statement on advanced practice registered nursing report of the APRN Consensus Work Group* (Draft). Washington, DC: Author.

American Association of Colleges of Nursing (AACN). (March 2007a). *Nursing shortage fact sheet.* Retrieved March 14, 2007, from http://aacn.nche.edu.

American Association of Colleges of Nursing (AACN). (2007b). *Consensus statement on advanced practice registered nursing report of the APRN Consensus Work Group* (Draft report, not for publication 2007). Washington, DC: Author.

American Association of Nurse Anesthetists (AANA). (2007). *Council on Accreditation of Nurse Anesthesia Educational Programs.* Retrieved March 17, 2007, from www.aana.com/credentialing.

American College of Nurse-Midwives (ACNM). (2006). *Position statement: Mandatory degree requirements for entry into midwifery practice.* Retrieved March 17, 2007, from www.acnm.org.

American Nurses Association (ANA). (1996). *Scope of practice and standards of advanced nursing practice.* Washington, DC: Author.

American Nurses Association (ANA). (2003). *Nursing's social policy statement* (2nd ed.). Washington, DC: Author.

Bodenheimer, T.S., & Grumbach, K. (2005). *Understanding health policy: A clinical approach* (4 ed., pp. 80-92). New York: McGraw-Hill/Appleton & Lange.

Buppert, C. (2002). *Avoiding malpractice. 10 rules, 5 systems, 20 cases.* Annapolis, MD: Law Offices of Carolyn Buppert.

Buppert, C. (2003). HIPAA patient privacy. *The American Journal for Nurse Practitioners, 7,* 17-22.

Buppert, C. (2004). *Nurse practitioner's business practice and legal guide* (2nd ed.). Boston: Jones & Bartlett.

Burroughs, R., Dmytrow, B., & Lewis, H. (2007). Trends in nurse practitioner professional liability: An analysis of claims with risk management recommendations. *Journal of Nursing Law, 11*(1), 53-60.

Cady, R.F. (2003). *The advanced practice nurse's legal handbook.* Baltimore: Lippincott-Williams & Wilkins.

Commission on Collegiate Nursing Education (CCNE). (1998). *Procedures for accreditation of baccalaureate and graduate nursing education programs.* Washington, DC: Author.

Deighton, B. (February 28, 2003). *The effect of the medical liability insurance crisis on physician supply and access to medical care.* Presented at the Georgia Health Strategies Council Meeting. Atlanta: Georgia Board for Physician Workforce.

Fang, D., Wisniewski, S.W., & Bednash, G.D. (2007). *2006-2007 Enrollment and graduations in baccalaureate and graduate programs in nursing.* Washington, DC: American Association of Colleges of Nursing.

Gelmon, S.B., O'Neil, E.H., Kimmey, J.R., & the Task Force on Accreditation of Health Professions Education. (1999). *Strategies for change and improvement: The report of the Task Force on Accreditation of Health Professions Education.* San Francisco: Center for the Health Professions, University of California at San Francisco.

Hamric, A.B. (1998). Using research to influence the regulatory process. *Advanced Practice Nursing Quarterly, 4,* 44-50.

Hamric, A.B. (2005). A definition of advanced practice nursing. In A.B. Hamric, J.A. Spross, & C.M. Hanson (Eds.), *Advanced practice nursing: An integrative approach* (pp. 85-108). Philadelphia: Saunders.

Hanson, C.M. (1998). Regulatory issues will lead advanced practice nursing challenges into the new millennium. *Advanced Practice Nursing Quarterly, 4,* v-vi.

Hanson, C.M., & Hamric, A.B. (2002). Reflections on the continuing evolution of advanced practiced nursing. *Nursing Outlook, 51*(5), 203-211.

Hodnicki, D.R. (1998). Advanced practice nursing certification: Where do we go from here? *Advanced Practice Nursing Quarterly, 4,* 34-43.

Huffstutler, S., Wyatt, T., & Wright, C.P. (2002). The use of handheld technology in nursing education. *Nurse Educator, 27,* 271-275.

Institute of Medicine (IOM), Committee on Quality of Healthcare in America. (1999). Kohn, L.T., Corrigan, J.M., & Donaldson, M.S. (Eds.). *To err is human: Building a safer health system.* Washington, DC: National Academies Press.

Institute of Medicine (IOM), Committee on Quality of Healthcare in America. (2001). *Crossing the quality chasm: A new health system for the 21st century.* Washington, DC: National Academies Press.

Johnson, J., Harper, D., Hanson, C., & Dawson, E. (2007). Forging a quality agenda, *American Journal of Nurse Practitioners, 11*(10), 10-19.

Klein, T. (2006). A new model for healthcare delivery. Working in a retail clinic: What nurse practitioners need to ask. *Medscape,*

Topics in Advanced Practice Nursing. Retrieved October 2, 2006, from www.medscape.com/article#544422_1.

Letz, K. (2002). *Business essentials for nurse practitioners: Essential knowledge for building your practice.* Fort Wayne, IN: Previcare Inc.

Lugo, N.R., O'Grady, E., Hodnicki, D, & Hanson, C. (2007). Ranking state NP regulation: Practice environment and consumer healthcare choice. *American Journal for Nurse Practitioners, 11*(4), 8-24.

National Association of Clinical Nurse Specialists (NACNS). (2004). *Statement on clinical nurse specialist practice and education.* Harrisburg, PA: Author.

National Council of State Boards of Nursing (NCSBN). (2002a). *Uniform advanced practice registered nurse licensure/practice requirements.* Chicago: Author.

National Council of State Boards of Nursing (NCSBN). (2002b). *Regulation of advanced practice nursing: 2002 national council of state boards of nursing position paper* (pp. 1-8). Chicago: Author.

National Council of State Boards of Nursing (NCSBN). (January 28, 2007). *A vision for the future regulation of advanced practice nursing* (Draft). Retrieved February 23, 2007, from www.ncsbn.org.

National Organization of Nurse Practitioner Faculties (NONPF), Practice Doctorate Task Force. (2003). The practice doctorate in nursing: Future or fringe. *Topics in Advanced Practice Nursing eJournal, 3*(2).

National Organization of Nurse Practitioner Faculties (NONPF), National Panel for NP Practice Doctorate Competencies. (2006). *Practice doctorate nurse practitioner entry level competencies.* Washington, DC. Retrieved June 14, 2007, from www.nonpf.org/NONPF2005/PracticeDoctorateResourceCenter/PDresource.htm.

National Task Force on Quality Nurse Practitioner Education. (1997). *Criteria for evaluation of nurse practitioner programs.* Washington, DC: Author.

National Task Force on Quality Nurse Practitioner Education. (2002). *Criteria for evaluation of nurse practitioner programs.* Washington, DC: Author.

O'Neil, E.H., & the Pew Health Professions Commission. (1998). *Recreating health professional practice for a new century.* San Francisco: Pew Health Professions Commission.

O'Sullivan, A., Carter, M., Marion, L., Pohl, J., & Werner, K. (2005). Moving forward together: The practice doctorate in nursing. *Online Journal of Issues in Nursing, 10*(3), Manuscript #4. Retrieved August 21, 2006, from www.nursingworld.org/OJIN.

Pearson, L. (2007). The Pearson Report: A national overview of NP legislation and health care issues. *American Journal for Nurse Practitioners, 11*(2), 10-99.

Rentmeester, K., & Kindig, D.A. (1994). *Physician supply by specialty in managed care organizations.* University of Wisconsin—Madison: School of Medicine.

Reel, S.J., & Abraham, I.L. (2007). *Business and legal essentials for nurse practitioners: From negotiating your first job through owning a practice.* St. Louis: Mosby.

Safriet, B. (1992). Health care dollars and regulatory sense: The role of advanced practice nursing. *Yale Journal of Regulation, 9,* 417-487.

Safriet, B. (1998). Still spending dollars, still searching for sense: Advanced practice nursing in an era of regulatory and economic turmoil. *Advanced Practice Nursing Quarterly, 4,* 24-33.

Safriet, B. (2002). Closing the gap between can and may in health care providers' scopes of practice: A primer for policymakers. *Yale Journal of Regulation, 19,* 301-334.

Seifert, P.C., & Hickman, D.S. (March 21, 2005). *Medscape, Topics in Advanced Practice Nursing eJournal, 5*(1). Retrieved April 9, 2007, from www.medscape.com.

Styles, M.M. (1998). An international perspective: APN credentialing. *Advanced Practice Nursing Quarterly, 4,* 1-5.

Summers, L., & Williams, D. (2003). Credentialing certified nurse-midwives and certified midwives. *Synergy, May-June,* 30-34.

Wilcox, P. (April 1995). *Advanced practice model response to needs of women at risk for female malignancies.* Abstract presented at the Oncology Nurses Society national conference, Anaheim, CA.

CHAPTER 22

Health Policy Issues in Changing Environments

Eileen T. O'Grady • Jean E. Johnson

INTRODUCTION

The purposes of this chapter are to (1) familiarize the advanced practice nurse (APN) with the policy process in order to help APNs be more effective in influencing policymakers; (2) provide information about specific programs that are a continual focus of policymaking; and (3) demonstrate policy in action through exemplars.

Powerful APN clinical experiences, when effectively communicated by APNs, will serve to deepen policymakers' understanding of the issues facing nurse providers and their patients. APN practice experiences offer poignant stories that enlighten policy issues by providing a human context while bringing nursing's value to the health policy arena. Most APNs in practice today have experienced the effects of ill-conceived policies that lead to needless poor health care. This practice experience, coupled with the ability to analyze the policy process, provides a strong foundation to propel APNs into politically competent action.

THE POLICY PROCESS

Policy as Historical Core Function in Nursing

Florence Nightingale spent much of her career in the halls of Parliament promoting policy change to improve quality, dignity, and equity, first for the Crimean War soldiers and later for the poor of London. Her 3 years of clinical practice gave her clinical expertise and credibility to assume the role of policymaker. She embraced that role because of her high degree of internal distress and concern about needless suffering and premature death of her patients. Empowered by her clinical practice during the Crimean War, she used data she collected to persuade Parliament to make needed military and civic law reforms that promoted health. In 1858, Nightingale became the first woman elected as a member of the Royal Statistical Society, and she later became an honorary member of the American Statistical Association (Gill & Gill, 2005). Her work and prestige were Victorian Era validations of the importance of using evidence to inform policy. Nightingale's activism presaged the APN role as patient advocate and policy shaper. She leveraged statistics and clinical expertise to become an effective advocate in influencing policy. She expected nurses to have a high degree of social interest and to be involved in the policymaking process.

This historic covenant with the public must be strengthened. APNs must deepen their commitment to and become masterful at critiquing, formulating, and influencing policies that interfere with human wholeness and health. We must substantively weave policy into the core APN role so that their experiences move APNs to become leaders and advocates for change.

Overview of the Health Policy Process: Politics Versus Policy

All policy involves decisions that influence the life of citizens on a daily basis. Longest (2006) defines health policy as the authoritative decisions pertaining to health or health care, made in the legislative, executive, or judicial branches of government, that are intended to direct or influence the actions, behaviors, or decisions of citizens.

Although there are many definitions of "policy" and "politics," *policy* generally refers to decisions resulting in a law or regulation. *Politics* refers to power relationships. It is the responsibility of a multitude of policymakers, whether mayors, county supervisors, government employees, legislators, governors, or presidents, to make health policy. Overall responsibility generally places authority with the legislative branch to craft laws, the executive branch to craft rules to implement the laws, and the judicial branch to interpret conflicts between the spheres of government or between citizens and a public or private entity. The U.S. government plays a substantial role in setting health policy, although to a far lesser degree than Canada or Britain, which have integrated, centralized, government-run health care systems. The U.S. government is a provider of health services via the prison system and Department of Veterans Affairs. However, health care delivery is still largely under private sector control, making U.S. health policy development incremental, fragmented, and decentralized.

Politics. Politics introduces non-rational, divisive, and self-interested approaches to policymaking, often along ideological lines. Any political maneuvering to enhance one's power or status within a group may be described as "politics." Politics is largely associated with a struggle for ascendancy among groups having different priorities and power relationships. Preferences and interests of stakeholders and political bargaining (favor swapping) are important and extremely influential political factors that overlie the policymaking process. The self-interest paradigm suggests that human motives in political arenas do not differ from those in the private marketplace. This behavioral assumption implies that it is rational for people and organizations to use the power of government to achieve what they cannot on their own. Ideally, elected officials seek office to serve the public interest, not their own. However, to be successful in the electoral process, they need electoral support through financial contributions, rendering them beholden to fundraising (Feldstein, 2006). Highly

politicized decisions may often create outcomes that have little to do with efficient use of scarce resources and what is best for the general public. These forces, which may or may not be based on evidence, contribute to the lack of coordination among health policies in the United States, making policy formulation highly complex and exceedingly interesting.

Policy Framework. Longest (2006) has conceptualized policymaking as an interdependent process that is depicted in Figure 22-1. The Longest Public Policy Process Model defines a policy formulation phase, implementation phase, and modification phase. This has immense utility for nursing because it amplifies the incremental and cyclical nature of policymaking, two of the most important features of the U.S. health policymaking process. Essentially, all health policy decisions are subject to modification because policymaking in the United States involves making decisions that are revisited when circumstances shift. Our system is not designed for big, bold reform. Rather, it considers intended or unintended consequences of existing policy and tweaks changes (Longest).

Federalism. To effectively influence policy, it is important to understand the process and the broad issues that influence health policy decisions, including

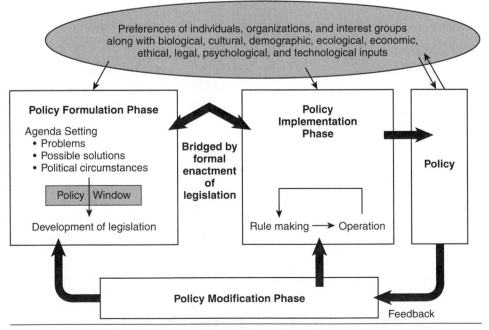

FIGURE **22-1: The Longest Public Policy Process Model.**

the tensions between the states and the federal government. The locus of responsibility between the states and the federal government is highly relevant to most health care programs such as Medicare, Medicaid, the State Children's Health Insurance Plan (SCHIP), and the creation of an interoperable health information technology system. Federalism is the allocation of "governing" responsibility between the states and federal government. The states and federal government have a complex relationship governing health policy, which explains a large part of our chaotic and fragmented approach to health care in place today.

The Constitution unambiguously gives the federal government absolute power to preempt state laws when it chooses to do so. However, the states are also granted unfettered authority such as regulation of health care plans (Litman & Robins, 1997). Ambiguity between state and federal authority allows states to experiment with policy solutions. The "states-as-learning-lab" concept has grown out of local health policy problems and enables states to experiment with innovative policy solutions that could not be done on a national level. Moreover, states have local health care problems, requiring local, flexible, and humane solutions. Many federal health policy decisions are devolving decision making to the states, as evidenced by the increase in Medicaid waivers and block grants. (A block grant is a large sum of money granted by the federal government to a state with only general provisions as to the way it is to be spent, contrasted with a categorical grant, which has more strict and specific provisions.) The most effective and innovative policy solutions are recognized by the National Governors Association Center for Best Practices, a clearinghouse for innovative policy solutions. Numerous state-based policies that are building an evidence base for nursing are featured on the Center's website *(www.nga.org)*. One example is the creation of the Michigan Nursing Corps to expand nursing school enrollments as a local response to the nursing shortage (National Governors Association, 2007). Because much of health care is experienced at the local level, APNs must be aware of the overlapping state and federal spheres of government and the tension between their authorities.

Incrementalism. While the policymaking process is a continuous, interrelated cycle, most efforts to change policy stem from the negative effects of an existing policy. The modification phase creates a feedback loop to the agenda-setting process. This concept of continuous, often modest modification of existing polices is known as *incrementalism*. Major

reforms of health policy are rarely seen, with the exception of Medicare, Medicaid, and the SCHIP. Minor changes of existing policies play out slowly over time and are therefore more predictable. Incrementalism promotes stability and stakeholder compromise. A good example of incrementalism is the gradual increase in federal spending for biomedical research from $300 in 1887 to more than $28 billion in 2007 going to the National Institutes of Health's (NIH's) 27 institutes and centers. Within that structure, the National Center for Nursing Research (NCNR) was created in 1985 by a congressional override of a presidential veto because of the influence of strong nurse leaders. In 1993, the NCNR was elevated to the Institute for Nursing Research with funding levels currently exceeding $138 million.

Agenda Setting. Agenda setting is a major component of the Longest policy formulation phase. With so many health policy problems in this country, why do some problems get attention while others languish at the bottom of the policy agenda for decades? Kingdon (1995) conceptualized an "open policy window" with three conditions streaming through the open window at once. First, the problem must come to the attention of the policymaker; second, it must have a menu of possible policy solutions that have the potential to actually solve the problem; and third, it must have the right political circumstances. If all three of these conditions occur simultaneously, the policy window opens and progress can be made on the issue. Conversely, once shut, this policy window (opportunity) may never open again.

Policy problems come to the attention of policymakers, either singly or collectively, through multiple ways, including constituents, litigation, research findings, market forces, fiscal environment, crisis, special interest groups, and the media. Wakefield (2004) identified nine policy dynamics particular to agenda setting. Each dynamic has one or more "accelerators" that drive agenda setting or trigger policymakers to take action on an issue (Table 22-1). The political circumstances that push problems onto the agenda must have a high degree of public importance and a low degree of stakeholder conflict surrounding the policy solution. If there is a great deal of stakeholder disagreement, competing proposals may be put forth, weakening the likelihood that the problem will be addressed. Strong health services research can provide the evidence base to help policymakers specify and therefore accelerate agenda setting (Longest, 2006).

Table 22-1 AGENDA-SETTING DYNAMICS

Dynamic	Activator	Examples
Constituents	The constituent can have enormous impact in agenda setting. When members of Congress learn from their constituents of deeply poignant tragedies that could have been prevented or lessened, they are moved to introduce legislation.	An automobile accident in a remote area killed three members of a family and seriously injured two. A Senator knew the family, which prompted introduction of the Wakefield Act, designed to improve pediatric emergency response in rural areas and to honor the family.
Litigation	Court decisions play an increasingly prominent role in setting health policy.	Medical malpractice decisions force states to consider new approaches to malpractice reform including the role of apology in malpractice litigation, mediation, health courts, and no-fault models.
Research findings	Health services research and IOM reports are particularly influential in clarifying issues and offering a menu of policy solutions. This policy impact is even more influential when the research findings are picked up by the lay media.	Early promising results from a CMS demonstration project on P4P accelerate development of policies that align payment incentives with quality health care.
Market forces	The fractured health care delivery system creates opportunities for unique and highly profitable businesses.	Rapid expansion of convenient care clinics appeals to both higher-income consumers willing to pay for convenience and uninsured consumers who have few alternatives. Promotes some physician groups to oppose this new model of care by emphasizing the importance of a "medical home."
Fiscal environment	Budget decisions vary based on whether the government is in deficit vs. surplus spending. Deficit spending restricts budgets to pay-as-you-go policy.	Deficit financing forces budgetary restrictions and demands paying for expenditures with funds that are made available as the program is in progress. The HRSA budget, which funds Title VIII nursing education grants, gets cut during a deficit period.
Special interest groups	HIV epidemic evolves from a rapidly progressive, acute, infectious terminal illness to a chronic illness, requiring a primary care and social services infrastructure.	Community Aids National Network, a unique consortium of pharmaceutical companies and AIDS advocates, shifted the Ryan White Care Act from an emergency funding program for communities overburdened by HIV/AIDS to modern, prevention-based programs (including antiretroviral therapy) and support services that enhance access to care. Strategies included highly effective, focused public advocacy campaigns directed at Congress and the public. (www.tiicann.org)
Crisis	Crisis can promote rapid-response policy change, usually centered on quality and access.	A hild on Medicaid dies as a result of an infection in an abscessed tooth that spread to his brain. His mother was unable to gain access to a dentist. Crisis prompts Medicaid agency to expand dental coverage.

AIDS, Acquired immunodeficiency syndrome; *CMS*, Centers for Medicare & Medicaid Services; *HIV*, human immunodeficiency virus; *HRSA*, Health Resources and Services Administration; *IOM*, Institute of Medicine; *P4P*, pay-for-performance; *VA*, Department of Veterans Affairs.

Table 22-1 AGENDA-SETTING DYNAMICS—CONT'D

Dynamic	Activator	Examples
Political ideology	The majority party (Democrats vs. Republicans) has a large impact on agenda setting.	A newly installed Democratic-controlled Congress prompts the introduction of many bills addressing stem cell research, which will, if passed, likely be vetoed by a Republican president.
Media	Lay press reporting on a health policy issue or crisis often compels policymakers to take action.	Major news outlet reports on deplorable outpatient care and facilities at Walter Reed Medical center for wounded Iraqi war veterans. Within days, congressional hearings on veterans' health care are held and scores of bills are introduced to improve veterans' care. Leaders are fired at the VA, and the story is headline news for weeks, prompting immediate physical plant and health care quality improvements

The Federal Budget Cycle. The budget process begins with the President's State of the Union address before the first Monday in February. The President's address highlights the Executive Branch's spending priorities for the upcoming fiscal year. The President's budget guides the activities of the Office of Management and Budget (OMB) staff, appointed by the President, to (1) create the budget; (2) communicate to Congress the President's overall federal fiscal policy; and (3) propose very specific spending recommendations for individual federal programs. The OMB ensures that all federal agency priorities, reports, testimony, and rules are consistent with the President's priorities. This budget is merely a suggestion until acted on by Congress. In February and March of each year, the House and Senate budget committees hold hearings on the proposed budget, and these joint conference committees hammer out differences. On April 15, Congress passes a House/Senate budget resolution, and no other spending bill can be considered until the budget resolution is adopted. Finally, the House and Senate appropriate or subdivide their allocations among the 13 appropriations subcommittees that have jurisdiction over specific spending legislation. The budget resolution is not an ordinary bill and therefore does not go to the President for his or her signature or veto. It requires only a majority vote to pass and is one of the few pieces of legislation that cannot be filibustered in the Senate.

If the appropriations process is not completed by October 1, then Congress must adopt a continuing resolution to provide stop-gap funding (Congressional Research Service, 2007). The federal budget process is not linear, in part because of the influence of stakeholders. Throughout the process, lobbyists and interest groups are vying to either keep their funding cycle level or increase it, depending on the fiscal and political circumstances.

The three largest entitlement programs (defined as federal programs that guarantee a certain level of benefits to citizens who meet the requirements set by law) are Medicare, Medicaid, and Social Security. These three entitlement programs consume two thirds of federal spending and do not go through the appropriations process because they are permanently enacted. All programs that fall into "discretionary" or "appropriated" spending must first be *authorized* by Congress. Once programs are authorized through legislation, Congress will then assign a funding amount, an entirely different procedure, called *appropriations* or spending legislation. All discretionary programs, such as the Nurse Reinvestment Act, must have their funding renewed each year to continue operating, and almost all health programs (other than Medicare and Medicaid) are discretionary. Altogether, discretionary programs make up one third of all federal spending and the President's budget spells out how much funding he or she recommends for each discretionary program.

Policy Formulation: How a Bill Becomes a Law

Figure 22-2 depicts a linear process for federal legislation; however, it is more of a choreography than a stepwise process. Only when each of the steps in the process is completed, can legislation be passed. Therefore very few legislative proposals introduced are ever enacted. The process begins with the introduction of a bill that is the result of legislators trying to address a policy problem. Getting involved in the process or policy solution at the conceptual phase, rather than responding to legislation already crafted, is extremely important because it maximizes influence. Any member of Congress can introduce legislation, which gets assigned a number and is posted with its status and list of co-sponsors at *thomas.loc.gov*. The legislation then gets referred to the committee of jurisdiction, referred to more than one committee, or split so that parts are sent to different committees.

Congressional Committees. Over 200 congressional committees and subcommittees are functionally structured to gather information; compare and evaluate highly specific legislative alternatives; identify policy problems and propose solutions; select, determine, and report measures for full chamber consideration; monitor executive branch performance (oversight); and investigate allegations of wrongdoing. Committee membership enables members of Congress to develop specialized knowledge of the matters under their jurisdiction. More than 13 committees and subcommittees have jurisdiction over health care. Woodrow Wilson said in 1885, "Congress in its committee rooms is Congress at work," which still rings true today (Wilson, 1913).

The first "action" that a committee can perform on a piece of legislation is to not take any action, which is equivalent to "killing it." If the committee chair chooses to act on the legislation, the federal agency that would be impacted by the legislation is queried for its opinions on the bill's merit. The bill is assigned to a subcommittee, and hearings may be held. Politically astute organizations will have developed relationships with committee staffers and seek invitations to testify before the committee. It is critical that the testimony has accurate data, is not purely

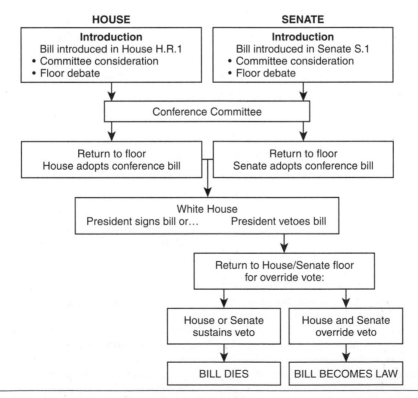

FIGURE **22-2:** The path of federal legislation. *H.R.1.,* House of Representatives introduced; *S.1.,* Senate introduced.

self-serving, and attempts to solve the problem at hand. Subcommittees report their findings to the full committee, who vote. The full committee will hold a "mark-up" session during which it will make revisions and additions. The House and Senate chambers must approve, change, or reject all committee amendments before conducting a final passage vote.

House or Senate Floor Action. The legislation is sent back to the whole House or Senate chamber for a vote, and if passed, it is then sent to the other chamber unless that chamber already has a similar measure under consideration. If either chamber does not pass the bill, then it dies. If the House and Senate pass the same bill, then it is sent to the President. If the House and Senate pass a different bill, which is more often the case, the bill goes to a conference committee. Members from the Senate and House form a conference committee and meet to work out the differences, with each chamber trying to maintain its version of the bill. Once the conference committee reaches a compromise, it prepares a written conference report, which is submitted to each chamber. The conference report must be approved by both the House and the Senate.

Presidential Action. A bill becomes law if signed by the President or if not signed within 10 days and Congress is in session. If Congress adjourns before the 10 days and the President has not signed the bill, then it does not become law (pocket veto). If the President vetoes the bill, it is sent back to Congress with a note listing his or her reasons. The chamber that originated the legislation can attempt to override the veto by a vote of two thirds of those present. If the veto of the bill is overridden in both chambers, then it becomes law. Once a bill is signed by the President or his or her veto is overridden by both houses, it becomes a law and is assigned an official number with *PL* (Public Law) preceding it.

The Interpretive Function of Rulemaking: Policy Implementation

Once the bill becomes public law, the legislative activities shift to policy implementation in the executive branch. Rulemaking launches the formal regulations process to fully operationalize what has been formulated by Congress. The executive agency responsible for implementing the law must make clear who is responsible for implementation and how it will be financed. The operational decisions are an important dimension of health policy and can have

an enormous impact on health care. Regulations can be added, deleted, or modified at any time, making rulemaking a continuous process. Each of the federal agencies has a number of public advisory bodies that inform the agency on rulemaking and policy. Serving on advisory bodies and engaging in the rulemaking process are key venues for APNs to influence policy.

Congressional Advisory Bodies. Congress created alternative bodies outside of the executive branch to assist with complex, high-conflict rulemaking or oversight. By way of example, Medicare is essentially undergoing constant rulemaking revision, so Congress created the Medicare Payment Advisory Commission (MedPAC), a freestanding advisory body to Congress on Medicare policy. Congress created a powerful tool for itself by creating the Government Accountability Office and Congressional Budget Office. Their sole purposes are to help Congress provide congressional oversight through detailed reports

Policy Modification. Almost every policy stems from a history of intended and unintended consequences, learned only through implementation of the policy. Appropriate policies at one time become highly inappropriate as time passes and economic, social, demographic, and commercial circumstances shift. Policy consequences are the reason that stakeholders and policymakers seek to continually modify policy. These policy changes can be driven by stakeholders when a policy negatively impacts a group or by members of Congress or rulemakers when policy does not meet its objective. Our system is based on continuous policy modification of a few policies initiated earlier. Understanding the process of policy modification or amendment of earlier polices is the key to mastering political competency.

Role of Public Comment. Public laws do not contain specific language about how the policy or program is to be carried out. The executive branch agency, usually the Department of Health & Human Services (DHHS) for health-related issues, must publish its proposed rules in the daily publication of the *Federal Register* seeking public comment. The public comment opportunity is usually limited to 60 days; however, stakeholder groups can exert an enormous degree of influence in the rulemaking process during this limited time period. APN organizations can powerfully influence rulemaking as evidenced by the American College of Nurse Practitioners in Exemplar 22-1.

EXEMPLAR 22-1   Focused Leadership for Medicare Reimbursement:
American College of Nurse Practitioners' Margaret Koehler, MSN, CRNP

Prior to 1997, federal law required Medicare and state Medicaid programs to cover health care services provided only by *some* APNs, including pediatric nurse practitioners, family nurse practitioners, and certified nurse midwives who practiced only in underserved or rural settings. No other APNs were authorized to receive payment unless the state chose to reimburse them. Essentially, many APNs had to link their services to physician services in order to receive Medicare reimbursement, rendering APN care invisible.

ACTIVATING THE GRASSROOTS
In 1997, Margie Koehler, President of the Maryland Nurse Practitioner Association and an NP at a Veterans Administration (VA) hospital in Baltimore saw a political window of opportunity. Within the context of the ACNP, Koehler built momentum to expand Medicare reimbursement to all APNs in all geographical settings. It became clear to Koehler that in order to expand the authorization for APN Medicare payment, bipartisan congressional support was needed, because only Democratic lawmakers in the House and Senate were supporting this idea at the time. With the help of professional lobbyists, Republican Senators became pivotal co-signers needed to pass legislation. To get the support of the Republican Senators, the grassroots APNs were activated nationally. Koehler identified and contacted each of the APN leaders who lived in the Senators' home states. She encouraged each of them to set up a meeting with their Senator in his or her state. She also provided talking points linked to evidence of access problems in each state, customizing the importance of the legislation to combat arguments against the legislation. She heavily coached the grassroots APNs, some of whom had never before approached an elected official, and encouraged them to get their patients to write letters to those Senators. Within 4 months, she raised $33,000 to help fund ACNP's bipartisan lobby team. She built coalitions across states and worked with many national nursing associations. Within 1 year, Medicare payment restrictions on APN services and practice settings were removed. Koehler had spearheaded a highly strategic and focused grassroots campaign that resulted in passage of the Health Care Incentive Act as part of the BBA of 1997.

INFLUENCING RULEMAKING
Once the legislation moved into the rulemaking phase, the CMS called for Public Comment on how to define and implement the BBA. Koehler again activated the large NP grassroots network she had developed to write letters detailing how APNs should be defined and qualified to bill Medicare. The CMS received scores of letters; portions of the letter from the ACNP were quoted and used as an evidence source in the published *Federal Register* final rules. Had this critical phase of policy development not been addressed by the APN community, any number of rules that adversely affect APNs and their patients could have been crafted. Today, APNs generally receive direct Medicare reimbursement for their services regardless of the setting.

LESSONS LEARNED
According to Koehler, the crucial factor in getting this legislation passed was the personal connection to APNs. She describes both encouraging and empowering techniques to engage practicing APNs in getting their Senators to support this legislation (ACNP, 2007). To underscore how important their contribution was in moving this legislation forward, she made personal follow-up calls with each state APN leader after he or she met elected officials. Essentially, she built momentum and obtained enormous buy-in from state APN leaders by way of personal relationship-building. This kind of focused energy can create a policy "win" for APNs, and Koehler demonstrated far-reaching political competence throughout.

Koehler has taken what she learned in this experience and applies it to her role in the VA Hospital in Baltimore. The skill set she learned from moving the Medicare legislation forward is applicable in all aspects of her professional life. She is skillful in knowing how to influence change in systems large and small by developing strategic partners, garnering buy-in, gaining the respect and credibility of those she is trying to influence, and acclimating to the role of change leader. This concept of leveraging change at the policy level requires strong leadership and relationship-building skills. To honor Koehler's effective leadership skills, the ACNP (2007) created an "Annual Margie Koehler Legislative Advocacy Award" for an APN who demonstrates strong policy leadership skills.

ACNP, American College of Nurse Practitioners; *APN,* advanced practice nurse; *BBA,* Balanced Budget Act; *CMS,* Centers for Medicare & Medicaid Services; *NP,* nurse practitioner.

CURRENT AND EMERGING HEALTH POLICY ISSUES RELEVANT TO ADVANCED PRACTICE NURSES: COST, QUALITY, AND ACCESS

Policy issues generally fall within the broad context of cost, quality, and access. The Cost-Quality-Access Schema (Figure 22-3) provides a context for health policy issues, whether at the international, national, state, local, community, institutional, or corporate level. All health policy issues and policy solutions can be framed in terms of increasing access to health care, increasing health care quality, or decreasing health care costs. These principal health policy drivers overlap and are inherently interdependent—a shift in one inevitably impacts the others. For example, the emphasis on lowering costs with managed care and capitation in the 1990s gave way to the recent emphasis on quality initiatives such as pay-for-performance (P4P). Cost, quality, and access issues are not tangential problems to our health care dilemma; they *are* the dilemma.

Health Care Costs

Costs of health care have risen faster than any other segment of our economy, and health care costs are consuming a greater proportion of the overall federal budget than ever before. The cost of health care is an important national issue because every dollar spent on health care is a dollar less spent on education, transportation, housing, food, and other essentials. Health care costs continue to increase as a percent of gross domestic product (GDP). In 1960, the United States spent approximately 5.2% of the GDP on health care, and this rate has risen steadily to 16% of the GDP in 2007 (Centers for Medicare & Medicaid Services [CMS] & Office of the Actuary, National Health Statistics Group, 2006). By 2016, it is estimated that health care will cost over $4.1 trillion and be nearly 20% of the GDP, representing $1 of every $5 spent in the United States (Poisal et al., 2007). On a per capita basis, health care spending is projected to be $12,782 per person in 2016 compared with $7,498 per person in 2006 (Heffler et al., 2005; Poisal et al.). Of the $2.1 trillion spent on health care in 2006, the federal, state, and local governments spent about $750 billion, representing 45% of the total costs. Because of the large investment, government has a keen interest in controlling costs and ensuring that the most efficient and effective care is delivered. See Figure 22-4 for expenditures on health care by source of funds. Figure 22-5 shows health care costs by service sector (National Center for Health Statistics, 2006).

The United States spends more than twice the portion of GDP than other major industrialized countries. When compared with other industrialized nations, the United States ranked number-one in health care costs and ranked lowest for healthy life expectancy, infant mortality, nursing home care, uninsured access to health care, and electronic information systems (Commonwealth Fund, 2007; World Health Organization [WHO], 2006). With regard to high cost and low health status, the United States is an astonishing outlier (Spitz & Abramson, 2005). These costs are rising because of exploding population growth; social, governmental, and business factors; and poor policies.

Factors Offsetting Cost

Cultural Context. Some of the costs are related to an American culture of prolonging life, no matter what the cost. The public is universally supportive of financing the health research enterprise through the NIH, making it politically unpalatable for politicians to rein in spending in this domain. Generally, Americans have a deep fascination with innovative technology, which creates demands for health technology that may carry great costs. We have a strong emphasis on individual autonomy that contributes to individuals wanting as much health care as possible.

Demographic Changes. The "baby boomer" generation has a level of income and living standard higher than previous generations and higher standards

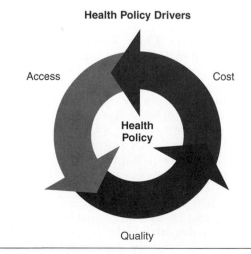

Health Policy Drivers

Access

Cost

Health Policy

Quality

FIGURE **22-3:** Cost-Quality-Access Schema.

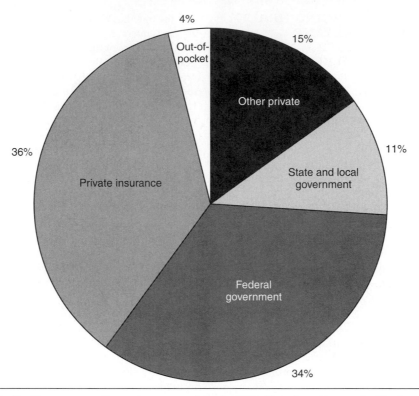

FIGURE 22-4: Health care expenditures by source of funds, 2004. (Data from Centers for Medicare & Medicaid Services, Office of the Actuary, National Health Statistics Group, National Health Accounts, *National health expenditures, 2006.*)

and expectations of health systems. As this generation becomes eligible for Medicare, more demands on the health care system aimed at improved quality of life are expected (Population Resource Center, 2008). Moreover, life expectancy is now at 78 years, and the fastest growing segment of the population is older than 85 years, most of whom have some form of chronic illness or disability (U.S. Department of Commerce, 2006). The ever-growing numbers of Americans who are overweight or obese and have lifestyles that bring on chronic illnesses are a major contributor to rising costs.

Technology. Unchecked and unplanned advances in technology have caused health care costs to soar in every health care sector. The profit potential for drug and device manufacturers is enormous, creating powerful incentives for innovations and expensive chronic disease management interventions. Some diseases have been redefined, and treatment has been recommended in the presymptomatic state. Many

screening tests have dubious benefits, such as total body scanning and prostate-specific antigen (PSA) screening in the asymptomatic population, further adding to the costs of health care.

Health Care Costs Invisible to Patient and Provider. Health care price increases have escalated faster than other sectors of the U.S. general economy because it is a "distorted" health care market. Third-party payers and tax exemptions remove the purchaser from health care cost decisions, so the person using the services is not directly paying for the services. This creates a perverse American imperative, "I want everything done," and further escalates the use of technology and services, irrespective of the cost-to-benefit ratio. Curtailing health care costs is difficult because there is a disconnect or "moral hazard" of insurance. Moral hazard refers to the additional health care that is utilized when persons become insured and care is paid for by a third party. Under conventional theory, health economists

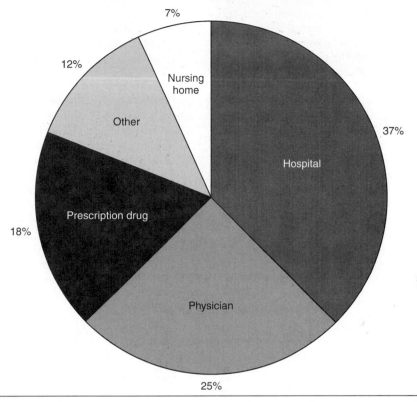

FIGURE 22-5: Health care expenditures by service sector, 2004. (Data from Centers for Medicare & Medicaid Services, Office of the Actuary, National Health Statistics Group, National Health Accounts, *National health expenditures, 2006*.)

regard this increase in use of services as inefficient because it creates demand for care that would not occur if patients were paying for care out of their pockets (Nyman, 2004).

Cost Containment. Policy approaches to contain costs have varied over the past three decades. The 1980s saw a strategy to limit payment to hospitals by establishing a set number of days for specific diseases, or diagnosis-related groups (DRGs). If hospitals could discharge patients before the allotted time frame for hospitalization, they made money; if not, they lost money. The efforts to limit hospital days spurred the development of more outpatient services including same-day surgery clinics and outpatient diagnostics. The advent of DRGs established payment based on fee schedules rather than charges by providers or institutions. In the 1990s, Congress and regulatory agencies fostered competition by imposing controls on physi-

cian payments. The competition came in the form of multiple options being available to organize health care delivery including point-of-service (POS) plans, preferred provider organizations (PPOs), and others. Purchasers (employers and government agencies) became a driving force that looked for the best buy among the health plans. The cost control that has recently been most contentious is the Medicare Sustainable Growth Rate (SGR) index implemented in 1998 that sets a target rate of growth on physician spending. Payment updates depend on whether actual spending is above or below the target. For the past 2 years, physician groups have had to go to Congress to enact legislation to prohibit the cut. Other cost-control measures include implementing a drug formulary to control prescription drug costs, more tightly managing chronic disease, and linking payment to quality measures. These cost-cutting measures directly affect APNs who are health care providers.

The 2000s introduced consumer-driven health care in which more of the financial burden rests on consumers who, it is hoped, will be more discriminating purchasers of health care. The newer payment structures, which force consumers to define their benefits package and pay for a larger percentage of care, have translated directly into increased burdens on family budgets. The Agency for Healthcare Research and Quality (AHRQ) Medical Panel Expenditure Survey (AHRQ, 2006a, 2006b) showed that 43% of Americans younger than 65 years had family-level out-of-pocket spending for health care and insurance of well over $2000 annually, with no sign of abatement. When rising premium costs associated with employer-based coverage are added into the equation, even more families are devoting a substantial share of their resources to health care expenses. These escalating costs are impacting the social fabric of the nation more broadly as health care costs are overwhelmingly responsible for the spike in bankruptcy filings (Himmelstein, Warren, Thorne, & Woolhandler, 2005). Rising health care costs are a driving force behind Americans' increasing dissatisfaction with the health care system. A survey conducted by the Commonwealth Fund (2006) found that Americans believe that steps should be taken to slow health care cost increases. Most adults are not satisfied with their health care costs. One third of Americans reported that they reduced their savings for retirement as a result of high costs, and one quarter had difficulty paying for basic necessities.

Government and private insurers have been largely ineffective at reining in health care costs, for a number of reasons. The summary of cost-control strategies (Table 22-2) has had only short-term or one-time-only impact on curtailing health care costs.

APNs have a social responsibility to establish and promote policies that work to control costs of health care. For those providing primary care, several studies

Table 22-2   SUMMARY OF COST-CONTROL STRATEGIES, 1980S TO 2000S

Cost-Control Strategy	Policy
Payment reforms	Limiting total increases in Medicare's PPS and RBRVS fee schedules instead of limiting cost-based reimbursement (PPS) for hospitals and RBRVS for physician payment Using capitation payments to incentivize providers to reduce costs and volume of services and cap total expenditures P4P financing to those health care systems that measure, report, and practice quality of care
Market reforms	Mergers that increase the economic power of insurers to set prices Contracting with only selected providers who agree to lower fees Credentialing providers in disease management so that purchasers steer patients to only those providers who demonstrate effective outcomes Competitive contracting (bidding out services to the lowest bidder) Profiling providers on the basis of the utilization and price, and eliminating the high-cost providers from the plan Using specific group rating instead of community rating (charging the enrolled group a premium based on the specific group's risks and utilization rather than on average risks and utilization of the community as a whole)
Utilization management	Requiring second opinions for expensive services such as surgery Concurrent and retrospective reviews resulting in denial of payments Practice guidelines, case management, disease management strategies, and other attempts to change the way health care is delivered
Reducing demands by shifting costs to consumers	Higher co-payments and deductibles Higher self-pay premiums Excluding services (contraception, transplant, infertility services) High-deductible health plans and health savings accounts for the self-insured, which creates a tax-free structure for health care costs

P4P, Pay-for-performance; *PPS*, prospective payment system; *RBRVS*, resource-based relative value scale.

show that good primary care can prevent costly hospitalizations, better management of chronic illnesses, and reduced use of emergency services (Brooten et al., 1986; Lenz, Mundinger, Kane, Hopkins, & Lin, 2004; Mondy, Cardenas, & Avila, 2003; Oakley et al., 1996). Those in acute care settings also have a contribution to make in decreasing length of stay, preventing complications, and ensuring adequate discharge planning (Brooten et al., 2001; Davidson, 2002; Pine, Holt, & Lou, 2003; Topp, Tucker, & Weber, 1998). In addition, a critical step is for APNs to obtain their own billing numbers so that data can be collected at a national and state level to show APN contributions to cost-savings.

Health Care Quality

One definition of health care quality specifies that the purpose of the health care system must be to continuously reduce the impact of illness, injury, and disability and to improve the health and functioning of the people (IOM, 2001). Quality of care has also been defined as "the degree to which health services for individuals and populations increase the likelihood of desired health outcomes and are consistent with current professional knowledge" (IOM, 2000, p. 4).

Quality-of-care issues have been conceptualized as problems related to underuse (providing too little care that is effective), overuse (providing care that is not effective or efficient), and misuse (providing care that is unsafe or inappropriate). Examples of this phenomenon include (1) underuse—the failure to give beta-blockers to patients who have had a myocardial infarction; (2) overuse—performing hysterectomies or doing cesarean sections when not needed; and (3) misuse—when antibiotics are prescribed for viral infections. Quality suffers when the following occur:

- Patients encounter long waiting times.
- Patients have difficulty getting referrals to needed specialty care.
- Treatment plans are not explained in understandable terms.
- Patient information gets lost.
- Substandard care or outright errors go unnoticed.
- Providers fail to provide preventive care or manage chronic conditions.
- Segments of the population endure disparities by race, income, and insurance status.
- Care is given outside of evidence-based standards and lacks personal attention and continuity in care.

Starfield (2000) succinctly described why the United States spends so much on health care and gets so little in return. The "inverse care law" describes it as those without insurance get too little necessary care, whereas those with insurance get too much unnecessary care. It is easy to see how systematic efforts to improve quality lead to increases in costs, at least initially. Overuse increases unnecessary costs, underuse raises the cost of care because late care is more costly than early care, and misuse raises costs as a result of higher complication rates. As costs rise, employers struggle to afford health insurance for their employees. As these rising health costs eat into employer profit margins, the benefits drop, co-payments are increased (costs shifted directly to consumers), or workers are laid off. Therefore conceptually, as health care costs increase, access to health care decreases (Center for Studying Health System Change [HSC], 2003).

Federal and state governments have had a broad interest in quality to ensure public safety as well as to promote best practices to get the most effective health care for the dollars spent. Although quality had been monitored through accreditation, certification, and licensing processes, there has been increased involvement in quality issues from purchasers, with those who pay the cost of health care—the federal government being the largest purchaser through Medicare, Medicaid, and the SCHIP (see the following discussion). The first direct incursion into health quality was a result of the enactment, in 1965, of the Medicare and Medicaid programs. The Health Care Financing Administration (HCFA), now the Center for Medicare & Medicaid Services (CMS), was charged with ensuring the effective and efficient use of public funds, including assessment of and ensuring the quality of care.

Although the quality-related function of HCFA/CMS initially grew slowly, it has accelerated rapidly since the late 1990s. Concerns about cost-containment strategies and competition in health care spurred public concern about quality. The emergence of competition and dominance of managed care with its perceived over-emphasis on cost set the stage for a backlash against the harmful effects of a sole focus on cost reduction over quality concerns. The expanded interest in quality was fueled by a series of reports from the Institute of Medicine (IOM) (2000, 2001), which marked the beginning of the modern quality movement in health care. Before those publications, there was implicit understanding that health care quality was universally high, based on the notion that health care professionals had high standards, were well-trained, and placed their patients before their own interests. Accrediting, certifying, and licensing bodies, whose standards were largely either decided by or dominated by input from the health professions in nursing, medicine, pharmacy, and others, were assumed to be adequate in ensuring health care quality

The first IOM report, "To Err is Human," (IOM, 2000) reviewed studies of medical errors and received widespread media attention with its estimation that between 50,000 and 100,000 Americans die each year from medical errors in hospitals (IOM, 2000). A second report, "Crossing the Quality Chasm," (IOM, 2001) noted that improving systems by creating valid and reliable measures of quality, providing feedback and benchmarking, and making other systems changes are the keys to improving quality. This report provided a framework for quality and defined six critical domains:

- Patient safety: providing services in a safe environment
- Effectiveness: providing interventions that have a good likelihood of improving health or function
- Patient centeredness: putting the needs of the patient at the center of the health system
- Efficiency: providing services in the most cost-effective manner
- Timeliness: providing services when they are really needed
- Equity: ensuring a just distribution of services based on health need rather than ability to pay

Subsequent IOM reports have looked at other aspects of the U.S. public health system including access to care, prioritizing several areas for quality improvement/action, health illiteracy, inappropriate mental and substance abuse care, and P4P (IOM, 2003, 2004a, 2004b, 2005, 2006, 2007). Business groups, such as Leapfrog, have united to demand more accountability and higher quality of care for their health care dollars and employees. This group of large employers seeks to use its collective purchasing power to push health providers to publicly report their quality and outcomes so that consumers and purchasing organizations can make informed health care choices.

The World Health Organization (WHO) (2006) cites various reasons for the United States ranking relatively low in quality among wealthy nations. The National Healthcare Disparities Report, developed by the AHRQ, is a national comprehensive analysis that looks at performance measures and differences in use

of health care services by various populations. Findings from these reports include these concerns:

- Some groups, such as Native Americans, rural African-Americans, and the inner-city poor, have extremely poor health, more characteristic of a poor developing country rather than a rich industrialized one.
- The human immunodeficiency virus (HIV) epidemic causes a higher proportion of death and disability to young and middle-aged Americans than in most other advanced countries.
- The United States is one of the leading countries for cancers relating to tobacco, especially lung cancer.
- The United States has a high coronary heart disease rate, which has dropped in recent years but remains high.
- The level of violence, especially of homicides, is fairly high when compared with that of other industrial countries.

Patient Safety. Patient safety is foundational to quality health care. Patients should be able to enter the health care system knowing that everything reasonable is being done to keep them safe from harm by the health care system itself. Public policy in safety is still, for the most part, mired in the belief that most harm to patients is the result of errors by "bad" health care providers and that malpractice is a major deterrent to such errors. There is strong evidence not only of the large number of adverse patient events but also of the fact that most adverse events are the result of systems failures rather than individual human error (IOM, 2000). The IOM report points out that all humans are subject to making errors and that the systems of care in which we work are the most important factors in determining which errors will occur. For example, a number of patients died because a gas other than oxygen was administered as ventilation during surgery. Blaming, firing, or educating the nurse anesthetist, anesthesiologist, or technician who connected the wrong tubing did little to change the error rate. These deaths were virtually eliminated when the connectors for oxygen to ventilators were made so that it is essentially impossible to connect any other gas to the machine. It should be noted that most errors (providing care in a manner that does not conform to acceptable practice) do not result in adverse events (harm to patients), and conversely, most adverse events are not the result of errors.

Existing APN research looking specifically at patient safety as a subset of health care quality is limited. According to "Crossing the Quality Chasm," the American health care system is in need of fundamental change because health care frequently harms and fails to deliver its potential benefits. Research must move beyond comparing APNs to physicians within the context of a health care system that is not built on a strong foundation of patient safety. Comparing APN to physician outcomes was an important validation of APN practice as these professions evolved. However, given the current mandate for fundamental system change, new research questions on APN practice as they relate to patient safety have emerged.

Advanced Practice Nurses and Quality.

Although nursing has only recently focused more seriously on quality from a policy perspective (e.g., the study by Mundinger and colleagues [2000]), seminal work on nursing outcomes has been supported by the National Institute of Nursing Research. Nursing staff levels have been related to patient mortality and morbidity in hospitals (Aiken, Clarke, Sloane, & Silber, 2002; Needleman, Buerhaus, Mattke, Stewart, & Selevinsky, 2001). In addition, in 2003, the National Quality Forum identified 15 nurse-sensitive measures (National Quality Forum, 2004). The American Nurses Association (ANA) is creating a report card for nursing care in hospitals called the *National Data on Nursing Quality Indicators,* with approximately 1000 hospitals participating in the data collection (American Nurses Association [ANA], 1996, 2007).

Although these studies are important, they represent only the beginning efforts of understanding the contribution of nurses to quality of care; much work needs to be done. There are no standardized nursing performance measures that are identified, collected, and reported for all hospitals in this country. As a result, no national or regional benchmarks exist by which the public or payers can compare the quality of nursing care, and nursing care in hospitals remains nearly invisible. The Robert Wood Johnson Foundation has recently invested in a project called *Interdisciplinary Nursing Quality Research Initiative* to expand the measures of nursing quality. This project focuses on hospital quality, but nursing home, home care, and ambulatory care need significant research in the area of measurement development.

One of the major barriers to conducting cross-national studies of APNs is the wide variation of nurse practice acts governing APN practice. An analysis of all 51 nurse practice acts suggests that state regulation of nurse practitioner practice varies widely, indicating the strong likelihood that, in some states, APNs cannot reach their full capacity to meet patients' needs. This wide variation also suggests that APN regulations have no evidence base and no patient-safety foundation and appear arbitrary. This lack of coherence makes it extremely difficult to conduct national studies on APN practice (Lugo, O'Grady, Hodnicki, & Hanson, 2007).

Measuring Quality.

Policymakers have moved to implement a public reporting system to ensure that consumers are informed in their decision to choose an institution or provider based on quality. Data generated from accreditation of health care institutions have been the basis for improved consumer information, now accessible at *Hospital Compare, Nursing Home Compare, Home Health Compare,* and *Health Plans Compare* (CMS, 2007; Department of Health & Human Services [DHHS], 2007; National Committee for Quality Assurance [NCQA], 2007). It is anticipated that, as consumers become more knowledgeable about quality, they will put pressure on employers to offer the best providers. In relation to health plans, children in health plans were nearly three times more likely to receive all recommended immunizations than 8 years ago and nearly 96% of heart attack patients were prescribed a beta-blocker, which was up from 62% in 1996 (NCQA, 2006). No data exist about office practice; however, the CMS has several demonstration projects underway in which physicians voluntarily report data. Although APNs are not recognized in the CMS projects, any reporting requirements instituted for outpatient practices will apply to APNs.

Many different types of organizations and agencies are currently influencing quality of care, thereby creating a complex landscape. Accrediting bodies such as The Joint Commission (TJC) accredit hospitals; state agencies examine nursing homes; and the National Committee for Quality Assurance (NCQA) accredits managed care organizations (MCOs). The primary driving organization for accreditation of health care institutions is the CMS because it administers the Medicare and Medicaid programs to ensure that they are paying for at least a minimum level of care. In addition to the CMS and the accrediting bodies, a number of organizations are dedicated to institutionalizing existing measures or developing new quality measures (e.g., the AHRQ) and private not-for-profit organizations (e.g., the National Quality Forum [NQF] and the NCQA). Professional associations are also involved in helping members improve care.

The linkage of incentive payments, also known as *pay-for-performance (P4P),* has existed in the private purchasing environment with over 100 health plans already having implemented P4P initiatives (Rowe, Cortese, & McGinnis, 2006). The federal government has now engaged in demonstration projects to test the effect of P4P on improving quality (CMS, 2006b). Payment to APNs in outpatient practices through federal, state, or private plans will be linked to quality with APNs measured in the same way that physicians are measured. Although nursing has had a commitment to quality of care as part of its heritage and day-to-day work, nursing in general has been slow to embrace the quality movement that encompasses development of measures. There is a vital need for APNs to take a leadership role in integrating existing measures into practices, creating and testing new measures, and implementing quality improvement programs in all practice settings.

Interdisciplinary Approach to Patient Care. APNs need to create interdisciplinary systems of care to reduce errors and enhance patient safety. Health systems must embrace a strong patient safety mission and culture, which will require strengthening clinical pass-offs, improving communications among provider groups, and practicing evidence-based health care. Dramatic improvement cannot be accomplished without interdisciplinary practice approaches; these will require revolutionary change to flatten the professional and cultural barriers between medicine and nursing (Health Resources and Services Administration [HRSA], COGME, and NACNEP, 2000). Policy can be used to encourage, foster, or mandate collaboration (see Chapter 10). There is no provider better positioned to bridge these disciplines than APNs, who, in some cases, share clinical and professional boundaries with medicine. While interdisciplinary practice is needed, it is crucial that APNs are separated out as distinct provider types in all interdisciplinary research, administrative, and clinical data sets. As more research is pursued within the context of interdisciplinary teams, APNs must not become invisible on the health care team. Building a strong evidence base on APN practice and patient safety will require adherence to methodological quality that explores APN practice within an interdisciplinary context.

Health Care Access

Access to health care is defined as "the timely use of personal health services to achieve the best health outcomes" (IOM, 1993).

Health care access is not simply owning health insurance coverage but also refers to an individual's ability to obtain appropriate health care services. *Access* is a broad term encompassing a set of more specific components describing the fit between the patient and the health care system. The specific dimensions are availability, accessibility, accommodation, affordability, and acceptability. Attaining access to care requires three distinct steps: gaining entry into the system; getting access to sites of care where patients can receive needed services; and finding providers who meet the needs of individual patients and with whom patients can develop a relationship based on mutual communication and trust (AHRQ, 2005). Health insurance allows a health care home to be established and makes an enormous difference in terms of the stage of illness that care is sought. Barriers to health care access, whether one is insured or not, include financial, geographical distance, organizational structure, lack of trust, delays, lost laboratory results, cultural and racial biases, and health care illiteracy. Regardless of the specific access barrier, an access problem is always a delay problem. Consider the following evidence of care process problems from the National Center for Health Statistics (2006) related to access:

- 40% of emergency department visits are not urgent; rather, they take place because patients do not have or cannot see a primary care provider.
- The percentage of people reporting an inability to obtain a timely appointment is as high as 33%.
- 43% of all adults reporting an urgent condition were unable to receive care when they wanted it (Institute for Healthcare Improvement [IHI], 2007).
- Among 18- to 64-year-olds, 7% did not get needed care, 10% received delayed care, and 9% did not get prescriptions filled because of cost.
- In looking at the effect of insurance on getting care, 20% of uninsured people younger than 65 years did not receive needed care because of costs compared with 2% of those who had insurance.

Access to health care has traditionally been provided through insurance, which is obtained primarily through employers. The employer-sponsored health insurance system, although still the dominant form of financing in the United States, is eroding. This decline is unequivocally affecting low-income working families because their employers do not sponsor insurance programs. We know that lack of insurance coverage overwhelmingly compromises the health status of the uninsured because they receive less preventive care, are diagnosed at a later state of illness, and once diagnosed, receive substandard therapeutic care. The consequences to those who forgo needed care are serious. The uninsured are more likely be hospitalized for an "avoidable" condition, to die in the hospital, to be born prematurely, and to experience premature death than the insured population (Kaiser Family Foundation, 2007).

Small businesses are not required to offer health insurance, and many larger companies are shifting more of the cost for health insurance to employees by requiring a larger contribution to the insurance plan, higher deductibles, and higher co-pays. As a result, the number of people lacking health insurance has continued to increase. The uninsured are primarily working families with low or moderate incomes, families for whom coverage is either not available in the workplace or not affordable (Commonwealth Fund, 2006).

Based on data from the Kaiser Family Foundation (2007), while the number of persons has grown, the percent of the population that are uninsured has remained relatively stable. One reason for this is, as private insurance coverage has decreased, more people have been covered by Medicaid or the SCHIP. The most likely to be uninsured are the poor and near poor (those with income levels <200% of the poverty level) and those who are between 18 and 24 years of age. Hispanic and African-Americans populations are most likely to be uninsured, because they are also more likely to be in a low-income group (AHRQ, 2005; Rhoades, 2005).

Some suggest that access to care is universal because even the uninsured can go to an emergency department (ED). However, the ED fails to provide basic primary care nor does it provide effective or efficient care. Self-pay and uninsured individuals using the ED as well as other services have to pay out of pocket for services, and the charge is usually at the full rate rather than a lower rate negotiated by insurers. This issue has created a sense of outrage among many policymakers because the poorest end up being charged the highest rates. The consequence of having the poorest individuals pay the larger share for health care, although an unintended consequence of our health care system, creates a dubious ethical foundation for practice and policy.

While affordability of insurance is a major access issue, geographical access is a perennial problem, with inner-city and rural areas often not having providers with the specific expertise needed. The lack of providers for rural and inner-city residents has plagued this country for decades, and significant gaps remain despite programs to attract people to underserved areas including loan repayment programs through states or the National Health Service Corps (NHSC). An estimated 50 million Americans live in communities that do not offer primary care services (National Health Service Corps [NHSC], 2003). Access to mental health care is an especially serious problem because mental health coverage has more restrictions than does coverage for physical complaints.

The insured population experiences access barriers differently. Once insured, the health care system is plagued by delays and long cycle times—delays of several weeks for appointments, long waits in EDs, extended waits when placed on hold, repeated phone calls to obtain test results or to have a question answered by a provider, and unreasonable wait times even when an appointment is scheduled. These delays adversely affect clinical outcomes, patient satisfaction, and costs, often impacting an organization's ability to attract and retain patients.

The states have recently taken action to expand access. Strategies include expanding existing programs to cover low-income adults, as well as children; creating an insurance pool for small businesses and the self-employed, with premium assistance for low-wage earners; and requiring employers to either provide health benefits or contribute to a fund to finance coverage for working people. For example, in 2006, Massachusetts' plan aimed to make health care coverage affordable for all uninsured residents. Employers must either provide benefits to workers or pay into a fund to finance coverage. State and federal dollars are used to subsidize care for the poor, and the state Medicaid program has been expanded to cover more uninsured children. California has proposed a universal coverage plan that includes premium subsidies for low-income individuals and a requirement that employers either provide insurance or pay a fee equal to 4% of employee earnings. Expanding access to APNs and removing their regulatory barriers have been central tenets to these state proposals.

Advanced Practice Nurses and Access. Access based on convenience as well as reasonable cost is the reason that convenient care clinics have rapidly expanded. APNs have been central to the success of these clinics that manage specific health problems in an easily accessible place. Based on recent data, these clinics have been well received in terms of satisfaction with the value of the care experience. Prices for visits as well as diagnostic tests are public information and are affordable by most. The clinics have provided the majority of their services to individuals who are well off and looking for convenience, as well as those who are uninsured and need affordable health care. While physician groups will continue to voice concerns about quality of care at the convenient care clinics, it is clear that the financial model is not one that they are embracing. The pricing structure of the clinics will provide care at lower costs than typical physician visits (Scott, 2006).

APNs have had a forceful voice to ensure access to comprehensive care. Access concerns by APNs are linked to the roots of advanced practice nursing. APN roles developed largely as a policy response to access problems for those in rural and other underserved areas. Much of the focus of the DHHS's Division of Nursing, which implements funds appropriated by Congress to support nursing education and special projects through Title VIII of the Nurse Practice Act, has been to support programs that increase the number of APNs with the specific purpose of enhancing access.

Any effort to improve access, by providing health insurance coverage or increasing the availability of providers in underserved areas, requires an increase in costs. Impacts on quality are generally positive because any care is better than no care and early care is better than delayed care. Policy options to expand access focus on the eligibility of publicly sponsored health insurance, the defined scope of benefits, and use of cost-sharing. The United States has the best health care in the world, provided the patient has the right disease and the right insurance and is in the right health care facility seeking treatment from the right provider mix. This overly stringent list of qualifiers creates enormous opportunities to improve quality, reduce the huge geographical variation in how care is delivered, and increase access to care.

Sources of Data That Inform Policy Decisions

Policy decisions are best made by informed decision makers. Accurate data are extremely important to policymakers. Congress has access to the Congressional Research Service (CRS) established in 1914 to serve members of Congress, their staff, and committees. The CRS provides nonpartisan policy analysis of any issue Congress requests. The staff members of the CRS come from a variety of backgrounds to bring multidisciplinary skills to a wide variety of issues. In addition, Congress has the Government Accountability Office (previously named the *General Accounting Office*) to provide nonpartisan analysis of ways to make government more effective. This office provides financial assessments of government programs with the intent of saving the American public from excessive costs.

The DHHS is the primary executive agency collecting and analyzing public health–related data. The major organizational entities that collect and analyze data are the Health Resources and Services Administration (HRSA), the National Center for Health Statistics (NCHS), the CMS, and the AHRQ. The HRSA maintains data related to the national nursing population including APNs.

In addition, the HRSA has a rich resource in the Area Resource File (ARF), which integrates information from more than 50 data sources including the U.S. Census Bureau, the Bureau of Labor Statistics, and the NCHS. The ARF provides information about health professions, health facilities, hospital utilization and expenditures, shortage areas and demographics, and economic indicators for communities (Quality Resource System, Inc, 2006).

The NCHS is the nation's principal health statistics agency that compiles information about the health status of the population and important subgroups. Data include information about health disparities, demographic information about specific populations, trends in health status, and health care delivery.

The CMS has numerous data that it collects and analyzes about Medicare, Medicaid, and the SCHIP. The primary data sources include claims data, provider information, and enrollment data. The AHRQ also has an important data set known as *Healthcare Cost and Utilization Project* that comprises several subsets of data. The Kaiser Family Foundation has a resource that lists the specific data sources available and a description of each (Henry J. Kaiser Family Foundation, 2007a). Data related to APNs is aggregated and includes CNMs, CRNAs, CNSs, and NPs; it is based on the use of billing numbers.

Over the past 20 years, the evolution of health services research (HSR), a distinct area of scholarship, has grown dramatically in both resources and influence and is currently funded publicly at $1.5 billion annually. HSR is important to APNs because it addresses questions that require observational or quasi-experimental design. This form of research includes determining the comparative effectiveness of interventions across a range of different settings, economic evaluation of different financing and organizational decisions, and qualitative designs that help us understand the *how* and *why* of social interactions (AcademyHealth, 2006). The HRS field is uniquely suited to exploring APN practice because it provides a mixing bowl of interdisciplinary perspectives working on similar problems. As HRS methods become increasingly more influential, APN research must be framed within a broader HSR and patient-safety context.

Advanced Practice Nurse Health Policy Issues

Medicare. Medicare was enacted in 1965 to provide health coverage to individuals 65 years of age and older and to those who are blind or disabled. Medicare now covers approximately 42 million Americans with a total expenditure in 2002 of $266 billion (Cubanski, Voris, Kitchman, Newman, & Potetz, 2005). Based on a 2006 report, the financial difficulties of Medicare will come sooner and be more severe than had been reported. Medicare costs are now projected to surpass Social Security expenditures in a little more than 20 years (Palmer & Saving, 2006).

Advanced Practice Nurse Medicare Payment. In August of 1997, Congress passed legislation that authorized nurse practitioners (NPs) to be reimbursed under Medicare Part B. NPs are reimbursed at the lesser of 80% of actual charges or 85% of the physician fee if billing on their own provider number or at the physician rate ($100%) if NP services are billed on the physician billing number as "incident to." APNs have regulatory authority to provide for and bill for services without direct supervision of a physician at the lower rate. APNs can also bill for services that are "incident to" APN care. For services to be billed "incident to," the following criteria must be met (DHHS, 2006):

- Must be an integral part, although "incident to" professional services
- Must be commonly rendered without charge or included in the bill
- Must be of a type commonly included in offices or clinic practices

- Must be furnished by the recognized practitioner or auxiliary personnel under the direct supervision of the provider

Certified nurse-midwives (CNMs) were recognized providers by Medicare in 1988 to care for the maternity needs of disabled women who qualified for coverage. In 1993, Congress recognized midwives to provide care for women needing services outside of the maternity cycle who were Medicare enrollees. CNMs have been pressing for equity in payment and have had several bills introduced into Congress, with the latest one in February 2007.

A major issue for certified registered nurse anesthetist (CRNA) billing has been a requirement for physician supervision. In 2000, HCFA (now CMS) developed new regulations that deferred to the states the decision about requiring physician supervision. To date, 14 states have waived the federal requirement and chose not to require physician supervision in order to pay CRNAs.

To receive payment from Medicare, APNs need to have a billing number and meet the following (see also Chapter 19):

- Hold an active license as a registered nurse, authorized to perform the services in the specific APRN role in the state where he or she practices
- Have a master's degree from an accredited educational institution
- Hold current certification from a nationally recognized certifying body
- Have physician collaboration

Medicaid. Medicaid is jointly funded by states and the federal government but managed by states. Medicaid is a larger program than Medicare in terms of the number of enrollees (53 million enrollees compared with 42 million in Medicare) and expenses ($305 billion in 2005) (Henry J. Kaiser Family Foundation, 2007b). A recent study suggests that Medicaid's share of national health spending will remain virtually unchanged until 2025 and then increase slowly through 2045 (Kronick & Rousseau, 2007).

The amount of federal Medicaid payments to a state for medical services depends on two factors. The first is the actual amount spent that qualifies as a match under Medicaid. The second factor is the federal medical assistance percentage (FMAP) for each state. The FMAP is computed from a formula that takes into account the average per capita income for each state relative to the national average. By law, the

FMAP cannot be less than 50%. Medicaid is administered by individual states, with substantial latitude, but states must offer coverage to specified groups to get federal matching dollars.

The Medicaid program is intended to cover poor children; however, older adults overwhelmingly dominate Medicaid spending. In fact, attempts to cut Medicaid costs have often been based on reducing "abuse" in the system by welfare mothers. Although children and mothers represent nearly 70% of Medicaid enrollees, they receive about 30% of the Medicaid funds. Conversely, older adults and disabled enrollees represent about 30% of the total enrollees but consume about 70% of the budget. The annual spending per child is estimated at $1,410 based on 2003 data compared with $11,659 for the disabled and $10,147 for older adults (Kaiser Commission on Medicaid and the Uninsured, 2006). The difference in amount per enrollee reflects the cost of long-term care for the disabled and older adult enrollees.

Policymakers have pursued a variety of strategies to contain the cost of Medicaid, mostly focused on the non–older adult portion of the program. Enactment of the Welfare Reform Act in 1996 prevented automatic enrollment in Medicaid for persons receiving cash assistance under a number of federal low-income assistance programs. The de-linking of Medicaid enrollment from cash assistance programs resulted in substantial decreases in the number of low-income, non–older adults enrolled in Medicaid. In addition, the Welfare Reform Act prohibited states from enrolling non-citizens in Medicaid other than in very limited situations. In addition, the Deficit Reduction Act (DRA) of 2005 (PL 109-171) makes it more difficult for families to "hide" or transfer assets in order to receive Medicaid support for nursing home care.

Payment from Medicaid was first obtained by CNMs. Currently, only specific groups of APNs are eligible for Medicaid reimbursement. These groups include pediatric NPs, family NPs, and CNMs. A major policy agenda of NPs is to extend Medicaid reimbursement to all APNs.

State Children's Health Insurance Program. The SCHIP was passed as a part of the Balanced Budget Act (BBA) as Title XXI of the Social Security Act. Enactment of this program occurred because of the recognition that 11 million children were uninsured (Congressional Budget Office, 1998). The SCHIP is intended to extend insurance to children in low-income families who have too much income to be eligible for Medicaid but not enough to be able to afford health insurance. Congress set aside $24 billion matching funds from general tax revenues over a 10-year period to create this program. Current data suggest that the SCHIP has covered approximately 6 million children. Like Medicaid, the SCHIP is a program in which federal funds must be matched by a set proportion of state funds and the program is managed by the states. Major efforts have been made to reach out to families and communities through schools, churches, and daycare centers to let parents know about the availability of coverage. A recent report suggests that 3.9 million children rely solely on the SCHIP coverage and another approximately 2 million uninsured children are eligible for the SCHIP but are not enrolled (Kenney & Cook, 2007).

APNs have been part of the effort in identifying and assisting enrollment of children who are eligible for the SCHIP. All states and territories have approved the SCHIP plans. However, some states were slow to implement the SCHIP because of the requirement for matching funds and the provisions requiring active enrollment efforts for both SCHIP- and Medicaid-eligible children. The SCHIP programs have been implemented through three different mechanisms. Nineteen states and territories have implemented the SCHIP as part of the Medicaid program; 16 have developed a separate child health insurance plan; and 21 have a combination plan.

Again in 2007, Congress addressed whether to continue the SCHIP program. Although the program is considered to be a success and there is bi-partisan support, there is disagreement about funding levels. Most estimates of the program cost indicate that maintaining the current coverage level will require increased funding. Without an increase in funds, many children could lose their coverage. However, the context of the SCHIP is changing and some states, such as Massachusetts, Minnesota, and Hawaii, have taken a broader view to provide insurance to children through universal coverage.

The SCHIP payments to APNs have presented some challenges. Although states recognize payment to family or pediatric NPs and CNMs through Medicaid, it has been difficult in some states, such as New York, for eligible APNs to get payment if the program was implemented under a separate state health plan and not through Medicaid. State and national organizations representing APNs have been active in working with these states to ensure access to APN care.

Health Disparities. Health disparities had been noted in the report of the Secretary's Task Force on Black and Minority Health in 1985 that led to the creation of the Office of Minority Health (OMH). The purpose of the Office is to improve health and safety of minority populations, specifically Native Americans and Native Alaskans, Asian-Americans, blacks/African-Americans, Hispanics/Latinos, and Native Hawaiians and other Pacific Islanders (see Figure 22-6 for percent of the population uninsured by race).

In 1999, Congress requested that the IOM study the issue of health disparities, which resulted in the 2002 report "Unequal Treatment: Confronting Racial and Ethnic Disparities in Health Care" (IOM, 2002). This report identified consistent variations in care based on race, even when insurance status, income, age, and severity of conditions were controlled. An example of the disparities is that minorities were not given the appropriate cardiac medications and were less likely to receive dialysis or kidney transplants and more likely to have amputation as a procedure for those with diabetes (IOM). In addition, the AHRQ has released an annual report on health care disparities for the past 3 years. The disparities go beyond those of race and ethnicity and examine disparities from the perspective of socioeconomics, as well as other vulnerable groups including women, children,

older adults, residents of rural areas, and individuals with special care needs.

Based on all reports, although there have been some successes on the disparities front, health disparities continue to exist. The AHRQ report found that among a core set of measures reflecting quality of care, poor people received lower quality of care on 85% of the measures compared with high-income people. For the set of access measures, disparities for blacks and Asians were decreasing but were increasing for Hispanics and poor people. KaiserNetwork.org is a website that has developed a link that provides weekly updates on activities related to health disparities *(www. kaisernetwork.org/daily_reports/rep_disparities).*

POLITICAL COMPETENCE IN THE POLICY ARENA

Health Policymaking: A Requisite Skill for Individual Advanced Practice Nurses

Early APNs prepared in continuing education and more recently in master's programs laid a strong foundation for the necessity of APN involvement in policy. The move to doctoral education raises this standard to a higher level. Policy competence is embedded in each of the clinical practice doctorate (Doctor of Nursing Practice [DNP]) competencies (as well as a stand-alone DNP competency, number 5),

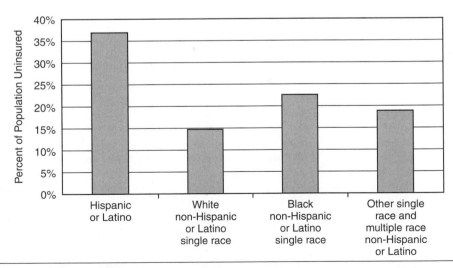

FIGURE 22-6: Percent of population (younger than 65 years) uninsured, by race/ethnicity, 2004. (Data from Centers for Medicare & Medicaid Services, Office of the Actuary, National Health Statistics Group, National Health Accounts, *National health expenditures, 2006.)*

requiring APNs to continuously incorporate policy strategies between the practice, research, and policy nexus in all practice settings (Table 22-3). As APNs move through DNP programs, policy analysis must be integrated into every course, content area, and project so that the DNP graduate has the ability to assume a broad leadership role on behalf of the public and the nursing profession. The solutions to today's social injustices, perverse financing, and uneven quality in the health care system are not simple. APNs are well positioned with clinical credibility to inform, design, and influence policy solutions, but this will happen *only* if they expand their scope of responsibility beyond the clinical setting.

Politically competent APNs serve as content experts with policymakers and their staff. Often policymakers are generalists who have to command expertise in a broad range of topics such as transportation, energy, agriculture, and tax policy. Serving as a resource to policymakers with evidence-based information and

helpful suggestions that are in the public interest is crucial. When serving in this capacity, it is important to avoid a self-serving posture. To effectively influence or participate meaningfully in policy development, APNs must be aware of the policymaking process (from conception to implementation) and the politically open windows of opportunity. Further, intentionally developing and maintaining strong relationships with policymakers and other health care interest groups are important APN activities. Policymakers seek advisement on highly specific policy modifications rather than on major reform recommendations. Elected officials turn over at a far greater rate than civil servants who make careers out of formulating and implementing health policy. Because of the longevity of their careers, developing strong, trustworthy relationships with the policymakers' staff members is important.

Another essential responsibility for APNs is to inform and contribute to the public discourse on

Table 22-3   HEALTH POLICY/POLITICAL DNP COMPETENCIES RELEVANT TO ALL APNs

DNP Essential	Requisite Policy Skill
1. Scientific underpinnings for practice	Analyze policy, practice of politics, political systems, and political behavior with nursing science to affect policy level change.
2. Organizational and systems leadership for quality improvement and systems thinking	Create and sustain coalitions on health care quality/ access improvement via an orientation to policy development, be it at institutional, community, corporate, regional, national, or international levels.
3. Clinical scholarship and analytic methods for evidence-based practice	Participate in design, translation, and/or dissemination of APN practice inquiry within the context of health services research. Employ research best practices to inform policymakers of APN practice and quality.
4. Information systems/technology and patient care technology for the improvement and transformation of health care	Overcome APN invisibility by ensuring the inclusion of nursing and APNs in all administrative and clinical data bases. Provide policy leadership to electronically link meaningful data on nursing activity to cost, quality, and health outcomes.
5. Health care policy for advocacy in health care	Engage in political activism and policy development, mentor activism, participate on boards that impact health policies.
6. Interprofessional collaboration for improving patient and population health outcomes	Build interdisciplinary coalitions as a powerful advocacy tool to promote positive change in the health care delivery system. Communicate across disciplines to build common ground.
7. Clinical prevention and population health for improving the nation's health	Promote the financing and delivery of evidence-based clinical preventive and population health services in all health policy arenas.
8. Advanced practice nursing	Function as content expert and policy change leader within area of mastery/APN specialization.

APN, Advanced practice nurse; *DNP,* Doctor of Nursing Practice.

important health policy issues, because APN interests and public interests are not at odds. Gaining public support and influencing public opinion can help get the attention of policymakers or propel issues onto the policy agenda. Submitting opinion-editorials (Op-Ed's) to major news outlets is one powerful way to do this. This requires writing that links the issues to the community, uses poignant stories to bring the problem to life, and incorporates evidence to build a strong case as to why a policy change is needed (see Box 22-1 for more suggestions). APNs must use their professional credentials and expertise with this sense of responsibility toward educating the public and must not hesitate to be active advocates based on their knowledge and experience.

APNs have numerous opportunities to serve on federal, corporate, and health-related advisory boards. Board membership is crucial to integrating APNs into policymaking. Often, APNs are appointed because they have strong working relationships with people who happen to be on boards and are familiar with the APN as a compelling knowledge source who is effective in groups. A definite set of behaviors is required to serve on national advisory or corporate boards, and a high degree of mastery is necessary to be re-appointed or invited back. Although the opportunities to directly serve in this capacity are limited to a few, it is possible to influence a board's policy recommendations by meeting with the agency staff, seeking invitations to testify before advisory boards, and meeting with members of boards (see Exemplar 22-2).

Barriers to Political Competence

Using Force Versus Power. Power accomplishes with ease what force, even with extreme effort, cannot. On the interpersonal front, it is important for APNs to avoid using force in advancing their positions in the policy arena. Doing so can diminish one's power. This is commonly done by nurses participating in interdisciplinary policy or problem-solving meetings. The twin approaches of being judgmental and parochial can quickly compromise effectiveness. *Judgementalism,* or criticizing other people or disciplines, distracts from effective problem-solving and in the process can reflect poorly on the judger, taking away the power to influence. When we diminish others or the work they do, we can provoke defensiveness and consequently limit ourselves and our capacity to influence others meaningfully. *Nursing parochialism* occurs when nurses present a narrow, restricted scope or outlook in which only nursing and nursing's interests are offered as solutions. These postures in the policy arena (or any other setting) do not build widebase support or strong relationships. APNs' potential impact on cost, quality, and access, if fully unleashed, is a powerful solution to some of the most perennial health care problems of our time. Power is characterized by humility and truth, which needs no defense or rhetoric—it is self-evident. Force is divisive and exploits people for individual or personal gain (Hawkins, 2002). For APNs to be effective in influencing policy, a great degree of maturity, discipline, restraint, and respect for self and others must be practiced. Many of these skills are highlighted in Exemplar 22-2 about Dr. Mary Wakefield.

Political Competence Through Organizational Unity. There are numerous ways for APN organizations to continuously exert influence on the policymaking process. Forming coalitions with other APNs and other nursing, health care, and consumer groups strengthens political effectiveness.

Box 22-1   Opinion-Editorial Suggestions

Opinion-editorials (Op-Ed's) are not formulaic; however, some general guidelines may enhance the potential for publication. Op-Ed's and letters to the editor are both unsolicited; however, letters to the editor are usually shorter and in direct response to a story/article previously written. Op-Ed's are longer opinion pieces usually related to some current event or news story. A strong, 750-word Op-Ed piece starts with the credentials and experience of the author. The policy problem is hooked to a leading current problem or news story. Add a poignant, specific story to describe how the problem impacts human beings. Offer policy solution(s) backed up by three points of evidence. Add a "to-be-sure" segment that anticipates and counters opponents' views and inoculates against those stakeholders who oppose your ideas. Finally, add a conclusion with possible action items for members of the public (e.g., call/write legislator). Ask at least five people with strong writing skills to critique the piece before submission.

EXEMPLAR 22-2   **Serving on a National Advisory Board:**
Mary Wakefield, RN, PhD, MedPAC Commissioner

The MedPAC is an independent federal body established to advise the U.S. Congress on issues affecting the Medicare program. This is an example of Congress creating an independent advisory body to inform them on the complex and highly contentious issues in the Medicare program. The Commission's 17 members bring diverse expertise in the financing and delivery of health care services. Commissioners are appointed to 3-year terms (subject to renewal) by the Comptroller General and are supported by an executive director and a staff of analysts.

MedPAC meets publicly to discuss policy issues and formulate its recommendations to the Congress. In the course of these meetings, Commissioners consider the results of staff research, presentations by policy experts, and public comments from interested parties. They meet with staff from congressional committees, CMS, health care researchers, health care providers, and beneficiary advocates.

To get appointed to MedPAC, individuals need broad-based support. In 1998, the ANA and the AACN strongly supported Dr. Mary Wakefield as a commissioner to MedPAC. Without the support of nursing organizations, she would not have been considered. More than that, Dr. Wakefield had a long history of developing strong relationships with individuals outside of nursing, including the rural health community and congressional policymakers who sent letters of endorsement for her appointment. Because of the strong relationships she had built and cultivated over years, those who knew her, trusted that she would serve from a universal posture of problem-solving—not make decisions solely to elevate the nursing discipline. Most federal advisory bodies do not have a nursing seat; rather, they are interested in individuals who have expertise in the nexus between practice, programs, and policy. Nurses who bring more than the nursing discipline as their sole area of expertise are better positioned for appointment. In this sense, MedPAC was able to "check off many boxes" with Dr. Wakefield, because she had expertise in public policy (she was the chief of staff to two Senators), rural health, and clinical nursing. Although the nursing community was pivotal in getting her appointed, she saw her responsibility as far broader than bringing nursing interests to the discussion.

GETTING INVITED BACK: SKILLS AND PERFORMANCE

Dr. Wakefield had served on President Clinton's Advisory Commission on Consumer Protection and Quality in the Health Care Industry and was noticed as an extremely effective commissioner. It is because of her impressive performance in that arena that she was supported for appointment to serve on MedPAC and went on to serve as a member of the IOM's committee that authored the highly influential and groundbreaking "To Err is Human" (IOM, 2000) and "Crossing the Quality Chasm" (IOM, 2001) reports.

As difficult as it was to get appointed to MedPAC, the real work began once she was sworn in as a commissioner. The commissioners were asked to serve by eliminating their self or special interest and turf battles. Serving on MedPAC required due diligence in terms of the amount of material she needed to read and fully comprehend. She spent an enormous amount of time poring over readings so that she could make valuable contributions to the discussion. This attention to detail was born out of a deep sense of responsibility that she did not want to squander.

According to Dr. Wakefield, it is important to serve in public venues with a great degree of humility. She identified a team of individuals with expertise in Medicare whose political agenda may have differed from hers, but she consulted them all along the way to gain insight and knowledge. While Dr. Wakefield was serving as an expert commission member, she had her own group of experts informing her. She did not presume to be an expert in all matters related to the Medicare program, so she sought out advice and then made a determination about how and whether to use that advice.

Content expertise is not the only skill set required to be effective on a federal commission or any interdisciplinary arena. Dr. Wakefield was extremely mindful of the commission process and carefully measured how she participated in the discussions to maximize "being heard." She did this using several strategies. Before each public meeting, she went "off-line" with MedPAC staff and other commissioners to get their take on contentious issues. She was careful to garner support and count votes before a vote was put on public record. She was cautious to lead only when she felt an important marker needed to be laid down. She never made off-the-cuff remarks for fear the public record could be used against nursing or other interests in

AACN, American Association of Colleges of Nursing; *ANA,* American Nurses Association; *CMS,* Centers for Medicare & Medicaid Services; *IOM,* Institute of Medicine; *MedPAC,* Medicare Payment Advisory Commission.

EXEMPLAR 22-2   **Serving on a National Advisory Board:**
Mary Wakefield, RN, PhD, MedPAC Commissioner—cont'd

the future. She continuously gauged the other commissioners, and if a physician made a point about nursing that she was going to make, she let that external validation stand as the comment supportive of nursing, rather than repeating the point. She often waited until all others spoke before she contributed to the discussion so that she could consider others' comments and respond to them in her remarks. She attributes her success to keeping cool, responding objectively and factually, and avoiding rhetorical, inflammatory comments and diminishing other disciplines. By participating in meetings with this respectful approach, deep content expertise, and focus on process, she was able to encourage others to support or "carry nursing's water."

Dr. Wakefield has witnessed nurses and other leaders who become shrill and consistently present positions that reflect pure self-interest in public arenas, whereby each person in the room knows what he or she will say *before* they speak. This is a posture she has worked hard to avoid. Dr. Wakefield was appointed and then re-appointed because of strong relationships built on trust and respect. She was able to demonstrate that nurses can solve problems in the health care system, not just for nurses' sake. She was successful because she saw that her responsibility as a commissioner was to bring a broader perspective on all of health care, not just nursing.

 EXEMPLAR 22-3   **Political Competence: AANA's Heroic Effort to Remove Supervisory Requirement**
Frank Purcell, AANA, On Participating in Pay-for-Performance Policy Development

IF YOU ARE NOT AT THE TABLE, THEN YOU ARE ON THE MENU
In 2000, the CMS, under the direction of the Clinton administration, published rules removing the requirement that CRNAs must be under the supervision of physicians in order to receive Medicare payment. When the Bush administration came into office in 2001, these final rules, which had not yet been implemented, were suspended and then re-

versed. The final rules that are still in place today state that the Medicare program requires CRNAs to practice under the supervision of a physician to receive Medicare payment. The rationale was that the administration wanted to give states more flexibility so that if states wanted to, they could opt out of the physician supervision requirement. Fourteen states have "opted-out" of the physician supervision requirement today.

AANA, American Association of Nurse Anesthetists; *CMS,* Centers for Medicare & Medicaid Services; *CRNA,* certified registered nurse anesthetist.

Although more than 120 diverse nursing organizations exist, none has a membership base that is more than a fraction of the more than 3 million nurses. Forming coalitions and strategic plans around policy reforms is necessary to maximize impact. APN organizational leaders can play a role in defining health policy problems and designing possible solutions. The APN movement has advanced tremendously; however, a greater degree of policy solidarity would significantly strengthen the political effectiveness of APN groups. APNs are characteristically pioneers, blazing new trails that have pushed the role and boundaries of nursing forward. As the number of APNs climbs to 250,000, their political influence will also grow.

Longest (2006) asserts that organizations that form *policy communities* (build coalitions) can exert enormous influence on the policy process. Policy communities comprise loosely structured, heterogeneous networks defined by the level of investment each group has around the issue. There is an enormous difference between sharing an investment in health policy issues and reaching concordance on policy positions. Reaching concordance in the development of policy positions is what adds great power to policy communities and is the organizational challenge for APN groups (Exemplar 22-3).

What is remarkable about the case history in Exemplar 22-3 is how a politically competent organization used the crisis to garner strength, professional unity, visibility, and strategic partners. After the favorable rules were suspended, the American Association of Nurse Anesthetists (AANA) began a wide-ranging effort to keep the physician requirement out of the final rules because of the strong evidence demonstrating that CRNAs are safe, effective providers without the oversight of another discipline. This rule would restrict access to anesthesia care, especially in rural and medically underserved areas, and add to the cost of care. This particular rulemaking process was especially active for the CMS because the opposition from the American Society of Anesthesiologists was strong. The AANA launched a grassroots response and identified key allies—most notably the Rural Health Association and the American Hospital Association, both of whom had policy interests in expanding access to anesthesia care. The ANA also invested its resources on behalf of the nation's nurse anesthetists and targeted political action committee (PAC) donations in this effort. Other APN groups were supportive, but the issue was only of tangential interest to certified nurse specialists (CNSs), NPs, and CNMs. There was a coordinated, targeted, nationwide effort by the AANA and their allies to educate legislators and CMS officials on the safety and value of CRNAs. They initiated a grassroots campaign and had CRNAs meeting with their congressional delegations all across the country, educating them on the role of CRNAs and how requiring physician supervision would restrict access and raise costs. Their PAC donations went from less than $100,000 in 2000 to over $1.5 million the following year.

Although the AANA was not able to change this unfavorable CMS ruling, they were able to demonstrate a high degree of political competence. First, 90% of the 36,000 CRNAs in the United States are members of the AANA, demonstrating internal cohesion, unity, strength, and credibility both within and outside the profession. This crisis strengthened their solid organizational foundation and energized practicing CRNAs to engage in policymaking. Today, the AANA has a sophisticated student acculturation program in which students are mentored and expected to be active in the association—a robust public policy program built on strong relationships and coalitions. Each election cycle (every 2 years) they raise over $1.5 million in their PAC, which is distributed equally among Democratic and Republican lawmakers. They are deeply involved in developing quality measures with the NQF and setting national P4P reporting and payment policy at the CMS. The AANA serves as an APN organizational exemplar as a highly effective, politically competent organization who knows how to corral its political power.

Moving Advanced Practice Nurses Forward in Health Policy

Two ways in which APNs can move the policy process forward are through research and the identification of strong policy initiatives. Findings on APN research must be published in journals outside of nursing to reach a broader policymaking and public audience. Key policymakers as well as the public must be made more aware of the contributions that APNs make in reducing health care costs and improving access and quality of care. Achieving broader recognition, reducing APN invisibility, and removing barriers to APN practice will be contingent upon APNs communicating methodologically sound APN research that produces results that are generalizable to the larger delivery system. In addition, APN-driven initiatives that positively impact health care reflect APNs' ability to change the system. The following sections provide examples of how this could be achieved.

Advanced Practice Nurse Policy Research Agenda. If APNs unite through organizations committed to policy solidarity, a more robust APN policy research agenda could be realized, providing a quality alliance to build a comprehensive and strategic APN research and policy agenda. The policy research agenda might include the following:
- Identify how APNs create value for payers to improve the quality in health care. Determine if APNs are a competitive advantage in the health care marketplace. Determine if APN practice demonstrates cost effectiveness and reduces errors and misuse/overuse of services.
- Identify the most reliable, valid, and feasible approach(es) to measure quality of care delivered by APNs.
- Determine how APN practice is most economically efficient and effective, and specify sectors (e.g., acute care, palliative care) or content areas (e.g., obesity, cardiac disease) in which APNs are most successful.
- Identify the outcomes of APN interventions targeted at changing patient behavior/lifestyle.

Do APNs uniquely or qualitatively employ effective strategies to prevent disease?

- Explore the most effective health care team composition for acute care, primary care, palliative care. Build an evidence base on interdisciplinary approaches or "collaboratories" to function as incubators and disseminators of team-delivered care.
- Identify how nurse state practice acts enhance or create barriers to safe, effective, and innovative APN-delivered care.
- Mount efforts to obtain demonstration funding through Medicare to expand graduate medical education (GME) to include interdisciplinary teams, including APNs in DNP programs, rather than just medical residents.
- Explore strategies for the cost savings of APN practice to be passed onto consumers, Medicare, and other payers.
- Identify the impact APNs have on vulnerable segments of the population including the uninsured, older adults, children, and rural dwellers.
- Identify how access and quality of care are impacted once a state has adopted the National Council of State Boards of Nursing's (NCSBN's) regulatory vision for APN practice, which eliminates regulatory barriers to APN practice.
- Determine if APN practice improves health care disparities—do improvements benefit minority populations preferentially?
- Expand the HRSA's National Sample Survey of RNs (NSSRN) (HRSA, 2004) to include a national sample of APNs and increase its frequency to every 2 years. This strategy would yield the timeliest APN workforce projections.
- Identify how APNs are reliably built into the ARF.

Advanced Practice Nurse Policy Initiatives. A number of policy initiatives would strengthen patient care quality, enhance access, and add to a more robust data collection system that could, overall, positively impact health care delivery. The following are policy initiatives that APN groups could unite to work toward resolving or creating:

- Eliminate all APN "incident-to" billing via Medicare.
- Develop a plan to include all APNs in Medicaid reimbursement.
- Create an action plan for highly qualified APNs to serve on convenient-care company

boards, health insurance and delivery system boards, and key federal and state health advisory boards.

- Encourage all of the nation's APNs to be identifiable and included in some quality measurement process in their practices (e.g., Healthcare Effectiveness Data and Information Set [HEDIS]).
- Develop a plan to include APNs in all health care quality initiatives including CMS demonstrations on P4P, the development of NQF quality measures, and private sector initiatives.
- Create a prominent award for APNs who serve as exemplars in health care quality. The alliance could award organizations or individual nurses who have had a major impact on quality improvement.

CONCLUSION

Political competency needs to be a part of every APN's professional role. Membership in professional organizations that advance issues critical to APN practice and the health of the nation are necessary for the continued viability of APNs. The first step to being involved in policy formulation is to be knowledgeable about the policy process and the current and emerging issues relevant to APNs. To be involved, APNs need to understand the details related to funding issues, measures of quality and how they reflect APN practice, and specific programs designed to improve access. The important lesson for APNs and policy is that a single person with deep understanding of an issue can make a difference. An individual backed by organizational strength, particularly by coalitions of organizations, can make an even more significant difference.

REFERENCES

AcademyHealth. (2006). Washington, DC: *AcademyHealth Report* (Issue 25, December). Retrieved March 1, 2007, from www. academyhealth.org/publications/academyhealthreports/ dec06.pdf.

Agency for Healthcare Research and Quality (AHRQ). (2005). *2005 National health disparities report* (No. 06-0017). Rockville, MD: Author.

Agency for Healthcare Research and Quality (AHRQ). (2006a). *Medical Expenditure Panel survey.* Rockville, MD: Author. Retrieved March 1, 2007, from www.ahrq.gov/data/mepsweb. htm.

Agency for Healthcare Research and Quality (AHRQ). (2006b). Out-of-pocket spending on health care rises sharply for American families. *AHRQ News and Numbers.* Rockville, MD: Author. Retrieved March 1, 2007, from www.ahrq. gov/news/nn/nn031506.htm.

Aiken, L., Clarke, S.P., Sloane, D.M., & Silber, J.H. (2002). Hospital nurse staffing and patient mortality, nurse burnout, and job satisfaction. *Journal of the American Medical Association, 288,* 1987-1993.

American College of Nurse Practitioners (ACNP). (2007). *Annual Margie Koehler Legislative Advocacy Award criteria.* Retrieved March 8, 2007, from www.acnpweb.org/i4a/pages/index.cfm?pageid=3312 - 43k.

American Nurses Association (ANA). (1996). *Nursing quality indicators: Definitions and implications* (#NP 108). Washington, DC: Author.

American Nurses Association (ANA). (2007). Nursing quality indicators for acute care settings. Silver Spring, MD. Retrieved February 10, 2007, from www.nursingworld.org/readroom/fssafe99.htm.

Brooten, D., Kumar, S., Brown, L.P., Butts, P., Finkler, S.A., Bakewell-Sachs, S., et al.(1986). A randomized clinical trial of early hospital discharge and home follow up of very low birth weight infants. *New England Journal of Medicine, 315,* 934-939.

Brooten, D., Youngblut, J.M., Brown, I., Finkler, S.A., Neff, D.F., & Madigan, E. (2001). A randomized trial of nurse specialist home care for women with high risk pregnancies, outcomes, and costs. *American Journal of Managed Care, 7*(8), 793-803.

Center for Studying Health System Change (HSC), Lesser, C.S., & Ginsburg, P.B. (2003). *Health care cost and access problems intensify* (Issue Brief No. 63). Retrieved June 14, 2007, from www.hschange.com/CONTENT/559/ - 84k.

Centers for Medicare & Medicaid Services (CMS). (2006b). *Demonstration projects and evaluation reports.* Retrieved July 25, 2006, from www.cms.hhs.gov/DemoProjectsEvalRpts/MD/itemdetail.asp?filterType=none&filterByDID=-99&sortByDID=3&sortOrder=ascending&itemID=CMS057286.

Centers for Medicare & Medicaid Services (CMS). (2007). *Nursing home compare.* Retrieved March 3, 2007, from www.medicare.gov/NHCompare/Home.asp?version=alternate&browser=IE%7C6%7CWinXP&language=English&defaultstatus=0&pagelist=Home&CookiesEnabledStatus=True.

Centers for Medicare & Medicaid Services (CMS) & Office of the Actuary, National Health Statistics Group. (2006). *National health expenditure data: Overview.* Retrieved January 11, 2008, from www.cms.hhs.gov/NationalHealthExpendData/Downloads/table.pdf.

Commonwealth Fund. (2006). *The 2006 Health Confidence Survey by the Employee Benefit Research Institute.* Retrieved March 21, 2006, from www.cmwf.org/surveys/surveys.htm.

Commonwealth Fund, Davis, K. Schoen, C., Schoenbaum, S.C., Doty, M.M., Holmgren, A.L., Kriss, J.L., et al. (2007). Mirror, mirror on the wall: An international update on the comparative performance of American health care. Retrieved February 10, 2007, from www.commonwealthfund.org/publications/publications_show.htm?doc_id=482678.

Congressional Budget Office. (1998). *Expanding health insurance coverage for children under Title XXI of the Social Security Act 1998.* Retrieved May 24, 2003, from www.cbo.gov/byclasscat.cfm?class-0&cat-9.

Congressional Research Service. (2007). *The congressional budget process: An overview.* Retrieved March 10, 2007, from www.rules.house.gov/archives/RS20368.

Cubanski, J., Voris, M., Kitchman, M., Newman, T., & Potetz, L. (2005). *Medicare chartbook* (No. 7284). Menlo Park, CA: The Henry J Kaiser Family Foundation.

Davidson, M. (2002). Outcomes of high-risk women cared for by certified nurse-midwives. *Journal of Midwifery & Women's Health, 1,* 46-49.

Department of Health & Human Services (DHHS). (2006). *Medicare benefit policy manual.* Washington, DC: Author.

Department of Health & Human Services (DHHS). (2007). *Hospital compare.* Retrieved March 7, 2007, from www.hospitalcompare.hhs.gov/Hospital/Home2.asp?version=alternate&browser=IE%7C6%7CWinXP&language=English&defaultstatus=0&pagelist=Home.

Feldstein, P. (2006). *The politics of health legislation: An economic perspective* (3rd ed.). Chicago: Health Administration Press.

Gill, C., & Gill, G. (2005). Nightingale in Scutari: Her legend re-examined. *Clinical Infectious Diseases, 40,* 1799–1805.

Hawkins, D. (2002). *Power vs. force: The hidden determinants of human behavior.* Australia: Hay House Publications.

Health Resources and Services Administration (HRSA), COGME, and NACNEP. (2000). *Collaborative education to ensure patient safety.* Retrieved March 15, 2007, from www.cogme.gove/jointmtg.pdf.

Health Resources and Services Administration (HRSA), Bureau of Health Professions. (2004). *The 2004 National Sample Survey of Registered Nurses.* Retrieved March 20, 2007, from http://bhpr.hrsa.gov/healthworkforce/reports/rnpopulation/preliminaryfindings.htm.

Health Resources and Services Administration (HRSA). (2006). *The registered nurse population: Findings from the March 2004 National Sample Survey of Registered Nurses.* Washington, DC: U.S. Department of Health & Human Services.

Heffler, S., Smith, S., Keehan, S., Borger, C., Kent, M., Clemens, M., et al. (2005). U.S. Health Spending Projections for 2004-2014. *Health Affairs, 24,* w74-w85.

Henry J. Kaiser Family Foundation. (2007a). *Data sources.* Retrieved March 15, 2007, from www.kaiseredu.org/research.asp?id=268#Dash_1_health_care.

Henry J. Kaiser Family Foundation. (2007b). *Total Medicaid spending FY2005.* Retrieved March 15, 2007, from www.statehealthfacts.org/cgi-.

Himmelstein, D., Warren, E., Thorne, D., & Woolhandler, S. (2005). Illness and injury as contributors to bankruptcy. *Health Affairs, 10,* w5-w63.

Institute for Healthcare Improvement (IHI). (2007). Cases for improvement. Retrieved April 14, 2007, from www.ihi.org/IHI/Topics/OfficePractices/Access/.

Institute of Medicine (IOM), Committee on Monitoring Access to Personal Health Care Services. (1993). In M. Millner (Ed.),

Access to health care in America. Washington, DC: National Academies Press.

Institute of Medicine (IOM). (2000). *To err is human: Building a safer health system.* Washington, DC: National Academies Press.

Institute of Medicine (IOM). (2001). *Crossing the quality chasm. A new health system for the 21st century.* Washington, DC: National Academies Press.

Institute of Medicine (IOM). (2002). Unequal treatment: Confronting racial and ethnic disparities in health care. Washington, DC: National Academies Press.

Institute of Medicine (IOM). (2003). *Priority areas for national action: Transforming health care quality.* Washington, DC: National Academies Press.

Institute of Medicine (IOM). (2004a). *Health literacy: A prescription to end confusion.* Washington, DC: National Academies Press.

Institute of Medicine (IOM). (2004b). *Insuring America's health: Principles and recommendations.* Washington, DC: National Academies Press.

Institute of Medicine (IOM). (2005). *Quality through collaboration: The future of rural health care.* Washington, DC: National Academies Press.

Institute of Medicine (IOM). (2006). *Improving the quality of health care for mental and substance-use conditions* (Quality Chasm series). Washington, DC: National Academies Press.

Institute of Medicine (IOM). (2007). *Rewarding provider performance: Aligning incentives in Medicare* (Pathways to Quality Healthcare series). Washington, DC: National Academies Press.

Kaiser Family Foundation, Commission on Medicaid and the Uninsured. (January 2007). *Health care coverage for low-income Americans: An evidenced-based approach to public policy.* Retrieved March 7, 2007, from www.kff.org/about/kcmu.cfm.

Kenney, G.M., & Cook, A. (February 2007). Coverage patterns among SCHIP-eligible children and their parents. *The Urban Institute*, No. 15.

Kingdon, J. (1995). *Agendas, alternatives, and public policies* (2nd ed.). New York: HarperCollins College Publishers.

Kronick, R., & Rousseau, D. (2007). Is Medicaid sustainable? Spending projections for the program's second 40 years. *Health Affairs (Project Hope), 26*(2), w271-w287.

Lenz, E.R., Mundinger, M.O., Kane, R.I., Hopkins, S.C., & Lin, S.X. (2004). Primary care outcomes in patients treated by nurse practitioners or physicians: Two-year follow up. *Medical Care Research and Review, 61*(3), 332-351.

Litman, T., & Robins, L. (1997). *Health politics and policy* (3rd ed.). Albany, NY: Delmar Publishers.

Longest, B. (2006). *Health policymaking in the United States* (4 ed.). Chicago, IL: Health Administration Press.

Lugo, N., O'Grady, E., Hodnicki, D., & Hanson, C. (2007). Ranking state NP regulation: Practice environment and consumer healthcare choice. *The American Journal for Nurse Practitioners, 11*(4), 8-9, 14-18, 23-24.

Mondy, C., Cardenas, D., & Avila, M. (2003). The role of an advanced practice public health nurse in bioterrorism preparedness. *Public Health Nursing (Boston, Mass.), 20*(6), 422-431.

Mundinger, M.O., Kane, R.I., Lenz, E.R., et al. (2000). Primary care outcomes in patients treated by nurse practitioners or physicians: A randomized trial. *JAMA, 283*(1), 59-68.

National Center for Health Statistics. (2006). *Health, United States, 2006.* With chartbook on trends in health of Americans. Hyattsville, MD: Department of Health & Human Services.

National Committee for Quality Assurance (NCQA). (2006). State of health care report. Washington, DC: Author.

National Committee for Quality Assurance (NCQA). (2007). *Report cards: Choosing quality health Care.* Retrieved March 14, 2007, from http://web.ncqa.org/tabid/60/Default.aspx.

National Governors Association. (2007). *Center for Best Practices.* Washington, DC. Retrieved March 20, 2007, from www.nga.org.

National Health Service Corps (NHSC). (2003). *The NHSC mission.* Retrieved March 14, 2007, from http://nhsc.bhpr.hrsa.gov/about/mission.asp.

National Quality Forum. (2004). *National voluntary consensus standards for nursing-sensitive care: An initial performance measure set.* Washington, D.C., National Quality Forum.

Needleman, J., Buerhaus, P., Mattke, S., Stewart, M., & Selevinsky, K. (2001). *Nurse staffing and patient outcomes in hospitals* (Report No. 230-99-0021). Washington, DC: Health Resources and Services Administration.

Nyman, J.A. (2004). Is "moral hazard" inefficient? The policy implications of a new theory. *Health Affairs, 23*(5), 194-199.

Oakley, D., Murray, M.E., Murtland, T., Hayashi, R., Andersen, H.F., Mayes, F., et al. (1996). Comparisons of outcomes of maternity care by obstetricians and certified nurse-midwives. *Obstetrics and Gynecology, 88*(5), 823-829.

Palmer, J.L., & Saving, T.R. (2006). *Status of the Social Security and Medicare programs: A summary of the 2006 annual reports.* Unpublished manuscript.

Pine, M., Holt, K.D., & Lou, Y.B. (April 2003). Surgical mortality and type of anesthesia providers. *AANA Journal, 71,* 109-116.

Poisal, J., Truffer, S., Smith, S., Sisko, A., Cowan, C., Keehan, S., et al. (2007). Health spending projections through 2016. Modest changes obscure Part D's impact. *Health Affairs, 26*(2), w242-w253.

Population Resource Center. (2008). The aging of America. Retrieved January 14, 2008, from www.prcdc.org/300million/The_Aging_of_America/.

Quality Resource System, Inc. (2006). *Area resource file: National county level health information resource database.* Retrieved June 29, 2007, from www.arfsys.com/.

Rhoades, J.A. (2005). *The uninsured in America, 2004.* Estimates for the civilian noninstitutionalized population under age 65 (Statistical Brief #842007). Rockville, MD: Agency for Healthcare Research and Quality.

Rowe, J.W., Cortese, D.A., & McGinnis, J.M. (2006). The emerging context for advances in comparative effectiveness assessment. *Health Affairs (Project Hope), 25*(6), w593-w595.

Scott, M.K. (2006). *Health care in the express lane: The emergence of retail clinics.* Oakland CA: California HealthCare Foundation.

Spitz, B., & Abramson, J. (2005). When health policy is the problem: A report from the field. *Journal of Health Politics, Policy and Law, 30*(3), 327-365, 367-373.

Starfield, B. (2000). Is U.S. health care really the best in the world? *Journal of the American Medical Association, 284,* 483-485.

Topp, R., Tucker, D., & Weber, C. (1998). Effect of clinical state case management/clinical nurse specialist patients hospitalized with congestive heart failure. *Nursing Case Management, 3*(4), 140-145.

U.S. Department of Commerce. (2006). *U.S. Census Bureau.* Retrieved March 7, 2007, from www.census.gov/Press-Release.

Wakefield, M. (2004). Government response: Legislation. In J. Milstead, *Health policy and politics: A nurses guide* (2nd ed., p. 68). Gaithersburg, MD: Aspen.

Wilson, W. (1913). *Congressional government.* Boston: Houghton Mifflin. Originally published 1885.

World Health Organization (WHO). (2006). *The World Health Report.* Retrieved February 27, 2007, from www.who.int/whr.

Strengthening Advanced Practice Nursing in Organizational Structures: Administrative Considerations

Brenda M. Nevidjon • Cynthia J. Simonson

INTRODUCTION

To say that the American health care system is in need of an overhaul is an understatement. It is the costliest system in the world and has poorer patient outcome results than many other countries. According to The Commonwealth Fund's report, "Mirror, Mirror on the Wall: An International Update on the Comparative Performance of American Health Care" (Davis et al., 2007), the United States lagged behind Australia, Canada, New Zealand, and the United Kingdom on quality, access, efficiency, equity, patient safety, and healthy lives. Of note, the United States is the only country in this comparison without universal health insurance. Although *Healthy People 2010* set clear goals to increase the quality and longevity of the public's health and to eliminate health disparities, results are thus far disappointing *(www.healthypeople.gov/)*. Over 45 million people in the United States are uninsured (ASPE Issue Brief, 2005). In general, care is episodic and disease-oriented even though many leading voices promote the importance of holistic care based on wellness, disease prevention, and effective management of chronic conditions. Not surprisingly, the state of the U.S. health care system is a recurring major platform issue during presidential election cycles.

In the midst of this chaos, advanced practice nursing continues its complex and, at times, controversial development. The most recent controversy has been the introduction of Doctor of Nursing Practice (DNP) degree and the recommendation that all advanced practice nurses (APNs) be prepared at this level by 2015 (American Association of Colleges of Nursing [AACN], 2004, 2006). APN history can be compared to a sine wave (see Chapter 1). Both clinical nurse specialists (CNSs) and nurse practitioners (NPs) have been in and out of demand as the health care system waxed and waned in its economic health. In the 1980s, administrators increased the number of CNS positions. In the turbulent 1990s, this number rapidly diminished as employers felt the impact of managed care and other payer changes. The number of NPs grew when managed care organizations

indicated they would need more primary care practitioners for their enrollees. The continuation of the CNS role, especially in acute care settings, was uncertain given the financial challenges faced by hospital administrators. Many CNSs quickly returned to school to prepare as NPs because administrators, often on the advice of consultants, eliminated hospital-based CNS positions in the early cycles of budget reductions. In response to these changes, schools of nursing eliminated CNS programs and ramped up programs to prepare more NPs. Since 2000, the acute care NP (ACNP) gained momentum as a solution for the decreasing numbers of medical residents in teaching hospitals. A change in the graduate medical education (GME) requirements has limited residents' work weeks to 80 hours, thus causing academic medical centers and teaching hospitals to seek new models of providing care to patients. Managed care did not penetrate the health care environment as originally expected, and nurse executives who eliminated CNS positions reintroduced them in the past few years because they saw the negative impact on basic nursing care that resulted from the lack of CNSs. Likewise, schools of nursing have increasingly reintroduced programs to prepare CNSs. During this time, physician organizations publicly challenged the competencies of APNs and conflict between nursing and medical organizations has intensified. The reaction to the DNP has been intense in some states as physician organizations have again questioned the competencies of APNs and sought legislative protection for the title "doctor" (Nelson, 2006; Phillips, Harper, Wakefield, Green, & Fryer, 2002).

Administrators who consider employing APNs in their health care organizations must deal with internal issues, such as how to define the value an APN will bring or how to identify what groups APNs might threaten within the organization. For organizations that support APN roles, the fiscal well-being of the organization and politics among the various clinicians can shape how APNs are included in the model of care. Numerous external factors also influence how advanced practice nursing is embraced and how care is delivered in all health care settings, whether community- or institution-based. Lack of consensus about the definition of roles, need for second licensure, reimbursement, prescriptive privilege, and scope of authority are some of the external national environmental issues that compound the internal issues about how organizations use APNs.

As changes regarding where and how health care is delivered continue, traditional and often inflexible organizational boundaries are disappearing. Administrators, partnering with clinicians, could lead the transformation of health care by building strong alliances among the health care professions to meet society's needs for accessible and affordable health care. However, Christensen, Bohmer, and Kenagy (2000) maintained that health care is the most entrenched, change-averse sector in the United States. They introduced the concept of *disruptive innovations* in health care—less expensive, simpler, and more convenient services that initially threaten the status quo but ultimately raise the quality of health care—and suggested that NPs are a disruptive innovation. As they noted, studies have shown that primary care NPs reliably diagnose and treat illnesses and spend more time counseling about prevention and wellness. However, numerous barriers, including resistance from health care organizations and restrictive state regulations, prevent NPs from working to their full potential.

In a more recent paper, Christensen, Baumann, Ruggles, and Sadtler (2006) again addressed the issue of lack of social change, including in health care, and identified that, rather than generating solutions, much of the financial investment goes to maintaining the status quo. They called the "MinuteClinic" a *catalytic innovator* and suggest that this model has great potential to increase access to health care. MinuteClinic, a privately owned network of primary care clinics located in retail outlets, promotes that it is staffed by NPs and lists a limited menu of services provided.

The purpose of this chapter is to outline the factors that contribute to the justification and use of APNs now and for the future. It provides information to help administrators in any setting champion the use of APNs in their organizations, whether introducing a new position or promoting a current one. The chapter also helps APNs understand the needs of administrators within complex health care systems and how to assist them in advocating for advanced practice roles in the organization. Factors such as

organizational culture, policy, and finance are discussed. As the authors' experiences have shown, when there is understanding and documentation of APNs' contributions, administrators sustain financial support for them.

Administrators also have the important responsibility to remain knowledgeable about APN roles and what these roles can accomplish for patient care and for organizations. In hospitals, the nurse administrator is a critical ally and key voice of support for APNs. A clearly articulated vision of advanced practice nursing by the nursing leadership of an organization will sustain commitment to the roles through difficult times. In other settings, physicians, physician executives, or business managers decide on the structure and function of APN roles. In any setting, collaboration is essential between APNs and administrators to define the expected contributions of the APN, including innovative practices, improved patient outcomes, cost savings, and revenue generation.

TRENDS DRIVING ADMINISTRATIVE DECISION MAKING

Administrators are bombarded daily with pressing decisions that can affect the organization's future. Some of the following trends are both challenges and opportunities in which administrators and APNs can partner to find creative solutions.

The Changing Health Care Environment

The health care system is an industry searching for definition. An increasingly diverse and demanding population now complicates the age-old dynamic tension inherent in a discussion of access, quality, and cost. Economics has been the driving force behind changes in the health care environment since the 1980s. Both private and governmental payers led initiatives aimed at reducing the costs of health care. Their key issues include cost containment, new forms of payment, consumer preferences, health reform efforts, and technological developments (Bodenheimer, 2005; Bodenheimer & Grumbach, 2005; Levit et al., 2003). Managed care was embraced in the 1990s as the way to contain costs. However, health care as a percentage of the U.S. gross national product (GNP) has continued to rise.

As shown in Box 23-1, many internal and external factors create opportunities for or impediments to the practice of nursing and the delivery of patient care. The external factors drive many of the internal

Box 23-1   Pressures on Health Care Administrators

EXTERNAL FACTORS	INTERNAL FACTORS
Managed care	Diminishing resources
Competition—market shifts	Restructuring work processes
Global pricing	Changes in skill mix
Emphasis on cost	Creation of new types of workers
Demand for outcomes data	Emphasis on customer service and patient satisfaction
Increased focus on patient satisfaction	Increased acuity in all settings
Insurers as driving forces regarding clinical decisions	Need for standard outcomes data, focus on evidence-based care
Emphasis on primary care	Enhanced training needs
Technological advances	Fewer workers through retirement, buy-out, termination
Increased Internet use	
Changing demographics	Cost of technology/automation
Shift to less-acute/ambulatory/home care	Emphasis on interdisciplinary efforts
Increased and/or changing regulatory requirements	Changing organizational structures
	Expanded scope of nurse executives
Licensing/credentialing requirements	Job/career insecurity
Changes in the medical profession	New reporting relationships
Better-informed consumers	Pressure to constrain wages
Federal and state health care initiatives	Multi-site practices, affiliations, networks
Labor shortages, multiple health care professions	Administration-physician relationships
Patient safety	Patient safety
Pay-for-performance initiative	24×7 coverage challenges including physicians no longer on call
Continued escalation of health care costs with declining reimbursement	Time pressures to see more patients in less time

factors. For example, the external payer environment has frequently led to reactive decisions about services and the future of specific disciplines in hospitals. However, the predicted restructuring of care delivery has not occurred as deliberatively, uniformly, or quickly throughout the country as one might think from media coverage of this issue (Burns & Pauly, 2002; Urden & Walston, 2001). Nonetheless, administrators have been challenged by decreasing reimbursement, increasing regulatory controls, increasing cost of technology, and increasing acuity of care. In hospitals, nurse administrators have responded by changing the skill mix of staff, developing cross-training programs, eliminating certain types of positions, and expanding the scope of middle managers. Commitment to CNSs and blended role APNs has varied throughout this time, particularly when the positions are fixed costs in a nursing department's budget. On the other hand, in ambulatory care settings, physician groups have increased service availability (access) by employing NPs. Other examples of how access has been increased are employment of gerontology NPs who coordinate care of patients in

skilled nursing facilities and employment of acute care NPs who coordinate care for a practice's hospitalized patients.

Population demographics are also affecting the health care environment, and administrators are strategically planning services to meet a variety of populations. The large generation of "baby boomers" is aging into the decades in which chronic diseases such as heart disease, cancer, and diabetes are more common. This has raised questions about hospital capacity, skilled nursing facilities, community care, and alternative care systems. It is likely that the traditional way of delivering care will not meet the increased demand brought by aging baby boomers. Immigration, particularly of Hispanics, will continue to challenge administrators. The 2000 U.S. census showed the shift occurring in the population, and Hispanics, as expected, exceeded African-Americans as the largest minority *(http://quickfacts.census.gov/qfd/states/00000. html)*. This has increased the need for providers with a multicultural philosophy and bilingual skills. Migrant health care clinics offer an opportunity for APNs and administrators to resolve the problem of overcrowded emergency departments. The number and needs of veterans are changing, and the Department of Veterans Affairs has redesigned its structure to create more options for care delivery.

Any and all of these changes in the health care environment can result in challenges for administrators, which can become opportunities for APNs. The wide variability of organizational structures and cultures provides rich settings in which APNs can practice.

Care Delivery Systems and Financial Pressures

The changing health care environment has led to changes in the structure of the care delivery system. Loose alliances of formerly competing organizations or formal contractual arrangements, such as integrated delivery networks (IDNs), have increased throughout the country. IDNs can be developed horizontally or vertically and be for-profit or not-for-profit. In a horizontal IDN, several like organizations form a legal entity. One example is an IDN of several hospitals, with one hospital usually being the tertiary or quaternary site. A vertical IDN, in contrast, brings together organizations from along the continuum of care. This network would include primary care, an acute care hospital, home health, a skilled nursing home, and perhaps even an insurance product. IDNs can cover a wide geographical area or consolidate care options in one city. It is more common to see one or two IDNs in a community than the several hospitals that once existed.

Ownership of the system may also be distant as regional consolidation occurs. In the case of national for-profit systems, such as Hospital Corporation of America (HCA) or Tenet, centralized administration exerts significant control over local operations. For-profit niche players, such as heart hospitals and cancer treatment facilities, have competed effectively against full-service institutions in many communities. Their strategy of having a joint venture with specialty physicians provides what physicians want—control and enhanced income. APNs are entering the specialty markets as major cost-effective members of the team. An example is US Oncology, a national health care services network for cancer care and research with services in 32 states. Built on a strategy of providing resources to oncologists, US Oncology routinely advertises for NPs whose scope of practice includes being an expert practitioner, educator/teacher, care manager, consultant, nurse researcher, and nurse leader *(www. usoncology.com/Home).*

Although the reorganization that is occurring should provide opportunities for APNs, support for their employment varies widely among managed care organizations (MCOs) and IDNs. Some of the reasons for this are that physicians do not want the competition, executives who set policy do not appreciate the benefits of APNs, and the managers who do know the benefits are usually not in positions of influence within the organization (Sinclair, 1997). Laurant and colleagues (2007) conducted a review of studies to evaluate the premise that NPs as primary care providers reduce costs and physicians' workload while maintaining quality of care. Their results suggest that NPs can achieve health outcomes equivalent to those of primary care physicians. Their work is an important document for APNs to use in educating employers and payers on the benefits of NPs as primary care providers.

The most effective way to employ APNs in IDNs is undetermined, but some characteristics of IDNs would indicate possibilities for APNs, particularly those in the blended CNS/NP role (see Chapter 15). These APNs are able to cross settings to follow specialty patients and are able to work with nurses in those multiple settings to meet the complex needs of these patients. Systematic planning and coordination of care across settings are necessary to ensure desired outcomes, patient satisfaction, and financial performance. APNs can fill gaps in services and cross boundaries. They can facilitate the integration of nursing into the overall mission of the organization and devise cost-effective and quality clinical program innovations. System-wide chief administrators, in particular, should find APNs to be excellent candidates for ensuring the standard of nursing practice across all sites, as demonstrated in Exemplar 23-1.

As the organizational structures for care delivery have been reshaped, the work and structures inside have been reshaped too. Some organizations have introduced a product line structure in which nursing is often decentralized. In a product line structure, services are integrated and coordinated by a defined focus. This focus could be age, as with children's services; gender, as with women's health services; or disease, as with cancer services. The structure may result in a marginalized nursing leadership that cannot advocate for appropriate patient care delivery models. However, a product line or decentralized structure does not necessarily indicate a lack of senior nursing voices. In fact, many product line administrators are nurses who have backgrounds in

EXEMPLAR 23-1   Identifying Opportunities for Advanced Practice Nurse Positions

In a large IDN, the chief nurse executive proposed that the cancer services unit employ a blended role APN to join oncologists in conducting consultative clinics in rural communities that were part of the IDN. Historically, the rural sites had designated a staff nurse to work with visiting oncologists, but the assignments were not consistent and the oncologists had expressed frustration. At first, the oncologists were uncertain about how the APN would function in the clinic. However, using skills in collaboration and negotiating entry to new organizations, the APN built credibility not only with the oncologists but also with the nurses and physicians at the rural sites. Originally, the APN accompanied the oncologist, but over time, her practice became increasingly independent. Typically, the oncologists evaluated patients with new diagnoses of cancer. The APN managed the care of patients receiving chemotherapy or those being followed up after completion of treatments. She also provided education for nurses in the rural sites and assisted in their development of chemotherapy administration skills. Because of her relationship with the comprehensive cancer center, she served as a source of information on clinical trials for the physicians in these communities. As the value of having a blended role APN available to patients with cancer in rural areas was recognized and the network of rural sites increased, the IDN cancer services hired an additional APN.

IDN, Integrated delivery network.

both advanced practice and administration. Product line structures can result in internal variability in advanced practice roles, with each product line defining positions differently, unless the organization develops linkages across product lines.

Financial Pressures and Reimbursement. Throughout the past several decades, pressures to reduce costs have resulted in fewer resources for patient care units, reductions in the overall number of hospital employees, changes in the skill mix of employees, and the introduction of new kinds of workers to provide direct and indirect patient care. An APN role that suffered through these changes is that of the CNS. Because the CNS was too often "all things to all people," the actual contributions made by the CNS to patient care have been underestimated. One of the more frequent administrative responses to budget pressures is to eliminate the position as a cost-containment initiative. However, the literature reveals that new and reconfigured roles for the CNS and other APNs emerged from the chaotic inpatient environment (McNatt & Eason, 2000; Naegle & Krainovich-Miller, 2001; Tobin, 2000; see also Chapter 18). The prediction that hospitals in the future will be purely intensive care facilities may create a justification for nurse administrators who are considering reintroduction of the CNS role. Having a CNS available to consult with staff about complex patient care situations will be increasingly necessary to support the staff at the bedside. The current foci of quality improvement and ensuring patient safely also are

creating opportunities for CNSs. Another emerging key role for APNs in hospitals is their leadership in achieving the American Nurses Credentialing Center (ANCC)–sponsored Magnet Recognition Program accreditation for the hospital. APNs not only directly contribute to meeting the Magnet standards but also are effective facilitators of various nursing governance groups (Exemplar 23-2).

As a result of turbulent health care reimbursement changes, physicians have experienced increased workloads with flat or decreased income. The Balanced Budget Act (BBA) (1997) decreased funding for GME, which is creating pressures on the competing missions of academic medical centers (Dickler & Shaw, 2000; Iglehart, 1999). Faculty are faced with the competing demands of seeing more patients while maintaining the teaching and research activities required for academic advancement. The decline in the number of residents and the restrictions on the number of hours they can work have prompted teaching hospitals to consider APNs and other alternative providers such as hospitalists. A role that has emerged in hospital settings is that of the ACNP (see Chapter 14). Although, historically, neonatal NPs were present in pediatric acute care settings, other NPs were not widely employed with other inpatient populations. Today, in contrast, ACNPs have roles with a wide variety of specialty services. As with other APN roles, the initial justification of these positions may be to substitute for physicians. For instance, in academic medical centers with reduced residency slots, ACNPs are being hired in to specialty medical practices. The

EXEMPLAR 23-2   Leading Institutional Initiatives

Coastal Community Hospital decided to apply for Magnet accreditation. The hospital has had a shared governance structure for several years and a flat administrative structure. The chair responsibilities of the research and clinical practice committees are shared by a CNS and a clinical nurse 4 (the hospital's clinical ladder has 4 levels). One of the measurement criteria for Magnet recognition is collaboration with nurse researchers and researchers from other disciplines. All the CNSs have appointments in the local school of nursing, and they collaborate with faculty in identifying clinical questions to study. They are skilled in using research findings to change practice and promote research use and development not only in nursing but also through interdisciplinary activities. They are well integrated into nursing governance and bridge the clinical arena and the academic program. The CNSs are respected clinical leaders in the organization, and thus the CNO has appointed several CNSs to key committees in which their leadership has been valuable. As the application document for Magnet is planned, the CNSs are assigned to lead teams preparing 4 of the 14 standards (research, ethics, education, collaboration) because of their expertise and are participants on other teams.

CNO, Chief nursing officer; CNS, clinical nurse specialist.

challenge to both APNs and administrators in these situations is to ensure that these roles are true APN roles and not simply physician substitutes. The challenge for administrators is that an APN's or hospitalist's salary is more expensive than that of a resident physician and there is no GME reimbursement. However, if the cost of educating and supervising the resident is factored in, the difference in cost may be slight. The dilemma for an APN is whether the role is purely substitution for the physician or is structured to allow the full benefit that an APN can provide. For instance, in critical care units, the ACNP can bring a distinct benefit to care delivery through advanced nursing skills of guidance and coaching, provision of continuity of care, and creative management of patient symptoms. Pioro and colleagues (2000) found that care delivered by an ACNP was associated with resource use and clinical and functional outcomes similar to care provided by attending and house staff physicians. Although such comparisons of APNs and physicians have been helpful in demonstrating the safety of APNs, the value-added component of advanced nursing needs to be emphasized in marketing these roles to administrators (see Chapter 24 for supporting research). The more recent focus on pay-for-performance (P4P), which links reimbursement to adherence to safety and quality measures, is not favored by physicians and also may disadvantage APNs in their ability to be compensated for their services because specialty NP data are not being captured (Bonis, 2005; Millenson, 2004; Thrall, 2004).

Subacute, transitional, or skilled nursing and hospice units exist today as freestanding organizations or within hospital systems. The goal of these units is to provide care in the most appropriate setting to meet patients' needs. In the process, it is expected that the cost of care will be reduced by enhancing efficiency, eliminating unnecessary activities, and reducing overhead costs. Nurse administrators face daily pressure to have models of care that will achieve those goals and help the organization be attractive to MCOs. They need clinical leaders who understand the continuum of patients' needs and who can develop appropriate services, an important niche for APNs, given their specialty skills. APNs will fulfill that need. Regardless of the care environment, APNs and administrators must work together to be successful in designing new nursing roles and to preserve and enrich nursing values and heritage within current and emerging systems.

APNs are eligible to receive direct reimbursement in the majority of states. However, obtaining reimbursement privileges from managed care and insurance organizations has been difficult. With the increase in IDNs, APNs may find that they are not recognized as primary care providers and thus are ineligible for reimbursement because they are not included on the provider list. However, state laws and private insurance companies tend to follow federal legislation, so gains at the national level are having a broader influence.

States have experimented with modifications to their Medicaid plans to improve access for their citizens. Historically, Medicaid enrollees have been predominantly women and children; currently, an increasing share of the funds covers services for people with chronic diseases and disabilities (Licking & Sampson, 1995). The State Children's Health Insurance Program (SCHIP), created by the BBA of 1997, provides grants to states to provide health insurance coverage to uninsured children up to 200% of the federal poverty level (FPL). Under Medicaid, family and pediatric NPs are recognized and reimbursed as primary care providers and health care organizations can employ them to meet the needs of these additional children. However, many of the SCHIP initiatives are underfunded or unfunded or have been subject to severe budget cuts because of state budget crises, and the predicted outcomes have not materialized (see *www.cms.hhs.gov/schip* and Chapter 22). Nurse administrators can and should advocate for APNs as programs and services are designed for vulnerable populations. Another population is older adults; an example is the APN-led geriatric service called *Evercare,* developed in 1987 by two nurse practitioners in Minnesota. Begun as a Medicare pilot program, it now has a range of Medicare, Medicaid, and private long-term care programs. Intensive primary and preventive services aim at avoiding acute illnesses and hospitalizations for seniors in nursing homes or living independently (Quaglietti & Anderson, 2002). Central to success of Evercare is a model of care that has a NP or care manager at the center of an integrated care team to coordinate care to achieve improved health outcomes for older adults, the disabled, and the chronically ill. Their studies have documented that this approach has reduced hospitalizations for nursing home residents by 45% and emergency department trips by 50%. Further information can be found at *www.evercarehealthplans.com.*

Health Care Professional Shortages

Since the early 2000s, the focus of most administrators has been on the registered nurse (RN) workforce and, more recently, on the nursing faculty shortage. In fact, the American Association of Colleges of Nursing (AACN) issues annual reports on the number of qualified applicants who have not been admitted to baccalaureate or graduate programs because of faculty shortages. Thus nurses seeking APN careers may face barriers to education if the faculty shortage worsens as predicted. Administrators face escalating contract labor costs to maintain services and again are making difficult decisions related to roles that are not direct care–related. However, they are also faced with issues of patient safety and quality of care. APNs can be a key resource in managing this complex scenario and improving the work environment (Disch, Walton, & Barnsteiner, 2001).

Nursing is not the only health care profession that is experiencing a shortage. A debate has evolved on whether a national physician shortage exists. The recent formation of the Council on Physician and Nurse Supply seeks to answer this question *(www.healthleadersmedia.com).* Regional shortages and specialty shortages, such as child and adolescent psychiatrists, have been documented (Croasdale, 2006). There is consensus that the number of primary care physicians is declining at a time when more are needed to care for an aging population. Fewer medical students are choosing to enter primary care as a career (Bodenheimer, 2006). The fact that increasing numbers of NPs and PAs are also entering specialty practices further complicates the deficit for primary care. Several other professions have shortages. For example, pharmacists, in demand by the retail pharmacy industry, are not filling hospital pharmacy vacancies. As the baby boomer health professionals retire, their positions will not necessarily be filled by members of the smaller Generation X that follows.

Quality and Safety

The Institute of Medicine's (IOM) report, "To Err is Human: Building a Safer Health System," (IOM, 2000) attracted national attention to the issues of safety in the health care system. The second report, "Crossing the Quality Chasm: A New Health System for the 21st Century" (IOM, 2001), focuses broadly on how to design the health care system to improve quality of care and ensure safety. Other studies have addressed questions about the outcomes of the 1990s' restructuring of hospitals and health systems and found mixed results for the desired outcomes (Burns & Pauly, 2002; Knox & Gharrity, 2002; Urden & Walston, 2001). APNs need to keep current with trends in redesign and restructuring so they can be effective advocates for patient care quality and safety. One challenge for administrators is achieving a balance between strengthening quality and containing costs. Data-driven care management through the use of evidence-based standards and technology enhances both safety and quality improvements but also has a high cost. The public has been greatly sensitized to this issue through several patient situations that gained national attention. Organizations must have safety and quality at the top of the priority list. APNs, particularly CNSs because of their systems perspective, are integral to quality and safety initiatives in their organizations (Exemplar 23-3).

EXEMPLAR 23-3 Moving into System Leadership

Susan is a cardiology CNS at a large academic medical center that is part of a six-hospital system that includes both academic and community cardiologists. The academic medical center and one of the community hospitals are known for their heart centers. Susan has been a CNS for 12 years, 7 of them at this medical center. In her CNS role, she served as a key leader for quality improvement initiatives across the system for the heart services. Two years ago, she decided to return to school for a DNP degree using the employee tuition benefit. As her capstone project, she reorganized and redesigned the congestive heart failure program that bridges the two heart centers and physician practices. One element of the project was defining the role and functions of the current NP staff. The outcomes of her project have been increased access for patients; increased satisfaction for patients, physicians, and staff; decreased ED visits; and decreased costs. Recently the CEO of the system added the position of Vice President, Quality and Service Improvement, to his executive team and reorganized resources for this new department. Because he had first-hand knowledge of Susan's capstone project, he invited her to apply for the position. During the interview process, Susan articulated the additional competencies and knowledge her DNP added to her strong clinical practice and was the preferred candidate. Susan realized that, although she would be giving up her APN position, she would be using all of her valuable CNS skills plus her DNP in the new position. After reflecting on the opportunity to lead a department whose influence would be across settings and institutions, Susan accepted this system level leadership position.

APN, Advanced practice nurse; *CEO,* chief executive officer; *CNS,* clinical nurse specialist; *DNP,* Doctor of Nursing Practice; *ED,* emergency department; *NP,* nurse practitioner.

Regulatory and Compliance Issues

Concern about the rising cost of medical care and health insurance premiums and the rising number of uninsured and underinsured continues to be part of the national conversation. Despite this, the health care system has changed little. Over the past 15 years, three pieces of federal legislation have made the most significant impact on the health care industry. The 1996 Health Insurance Portability and Accountability Act (HIPAA) increased flexibility in coverage. The 1997 BBA affected reimbursement *(www.cms.gov)* and also created the SCHIP. The passage of the Medicare Prescription Drug, Improvement, and Modernization Act of 2003, Part D, greatly expanded coverage for medications as well as directed the IOM to develop a strategy for aligning payment and clinical performance (Kennerly, 2007; Millenson, 2004; see also Chapter 22). Other legislation that affected the role of APNs in larger organizations included the past change by the Centers for Medicare & Medicaid Services (CMS) from cost-based hospital payment to prospective payment (diagnosis-related groups [DRGs]) and legislation limiting the number of hours residents in teaching hospitals can work (Buppert, 2005a). Such legislation has influenced the level of APN reimbursement within health care organizations and has affected administrators' views of the cost-effectiveness of APNs. The most important regulations affecting APN roles remain those related to each state's determination of APN scope of practice. Scope determines the services an APN can provide and, hence, what may be billed (see Chapter 21).

Administrators must look at APNs from both a revenue-producing perspective and a cost-saving perspective. Given the continuing concern about rising costs, providers are under increasing pressure to be accountable for evidence-based, cost-effective care. Many legislative bodies, regulatory agencies and organizations such as The Joint Commission (TJC), the National Committee for Quality Assurance (NCQA), CMS, and insurers are rapidly developing quality indicators that health care organizations are required or encouraged to meet to be able to participate in their programs (Bonis, 2005; Thrall, 2004). Many payers are beginning to provide incentive payments for organizations that exceed their specified quality indicators (Bonis; Millenson, 2004; Thrall). Although these quality-based P4P plans currently do not put the organization's reimbursement at risk, this may change in the future. In short, documenting quality matters. Organizations must be flexible, provide high-quality care, and be cost-effective. APNs have demonstrated the ability to provide high-quality care very cost-effectively (Cowan et al., 2006; Mezey et al., 2005; Naylor et al., 2004). These considerations impact how administrators develop, redefine, or justify APN roles.

COMMON PROBLEMS AND STRATEGIES FOR SOLVING THEM

There are compelling reasons for administrators to consider advanced practice nursing roles as the answers to many of the important challenges of today's health care environment. Box 23-2 lists some of the characteristics that provide justifications for advanced practice nursing roles. Descriptions of the core competencies of APNs and other attributes that make them invaluable to administrators can be found in Chapter 3 and in the role chapters in Part III. Many of the variables that contribute to the success of APN roles are within the control of the administrator, so the needs and concerns of the administrator are important. Likewise, many of the variables that are within the control of the APN can contribute to the administrator's success. The next sections are relevant for both administrators and APNs.

Box 23-2 JUSTIFICATION FOR ADVANCED PRACTICE NURSE ROLES

- Use of theory-based and evidence-based clinical care
- Knowledge of clinical practice, including both medical and nursing perspectives
- Knowledge of health care systems
- Ability to develop and integrate practice within organizations, communities, and systems
- Ability to make independent judgments and ethical decisions
- Ability to practice in multiple care settings, such as tertiary, hospice, and home care
- Flexibility
- Ability to identify the nature and costs of nursing interventions and their effects on patient outcomes
- Expertise in specific clinical specialty areas, such as pain management and women's health
- Ability to translate research into practice
- Ability to analyze care for not only an individual but also a population
- Skill in educating staff
- Organizational need for APN core competencies, such as skilled guidance and coaching, interdisciplinary collaboration, consultation, and leadership
- Skill in working with underserved and culturally diverse populations

---

Developing a Climate of Support for Advanced Practice Nurses

Abdellah (1997) described APNs worldwide and noted that their frustrations included balancing components of and defending their roles, lack of involvement in decision making, and lack of authority to make change. The last two are an alert, particularly to nurse administrators. They indicate that nurse administrators may be missing an opportunity to position APNs effectively within the nursing organization. However, they may also indicate that APNs have not been assertive in taking a leadership role. Richmond and Becker (2005) identified nine characteristics of an APN-friendly culture, noting that these cultures must be developed and do not occur by chance. Given today's health care climate, clinical and systems leadership are essential for redesigning care delivery (see Chapter 9). The move to doctoral education for APNs should strengthen their systems leadership abilities, since this is a strong theme of the DNP *Essentials* competencies (AACN, 2006). APNs should be the administrator's designees to lead redesign efforts because they are the experts in direct patient care and they interact with patients along the continuum of care. They are also ideal candidates to lead an interdisciplinary team in performance improvement initiatives.

Administrators want APNs who are able to build partnerships and work comfortably in interdisciplinary teams. Support from physician and nurse colleagues tops the list of factors that help or hinder an APN. Acceptance by colleagues creates a successful environment in which to develop a practice. The opposite holds if support and acceptance are absent. Resistance to the role may be the result of misconceptions about APN roles or concerns about reimbursement. Administrators and APNs must give attention to key factors for success such as the APN's own confidence in his or her ability, the APN's skill in building collaborative relationships, autonomy coupled with clear expectations of the position, and being positioned organizationally so that staff recognize the value of the APN. Mitigating inhibiting factors also enhances the APN's opportunity for success. Inhibitors can include lack of orientation to the organization, lack of resources for the APN, or nonaligned expectations of the administrator, APN, practice colleagues, and staff.

Modulating Interprofessional and Intraprofessional Tensions

Interprofessional tensions can limit the effectiveness of APNs and must be recognized and addressed. Whatever the specific practice role, APNs have experienced tensions with other professions and within nursing (see Chapter 1). Several studies document the problem of collaborative tensions among health care providers that make APNs feel undervalued (Baggs, 2005; Gardner, 2005; Lindeke & Sieckert, 2005). Physicians, nurses, and administrators all contribute to this dynamic. These tensions can influence the commitment of administrators to APN roles. Each organization is different and may face specific challenges because of structure or personalities involved, but there are many common pitfalls that APNs and administrators should be aware of and make plans to resolve. These are different for novice versus experienced APNs and newly created versus existing roles.

Novice APNs need extra support from administrators to help them fully understand their roles and concentrate on performing advanced practice activities rather than performing more comfortable RN activities. If novice APNs are familiar to the staff with whom they will be working, it may be difficult to change roles or have the other staff accept them as an APN. Novice APNs may be slower and need more consultation and support in their patient care and may be seen as not able to carry a full load. This can present a problem in busy primary care practices in which time is revenue. Both novice and experienced APNs coming into new roles or organizations may face turf issues. Because of the flexible nature of the APN role, this can be felt from both the RNs and physicians in the practice. Introducing an APN role where none has existed may cause tension in long-term, established professional relationships between RNs and physicians. Turf issues may also occur between others in the practice who may be competing for the same patient visits, including other APNs, physician assistants (PAs), or physicians. Tension between APNs and PAs may arise because of their different professional approach to similar positions.

Administrators also face tension wanting to employ APNs and dealing with insurers who do not want to reimburse for their services. This is a key issue for health care administrators and can also be an issue for employer benefits managers. When there is conflict and lack of clarity about a role, administrators may shy away from introducing the role into an organization, even if there is a good business case. The administrator should be the voice to influence decisions but may also be someone who does not understand the value of the various APN roles. Thus APNs must build meaningful working relationships with key administrators. This includes assessing the administrator's understanding of the APN's potential contributions

and undertaking sustained efforts to educate and inform the administrator about advanced practice if necessary. Partnerships between administrators and APNs can lead to innovative solutions to the stresses experienced in health care organizations.

Confusion among physicians and other staff and colleagues about the specific nature of advanced practice nursing roles may stop them from giving support. Administrators and APNs can alleviate this confusion in a number of ways. These include providing information and research data regarding the attributes of APN roles and the benefits of collaboration for clinical practice, research activities, and teaching responsibilities. Introducing APN students and faculty into the clinical setting can assist providers in other disciplines to understand APN roles. The administrator needs to demonstrate the positive value APNs add to patient care. The importance of using appropriate data to support one's point of view cannot be overemphasized. The demonstration of successful role implementation is the most powerful means by which administrators and APNs can garner organizational support. Building institutional success stories can be most helpful to administrators.

Regardless of the organization and its structure, the administrator is influential in preparing the organization for successful implementation of any APN role. The administrator can broker relationships, making sure the APN is introduced effectively in the organization by using formal communication tools such as newsletters and by setting up meetings with key individuals during the APN's orientation. The administrator can align resources that help an APN achieve the expected outcomes, such as arranging for access to current technology versus providing a "hand-me-down" computer from another employee in the organization. Such actions demonstrate how the organization values the APN's contribution. Administrators also need to ensure that there is a strong and senior voice for nursing in the credentialing and privileging process to facilitate advocating for privileges, including admitting privileges, for APNs.

Interprofessional tension also occurs on a more global level. Although many physicians have been strong supporters of APNs, tensions over control of practice and reimbursement for services continue (Phillips et al., 2002). The American Medical Association (AMA) continues to struggle to protect its perceived turf by working for policy and legislative measures to control and limit the practice of nonphysician health care providers. At its annual meeting in June of 2006, the AMA approved and adopted Resolution 211, "Need to Expose and Counter Nurse Doctoral Programs [NDP] Misrepresentation." Positing that "nurses and other non-physician providers who hold doctoral degrees and identify themselves as 'doctors' will create confusion, jeopardize patient safety and erode the trust inherent in the true patient-physician relationship," the resolution calls for the AMA to work with state attorneys general "to identify and prosecute individuals who misrepresent themselves as physicians" and to counter misrepresentation by nurse doctoral programs (Nelson, 2006). According to Phillips and colleagues (2002):

> Turf battles interfere with joint advocacy for needed health system change and delay development of interdisciplinary teams that could help patients. A combined, consistent effort is urgently needed for studying, training, and deploying a collaborative, integrated workforce aimed at improving the health care system of tomorrow. The country can ill afford doctors and nurses who ignore one another's capabilities and fail to maximize each other's contributions cost-effectively. (p. 133)

Maximizing "Profitability"

Decreasing reimbursement from third-party payers over the past few years has increased pressure on administrators and clinicians to maximize profitability while maintaining ethical billing practices. All health care providers must adjust to practicing in an era of finite resources. Although most providers do not like to think of health care as a business (Bodenheimer & Grumbach, 2005), that attitude must change to survive in today's health care environment. Therefore it is important that APNs have a basic understanding of business principles (see Chapter 19). APNs must be knowledgeable about the operations and finances of their practice group or institution, such as where revenues come from and the costs associated with providing health care. APNs must be aware of the financial consequences of their practice style and be willing to work with administrative staff to improve their "profitability" to the organization.

One method of maximizing profitability is to maximize revenue. APNs must pay special attention to the different payer types found in their patient population. What percentage of the patients have Medicaid, Medicare, managed care, point of service (POS), preferred provider organization (PPO), health maintenance organization (HMO), or fee for service? Are any patients self-pay? APNs should familiarize themselves

with the specific services covered by their largest third-party payers and use this information to develop programs or services to maximize payments from those payers. For example, many managed care plans cover health promotion and disease prevention. Based on the level of financial risk the practice assumes (e.g., under a capitated payment system), developing a method to track glucose control for all diabetics in the practice along with strategies to reduce diabetic complications may be cost-effective (Litaker et al., 2003). In some fee-for-service plans, preventive medicine services are not covered benefits and these same strategies may not be as cost-effective.

APNs must understand the different reimbursement mechanisms. Whereas Medicare allows direct reimbursement for services rendered by APNs, Medicaid, MCOs, and private payers may or may not follow suit. Some private insurance companies recognize NPs as participating providers in their health plans. APNs should obtain their own individual provider number with each plan to bill for their services and generate revenue. (See Chapter 19 and specific roles chapters in Part III for further discussion of reimbursement by advanced practice nursing specialty.)

A key factor in revenue maximization is the concept of time. The only thing APNs have to "sell" is their expertise and time. For APNs in primary care practices, an open slot in an appointment schedule is a lost revenue opportunity that cannot be retrieved. Making sure that the APN's schedule is full, ensuring that the system for care is set up in a way that maximizes efficiency, and concentrating on billable functions rather than activities that can be accomplished by a non-reimbursable staff member can enhance revenue. One method for ensuring a full schedule is for the APN to develop his or her own patient following or practice, such as seeing all breast-feeding mothers or developing a nurse-run pacemaker clinic. APNs can be powerful practice builders with their ability to attract patients and referral sources. By establishing a patient and referral base, the APN becomes a valuable asset to the practice or institution. Marketing the unique skills of the APN or his or her expertise as a clinician can also help build the practice. One way this can be accomplished is by developing a schedule template that allows the APN to be more available for urgent care or same-day patient appointments. Patients who have positive experiences are much more likely to return to the APN for subsequent appointments.

All third-party payers require that any service rendered be properly coded to be paid. Coding all patient encounters accurately requires familiarity with the International Classification of Diseases, 9th Revision (ICD-9) diagnostic codes and Current Procedural Terminology (CPT) billing codes (Buppert, 2005b; see also Chapter 19). Coding is now routinely taught in advanced practice nursing programs. Unfortunately, many APNs undercode or do not include all applicable diagnostic codes, which loses revenue for the practice. Asking the person who does the billing to informally audit the APN's charts to determine whether the appropriate billing and diagnostic codes are routinely selected can be a good way to ensure accuracy (Henley, 2003). A related concept is resource-based relative value units (RVUs). RVUs are non-monetary, numeric values that Medicare has developed to represent the relative amount of provider time, resources, and expertise needed to provide various services to patients. RVUs are assigned to each CPT code and provide administrators with a tool to assess provider productivity.

Another strategy for maximizing profitability is reducing costs. Eliminating ineffective and inappropriate care and administrative waste can be a painless cost-control method that does not adversely affect the quality of care provided to individual patients. APNs can be leaders in this effort and ensure that the chosen cost-control strategies do not adversely affect the quality of patient care.

Developing Policies, Procedures, and Protocols

Whatever the practice setting, administrators value and require policies, procedures, and protocols to guide and standardize practice. As the health care environment has become increasingly litigious, policies, procedures, and protocols have become the infrastructure for safety and quality. APNs can bring their expert knowledge to the development of general institution-wide policies and procedures, as well as those that specifically address advanced practice. In a hospital setting, an APN may be the best choice to lead the clinical practice council or the product selection committee. Administrators can also recruit APNs to ensure that translating health policy regulations into the practice setting does not compromise clinical care.

Compliance with Regulatory Agencies

The health care environment has many regulatory influences that affect everything from reimbursement to worker safety (Table 23-1). Whether the APN is an employee or an employer, awareness of regulations that direct clinical practice and business operations is critical. Many hospitals do not take advantage of the potential scope of advanced practice nursing because there is not a champion who understands the regulatory arena for APNs. For example, under Medicare, APNs can be reimbursed "incident to" the services of a physician at 100% of the physician fee schedule if all of the "incident to" rules are followed, or they may apply for their own Medicare provider identification number and be reimbursed directly at 85% of the physician fee schedules (see Chapter 19).

Many managed care plans monitor health care providers' performance in providing care. Individual providers track performance-related information. A provider profile presents summarized statistics to reflect provider performance in the form of rates and averages pertaining to the care rendered to a specific population. Pharmacy claims are an important source of profiling information. They allow a health plan to measure preventive care and long-term management of chronic disease (e.g., prescription of inhaled steroids for patients with asthma). Measures of resource utilization are another common indicator used, such as the number of emergency department visits or the number of days of hospitalization for patients in the provider's panel. Measures that directly address quality of care have gained a more prominent place in provider profiling in the past several years. Many of these measures are required for external reporting of total plan performance. A common measurement tool is the Healthcare Effectiveness Data and Information Set (HEDIS). Among the key areas of HEDIS reporting are immunization rates, mammography rates, cervical screening rates, and treatment of patients with a chronic disease such as asthma or diabetes. APNs need to be aware of the measures used to evaluate their effectiveness as providers in a practice (see Chapter 25).

The National Practitioner Databank was established under the Healthcare Quality Improvement Act of 1986. The intent is to improve the quality of health care by encouraging hospitals and other health care agencies to restrict the ability of incompetent health care providers to move from state to state without disclosure or discovery of previous malpractice. It is primarily a flagging system intended to facilitate a comprehensive review of health care practitioners' professional credentials. Hospitals must query practitioners when they apply for privileges and every 2 years for practitioners who are on the

Table 23-1 KEY REGULATORY AGENCIES

Acute Care or Inpatient Settings	Outpatient or Community-Based Settings
The Joint Commission (TJC): TJC is an independent not-for-profit organization that evaluates the quality and safety of care provided by health care organizations. TJC has specific regulations that must be adhered to in order for the institution to be accredited. Website: www.jointcommission.org	TJC accredits ambulatory organizations also.
	Healthcare Effectiveness Data and Information Set (HEDIS): HEDIS is a tool used by more than 90% of America's health plans to measure performance on important dimensions of care and service. It is a set of standardized measures that specifies how health plans collect, audit, and report on their performance in important areas ranging from breast cancer screening, to helping patients control their cholesterol, to customer satisfaction. Website: www.ncqa.org/tabid/59/Default.aspx
	National Committee for Quality Assurance (NCQA): NCQA is a consumer-driven, nonprofit organization that accredits health plans. Plans are being made to accredit group practices. Website: www.ncqa.org
Health Insurance Portability and Accountability Act (HIPAA): Title I of HIPAA protects health insurance coverage for workers and their families when they change or lose their jobs. Title II of HIPAA requires the Department of Health and Human Services to establish national standards for electronic health care transactions and national identifiers for providers, health plans, and employers. It also addresses the security and privacy of health data. Website: www.cms.hhs.gov/hipaa	HIPAA rules apply to outpatient settings as well as inpatient settings
Centers for Medicare & Medicaid Services (CMS): CMS is the federal agency that administers the Medicare and Medicaid programs. Both programs have regulations that affect the care of patients covered under these plans. Website: www.cms.hhs.gov	CMS rules apply to outpatient settings as well as inpatient settings.

medical staff or hold privileges. State licensing boards may query at any time. Health care practitioners may self-query at any time (see *www.npdb-hipdb.com*).

Ensuring Patient Safety

In the IOM's 2003 report, "Health Professions Education: A Bridge to Quality," the five core competencies that all health care clinicians should have are outlined (IOM, 2003). The five competencies are providing patient-centered care, working in interdisciplinary teams, employing evidence-based practice, applying

quality improvement, and utilizing informatics. They are each prominently featured in the DNP *Essentials* as well (AACN, 2006).

APNs can be the champions for safety and quality initiatives in organizations. Because of the admission of more patients with acute and complex illnesses and the issues related to nursing staffing, APNs in hospitals can provide the expertise needed to identify performance improvement initiatives and to lead those initiatives. By virtue of education and experience, APNs should be role models of the five competencies, and administrators can turn to them as internal consultants rather than hiring external ones. While the national attention to safety and quality has focused primarily on the hospital environment, community practices also need to have ongoing performance improvement as part of their agenda. The HEDIS supports this at the community level.

Technology and Informatics

Technology and advances in the understanding of disease, especially through genetics, have affected the cost of care and have led to changes in the care environment. The rate of discovery in the past two decades has been incredible and has translated new knowledge into clinical treatment. Advances in electronic communication—in particular, access to the Internet—have meant immediate worldwide information distribution. Patients and their families can obtain in-depth details about their diseases in a matter of minutes and come to their providers with more information than the providers may have. All websites with medical information are not accurate, however, and providers may find they are spending increased time correcting misinformation. With a more informed public, providers encounter patients who expect more time to discuss their disease and treatment options. At the same time, payers may be restricting access to certain technologies and pressuring providers to see more patients.

Organizations diligently deliberate choices of clinical and information technology because the demands are endless and the financial resources are not. Administrators often face difficult decisions related to capital expenditures. APNs can advocate for both clinical and informatics technology and are excellent members of committees that evaluate requests. Because they have a broad view of the organization and the patients being cared for, APNs can relate technology to work flow and identify cost/benefit factors. For example, handheld devices or personal digital assistants (PDAs) can store reference books, calculate complex medical results, keep track of patients and procedures, and serve as daily planners. There are even programs that create prescriptions to be automatically sent to a pharmacy or calculate CPT codes for billing.

STRATEGIES TO STRENGTHEN ADVANCED PRACTICE NURSING ROLES

Unless an APN establishes an independent practice, administrators decide whether to create a new APN role, whether to eliminate one, whether to transform the role, or whether to keep it as it is. They also can influence how an advanced practice nursing position is compensated and what resources will be made available for the APN. Thus, by understanding the needs of administrators, APNs can cultivate champions within an organization for their roles. Likewise, by understanding the contributions APNs can make, administrators can most effectively position APNs as leaders and achieve success in fulfilling the organization's mission.

An administrator can assess the organization's need for an APN and determine which advanced practice role will fulfill the need. Involving stakeholders in planning for the new position ensures commitment to the person who is hired. A well-developed position description and agreed-upon reporting relationships establish the foundation for the APN and facilitate entry to the organization. The process of recruiting the best APN includes a comprehensive interview process to ensure that all stakeholders have an opportunity for input about their expectations. Finally, an orientation to the organization, including communication about the expectations of the APN, is necessary to foster success.

Considerations When Applying for a Position

APNs must consider many factors when applying for a position in an organization or practice (Box 23-3; see also Chapter 20). Although it may seem that many of these factors relate to larger organizations, they can be equally important when an APN is considering entering a primary care practice or physician group. For example, being knowledgeable about the regulatory conditions in a particular state is important if the APN is considering relocation. Some states are more supportive of advanced practice nursing than others. Once the APN understands the state's regulatory environment, learning the conditions specific to a position is critical.

The leadership of an organization provides the vision and shapes the culture for nursing practice within hospitals, community-based practices, and many other health care organizations. Although physician private practice groups may not be as formal as other health care organizations, the APN candidate needs to know who the leadership is and their philosophy about advanced practice nursing. The organization's mission and vision can alert an APN candidate to the potential support for the role. Organizations with a strong community focus may

Box 23-3 ORGANIZATIONAL CONSIDERATIONS FOR ADVANCED PRACTICE NURSES
WHEN APPLYING FOR A POSITION

- Organization's mission, structure, strategic priorities, culture
- Nursing philosophy, share of organizational power, definition of APN roles
- Knowledge of who are the key supporters and alliances for the position
- Commitment to interdisciplinary care and continuous improvement principles
- Communication and collaborative processes among providers, administrators, and APNs
- Data that support the position, expected outcomes
- Reporting relationship, opportunities/ability to negotiate APN responsibilities
- Credentialing requirements
- Reimbursement potential, financial objectives
- Resources, other APNs
- Models of care delivery, clinical programs, patient populations
- State regulations for APNs

APN, Advanced practice nurse.

be seeking to develop APN-run clinics. Academic organizations—with their triple mission of patient care, teaching, and research—may seek doctorally prepared CNSs to influence the advancement of all nursing practice. IDNs may create a blended APN role that crosses boundaries of the discrete entities within the network to ensure a consistent standard of care for patients.

In assessing an organization, an APN applicant needs to evaluate how firmly established the APN role is by administrators, whether nurses or not. Administrators must recognize that advanced practice nursing is central to quality of care, access to care, and cost containment. However, administrators are also faced with pressures of balancing cost and quality and a workforce shortage. APNs provide the clinical surveillance within an organization. They are able to see patterns of care, as well as assess and meet the individual needs of patients. Because APNs are able to move throughout the care continuum, they can collaborate with administration to identify ways to manage resources effectively. Also, they are able to address development needs among the nursing staff. When administrators understand this, it is easy to maintain a commitment to advanced practice even in difficult times. For example, one author (B.M.N.) refused to eliminate the CNS role in her organization, even though consultants were suggesting to administration that this was an easy budget cut.

An important consideration for an APN applying for a position with a corporate MCO is that the central operation's office and high-level administrators who control policy and budget may be several states away and virtually inaccessible. APNs need to assess for dissonance between midlevel management at the local level and the centralized hierarchy. In such structures, final decisions usually come from the central administration and there may not be a nursing administrator to serve as a champion.

A candidate should assess how members of the organization understand the mission and vision and how an APN contributes to achieving them. Likewise, the nurse administrator will evaluate the APN candidate as to his or her interpretation and understanding of the organization and its goals. The nurse administrator will look for the fit between the mission and vision of the organization and the APN's personal abilities and reasons for seeking the position. In the interview process, the selection committee and hiring administrator will also evaluate the candidate's ability to negotiate the political environment of the organization, particularly if the position is new.

When an APN considers a position, he or she must evaluate the collaborative atmosphere of the organization, regardless of whether it is a large and complex system or a small group practice. The advertising of a position does not necessarily mean that all the people within the organization embrace an advanced practice nursing role. Learning about the partnerships that exist and seeking examples of past successes can be helpful in understanding who may be champions of the role. A champion is not found just in the physician or nursing arenas. Strategic alliances can be formed with any of the organization's formal and informal leaders. They are more likely to be supporters if they understand the purpose of the position and, as appropriate, participate in the interviewing process.

In an organizational culture with open and honest communication, the administrator and APN can identify key leaders and anticipate their needs for specific information. All organizations may not have that culture, and the administrator can help the APN understand the politics. Other APNs in the organization can also help a new APN by introducing the new APN to key leaders. Partnering with supporters builds a strong network that can prevent an APN from being seen as an intruder.

The "Fit" of the Advanced Practice Nurse Within the Organization

The requirements of the position will determine the educational preparation and previous work experiences needed by the APN. For example, an organization seeking ways to maximize its reimbursement potential may develop NP and certified nurse-midwife (CNM) positions to achieve this goal. The goals and objectives of the position determine the APN's responsibilities, such as primary care delivery, consultation, program planning, staff development, clinical research, and expansion of patient services. The nature of the clinical program will determine the selection of the appropriate APN role. The number and type of other disciplines and professionals within the practice setting are other considerations. A CNS position may be selected to enhance staff nurses' clinical and communication skills within a clinical program that includes physicians, PAs, and ACNPs. A blended role CNS/NP may be desired if the purpose is to manage the care of a group of patients across multiple settings in an IDN. A certified registered nurse anesthetist (CRNA) may be hired to cost-effectively enhance the day surgery program. The purpose of a position will also determine the licensure and credentialing requirements (see Chapter 21).

Delineation of roles and clear communication and reporting structures strengthen these relationships. The emerging focus on advanced practice nursing within the context of work redesign affects other care providers in different ways. In some organizations, APNs are assuming functions previously performed by other professionals, including physicians, social workers, and clinical dietitians. Because APNs potentially affect the practice of other care providers, having well-defined expectations modulates what can become turf issues. The broadest communication of the APN's responsibilities and goals helps ensure the APN's success. The administrator can minimize the potential for these disputes by maintaining the focus of decision making on patient care requirements and how to address them in the most cost-effective and efficient manner with the best possible outcomes. Sincerely expressed respect for the work of other professionals, coupled with sensitivity and diplomacy, can minimize the potentially negative effects of these negotiations.

APNs may align with medicine's organizational structure and discount their nursing connection. APNs need to seek collaborative relationships within the nursing organizational structure because nursing leaders can be essential advocates for APNs. For example, although CRNAs have worked for many years with their physician colleagues, many occasions of conflict have occurred between the two, and for this reason, organizations and practices may have concerns about hiring CRNAs. Anesthesia is a recognized specialty in both medicine and nursing. Approximately 80% of CRNAs work as partners in care with anesthesiologists, while the remaining 20% function as sole anesthesia providers working and collaborating with surgeons and other licensed physicians (see Chapter 17). When anesthesia is administered by a CRNA, it is recognized as the practice of nursing; when it is administered by an anesthesiologist, it is recognized as the practice of medicine. In a hospital that employs CRNAs, the nurse administrator can be an effective voice in collaboration with them if interprofessional tensions arise.

Organization Entry and Success

How an APN is introduced in the organization sets the stage for the APN's success. Being educated about organizational culture and politics, as well as being given the usual basic information of orientation, prepares the APN for the work environment. Larger organizations usually have well-developed orientation plans in place that introduce new employees to the organizational culture. However, even a small primary care practice needs to develop an orientation plan for a new APN. The APN and administrator should collaborate in establishing goals and mutually clear expectations to lay foundation. In big HMOs, APNs need to understand structure of the organization and chain of command. Early identification of performance measures to define success is also important. Success may be defined as shorter waiting times for a new patient appointment, higher patient satisfaction scores, or decreased lengths of stay in an inpatient unit. It can mean developing a new home care service for seniors who cannot travel to office practices or designing a clinical advancement program for staff nurses.

Whether the new position is in a private practice or in a hospital, establishing credibility as a clinician begins as soon as the APN joins the organization. Once physicians, administrators, nurses, and other staff have confidence in the APN's abilities and judgment as a clinician, they will begin to offer support for the APN's efforts. As a new employee in an institution, the most important priority for the APN is to establish a clinical practice and gain the respect of colleagues. One of the ways an administrator can expedite an APN's transition into the organization is to set up a peer review system for the first 30 to 90 days of employment. For example, a senior provider in a clinic practice can review the charts of patients who have been seen by the new APN. This is usually an expeditious way for the new APN to gain the confidence and trust of the other providers in the practice. Once the other providers have confidence in and respect for the APN, they will be more apt to support changes that remove barriers to the APN's practice. Another method for building credibility is reporting and tracking satisfaction scores of patients who have been cared for by the APN. Randomized clinical trials in which NPs were compared with primary care physicians revealed no major differences in selected patient outcomes and high patient satisfaction with NP care (see Chapter 24). The APN can also become a resource for the practice by training other staff or providers in the practice. As the APN gains credibility with administrators, the potential for the APN to become an influential leader in the organization is enhanced.

In most institutions and larger practices, committees make decisions about practice management. APNs should apply to be members on the different committees in the practice and the institution. Common committees are customer satisfaction, performance improvement, product/technology evaluation, practice management, utilization review, credentialing, and the executive committee. As a committee member, it is the responsibility of the APN to have an understanding of the economics of providing health care in the institution and a willingness and desire to participate in finding solutions to provide care cost-effectively. Institutions and practices cannot remain open unless they remain solvent. It is critical that APNs remain cognizant of the dual responsibility and goal of providing quality care in the most cost-effective manner possible.

Most primary care practice sites have a designated medical director whose role is to be the administrator of the practice at each clinic. In many institutions, one of the requirements for becoming a medical director is being a physician. If the requirements are restrictive, APNs can lobby to have them changed to be more inclusive. If the bylaws are successfully changed, APNs can apply for the position. One approach is to make the changes in stages. The APN can begin as an associate medical director or co–medical director. APNs have the skills and knowledge to be leaders in primary care practices.

Reporting Relationships

Models of practice can be seen as a matrix built on degree of autonomy, type of practice ownership, and practice setting. Different combinations of these factors can yield myriad forms of practice models, from a solo clinical practice to a practice performing physical examinations for an insurance company. The type of practice model and size of the organization are major factors affecting reporting relationships. This, in turn, influences many aspects of the APN's role.

There is no singular reporting structure for APNs, regardless of the organization. APNs may report to another APN in organizations with many APNs, to a nursing director responsible for an acute care area, to a physician, or to a practice manager in a community-based agency. APNs may have dual reporting relationships that include a clinical reporting relationship and an administrative relationship. Nursing administrators and physicians may have differing or competing expectations of APN roles. Dual reporting relationships may be helpful in maximizing support for the role and in clarifying expectations (Bryant-Lukosius & Dicenso, 2004). APNs with these reporting relationships must be clear about the need to have consensus from both sides when resolving role conflicts. Specific roles, legal requirements, and other variables in the organization will shape the reporting relationship. For instance, NPs, CNMs, and CRNAs who practice in hospital settings must obtain privileges through the credentialing committee, which may require a designated physician supervisor/collaborator. Recent improvements in direct reimbursement for APNs may change the requirements for a physician supervisor/collaborator, but the authors' experience is that most hospital risk managers still expect this supervision/collaboration if APNs seek hospital privileges. Some APNs may also be accountable to a nurse administrator. Whereas acute care CNSs are unlikely to need formal credentialing or require a collaborating physician, blended role CNS/NPs or CNSs in a physician practice may require both. The individual to whom the APN reports can indicate the importance of the position, but this should not be overvalued. Access to key leaders may be more important than where an APN is listed on an organizational chart. The degree of supervision desired may change as the APN becomes more experienced. A novice APN may benefit from a practice that offers more supervision and collaboration. A very experienced APN may be more comfortable in a more independent model of practice. APNs should carefully examine a potential practice setting before accepting a job offer. They should consider how the job is positioned in the organization and the position or individual to whom the APN is accountable.

Parrinello (1995) described three models of APN practice: the physician practice model, the nursing model, and the joint practice model. In the physician practice model, the APN typically joins a group practice and reports to a physician. In the nursing model, usually seen in hospitals, the APN typically reports to a nurse administrator and works with a specific group of patients, physicians, or units. This is the traditional CNS structure, but it is also often used with ACNPs, such as those in intensive care units. The joint practice model is a cohesive physician and nurse care delivery model in which the funding for the APN is a private enterprise between stakeholders or a combination of nursing/hospital and professional revenue funds. An additional model is the independent contractor model, in which the APN establishes a private business and serves as both administrator and clinical provider to patients (see Chapter 20). The business may also be consultative, in which the APN provides educational and project consultation to an organization. Table 23-2 outlines some of the advantages and disadvantages of each model.

Resources

To succeed, APNs need resources. The APN needs to negotiate at the time of hire for salary, benefits, and resources needed to practice effectively. Some are as simple as adequate space for direct and indirect patient care activities. Common practice-related expenses are telephone lines, computer, malpractice insurance, and a beeper for answering pages. In primary care practices, employment of a medical assistant or RN to admit patients to examination rooms, a medical billing person, and a receptionist are also needed resources. The organization needs to assure the APN of appropriate salary support and opportunities for raises or sufficient opportunities to generate income through professional fees. Assistive staff, such as clinical assistants, secretarial support, and data entry personnel, may be required. Access to automated systems is essential in today's environment. Financial and administrative support for continuing education opportunities in both academic and nonacademic programs are essential for maintaining skills. Asking to see a budget for the APN position is an easy way to evaluate whether the organization has planned for the needed resources. Finally, routine and regular contact with the administrator ensures that ongoing and new resources are provided (see Chapter 19).

Table 23-2   MODELS OF PRACTICE IN ORGANIZATIONS

Model	Advantages	Disadvantages
Physician Practice Model	Funding linked to the success of the group practice, not nursing budget; clinical work closely linked with physicians and clearly defined	Potential conflict in definition of collaboration versus supervision; isolation from nursing colleagues
Nursing Model	Clear identification with nursing, credibility with staff, focus on broader advanced practice nurse skills	Potential for decreased collaboration with physicians; risk for losing continued funding within the large nursing budget
Joint Practice Model	Captures the best of physician- and nursing-based models; interdependency is recognized	Complexity of a matrix structure and potential to be caught between two supervisors
Independent Contractor Model	Autonomy, minimal bureaucracy	Isolation, financial risk, professional liability

Measuring the Impact of Advanced Practice Nurses

During the turmoil of the changing health care payer environment, much has been written about the value of NPs to provide primary care. The lay media and the professional literature have viewed the use of this APN role as a way to increase access to care and to control costs. However, the literature also reinforces the necessity of measuring the impact of all advanced practice roles on the cost and quality of care (Jackson et al., 2003; see also Chapter 24). By demonstrating their ability to deliver high-quality, cost-effective care, APNs show their value and secure a position in the health care marketplace. Box 23-4 lists web-based resources APNs and administrators can use to develop measurement and monitoring strategies.

Carroll and Fay (1997) reviewed the challenges APNs and administrators face in measuring the impact of advanced practice nursing. They discussed several considerations:

- Defining the scope of practice of the APN
- Building consensus about the definition and the relationship of structure, process, and outcome variables (see Chapter 24)
- Designating the settings and systems of practice
- Influencing stakeholders
- Ensuring the scientific rigor of a study

In making informed decisions about the employment of APNs in an organization, an administrator will often search the literature for studies that document cost and quality outcomes of employing APNs.

Administrators are inundated with a tremendous amount of information, so it is helpful to the administrator when APNs summarize articles, particularly reports about outcomes and cost savings attributed to APNs, that the administrator can use.

Evaluation strategies have typically focused on specific components of an APN's role. Chapter 24 details comprehensive models for evaluating the impact of APNs and examines the growing research literature supporting the varied outcomes of advanced practice nursing. Administrators need to consider allocation of resources to support APNs in practice evaluation beyond the basics required by regulatory agencies or performance management systems. In too many settings, APN evaluation is limited to a perfunctory annual performance appraisal. The absence of evaluative data in such evaluations weakens support for these roles; particularly in times of economic down-turn for the institution, lack of these data can jeopardize the APN's continued employment.

In any organization, a clear definition of the APN roles, the roles' objectives, and the time frame for achieving them is required to measure and monitor APN contributions. The APN and the person or persons to whom the APN is accountable must understand these factors. Ongoing communication to ensure consensus between APNs and administrators about performance and achievement of objectives is a key step in measuring the value of the role. Formal goal setting and review of performance according to the organization's performance management system should be done annually.

Box 23-4   RESOURCES FOR SAFETY AND QUALITY MEASUREMENT

Agency for Healthcare Research and Quality: www.ahrq.gov
American Nurses Association: www.nursingworld.org
American Society for Quality: www.asq.org
Healthcare Effectiveness Data and Information Set (HEDIS): http://web.ncqa.org/tabid/59/Default.aspx
Institute for Healthcare Improvement: www.ihi.org
Institute of Medicine: www.iom.edu
International Council on Nursing: www.icn.ch
The Joint Commission: www.jointcommission.org
Leap Frog Group: www.leapfroggroup.org

Medical Group Management Association: www.mgma.com
National Association for Healthcare Quality: www.nahq.org
National Guideline Clearinghouse: www.guideline.gov/index.asp
Medical Outcomes Trust: www.outcomes-trust.org
Health Outcomes Institute: www.health-outcomes-institute.com
Foundation for Accountability: www.facct.org
National Healthcare Practitioner Databank: www.npdb-hipdb.com

In a primary care practice, deciding the appropriate number of patients for whom the APN is responsible is based on the context and nature of the clinical practice and forms the basis for one measure— productivity. NPs and PAs believed that 81% to 91% of the patients they saw were appropriately cared for and did not require the services of a physician (Grumbach, Hart, Mertz, Coffman, & Palazzo, 2003). Other factors that influence this number include the organization's standards of practice and the number and diversity of other staff members within the clinical practice. Litaker and colleagues (2003) demonstrated the benefits of a NP–Doctor of Medicine (MD) team in chronic disease management: "…nurse practitioners have much to offer as partners in complementing physician-based practice at a time when high quality health care, documentable outcomes, and affordable costs occupy the minds of consumers and insurers" (p. 234).

As health care administrators know, listening to patients' concerns regarding the operation of a practice is instructive. Besides receiving quality patient care and having confidence in the providers in the practice, patients choose to remain with a practice for many other reasons. Patient satisfaction surveys are a valuable means of obtaining feedback about how patients perceive the practice and what areas need improvement. Many standard surveys are available. An example used by many large clinics and hospitals is the Press Ganey survey *(www.pressganey.com)*. This survey, like others, measures a variety of factors that patients are concerned about including ability to schedule an appointment quickly and conveniently when needed, ability to obtain refills in a timely manner, adequate parking facilities, waiting time in the office and examination room before being seen, waiting time on-hold trying to get an appointment, being able to speak with a real person, friendliness and efficiency of the front and back office, clinic location, office hours, and environment. Common provider factors that patients identified in this survey included being listened to, having their questions answered, and having confidence in the provider. APNs tend to score well on patient satisfaction surveys. In practices that use patient satisfaction surveys, positive scores increase the value of the APN to the practice. However, it is most helpful if the generic surveys can be modified to contain specific items that are more reflective of advanced practice nursing strengths and areas of emphasis. Data do not indicate that generic patient satisfaction instruments demonstrate significant differences between APNs and physicians

(Girouard, 2000; Mundinger et al., 2000). Litaker and colleagues (2003) found that two satisfaction subscales more sensitive to APN practice were higher for MD-NP care teams than for MD only. Smaller practices can develop their own survey instrument if necessary.

CONSIDERATIONS FOR THE FUTURE

The turmoil of the current health care environment is expected to continue. This holds both opportunities and threats for APNs. The passage of the BBA in 1997 was a critical step in expanding practice options for NPs and CNSs (Keepnews, 1998), since direct billing by these APNs identifies the types of patients they see. The BBA also defined CNS practice for the first time in Medicare law, which gave CNSs the opportunity to serve Medicare beneficiaries. However, the BBA also affected physicians, and APNs are finding increased competition with physicians who are struggling to maintain their practices and their income. In addition, the rising cost of malpractice insurance is part of the turmoil in the health care environment for both physicians and APNs.

A theme throughout this chapter has been reimbursement. Given the increasing pressure on institutions and practices to sustain financial viability, APNs and administrators must work together to maximize reimbursement for APN services (see Chapter 19).

It is essential that APNs define the value-added services they provide that complement both physician and nursing practices. As seen in Litaker and colleagues' study (2003), analyses of NP-physician collaborative practice show that patients benefit from the combination of complementary skill sets. Several studies of NP-physician teams have demonstrated cost and quality-of-care improvements in nursing homes, as well as in primary care, emergency, obstetrical, and surgical inpatient settings (Burl, Bonner, Rao, & Khan, 1998; Grumbach & Bodenheimer, 2004; Horrocks, Anderson, & Salisbury, 2002; Jackson et al., 2003; Naylor et al., 2004). Disease prevention and management of chronic conditions also benefit from NP-physician teams (Phillips et al., 2002). Studies have shown that physicians who work with NPs report improved job satisfaction, reduced workloads, and increased ability to offer a higher standard of care (Koperski, Rogers, & Drennan, 1997).

Berger and colleagues (1996) defined several future roles to promote the optimal use of knowledge, skills, and abilities of APNs. The reality of the marketplace is that confusion continues regarding APN definitions and roles. New titles and role definitions that do not fit the definition of advanced practice nursing continue to arise. The promotion of the DNP as the terminal degree for advanced practice, with a broad definition that includes non-APN roles, further confounds the problem (see Chapter 3). One rationale for the DNP is the increasingly complex health care needs of the community and organizations seeking ways to deliver quality and safe care cost-effectively. Whether new job titles will be needed for the DNP-prepared APNs of the future is uncertain, but during a state of major change, more roles and titles are likely to develop (see Chapters 3 and 18). All executives, but nurse administrators in particular, can assist in reducing the confusion about APN roles by not introducing more nomenclature into the job lexicon. Increasing clarity about the advanced practice nursing roles described in this text is an important responsibility of administrators, as well as other nursing leaders.

Achieving such clarity will require that educational programs, whether formal education or continuing education, prepare nursing administrators to understand advanced practice nursing. As APN roles become more prevalent, administrators need program content on APN roles and outcomes. Further, managing a differentiated workforce requires attention to organizational positioning of APNs to maximize their contributions. This need is complicated by the fact that non-nurse administrators supervise APNs in many settings. Faculty in both nursing administration programs and health care administration programs need to educate their students so that administrators are in a better position to promote and preserve advanced practice nursing.

This chapter has emphasized that APNs must become more knowledgeable about the "business" of health care and learn to speak the language of administrators. As early as 1989, Brown described the need for CNSs to serve as "shuttle diplomats" who interpret economic realities and administrative decisions to nursing staff and clinical realities to administrative staff. Brown (1989) described the CNS as able to be "the person in the middle, a person expected and required to speak the language of both subcultures, understand the issues and dilemmas of each, and participate in the problem-solving of both arenas" (p. 285). The need for shuttle diplomacy by all APNs, particularly those working in large, complex organizations, has never been more critical, especially in relating clinical activities to institutional costs. Administrators must help APNs

develop their knowledge and skills through a comprehensive orientation and ongoing educational support. Likewise, APNs can educate administrators about the clinical impact of organizational initiatives through e-mail briefs or in face-to-face meetings. The era of APNs being able to self-define their positions and be vaguely accountable within an organization is over. In addition, changes in the organizational structures that support care delivery can present advantages for advanced practice nursing. APNs need to view the development of IDNs or community-based programs as realms in which they can advance their services and create new opportunities.

The APN's direct clinical practice is the foundation for advanced practice nursing success in the twenty-first century. As noted throughout this book, clinical care is increasingly complex; the aging population is living longer with multisystem chronic illnesses; increases in technology continue; and burgeoning research findings, particularly in genetics research, need to be incorporated into clinical care. Having a strong expert clinical practice base is critical for APNs to enact the clinical leadership and critical thinking skills so valued by administrators. The characteristics of APN direct clinical practice noted in Chapter 5 (use of a holistic perspective, formation of partnerships with patients, expert clinical thinking and skillful performance, use of reflective practice, use of research evidence, and diverse health and illness management approaches) are the sources of the APN's value-added contributions to patient care. Core competencies (see Chapter 3) emanate from this practice expertise. On the one hand, administrators must be careful not to overload APNs with committee and project work to the extent that they lose these skills or become less visible in key practice arenas. On the other hand, the additional education that DNP programs offer can enhance APN preparation as organizational leaders of change. Thus APNs can be increasingly influential not only at the individual patient level but also at the system level. Both administrators and APNs must be careful not to weaken the APN's practice strength, which remains the reason that most positions were established. APNs must also be vigilant in communicating with their administrators when nonclinical activities require them to compromise their practice expertise.

As discussed in Chapters 9 and 22, the role of political activist is one that APNs should embrace. Certainly, APNs need to follow national and state legislation closely and make their views known. They can also be valuable educators of politicians and their staffs about the issues faced by patients and by nurses in advanced practice. Many of the APN's clinical skills, such as communication, conflict resolution, and critical thinking, transfer well into the political arena. Administrators should be allies to APNs in the political arena to present a strong, united voice for nursing.

SUMMARY

APNs and organizational leaders—whether nurse executives, administrators, or physicians—should think in terms of the skills that APNs bring to an organization, especially as changes continue in the provision and the location of care delivery within an organization and within the community. APNs should promote their skills as new opportunities and new relationships emerge, and administrators should assist them in doing so. A collaborative effort between the administrative team and APNs greatly enhances the potential for successful implementation of advanced practice nursing and reduces the potential for interprofessional tensions. Furthermore, the community's and the organization's needs and strategic imperatives are the context for current and future job-related opportunities for APNs. By committing to the mission and objectives of the organization and consistently developing and expanding their skills, APNs ensure their place in the future of health care delivery.

REFERENCES

Abdellah, F.G. (1997). Managing the challenges of role diversification in an interdisciplinary environment. *Military Medicine, 162,* 453-458.

American Association of Colleges of Nursing (AACN). (2004). *Position statement on the practice doctorate in nursing.* Washington, DC: Author.

American Association of Colleges of Nursing (AACN). (2006). *The essentials of doctoral education for advanced nursing practice.* Washington, DC: Author.

ASPE Issue Brief. (2005). *Overview of the uninsured in the United States: An analysis of the 2005 current population survey.* Retrieved May 12, 2007, from http://aspe.hhs.gov/search/health/reports/05/uninsured-cps/index.htm.

Baggs, J.G. (January 31, 2005). Overview and summary—Partnerships and collaboration: What skills are needed? *Online Journal of Issues in Nursing, 10*(1). Retrieved May 12, 2007, from www.nursingworld.org/ojin/topic26/tpc26ntr.htm.

Berger, A.M., Eilers, J.G., Pattrin, L., Rolf-Fixley, M., Pfeifer, B.A., Rogge, J.A., et al. (1996). Advanced practice roles for nurses in tomorrow's healthcare systems. *Clinical Nurse Specialist, 10,* 250-255.

Bodenheimer, T. (2005). High and rising health care costs. Part 1. Seeking an explanation. *Annals of Internal Medicine, 142,* 847-854.

Bodenheimer, T. (2006). Primary care: Will it survive? *The New England Journal of Medicine, 355,* 861-864.

Bodenheimer, T., & Grumbach, K. (2005). *Understanding health policy: A clinical approach* (4th ed.). New York: Appleton & Lange.

Bonis, P.A. (2005). Quality incentive payment systems: Promise and problems. *Journal of Clinical Gastroenterology, 39* (4 Suppl. 2), S176-182.

Brown, S.J. (1989). Supportive supervision of the CNS. In A.B. Hamric & J.A. Spross (Eds.), *The clinical nurse specialist in theory and practice* (2nd ed., pp. 285-298). Philadelphia: Saunders.

Bryant-Lukosius, D., & Dicenso, A. (2004). A framework for the introduction and evaluation of advanced practice nursing roles. *Journal of Advanced Nursing, 48,* 530-540.

Buppert, C. (2005a). Capturing reimbursement for advanced practice nurse services in acute and critical care: Legal and business considerations. *AACN Clinical Issues, 16,* 23-35.

Buppert, C. (2005b). *The primary care provider's guide to compensation and quality* (2nd ed.). Boston: Jones & Bartlett.

Burl, J.B., Bonner, A., Rao, M., & Khan, A.M. (1998). Geriatric nurse practitioners in long-term care: Demonstration of effectiveness in managed care. *Journal of the American Geriatrics Society, 46,* 506-510.

Burns, L.R., & Pauly, M.V. (2002). Integrated delivery networks: A detour on the road to integrated health care? *Health Affairs, 21*(4), 128-143.

Carroll, T.L., & Fay, V.P. (1997). Measuring the impact of advanced practice nursing on achieving cost-quality outcomes: Issues and challenges. *Nursing Administration Quarterly, 21,* 32-40.

Christensen, C., Baumann, H., Ruggles, R., & Sadtler, T. (2006). Disruptive innovation for social change. *Harvard Business Review, 84,* 94-101.

Christensen, C., Bohmer, R., & Kenagy, J. (2000). Will disruptive innovations cure health care? *Harvard Business Review, 78,* 102-112.

Cowan, M.J., Shapiro, M., Hays, R.D., Afifi, A., Vazirani, S., Ward, C.R., et al. (2006). The effect of a multidisciplinary hospitalist/physician and advanced practice nurse collaboration on hospital costs. *Journal of Nursing Administration, 36,* 79-85.

Croasdale, M. (2006). *Work force studies find scattered physician shortages.* Retrieved May 9, 2007, from www.ama-assn.org/amednews/2006/08/14/prsb0814.htm.

Davis, K., Schoen, C., Schoenbaum, S.C., Doty, M.M., Holmgren, A.L., Kriss, K.L., et al. (2007*). Mirror, mirror on the wall: An international update on the comparative performance of American health care,* The Commonwealth Fund. Retrieved May 9, 2007, from www.commonwealthfund.org.

Dickler, R., & Shaw, G. (2000). The Balanced Budget Act of 1997. Its impact on U.S. teaching hospitals. *Annals of Internal Medicine, 132,* 820-823.

Disch, J., Walton, M., & Barnsteiner, J. (2001). The role of the clinical nurse specialist in creating a healthy work environment. *AACN Clinical Issues, 12,* 345-355.

Gardner, D. (January 31, 2005). Ten lessons in collaboration. *Online Journal of Issues in Nursing, 10*(1), Manuscript 1. Retrieved May 12, 2007, from www.nursingworld.org/ojin/topic26/tpc26_1.htm.

Girouard, S.A. (2000). New directions for the advanced practice nurse in health care quality: Performance and outcome improvement. In A.B. Hamric, J.A. Spross, & C.M. Hanson (Eds.), *Advanced nursing practice: An integrative approach* (2nd ed., pp. 755-794). Philadelphia: Saunders.

Grumbach, K., & Bodenheimer, T. (2004). Can health care teams improve primary care practice? *JAMA, 291,* 1246-1251.

Grumbach, K., Hart, G., Mertz, E., Coffman, J., & Palazzo, L. (2003). Who is caring for the underserved? A comparison of primary care physicians and non-physician clinicians in California and Washington. *Annals of Family Medicine, 1,* 97-104.

Henley, D. (2003). Coding better for better reimbursement. *Family Practice Management, 10,* 29-35.

Horrocks, S., Anderson, E., & Salisbury, C. (2002). Systematic review of whether nurse practitioners working in primary care can provide care equivalent to doctors. *British Medical Journal, 323,* 819-823.

Iglehart, J.K. (1999). Support for academic centers: Revisiting the 1997 Balanced Budget Act. *The New England Journal of Medicine, 341*(4), 299-304.

Institute of Medicine (IOM). (2000). *To err is human: Building a safer health system.* Washington, DC: National Academies Press.

Institute of Medicine (IOM). (2001). *Crossing the quality chasm: A new health system for the 21st century.* Washington, DC: National Academies Press.

Institute of Medicine (IOM). (2003). *Health professions education: A bridge to quality.* Washington, DC: National Academies Press.

Jackson, D.J., Lang, J.M., Swartz, W.H., Ganiats, T.G., Fullerton, J., Ecker, J., et al. (2003). Outcomes, safety, and resource utilization in a collaborative care birth center program compared with traditional physician-based perinatal care. *American Journal of Public Health, 93,* 999-1006.

Keepnews, D. (1998). New opportunities and challenges for APRNs. *American Journal of Nursing, 98,* 62-64.

Kennerly, S. (2007). The impending reimbursement revolution: How to prepare for future APN reimbursement. *Nursing Economic$, 25,* 81-84.

Knox, S., & Gharrity, J. (2002). Transitions in American hospitals: The necessary reshaping is taking place. "Turnaround" processes in organizations. *JONA's Healthcare Law, Ethics, and Regulation, 4,* 13-17.

Koperski, S., Rogers, S., & Drennan, V. (1997). Nurse practitioners in general practice: An inevitable progression? *British Journal of General Practice, 47,* 696-698.

Laurant, M., Reeves, D., Hermens, R., Braspenning, J., Grol, R., & Sibbald, B. (2007). *Substitution of doctors by nurses in primary care* (review). The Cochrane Collaboration, John Wiley & Sons. Retrieved May 9, 2007, from www.thecochranelibrary.com.

Levit, K., Smith, C., Cowan, C., Lazenby, H., Sensenig, A., & Catlin, A. (2003). Trends in U.S. health care spending, 2001. *Health Affairs, 22,* 154-164.

Licking, M., & Sampson, D. (1995). HCFA regulations and financing. *Nurse Practitioner, 20*(12), 6-9.

Lindeke, L., & Sieckert, A. (January 31, 2005). Nurse-physician workplace collaboration. *Online Journal of Issues in Nursing, 10*(1), Manuscript 4. Retrieved May 12, 2007, from www.nursingworld.org/ojin/topic26/tpc26_4.htm.

Litaker, D., Mion, L., Planavsky, L., Kippes, C., Mehta, N., & Frolkis, J. (2003). Physician–nurse practitioner teams in chronic disease management: The impact on costs, clinical effectiveness, and patients' perception of care. *Journal of Interprofessional Care, 17,* 223-237.

McNatt, G.E., & Eason, A. (2000). The role of the advanced practice nurse in the care of organ transplant recipients. *Advances in Renal Replacement Therapy, 7,* 172-176.

Mezey, M., Burger, S.G., Bloom, H.G., Bonner, A., Bourbonniere, M., Bowers, B., et al. (2005). Experts recommend strategies for strengthening the use of advanced practice nurses in nursing homes. *Journal of the American Geriatric Society, 53,* 1790-1797.

Millenson, M.L. (2004). Pay for performance: The best worst choice. *Quality & Safety in Health Care, 13,* 323-324.

Mundinger, M.O., Kane, R.L., Lenz, E.R., Totten, A.M., Tsai, W.U., Cleary, P.D., et al. (2000). Primary care outcomes in patients treated by nurse practitioners or physicians. *Journal of American Medical Association, 283,* 59-68.

Naegle, M.A., & Krainovich-Miller, B. (2001). Shaping the advanced practice psychiatric–mental health nursing role: A futuristic model. *Issues in Mental Health Nursing, 22,* 461-482.

Naylor, M.D., Brooten, D., Campbell, R., Maislin, G., McCauley, K.M., & Schwartz, J.S. (2004). Transitional care of older adults hospitalized with heart failure: A randomized, controlled trial. *Journal of the American Geriatric Society, 52,* 675-684.

Nelson, R. (2006). Protecting patients or turf? The AMA aims to limit nonphysician health care professionals. *American Journal of Nursing, 106,* 25-26.

Parrinello, K.M. (1995). Advanced practice nursing: An administrative perspective. *Critical Care Nursing Clinics of North America, 7,* 9-16.

Phillips, R., Harper, D., Wakefield, M., Green, L., & Fryer G. (2002). Can nurse practitioners and physicians beat parochialism into plowshares? *Health Affairs, 21,* 133-142.

Pioro, M., Landefeld, C., Brennan, P., Fortinsky, R., Kim, U., & Rosenthal, G. (2000). Outcome based trial of an inpatient nurse practitioner service for general medical patients. *Journal of Evaluation in Clinical Practice, 7,* 21-33.

Quaglietti, S., & Anderson, B. (2002). Developing the adult NP's role in home care. *Nurse Practitioner, 27,* 14, 81-82.

Richmond, T., & Becker, D. (2005). Creating an advanced practice nurse-friendly culture: A marathon, not a sprint. *AACN Clinical Issues, 16*(1), 58-66.

Sinclair, B.P. (1997). Advanced practice nurses in integrated health care systems. *Journal of Obstetric, Gynecologic, and Neonatal Nursing, 26,* 217-223.

Thrall, J.H. (2004). The emerging role of pay-for-performance contracting for health care services. *Radiology, 233,* 637-640.

Tobin, C.T. (2000). A rainbow of opportunities: Advanced practice. *Diabetes Educator, 26,* 216, 326-327.

Urden, L., & Walston, S. (2001). Outcomes of hospital restructuring and reengineering: How is success or failure being measured? *Journal of Nursing Administration, 31,* 203-209.

CHAPTER 24

Outcomes Evaluation and Performance Improvement: An Integrative Review of Research on Advanced Practice Nursing

Gail L. Ingersoll

INTRODUCTION

Increased health system accountability and changes in the organization, delivery, and financing of health care are prompting the need for accurate assessments of advanced practice nurse (APN) performance. Employers, consumers, insurers, and others are calling for APNs to justify their contribution to health care and to demonstrate the value they add to the system. This verification of APNs' contributions requires an assessment of the structures, processes, and outcomes associated with APN performance and the care delivery systems in which they practice.

Assessment of individual APN impact occurs at multiple levels, with supporting evidence collected during annual performance reviews, outcomes measurement activities, process improvement analyses, and program evaluations, as well as small- and large-scale clinical, health systems, and outcomes research. At the least, individual performance review and outcomes measurement are required of all APNs, regardless of practice setting, population served, or previous experience with impact assessment.

Outcomes evaluation and ongoing performance assessment are essential to the survival and success of advanced practice nursing. The importance of this dimension of advanced practice is highlighted repeatedly in the American Association of Colleges of Nursing's (AACN) *The Essentials of Doctoral Education for Advanced Nursing Practice.* Incorporated within each essential competency is a discussion of the need to evaluate the effect of APN action and decision making on care delivery outcome (AACN, 2006).

This chapter focuses on measuring and monitoring the quality of care delivered and the outcomes achieved by APNs. Performance indicators are discussed at two levels—the aggregate level, where evidence addresses APN role impact; and the individual level, with activities directed at the outcomes of a single APN's practice. The chapter defines key terms and describes frameworks for quality and outcomes assessment. APN outcomes research is reviewed extensively, and recommendations are made for further

study. Readers will find several APN-sensitive outcome indicators relevant to their practice and a number of strategies for evaluating and improving individual performance. Finally, the chapter discusses steps APNs can take to develop an individualized, goal-focused monitoring plan to facilitate annual performance review.

REVIEW OF TERMS

Numerous interrelated terms are used to define and describe the components of performance appraisal and outcomes assessment. The principal terms used in this chapter are defined as follows:

Benchmark: A point of reference for comparison. Benchmarking requires an assessment of the processes used by high-performing practitioners or organizations to achieve their outcomes, as well as the strategies and systems used to attain and then sustain performance excellence (Mathaisel, Cathcart, & Comm, 2004). It is the process used to compare an individual's (or organization's) outcomes with those of high performers. Four phases are involved in the benchmarking process for APNs: (1) the conduct of a comprehensive self-assessment of current processes and outcomes of care, including comparisons of performance across internal departments and documentation of baseline data; (2) the identification of comparable providers whose outcomes are superior to those of the benchmarking APN; (3) an analysis of the differences between the processes used by the high performers and the benchmarking APN, with the establishment of goals for improved performance by the benchmarking practitioner; and (4) the implementation of best practice processes and the monitoring of results over time (DeLise & Leasure, 2001).

A *performance benchmark* is defined in health care as an ideal target that has been achieved by some group or organization known for its quality of services. This process-focused benchmark serves as the gold standard against which others are compared. Some evaluators also use this term to denote achievement of an intermediate outcome (e.g., attainment of desired best practice performance).

Disease management: An organized process focusing on the patient's disease as the target of interest, with improvements in outcomes seen as a result of attention to the attributes or characteristics of the disease. The intent is the same as *outcomes management*—to take some action/intervention to achieve a desired effect. The principal difference is the focus, with disease management directed at the patient's underlying condition and outcomes management focused on any observed effect of treatment. Assessments of disease management effectiveness should indicate clearly what changes in care delivery affected the disease process or symptoms seen.

In health insurance plans targeted at cost containment, the monitoring of disease management activities usually includes a review of medical provider profiling reports. For example, an annual provider profile might include a list of patients treated for asthma, the asthma patients' total number of office and emergency department (ED) visits within a year's period, the number of filled prescriptions for inhaled corticosteroids, and whether the patients had an influenza or pneumococcal vaccine (Lind, 2001). Similar data can be used to profile APN practices and to lay a foundation for the APN's effectiveness in disease management activities.

Effectiveness: The extent to which interventions or actions taken in *clinical* settings perform as desired with defined populations (Armenian & Shapiro, 1998). Indicators of program or intervention effectiveness are commonly included in assessments of cost outcomes (e.g., cost-effectiveness analysis). In *cost-effectiveness analysis*, outcomes are measured both in terms of dollars expended and beneficial effects achieved (often for which no dollar amount can be readily assigned) (Hargreaves, Shumway, Hu, & Cuffel, 1998). This measurement approach is different from cost-*benefit* analysis, in which dollars are used to compare money spent with money saved. In clinical

practice, cost-benefit analyses are rarely possible for determining which program or intervention is most useful for achieving outcomes.

Efficiency: The effects achieved by some intervention in relation to the effort expended in terms of money, resources, and time. In outcomes assessment, efficiency measures are used to compare two equally effective interventions (Hargreaves et al., 1998), and for care providers, often include productivity considerations. In such cases, costs of care, treatment patterns, service volumes, and time required are usually compared (Armenian & Shapiro, 1998).

Evidence-Based Practice: The integration of research findings (evidence) into clinical decision-making and care delivery processes. *Best evidence* for clinical practice is derived from methodologically sound research that is theory-derived, consistent with patient needs and preferences (Ingersoll, 2000), and clinically relevant to the population of interest. The findings of these investigations support and enhance the clinician's clinical expertise—they do not replace it. This is particularly true for decisions concerning individual patients, in which personal characteristics and circumstances may differ from those of the populations studied.

When available, evidence-based information should be used in the selection of process of care measures (e.g., percent of eligible acute myocardial infarction patients receiving aspirin at time of arrival to hospital). Evidence-based data are useful also in the development of *practice guidelines*, which are "systematically developed statements to assist practitioner and patient decisions about appropriate health care for specific clinical circumstances" (Institute of Medicine [IOM], 2001, p.151). Although evidence-based guidelines can influence both the ways in which providers practice and the methods they use to evaluate quality of care, some reports suggest that clinicians fail to use the evidence currently available (McGlynn et al., 2003) and that this failure results in serious negative outcomes for patients (IOM). Ultimately, an individual provider's performance and health care outcome will be evaluated by the extent to which that practice complies with and supports evidence-based guidelines and best practice decision making. APNs also will be held accountable for best practice expectations by courts of law, which increasingly are basing malpractice decisions on performance according to evidence-based standards (Brent, 2001).

Impact Analysis: An assessment of the magnitude of some intervention or change (e.g., APN care delivery) on recipients, programs, policies, and stakeholders. An impact analysis also may be performed before the introduction of an intervention to determine whether a proposed action theoretically should produce better results than an alternative or the current standard of care. Some evaluators differentiate *impact analysis* from *outcomes analysis* by the length of time required to achieve an effect, with impact analysis denoting longer-term changes (Krueger, n.d.). In most cases, however, the term *impact analysis* is a more global statement for assessment of some intervention effect.

Metric: Also described as measures or key performance indicators (KPIs), metrics are parameters for what will be accomplished by a program, how its impact will be evaluated, and what will constitute evidence of success (Robertson, 2003). Although the word *metric* is a bit more expansive than the terms *measure* and *indicator*, in many cases the terms are used interchangeably (Ingersoll, 2006b).

Outcome: A change or result in the recipient of some intervention or action. Recipients may be patients, families, students, other care providers, communities, and, in some cases, organizations if the organization as a whole is the recipient of the intervention. Outcomes may be intended or unintended; both should be assessed in a comprehensive outcomes assessment.

Most definitions of *outcome* have evolved from the original writings of Donabedian (1966, 1980), who defined an outcome as a change in a patient's current and future health that can be attributed to some alteration in delivery of health care. His definition focused exclusively on the patient and incorporated physiological, attitudinal (patient satisfaction), acquisition of health-related knowledge, and health-related behavioral change in his measurement recommendations. This definition is particularly relevant to APNs, whose actions directly or indirectly affect patients and families.

Outcome(s) Assessment: An evaluation of the observed results of some action or intervention for recipients of services. Outcome assessments provide the data needed to support or refute the perceived beneficial effect of some clinical decision, care delivery process, or targeted action.

Outcome Indicators or Measures: Observable, measurable evidence of the effect of some intervention or action on the recipient of services. Although some authors distinguish between *indicators* and *measures,* usually the terms are used interchangeably, as they are in this chapter. Outcome indicators denote changes in the *recipient* of the service or action—*not the provider.* Acceptable measures should vary sufficiently to allow for the assessment of intra- and inter-individual differences across providers, employers, insurers, and circumstances. They focus on changes over time and measure some aspect of behavior, cognitive, or psychosocial process, or physiological response (Bloch, 1975). An essential attribute of an outcome indicator is its implied or explicit causal link to an intervention or action. One of the challenges for APNs is determining which of several measures is the most reliable, valid, and sensitive to individual or program effect. In selecting indicators, APNs must consider the resources needed to collect the data, the time required to do so, and the fit between the data and the organization's mission.

The most desirable indicators of care delivery outcome are suitable to the population or target of interest, are not overly costly to collect, and are sensitive to changes within and across individuals or departments. They can be global (applicable to any population or care delivery environment) or population-specific. The more global the indicator, the more difficult is the determination of its relationship to APN intervention or action. The more specific the indicator, the less generalizable it is to other groups or circumstances. For example, "patient satisfaction" is a global indicator that is relevant to all patients but is influenced by a number of factors and a variety of care providers. As a result, distinguishing the APN's impact from everyone else's is difficult. On the other hand, the outcome indicator "birth complications" is specific to newborns, making it relevant only to APNs serving that particular patient population.

Intermediate Outcome Indicators: Observable evidence of some movement toward the achievement of a desired outcome. These indicators assist in determining whether any progress is being made in response to some intervention. They are most useful when the desired outcome is long-range or multidimensional and preliminary actions or changes are required before the final outcome is achieved.

Because APNs often influence patient outcome through indirect means, intermediate outcome indicators may be a useful way for measuring progress toward an overall goal of improving patient care. For instance, many APN role responsibilities include the mentoring of other nursing staff or the management of interdisciplinary teams. As a result, changes in team member behavior or staff nurse performance may be an indication of APN effect. When possible, the proposed relationships between the intermediate outcome and the subsequent patient outcome should be clearly described.

Outcome(s) Management: Deliberate care delivery actions designed to achieve desired outcomes through the application of outcomes research to practice (adapted from Powell, 2000). Outcome management is directed toward the refinement of care delivery processes for the purpose of maximizing care delivery outcome. According to Ellwood (1988), a comprehensive outcomes management program (1) emphasizes the use of standards to select appropriate interventions, (2) measures both disease-specific and generic, behaviorally-focused or perception-focused outcomes, (3) pools clinical and outcomes data for groups of patients, and (4) analyzes and disseminates information to decision makers. Decision-making action for individual patients is not necessarily the goal of outcomes management programs. Rather, the intent is directed toward the improvement of care to aggregate populations.

Outcome(s) Measurement: The collection and reporting of information about an observed effect. Outcomes measurement involves the identification of reliable and valid outcome measures, the selection of appropriate measurement methods, and attention to the timing of data collection. Outcome findings may be influenced by the amount of time elapsed since an intervention and what transpires during that period. They also may be affected by the circumstances evident at the time of data collection.

Outcome(s) Research: The use of rigorous scientific methods to measure the effect of some intervention on some outcome or outcomes (Ingersoll, 1998). It is directed toward populations of patients and is designed to establish care delivery standards or policy statements about best practice. The term *outcomes* research is a fairly new one, with previous studies focusing on cause (intervention) and effect (outcome) relationships. In many respects, the intent of the research (interventional vs. outcomes) is the same—to demonstrate causal connections between some change in clinical practice and the outcomes observed. Because of its focus on formal research investigations, usually involving randomized controlled (or clinical) trials (RCTs), the term should not be used synonymously with the terms *outcome evaluation* or *outcome management.*

Performance (Process) Improvement: Activities designed to increase the quality of services provided. The focus of attention shifts to the actions taken by the provider rather than the outcomes achieved. Although outcomes may be monitored to determine whether the change in process produces a desired effect, primary attention is on the interventions (care delivery processes) delivered. Clearly linked with these actions is outcomes evaluation, which focuses on the *impact* of care delivery processes and the identification of areas of needed improvement.

Subsumed within performance improvement activities are those associated with quality improvement initiatives, also described by some as continuous quality improvement (CQI) or total quality management (TQM). Although subtle distinctions are assigned to each of these terms, the focus and the intent are the same—to ensure the delivery of care that is appropriate, safe, competent, and timely and to maximize the potential for favorable patient outcome. In most instances, the measurement of performance is guided by the use of established indicators of best practice, such as national guidelines for care. These performance indicators may be internally derived or externally developed by expert panels who use existing evidence to specify which indicators are most reasonable and which targets are most desirable for achievement.

Performance Evaluation (Assessment): Assessment of individual achievement and the attainment of personal, professional, and organizational goals. Performance assessment activities for APNs include those associated with evaluating and improving day-to-day interactions with individual patients and health care colleagues and those involving the measurement of APN impact on populations, organizations, and communities. During these self-assessment and peer- or supervisor-initiated reviews, areas for improvement are defined. These performance improvement activities may be directed toward technical skills enhancement, interpersonal style, productivity specifications, professional development, or other individual APN actions linked to improved processes of care or care delivery outcome. In this case, the focus is on the APN's behaviors, with specific goals for improved performance identified for the upcoming quarter or year.

Process Indicator/Measure: A measure of visible behavior or action that a care provider undertakes to deliver care. Process indicators measure what care providers do during their interactions with patients and are necessary for demonstrating a cause-and-effect relationship between intervention and outcome.

Process-As-Outcome Indicators: The incorrect use of process indicators as evidence of improved patient or organizational outcome. A common example of a process-as-outcome indicator is nursing documentation, which often is identified in research reports and program evaluations as a desired *outcome* for some targeted intervention. The assumption is that improved documentation provides evidence of the delivery of better quality care, which

should result in improved patient outcome. The problem is that process-as-outcome indicators focus on the *care providers* and actions taken, not the *recipient* of services. There is no guarantee that the processes of care observed (or documenting their occurrence) will result in the desired outcome. Although process actions should be described fully and included in any discussion of how some program or action is expected to result in some care delivery outcome, they should not be identified as outcome indicators. At best, they are indications of intermediate effect, or process improvement; they are not acceptable outcomes by themselves. For example, any changes in documentation frequency, accuracy, or consistency must be tied to the changes in outcomes expected at the patient or organizational level.

For some APNs, particularly clinical nurse specialists (CNSs), whose role responsibilities include mentoring and teaching others, the *recipient* of the APN's intervention may be a staff member or group of staff members. In this case, assessment of the CNS's impact may include an evaluation of change in staff nurse performance or level of understanding. This is a legitimate and acceptable indicator of APN effect. Ideally, the assessment should follow the performance changes by staff nurses with an evaluation of the impact of the staff's improved performance on organizational or patient outcomes. The overall impact of the change in staff nurse performance or level of understanding may be increased patient satisfaction with care, reduced incidence of adverse events, reduced length of stay, or reduced cost of care.

Program Evaluation: An assessment of a program's overall worth or benefit. In most cases, program evaluations are designed to provide decision makers with information about the costs and benefits of some program or service. They provide an indication of indirect APN impact when the APN designs or assists in the implementation and maintenance of some educational or health services program. Program evaluations also may determine the direct effect of APN performance when the APN's care delivery actions are the principal component of the program. Because programs generally involve multiple components, however, isolating the APN's impact is often difficult.

Program evaluations can be as simple or as rigorous as any other investigation and require the same types of planning and attention to detail that are demanded of all research or outcomes assessment projects. Ideally, program evaluations begin at the time the programs are designed. They may include the collection of both qualitative and quantitative data to ensure that the program's evolutionary process is described and its anticipated and unanticipated effects are assessed.

Proxy Indicators: An indirect measure of some anticipated outcome that is used when a direct measure cannot be obtained or when an accurate indicator has not been identified. An example of a proxy indicator is the collection of self-report data from parents or spouses when patients are unable to respond to questions about perceptions of care or previous health. In the acute care hospital setting, case mix index, patient age, and co-morbidity often are used as proxy indicators of risk adjustment for given clinical populations, simply because more direct indicators are not readily accessible.

Quality of Care: The degree to which health services for individuals and populations increase the likelihood of desired health outcomes and are consistent with professional knowledge (IOM, 2001, p. 232). Quality of care is a dimension of the *process* of care; it is not an *outcome*. Outcomes should be assessed in evaluating quality of care to provide an indication of changes to the recipient of care that were achieved during the care delivery process.

Risk Adjustment: A process used to standardize groups according to some characteristic that might unduly influence an outcome. For example, the number and severity of co-morbid conditions may make one person less likely to achieve a favorable outcome simply because of physiological state, even when the best possible care is delivered. If patients with similarly high numbers of co-morbid conditions are not standardized against other patients without those same conditions, an incorrect impression of intervention effect may occur. Those persons with fewer co-morbid conditions, who

happen to be treated by one provider, may have better outcomes than patients with a greater number of co-morbid conditions, who happen to be treated by another. Comparing the outcomes of the two providers would erroneously suggest that one provider gives better quality care, when in fact the difference is the result of the patients' underlying conditions and the influence of those underlying conditions on the individuals' ability to achieve an outcome.

Standards: A profession's authoritative statements that describe the responsibilities of its practitioners (American Nurses Association [ANA], 2004, p. 13). Standards define the boundaries and essential elements of practice and link nursing care, quality, and competence through their delineation of nursing practice components (Dozier, 1998). They also serve as a criterion for the establishment of practice-related rules, conditions, and performance requirements (Ingersoll, 2006a). Standards focus on the *processes* of care delivery.

Structural Indicators: Measures of human, technical, and other resources used in the process of delivering care. These structures focus on the characteristics of the setting, system, or care providers and include such elements as numbers and types of providers, provider qualifications, agency policies and procedures, characteristics of patients served, and payment sources. Examples of structural indicators are ratio of registered nurses (RNs) or APNs to total nursing staff, nurse-to-patient ratio, nursing care hours per patient day, nursing injury rates, and attrition rates. The assumption underlying these measures is that the provision of adequate structures results in adequate outcomes. Although structural indicators provide important information about the impact of APN practice, they cannot stand alone.

CONCEPTUAL MODELS OF CARE DELIVERY IMPACT

Because APNs usually work with other health professionals, their influence on care delivery outcome is difficult to assess. They may have a direct effect through their interactions with patients and families, and/or they may have an indirect effect through their enhancement of the performance of others. Moreover, a number of factors influence APN practice irrespective of the direct or indirect efforts of APNs.

Measurement of the full range of APN effect also may be hampered by the organizational or clinician's philosophy underlying the care delivery process. For example, Murphy and Fullerton (2001) note that a hallmark of midwifery practice is the "advocacy of non-intervention in the absence of complications" (p. 274). Measuring this advocacy process is difficult, and relating it to observed care delivery outcomes is even harder. Linking *non*-interventions to outcomes, likewise, is a challenge.

Quality of Care Models

Much of the difficulty associated with measuring APN impact can be minimized through the use of a conceptual model to guide assessment and monitoring activities. A number of outcomes measurement and role impact models have been proposed, with several of these evolving from an original quality of care framework proposed by Donabedian (1966; 1980). Donabedian posited that quality is a function of the structural elements of the setting in which care is provided, the processes used by care providers, and the changes to the recipients of care (i.e., the outcomes). Applying these concepts to APN practice, structural variables relate to the components of a system of care. Process variables pertain to the behavior or actions of the APN or the activities of an APN-directed educational or care delivery program. Interactions among structure and process variables result in outcomes. Structure, process, and outcome variables can be studied independently or as a model for overall APN practice. The more complete the model (e.g., the inclusion of all or at least two of the components), the more likely is the successful isolation of the APN's impact on care delivery outcome.

Value of Care Model

Byers and Brunell (1998) used Donabedian's model to describe what they defined as the APN's value to the health delivery system. In their approach, value is equivalent to quality divided by cost. According to Byers and Brunell, structural factors refer to the characteristics of the APN and the practice setting. The stronger the structural elements of the setting or the provider, the greater the likelihood an APN can provide quality care and achieve desired outcomes. In this model, process elements include not only what the APN does but also whether the actions are appropriate and indicated for the circumstance. Ideally, process

activities are guided by best practice evidence. Outcomes in this model are defined by evidence-based standards and are compared with benchmarks for determining APN impact. Byers and Brunell's model categorizes APN-sensitive outcomes as short-term clinical outcomes, long-term clinical outcomes, perceived outcomes, patient/family satisfaction with care versus need, functional status, and resource utilization. The patient/family satisfaction with care-versus-need outcome represents a fairly new approach to measuring patient and family satisfaction. It incorporates a comparison between an individual's perception of the value of (or need for) an intervention or structural characteristic and the individual's level of satisfaction with it. For example, if an item is not perceived as valuable, or *needed* by patients, its satisfaction rating may not be particularly useful for assessing whether an individual's needs are met. On the other hand, if a patient or family member rates an item as highly valued or needed, the satisfaction rating provides a better indication of how well the service provided met what the patient or family expected.

Outcomes Evaluation Model

A second Donabedian-guided model was designed by Holzemer (1994) and adapted by others (Cohen, Saylor, Holzemer, & Gorenberg, 2000; Mitchell, Ferketich, & Jennings, 1998; Radwin, 2002; Wong, Stewart, & Gilliss, 2000). The value of this model is its program planning structure, which helps identify essential components of any outcomes evaluation plan. In Holzemer's model, essential outcomes measurement components are defined in a table consisting of inputs/context (structure), processes, and outcomes, which are identified along the horizontal axis.

For the APN, the patient is any recipient of APN services (e.g., patients, families). The provider is the person (APN) or the interdisciplinary group providing the service and potentially could include trained community laypersons who assist with the provision of services. The setting is the local environment in which the services are delivered and includes the resources available to provide the care. Table 24-1 contains an application of Holzemer's (1994) model to APN outcomes assessment planning. Included in the table are potential variables that may facilitate assessment of APN impact. Additional variables would be selected based on specialty service, population specifics, and additional characteristics of the provider, patient, or environment.

Table 24-1   ADVANCED PRACTICE NURSE OUTCOMES PLANNING GRID*

	Inputs/Context (Structure)	Processes	Outcomes

Patient	Age
	Gender
	Ethnicity
	Marital status/social
	  supports
	Educational background
	Health status (current &
	  past)
	Previous experience with
	  health system
	Special needs (e.g., visual,
	  literacy, hearing)
	Expectations of provider &
	  health system
	Access to care
	Insurance coverage
		Performance of self-care
		  behaviors
		Ability
		Willingness
		Family involvement in care
		  delivery process
		Use of alternative or com-
		  plementary therapies
			Generic
			  Physical health
			  Mental health
			  Symptom control
			  Functional status
			  Perceived well-being
			  Satisfaction with care
			  Adherence to treatment
			    regimen
			Knowledge of condition,
			  treatment program, &
			  expected outcomes
			Specific (dependent on
			  patient condition & need;
			  representative examples)
			  Serum glucose level
			  Birth weight
			  Reinfarction rate
			  Transplant rejection rate
			  Smoking quit rate
			  Length of stay
			  Ventilator days
			  Wound closure/healing

APN
  Provider
	Educational preparation
	Specialty focus
	Years of experience
	Level of self-esteem
	Resourcefulness
	Assertiveness
		Expert practice
		Collaboration
		Communication patterns
		Interactions with other care
		  providers & staff
		Expert coaching
		Consultation
		Clinical & professional
		  leadership
		Ethical decision making
		Evidence-based practice
		Case management
		Care delivery according to
		  practice standards
		Documentation
			Productivity

For APNs involved in quality improvement, the Quality Health Outcomes Model (QHOM) (Figure 24-1) is particularly relevant (Mitchell et al., 1998). This model provides a structure for studying complex relationships among patient, provider, and system level variables. As a result, studies guided by the model may better inform our understanding of patient outcomes. It focuses on the individual, organization, and group dimensions of the health care system that influence and are influenced by care delivery interventions and outcomes and defines the patient as the individual, family, or community receiving the care provider's services.

Mitchell and colleagues' model (1998) extends Holzemer's work (1994) by suggesting that the relationships between model components are reciprocal and that interventions never affect outcomes directly but do so through their interactions with the system and the patient. As a result, all assessments of APN impact must include information about both the

Table 24-1 ADVANCED PRACTICE NURSE OUTCOMES PLANNING GRID*—CONT'D

	Inputs/Context (Structure)	Processes	Outcomes
Setting	Geographical location (rural, urban, mixed)	Care provider credentialing process	Length of stay
	Type of facility (academic health center, acute care, clinic, industry)	Quality improvement process	Staff turnover rate
	Diagnostic equipment	Communication patterns	Cost of services
	Organizational culture & philosophy	Governance process	New program development
	Administrative structure	Care provider documentation process	Revenue generated
	State regulations on advanced practice	Annual performance review process	Community satisfaction
	Policies & procedures	Provider credentialing process	Provider satisfaction
	Patient mix		Staff satisfaction
	Type of care delivery model		
	Availability of other services in vicinity		
	Credentialing agency requirements		
	State health department regulations		
	Annual goals		
	Annual budget		

Adapted from Holzemer, W.L. (1994). The impact of nursing care in Latin America and the Caribbean: A focus on outcomes. *Journal of Advanced Nursing, 20,* 5-12.

*Components are not exhaustive of APN-related outcomes planning but serve as a guide for planning activities.

APN, Advanced practice nurse.

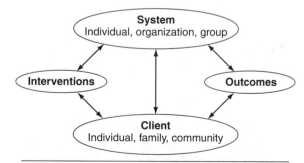

FIGURE **24-1:** Mitchell, Ferketich, and Jennings' **Quality Health Outcomes Model (QHOM).** This model proposes two-direction relationships among components, with interventions always acting through characteristics of the system and of the patient. (From Mitchell, P.H., Ferketich, S., & Jennings, B.M. [1998]. Quality Health Outcomes Model. American Academy of Nursing Expert Panel on Quality Health Care. *Image: The Journal of Nursing Scholarship, 30,* 43-46.)

system and the individual targeted for the intervention. By proposing a model that allows for multiple inputs at the level of patient, personnel, and system, the authors suggest that the model allows evaluators to analyze the contribution of specific variables to patient outcomes. Because the model incorporates organization/system level influences, it can guide studies of system level interventions such as program initiatives or reimbursement changes, the results of which can be used to influence health policy.

Radwin (2002) refined this model further by proposing that patient characteristics can best be understood in terms of state and trait, arguing that nursing interventions cannot influence trait variables such as age or gender (which may exert influences on health outcomes) (Figure 24-2). Consequently, this model distinguishes between those patient characteristics that are reciprocal to other model components (state characteristics, which change over time) and those

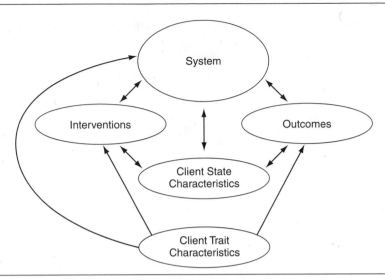

FIGURE **24-2:** Radwin's **Refined Quality Health Outcomes Model (QHOM).** (From Radwin, L. [2002]. Refining the Quality Health Outcomes Model: Differentiating between client trait and state characteristics. *Nursing Outlook, 50*[4], 168-169.)

that are not (trait characteristics, which do not change). Neither Mitchell and colleagues' model (1998) or Radwin's model has been tested yet, making their usefulness for assessment of APN impact uncertain. Nonetheless, they provide a useful framework for considering the various attributes of the individual and the organization that may influence APN effect.

Nursing Role Effectiveness Model

Sidani and Irvine (1999) proposed a conceptual model designed to facilitate the evaluation of the acute care nurse practitioner (ACNP) role in acute care settings (Figure 24-3). This model, which was adapted from their original nursing role effectiveness model, also is a derivative of Donabedian's framework, with components focusing on structure (patient, ACNP, and organization), process (ACNP role components, role enactment, and role functions) and outcome (goals and expectations of the ACNP role). A concern with this model is the use of the term *goals and expectations* for outcome and the focus on quality of care (which is a dimension of care delivery process rather than outcome). Four process mechanisms within the direct care component are expected to achieve patient and cost outcomes. These mechanisms are (1) providing comprehensive care, (2) ensuring continuity of care, (3) coordinating services, and (4) providing care in

a timely way (Sidani & Irvine). According to Sidani and Irvine, selection of outcome indicators is guided by the role and functions assumed by the ACNP, by the ways in which the role is enacted, and by the ACNP's particular practice model. Like the models before it, the usefulness of this framework for determining APN impact is limited by its virtual absence of testing in clinical settings.

THE EVIDENCE THUS FAR

A review of the literature suggests that increased attention is being given to the assessment of APN performance. Before the 1990s, most reports of APN performance were descriptive in nature, with limited use of the experimental or quasi-experimental designs that allow for comparisons across studies. In a meta-analysis of nurse practitioner (NP) and certified nurse-midwife (CNM) performance in primary care, Brown and Grimes (1995) identified 210 studies pertaining to NPs and CNMs. Of this number, only 53 met study inclusion criteria, which required evidence of NP or CNM intervention, data from patients in the United States or Canada, presence of a control group, measures pertaining to process of care or clinical outcome, use of an experimental or quasi-experimental design, and data availability to support the calculation of effect size to determine the magnitude of the effect. Outcome indicators

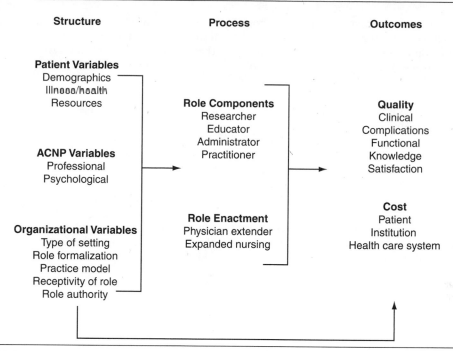

FIGURE 24-3: Sidani and Irvine's **Nursing Role Effectiveness Model (NREM)** for acute care nurse practitioners. *ACNP,* Acute care nurse practitioner. (From Sidani, S., & Irvine, D. [1999]. A conceptual framework for evaluating the nurse practitioner role in acute care settings. *Journal of Advanced Nursing 30*[1], 58-66.)

varied across studies, and cause-and-effect relationships between type of care provider (APN or physician) and outcomes observed were not substantiated. Outcomes measured for NPs reflected more generic indicators of provider impact (e.g., patient compliance, patient satisfaction, functional status, and use of EDs), whereas CNM outcomes were more reflective of specialized practice and included number of cesarean sections, spontaneous vaginal deliveries, incidence of fetal distress, birth weight, and 1-minute Apgar scores. Findings suggested that NPs requested more laboratory testing than physicians did and had more favorable outcomes pertaining to patient satisfaction, health promotion behaviors, time spent with patients, and number of hospitalizations. CNMs used less anesthesia, analgesia, intravenous fluids, and fetal monitoring and performed fewer episiotomies, forceps deliveries, and amniotomies. Their patients also were more likely to have spontaneous vaginal deliveries, although these were accompanied by an increased number of perineal lacerations.

Since 1998, APN performance and impact have been investigated in a number of locales. For purposes of summarization, studies have been categorized according to whether they focused on role descriptions or practice characteristics, care delivery processes, process (or performance) improvement activities, program evaluation, disease management activities, outcomes management programs, or outcomes research.

Role Description Studies

Role description studies focus on defining and describing role components and job attributes of APNs. These foundational studies assist in identifying the direct and indirect APN actions that potentially influence care delivery outcome. As such, they provide information about the structure or process components of Donabedian's model (1966, 1980). Without information about the outcomes associated with the characteristics and role behaviors identified in these studies, however, little can be said about their impact on patient care. What these studies provide is evidence to guide the development of theories about which characteristics of APN practice or aspects of the APN role contribute to care delivery outcome. For example, do the APN's expert coaching or collaboration processes contribute to more favorable outcomes when compared with care providers whose use of these processes is less apparent?

Role description studies have explored the role and patient characteristics of **psychiatric mental health APNs** (Campbell, Musil, & Zauszniewski, 1998), **ACNPs** (Irvine et al., 2000; Kannusamy, 2006; Kleinpell, 1998, 2005; Kleinpell-Nowell, 2001; Lambing, Adams, Fox, & Divine, 2004; Rosenfeld, McEvoy, & Glassman, 2003; Sidani et al., 2000), **CNSs** (Darmody, 2005; Scott, 1999), **neonatal nurse practitioners (NNPs)** (Beal et al., 1999), **pediatric nurse practitioners (PNPs)** (Brady & Neal, 2000; Jackson et al., 2001), **primary care NPs** (Edwards, Oppewal, & Logan, 2003; Holcomb, 2000; Hooker & McCaig, 2001; Kane, Flood, Keckhafer, & Rockwood, 2001; Kane, Keckhafer, Flood, Bershadsky, & Siadaty, 2003; Moody, Smith, & Glenn, 1999; Way, Jones, Baskerville, & Busing, 2001), **certified registered nurse anesthetists (CRNAs)** (McAuliffe & Henry, 1998), **CNMs** (Stuart & Oshio, 2002), **APNs working in gastroenterology** (Hillier, 2001) and **acute pain services** (Musclow, Sawhney, & Watt-Watson, 2002), and **NPs based in hospital outpatient clinics** (Lin, Hooker, Lenz, & Hopkins, 2002), **ambulatory services** (Mills & McSweeney, 2002; Mills, McSweeney, & Lavin, 1998; Reavis, 2004; Williams & Sidani, 2001), **faculty practice sites** (Barton, Baramee, Sowers, & Robertson, 2003), **local health departments** (Hughes, 2000), and **home health agencies** (Dick & Frazier, 2005). APN activities have been directed primarily toward the oversight and management of patients' needs, followed by administrative, teaching, research, program development, process improvement, and miscellaneous other demands. Some differences existed for locale and educational preparation (Hughes) and whether the APN was an NP or CNS (Becker, Kaplow, Muenzen, & Hartigan, 2006; Lincoln, 2000; Mick & Ackerman, 2000). Studies comparing NPs with physician assistants (PAs) also have found differences between these two roles (Lin et al.; Mills & McSweeney).

The role of APNs also has been explored in a grounded theory study by Ball and Cox (2003), who interviewed 39 CNSs, NPs, consultants, and coordinators from Australia, Canada, New Zealand, and the United States. The investigators identified three strategic activities that APNs believe contribute to restoring patients' health, which were defined as improving patient care, continuity of care, and patient education. These activities in combination with one another are expected to prepare patients for transition (to home or independence), to produce high levels of satisfaction with service, and to enable independence through a clear understanding of illness and health-promoting behaviors.

Role Perception/Acceptance Studies

Studies examining the acceptance of APNs have been conducted since the various roles were introduced and generally involve surveys of staff nurses, administrators, patients, and other care providers. The contribution of role perception studies to the assessment of APN impact lies with their potential for clarifying which contextual (structural) factors influence APN ability to perform maximally. If the environment in which an APN practices does not support the APN's delivery of services or if colleagues view the APN's performance as unsatisfactory or unacceptable, outcomes may be affected. These studies identify potential confounding factors that may need to be controlled when measuring APN effect.

Overall perception of APN performance has been favorable, with most care providers and patients rating the performance and contribution of APNs highly (Allen & Fabri, 2005; Baldwin et al., 1998; Gooden & Jackson, 2004; Mitchell, Dixon, Freeman, & Grindrod, 2001). Concerns expressed have focused on the proficiency of APNs taking call, covering in EDs, conducting hospital rounds, and spending time with patients (Marsden & Street, 2004). In one study, physician perceptions about the role differed according to previous experience working with NPs and location of practice (Aquilino, Damiano, Willard, Momany, & Levy, 1999). In another, emergency medical residents were unwilling to be treated by an APN for acute illness or injury. Some reported they would do so if the illness or injury was minor and the APN could treat the resident's condition sooner than an attending physician. An additional finding in this study was resident concern over threat to practice, with one third of respondents perceiving ED APNs as a professional threat (Larkin, Kantor, & Zielinski, 2001).

APN role receptivity studies also have explored physician acceptance of specialized diagnostic screening and invasive interventions by APNs. In a study of skin cancer screening, between 60% and 70% of family physicians and internists were supportive of NP screening (Oliveria, Altman, Christos, & Halpern,

2002). Similar findings were noted for the acceptance of NP and CNM involvement in medical abortions (Beckman, Harvey, & Satre, 2002).

A phenomenological design was used to assess families' perceptions of the "essence" of NNP care (Beal & Quinn, 2002). Themes identified included being positive and reassuring, being present, caring, translating information, and making parents feel at ease. In this same study, expert practitioner ability was identified as an expectation families had of all care providers, regardless of background (medical or nursing) or level of practice (staff nurse or APN). Expectations for the NNP focused on interpersonal style and effectiveness of interactions with families. An important pragmatic implication of this study's findings is the potential difficulty in placing a dollar amount on APN behavior. Because much of health care practice is reimbursement-driven, intangible provider attributes such as interpersonal competence often go unrecognized or are disregarded in provider payment decisions. This is a serious concern because patient and family perceptions of intangible processes often influence overall impressions of care delivery experience and may contribute to more tangible outcomes. APN competencies as value-added complements to medical care are invisible. Additional research is needed to clarify the magnitude and the importance of this link.

A caution with each of these studies is the potential for respondent bias, with persons unfamiliar with the role less likely to respond. In addition, many of the investigations are site-specific, making them more useful for individual performance improvement activities than for global indication of APN acceptance.

Care Delivery Process Studies

Studies evaluating care delivery processes often occur in combination with role definition research. The distinction between these studies and role definition explorations is their attention to what APNs *do* as part of their roles. Examples include the delivery of preventive services (Carroll, Robinson, Buselli, Berry, & Rankin, 2001; Johnson, 2000; Sheahan, 2000; Windorski & Kalb, 2002; Zapka et al., 2000), the inclusion of alternative treatments in care delivery processes (Sohn & Cook, 2002), the management of ED patients (Mabrook & Dale, 1998), the ordering of antibiotics (Goolsby, 2007), diagnostic tests and invasive and noninvasive procedures (Cole & Ramirez, 2000; Sole, Hunkar-Huie, Schiller, & Cheatham, 2001; Venning, Durie, Roland,

Roberts, & Leese, 2000), the inclusion of physical activity and physical fitness counseling in primary care practices (Buchholz & Purath, 2007), and the use of collaboration in caring for high-risk patients (Brooten et al., 2005). In these descriptive studies, information is provided about the direct and indirect actions APNs take during the delivery of care. No statements can be made about the relationships between any of these processes and care delivery outcomes, however, although some hypotheses can be proposed based on study findings. As a result, these studies are useful as a preliminary step toward outcomes assessment.

In some studies, APN care delivery processes were compared with those of physicians and other care providers. These studies found that NPs were more likely than physicians and other community health providers to spend more time with patients (Seale, Anderson, & Kinnersley, 2005; Venning et al., 2000), nursing staff, and other disciplines (Hoffman, Tasota, Scharfenberg, Zullo, & Donahoe, 2003); to informally manage patient care needs (Sidani et al., 2006a; Sidani et al., 2006b); to discuss treatment options (Seale, Anderson, & Kinnersley, 2006); and to discuss and encourage smoking cessation (Sheahan, 2000; Zapka et al., 2000) (although this prevention-focused activity may not extend to other health risks [Sheahan]). No differences were seen for the treatment of febrile infants (Badger, Lookinland, Tiedeman, Anderson, & Eggett, 2002) or the timing and initiation of collaborative action to discuss patient concerns (Brooten et al., 2005). In one study, NPs were more likely to provide structural support for the emergency management of closed musculoskeletal injuries, although other interventions were similar to those of physician providers (Ball, Walton, & Hawes, 2007). In another study, residents spent significantly more time on coordination of care than NPs did (Sidani et al., 2006a; Sidani et al., 2006b). It is interesting to note that, despite this difference, patients managed by NPs reported higher levels of coordination than those overseen by residents.

Other process-focused studies have focused on CNM visit scheduling (Walker et al., 2002) and communication styles between CNMs and physicians, with both groups using informational styles during interactions with patients (Lawson, 2002). Intra-individual differences were noted for the CNM providers, however, suggesting they changed to a more controlling communication style with certain patients. Contrary to the researcher's expectations, communication style was not related to patient-perceived support for autonomy or patient satisfaction.

Process-focused studies also have explored APN use of clinical practice guidelines during the management of symptoms in oncology patients (Cunningham, 2006), NP health counseling behaviors (Lin, Gebbie, Fullilove, & Arons, 2004), and prescriptive writing patterns (Campbell et al., 1998; Hamric, Lindebak, Worley, & Jaubert, 1998; Shell, 2001). These latter studies provide clear evidence to counter early concerns about the potential for NPs to overprescribe. In one study of mental health NPs, however, an analysis of prescribing patterns for managing depression suggested that the NPs overused drugs that are considered less desirable, discontinued medications prematurely, and minimized important patient characteristics such as age when prescribing (Shell).

These process-focused investigations highlight some of the APN activities that are expected to contribute to care delivery outcome. Because most of the studies did not assess the relationship between process of care and any specific outcome, however, little is known about the actual impact of these actions on recipients of care. Some information about this potential relationship was provided in two reports of a process analysis conducted as part of a randomized clinical trial of APN impact on early discharge of very-low–birthweight infants (Brooten, Gennaro et al., 2002); women with unplanned cesarean birth, high-risk pregnancy, and hysterectomy; and older adults with cardiac diagnoses (Brooten, Youngblut, Deatrick, Naylor, & York, 2003). (Most of these studies used *CNSs,* although later reports by these authors used the generic term *APN.*) During each of these investigations, protocols were used to guide APN care delivery; APNs also recorded what was done during their interventions, the number of patient contacts made, the time spent during contacts, patient outcomes, and health care costs. In the study of mothers and infants, the majority of APN time was spent on assessment activities (69%), with the remaining time devoted to interventions (Brooten, Gennaro et al.). Assessments of infants focused on physical status, whereas assessments of mothers were directed at coping, health care, availability of support systems, and home environment. Assessments of mothers also addressed caretaking skills, understanding of procedures and medications, knowledge of infant growth and development, and recognition and prevention of infection. Intervention activities were devoted primarily to teaching, followed by liaison or consultation, and encouragement of self- or infant care.

In the combined analysis, surveillance was identified as the most common intervention, with APNs spending the greatest amount of time on monitoring signs and symptoms of physical problems (Brooten et al., 2003). An important finding of this second analysis was the relationship between magnitude of APN interaction and improvement in patient and cost outcomes. The greater the amount of time spent by the APN, the better the outcomes. A second important finding was the difference in outcomes seen and the amount of APN involvement required across patient populations. This finding reinforces the importance of carefully describing the makeup of the patient population, the care delivery setting (both of which are contextual or structural components of the quality of care framework), and the processes of care when measuring APN impact. Without this information, Brooten and colleagues might have erroneously concluded that some APNs performed better than others, when in fact the differences were the result of patient condition and need.

Although no statement can be made as to which of the APNs' activities contributed specifically to the favorable outcomes seen, the inclusion of a process assessment component provides preliminary indication of a cause-and-effect relationship between APN practice and patient outcome. Additional research is needed to determine whether selected aspects of the process are more important or if favorable outcomes are achieved only through a combination of APN actions.

Process-as-Outcome Studies

Ongoing confusion about the use of process indicators to denote outcomes achieved is evident in the literature. Among those processes proposed or examined by authors are resolution of nursing problems (Kleinpell-Nowell & Weiner, 1999), completeness of admission note (Rudy et al., 1998), collaboration among care providers, providers' recommendations for care based on need, and frequency and type of procedures ordered (Ingersoll, McIntosh, & Williams, 2000).

Among the process-as-outcome studies reported in the literature are a few that have explored whether the availability of clinical guidelines improves primary care provider documentation of preventive and screening services (Gray, 1998; Windorski & Kalb, 2002). Improved documentation was seen with the use of guidelines; when not used, the frequency of screening behaviors was less than desired. In one study, NPs reported rarely ordering cholesterol screening in children unless some evidence of family history for premature heart disease, stroke, or hypercholesterolemia was present (Windorski & Kalb)—a practice that clearly conflicted with recommended standards.

Studies that focus exclusively on processes as indicators of outcome are rarely seen. More commonly, investigators mistakenly report some process as an outcome—that is, as an indication of intervention effect. For example, Rudy et al. (1998) identified completeness of admission note as one of seven clinical outcome indicators for their comparison of ACNP, PA, and medical resident practice. In this case, the completeness of an admission note measures care provider performance; it is not a measure of the care received by patients, and there are no data to support the proposed causal link with a true clinical outcome, such as pain intensity or complication rate. A second example is evident in a report by Kinnersley et al. (2000), who described secondary outcomes of a comparison between NP and general practitioner consultations as length of consultation, information provided, resources used (prescriptions, investigations, referrals), and follow-up consultations—all of which are structure (e.g., resources used) and process indicators (e.g., information given, referrals made). However, these researchers did collect information about patient satisfaction, resolution of symptoms and concerns, and patients' intentions to deal with future similar illnesses, which constitute reasonable clinical outcome indicators. The ability to accurately measure patient intention to deal with future similar illnesses is questionable, however, and the authors provided no information about how they did this.

An example of a case in which all the indicators described as outcomes were actually process focused involved a retrospective medical record review of ACNP versus resident performance on patients admitted for cardiac catheterization (Reigle, Molnar, Howell, & Dumont, 2006). In this study, outcome indicators were defined as documentation of education and counseling for risk factors and discharge prescribing practices. Both these measures are indicators of care provider performance (process) rather than patient outcome. Findings demonstrated that ACNPs provided more education and counseling concerning dyslipidemia, exercise, and diabetes; counseling for hypertension and smoking was comparable for both groups. The ACNPs also provided

more appropriate medication prescriptions for management of heart disease post-discharge.

Process (Performance) Improvement Activities

Few reports of process improvement activities specifically mention the involvement of APNs or their probable impact on care delivery outcome. In one approach, an individual APN served as the process improvement intervention (Counsell & Gilbert, 1999). The difficulty with this report is the limited information concerning how the outcome data were collected and analyzed and how any variables unrelated to APN intervention were considered in the data interpretation process.

The use of interdisciplinary rounds as a process improvement approach was described by Halm and colleagues (2003). In this case, a CNS oversaw the shift of unit-based patient rounds to an interdisciplinary approach that involved all disciplines in the review and discussion of care delivery decisions. No information was provided about the impact of this change at the hospital involved. Instead, the authors reported the findings of an Internet survey of APNs who summarized the processes they used to measure the impact of interdisciplinary rounds on patient outcomes and the outcomes APNs recommended for measurement of effect. Several of the outcome indicators suggested are measures of process rather than outcome, however (e.g., case finding, consults/referrals, accomplishment of plan for patient, continuity of care, ethical issues addressed, quality initiatives for population, evidence-based protocols). Although these may indeed be useful indicators of improved processes of care and the potential for better care delivery outcomes, they should not be labeled as patient/family outcome indicators.

In a third study, an NP-managed performance improvement intervention model achieved improved outcomes through a process designed to facilitate compliance with community-acquired pneumonia (CAP) guidelines (Gross et al., 2004). Quarterly performance measurement data demonstrated improvements in each of the performance measures for prevention of CAP. The program also resulted in a reduction in patient length of stay and cost of care.

Disease Management Activities

Formal reports of the APN's role in disease management initiatives are few. The failure to identify disease management analyses may, in part, be because of their close linkages with other intervention and assessment activities. One example describes an ACNP disease management program for patients admitted to hospital for uncomplicated heart failure (Dahle, Smith, Ingersoll, & Wilson, 1998). In this case, the ACNP used disease-specific protocols to manage and monitor the care of hospitalized patients. Before the ACNP's arrival, disease management processes were managed by hospital residents who rotated through the cardiac service on a monthly basis. The ACNP's impact on organizational and patient outcomes was assessed by comparing administrative databases for the year before and after the ACNP's assumption of care. Overall costs, ancillary service costs, and use of electrocardiogram and respiratory care services declined significantly after the ACNP arrived. Mortality rates and lengths of stay were comparable before and after the disease management activities of the ACNP. Although there was no difference in patient outcomes, the ACNP did have an impact on the resources used, which would be considered an organizational outcome.

The report of an outpatient NP case manager for patients with cardiovascular disease also constitutes a disease management approach (Dougherty, Spertus, Dewhurst, & Nichol, 2000), although it is not described as such in the article. The authors focused their attention on the case management aspects of the NP role instead, which they described as assessing the patient's needs for specific services and facilitating access to each of these. In this situation, case management was used to provide the services required to manage the disease of the targeted group. A concern with this report is the authors' contention that they evaluated the impact of case management on patient outcomes, when, in fact, they evaluated the effect of different medication administration approaches. The case management process, per se, was not the intervention of interest. Consequently, the outcome findings reported by the authors provide no indication of whether that approach to disease management is better than any other.

A description of an APN-directed work site disease management program also is available (Carioti, Lavigne, Stone, Tortoretti, & Chiverton, 2001). In this case, 54 employees were surveyed about their perceptions of disease control, behavioral change, and understanding of disease condition after program completion. A majority of respondents (who were primarily educated white males managed for hypertension, dyslipidemia, and diabetes) reported behavioral changes as a result of the program. Those who

were managed for dyslipidemia and for hypertension also reported greater understanding of their disorders. Participants with asthma reported no change in level of understanding or initiation of behavioral change. Overall, participants were highly satisfied with the program. Because the outcome indicators were self-reports of perceived changes that were measured post-intervention only, caution is required when considering the impact of this intervention. Additional indicators, including those that could validate self-reports, are desirable. Moreover, the collection of data before the intervention and at longer intervals after program completion would help ensure that the behavioral and perceptual changes did, in fact, occur and that the impact was sustained long enough to achieve a true outcome effect. Blood pressure, lipid level, pulmonary function, medication intake, blood glucose level, and other quantifiable measures collected longitudinally would assist with validation of self-reports.

Outcomes Management Activities

Reports of APN-directed outcomes management programs also are few in number. Several descriptions of program development activities are available, with each of these highlighting the steps necessary to successfully design and implement such programs (Davidson, 1999; Peters, Cowley, & Standiford, 1999). The long-term impact of these programs is rarely described, although one program did reduce cesarean section rates in an obstetrical department by 6% over a 3-year period (Peters et al.).

The results of an outcomes management approach at an academic health science center have been described (Russell, VorderBruegge, & Burns, 2002). In this outcomes-managed model, two ACNPs served as outcomes managers for a population of neuroscience patients. The impact of the model was assessed through a retrospective medical record review of outcomes directly linked to daily management by and interventions of the APNs. A significant reduction in length of hospital stay was seen for patients at risk. Reductions in intensive care unit (ICU) length of stay and incidence of urinary tract infection and skin breakdown also were evident, with overall cost savings approaching $2.5 million for a 1-year period.

This outcomes management approach was applied to the care of ICU patients requiring mechanical ventilation for longer than 3 days (Burns & Earvin, 2002; Burns et al., 2003). In this study, four ACNPs managed and monitored care delivery using evidence-based weaning trial and sedation withdrawal guidelines. Number of ventilator days, ICU and hospital lengths of stay, and mortality rates all declined significantly after the outcomes management process was implemented. In addition, total costs attributed to this population declined by $3 million during the first year of the ACNP outcomes management intervention.

An NP-directed outcomes management program for patients with coronary heart disease also resulted in favorable outcomes (Allen et al., 2002). In this comparison of NP-managed care with usual care plus feedback about lipid levels, NP-managed patients achieved low-density lipoprotein (LDL) cholesterol levels that were significantly better than for patients in the usual care group. NPs achieved these outcomes through the management of patients' lipid levels, the provision of individualized lifestyle modifications, and the oversight of lipid-reducing medication use for 1 year after discharge from hospital.

Outcomes Research

Outcomes research has investigated care delivery outcomes across providers and between different APN types. In most cases, physician groups (including medical residents) have been used for comparison. This process is a concern because it implies that physician practice is the gold standard for APNs and that it encompasses the full range of APN activity. Actually, physician practice overlaps in some respects and diverges in others. In the process studies reviewed earlier, APNs routinely used strategies that either were not considered by physicians or were not incorporated to the extent evident in APN practice. Ideally, attention should be directed at indicators that accurately measure all care providers' impact as well as those that can serve as benchmarks for APN practice alone.

In a study to investigate which outcome indicators APNs routinely used or would recommend using for measurement of APN impact, Ingersoll et al. (2000) employed a Delphi survey method with 177 APNs in Tennessee. The top 10 APN-sensitive outcome indicators selected (in descending order) were satisfaction with care; symptom reduction or resolution; perception of being well cared for; compliance/adherence with treatment plan; knowledge level of patients and families; trust of care provider; collaboration among care providers; care provider recommendation according to need; frequency and type of procedures ordered; and quality of life. Of note in this listing is the inclusion of three process indicators (collaboration, care

provider recommendation, and procedures ordered), which would not reflect the APN's impact on outcomes.

In this section of the review of literature, studies that measured the actual effect of APN practice on outcomes are reviewed. These studies are further divided into those that compare APN outcomes with outcomes of other provider groups (e.g., physician), those that compare APN outcomes with outcomes of usual care, and those without comparison groups that measure outcomes before and after the introduction of an APN. Because of the increase in such research, this section includes representative reports highlighting the indicators measured in outcomes studies, the limitations evident in some of the research, and the findings described.

Studies Comparing Advanced Practice Nurse and Physician Outcomes. Studies comparing APNs with medical practitioners have been reported in the United States, Canada, the British Isles, Europe, Australia, the Middle East, and elsewhere. Caution is needed when comparing these studies, however, because educational requirements for advanced practice differ by country. Graduate education is now the standard in the United States and is moving in that direction throughout Canada. In the British Isles and in other countries, certificate programs are often the norm. In addition, some reports label nurses as *specialists* or *advanced practitioners* solely because of their number of years of experience in the clinical setting (Chang et al., 1999; Sakr et al., 1999) or because their role behaviors are "typical" of APNs (Oddi & Cassidy, 1998).

Nurse Practitioner Outcomes. Most studies of APN versus physician practice have compared NPs with primary care physicians. In a systematic review of this research conducted between 1966 and 2001, randomized controlled trials and studies with prospective experimental designs were reviewed if they included patient satisfaction, health status, health service costs, or process of care measures (Horrocks, Anderson, & Salisbury, 2002). In addition to searching electronic databases for studies from developed countries, investigators contacted schools of nursing offering NP training programs and authors of identified studies. When the study reports did not specify whether the nurse providing the care was an NP, the investigators used specific criteria to determine whether the study should be included. This process is a limitation and may have resulted in the inclusion of studies that should not have been considered. Thirty-five of 119 potential studies met review inclusion criteria, although none included sufficient information to compare health care costs. Overall, the research demonstrated that patient satisfaction with care provider was significantly greater for NPs. No differences were seen for health status or quality of life. Process indicators suggested NPs spent more time with patients, identified physical abnormalities more often, communicated more effectively, and recorded in the medical record more completely than physicians did. The ordering and the interpreting of x-ray films were comparable across groups. Evident from this review is the need for additional rigorous research concerning APN impact. Only 29.4% of studies comparing NP with primary care physician outcomes were sufficiently designed to meet the review's inclusion criteria. Without this level of comparison, few recommendations can be made about which indicators are most reflective of and sensitive to APN practice.

Studies also have compared NP performance with that of medical residents (see Table 24-2), with findings consistently reporting equivalent or better outcomes. In one descriptive comparison study, however, lengths of stay and total costs were higher for the NP group (Lambing et al., 2004). Information about the calculations used to compute cost is limited. In addition, the patient mix for the NPs was sicker, which may have contributed to the differences seen. The investigators noted that differences were likely the result of the NPs consulting more often with other providers, resulting in additional care provider charges. Laboratory and radiology costs were comparable, and when the costs were reported as mean (average) charge per patient day, the costs were less for NPs.

Two randomized controlled trials of NP and primary care physician practice include one from the United States (Mundinger et al., 2000) and one from Wales and England (Kinnersley et al., 2000). In both studies, over 1000 patients were randomized to either NP or primary care physician practice. In the Mundinger and colleagues' study, health status, patient satisfaction, service utilization, and physiological test results were comparable for NP and physician groups. Similar results were seen in the Kinnersley and colleagues' study, although patients in that sample were significantly more satisfied with the care provided by NPs and reported receiving more information about their illnesses.

Several studies also have compared physician practice alone with physician practice in collaboration with an NP. In a retrospective review of the outcomes of cardiovascular surgeon alone versus cardiovascular surgeon plus ACNP, postoperative lengths of stay were shorter for the collaborate group (Meyer & Miers, 2005). Collaborative care also resulted in lower cost of care, with organizational savings estimated at over $3 million per year. A second study found similarly favorable findings for NP/physician teams overseeing patients with hypertension and diabetes mellitus (Litaker et al., 2003). A third study comparing outcomes of physician-only care with outcomes of NP/physician care for nursing home residents demonstrated equivalent findings for both groups. ED visits, ED and hospital costs, lengths of stay, and number of hospitalizations all were comparable. The sole difference pertained to the frequency of acute visits, which were higher for the NP/physician group (Aigner, Drew, & Phipps, 2004). Because the increased acute visit frequency was solely related to NP inpatient oversight (with no charges incurred per visit), however, no differences in cost were seen. Had the NP visits resulted in a charge per visit, the costs between the groups might have differed considerably, although the authors suggest that the lower salary costs of the NPs (compared with physician visit) would have offset this rise.

Acute Care Nurse Practitioner Outcomes. Rudy and colleagues (1998) used a longitudinal, matched group design to compare ACNP/PAs' with resident physicians' outcomes at two medical centers. Outcomes data were collected from the medical records of patients overseen by ACNPs, PAs, and medical residents. During the 14-month period of the study, patient outcomes (length of stay, mortality, adverse drug reaction, readmission to the hospital within 2 weeks) were comparable across care providers. A shortcoming of this study is the mixing of ACNP and PA providers, which suggests these two groups have comparable education, skill, and practice. Because of the distinctions between ACNPs and PAs, outcomes assessment initiatives should measure their impact separately.

Comparable outcomes were seen in a study of ACNPs in a subacute ICU (Hoffman, Tasota, Zullo, Scharfenberg, & Donahoe, 2005). In this study, workload, demographic, and medical conditions of patients were comparable for APN/attending physician and resident/attending physician teams. Readmissions to ICU, mortality rates, duration of mechanical ventilation, and weaning status at discharge were comparable. The reintubation rate was higher for patients cared for by the physician group, even though patient acuity was comparable for both groups.

Clinical Nurse Specialist Outcomes. Favorable outcomes have been seen for cancer patients managed by CNSs in outpatient settings (McCorkle et al., 1989; Moore et al., 2002). In the Moore and colleagues' study, CNSs managed patient care in nurse-led clinics and then contacted patients by phone for follow-up assessment. CNS-managed patients with a diagnosis of lung cancer had significantly better levels of emotional functioning and less peripheral neuropathy than patients managed by physicians. CNS-managed patients also were significantly more likely to die at home than were patients treated by physicians. Costs of care were comparable for both groups. In the McCorkle and colleagues' study, patients with lung cancer were randomly assigned to one of three treatment groups. The first group received specialized home care provided by CNSs, the second received standard home care consisting of service delivery from an interdisciplinary team, and the third received care provided at a medical provider's office. Patients managed in physician offices had significantly more symptom distress and became more dependent earlier in their treatment period than either of the home care groups (standard or specialized). Patients managed by the CNSs had significantly fewer hospitalizations and, although not significant, also had shorter lengths of stay. Patients managed by the standard approach and during physician office visits had lengths of hospital stay averaging 73 days longer than patients overseen by CNSs. Although dated and limited by high attrition rates, this study is relevant because of its use of a true experimental design and its inclusion of two types of home care oversight in its investigation.

Certified Nurse-Midwife Outcomes. A large, prospective study of planned home births was conducted to compare CNM outcomes with those achieved for all singleton, vertex births at greater than 37 weeks' gestation (Johnson & Daviss, 2005). Women who started the birthing process at home were older, of lower socioeconomic status but higher education, and less likely to be African-American or Hispanic. Medical interventions for home births were significantly fewer than for hospital births. Intrapartum

and neonatal mortality rates were comparable for hospital and home births, and mothers' satisfaction with care was high for the home birth group, with over 97% of mothers reporting they were extremely or very satisfied with the care received.

A second study of CNM outcomes used an optimality index (OI) to compare midwifery and physician practices according to extent of preexisting health status at time of treatment (Cragin & Kennedy, 2006). The OI contained a list of 40 care delivery processes and outcome measures pertaining to pregnancy, parturition, neonatal condition, and maternal postpartum condition, which were scored according to level of optimality (0=non-optimal; 1=optimal). Women cared for by physicians were 1.7 times as likely as those cared for by CNMs to have a cesarean section during delivery. Women seen by physicians in this study had a significantly greater proportion of chronic illness and drug abuse, although these differences did not explain the higher rate of cesarean section for the group.

Certified Registered Nurse Anesthetist Outcomes. Three studies of CRNA impact compared CRNA outcomes with those of anesthesiologists. One of these estimated costs based on cases from four anesthesia services at four different hospitals: a large academic medical center, a large community hospital, a medium-size community hospital, and a small community hospital (Cromwell & Snyder, 2000). Labor cost projections for 10,000 anesthetics delivered per year demonstrated that an all–CRNA care delivery model cost less than half of an all-anesthesiologist model. The cost savings for a mixed model composed of anesthesiologists and CRNAs in ratios of 1:1 to 1:4 ranged from 33% to 41% of the total costs for an all-anesthesiologist model. In the second study, risk-adjusted mortality rates of patients undergoing carotid endarterectomy, cholecystectomy, herniorrhaphy, hysterectomy, knee replacement, laminectomy, mastectomy, or prostatectomy were compared for CRNAs and anesthesiologists (Pine, Holt, & Lou, 2003). Medicare data were analyzed for a 3-year period, with no differences seen for type of anesthesia provider. The third study examined obstetrical care anesthesia outcomes between hospitals employing CRNAs only and those employing anesthesiologists only (Simonson, Ahern, & Hendryx, 2007). Although the investigators of this study stressed the focus of the comparison on the differences between hospitals rather than care providers, the findings are relevant to the discussion of APN outcomes. Hospitals with

CRNA-only staffs had significantly fewer complications, although this difference disappeared when the complication rates were risk-adjusted. This risk-adjustment process included examining information about the impact of co-morbid conditions, hospital size, teaching status, and patient transfers on development of complications. The demonstration of equivalent outcomes for CRNAs and anesthesiologists provides additional evidence concerning the quality of care provided by APNs.

Neonatal Nurse Practitioner Outcomes.

NNP resuscitation effectiveness was compared with that of junior medical staff in one institution in which a resuscitation team was introduced into the neonatal intensive care unit (NICU) (Aubrey & Yoxall, 2001). In this study, NNP and medical resident intubation rates were similar, although NNPs intubated infants more quickly and administered surfactant earlier. Survival rates and adverse events for infants were comparable for both groups. The earlier intubation timing and the administration of surfactant suggested that the NNPs were more familiar with the institution's best practice protocols, which stressed early intubation and early administration of surfactant for at-risk neonates.

An interesting and noteworthy finding of this study is the failure of the NNPs' improved care delivery processes (earlier intubation and administration of surfactant) to achieve better patient outcomes. This finding highlights the difficulty in identifying which factor or combination of factors contributes to the achievement of improved care delivery outcome. Clearly, factors other than timing of intervention and administration of surfactant were influencing the outcomes achieved. A strength of this study is its comparison of resuscitation process (reflected by frequency of intubation, timing of intubation, and administration of surfactant) with resuscitation outcome (infant survival rate and frequency of adverse events). Any time information is included about the comparability of or differences in actions taken during the delivery of care, the degree of comfort with probable cause/effect relationships is increased.

Another study compared NNP outcomes with those of other care providers, including PAs and resident physicians. In this study, chart reviews assessing care delivery outcomes found comparable morbidity and mortality rates, costs of care, and lengths of stay in the NICU and the hospital as a whole (Karlowicz & McMurray, 2000). Favorable outcomes also were

seen for PNPs when compared with those of trauma service residents (Fanta et al., 2006). Patients overseen by the PNP group had significantly shorter lengths of stay and reported significantly higher levels of satisfaction.

Studies Comparing Advanced Practice Nurse and Physician Productivity. One of the most difficult and contentious elements of APN outcomes measurement is the assessment of APN productivity, which is an organizational rather than patient outcome. Productivity is an indication of care provider efficiency rather than skill or capability and, as such, does not provide any guarantee of quality patient care. The issue with productivity is that reimbursement practices and the income generated by care providers are directly tied to productivity levels. Because APNs spend more time with patients, their overall productivity levels may result in changes in potential income for the organization or practice. Until reimbursement decisions are shifted to a care delivery outcomes approach, this will continue to be a problem for APNs.

Relative Work Value of Advanced Practice Nurses.

Payment for services provided to Medicare patients is based on a resource-based relative work value (RBRV) scale methodology, which incorporates an estimate for the amount of work, practice expense, and professional liability insurance associated with various procedures. The total relative value of each procedure is multiplied by a standard dollar conversion factor to determine the allowable service charge care providers may request for reimbursement of services (Sullivan-Marx & Maislin, 2000). Until 1994, all RBRVs were calculated solely on physician data. Since that time, NP data have been used to adjust the RBRVs for some payment codes, although considerable work is needed to clarify how NPs' work values differ from physicians' (Sullivan-Marx & Maislin).

Sullivan-Marx and Maislin (2000) and Sullivan-Marx, Happ, Bradley, and Maislin (2000) have begun to explore this issue. In a mailed survey to expert practitioners, NPs quantified both the time and complexity of the work required to provide care during three office encounter vignettes. In quantifying the time required, NPs estimated pre-service, intra-service, and post-service time in minutes. Complexity was measured by assessing mental effort, technical skill, and physical effort, and the psychological stress associated with an iatrogenic event related to the current procedural technology (CPT) code associated with the vignette. In all cases, NPs estimated relative work values comparable to those established for physician practice, suggesting that their practice patterns were similar for the scenarios described. Because the CPT codes and descriptors were designed with physicians in mind, however, other activities by APNs may not have been included in the estimation process. Until these are well defined and marketed by APNs, this process will continue to potentially underrepresent the APN's actual relative value in the delivery of care.

Studies Comparing Advanced Practice Nurse and Usual Practice Outcomes. Some of the strongest APN outcomes research has focused on the impact of early hospital discharge using a CNS-directed discharge planning and home follow-up intervention (Brooten, Naylor et al., 2002). This care delivery model has been tested with high-risk childbearing women (York et al., 1997), with older postsurgical cancer patients (McCorkle et al., 2000), and with older adults (Naylor et al., 1999 [this report used the term *APN*, so NPs, as well as CNSs, may have been interveners]). In each of these investigations, a randomized controlled clinical trial design was used to compare CNS outcomes with those seen with usual care. In all cases, outcomes were superior for the CNS intervention groups. Cost of care for CNS-directed services was 44% less than for standard care (York et al.). Most of the cost savings for the older adult group were the result of a significant reduction in the number of readmissions for APN-managed patients (Naylor et al.).

Other studies comparing APN outcomes with those of standard care have been conducted in long-term care facilities (Ryden et al., 2000), with recently diagnosed women with cancer (Ritz et al., 2000), with patients with coronary heart disease (Allen et al., 2002), with caregivers of rural older adults (Dellasega & Zerbe, 2002), with postoperative coronary revascularization patients with hypercholesterolemia (Paez & Allen, 2006), and with rehabilitation patients discharged from an acute care facility (Rawl, Easton, Kwiatowski, Zemen, & Burczyk, 1998). In the long-term care facility, gerontological CNSs used evidence-based protocols to manage newly admitted patients at risk for incontinence, pressure ulcers, depression, and aggressive behavior (Ryden et al.). Care delivery outcomes were compared with those at a site where residents received usual care. Findings suggested CNSs influenced care

delivery outcomes through direct and indirect means, with reductions seen in the number of episodes of urinary incontinence, the incidence of pressure ulcers, and the frequency of aggressive behavior. An overall 6-month composite change score also was significantly higher for patients managed by the CNSs. Missing from this report is an indication of how the direct versus indirect activities of the CNS influenced outcomes seen. This component of impact assessment studies is difficult to determine, although steps in this direction are needed to clarify how the APN improves care delivery through direct intervention as well as through the improved performance of others.

In the study of APN (type of provider not specified) impact on early adjustment to diagnosis of breast cancer, inclusion of an APN in delivery of services resulted in improved quality of life, less uncertainty, and decreased mood disturbances (Ritz et al., 2000). Overall costs of care were comparable for usual services and for those that were APN-enhanced, suggesting that this approach is cost-effective for improving care delivery outcomes in recently diagnosed women. Findings with rehabilitation patients were less conclusive. Although anxiety and number of post-discharge phone calls declined significantly in experimental but not control groups, other measured outcomes demonstrated no difference (Rawl et al., 1998).

The study of postoperative patients with hypercholesterolemia involved a randomized clinical trial designed to compare the cost-effectiveness of services provided by an NP with that of usual care enhanced by feedback to primary care provider (Paez & Allen, 2006). The incremental costs associated with the oversight of the NP included the costs of the NP's time and the lipid-lowering medications and laboratory monitoring activities of the NP. At 12 months after surgery, the incremental costs of the NP-managed group were $26 per mg/dL of cholesterol outcome and $39 per percent reduction in mg/dL of lipid level. NP management was most intensive during the first 6 months of the year and medication costs were highest during this period when NPs titrated dosages to achieve maximum effect. Although more costly during this initial period than for the usual care group, the ultimate outcome of achieving better lipid management offset the extra cost.

Studies Using Non-Comparison Groups. A number of studies have compared care delivery outcomes before and after the APN's introduction into clinical practice. In many of these studies, a pre-/post-intervention approach was used to test for differences. A weakness of these studies is the frequent reliance on retrospective reviews of medical records for evidence of outcomes before the APN's arrival. The absence of a comparison group also makes confirmation of the relationship between APN and outcome difficult. Nevertheless, the studies do provide useful information for further exploration in controlled trials and should be viewed as preliminary indications of possible effect. One such study compared the length of stay, patient satisfaction, use of laboratory tests (a process-as-outcome indicator), and overall costs for the year before ACNP arrival with 16 months after (Sarkissian & Wennberg, 1999). Reductions in length of stay, less use of laboratory tests, and a significant decline in overall costs of services followed the arrival of the ACNP. Satisfaction, which was measured in the post-arrival period only, was high. Similarly high ratings were seen in a prospective, non-comparison study of psychiatric CNSs (Baradell & Bordeaux, 2001). Patients in this study also reported significant improvements in clinical symptoms and quality of life.

Several other studies have focused solely on patient or staff satisfaction with APN practice as an indicator of care provider effect (Benkert et al., 2002; Bryant & Graham, 2002; Knudtson, 2000; Stutts, 2001). In many cases, these studies used questionnaires with limited reliability and validity estimates and included single-site samples of patients. In most instances, no comparison groups were available. Because of the methodological issues associated with the measurement of satisfaction, reliance on this outcome indicator alone is generally not sufficient for assessing APN impact. Patient satisfaction data are often skewed, with only the most satisfied or dissatisfied patients responding. In addition, general satisfaction measures may not be sufficiently sensitive to detect differences across APN providers. Their use should not be avoided altogether, however, because they do offer one indication of care provider impact. When serious problems with delivery of services occur, satisfaction levels drop. In stable environments, the variation may not be sufficient to detect differences across care providers.

A more comprehensive summary of APN outcome studies published since 1998 and organized by outcome indicators is provided in Table 24-2. Only studies that contained sufficient information about how the outcomes were measured and when they were measured in relation to APN intervention are included in the table. Also excluded are studies in which APNs and PAs were linked together as providers of care and studies in which the APNs were not prepared at the master's or higher level.

Program Evaluation

Differentiating program evaluation initiatives from outcomes research is difficult, especially if an APN has been actively involved in developing and implementing the program. In most cases, outcome measures are used to assess program impact, contributing further to the confusion. For purposes of this review, program evaluation reports are those in which the authors described the activity as an evaluation, those in which the APN activity was one component of several initiatives designed to provide some service or influence some outcome, and those in which the purpose of the assessment was to determine the worth or value of the intervention for purposes of decision making. Table 24-3 on pp. 715-716 highlights the variety of program foci and the patient populations involved in these program evaluations.

In keeping with the primary purpose of evaluations, which is to inform decision makers, many of the evaluations reported in the literature are of limited duration and locally focused. The evaluation designs also vary considerably. Although these limitations may be reasonable for purposes of decision making by APNs or organizations performing the evaluations, caution must be used when applying these findings to any other APN practice in any other setting. When reviewing program evaluations, careful attention should be paid to the evaluation method used (which can range from descriptive to randomized clinical trial), the population targeted, the organization involved, the data collection time frame, and the type of data collected.

Three other reports of APN impact provide representative examples of rarely performed but highly desirable first steps in APN program implementation and outcome evaluation activities: feasibility/pilot studies and instrument sensitivity testing. In two of these studies, pilot testing was done with a small sample of the population targeted for APN-directed care (Anetzberger, Stricklin, Gaunter, Banozic, & Laurie, 2006) or program development (Barnason, Merboth, Pozehl, & Tietjen, 1998). *Feasibility/pilot studies* are useful for preventing the implementation of interventions that will not be received favorably by targeted recipients or stakeholders (e.g., other care

Text continues on p. 716.

Table 24-2   ADVANCED PRACTICE NURSE–SENSITIVE OUTCOME INDICATORS TESTED IN PRACTICE*

Outcome Indicator	Authors (Year)	Study Design	Focus of Indicator: Population Generic, Population Specific, or Organizational	Findings
Activities of daily living (ADL)	Leveille et al. (1998)	Randomized Controlled Trial	Population Generic	Significantly improved over control group
	Neff et al. (2003)	Quasi-experimental Comparison	Population Generic	Significantly improved over control group
Adverse events/unplanned incidents, including drug reactions	Rudy et al. (1998)	Comparative Analysis	Population Generic Organizational	Comparable to residents
	Simonson et al. (2007)	Retrospective Comparison		Comparable to anesthesiologists
Affect	Ryden et al. (2000)	Quasi-experimental Comparison	Population Generic	Significantly improved over control group
Aggressive behavior	Ryden et al. (2000)	Quasi-experimental Comparison	Population Generic	Significantly improved over control group
Alcohol consumption	Ockene et al. (1999)	Program Evaluation	Population Specific	Significantly improved over control group
Anxiety/depression; mental health status; emotional state	Corner et al. (2003)	Case Study	Population Generic	Decreased over time
	Krichbaum et al. (2005)	Quasi-experimental Repeated Measures		Significantly better than control group
	Lenz et al. (2004)	Longitudinal Follow-up Study		Comparable to physicians
	Leveille et al. (1998)	Randomized Controlled Trial		Comparable to control group

Continued

APN, Advanced practice nurse; *CRNA,* certified registered nurse anesthetist; *GNP,* geriatric nurse practitioner; *ICU,* intensive care unit; *MD,* Doctor of Medicine; *NP,* nurse practitioner.

NOTE: Some indicators that were used with specific populations in studies have been labeled as *generic* because they can be applied to multiple patient groups.

*Published studies since 1998.

†Constitute both a process (action by provider) and an outcome (condition or response in patient).

Definition of terms for the focus of the indicator:

Population Generic—indicators that could be used with any patient population.

Population Specific—indicators that are relevant to specific populations only.

Organizational—indicators that focus on the outcomes of the setting rather than the patient.

Table 24-2 ADVANCED PRACTICE NURSE–SENSITIVE OUTCOME INDICATORS TESTED IN PRACTICE*—CONT'D

Outcome Indicator	Authors (Year)	Study Design	Focus of Indicator: Population Generic, Population Specific, or Organizational	Findings
Anxiety/depression; mental health status; emotional state—cont'd	McCorkle et al. (2007)	Secondary Data Analysis		Comparable to control group
	McMullen et al. (2001)	Program Evaluation		Comparable to physician service
	Moore et al. (2002)	Randomized Controlled Trial		Significantly better than physicians
	Naylor & McCauley (1999)	Randomized Controlled Trial		Comparable to control group
	Neff et al. (2003)	Quasi-experimental Comparison		Significantly better (depression) than control group
	Rawl et al. (1998)	Randomized Controlled Trial		Significantly better than control group
	Ritz et al. (2000)	Randomized Controlled Trial		Significantly better than control group
	Ryden et al. (2000)	Quasi-experimental Comparison		Comparable to control group
Apgar score	Murphy & Fullerton (1998)	Survey	Population Specific	Low incidence of low score
Autonomous decision making (patient perceived)	Lawson (2002)	Survey	Population Generic	Comparable to physicians
Blood pressure	Krein et al. (2004)	Randomized Controlled Trial	Population Generic	Comparable to control group
	Lenz et al. (2004)	Longitudinal Follow-up Study		Comparable to physicians
	Litaker et al. (2003)	Randomized Controlled Trial		Comparable to control group
	Mundinger et al. (2000)	Randomized Controlled Trial		Comparable to physicians
	Scisney-Matlock et al. (2004)	Randomized Controlled Trial		Comparable to physicians

Indicator	Author	Design	Population	Findings
Caregiver psychosocial status	Dellasega & Zerbe (2002)	Randomized Controlled Trial	Population Generic	Significantly better than control group
Cesarean delivery†	Jepson et al. (1999)	Randomized Controlled Trial		Comparable to control group
	Cragin & Kennedy (2006)	Prospective Descriptive Cohort	Population Specific	Significantly lower than physician group
Cholesterol	Allen et al. (2002)	Randomized Controlled Trial	Population Generic	Significantly better than usual care group
Complication rate	Krein et al. (2004)	Randomized Controlled Trial		Comparable to control group
	Rawl et al. (1998)	Randomized Controlled Trial	Population Generic	Comparable to control group
	Wheeler (1999)	Medical Record Review		Trend for fewer with APN present on patient unit
Cost of care	Aigner et al. (2004)	Medical Record Review	Population Generic	NP/MD team comparable to physicians alone
	Burl et al. (1998)	Administrative Database Review		GNP/MD team significantly less than physician alone
	Burns et al. (2003)	Pre/Post‡ Comparison		Significantly reduced with APN outcomes management
	Carr (2000)	Administrative Database Review		Significantly less than physicians
	Cromwell & Snyder (2000)	Case Study Cost Comparison		Significantly less with CRNA team model
	Dahle et al. (1998)	Pre/Post Comparison		Significantly less than physicians
	Karlowicz & McMurray (2000)	Medical Record Review		Comparable to residents
	Lambing et al. (2004)	Descriptive Comparison		Significantly more than physicians overall; less for charges per patient day

Continued

APN, Advanced practice nurse; *CRNA*, certified registered nurse anesthetist; *GNP*, geriatric nurse practitioner; *ICU*, intensive care unit; *MD*, Doctor of Medicine; *NP*, nurse practitioner.

NOTE: Some indicators that were used with specific populations in studies have been labeled as *generic* because they can be applied to multiple patient groups.

*Published studies since 1998.

†Constitute both a process (action by provider) and an outcome (condition or response in patient).

Definition of terms for the focus of the indicator:

Population Generic—indicators that could be used with any patient population.

Population Specific—indicators that are relevant to specific populations only.

Organizational—indicators that focus on the outcomes of the setting rather than the patient.

Table 24-2 ADVANCED PRACTICE NURSE–SENSITIVE OUTCOME INDICATORS TESTED IN PRACTICE*—CONT'D

Outcome Indicator	Authors (Year)	Study Design	Focus of Indicator: Population Generic, Population Specific, or Organizational	Findings
Cost of care—cont'd	Naylor et al. (1999)	Randomized Controlled Trial		Significantly less than control group
	Paez & Allen (2006)	Randomized Controlled Trial		Incremental costs offset by improved outcome
	Ritz et al. (2000)	Randomized Controlled Trial		Comparable to control group
	Roblin, Howard et al. (2004)	Predictive Modeling		Significantly less than for physicians
	Russell et al. (2002)	Outcomes Management Program		Average cost per patient day reduced
	Sarkissian & Wennberg (1999)	Pre/Post Comparison		Significantly reduced
	Stone et al. (2000)	Cost Estimation		Less than physicians, when adjusted for productivity
	Topp et al. (1998)	Administrative Database Review		Significantly lower than comparison group
	Venning et al. (2000)	Randomized Controlled Trial		Comparable to residents
Disability (bed) days	Leveille et al. (1998)	Randomized Controlled Trial	Population Specific	Significantly less than control group
Discharge disposition	Hoffman et al. (2005)	Quasi-experimental Longitudinal Comparison	Organizational	Comparable to physicians
Disease activity	Tijhuis et al. (2003)	Randomized Controlled Trial	Population Generic	Comparable to multidisciplinary teams
Emergency department use	Aigner et al. (2004)	Medical Record Review	Population Generic	NP/MD team comparable to physicians alone
	Lenz et al. (2004)	Longitudinal Follow-up Study		Comparable to physicians
	Leveille et al. (1998)	Randomized Controlled Trial		Comparable to control group
	Mundinger et al. (2000)	Randomized Controlled Trial		Comparable to physicians

Indicator	Citation	Study Type	Population	Finding
Episiotomy, with & without laceration†	Murphy & Feinland (1998)	Observational Cohort Study	Population Specific	Low incidence
Functional status/ability	Bula et al. (1999)	Secondary Analysis	Population Generic	Significantly better than control group
	Lenz et al. (2004)	Longitudinal Follow-up Study		Comparable to physicians
	Leveille et al. (1998)	Randomized Controlled Trial		Significantly better than control group
	Mundinger et al. (2000)	Randomized Controlled Trial		Comparable to physicians
	Naylor & McCauley (1999)	Secondary Data Analysis		Comparable to control group
	Naylor et al. (1999)	Randomized Controlled Trial		Comparable to control group
	Rawl et al. (1998)	Randomized Controlled Trial		Comparable to control group
	Tijhuis et al. (2003)	Randomized Controlled Trial		Comparable to multidisciplinary teams
Glucose level, serum	Brown et al. (2001)	Program Evaluation	Population Specific	Significantly improved over time
Health state	Dellasega & Zerbe (2002)	Randomized Controlled Trial	Population Generic	Comparable to control group
	Tijhuis et al. (2003)	Randomized Controlled Trial		Comparable to multidisciplinary teams
HbA$_{1c}$	Lenz et al. (2004)	Longitudinal Follow-up Study	Population Specific	Comparable to physicians
	Litaker et al. (2003)	Randomized Controlled Trial		Comparable to control group
Hospitalizations, including readmissions†	Dahl & Penque (2001)	Program Evaluation	Population Generic	Significantly fewer than before program
	Kane et al. (2003)	Quasi-experimental Comparison		Significantly fewer than controls

Continued

APN, Advanced practice nurse; *CRNA,* certified registered nurse anesthetist; *GNP,* geriatric nurse practitioner; *ICU,* intensive care unit; *MD,* Doctor of Medicine; *NP,* nurse practitioner.

NOTE: Some indicators that were used with specific populations in studies have been labeled as *generic* because they can be applied to multiple patient groups.

*Published studies since 1998.

†Constitute both a process (action by provider) and an outcome (condition or response in patient).

Definition of terms for the focus of the indicator:

Population Generic—indicators that could be used with any patient population.

Population Specific—indicators that are relevant to specific populations only.

Organizational—indicators that focus on the outcomes of the setting rather than the patient.

Table **24-2** Advanced Practice Nurse–Sensitive Outcome Indicators Tested in Practice*—cont'd

Outcome Indicator	Authors (Year)	Study Design	Focus of Indicator: Population Generic, Population Specific, or Organizational	Findings
Hospitalizations, including readmissions†—cont'd	Lambing et al. (2004)	Descriptive Comparison		Comparable to physicians
	Lenz et al. (2004)	Longitudinal Follow-up Study		Comparable to physicians
	Leveille et al. (1998)	Randomized Controlled Trial		Significantly fewer than controls
	McCorkle et al. (2000)	Randomized Controlled Trial		Comparable to control group
	Mundinger et al. (2000)	Randomized Controlled Trial		Comparable to physicians
	Naylor & McCauley (1999)	Secondary Data Analysis		Comparable to control group
	Naylor et al. (1999)	Randomized Controlled Trial		Significantly fewer than control group
	Neff et al. (2003)	Quasi-experimental Comparison		Significantly fewer than control group
	Rawl et al. (1998)	Randomized Controlled Trial		Comparable to control group
	Rudy et al. (1998)	Comparative Study		Comparable to residents
Incontinence, control of	Ryden et al. (2000)	Quasi-experimental Comparison	Population Specific	Significantly better than control group
Length of stay	Aigner et al. (2004)	Medical Record Review	Population Generic Organizational	NP/MD team comparable to physicians alone
	Burns et al. (2003)	Pre/Post Comparison		Significantly shorter with APN outcomes management
	Carr (2000)	Administrative Database Review		Significantly shorter than physicians
	Dahl & Penque (2001)	Program Evaluation		Significantly shorter than before program (overall)
	Dahle et al. (1998)	Pre/Post Comparison		Comparable to physicians
	Fanta et al. (2006)	Randomized Controlled Trial		Significantly shorter than for residents

Indicator	Population	Study	Design	Findings
		Gross et al. (2004)	Pre/Post Comparison	Significant reduction over time
		Karlowicz & McMurray (2000)	Medical Record Review	Comparable to residents
		Lambing et al. (2004)	Descriptive Comparison	Significantly longer than physicians
		Leveille et al. (1998)	Randomized Controlled Trial	Comparable to control group
		Naylor & McCauley (1999)	Secondary Data Analysis	Comparable to control group
		Naylor et al. (1999)	Randomized Controlled Trial	Significantly shorter than control group
		Neff et al. (2003)	Quasi-experimental Comparison	Significantly shorter than control group
		Rideout (2007)	Pre/Post Comparison	No difference pre to post
		Rudy et al. (1998)	Comparative Study	Comparable to residents
		Russell et al. (2002)	Outcomes Management Program	Significantly reduced
		Sarkissian & Wennberg (1999)	Pre/Post Comparison	Significantly reduced
		Topp et al. (1998)	Administrative Database Review	Significantly shorter for units with APN
		Wheeler (1999)	Medical Record Review	Significantly shorter than comparison group
Length of survival/ survival rate	Population Generic	Bula et al. (1999)	Secondary Data Analysis	Comparable to control group
		Karlowicz & McMurray (2000)	Medical Record Review	Comparable to residents
		McCorkle et al. (2000)	Randomized Controlled Trial	Significantly greater for APN-directed home care

Continued

APN, Advanced practice nurse; *CRNA*, certified registered nurse anesthetist; *GNP*, geriatric nurse practitioner; *ICU*, intensive care unit; *MD*, Doctor of Medicine; *NP*, nurse practitioner.

NOTE: Some indicators that were used with specific populations in studies have been labeled as *generic* because they can be applied to multiple patient groups.

*Published studies since 1998.

†Constitute both a process (action by provider) and an outcome (condition or response in patient).

Definition of terms for the focus of the indicator:

Population Generic—indicators that could be used with any patient population.

Population Specific—indicators that are relevant to specific populations only.

Organizational—indicators that focus on the outcomes of the setting rather than the patient.

Table 24-2   Advanced Practice Nurse–Sensitive Outcome Indicators Tested in Practice*—cont'd

Outcome Indicator	Authors (Year)	Study Design	Focus of Indicator: Population Generic, Population Specific, or Organizational	Findings
Mechanical ventilation duration & weaning	Burns et al. (2003)	Pre/Post Comparison	Population Specific	Significantly reduced with APN outcomes management
	Hoffman et al. (2005)	Quasi-experimental Longitudinal Comparison		Comparable to physicians
Morbidity	Murphy & Fullerton (1998)	Survey	Population Generic Organizational	Low incidence
Mortality	Aubrey & Yoxall (2001)	Medical Record Review	Population Generic Organizational	Comparable to residents
	Burns et al. (2003)	Pre/Post Comparison		Significantly reduced with APN outcomes management
	Dahl & Penque (2001)	Program Evaluation		Significantly less than before program
	Dahle et al. (1998)	Pre/Post Comparison		Comparable to physicians
	Hoffman et al. (2005)	Quasi-experimental Longitudinal Comparison		Comparable to physicians
	Karlowicz & McMurray (2000)	Medical Record Review		Comparable to residents
	Lambing et al. (2004)	Descriptive Comparison		Comparable to physicians
	Murphy & Fullerton (1998)	Survey		Low incidence
	Pine et al. (2003)	Medicare Database Review		Comparable to anesthesiologists
	Rudy et al. (1998)	Comparative Study		Comparable to physicians
	Simonson et al. (2007)	Medical Record Review		Comparable to anesthesiologists
Nurse satisfaction	McMullen et al. (2001)	Program Evaluation	Population Specific Organizational	Highly satisfied
	Rideout (2007)	Pre/Post Comparison		Highly satisfied post-intervention (no pre-intervention data)

	Study	Study Type	Population	Findings
Optimality of services†	Shebesta et al. (2006)	Survey		Highly satisfied
	Stolee et al. (2006)	Survey		Comparable to/significantly greater than residents
	Cragin & Kennedy (2006)	Descriptive Cohort Study	Population Specific	Significantly greater than physicians
Patient/family satisfaction	Benkert et al. (2002)	Survey	Population Generic	Scores influenced by number of visits, type of contact, and respondent characteristics
	Brown et al. (2001)	Program Evaluation		Highly satisfied
	Bryant & Graham (2002)	Survey		Highly satisfied
	Chang et al. (1999)	Randomized Controlled Trial		Comparable to physicians
	Fanta et al. (2006)	Survey		Comparable to or significantly greater than residents
	Green & Davis (2005)	Randomized Controlled Trial		Highly satisfied
	Hamric et al. (1998)	Demonstration Project Evaluation		Highly satisfied
	Kinnersley et al. (2000)	Randomized Controlled Trial		Significantly greater than general practitioners
	Knudtson (2000)	Survey		Highly satisfied
	Krein et al. (2004)	Randomized Controlled Trial		Significantly greater than controls
	Lenz et al. (2004)	Longitudinal Follow-up Study		Comparable to physicians
	Litaker et al. (2003)	Randomized Controlled Trial		Significantly greater than controls

Continued

APN, Advanced practice nurse; CRNA, certified registered nurse anesthetist; GNP, geriatric nurse practitioner; ICU, intensive care unit; MD, Doctor of Medicine; NP, nurse practitioner.

NOTE: Some indicators that were used with specific populations in studies have been labeled as *generic* because they can be applied to multiple patient groups.

*Published studies since 1998.

†Constitute both a process (action by provider) and an outcome (condition or response in patient).

Definition of terms for the focus of the indicator:

Population Generic—indicators that could be used with any patient population.

Population Specific—indicators that are relevant to specific populations only.

Organizational—indicators that focus on the outcomes of the setting rather than the patient.

Table 24-2   ADVANCED PRACTICE NURSE–SENSITIVE OUTCOME INDICATORS TESTED IN PRACTICE*—CONT'D

Outcome Indicator	Authors (Year)	Study Design	Focus of Indicator: Population Generic, Population Specific, or Organizational	Findings
Patient/family satisfaction—cont'd	McMullen et al. (2001)	Program Evaluation		Significantly greater for communication rate than physician services
	Moore et al. (2002)	Randomized Controlled Trial		Significantly greater than physicians
	Mundinger et al. (2000)	Randomized Controlled Trial		Comparable to control group
	Roblin, Becker et al. (2004)	Survey		Significantly greater than physicians
	Sarkissian & Wennberg (1999)	Post-intervention, Non-comparison Survey		Highly satisfied
	Scisney-Matlock et al. (2004)	Quasi-experimental Comparison		Significantly greater than physicians
	Sidani et al. (2006a; 2006b)	Cross-sectional Comparison		Significantly greater than residents
	Stutts (2001)	Program Evaluation		Improved with program
	Venning et al. (2000)	Randomized Controlled Trial		Significantly greater than general practitioners
Perineal lacerations	Murphy & Feinland (1998)	Observational Cohort Study	Population Specific	Low incidence
Physician satisfaction/ perception of APN performance	Brown et al. (2001)	Program Evaluation	Organizational	Highly satisfied
	Hamric et al. (1998)	Demonstration Project Evaluation		Highly satisfied
	McMullen et al. (2001)	Program Evaluation		Highly satisfied
	Rideout (2007)	Pre/Post Comparison		Highly satisfied post (no pre data)
	Stutts (2001)	Program Evaluation		Mixed response
Post-discharge phone contact (for questions)	Rawl et al. (1998)	Randomized controlled trial	Population Specific	Significantly fewer than control group

Indicator	Author (Year)	Study Type	Category	Results
Pressure ulcers; skin breakdown	Russell et al. (2002)	Outcomes Management Program	Population Specific	Significantly reduced
	Ryden et al. (2000)	Quasi-experimental Comparison		Significantly less than control group
Pulmonary function	Lenz et al. (2004)	Longitudinal Follow-up Study	Population Specific	Comparable to physicians
	Rideout (2007)	Pre/Post Comparison		No difference pre/post
Quality of life	Corner et al. (2003)	Case Study	Population Generic	Initial improvement, with decline by end of study
	Hamilton & Hawley (2006)	Retrospective Review		Significant improvement over time
	Kutzleb & Reiner (2006)	Quasi-experimental Comparison		Significantly better than control group
	Moore et al. (2002)	Randomized Controlled Trial		Comparable to physicians
	Ritz et al. (2000)	Randomized Controlled Trial		Significantly better than control group (for some dimensions)
	Tijhuis et al. (2003)	Randomized Controlled Trial		Comparable to multidisciplinary teams
Readmission to ICU, unplanned	Hoffman et al. (2005)	Quasi-experimental Longitudinal Comparison	Organizational	Comparable to physicians
Smoking cessation	Gebaur et al. (1998)	Program Evaluation	Population Generic	Significantly greater than control group
Status of presenting condition	Hamric et al. (1998)	Demonstration Project Evaluation	Population Generic	Improved following initiation of APN prescription writing
Symptom control	Corner et al. (2003)	Case Study	Population Generic	No change over time
	Moore et al. (2002)	Randomized Controlled Trial	Population Specific (depending on symptom)	Comparable to physicians; neuropathy significantly less

Continued

APN, Advanced practice nurse; *CRNA,* certified registered nurse anesthetist; *GNP,* geriatric nurse practitioner; *ICU,* intensive care unit; *MD,* Doctor of Medicine; *NP,* nurse practitioner.
NOTE: Some indicators that were used with specific populations in studies have been labeled as *generic* because they can be applied to multiple patient groups.
*Published studies since 1998.
†Constitute both a process (action by provider) and an outcome (condition or response in patient).
Definition of terms for the focus of the indicator:
Population Generic—indicators that could be used with any patient population.
Population Specific—indicators that are relevant to specific populations only.
Organizational—indicators that focus on the outcomes of the setting rather than the patient.

Table 24-2   ADVANCED PRACTICE NURSE–SENSITIVE OUTCOME INDICATORS TESTED IN PRACTICE*—CONT'D

Outcome Indicator	Authors (Year)	Study Design	Focus of Indicator: Population Generic, Population Specific, or Organizational	Findings
Time to service delivery†	Reigle et al. (2006)	Medical Record Review	Population Generic Organizational	Significantly less than physicians
Transfer to acute setting†	Murphy & Fullerton (1998)	Survey	Population Generic Organizational	Low incidence
Urinary tract infection	Russell et al. (2002)	Outcomes Management Program	Population Generic	Significantly reduced
Visits to care provider	Leveille et al. (1998) Mundinger et al. (2000)	Randomized Controlled Trial Randomized Controlled Trial	Population Generic	Comparable to control group Comparable to physicians
Weight	Rideout (2007)	Pre/Post Comparison	Population Generic	No difference pre/post

APN, Advanced practice nurse; *CRNA*, certified registered nurse anesthetist; *GNP*, geriatric nurse practitioner; *ICU*, intensive care unit; *MD*, Doctor of Medicine; *NP*, nurse practitioner.
NOTE: Some indicators that were used with specific populations in studies have been labeled as *generic* because they can be applied to multiple patient groups.
*Published studies since 1998.
†Constitute both a process (action by provider) and an outcome (condition or response in patient).
Definition of terms for the focus of the indicator:
Population Generic—indicators that could be used with any patient population.
Population Specific—indicators that are relevant to specific populations only.
Organizational—indicators that focus on the outcomes of the setting rather than the patient.

Table 24-3   ADVANCED PRACTICE NURSE–DIRECTED PROGRAM EVALUATIONS

Authors (Year)	Focus of Evaluation	Target Population	Findings
Allen & Fabri (2005)	Perceptions about impact of role	Older patients and their care providers	Themes focused on holistic health assessment; patient and caregiver values; symptom management; assistance with supplies; education; advocacy; collaboration
Anetzberger et al. (2006)	Achievement of program goals: service to at-risk groups and improved outcomes	High-risk older adults	Completed over 1600 visits to targeted population; number of referrals doubled; patients highly satisfied with service
Barnason et al. (1998)	Self-study pain management program	Staff nurses Hospitalized patients	Staff knowledge level improved; post-intervention patient pain satisfaction ratings favorable
Brown et al. (2001)	Diabetes care delivery	Primary care patients	Mean HbA_{1c} levels declined significantly; weight declined significantly; patient satisfaction high
Capezuti et al. (2007)	Consultation and educational services re: siderail use	Long-term care nursing staff and patients	Reduction in siderail use varied by site; falls significantly reduced for site with reduced use of rails
Carioti et al. (2001)	Work site disease management program	Employees	Significant self-reported change in behaviors related to hypertension, dyslipidemia, and diabetes; employees highly satisfied with program
Dahl & Penque (2001)	Service delivery and cost of care	Inpatients with diagnosis of heart failure	Significant reduction in length of stay, mortality, and 30-day readmission rate
DeJong & Veltman (2004)	Screening program with smoking cessation counseling	Persons with chronic obstructive pulmonary disease	Significant reduction in smoking frequency
Dickerson et al. (2006)	Support groups	Patients receiving implantable cardioverter defibrillators	No difference in quality-of-life scores for support group attendees
Gebaur et al. (1998)	Smoking cessation program	Pregnant women	Significant reduction in number of cigarettes smoked per day and blood cotinine levels
Gross et al. (2002)	Use of telemetry resources	Inpatients receiving telemetry monitoring	Significant reduction in hours of telemetry use with no increase in adverse effect
Gross et al. (2004)	Quality improvement program	Inpatients with community-acquired pneumonia	Increased compliance with vaccine screening procedures; reduced length of stay; reduced readmission rate; reduced cost per case
Hamilton & Hawley (2006)	Outpatient management of anemia	Patients with chronic renal disease	Significant improvement in quality of life

Continued

Table 24-3   ADVANCED PRACTICE NURSE–DIRECTED PROGRAM EVALUATIONS—CONT'D

Authors (Year)	Focus of Evaluation	Target Population	Findings
Intili & Laws (2003)	Urgent care clinic	Hotel employees	Reduced cost of services
Krichbaum et al. (2005)	Two-tiered care delivery model	Long-term care patients	Significant reductions in depression and improvements in outlook
Kutzleb & Reiner (2006)	Patient education program	Patients with heart failure	Significant improvement in quality of life
Leveille et al. (1998)	Prevention program	Frail older adults	Significant reductions in hospital days and use of psychoactive medications; significantly better physical function
McMullen et al. (2001)	NP/attending physician collaboration	Inpatient medical patients	Significantly better physical health scores; staff and physician satisfaction high
Ockene et al. (1999)	Brief counseling intervention	High-risk drinkers	Significant reduction in alcohol consumption
Rideout (2007)	Care coordination	Hospitalized children with cystic fibrosis	Timeliness of nutrition and social work consultation improved significantly; LOS declined by 1.35 days
Small et al. (2000)	Debriefing sessions	Postpartum women	No impact on maternal depression
Stolee et al. (2006)	Role of NP	Long-term care nursing employees	Perception of positive impact; majority of staff reported improved skill level
Wagner et al. (2007)	Consultation and educational services re: siderail use	Long-term care patients	Median number of recommendations per resident was 5; median cost of intervention per resident was $135

LOS, Length of stay; *NP,* nurse practitioner.

providers, community leaders). They also help identify unforeseen barriers that might interfere with the introduction of new programs and the assessment of their impact. In addition, they clarify the direct and indirect costs of program implementation and maintenance and uncover the strategies required to implement a new process and evaluate its results. In Anetzberger and colleagues' study, pilot evaluation activities focused on whether a primary care program offered in patients' homes met its goals of meeting community service needs and achieving positive patient outcomes. Medical record review, surveys, and interviews were used to collect data. An 8-month period of data collection demonstrated that the number of visits exceeded initial projections and improvements were seen in outcomes measured (satisfaction, func-

tional status). The pilot study also determined that over one half to two thirds of patients interviewed or surveyed would not have received needed care without the services provided by the program. An important aspect of this study's pilot purpose was the identification of problems with missing data that would need to be addressed in a larger, longer-term evaluation.

In Baranson and colleagues' pilot study (1998), data were collected from a convenience sample of nurses receiving an evidence-based educational intervention designed to improve nurses' pain management of hospitalized patients and from patients who received analgesics for pain. The study determined that almost half of patients continued to receive intramuscular pain medication despite its being the least desirable option. It also found that nurses' level of knowledge increased significantly after the educational program. The authors reported plans to use the pilot study's findings to refine the educational program offered, to promote the use of a pain assessment record, and to continue to measure patient perception of nursing staff management of pain.

Instrument sensitivity testing is also a common component of pilot studies and was undertaken in a feasibility/pilot study by Beeber and Charlie (1998). Instrument sensitivity testing provides information about the usefulness and appropriateness of the data collection tools selected. In this study, the investigators tested instruments used previously in a variety of studies to confirm their sensitivity to changes in the outcomes proposed for the targeted intervention group. Data from the pilot study supported reliability and validity estimates from other research. The study also demonstrated that patients were willing to complete questionnaires concerning their level of satisfaction with mental health counseling services, an important consideration before initiating a long-term study of patient satisfaction with APN-directed care.

Cost Analyses. Comprehensive cost analyses of program performance are few, with most discussions reflecting charges associated with services rather than true cost of care. Two comprehensive cost analyses of APN-managed care facilities were identified in the literature. The first study focused on the delivery of services to low-risk pregnant women with CNM provider costs in a freestanding clinic compared with physician costs for care delivered in a hospital setting (Stone, Zwanziger, Walker, & Buenting, 2000). In both cases, costs were estimated according to maternity episode, with direct prenatal and childbirth costs calculated from institutional reports, census reports, office profit-and-loss statements, and billing records. A sensitivity analysis was performed to determine the effect of patient volume on cost of care. The costs of the CNMs' prenatal services were significantly higher than the physicians' costs; childbirth costs were significantly less. When combined over the episode of care, costs were comparable for both provider types.

The second study, costs of care for inpatients managed by physicians compared with that of NP/physician provider teams, examined direct care costs and costs associated with services provided outside the inpatient admission (Ettner et al., 2006). These indirect costs included hospitalizations other than the study

investigational one, nursing home stays, emergency department visits, primary care physician visits, other care provider visits, and formal home care services. The additional costs associated with NP involvement in inpatient care were more than offset by savings in indirect costs. The NP/physician model of care resulted in approximately $975 saved per patient (Ettner et al.). In a companion article based on the same study, the NP/physician model also resulted in significant reductions in lengths of stay and comparable readmission rates and mortality outcomes (Cowan et al., 2006).

Summary of the Research Thus Far

The evidence concerning APN impact on individual patient and organizational outcomes suggests that the quality of care APNs deliver is comparable or superior to that of other care providers in the specialty. A variety of studies have explored the direct and indirect processes APNs use to manage patient care and the outcomes achieved. All have determined that APN practice overlaps other care providers in some respects and differs in others. These distinctions and their potential to confound comparisons with other care providers contribute to the complexity inherent in measuring APN effect. Moreover, the limited research linking specific APN processes to care delivery outcomes makes it difficult to determine which role components achieve the effect. Difficult or not, a clear distinction is needed if APNs are ever to receive the recognition they deserve or the financial reimbursement they are due.

This review of APN outcomes research suggests that the quality and quantity of research pertaining to APN outcomes has improved over time, with initial studies focusing primarily on role description and acceptance issues and more recent studies addressing performance and outcome considerations between APN and other provider groups. A variety of research designs are now being used to measure APN impact, with an increasing number of investigators using prospective designs and including comparison groups. Although medical record reviews continue to provide much of the data for these comparison studies, methods to control for differences in patient populations and the use of more sophisticated data analysis techniques are providing more reliable, replicable, and generalizable information.

Despite these improvements, intensive work is needed in several areas. The first of these involves the consistent use of a set of core outcome indicators relevant to and sensitive to differences in APN practice.

To achieve this goal, national leadership groups should assume responsibility for coordinated efforts to evaluate APN outcomes, with recommendations for which indicators to choose and the allocation of funds to support the central collection and dissemination of research findings. Collaborations between APNs and nurse researchers and the development of outcomes consortia also will facilitate this process. Bringing together clinical practice and research design and measurement experts from multiple locations and specialties is the best approach for identifying the most reliable and valid indicators of APN effect. Networks of APN groups and institutions in which APNs practice can also promote the collection of comparable data and the sharing of results for comparisons across groups, specialties, and locales. This approach is particularly important for APNs whose practices are too small to generate the data needed to influence policymakers and decisions about which performance measures to reward. A recommendation is to begin small, selecting evidence-based indicators that appear to be the most reliable, valid, and sensitive to differences in APN practice. Other indicators can be added as further investigations demonstrate evidence of cause and effect between APN practice and care delivery outcome. Ideally, these data should be relatively inexpensive to collect and the reporting methods should be comparable across sites. Table 24-2 lists the numerous APN-sensitive outcome indicators that have been used in previous studies.

Second, there is an urgent need to reexamine reimbursement practices that reinforce productivity levels according to physician performance. Process-focused and cost-effectiveness studies demonstrate that APNs take more time with patients and, as such, are at risk for failing to meet organizational or group practice productivity standards based on the medical model. Because research has not compared different types of productivity estimations, the true magnitude and impact of APN efficiency is not known. A shift in focus from time spent during individual patient interaction to one that considers total time spent during episode of care (as was done by Ettner et al., 2006, and Stone et al., 2000) might be more realistic for measuring and comparing APN practice. In the episode-of-care approach, total time and resources used per episode are preferable indicators of productivity. In this case, the extra time spent by APNs and the number of interactions with patients at the outset of service may eliminate the need for longer-term, sustained interactions that occur when patients and families are not sufficiently prepared to manage their health care needs. In addition, the increased time spent in education and counseling in the initial phase may eliminate the need for more costly care over the course of the episode. At this time, the evidence is insufficient to determine whether this or alternative approaches to productivity measurement more accurately assess the efficiency and benefits of APN practice.

Closely linked with this issue is the third need, which is to determine whether the increased patient and family satisfaction evident when APNs spend extra time also contributes to improvements in longer-term care delivery outcomes. Because APNs spend more time with patients and provide additional teaching and healthy behaviors counseling, their impact may be most evident in the long-term prevention of diseases and the adverse outcomes commonly associated with poor health behaviors. Studies thus far have followed patient outcomes for relatively short periods—usually 6 months to 1 year post-APN intervention. Additional longitudinal studies are needed to determine the true long-term impact of these early outcomes on overall lifestyle, quality of life, and health.

Fourth, additional research is needed to compare APNs with other APN providers. To date, the focus has been directed at comparisons of APNs with physicians, medical residents, or PAs. Although these studies are useful, evidence is unavailable concerning which outcome indicators are most sensitive to differences in APN practices.

Fifth, this review makes evident the pressing need to explore the value-added impact of APNs in collaborative practice with physicians and other care providers. Some preliminary work has begun in this regard, but additional work is necessary. Because APNs and physicians bring different perspectives about care and demonstrate distinct but complementary behaviors, studies are needed to determine how these combined practices reinforce and maximize the beneficial effects of one another. Such studies may generate the data needed to demonstrate the value-added benefits of combining APN and physician practices. By documenting favorable outcomes when a collaborative APN/physician approach is used, the profession can more effectively argue for altered reimbursement procedures and make visible the contributions of APNs to the public.

The literature also highlights the difficulties evident in generating widespread interest in measuring care delivery outcomes. Many APNs view the ongoing assessment of care delivery impact as an additional burden to an already full agenda. This problem was highlighted in a survey of oncology APNs who identified critical issues that warranted planning for future nursing society projects (Lynch, Cope, & Murphy-Ende, 2001). Only 2% of respondents included outcomes management as important content for APN programs. At the same time, outcomes documentation was identified as one of the top five priority issues for oncology APNs. Clearly, the foundational work pertaining to outcomes assessment needs to begin during graduate education. Because APN outcome measurement activities begin immediately upon hire, preparation for identifying target outcomes, collecting data, and managing and reporting findings is the minimum information required in graduate programs. In addition to clinically focused outcomes content, several individuals and groups are recommending including content on health care financing, health care information systems, database query, and statistics, particularly in DNP education for APNs (AACN, 2006; Mahn & Zazworsky, 2000). Without these skills at the outset, APNs are likely to be ill-prepared to succeed in today's outcomes-driven environment.

The research to date suggests that APNs can contribute to the field of outcomes assessment in several ways. One of the simplest and most common mechanisms for monitoring APN practice is the routine documentation of what the APN does. This includes patient-specific documentation in medical records, process improvement reporting for groups of patients, descriptions of new program initiatives, annual performance self-assessment summaries, and published reports of projects, programs, evaluations, or research studies. The documentation of APN work should be considered an inherent job responsibility that contributes to the quantification of role impact, effectiveness, and value. It is the basic starting point for measuring care delivery outcome. APN impact assessments can range from individual performance review to large scale, multi-site studies. In each of these situations, however, the common denominator is the consistency and quality of the process and outcome measures used.

Because standardized approaches to reporting APN work and care delivery impact are unavailable at this time, health care organizations with more than one APN should ensure that comparable reporting mechanisms are used and that both generic (organization-wide) and specific (population-focused) indicators are included to evaluate overall effect. Ideally, decisions about which outcomes to measure and determinations about how to monitor care delivery processes should be driven by existing evidence and expert panel standards or recommendations.

USING EVIDENCE TO GUIDE INDIVIDUAL ADVANCED PRACTICE NURSE PERFORMANCE REVIEW

Descriptions of recommended methods for applying evidence to *individual* APN performance assessment are notably absent in the literature. The few articles available stress the importance of clearly defined role components, clarification of the responsibilities of other health team members, the environmental factors that affect role implementation, the identification of stakeholder expectations, and the predetermination of outcome-based goals (Bryant-Lukosius, DiCenso, Browne, & Pinelli, 2004). Initial evaluations of any APN role should center on outcomes related to safety, efficiency, acceptance, satisfaction, cost, and actualization of role components (Bryant-Lukosius & DiCenso, 2004).

Advanced Practice Role Considerations

Minimum expectations for APN performance review include the confirmation of performance according to scope of practice specifications and regulatory requirements, which is an expectation of accrediting and certification agencies, licensing organizations, individual organizations, and consumers. In addition, professional standards specify performance expectations, delineate procedures and processes to be followed, and promote the measurement of services and outcomes of care (Beaudin, 1998). They can be general, such as those associated with an advanced practice specialty (e.g., pediatrics, acute care, primary care), or they can focus on a specific activity, care delivery process, disease, or condition (e.g., pain management, diabetes). Often they are prepared by professional organizations and use expert panels to develop practice statements. As an example, the National Association of Pediatric Nurse Practitioners (2004) includes in its standards document a definition of the role, a statement concerning educational preparation requirements, a summary of practice parameters and expectations for assessment and diagnosis of patients, appropriate interventions, methods for evaluating practice, collaborative responsibilities, professional accountability, continued competence, and quality assurance.

The Oncology Nursing Society's (ONS) statement on standards incorporates similar information and includes a standard specifically devoted to self-evaluation (ONS, 2003). This standard speaks to (1) the APN's self-evaluation of practice according to institutional, state, and federal laws and regulations, and patient and family outcomes; (2) the APN's regular solicitation of feedback concerning practice and role performance from colleagues and customers; and (3) the APN's participation in the appraisal of others to further enhance the overall performance and effectiveness of the health care team.

Essential Elements of Advanced Practice Nurse Performance Review

The onus for performance evaluation is on both the APN and the hiring organization or practice. Although states and accrediting bodies hold the organization accountable for ensuring that its practitioners are in compliance with laws and expectations for confirmation of competency, the individual APN is equally accountable for guaranteeing that regulations and requirements are met. As a result, the APN is best served by paying close attention to performance review expectations and collecting tangible evidence to demonstrate behaviors that support individual, organizational, and certification body goals and expectations.

Smolenski (2005) recommends starting a credentialing file as soon as possible after graduation to ensure that all documents are retained and available to support job application and ongoing performance review. She also proposes that APNs develop a method for keeping track of certification and license renewal dates and attendance at educational offerings that support continued competence. Beginning this process at the time of hire or the first day of each year facilitates self-assessment reporting and preparation for recertification.

Essential elements of the performance review include a self- and peer-assessment and a review by the person with overall responsibility for administrative oversight of the APN's performance. Evidence in the form of documentation of continued competence (e.g., continuing education, certification, course enrollment), practice according to standards and organizational expectations, and contribution to the community and profession should be incorporated into each assessment process. Also included are goals (both achieved and established for the next evaluation period), productivity measures, and outcomes achieved.

Depending on the role and practice site of the APN, additional elements may be required. Before hire, APNs applying for positions in existing health care organizations should request to see the performance evaluation tool that will be used to assess performance in the role.

The Evaluation Process

Unfortunately, most performance evaluations are a once-a-year event, with the APN conducting a self-assessment, asking for peer input, and meeting with the direct supervisor during scheduled meetings. Ideally, performance evaluation should be an ongoing process, with at least quarterly self- and other-directed checks of performance and achievement of individual and organizational goals. These sessions should include discussions about workload and productivity issues, if any, for purposes of identifying additional resource needs or developmental strategies for addressing each. In all cases, the process and the mutual decisions of the APN and supervisor should be documented and used to monitor improvement or sustained high performance.

Performance Review Components

Self-Assessment. One of the most difficult expectations for many APNs is the self-rating and review of personal performance. Much of this difficulty is the result of unclear performance expectations, trouble quantifying such intangible activities as support and coordination of services, and lack of time to reflect upon and carefully document all but immediate performance and outcome indicators. These problems can best be addressed through the careful documentation of activities and achievements as they occur throughout the year. The designation of specific goals and performance targets facilitates determining whether or not individual performance is meeting or exceeding expectations. In all cases, the self-rating of performance should be based on a comparison of expected versus actual outcome.

Peer Review. Peer review of APN performance is an essential dimension of confirmation of practice according to standards. The peer reviewer should be someone with the same or higher level of educational preparation, clinical experience, and focus (Briggs, Heath, & Kelley, 2005). The reviewer also needs to have a clear understanding of practice and role expectations. Physicians are not considered peer reviewers, although their input may be useful for confirming collaborative relationships and membership on interdisciplinary teams. Their input into the performance evaluation process should be requested, with clear specification of the evaluation criteria to which they are expected to respond.

Essential to the peer review process is the early development of a statement concerning the purpose of the peer review (Briggs et al., 2005). This statement guides the APN's selection of peer reviewers and clarifies the boundaries and expectations of the peer review process. It also makes clear to the peer reviewer the extent to which the peer review will be factored into the overall performance evaluation. Included in the peer review assessment is attention to clinical competence, interpersonal style, ability to work with individuals and teams, performance according to

Box 24-1   SAMPLE RATING FORMAT PEER OR CUSTOMER EVALUATION TOOL

Please evaluate using the 1-5 scale as indicated below.

5	**Excellent/Exceptional**	Consistently performs in an exceptional manner that far exceeds performance standards
4	**Exceeds Standards**	Performs in a manner that exceeds expected performance standards
3	**Meets Standards**	Consistently performs in a manner that meets expected performance standards
2	**Needs Improvement**	Performs in a manner that needs improvement—identified area for growth
1	**Unsatisfactory/Does not meet**	Performs in a manner that does not meet expected performance standards

	THIS APN CONSISTENTLY:	**Rating**

Evidence-Based Clinical Practice

Coordinates/facilitates care for individual patients and populations.
Is able to prioritize and respond to multiple demands of role in a timely, organized and competent manner.
Communicates patient or other information accurately and completely to appropriate group(s).
Demonstrates/develops/enforces safety practices by adhering to guidelines, policies, practice standards and precautions and patient safety standards.
Provides/promotes patient care in a competent and efficient manner.
Uses the best evidence available in clinical decision making.
Contributes effectively to the interdisciplinary care delivery process.
Stays current in field and shares knowledge and experience with others.

Service Excellence

Demonstrates the ability to work well with other members of the healthcare team.
Shows respect and uses effective communication with patients, their families and members of the healthcare team.
Treats customers with courtesy and respect.
Incorporates customer service values and behaviors into practice.
Resolves individual, clinical care issues, and consumer complaints and difficult situations effectively.

Professional Development

Utilizes peer feedback to enhance professional growth.
Serves as a mentor for others.
Disseminates information to others through presentations, publications, and other forums.
Participates in unit/hospital/institutional committees. Participates in professional/community activities.

Describe one area of strength for this individual:
Describe one area for growth for this individual:

© 2006, Office of Nursing Accreditation and Advancement, Strong Memorial Hospital, University of Rochester Medical Center.
APN, Advanced practice nurse.

Box 24-2   SAMPLE OF WRITTEN NARRATIVE FORMAT FOR PEER OR CUSTOMER EVALUATION INPUT

Please provide an assessment of _____ _____ performance over the past year concerning the following. Please include examples, where possible, to support statements made:

1. Provides safe, effective care to individuals and their families.

2. Works effectively with others, and respects diverse viewpoints.

3. Uses the best available evidence to support clinical decision making.

4. Treats customers with courtesy and respect.

5. Stays current, and shares knowledge with other members of the health care team.

6. Maintains a high level of competence through the use of feedback and participation in educational programs.

7. Serves as a resource and mentor for others.

8. Contributes to the profession through the regular dissemination of information through publications, presentations, and involvement in professional organizations.

Describe one area of particular strength for this individual.

Describe one area for growth for this individual.

NOTE: With the open text format, the criteria may be a bit more expansive than with the rating format, and the number of behaviors included should be fewer. It will take the evaluator more time to write a narrative about the behaviors than it will to complete a rating scale.

standards, continued professional development, and contribution to the profession as a whole. The format of the review may be structured, with specific evaluation criteria and a rating scale included, or it may be unstructured, with general performance evaluation criteria identified for written comment. An example of each approach, using the same performance expectation, is provided in Boxes 24-1 and 24-2.

Customer Review. Additional input should be obtained from the individuals and groups who interact with and receive services from the APN. This might include physician collaborators, other health care professionals, nursing staff, patients, families, and community members. If routine methods are used to collect satisfaction-with-service data, this information can be incorporated here. In some cases, requests for input will need to be solicited from targeted groups or individuals. When this is done, information should be provided concerning the performance behaviors for which information is sought. Input may be given in the form of a letter describing impressions of overall performance or through the use of a more formal rating tool that specifies the attributes to be evaluated. Sufficient time should be given to the evaluators to ensure they can carefully

reflect on the performance criteria and provide examples to substantiate their comments or ratings. Unsolicited feedback from customers also may be received throughout the year, and this information should be summarized or copies included as exemplars of APN impact.

Supporting Evidence. Clearly defining the evidence to support APN performance review is a critical aspect of both planning for the review and conducting a review that is accurate and useful and meets individual and organizational needs. Using a goal-focused approach to the identification of performance indicators is likely to be the most effective method for APNs, although any theory-derived approach can be used. With the goal-focused approach, the APN identifies performance and project goals for the year and then determines what evidence is required to document achievement of short-term (quarterly) and long-term (annual or multiple year) outcomes. Due dates, indicators, and achievement targets are included in the plan. Also included may be notations describing what degrees of variance in performance outcome constitute immediate action. Goals should be specific to the role, measurable, and feasible. Table 24-4 provides an example of how an

Table 24-4   GOAL-FOCUSED EVALUATION PLAN

Goal #1: Develop and sustain therapeutic relationships and partnerships with patients (individual, family, or group) and other professionals to facilitate optimal care and patient outcomes (Essential Competency 8.3 of DNP Program Graduates [AACN, 2006]).

Process Indicators	Data Collection Time Frame	Outcome Indicators	Data Collection Time Frame
1.1 Documentation in medical record of inclusion of patient/family input into decisions	Monthly	1.1 Patient/family satisfaction with inclusion in decision-making processes (rating >4.5 out of maximum score of 5)	Quarterly
1.2 Number of family meetings	Quarterly	1.2 Patient/family satisfaction with inclusion in care planning (rating >4.5 out of maximum score of 5)	Quarterly
1.3 Number of interdisciplinary care planning meetings	Quarterly	1.3 Interdisciplinary team member satisfaction with collaborative decision making (rating >4.5 out of maximum score of 5)	Annually
1.4 Frequency of nursing staff involvement in care planning decisions	Quarterly	1.4 Staff nurse satisfaction with inclusion in care planning for patients (rating >4.5 out of maximum score of 5)	Annually

Goal #2: Disseminate findings from evidence-based practice and research to improve health care outcomes (Essential Competency 3.7 of DNP Program Graduates [AACN, 2006]).

Process Indicators	Data Collection Time Frame	Outcome Indicators	Data Collection Time Frame
2.1 Number of articles reviewed for application to clinical practice	Quarterly	2.1 Number of publications	Annually
2.2 Number of journal club sessions held for discussion of application of evidence to practice	Quarterly	2.2 Participant satisfaction with journal club experience/preparation for publication	Annually
2.3 Number of requests for assistance with review of evidence for application to clinical practice	Quarterly	2.3 Number of consultations provided concerning application of evidence to clinical practice	Annually

APN might use two of the proposed expectations for the DNP (AACN, 2006) as a format for individual goal specification and performance measurement.

The evaluation plan is updated and revised as role components change and as individual and organizational goals are met. Throughout the process, however, the evaluation plan sets the stage for what is done, what is monitored, and what is reported to demonstrate APN impact on care delivery outcome.

Supporting evidence may be drawn from a variety of sources and may include information collected by the APN and the organization. The following are examples of evidence monitored and reported by APNs:

- Number and type of consultations provided (and for whom)
- Number and focus of care conferences led
- Number and type of procedures performed
- Number and type of patients seen

- Number of presentations and publications completed
- Number and type of performance improvement and/or research projects undertaken
- Number and location (regional, national) of conferences attended and other activities designed to maintain competence
- Patient length of stay (specialty area, if relevant, and overall)
- Mortality rate for population served
- Adverse event prevalence rate or cases per 1000 patient days
- Revenue generated through provision of chargeable services and procedures

Collating the Evidence

Essential to any effective performance review is the presentation of information that is timely, relevant, and easy to decipher. Using a goal-focused approach helps, as does the use of a portfolio that provides representative examples of data and activities that support self-assessment ratings and descriptions of performance and outcomes achieved. Using the process and outcome indicators in Table 24-4 as an example, portfolio components might be divided according to goals (or according to organization-required performance indicators such as evidence-based clinical practice, service excellence, and professional development as identified in Box 24-1). In the goals example, one segment of the portfolio would be devoted to developing and sustaining therapeutic relationships and another to disseminating findings. In the first goal's process-related activities, portfolio documents might include reports of medical record audits and de-identified samples of documentation that support inclusion of the patient and family in decision making, tables or graphs by quarter denoting number of family meetings and interdisciplinary care meetings, along with representative samples of meeting minutes. Outcome data, likewise, can be presented in visual formats that demonstrate consistency or improvement over time. When data suggest areas in need of improvement, these should be addressed by an action plan with specific targets and time frame for improvement. Activities directed at the second goal can be supported by providing a list of publications and presentations, denoting titles of topics and number of persons attending (if available). Copies of abstracts and publications can be included in this section along with evaluation summaries for presentations and consultation services. Each item included in the portfolio should be clearly linked to role performance expectations and progress toward individual and organizational goals.

Resource Needs

Carefully monitoring and managing APN performance data necessitate the allocation of resources to support the time and effort required for this essential care delivery process. Among the resources needed are a computer and software that support data management, manipulation, and reporting procedures. Also needed are access to relevant databases and assistance with analysis and report generation. Time is one of the most essential resource needs, and APNs should negotiate for the time to collect, enter, analyze, and report data that support productivity and outcomes achieved. Monitoring the actual time devoted to performance evaluation activities is useful for renegotiating allocated percent effort when productivity or role responsibilities change.

Essential to the evaluation process is proactive action by the APN who collects data in an ongoing fashion; identifies clear, measurable goals; and uses feedback to inform and identify ways by which to improve service to others. When done successfully, with careful planning and input from others, the APN performance evaluation process can be an excellent method for ensuring individual competence and professional growth and advancement. It also can guarantee that the quality of care provided to patients and families and the impact of the APN on the health care system are outstanding at all times.

SUMMARY

The issues facing the profession in relation to justifying the use of APNs and measuring the effect of APN practice on patients and health care systems are similar to but distinct from those faced by individual APNs evaluating the outcomes of their particular practice. This chapter has examined both sets of issues. It is apparent that the need for well-designed, longitudinal assessments of APN impact has never been stronger. Because reimbursement decisions are driven by evidence of provider performance, APNs without reliable and valid data to substantiate their impact will struggle for equitable reimbursement for services. Moreover, reimbursement decisions made solely on the basis of physician-derived outcome indicators seriously limit the understanding of APN impact on patient care (Mason, Cohen, O'Donnell, Baxter, & Chase, 1997). Furthermore, the magnitude of APN contribution to care is often lost because managed care organizations, among others, regularly attribute all outcomes to the collaborating physician (Mason et al., 1999). This invisibility in the health care system further threatens the recognition of APNs as viable, important providers of health care services.

Addressing the need for inclusion of APN-sensitive outcome indicators will require focused attention on the development of electronic information systems that support the identification and tracking of APN outcome data. A first step in this process is national agreement on a core set of outcome indicators relevant to APNs and the initiation of standards that support the collection of APN-sensitive data. Until health care organizations and reimbursement agents begin demanding data to substantiate individual APN and APN group provider performance, no widespread action is likely.

This chapter highlights several frameworks for measuring and monitoring APN practice. Other approaches also are available, and the APN should begin the process by selecting one and refining it to meet individual and organizational needs. The best approach is to begin small and expand activities over time. Networking with other APNs is useful for identifying beneficial outcomes and for sharing personal experiences about what does and does not work when integrating outcomes measurement into busy practices.

This discussion also illustrates the interconnectedness of outcomes measurement with every other aspect of the APN role. Effective outcomes measurement and outcomes-focused performance review require APNs to work collaboratively with others, to plan and organize processes of care and assessment of quality in highly complex health services environments, and to expose their individual practices to the scrutiny of others. Experience with organizational change behaviors and a willingness to seek information and assistance from others will help with this process. In the end, the quality and value of care will improve, as will the community's recognition of the APN's impact on outcomes of care.

REFERENCES

Aigner, M.J., Drew, S., & Phipps, J. (2004). A comparative study of nursing home resident outcomes between care provided by nurse practitioners/physicians versus physicians only. *Journal of the American Medical Directors Association, 5,* 16-23.

Allen, J.K., Blumenthal, R.S., Margolis, S., Young, D.R., Miller, E.R., & Kelly, K. (2002). Nurse case management of hypercholesterolemia in patients with coronary heart disease: Results of a randomized clinical trial. *American Heart Journal, 144,* 678-686.

Allen, J., & Fabri, A.M. (2005). An evaluation of a community aged care nurse practitioner service. *Journal of Clinical Nursing, 14,* 1202-1209.

American Association of Colleges of Nursing (AACN). (2006). *The essentials of doctoral education for advanced nursing practice.* Washington, DC: Author.

American Nurses Association (ANA). (2004). *Scope and standards for nurse administrators* (2nd ed.). Silver Spring, MD: Author.

Anetzberger, G.J., Stricklin, M.L., Gaunter, D., Banozic, R., & Laurie, R. (2006). VNA Housecalls of Greater Cleveland, Ohio: Development and pilot evaluation of a program for high-risk older adults offering primary medical care in the home. *Home Health Services Quarterly, 25,* 155-166.

Aquilino, M.L., Damiano, P.C., Willard, J.C., Momany, E.T., & Levy, B.T. (1999). Primary care physician perceptions of the nurse practitioner in the 1990s. *Archives of Family Medicine, 8,* 224-227.

Armenian, H.K., & Shapiro, S. (1998). *Epidemiology and health services.* New York: Oxford University Press.

Aubrey, W.R., & Yoxall, C.W. (2001). Evaluation of the role of the neonatal nurse practitioner in resuscitation of preterm infants at birth. *Archives of Disease in Childhood, 85,* F96-F99.

Badger, M.J., Lookinland, S., Tiedeman, M., Anderson, V., & Eggett, D. (2002). Nurse practitioners' treatment of febrile infants in Utah: Comparison to physician practice nationally. *Journal of the American Academy of Nurse Practitioners, 14,* 540-553.

Baldwin, K.A., Sisk, R.J., Watts, P., McCubbin, J., Brockschmidt, B., & Marion, L.N. (1998). Acceptance of nurse practitioners and physician assistants in meeting the perceived needs of rural communities. *Public Health Nursing, 15,* 389-397.

Ball, C., & Cox, C.L. (2003). Restoring patients to health: Outcomes and indicators of advanced nursing practice in adult critical care, Part 1. *International Journal of Nursing Practice, 9,* 356-367.

Ball, S.T.E., Walton, K., & Hawes, S. (2007). Do emergency department physiotherapy practitioners, emergency nurse practitioners and doctors investigate, treat and refer patients with closed musculoskeletal injuries differently? *Emergency Medicine Journal, 24,* 185-188.

Baradell, J.G., & Bordeaux, B.R. (2001). Outcomes and satisfaction of patients of psychiatric clinical nurse specialists. *Journal of the American Psychiatric Nurses Association, 7*(3), 77-85.

Barnason, S., Merboth, M., Pozehl, B., & Tietjen, M.J. (1998). Utilizing an outcomes approach to improve pain management by nurses: A pilot study. *Clinical Nurse Specialist, 12,* 28-36.

Barton, A.J., Baramee, J., Sowers, D., & Robertson, K.J. (2003). Articulating the value-added dimension of NP care. *Nurse Practitioner, 28,* 34-40.

Beal, J.A., & Quinn, M. (2002). The nurse practitioner role in the NICU as perceived by parents. *MCN, The American Journal of Maternal/Child Nursing, 27,* 183-188.

Beal, J.A., Richardson, D.K., Dembinski, S., Hipp, K.O., McCourt, M., Szlachetka, D., et al. (1999). Responsibilities, roles & staffing patterns of nurse practitioners in the neonatal intensive care unit. *MCN, American Journal of Maternal Child Nursing, 24,* 168-175.

Beaudin, C.L. (1998). Outcomes measurement: Application of performance standards and practice guidelines in managed behavioral healthcare. *Journal of Nursing Care Quality, 13*(1), 14-26.

Becker, D., Kaplow, R., Muenzen, P.M., & Hartigan, C. (2006). Activities performed by acute and critical care advanced practice nurses: American Association of Critical-Care Nurses study of practice. *American Journal of Critical Care, 15,* 130-148.

Beckman, L.J., Harvey, S.M., & Satre, S.J. (2002). The delivery of medical abortion services: The views of experienced providers. *Women's Health Issues, 12,* 103-112.

Beeber, L.S., & Charlie, M.L. (1998). Depressive symptom reversal for women in a primary care setting: A pilot study. *Archives of Psychiatric Nursing, 12,* 247-254.

Benkert, R., Barkauskas, V., Pohl, J., Corser, W., Tanner, C., Wells, M., et al. (2002). Patient satisfaction outcomes in nurse-managed centers. *Outcomes Management, 6,* 174-181.

Bloch, D. (1975). Evaluation of nursing care in terms of process and outcome: Issues in research and quality assurance. *Nursing Research, 24,* 256-263.

Brady, M.A., & Neal, J.A. (2000). Role delineation study of pediatric nurse practitioners: A national study of practice and responsibilities and trends in role functions. *Journal of Pediatric Health Care, 14,* 149-159.

Brent, N.J. (2001). Are ignoring best practice changes putting your agency at legal and financial risk? *Home Healthcare Nurse, 19,* 721-724.

Briggs, L.A., Heath J., & Kelley, J. (2005). Peer review for advanced practice nurses. What does it really mean? *AACN Clinical Issues, 16,* 3-15.

Brooten, D., Gennaro, S., Knapp, H., Jovene, N., Brown, L., & York, R. (2002). Functions of the CNS in early discharge and home follow-up of very low birthweight infants. *Clinical Nurse Specialist, 16,* 85-90.

Brooten, D., Naylor, M.D., York, R., Brown, L.P., Munro, B.H., Hollingsworth, A.O., et al. (2002). Lessons learned from testing the quality cost model of advanced practice nursing (APN) transitional care. *Journal of Nursing Scholarship, 34,* 369-375.

Brooten, D., Younblut, J., Blais, K., Donahue, D., Cruz, I., & Lightbourne, M. (2005). APN-physician collaboration in caring for women with high-risk pregnancies. *Journal of Nursing Scholarship, 37,* 178-184.

Brooten, D., Youngblut, J.M., Deatrick, J., Naylor, M., & York, R. (2003). Patient problems, advanced practice nurse (APN) interventions, time and contacts among five patient groups. *Journal of Nursing Scholarship, 35,* 73-79.

Brown, A.W., Wolff, K.L., Elasy, T.A., & Graber, A.L. (2001). The role of advanced practice nurses in a shared care diabetes practice model. *Diabetes Educator, 27,* 492-500.

Brown, S.A., & Grimes, D.E. (1995). A meta-analysis of nurse practitioners and nurse midwives in primary care. *Nursing Research, 44,* 332-339.

Bryant, R., & Graham, M.C. (2002). Advanced practice nurses: A study of client satisfaction. *Journal of American Academy of Nurse Practitioners, 14,* 88-92.

Bryant-Lukosius, D., & DiCenso, A. (2004). A framework for the introduction and evaluation of advanced practice nursing roles. *Journal of Advanced Nursing, 48,* 530-540.

Bryant-Lukosius, D., DiCenso, A., Browne, G., & Pinelli, J. (2004). Advanced practice nursing roles: Development, implementation and evaluation. *Journal of Advanced Nursing, 48,* 519-529.

Buchholz, S.W., & Purath, J. (2007). Physical activity and physical fitness counseling patterns of adult nurse practitioners. *Journal of the American Academy of Nurse Practitioners, 19,* 86-92.

Bula, C.J., Berod, A.C., Stuck, A., Alessi, C.A., Aronow, H.U., Santos-Eggimann, B., et al. (1999). Effectiveness of preventive in-home geriatric assessment in well functioning, community-dwelling older people: Secondary analysis of a randomized trial. *Journal of the American Geriatrics Society, 47,* 389-395.

Burl, J.B., Bonner, A., Rao, M., & Khan, A.M. (1998). Geriatric nurse practitioners in long-term care: Demonstration of effectiveness in managed care. *Journal of the American Geriatrics Society, 46,* 506-510.

Burns, S.M., & Earvin, S. (2002). Improving outcomes for mechanically ventilated medical intensive care unit patients using advanced practice nurses: A 6-year experience. *Critical Care Nursing Clinics of North America, 14,* 231-243.

Burns, S.M., Earven, S., Fisher, C., Lewis, R., Merrell, P., Schubart, J.R., et al. (2003). Implementation of an institutional program to improve clinical and financial outcomes of mechanically ventilated patients: One-year outcomes and lessons learned. *Critical Care Medicine, 31,* 2752-2763.

Byers, J.F., & Brunell, M.L. (1998). Demonstrating the value of the advanced practice nurse: An evaluation model. *AACN Clinical Issues, 9,* 296-305.

Campbell, C.D., Musil, C.M., & Zauszniewski, J.A. (1998). Practice patterns of advanced practice psychiatric nurses. *Journal of American Psychiatric Nurses Association, 4,* 111-120.

Capezuti, E., Wagner, L.M., Brush, B.L., Boltz, M., Renz, S., & Talerico, K.A. (2007). Consequences of an intervention to reduce restrictive side rail use in nursing homes. *Journal of the American Geriatrics Society, 55,* 334-341.

Carioti, C.A., Lavigne, J.E., Stone, P., Tortoretti, D.M., & Chiverton, P. (2001). Work site disease management outcomes: Expanding the role of the APN. *Outcomes Management for Nursing Practice, 5,* 179-184.

Carr, C.A. (2000). Charges for maternity services: Associations with provider type and payer source in a university teaching hospital. *Journal of Midwifery & Women's Health, 45,* 378-383.

Carroll, D.L., Robinson, E., Buselli, E., Berry, D., & Rankin, S.H. (2001). Activities of the APN to enhance unpartnered elders self-efficacy after myocardial infarction. *Clinical Nurse Specialist, 15,* 60-66.

Chang, E., Daly, J., Hawkins, A., McGirr, J., Fielding, K., Hemmings, L., et al. (1999). An evaluation of the nurse practitioner role in a major rural emergency department. *Journal of Advanced Nursing, 30,* 260-268.

Cohen, J., Saylor, C., Holzemer, W.L., & Gorenberg, B. (2000). Linking nursing care interventions with client outcomes: A community-based application of an outcomes model. *Journal of Nursing Care Quality, 15*(1), 22-31.

Cole, F.L., & Ramirez, E. (2000). Activities and procedures performed by nurse practitioners in emergency care settings. *Journal of Emergency Nursing, 26,* 455-463.

Corner, J., Halliday, D., Haviland, J., Douglas, H.R., Bath, P., Clark, D., et al. (2003). Exploring nursing outcomes for patients with advanced cancer following intervention by Macmillan specialist palliative care nurses. *Journal of Advanced Nursing, 41,* 561-574.

Counsell, C., & Gilbert, M. (1999). Implementation of a nurse practitioner role in an acute care setting. *Critical Care Nursing Clinics of North America, 11,* 277-282.

Cowan, M.J., Shapiro, M., Hays, R.D., Afifi, A., Vazirani, S., Ward, C.R., et al. (2006). The effect of a multidisciplinary hospitalist/physician and advanced practice nurse collaboration on hospital costs. *Journal of Nursing Administration, 36,* 79-85.

Cragin, L., & Kennedy, H.P. (2006). Linking obstetric and midwifery practice with optimal outcomes. *Journal of Obstetric, Gynecologic, & Neonatal Nurses, 35,* 779-785.

Cromwell, J., & Snyder, K. (2000). Alternate cost-effective anesthesia care teams. *Nursing Economic$, 18,* 185-193.

Cunningham, R.S. (2006). Clinical practice guideline use by oncology advanced practice nurses. *Applied Nursing Research, 19,* 126-133.

Dahl, J., & Penque, S. (2001). The effects of an advanced practice nurse–directed heart failure program. *Dimensions of Critical Care Nursing, 20,* 20-28.

Dahle, K.L., Smith, J.S., Ingersoll, G.L., & Wilson, J.R. (1998). Impact of a nurse practitioner on the cost of managing inpatients with heart failure. *American Journal of Cardiology, 82,* 686-688.

Darmody, J.V. (2005). Observing the work of the clinical nurse specialist: A pilot study. *Clinical Nurse Specialist, 19,* 260-268.

Davidson, J.U. (1999). Blending case management and quality outcomes management into the family nurse practitioner role. *Nursing Administration Quarterly, 24*(1), 66-74.

DeJong, S.R., & Veltman, R.H. (2004). The effectiveness of a CNS-led community-based COPD screening and intervention program. *Clinical Nurse Specialist, 18,* 72-79.

DeLise, D.C., & Leasure, A.R. (2001). Benchmarking: Measuring the outcomes of evidence-based practice. *Outcomes Management for Nursing Practice, 5*(2), 70-74.

Dellasega, C., & Zerbe, T.M. (2002). Caregivers of frail rural older adults: Effects of an advanced practice intervention. *Journal of Gerontological Nursing, 28*(10), 40-49.

Dick, K., & Frazier, S.C. (2005). An exploration of nurse practitioner care to homebound frail elders. *Journal of American Academy of Nurse Practitioners, 18,* 325-334.

Dickerson, S.S., Wu, Y.W.B., & Kennedy, M.C. (2006). A CNS-facilitated ICD support group: A clinical project evaluation. *Clinical Nurse Specialist, 20,* 116-153.

Donabedian, A. (1966). Evaluating the quality of medical care. *Milbank Quarterly, 44,* 166–206.

Donabedian, A. (1980). *Explorations in quality assessment and monitoring: The definition of quality and approaches to its assessment.* Ann Arbor, MI: Health Administration Press.

Dougherty, C.M., Spertus, J.A., Dewhurst, T.A., & Nichol, W.P. (2000). Outpatient nursing case management for cardiovascular disease. *Nursing Clinics of North America, 35,* 993-1003.

Dozier, A.M. (1998). Professional standards: Linking care, competence, and quality. *Journal of Nursing Care Quality, 12*(4), 22-29.

Edwards, J.B., Oppewal, S., & Logan, C.L. (2003). Nurse-managed primary care: Outcomes of a faculty practice network. *Journal of American Academy of Nurse Practitioners, 12,* 563-569.

Ellwood, P.M. (1988). Outcomes management. A technology of patient experience. *New England Journal of Medicine, 318,* 1549-1556.

Ettner, S.L., Kotlerman, J., Abdelmonem, A., Vazirani, S., Hays, R.D., Shapiro, M., et al. (2006). An alternative approach to reducing the costs of patient care? A controlled trial of the multi-disciplinary doctor-nurse practitioner (MDNP) model. *Medical Decision Making, 26,* 9-17.

Fanta, K., Cook, B., Falcone, R.A. Jr., Rickets, C., Schweer, L., Brown, R.L., et al. (2006). Pediatric trauma nurse practitioners provide excellent care with superior patient satisfaction for injured children. *Journal of Pediatric Surgery, 41,* 277-281.

Gebaur, C., Kwo, C.Y., Haynes, E.F., & Wewers, M.E. (1998). A nurse-managed smoking cessation intervention during pregnancy. *Journal of Gynecologic & Neonatal Nursing, 21,* 47-53.

Gooden, J.M., & Jackson, E. (2004). Attitudes of registered nurses toward nurse practitioners. *Journal of American Academy of Nurse Practitioners, 16,* 360-364.

Goolsby, M.J. (2007). Antibiotic-prescribing habits of nurse practitioners treating adult patients: Antibiotic use and guidelines survey adult. *Journal of the American Academy of Nurse Practitioners, 19,* 212-214.

Gray, M. (1998). The impact of the "Put Prevention into Practice" initiative on pediatric nurse practitioner practices. *Journal of Pediatric Health Care, 12,* 171-175.

Green, A., & Davis, S. (2005). Toward a predictive model of patient satisfaction with nurse practitioner care. *Journal of American Academy of Nurse Practitioners, 17,* 139-148.

Gross, P.A., Aho, L., Ashtyani, H., Levine, J., McGee, M., Moran, S., et al. (2004). Extending the nurse practitioner concurrent intervention model to community-acquired pneumonia and chronic obstructive pulmonary disease. *The Joint Commission Journal on Quality and Safety, 30,* 377-386.

Gross, P.A., Patricio, D., McGuire, K., Skurnick, J., & Teichholz, L.E. (2002). A nurse practitioner intervention model to maximize efficient use of telemetry resources. *The Joint Commission Journal on Quality Improvement, 28,* 566-573.

Halm, M.A., Gagner, S., Goering, M., Sabo, J., Smith, M., & Zaccagnini, M. (2003). Interdisciplinary rounds. Impact on patients, families, and staff. *Clinical Nurse Specialist, 17,* 133-142.

Hamilton, R., & Hawley, S. (2006). Quality of life outcomes related to anemia management of patients with chronic renal failure. *Clinical Nurse Specialist, 20,* 139-143.

Hamric, A.B., Lindebak, S., Worley, D., & Jaubert, S. (1998). Outcomes associated with advanced nursing practice prescriptive authority. *Journal of the American Academy of Nurse Practitioners, 10,* 113-118.

Hargreaves, W.A., Shumway, M., Hu, T.W., & Cuffel, B. (1998). *Cost-outcome methods for mental health.* New York: Academic Press.

Hillier, A. (2001). The advanced practice nurse in gastroenterology: Identifying and comparing care interactions of nurse practitioners and clinical nurse specialists. *Gastroenterology Nursing, 24,* 239-245.

Hoffman, L.A., Tasota, F.J., Scharfenberg, C., Zullo, T.G., & Donahoe, M.P. (2003). Management of patients in the intensive care unit: Comparison via work sampling analysis of an acute care nurse practitioner and physicians in training. *American Journal of Critical Care, 12,* 436-443.

Hoffman, L.A., Tasota, F.J., Zullo, T.G., Scharfenberg, C., & Donahoe, M.P. (2005). Outcomes of care managed by an acute care nurse practitioner/attending physician team in a subacute medical intensive care unit. *American Journal of Critical Care, 14,* 121-132.

Holcomb, L.O. (2000). A Delphi survey to identify activities of nurse practitioners in primary care. *Clinical Excellence in Nursing Practice, 4,* 163-172.

Holzemer, W.L. (1994). The impact of nursing care in Latin America and the Caribbean: A focus on outcomes. *Journal of Advanced Nursing, 20,* 5-12.

Hooker, R.S., & McCaig, L.F. (2001). Use of physician assistants and nurse practitioners in primary care, 1995-1999. *Health Affairs, 20,* 231-238.

Horrocks, S., Anderson, E., & Salisbury, C. (2002). Systematic review of whether nurse practitioners working in primary care can provide equivalent care to doctors. *British Medical Journal, 324,* 819-823.

Hughes, W.J. (2000). Health department nurse practitioners as comprehensive primary care providers. *Family & Community Health, 23*(1), 50-65.

Ingersoll, G.L. (1998). Administrative issues in the measurement and management of outcomes. *Applied Nursing Research, 11,* 93-97.

Ingersoll, G.L. (2000). Evidence based nursing: What it is and what it isn't. *Nursing Outlook, 48,* 151-152.

Ingersoll, G.L. (2006a). *Using evidence to define and monitor standards of practice* [online]. Indianapolis, IN: Sigma Theta Tau, International.

Ingersoll, G.L. (2006b). *Using evidence to improve organizational performance and outcomes* [online]. Indianapolis, IN: Sigma Theta Tau, International.

Ingersoll, G.L., McIntosh, E., & Williams, M. (2000). Nurse-sensitive outcomes of advanced practice. *Journal of Advanced Nursing, 32,* 1272-1281.

Institute of Medicine (IOM). (2001). *Crossing the quality chasm: A new health system for the 21st century.* Washington, DC: National Academies Press.

Intili, H., & Laws, C. (2003). Delivering health care in a large urban hospital. *AAOHN Journal, 51,* 306-309.

Irvine, D., Sidani, S., Porter, H., O'Brien-Pallas, L., Simpson, B., Hall, L.M., et al. (2000). Organizational factors influencing nurse practitioners' role implementation in acute care settings. *Canadian Journal of Nursing Leadership, 13*(3), 28-35.

Jackson, P.L., Kennedy, C., Sadler, L.S., Kenney, K.M., Lindeke, L.L., Sperhac, A.M., et al. (2001). Professional practice of pediatric nurse practitioners: Implications for education and training of PNPs. *Journal of Pediatric Health Care, 15,* 291-298.

Jepson, C., McCorkle, R., Adler, D., Nuamah, I., & Lusk, E. (1999). Effects of home care on caregivers' psychosocial status. *Image: Journal of Nursing Scholarship, 31,* 115-120.

Johnson, J.E. (2000). Assessment of older urban drivers by nurse practitioners. *Journal of Community Health Nursing, 17,* 107-114.

Johnson, K.C., & Daviss, B.A. (2005). Outcomes of planned home births with certified professional midwives: Large prospective study in North America. *British Medical Journal, 330,* 1416-1422.

Kane, R.L., Flood, S., Keckhafer, G., & Rockwood, T. (2001). How EverCare nurse practitioners spend their time. *Journal of American Geriatrics Society, 49,* 1530-1534.

Kane, R.L., Keckhafer, G., Flood, S., Bershadsky, B., & Siadaty, M.S. (2003). The effect of EverCare on hospital use. *Journal of the American Geriatrics Society, 51,* 1427-1434.

Kannusamy, P. (2006). A longitudinal study of advanced practice nursing in Singapore. *Critical Care Nursing Clinics of North America, 18,* 545-551.

Karlowicz, M.G., & McMurray, J.L. (2000). Comparison of neonatal nurse practitioners' and pediatric residents' care of extremely low-birth-weight infants. *Archives of Pediatric & Adolescent Medicine, 154,* 1123-1126.

Kinnersley, P., Anderson, E., Parry, K., Clement, J., Archard, L., Turton, P., et al. (2000). Randomised controlled trial of nurse practitioner versus general practitioner care for patients requesting "same day" consultations in primary care. *British Medical Journal, 320,* 1043-1048.

Kleinpell, R.M. (1998). Reports of role descriptions of acute care nurse practitioners. *AACN Clinical Issues, 9,* 290-295.

Kleinpell, R.M. (2005). Acute care nurse practitioner practice: Results of a 5-year longitudinal study. *American Journal of Critical Care, 14,* 211-221.

Kleinpell-Nowell, R. (2001). Longitudinal survey of acute care nurse practitioner practice: Year 2. *AACN Clinical Issues, 12,* 447-452.

Kleinpell-Nowell, R., & Weiner, T.M. (1999). Measuring advanced practice nursing outcomes. *AACN Clinical Issues, 10,* 356-368.

Knudtson, N. (2000). Patient satisfaction with nurse practitioner service in a rural setting. *Journal of American Academy of Nurse Practitioners, 12,* 405-412.

Krein, S.L., Klamerus, M.L., Vijan, S., Lee, J.L., Fitzgerald, J.T., Pawlow, A., et al. (2004). Case management for patients with poorly controlled diabetes: A randomized trial. *American Journal of Medicine, 116,* 732-739.

Krichbaum, K., Pearson, V., Savik, K., & Mueller, C. (2005). Improving resident outcomes with GAPN organization level interventions. *Western Journal of Nursing Research, 27,* 322-337.

Krueger, R.A. (n.d.). *Outcome evaluation.* Retrieved February 20, 2007, from www.tc.umn.edu/~rkrueger/evaluation_oe.html.

Kutzleb, J., & Reiner, D. (2006). The impact of nurse-directed patient education on quality of life and functional capacity in people with heart failure. *Journal of American Academy of Nurse Practitioners, 18,* 116-123.

Lambing, A.Y., Adams, D.L.C., Fox, D.H., & Divine, G. (2004). Nurse practitioners' and physicians' care activities and clinical outcomes with an inpatient geriatric population. *Journal of American Academy of Nurse Practitioners, 16,* 343-352.

Larkin, G.L., Kantor, W., & Zielinski, J.J. (2001). Doing unto others? Emergency medicine residents' willingness to be treated by moonlighting residents and nonphysician clinicians in the emergency department. *Academic Emergency Medicine, 8,* 886-892.

Lawson, M.T. (2002). Nurse practitioner and physician communication styles. *Applied Nursing Research, 15,* 60-66.

Lenz, E.R., Mundinger, M.O., Kane, R.L., Hopkins, S.C., & Lin, S.X. (2004). Primary care outcomes in patients treated by nurse practitioners or physicians: Two-year follow-up. *Medical Care Research and Review, 61,* 332-351.

Leveille, S.G., Wagner, E.H., Davis, C., Grothaus, L., Wallace, J., LoGerfo, M., et al. (1998). Preventing disability and managing chronic illness in frail older adults: A randomized trial of a community-based partnership with primary care. *Journal of American Geriatrics Society, 46,* 1191-1198.

Lin, S.X., Gebbie, K.M., Fullilove, R.E., & Arons, R.R. (2004). Do nurse practitioners make a difference in provision of health counseling in hospital outpatient departments? *Journal of American Academy of Nurse Practitioners, 16,* 462-466.

Lin, S.X., Hooker, R.S., Lenz, E.R., & Hopkins, S.C. (2002). Nurse practitioners and physician assistants in hospital outpatient departments, 1997-1999. *Nursing Economic$, 20,* 174-179.

Lincoln, P.E. (2000). Comparing CNS and NP role activities: A replication. *Clinical Nurse Specialist, 14,* 269-277.

Lind, P. (2001). Disease management: Applying systems thinking to quality patient care delivery. In E. Cohen & T. Cesta (Eds.), *Nursing case management: From essentials to advanced practice applications* (3rd ed., pp. 37-48). St. Louis: Mosby.

Litaker, D., Mion, L.C., Planavsky, L., Kippes, C., Mehta, N., & Frolkis, J. (2003). Physician-nurse practitioner teams in chronic disease management: The impact on costs, clinical effectiveness, and patients' perceptions of care. *Journal of Interprofessional Care, 17,* 223-237.

Lynch, M.P., Cope, D.G., & Murphy-Ende, K. (2001). Advanced practice issues: Results of the ONS advanced practice nursing survey. *Oncology Nursing Forum, 28,* 1521-1530.

Mabrook, A.F., & Dale, B. (1998). Can nurse practitioners offer a quality service? An evaluation of a year's work of a nurse led minor injury unit. *Journal of Accident & Emergency Medicine, 15,* 266-268.

Mahn, V., & Zazworsky, D. (2000). The advanced practice nurse case manager. In A.B. Hamric, J.A. Spross, & C.M. Hanson (Eds.), *Advanced nursing practice: An integrative approach* (2nd ed., pp. 549-606). Philadelphia: Saunders.

Marsden, J., & Street, C. (2004). A primary health care team's views of the nurse practitioner role in primary care. *Primary Health Care Research and Development, 5,* 17-27.

Mason, D.J., Alexander, J.M., Huffaker, J., Reilly, P.A., Sigmund, E.C., & Cohen, S.S. (1999). Nurse practitioners' experiences with managed care organizations in New York and Connecticut. *Nursing Outlook, 47,* 201-208.

Mason, D.J., Cohen, S.S., O'Donnell, J.P., Baxter, K., & Chase, A.B. (1997). Managed care organizations' arrangements with nurse practitioners. *Nursing Economic$, 15,* 306-314.

Mathaisel, D.F.X., Cathcart, T.P., & Comm, C.L. (2004). A framework for benchmarking, classifying, and implementing best sustainment practices. *Benchmarking: An International Journal, 11,* 403-411.

McAuliffe, M.S., & Henry, B. (1998). Survey of nurse anesthesia practice, education, and regulation in 96 countries. *AANA Journal, 66,* 273-286.

McCorkle, R., Benoliel, J.Q., Donaldson, G., Georgiadou, F., Moinpour, C., & Goodell, B. (1989). A randomized clinical trial of home nursing care for lung cancer patients. *Cancer, 64,* 1375-1382.

McCorkle, R., Dowd, M.F., Pickett, M., Siefert, M.L., & Robinson, J.P. (2007). Effects of advanced practice nursing on patient and spouse depressive symptoms, sexual function, and marital interaction after radical prostatectomy. *Urologic Nursing, 27,* 65-77.

McCorkle, R., Strumpf, N.E., Nuamah, I.F., Adler, D.C., Cooley, M.E., Jepson, C., et al. (2000). A specialized home care intervention improves survival among older post-surgical cancer patients. *Journal of the American Geriatrics Society, 48,* 1707-1713.

McGlynn, E.A., Asch, S.M., Adams, J., Keesey, J., Hicks, J., DeCristofaro, A., & Kerr, E.A. (2003). The quality of health care delivered to adults in the United States. *New England Journal of Medicine, 348,* 2635-2645.

McMullen, M., Alexander, M.K., Bourgeois, A., & Goodman, L. (2001). Evaluating a nurse practitioner service. *Dimensions of Critical Care Nursing, 20,* 30-34.

Meyer, S.C., & Miers, L.J. (2005). Cardiovascular surgeon and acute care nurse practitioner: Collaboration on postoperative outcomes. *AACN Clinical Issues, 16,* 149-158.

Mick, D.J., & Ackerman, M.H. (2000). Advanced practice nursing role delineation in acute and critical care: Application of the Strong Model of advanced practice. *Heart & Lung: Journal of Acute & Critical Care, 29,* 210-221.

Mills, A.C., & McSweeney, M. (2002). Nurse practitioners and physician assistants revisited: Do their practice patterns differ in ambulatory care? *Journal of Professional Nursing, 18,* 36-46.

Mills, A.C., McSweeney, M., & Lavin, M.A. (1998). Characteristics of patient visits to nurse practitioners and physician assistants in hospital outpatient departments. *Journal of Professional Nursing, 14,* 335-343.

Mitchell, J., Dixon, H.L., Freeman, T., & Grindrod, A. (2001). Public perceptions of and comfort level with nurse practitioners in family practice. *Canadian Nurse, 97,* 21-26.

Mitchell, P.H., Ferketich, S., & Jennings, B.M. (1998). Quality health outcomes model. American Academy of Nursing Expert Panel on Quality Health Care. *Image: Journal of Nursing Scholarship, 30,* 43-46.

Moody, N.B., Smith, P.L., & Glenn, L.L. (1999). Client characteristics and practice patterns of nurse practitioners and physicians. *Nurse Practitioner, 24,* 94-103.

Moore, S., Corner, J., Haviland, J., Wells, M., Salmon, E., Normand, C., et al. (2002). Nurse led follow up and conventional medical follow up in management of patients with lung cancer: Randomized trial. *British Medical Journal, 325,* 1145-1147.

Mundinger, M.O., Kane, R.L., Lenz, E.R., Totten, A.M., Tsai, W.U., Cleary, P.D., et al. (2000). Primary care outcomes in patients treated by nurse practitioners or physicians. *Journal of American Medical Association, 283,* 59-68.

Murphy, P.A., & Feinland, J.B. (1998). Perineal outcomes in a home birth setting. *Birth, 25,* 226-234.

Murphy, P.A., & Fullerton, J.T. (1998). Outcomes of intended home births in nurse-midwifery practice: A prospective descriptive study. *Obstetrics & Gynecology, 92,* 461-470.

Murphy, P.A., & Fullerton, J.T. (2001). Measuring outcomes of midwifery care: Development of an instrument to assess optimality. *Journal of Midwifery & Women's Health, 46,* 274-284.

Musclow, S.L., Sawhney, M., & Watt-Watson, J. (2002). The emerging role of advanced nursing practice in acute pain management throughout Canada. *Clinical Nurse Specialist, 16,* 63-67.

National Association of Pediatric Nurse Practitioners. (2004). *Scope and standards of practice.* Retrieved June 28, 2007, from www.napnap.org/Docs/FinalScope2-25.pdf.

Naylor, M.D., Brooten, D., Campbell, R., Jacobsen, B.S., Mezey, M.D., Pauly, M.V., et al. (1999). Comprehensive discharge planning and home follow-up of hospitalized elders: A randomized clinical trial. *Journal of American Medical Association, 281,* 613-620.

Naylor, M.D., & McCauley, K.M. (1999). The effects of a discharge planning and home follow-up intervention on elders hospitalized with common medical and surgical cardiac conditions. *Journal of Cardiovascular Nursing, 14,* 44-54.

Neff, D.F., Madigan, E., & Narsavage, G. (2003). APN-directed transitional home care model: Achieving positive outcomes for patients with COPD. *Home Healthcare Nurse, 21,* 543-550.

Ockene, J.K., Adams, A., Hurley, T.G., Wheeler, E.V., & Hebert, J.R. (1999). Brief physician and nurse practitioner–delivered counseling for high-risk drinkers: Does it work? *Archives of Internal Medicine, 159,* 2198-2205.

Oddi, L.F., & Cassidy, V.R. (1998). The message of SUPPORT: Change is long overdue. *Journal of Professional Nursing, 14,* 165-174.

Oliveria, S.A., Altman, J.F., Christos, P.J., & Halpern, A.C. (2002). Use of nonphysician health care providers for skin cancer screening in the primary care setting. *Preventive Medicine, 34,* 374-379.

Oncology Nursing Society (ONS). (2003). *Statement on the scope and standards of advanced practice nursing in oncology* (3rd ed.). Pittsburgh: Author.

Paez, K.A., & Allen, J.K. (2006). Cost-effectiveness of nurse practitioner management of hypercholesterolemia following coronary revascularization. *Journal of American Academy of Nurse Practitioners, 18,* 436-444.

Peters, C., Cowley, M., & Standiford, L. (1999). The process of outcomes management in an acute care facility. *Nursing Administration Quarterly, 24*(1), 75-89.

Pine, M., Holt, K.D., & Lou, Y.B. (2003). Surgical mortality and type of anesthesia provider. *AANA Journal, 71,* 109-116.

Powell, S.K. (2000). *Advanced case management: Outcomes and beyond.* Philadelphia: Lippincott.

Radwin, L. (2002). Refining the Quality Health Outcomes Model: Differentiating between client trait and state characteristics. *Nursing Outlook, 50,* 168-169.

Rawl, S.M., Easton, K.L., Kwiatkowski, S., Zemen, D., & Burczyk, B. (1998). Effectiveness of a nurse-managed follow-up program for rehabilitation patients after discharge. *Rehabilitation Nursing, 23,* 204-209.

Reavis, C. (2004). Nurse practitioner–delivered primary health care in urban ambulatory care settings. *American Journal for Nurse Practitioners, 8*(5), 41-49.

Reigle, J., Molnar, H.M., Howell, C., & Dumont, C. (2006). Evaluation of in-patient interventional cardiology. *Critical Care Nursing Clinics of North America, 18,* 523-529.

Rideout, K. (2007). Evaluation of a PNP care coordinator model for hospitalized children, adolescents, and young adults with cystic fibrosis. *Pediatric Nursing, 33,* 29-34, 48.

Ritz, L.J., Nissen, M.J., Swensen, K.K., Farrell, J.B., Sperduto, P.W., Sladek, M.L., et al. (2000). Effects of advanced nursing care on quality of life and cost outcomes of women diagnosed with breast cancer. *Oncology Nursing Forum, 27,* 923-932.

Robertson, J. (2003). *Metrics for knowledge management and content management.* Retrieved February 20, 2007, from www.steptwo.com.au/papers/kmc_metrics/index.html.

Roblin, D.W., Becker, E.R., Adams, K.E., Howard, D.H., & Roberts, M.H. (2004). Patient satisfaction with primary care: Does type of practitioner matter? *Medical Care, 42,* 579-590.

Roblin, D.W., Howard, D.H., Becker, E.R., Adams, E.K., & Roberts, M.H. (2004). Use of midlevel practitioners to achieve labor cost savings in the primary care practice of an MCO. *Health Services Research, 39,* 607-625.

Rosenfeld, P., McEvoy, M.D., & Glassman, K. (2003). Measuring practice patterns among acute care nurse practitioners. *Journal of Nursing Administration, 33,* 159-165.

Rudy, E.B., Davidson, L.J., Daly, B., Clochesy, J.M., Sereika, S., Baldisseri, M., et al. (1998). Care activities and outcomes of patients cared for by acute care nurse practitioners, physician assistants, and resident physicians: A comparison. *American Journal of Critical Care, 7,* 267-281.

Russell, D., VorderBruegge, M., & Burns, S.M. (2002). Effect of an outcomes-managed approach to care of neuroscience patients by acute care nurse practitioners. *American Journal of Critical Care, 11,* 353-364.

Ryden, M.B., Snyder, M., Gross, C.R., Savik, K., Pearson, V., Krichbaum, K., et al. (2000). Value-added outcomes: The use of advanced practice nurses in long-term care facilities. *The Gerontologist, 40,* 654-662.

Sakr, M., Angus, J., Perrin, J., Nixon, C., Nicholl, J., & Wardrope, J. (1999). Care of minor injuries by emergency nurse practitioners or junior doctors: A randomized controlled trial. *The Lancet, 354,* 1321-1326.

Sarkissian, S., & Wennberg, R. (1999). Effects of the acute care nurse practitioner role on epilepsy monitoring outcomes. *Outcomes Management for Nursing Practice, 3,* 161-166.

Scisney-Matlock, M., Makos, G., Saunders, T., Jackson, F., & Steigerwalt, S. (2004). Comparison of quality-of-hypertension care for groups treated by physician versus groups treated by physician-nurse team. *Journal of the American Academy of Nurse Practitioners, 16,* 17-23.

Scott, R.A. (1999). A description of the roles, activities, and skills of clinical nurse specialists in the United States. *Clinical Nurse Specialist, 13,* 183-190.

Seale, C., Anderson, E., & Kinnersley, P. (2005). Comparison of GP and nurse practitioner consultations: An observational study. *British Journal of General Practice, 521,* 938-943.

Seale, C., Anderson, E., & Kinnersley, P. (2006). Treatment advice in primary care: A comparative study of nurse practitioners and general practitioners. *Journal of Advanced Nursing, 54,* 534-541.

Sheahan, S.L. (2000). Documentation of health risks and health promotion counseling by emergency department nurse practitioners and physicians. *Journal of Nursing Scholarship, 32,* 245-250.

Shebesta, K.F., Cook, B., Rickets, C., Schweer, L., Brown, R.L., Garcia, V.F., et al. (2006). Pediatric trauma nurse practitioners increase bedside nurses' satisfaction with pediatric trauma patient care. *Journal of Trauma Nursing, 13,* 66-69.

Shell, R.C. (2001). Antidepressant prescribing practices of nurse practitioners. *Nurse Practitioner, 26*(7), 42-47.

Sidani, S., Doran, D., Porter, H., LeFort, S., O'Brien-Pallas, L.L., Zahn, C., et al. (2006a). Outcomes of nurse practitioners in acute care. *Internet Journal of Advanced Nursing Practice, 8*(1).

Sidani, S., Doran, D., Porter, H., LeFort, S., O'Brien-Pallas, L.L., Zahn, C., et al. (2006b). Processes of care: Comparison between nurse practitioners and physician residents in acute care. *Nursing Leadership, 19,* 69-85.

Sidani, S., & Irvine, D. (1999). A conceptual framework for evaluating the nurse practitioner role in acute care settings. *Journal of Advanced Nursing, 30*(1), 58-66.

Sidani, S., Irvine, D., Porter, H., O'Brien-Pallas, L., Simpson, B., McGillis-Hall, L., et al. (2000). Practice patterns of acute care nurse practitioners. *Canadian Journal of Nursing Leadership, 13*(3), 6-12.

Simonson, D.C., Ahern, M.M., & Hendryx, M.S. (2007). Anesthesia staffing and anesthetic complications during cesarean delivery: A retrospective analysis. *Nursing Research, 56,* 9-17.

Small, R., Lumley, J., Donohue, L., Potter, A., & Waldenstrom, U. (2000). Randomised controlled trial of midwife led debriefing to reduce maternal depression after operative childbirth. *British Medical Journal, 321,* 1043-1047.

Smolenski, M.C. (2005). Credentialing, certification, and competence: Issue for new and seasoned nurse practitioners. *Journal of American Academy of Nurse Practitioners, 17,* 201-204.

Sohn, P.M., & Cook, C.A.L. (2002). Nurse practitioner knowledge of complementary alternative health care: Foundation for practice. *Journal of Advanced Nursing, 39,* 9-16.

Sole, M.L., Hunkar-Huie, A.M., Schiller, J.S., & Cheatham, M.L. (2001). Comprehensive trauma patient care by nonphysician providers. *AACN Clinical Issues, 12,* 438-446.

Stolee, P., Hillier, L.M., Esbaugh, J., Griffiths, N., & Borrie, M.J. (2006). Examining the nurse practitioner role in long-term care. *Journal of Gerontological Nursing, 32*(10), 28-36.

Stone, P.W., Zwanziger, J., Walker, P.H., & Buenting, J. (2000). Economic analysis of two models of low-risk maternity care: A freestanding birth center compared to traditional care. *Research in Nursing & Health, 23,* 279-289.

Stuart, D., & Oshio, S. (2002). Primary care in nurse-midwifery practice: A national survey. *Journal of Midwifery & Women's Health, 47,* 104-109.

Stutts, A. (2001). Developing innovative care models: The use of customer satisfaction scores. *Journal of Nursing Administration, 31,* 293-300.

Sullivan-Marx, E.M., Happ, M.B., Bradley, K.J., & Maislin, G. (2000). Nurse practitioner services: Content and relative work value. *Nursing Outlook, 48,* 269-275.

Sullivan-Marx, E.M., & Maislin, G. (2000). Comparison of nurse practitioner and family physician relative work values. *Journal of Nursing Scholarship, 32,* 71-76.

Tijhuis, G.J., Zwinderman, A.H., Hazes, J.M.W., Breedveld, F.C., & Vlieland, P.M.T. (2003). Two-year follow-up of a randomized controlled trial of a clinical nurse specialist intervention, inpatient, and day patient team care in rheumatoid arthritis. *Journal of Advanced Nursing, 41,* 34-43.

Topp, R., Tucker, D., & Weber, C. (1998). Effect of a clinical case manager/clinical nurse specialist on patients hospitalized with congestive heart failure. *Nursing Case Management, 3,* 140-147.

Venning, P., Durie, A., Roland, M., Roberts, C., & Leese, B. (2000). Randomised controlled trial comparing cost effectiveness of general practitioners and nurse practitioners in primary care. *British Medical Journal, 320,* 1048-1053.

Wagner, L.M., Capezuti, E., Brush, B., Boltz, M., Renz, S., & Talerico, K.A. (2007). Description of an advanced practice nursing consultative model to reduce restrictive siderail use in nursing homes. *Research in Nursing & Health, 30,* 131-140.

Walker, D.S., Day, S., Diroff, C., Lirette, H., McCully, L., Mooney-Hescott, C., et al. (2002). Reduced frequency prenatal visits in midwifery practice: Attitudes and use. *Journal of Midwifery & Women's Health, 47,* 269-277.

Way, D., Jones, L., Baskerville, B., & Busing, N. (2001). Primary health care services by nurse practitioners and family physicians in shared practice. *Canadian Medical Association Journal, 165,* 1210-1214.

Wheeler, E.C. (1999). The effect of the clinical nurse specialist on patient outcomes. *Critical Care Nursing Clinics of North America, 11,* 269-275.

Williams, D., & Sidani, S. (2001). An analysis of the nurse practitioner role in palliative care. *Canadian Journal of Nursing Leadership, 14*(4), 13-19.

Windorski, S.K., & Kalb, K.A. (2002). Educating NPs to educate patients: Cholesterol screening in pediatric primary care. *Journal of Pediatric Health Care, 16,* 60-66.

Wong, S.T., Stewart, A.L., & Gilliss, C.L. (2000). Evaluating advanced practice nursing through use of a heuristic framework. *Journal of Nursing Care Quality, 14*(2), 21-32.

York, R., Brown, L.P., Samuels, P., Finkler, S.A., Jacobsen, B., Persely, C.A., et al. (1997). A randomized trial of elderly discharge and nurse specialist transitional follow-up care for high-risk childbearing women. *Nursing Research, 46,* 254-261.

Zapka, J.G., Pbert, L., Stoddard, A.M., Ockene, J.K., Goins, K.V., & Bonollo, D. (2000). Smoking cessation counseling with pregnant and postpartum women: A survey of community health center providers. *American Journal of Public Health, 90,* 78-84.

CHAPTER 25

Outcomes Evaluation and Performance Improvement: Using Data and Information Technology to Improve Practice

Vicky A. Mahn-DiNicola

INTRODUCTION

The current emphasis on patient safety and improving health care quality has led to increased public reporting of quality indicators. Health care systems want to demonstrate to payers and the public that they are meeting these evidence-based benchmarks so that they will be "paid for performance." The notion of "pay for performance" (or P4P) is a key driver of continuous quality improvement (CQI), systems redesign, and financial sustainability in the organizations in which advanced practice nurses (APNs) are employed. APNs are expected to understand and participate in these efforts to improve the quality and safety of care and maximize reimbursement. Therefore it is critical that APNs develop competency in quality improvement strategies and systems thinking (see Chapters 8 and 9). They must also become proficient in the use of tools and information systems that support quality improvement (QI) and system redesign efforts.

If readers have participated in the adoption of electronic medical records (EMRs) or computerized provider order entry (CPOE) systems, they have already experienced some of the benefits and challenges of adopting health information technology (HIT) to improve patient care. APNs in practice will need to master the basics of HIT and learn ways to keep up to ensure they remain value-added contributors to the health care systems in which they work. Both the APN competencies described in this chapter and the *Essentials of Doctoral Education for Advanced Nursing Practice* (American Association of Colleges of Nursing [AACN], 2006) address the need for APNs to be proficient in quality improvement strategies, informatics, and systems thinking. The Doctor of Nursing Practice (DNP)–prepared APN is expected to be more expert at these competencies than the APN who is master's prepared. In addition, the Institute of Medicine's report entitled *Health Professions Education: A Bridge to Quality* (2003) calls for nursing education that prepares individuals for practice with interdisciplinary, information systems, quality improvement, and patient safety expertise.

Developing such expertise in today's academic arena is a challenge. Academic institutions that prepare APNs must seek alliances with practice environments that not only exemplify or aspire to the best in professional nursing practice but also are "learning organizations" (see Chapter 9) that are fully invested in the QI process. Institutional commitments to adopting best practices and CQI are essential if health care systems are to keep pace with new developments in performance measurement and outcomes evaluation. In addition, a robust, integrated, and reliable information systems infrastructure is essential to assist the APN student and graduate to achieve competencies in informatics and system evaluation.

Addressing the need for inclusion of APN-sensitive processes of care and outcome indicators will require focused attention on development of electronic information systems that identify and track APN data. A first step in this process is national agreement on a core set of outcome indicators relevant to APNs and the initiation of standards that support the collection of APN-sensitive data. Until then, it is likely that the process and outcome indicators used by APNs in the evaluation of their practice will be "shared" indicators that are also reflective of medical and professional nursing practice, making it difficult to attribute outcomes solely to APN practice.

This chapter provides the reader with a background on regulatory policies and patient safety initiatives that are driving both the adoption of HIT, as well as performance improvement activities and payment structures. Specific informatics skills that APNs need now and in the future are presented, along with strategies to implement HIT to evaluate patient care and evaluate APN practice. Finally, the author describes several frameworks for measuring and monitoring APN practice.

REGULATORY INITIATIVES THAT DRIVE PERFORMANCE IMPROVEMENT

Health care regulatory requirements imposed by The Joint Commission (TJC), the Centers for Medicare & Medicaid Services (CMS), the National Quality Forum (NQF), and other agencies have driven and will continue to drive much of the performance improvement activities within health care settings.

Acute Care Hospitals

In 1997, TJC established requirements for hospitals to contract with selected performance measurement system vendors for the purposes of collecting and submitting performance measurement data to be used in the accreditation process. This initiative, known as *ORYX®*, was described as "voluntary"; however, there is little argument that this was a requirement for those hospitals wishing to be accredited under TJC's umbrella. Beginning in 2000, the ORYX® initiative expanded to include the collection and reporting of selected "core measures," which reflect evidence-based practices and outcomes in high-risk, high-volume populations. This program has since expanded to include acute myocardial infarction (AMI), heart failure (HF), pneumonia, the Surgical Care Improvement Project (SCIP), pregnancy-related conditions, children's asthma care (CAC), and hospital-based inpatient psychiatric services (HBIPS). This initiative was subsequently embraced by CMS in a program called *Reporting Hospital Quality Data for Annual Payment Updates (RHQDAPU),* a mandate that requires hospitals to submit a subset of measures reflecting their performance data for AMI, HF, SCIP, and pneumonia populations. (See *www.cms.gov* for a full review of measures required for RHQDAPU.) Hospitals failing to meet the requirements for data submission lose a percentage of their Medicare Annual Payment Update (APU), which in some cases amounts to $1 million or more. Although this program was also described as "voluntary," few hospitals across the country fail to meet these requirements for obvious reasons.

During this early period, the emphasis was on "pay for reporting." The objective was to submit data to the CMS clinical data warehouse within the required quarterly time frames and to ensure that the data met specific quality standards. Hospitals failing to achieve an interrater reliability score of 80% or higher were subject to the withholding of a percentage of their APU. This emphasis on complete and accurate data abstraction continues to be pivotal to health care systems, and more and more clinical resources are being committed to collecting the required performance data.

In 2002, the Hospital Quality Alliance (HQA) endorsed selected core measures for public disclosure in a "report card" format, and the emphasis shifted from "pay for reporting" to "public transparency" of health care quality indicators. Individual hospital performance data are now published on HQA, CMS, and TJC websites for consumers to review and evaluate whether their local hospitals comply with evidence-based best practices. These measures, now referred to as the *National Hospital Quality Measures (NHQM),* continue to expand and grow, with additional measure sets being developed for venous thromboembolism prevention (scheduled for release in 2009) and the nursing-sensitive care measure set (preliminarily scheduled for release in 2009).

Public transparency of NHQM measures has raised the bar on performance; however, actual P4P has not yet become a direct motivator for improvement, although that is likely to change as early as October 2008. A value-based purchasing (VBP) model proposed by CMS (2007) will link payment more directly to performance. Under this proposed model, the hospital's APU would be allocated in accordance with its performance scores against national benchmarks. Only hospitals that score in the top 10th percentile of performance for all required measures would receive their full APU. This model, if adopted, would have significant financial implications for those health care systems that are still working to achieve benchmark performance or that maintain substandard performance over time.

In addition to the proposed VBP model for Medicare reimbursement to hospitals, additional regulatory changes mandate reduced Medicare reimbursement on selected conditions not present on admission. These changes target conditions that could have been prevented through application of evidence-based guidelines and for which the cost/volume burden is high. These conditions include catheter-associated urinary tract infection, decubitus ulcers, objects left in the body after surgery, blood incompatibility, air embolus, and central venous catheter infections. Additional complications of care such as mediastinal infections after coronary artery bypass graft (CABG) surgery and hospital-acquired injuries have also been selected pending final diagnostic coding changes (retrieved September 8, 2007, from *www.cms.hhs.gov/AcuteInpatientPPS/downloads/CMS-1533-FC.pdf*, p. 368). Although the initial implementation of reduced payments for such conditions will be limited to these conditions, two things are clear. First, this is a trend likely to continue, with additional conditions being added in future years. Second, the majority of these complications, whether they occur or are avoided, are directly related to the contributions of professional nursing care. APNs have the knowledge and skill to lead efforts to prevent such complications, either through direct practice or system interventions.

The implications of moving toward direct P4P are staggering in terms of the commitment hospitals will have to make to create or enhance their HIT infrastructures and dedicate resources to collect these required data. In an unpublished survey conducted by ACS MIDAS+, an ORYX® performance measurement system vendor serving over 500 hospitals nationally, smaller hospitals averaged 1.5 full time equivalent (FTE) positions toward data abstraction efforts and quality oversight of three measure sets in 2005. Larger hospital systems employed as many as 4.5 FTEs to complete data abstraction and quality oversight for NHQM measures, which does not include the upstream efforts to educate clinicians about required changes in documentation and care delivery standards, which is where APNs are affected. Having an idea of the resources needed for these efforts is useful since APNs are likely to be involved in efforts to "ramp up" their system's QI and HIT activities.

Across the country, significant resources are devoted to improving provider and hospital staff compliance with selected drug-ordering practices, timeliness of treatment interventions and diagnostics, and patient educational strategies. To achieve competitive performance scores, the data collection effort has started to shift from a retrospective review (meaning data abstraction occurred after the patient was discharged and the medical record was coded with final International Classification of Diseases, 9th revision, [ICD-9] diagnoses), to a concurrent review process; this is so that hospital staff and medical providers have the opportunity to ensure that all patients receive the right care before discharge and provider or hospital performance measurement scores remain high.

The author has observed that many APNs nationwide are now engaged in efforts to monitor direct care for compliance with the standards of care reflected in these various performance measurement systems. APNs are participating in quality improvement committees; workflow and system redesign efforts; and the selection, design, and evaluation of information systems supporting data collection efforts. For example, adult nurse practitioners (NPs) and clinical nurse specialists (CNSs) are likely to find themselves accountable for making rounds on AMI, HF, pneumonia, and surgical populations to ensure that the patients have received appropriate and timely medications, that assessments and interventions have been completed, and that care has been sufficiently documented in the medical record. Selected examples of possible APN interventions in achieving excellence in the NHQM measures and preventing complications of care are presented in Box 25-1.

At most acute care hospital settings, NHQM data are now included in individual provider profiles and evaluated at the time of reappointment. However, the issues of provider attribution are difficult to address in an acute care hospital environment in which so many providers contribute to the management of a single patient's care episode. For example, medical orders for a patient with HF who is eligible for angiotensin-converting enzyme (ACE) inhibitors at discharge could be written by the patient's physician, a cardiac specialist, a hospitalist, or an acute care NP (ACNP) who is accountable for overseeing the cardiac medical population. In the absence of a CPOE system, most information or clinical documentation systems do not capture the provider responsible for ordering individual medications or nonprocedural treatments. In reality, patient care is moving toward an interdisciplinary model of care in which the "whole team" shares responsibility for the outcome (Mahn-DiNicola, 2004).

What is clear is that in order for hospitals to improve and maintain their performance, underlying care delivery systems must be redesigned; it is not simply a matter of enforcing compliance. Barriers to care occur at a systems level and require an integrated approach to CQI. To accelerate improvement, integrated CQI approaches must consider the following: provider expertise and the degree of autonomy inherent in clinical practice; organizational culture and theory; effective strategies for disseminating new knowledge; leadership commitment; and CQI principles and practices (Shortell, Bennet, & Byck, 1998). Achieving these goals requires resources. APNs, by virtue of their competencies in both practice and systems, can provide much-needed leadership in improving care processes and establishing effective infrastructures that support

Box 25-1   ADVANCED PRACTICE NURSING INTERVENTIONS AFFECTING CLINICAL
OUTCOMES AND PATIENT SAFETY

- Collaborate with physician or write orders to administer influenza or pneumococcal vaccinations upon discharge for appropriate pneumonia patients.
- Collaborate with physician or write orders to administer prophylactic antibiotics within 1 hour of surgery start time.
- Collaborate with physician or write orders to discontinue prophylactic antibiotics within 24 hours of surgery end time (48 hours if cardiac surgery).
- Collaborate with nursing staff to ensure discharge medications are appropriately documented in the patient's take-home materials and that they match discharge medications listed in the medical record.
- Review AMI patients who experienced delays in receiving PCI within 90 minutes of arrival, and facilitate systemwide improvements to remove barriers to timely arrival to the cath lab.

- Participate on an interdisciplinary team to redesign documentation systems to ensure that the medical record captures the necessary information required for data abstraction.
- Participate on an interdisciplinary team to develop standardized order sets and policies and procedures to support the implementation of best practices to prevent catheter-associated UTIs and ventilator-associated pneumonias.
- Attend classes to maintain expertise in current data abstraction requirements and inclusion and exclusion criteria described in each of the NHQM algorithms.
- Provide expert guidance and coaching as to why a given patient did or did not meet the standard of care being captured in a NHQM measure; in other words, why a particular patient became an "opportunity for improvement."

AMI, Acute myocardial infarction; *cath lab,* cardiac catheterization laboratory; *NHQM,* National Hospital Quality Measures; *PCI,* percutaneous coronary intervention; *UTI,* urinary tract infection.

care delivery and performance outcomes that will ensure maximum reimbursement. Exemplar 25-1 illustrates an APN influencing both practice and systems by exercising leadership, QI, systems thinking, and use of informatics.

Home Health Settings

In 2000, as part of a broad QI initiative, the federal government began requiring that every Medicare-certified home health agency complete and submit health assessment information for their clients. A valid and reliable instrument called the *Outcome and Assessment Information Set (OASIS)* is used to collect and report performance data by home health agencies. Since Fall 2003, CMS has maintained a website *(www. medicare.gov)* on which it posts a subset of OASIS-based quality performance information showing how well home health agencies meet benchmarks for improving or maintaining patients' ability to function. These measures, listed in Box 25-2, reflect how well homebound patients perform activities of daily living (ADL); there are also several use-of-service measures reflecting rehospitalization and emergent care. These measures are currently reported on the Home Health Compare website *(www.cms.hhs.gov/HomeHealthQualityInits,* retrieved July 5, 2007).

APNs employed by a home health agency will likely find themselves responsible for data collection activities associated with these reporting requirements, as well as improving documentation systems that reflect the care delivery necessary to achieve acceptable performance in these areas. For example, graduate CNS students who were also employed as home health nurses created a presentation for the agency's board of directors that demonstrated the differences in reimbursement capture for the same patient when the OASIS assessment was performed by a novice staff nurse versus an expert/APN nurse. The expert's initial OASIS assessments were more complete, identified more problems earlier, and permitted interventions that prevented complications. Using an APN creates the potential for fewer complications and higher reimbursement capture. This presentation illustrated to the board members the significance of advanced knowledge and skills in achieving clinical and financial outcomes (J.A. Spross, V. Erickson, & R. Unnold, personal communication, August 10, 2007).

Nursing Home Settings

In November 2002, the CMS began a national Nursing Home Quality Initiative Pilot to adopt a set of improved nursing home quality measures, which have

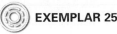

Judy is an adult nurse practitioner at a 425-bed community hospital that is part of a 27-hospital health care system in Southern California. Her principal accountabilities are managing care on an interdisciplinary team for a medical and surgical cardiac population. In addition to Judy's clinical role, she also has oversight for data collection of registry information for the STS's database, developed by Duke University. She also has responsibility for collecting NHQM data required by TJC and the CMS in the AMI, HF, and cardiac surgical populations.

In a typical day, as Judy makes rounds on patients, she uses a paper tracking tool to collect information required by the STS registry. She uses a second data collection worksheet to collect data required by the CMS and TJC. At a later date, either she or an RN quality specialist enters the STS data into an electronic access database for future submission to STS and enters the NHQM data into a separate care management system for later submission to the hospital's contracted vendor for NHQM. Judy collects data concurrently while patients are still in the hospital and intervenes as necessary to ensure that all standards of care are being met and that appropriate interventions have been ordered in a timely fashion. Ultimately, her goal is to ensure the highest levels of performance for measures that are being publicly reported to TJC and the CMS, which ultimately will be tied to the hospital's Medicare annual payment updates once P4P arrives.

Recently, Judy has been asked to participate on an interdisciplinary team that is piloting the use of tablet PC technology connected to a wireless network system in the hospital to streamline data collection efforts associated with all registry data and NHQM data across the corporation. The tablet PC uses a mobile data capture software system called *Mi-Forms* (see *www.mi-forms.com*). The first challenge for the team is to design a comprehensive data collection form that can be used at the bedside. Judy is instrumental in identifying all the data elements that have to be collected by both the STS and NHQM. She notes that many data elements are redundant and do not have to be collected twice. Further, she points out to the team that several of the data elements required on the data collection forms are essentially "administrative data," such as patient name, age, race, ethnicity, admission status, payer, and Medicare HIC number. She wonders whether any of these data elements might be "auto-populated" into the Mi-Form on the tablet PC so as to avoid duplicative data entry steps. The team decides to invest in an electronic interface from the hospital's ADT system and to develop a patient look-up system directly from the tablet PC so that patient data can be automatically entered into the form.

After several weeks of designing the form and creating consensus with other clinicians across the organization who are responsible for collecting similar data, Judy is ready to pilot the form in a live clinical environment. She quickly discovers that the data variables related to medications are organized inefficiently on the form. Instead of having all medications grouped together in one place on the form, she recommends that it would be more efficient to group medications required within the first 24 hours of arrival, such as aspirin or beta-blockers, on the first tab of the form and to group medications required at discharge on the last tab of the form. In this manner, the data collection flow coincides with the patient's progress through the episode of care. The modifications to the form are completed within 4 hours by a technical member of the committee so that Judy can continue piloting the form.

On the third day of piloting the form, Judy follows a patient to the cath lab. During her data entry onto the tablet PC, she notices that the data she entered is being lost because of interference with the wireless network from the cath lab equipment. She contacts the IT leader on the committee, who realizes that a real-time wireless connection to the database will not work in their hospital environment. A decision is made to change to an upload system, whereby at the end of Judy's rounds, she will simply dock the PC into a docking station in her office and upload the data collected thus far directly into the database.

Judy offers additional suggestions for improving the data collection flow, such as adding "branching logic" in the form so that certain questions either appear or grey out, depending upon previous responses. In addition, she suggests various data validation rules to prevent inappropriate data entry, such as entering a date of surgery that is before the date of admission.

Judy understands that the reliability of the data entered into the forms must also be verified before the technology can be broadly adopted across the organization. She consults with the RN quality specialist to design an inter-rater reliability study, in

---

ADT, Admission-discharge-transfer; *AMI,* acute myocardial infarct; *cath lab,* cardiac catheterization laboratory; *CMS,* Centers for Medicare & Medicaid Services; *HF,* heart failure; *HIC,* health insurance claim; *IT,* information technology; *NHQM,* National Hospital Quality Measures. *P4P,* pay-for-performance; *PC,* personal computer; *RN,* registered nurse; *STS,* Society of Thoracic Surgeons; *TJC,* The Joint Commission.

Continued

EXEMPLAR 25-1   **Advanced Practice Nurse Role in Leveraging Technology Solutions to Improve Care—cont'd**

which several patient records will be re-abstracted by experts in the STS and NHQM data sets, to ensure that the data collected by Judy on the tablet PC are complete, accurate, and consistent with the data abstraction requirements defined by the STS, the CMS and TJC.

After several weeks of collecting the data using the tablet PC technology, word has quickly spread throughout the organization of how efficient the data collection process is for capturing the STS and NHQM data. In addition, performance data are now immediately available within the care management system because delays in data entry

have been eliminated. The RN quality specialist no longer spends time entering data. Instead, she is able to direct her efforts to disseminating more concurrent performance information to the various committees and departments within the hospital and participating on quality improvement teams, which she did not have time for previously. Performance continues to improve in all areas, and the technology is now being expanded to additional registries and NHQM topics. Judy continues to provide expert guidance and coaching to nursing colleagues new to this approach across the organization.

ADT, Admission-discharge-transfer; *AMI,* acute myocardial infarct; *cath lab,* cardiac catheterization laboratory; *CMS,* Centers for Medicare & Medicaid Services; *HF,* heart failure; *HIC,* health insurance claim; *IT,* information technology; *NHQM,* National Hospital Quality Measures. *P4P,* pay-for-performance; *PC,* personal computer; *RN,* registered nurse; *STS,* Society of Thoracic Surgeons; *TJC,* The Joint Commission.

 Box 25-2   OASIS-BASED HOME HEALTH QUALITY MEASURES

- Improvement in ambulation/locomotion
- Improvement in bathing
- Improvement in transferring
- Improvement in management of oral medication
- Improvement in pain occurring with activity
- Acute care hospitalization
- Emergent care
- Discharge to community
- Improvement in dyspnea
- Improvement in urinary incontinence

OASIS, Outcome and Assessment Information Set.

since been finalized. Data are collected through a process of state inspections as well as by nursing home staff, using the Minimum Data Set (MDS) assessment form. An MDS assessment is performed at admission, quarterly, annually, and whenever the resident experiences a significant change in status. For residents in a Medicare Part A stay, the MDS is also used to determine the Medicare reimbursement rate; for these residents, assessments are performed on the 5th, 14th, 30th, 60th, and 90th day after admission. Box 25-3 lists the enhanced chronic care measures that are currently posted on the Nursing Home Compare website (*www.medicare.gov/NHCompare,* retrieved July 5, 2007) for long-term care patients.

Primary Care and Outpatient Settings

Legislation has been proposed that will authorize a similar VBP model for reimbursement in hospital outpatient services (scheduled implementation by October 2009) and ambulatory surgery centers (scheduled implementation by October 2010). In addition, the Physician Quality Reporting Incentive (PQRI) measures have been established under the Tax Relief and Health Care Act of 2006. This legislation authorized the establishment of a physician quality reporting system by the CMS and established a financial incentive for eligible professionals to participate in a voluntary quality reporting program. Eligible professionals who successfully reported a designated set of quality measures on claims for dates of service from July 1 to December 31, 2007, earned a bonus payment, subject to a cap of 1.5% of total allowed charges for covered Medicare physician fee schedule services. There are 74 measures that have been established as part of the PQRI measure set. Many of these are clearly relevant to APNs who monitor or manage a variety of diseases and chronic conditions (e.g., hemoglobin A_{1c}, future fall risk). See a complete list of PQRI measures at *www.cms.hhs.gov/PQRI/Downloads/PQRIMeasuresList.pdf,* retrieved August 11, 2007. It is likely that APNs will share responsibilities for data collection efforts associated with the capture of this information and will share accountability for achieving performance outcomes for these metrics.

Box 25-3   CHRONIC CARE MEASURES FOR LONG-TERM CARE

- Percent of residents given influenza vaccination during the flu season
- Percent of residents who were assessed and given pneumococcal vaccination
- Percent of residents whose need for help with daily activities has increased
- Percent of residents who have moderate to severe pain
- Percent of high-risk residents who have pressure sores
- Percent of low-risk residents who have pressure sores
- Percent of residents who were physically restrained
- Percent of residents who are more depressed or anxious

- Percent of low-risk residents who lose control of their bowels or bladder
- Percent of residents who have/had a catheter inserted and left in their bladder
- Percent of residents who spent most of their time in bed or in a chair
- Percent of residents whose ability to move about in and around their room got worse
- Percent of residents with a urinary tract infection
- Percent of residents who lose too much weight
- Percent of short-stay residents who had moderate to severe pain
- Percent of short-stay residents with delirium
- Percent of short-stay residents with pressure sores

Regardless of setting, these various initiatives are pressing APNs to contribute not only to the achievement of direct practice outcomes but also to QI strategies undertaken by the health care organization to secure maximum reimbursement and market share in this competitive health care environment.

QUALITY IMPROVEMENT AND DATA ANALYTICAL COMPETENCIES REQUIRED FOR ADVANCED PRACTICE NURSING

Quality Improvement

APNs must be able to effectively participate in and lead interdisciplinary teams toward data-based conclusions and process improvements. This discussion elaborates on Competency II of the research competencies described in Chapter 8—evaluation of practice. Data analysis is a specific skill for research Competency II and requires the ability to manipulate and interpret raw data, query information within a database containing clinical or financial information, and utilize an information system to collect data and trend performance. Historically, most APNs did not need this level of skill in a direct practice role. However, the environments in which APNs are practicing have changed. The purpose of this section is to elaborate on these specific skills that APNs need in order to be knowledgeable participants and leaders in CQI efforts. APN students need content on CQI knowledge and skills. Graduate APNs should seek additional CQI training through reading, continuing

education, and participation in formal QI training programs. A health care system's approach to CQI should be included in an APN's orientation. If such programs are not in place, APNs are strongly encouraged to include formal QI training in their performance and learning objectives within the first year of hire and to identify opportunities to initiate modest QI initiatives.

Continuous Quality Improvement Frameworks. There are numerous frameworks and related strategies for improving performance and evaluating outcomes in today's health care system. Some of these include the "Plan-Do-Study-Act" (PDSA) model used by the Institute for Healthcare Improvement (IHI), Six Sigma, and Lean Manufacturing techniques. APNs can examine selected frameworks to understand the "how-to" mechanics of creating a health care system that is safe, effective, patient-centered, timely, efficient, and equitable. In many cases, the employer will have selected a framework or philosophy that guides CQI efforts across the organization. Many of these methodologies have evolved from the work of Dr. W. Edwards Deming and Dr. Joseph M. Juran, both considered to be forefathers of modern day statistical process control theory. The reader is referred to the work of Marash, Berman, and Flynn (2003) for a comprehensive overview of traditional QI methodologies. The author relies primarily on PDSA and traditional CQI frameworks to inform this section.

All QI frameworks have these common features: the phenomenon that is the focus of a QI effort must be measurable and once measured, analysis is applied in a systematic way to improve, if not transform, health care. Such activities are referred to as *data analytics*. Regardless of the type of QI approach an organization selects, the APN should be competent in a variety of specific techniques, tools, and methodologies that are used to evaluate process performance and outcomes. Most approaches involve the use of different types of charts and analysis tools to examine findings and establish linkages. Some charts are easy to learn, such as flow charts. Other charts, such as Pareto charts, statistical process control charts, scatter diagrams, and cause-and-effect diagrams (also referred to as *fishbone* or *Ishikawa diagrams*), require specific training and expertise in statistical software. There are software packages that perform analyses and create charts, including SAS (see *www.sas.com/index.html*), SPSS (see *www.spss.com/*), Statit (see *www. statit.com*), and QI Macros, an easy-to-use software program that works with Microsoft Excel and can be downloaded from the Internet at a reasonable cost (see *www.qimacros.com/*). APNs will need to become familiar with the software used in their agencies to conduct CQI analyses and reports. A summary of tools for process improvement are presented in Table 25-1. APNs prepared at a master's level should achieve beginning level competencies with these tools, including the ability to interpret the data in such reports and effectively participate on teams using CQI techniques. DPN-prepared APNs should achieve mastery, with full accountability for planning the CQI project; selecting and using appropriate tools and techniques, including being able to enter data and run the reports; synthesizing information from the reports; and coaching others in deriving meaning from the information and making decisions.

QI training typically includes techniques for analyzing how people and processes work. Root cause analysis is one popular approach to identifying underlying causes of problems and process failures within the health care system. This approach may be particularly useful for examining adverse events and other patient safety issues. An excellent root cause analysis of suboptimal pain management using a fishbone diagram will give the reader an idea of how to apply this technique to a clinical problem (Berry & Dahl, 2000). A comprehensive introduction to QI charts and tools and their specific applications to case, disease, and population management may be found in *Advanced Case Management: Outcomes and Beyond* (Powell, 2000).

Data and Outcomes Management

Outcomes management refers to the application of outcomes research in practice to produce desirable outcomes in a clinical setting (Powell, 2000). Therefore this author proposes an expanded definition of outcomes management to include evaluation of practice: *the ability to manage data and information effectively in order to assess, plan, implement, and evaluate strategies to improve care processes and outcomes and maximize care efficiency for individuals and populations*. This definition is congruent with the nursing process and describes the process used by APNs to evaluate program effectiveness and continuously improve performance.

APNs are accustomed to recognizing and acting on clinical patterns they observe within and across patients. Similarly, as APNs work with data as part of their CQI responsibilities, they learn to recognize meaningful patterns within and across clinical datasets and reports. This skill is as important in CQI as it is in the delivery of direct care. Only after patterns in the data are identified do certain questions emerge about the meaning of such patterns, which often leads to further data queries. This process, often referred to as *data mining*, is a dynamic one that requires direct access to raw data and rapid report turnaround time.

To develop skill in data mining, APNs should learn what types of information management systems are available in their organizations and request training in how to use these systems. At the least, they need to become familiar with the types of data and reports available from the systems so that they can request information from designated experts. Information systems that are most likely to contain data needed for outcomes management include but are not limited to dedicated case or care management systems; medical records coding systems; billing and claims data; pharmacy, risk, quality, and claims management systems; and infection control, nursing acuity, and cost accounting systems. Exemplar 25-2 illustrates this pattern-recognition skill when an APN is given a summary report versus a data spreadsheet containing the actual encounter level detail used to create the summary report.

Common Performance Measures. In addition to recognizing patterns in data, APNs should be familiar with common performance measures that are used to evaluate care and determine whether benchmarks have been met. Commonly used indicators,

Table 25-1   CONTINUOUS QUALITY IMPROVEMENT TOOLS AND TECHNIQUES FOR PROCESS IMPROVEMENT

Tools and Techniques	Primary Function	Benefits
Flowchart	Displays the process	Facilitates understanding of the process Identifies stakeholders Clarifies potential gaps and system breakdowns
Run Chart	Displays performance over time	Increases understanding of the problem Identifies changes over time
Control Chart	Displays how predictable the process is over time	Identifies change in the process as a result of intentional or non-intentional changes in the process Identifies opportunities for improvement
Pie Chart	Displays the percentage each variable contributes to the whole	Identifies variables affecting process Increases understanding of the problem
Bar Chart	Compares categories of data during a single point in time	Increases understanding of the problem Identifies differences in variables Compares performance with known standards
Pareto Chart	Identifies the most frequent trend within a data set	Identifies principal variables impacting the process Identifies opportunities for improvement
Cause and Effect	Displays multiple causes of a problem	Identifies root causes Identifies variables affecting the process Identifies opportunities for improvement Plans for change
Scatter Diagram	Displays relationship between two variables	Increases understanding of the relationship between multiple variables
Brainstorming	Rapidly generates multiple ideas	Promotes stakeholder buy-in Increases understanding of the problem Identifies variables affecting the process
Multi-voting	Consolidates ideas	Achieves consensus among stakeholders Prioritizes improvement strategies
Nominal Group Technique	Rapidly generates multiple ideas and prioritizes them	Identifies the problem Achieves consensus among stakeholders Prioritizes improvement strategies Plans for change
Root Cause Analysis	Identifies the cause of the problem	Increases understanding of the problem Identifies multi-cause variables affecting the process Identifies opportunities to improve Plans for change
Force Field Analysis	Identifies driving and restraining forces that impact proposed change	Identifies and lists variables affecting process Plans for change
Consensus	Generates agreement among stakeholders	Increases understanding of the problem Reduces resistance to change Plans for change

Adapted from Powell, S.K. (2000). *Advanced case management: Outcomes and beyond.* Philadelphia: Lippincott. Used with permission.

EXEMPLAR 25-2   **Advanced Practice Nurse Role in Data Analysis to Influence Decision Making**

Figure 25-1 illustrates the "summary report," which provides useful administrative information. However, the APN cannot identify clinically relevant patterns in the data that are opportunities for improvement. In addition, the APN requires additional information, including national comparison data or benchmarks, to determine if the LOS, readmission rates, mortality rates, and charges are in alignment with other organizations similar to the APN's. In contrast, raw data provided to the APN in a spreadsheet, such as the one illustrated in Figure 25-2 (p. 744), allow APNs to immerse themselves in data to find unexpected pieces of information about the population that may not have been part of their original report request. (Electronic source data most commonly available from health care information systems are outlined in Box 25-6 on p. 763). With the use of Excel, the data can be sorted, filtered, grouped, and organized using spreadsheet functions to identify meaningful patterns in resource utilization, complications of care, variations in physician practice, and patient characteristics that affect severity of illness or intensity of service.

Formerly, the APN sorted patients using the following criteria: whether they were admitted through the ED, admitting times (in ascending order), and time of arrival at ED (to see the distribution of arrivals) (see Figure 25-2). Using this simple approach, she was able to determine that the peak time of day in which admissions were occurring was between 1400 and 2200. When she used an Excel tool to sort the data by day of week (not shown), the APN noted that fewer patients were admitted over the weekend, with the largest spike occurring on Mondays. The APN inferred that patients delayed reporting symptoms until the doctor's office opened on Monday and that by the time physicians returned the calls on Monday, the patients' symptoms had worsened, requiring more urgent medical intervention in the ED. The APN leveraged this information, along with additional data from patients admitted with chest pain who had similar utilization patterns, to build support for an ED-based "CHF and Chest Pain Clinic" at the hospital, staffed heaviest in the late afternoon and evening hours, which could accommodate this volume and more efficiently manage, treat, and triage patients with CHF and chest pain. A community-wide marketing plan was implemented to inform both the public and providers across the community of this service.

APN, Advanced practice nurse; *CHF,* congestive heart failure; *ED,* emergency department; *LOS,* length of stay.

including some of their strengths and limitations, are discussed below.

Average Length-of-Stay Indicators. When analyzing patterns of acute care hospital utilization, the APN should evaluate patterns in length-of-stay (LOS) data in relation to other variables that influence LOS for a given population. These include the following:

- Admission volume (larger population denominators tend to reflect shorter LOS)
- Readmission rates (evaluate readmissions for any condition, including conditions different from the index admission, within 15 and 31 days of discharge)
- Percentage of patients discharged alive with an LOS of 1 to 2 days (this reflects the percentage of patients who may not have been as acutely ill and therefore may have been admitted to the hospital unnecessarily)
- Percentage of patients who are discharged to other places of care along the continuum

other than home or death (this reflects the degree to which patients are transitioned to alternative levels of care)
- Complication rates or unexpected adverse medical outcomes (this reflects quality of care and the degree of successful acute care complication management)
- Severity of illness (this reflects preexisting conditions, co-morbidities, and physiological variables of the population)

The relative "goodness or badness" of LOS performance must be interpreted within the context of the health care organization's reimbursement structure and patient outcomes achieved. LOS cannot stand alone. For example, organizations that have exemplary average LOS (ALOS) performance but who have a higher proportion of patients who are readmitted within 15 days of discharge may actually have greater problems with ineffective resource utilization than hospitals with slightly higher LOS but lower readmission rates. In addition, competitive ALOS performance may be achieved as a result of aggressive transition

Utilization Profile: CHF MS-DRGs 291, 292, 293
USA Memorial Hospital
Start month 1/2006   End month 6/2006

Total Volume	240
Mean LOS	5.6
Median LOS	5.0
Std. Deviation	3.83
Max LOS	21
Total Charges	$3,501,338.58
Total Costs	$949,625.00
Average Charge/Case	$14,588.88
Average Cost/Case	$3,956.77
31-day readmission rate	11.57%
Mortality rate	9.56%

Admission Source
Emergency department   80% (192/240)
Physician office   17% (40/240)
SNF   2%   (5/240)

FIGURE 25-1: Sample data summary report for congestive heart failure. *CC,* Complications and co-morbidities; *CHF,* congestive heart failure; *DRG,* diagnosis-related group; *LOS,* length of stay; *Max,* maximum; *MCC,* major complications and co-morbidities; *MS-DRG 291,* heart failure and shock with MCC; *MS-DRG 292,* heart failure and shock with CC; *MS-DRG 293,* heart failure and shock without CC/MCC; *SNF,* skilled nursing facility; *Std.,* standard.

plans to move patients to other points of care along the continuum. As long as the costs of providing care at these alternative care settings (e.g., skilled nursing facility [SNF], acute rehabilitation, long-term care [LTC]) do not outweigh the minimal costs associated with a few more end-hospital days of bed, board, and recuperative nursing care, then the LOS is commendable. As soon as such aggressive transition planning begins to cost the health care system more than it would to keep the patient in the acute care environment and does not offer significant advantages to the patient, the organization may well be satisfied with a slightly higher LOS performance versus such an arbitrary marker of success. Of course, LOS performance can also be affected by adverse medical outcomes and

unexpected changes in the disease trajectory. For these situations, the APN's skill in acute care complication management, which also involves the ability to see patterns in the data and apply best practice research, will be instrumental in improving outcomes (see Chapter 24 for research-based examples).

Shared Accountability for Managing Utilization

APNs are often charged with designing and producing reports on team outcomes for administrators and clinicians at the organizational, departmental, and practice levels. For example, if a hospital working in cooperation with a managed care plan is striving to decrease inpatient admissions, bed-days per 1000 covered lives, and costs of delivering care, both hospital- and community-based APNs will share accountability with the product line administrators to achieve related goals and financial targets at the department and practice levels. Hospital-based APNs who provide care to and are charged with monitoring a specific clinical population within the product line, such as AMI and CHF patients within a cardiovascular product line, may implement specific interventions, such as a CHF admission protocol, standard order sets, or best practice guidelines, and then report to the cardiovascular product line director on the reduced numbers of unnecessary CHF admissions and critical care bed-days by payer. In contrast, a community-based APN may give a report to the same cardiovascular product line director on the reduced CHF readmission rate by payer. Both clinical and community APNs would provide reports that product line directors could translate to determine the reductions in costs by payer. Below are some common formulas used by payers and providers to evaluate utilization. The formula is presented first, followed by an explanation.

Common Utilization Measures
Bed Days per 1000 Covered Lives
Calculation:

$$ x = \frac{\text{Sum of all inpatient days for a selected health plan}}{\text{Total count of members enrolled in the health care plan}} $$

Example:
- 182 total inpatient days during the month of January
- 12,845 members enrolled in January
  $\sqrt{}$ 182 ÷ 12,825 = 0.01419

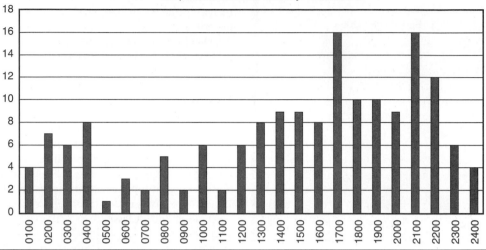

FIGURE **25-2:** Histogram of admission times to emergency department. *CHF,* Congestive heart failure; *ED,* emergency department. (Sample data reprinted with permission ACS MIDAS+, Tucson, AZ.)

√ 0.01419×1000=14.19 days in January per 1000*
√ 14.19×12 months=170.28 days/1000
(annualized)

One of the most common markers of utilization of hospital services is bed-days per 1000 covered lives. This measure is widely used by executives to monitor "the big picture." As an industry standard, this measure gives health care providers and managed care organizations the ability to compare utilization of inpatient days with a common denominator. Determination of whether bed-days are within acceptable ranges of performance may be based on comparative data or medical management guidelines, such as Milliman and Robertson, Inc. Health Care Management Guidelines® *(www. milliman. com)* which lists expected bed-day ranges for a wide variety of diagnosis-related group (DRG) and ICD-9 diagnosis codes in various managed care market environments. The calculation of bed-days is a function of both LOS and admission frequency. Therefore, if bed-days per 1000 covered lives are higher than desired, the APN will need to ascertain whether bed-days are higher as a result of excess hospital admissions or whether they are a result of a longer LOS. These are important data, because interventions to reduce admissions are very different from

those needed to reduce LOS within the acute care environment. The formula for inpatient admissions is presented below.

Inpatient Admissions per 1000 Covered Lives
Calculation:

$$x = \frac{\text{Total number of admissions}}{\text{Total count of members enrolled in the health care plan}}$$

Example:
- 67 patients admitted during the month of January
- 12,845 members enrolled in January
  √ 67÷12,825=0.00522
  √ 0.00522×1000=5.22 admits per 1000 lives*
  √ 5.22×12 months=62.7 per 1000 lives per year (annualized)

Inpatient admissions are widely used by executives to monitor overall utilization of inpatient services. Similar to bed-days, industry standards exist for various case types for both commercial and Medicare populations. This allows APNs to benchmark their organization's utilization against similar markets.

Cost per Patient Day
Calculation:

$$x = \frac{\text{Total direct costs}}{\text{Total patient days}}$$

Example:
- $286,342.21 direct costs assigned to a cardiac medical unit during the month of June
- 1908.9 patient days in June
  - √ $286,342.21÷1908.9=$150.00/patient day in June

Cost per patient day is typically used to describe incremental costs of care associated with a particular unit or point of service and helps mid-level managers make budgeting and financial projections. APNs can use this calculation also to report savings accrued when patients are redirected to alternative levels of care as a result of changes made in care delivery processes.

Cost per Discharge and Severity-Adjusted Data
Calculation:

$$x = \frac{\text{Sum of total costs accrued from admission to discharge}}{\text{Count of all patients discharged in the population of interest}}$$

Example:
- Total costs for patients discharged with MS-DRGs 291 + 292 + 293 (CHF) = $3,538,784
- Total number of patients discharged with MS-DRGs 291 + 292 + 293 = 914
  - √ $3,538,784÷914 = $3,871.75 per case

Cost per discharge is often used to evaluate cost of care trends for a particular case type or population over time. It is reported as an average. This measure is even more meaningful when the population of interest is risk- or severity-adjusted. The terms *risk adjustment* and *severity adjustment* are often used synonymously. However, the most clinically valid severity-adjustment methodologies imply a calculation of expected values based on each individual subject's physiological risk factors as compared with those of a normative population. Less rigorous severity-adjustment methodologies assign individual subjects to stratification subgroups based on related demographics, such as region, hospital bed size, or hospital case mix index. In the case of a CHF population, a meaningful indication of cost of care would be severity-adjusted costs that were calculated for each

of the four levels of New York Heart Association (NYHA) classifications of heart failure. However, obtaining the data necessary to severity-adjust a population based on physiological variables requires a dedicated medical record review effort and is often not sustainable over time. For example, specific clinical variables such as ejection fraction, laboratory values indicating renal function, and smoking history for individual patients may be required to calculate a severity-adjusted cost per discharge. However, typically these variables are not readily available in the HIT system, or if they are, they require costly integration of disparate HIT systems to acquire. For this reason, many heath care organizations invest in automated risk-adjustment methodologies that use more widely available coded claims data. For example, the 3M™ APR DRG Classification System uses ICD-9 diagnosis and procedure coding, along with other commonly available demographical information to risk-adjust patients into varying levels of intensity and severity.

In fiscal year 2008, CMS adopted Medicare severity-adjusted diagnosis-related groups (MS-DRGs), which stratify selected case types into those with major complications and co-morbidities, those with complications and co-morbidities, and those with none. This new DRG taxonomy will greatly facilitate the ability to obtain "severity-adjusted" data from administrative data that are commonly available in all HIT systems and available in the public domain at no cost.

Mean Cost per Covered Life
Calculation:

$$x = \frac{\text{Cost of all care provided over course of year to all enrollees}}{\text{Count of all enrollees in the health plan}}$$

Example:
- Total cost of care provided by health plan = $18,487,234
- Total number of enrollees during the year=2421
  - √ $18,487,234÷2421=$7636.20 per enrollee

The calculation of mean cost per covered life is a difficult measure to capture for most health care organizations because it requires claims data from the payers to determine all costs associated with care across the continuum. Ideally, this would include claims data from inpatient, emergency, outpatient, skilled nursing, rehabilitation, hospice, physician office visit, home health care, and pharmaceutical services. Despite the difficulty in gathering the data necessary to produce this measure, it is of particular interest to administrators in capitated environments because it illustrates cost shifting that results when patients are redirected to alternative levels of service. It is an important fiscal measure for APNs who practice in integrated health care delivery systems.

Readmission Rates
Calculation:

$$x = \frac{\text{Count of all non-elective inpatient encounters within 15 days of discharge}}{\text{Count of all inpatients discharged alive with MS-DRGs } 291 + 292 + 293}$$

Example:
- The denominator identifies the population of interest. In this example, 914 patients had an inpatient hospital admission for heart failure as identified by MS-DRGs 291, 292, and 293 and were discharged alive. Patients who expired during their first (index) admission were excluded from the population.
- The numerator identifies the number of patients readmitted within 15 days of discharge. In this example, 82 of 914 patients had a return inpatient admission with any diagnosis (not just limited to heart failure) within 15 days of discharge from their index encounter. Patients who were admitted for "elective" or outpatient procedures were excluded from the count.
  √ $82 \div 914 = .089$
  √ $.089 \times 100 = 8.9\%$ readmission rate

The readmission rate is one of the most commonly calculated indicators in case management and population-based outcome management; however, it remains one of the most controversial because of differing methodologies for computing the measure. Readmission rates are valuable because they are viewed as an indicator of the effectiveness of the treatment plan and the patient's readiness for discharge. Patients who are discharged too early or with insufficient supports in place tend to "bounce back in" and are considered management failures, although in some cases the natural disease trajectory and unforeseeable complications contribute to the readmission.

When calculating readmission rates, most hospitals rely on their HIT systems to identify these occurrences;

however, the APN should be aware of several problems associated with the computation of readmission rates using administrative claims data. First, most hospital HIT systems cannot look forward from the date of discharge and track a true readmission rate that occurs in the future. In reality, the majority of HIT systems actually look backward from the date of discharge and count patients who had any inpatient encounter before the specified date; what is essentially being measured is a "preadmission rate," which is often used as a proxy measure for readmission. As a result, many hospitals still devote time to reviewing charts and collecting readmission statistics manually. In addition, there appears to be some debate about whether to count only patients who were readmitted for the same diagnosis they had during their index admission or whether to count readmissions regardless of the clinical reason for returning, as long as it was not for an elective procedure or outpatient visit. Although some hospital and case management HIT systems can provide "true" readmission rates by looking forward in the database, the APN must know how the index encounters (the ones on which the calculation is based) are being identified and must have a clear understanding of how readmissions are being quantified at their organizations.

Once readmission rates are obtained, it may be quite informative for the APN to view readmission patterns sorted by elapsed days between discharge and readmission. Figure 25-3 illustrates a histogram of 30-day readmission patterns. Although the overall readmission rate is reported to be 13.2%, what is most significant is that 75 of 164 (46%) of all readmissions occurred within the first 7 days after discharge. This information provides the APN with greater insight into where in the process to intervene. In this example, information was used to shift the standard post-discharge home health or case management follow-up visit for CHF patients from 1 to 2 weeks after discharge to 1 to 2 days after discharge (Lamb, Mahn, & Dahl, 1996).

Productivity and Acuity Considerations
The nursing case management literature offers several models of tracking and monitoring productivity and acuity measures that may be helpful to APN practice. A study by Papenhausen (1996) demonstrated that community nurse case managers spent their visit time performing the following intervention activities: 30% assessing and monitoring, 17% teaching and informing, 7% in direct service, 23% supporting and sharing, and 11% exploring alternatives and goal setting. Brooten,

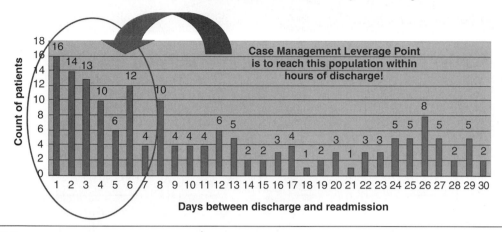

Readmission Patterns Sorted by Elapsed Days Between Discharge and Readmission

75/164 (46%) of all readmissions occur within 7 days of discharge

FIGURE 25-3: Histogram of readmission rates reveals leverage points for case management. (Copyright 1998-2007 by ACS MIDAS+, Tucson, AZ.)

Youngblut, Deatrick, Naylor, and York (2003) demonstrated that APN interventions were directly linked to improved patient outcomes and reduced health care costs in maternal/child, high-risk newborn, hysterectomy, and cardiac medical and surgical populations. In this study, the APN intervention of surveillance was the predominant APN function (48.1% to 65.4%) across all populations studied, followed by health teaching, guidance, and counseling (12.5% to 35.8%) and case management functions (12.9% to 24.9%). Treatments and procedures (0.1% to 0.6%) were the least dominant functions. Patient groups with more APN time and contacts per patients had greater improvements in patient outcomes and savings in health care charges even after costs for APN services were accounted for.

When APNs have this type of information, they can establish targets with administrators and contracted providers related to productivity and contract accountability. Productivity information and cost-benefit analyses enable the organization or practice to negotiate better contracts for its services.

Acuity addresses the level and complexity of care for patients managed by APNs. This information must be captured to demonstrate the costs and benefits of APN interventions. For example, Ward and Rieve (1997) illustrated an acuity-based framework for case managers in a disease management/episodic-based case management (CM) model. In this model, patients at the lowest levels of complexity and risk, requiring only 1 to 2 hours of CM intervention, are assigned an acuity level of 1. Patients requiring extensive diagnostic testing, multiple complex treatments, and over 15 hours of CM intervention are assigned an acuity level of 5. As APNs reflect on these best practices, an acuity schema may evolve to identify those patients who need a higher level of care associated with APN interventions.

Organizing Multi-Series Site Information to Evaluate Care Across the Continuum

The APN who is evaluating outcomes for a clinical population cared for at multiple points of service and over time must understand that the information needed to conduct such an analysis will reside in multiple data collection points and information systems. For the outcome management plan to be successful, the APN must bring the plan together into an organized framework. This is helpful not only for coordinating the data collection efforts needed to conduct a population-focused outcomes evaluation plan but also for communicating the information needs to the various information systems staff who support and control information throughout the care continuum. Data drawn from multiple points of service are called *multi-series information (MSI)*.

One way to effectively communicate a multi-series evaluation plan is by using a conceptual data plan wheel, illustrated in Figure 25-4. The wheel illustrates a plan for a population with CHF cared for in an

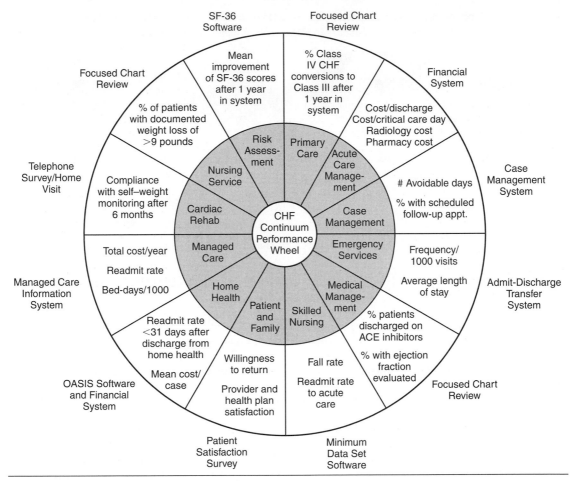

FIGURE 25-4: Conceptual data plan for coordinating cross-continuum outcomes data for patients with congestive heart failure. *ACE,* Angiotensin-converting enzyme; *apt,* appointment; *CHF,* congestive heart failure; *OASIS,* Outcome and Assessment Information Set; *Rehab,* rehabilitation. (Copyright 1998-2007 by ACS MIDAS+, Tucson, AZ.)

integrated delivery network (IDN). The central circle indicates that CHF is the focus of the performance evaluation plan. The wedges within the second circle identify points of service delivery (e.g., primary care) to CHF patients, specific care processes (e.g., risk assessment), and care focus (e.g., patient and family) that are being monitored. Key outcome measures for each of these aspects of service delivery are specified in the third circle. The sources of data for each measure that will be used to evaluate the care of CHF patients are indicated on the perimeter of the wheel, and analysis of these data can be used to create a "scorecard" for CHF patients. The CHF conceptual data plan addresses several processes and outcomes of

interest to multiple stakeholders across the care continuum. This particular scorecard permits one to examine the impact of selected interventions on patient outcomes and resource utilization. It also illustrates that the information needed to create a data plan and analyze the data across multiple information systems and multiple points of service may not be readily available to the APN who is accountable for the evaluation plan. Because the information associated with each point of service is generally considered to be proprietary to that service, the combined efforts of the stakeholders themselves are necessary to ensure that the information required to carry out the evaluation plan is available. A well-designed conceptual data plan can become a means to determine an organization's clinical effectiveness, cost effectiveness, and overall efficiency of managing the population for whom the APN is responsible.

Organizational Structures and Cultures That Optimize Performance Improvement

APNs who practice in a hospital or IDN setting may find that their span of influence crosses many units, departments, and points of service within the system. Thus it is important to consider carefully the reporting structures that will best support their role. In many organizations, APNs report to nurse or medical executives (see Chapter 23). APNs with a case management component to their practice may be based in the following departments: nursing, medical group, home health, quality and performance improvement, utilization resource management, social work, or even finance or information systems, though these last three are less common.

Regardless of organizational placement, APNs should seek to work within a reporting structure that supports "whole-system" thinking and places a high value on innovation and process improvement. APNs should avoid reporting structures that constrain their practices to one unit's or department's interests or seem to place a particular emphasis on task-oriented activities. Optimally, the organization and its administrators should recognize that the APN is in a unique position to promote excellence in clinical practice and system performance. To achieve such outcomes, the APN may at times require both the formal and the tacit authority that come with the position and title of those to whom the APN reports. Those who lead APNs must be prepared to "take the heat," if necessary, for changes that are perceived as coming from the APN. Although APNs will not need daily, or even weekly, supervision, they will need to be kept abreast of organizational issues that are likely to affect the practice and business environment (see Chapter 23). The APN should have routine briefing sessions scheduled with his or her immediate supervisor to clarify goals and expected outcomes, identify any resource needs, discuss any barriers, and exchange information relating to pending contracts, changes in the product line, medical practice issues, or staff education needs. Active membership on key medical and quality oversight committees and direct access to administrative decision makers are imperative. Such access affords APNs the opportunity to integrate clinical expertise with communication, negotiation, and leadership skills to promote effective and efficient clinical processes. For those APNs who contract independently, becoming familiar with the organizational structure and culture and becoming a trusted insider to the organization will be critical to successful contracting and service delivery (see Chapters 19 and 20).

EVOLVING INFORMATION TECHNOLOGIES THAT AFFECT ADVANCED PRACTICE NURSING

Regardless of setting, the increasingly sophisticated use of technology in health care environments mandates APNs' familiarity with and ability to use information systems and other technologies to support and improve patient care. The delivery of clinical care depends on many technologies—from software applications listing medications and their side effects to evidence-based guidelines and critical pathway tools. For APNs prepared at the DNP level, the expectation is that the APN is prepared to "apply new knowledge, manage individual and aggregate level information, and assess the efficacy of patient care technology appropriate to a specialized area of practice." DNP graduates also design, select, and use information systems technology to evaluate programs of care, outcomes of care, and care systems. Indeed, these expectations for being fluent in the use of technology are reflected in virtually every DNP Competency (AACN, 2006). This section discusses key information technology (IT) resources that APNs can use to guide and direct patient care at individual and systems levels.

Evidence-Based Practice

APNs must be able to review and synthesize evidence and assist other health care team members to draw meaningful conclusions and see potential applications to their own practices (see Chapter 8). Presenting such information to interdisciplinary providers should be done in a nonjudgmental and nonpunitive manner for the sole purpose of supporting and providing safe, effective, quality care and improving outcomes in both individual patients and aggregate populations. The APN should understand the strengths and limits of evidence-based practice, particularly for uncommon diseases for which evidence of effective interventions is neither available nor feasible to collect.

Box 8-3 in Chapter 8 lists a number of web-based services designed to provide clinicians with up-to-date reviews, guidelines, and other evidence-based information. One technology strategy to assist APNs with early and rapid access to best practice literature is the use of web-based services that are tied to specific clinical disease states, surgical procedures, and nursing/medical diagnoses. For example, the ZynxEvidence™ system *(www.zynx.com)* offers rapid access to current best practice literature and provides meta-analyses supporting diagnostic and treatment decisions for over 150 disease states. In addition, the system can be used to predict cost and quality outcomes likely to be gained from more efficient resource utilization and adherence to best practice strategies. Box 25-4 provides the reader with additional online sources of evidence-based practice literature that are potentially useful to APNs engaged in CQI activities.

Keeping up with advances in the health care industry is no easy task. Masys (2002) described the flood of information and information technologies that clinicians face. In the National Library of Medicine's MEDLINE database, which contains bibliographical records for over 12 million articles dating from 1966 to the present, an estimated 400,000 new entries are added yearly. According to Masys, "a conscientious practitioner who reads two articles each evening will, at the end of the year, be approximately 550 years behind in keeping up with the literature" (p. 35). This observation is highly relevant to creating safer and more effective care delivery systems. Numerous studies cited by the IOM (2001) demonstrate that there is an unacceptably slow adoption rate of new evidence-based best practices. According to Christopher J. Heller, MD, FACS (personal communication, 2005), even the most-understood practice of administering beta-blockers to post–myocardial infarction patients took over 17 years to reach broad adoption (defined as ≧90% of patients discharged in the United States with a diagnosis of AMI receiving beta-blockers at discharge when clinically indicated).

Delays in the adoption of new best practices cannot be attributed solely to the failure to disseminate information in a timely fashion. Such delays are often the result of traditional practice models, which rely on clinical decision making by autonomous practitioners. Health care professionals too often depend on their training, memory, and personal experience rather than on a decision-making process supported by a computer-based clinical decision support system or grounded in evidence-based practice.

Computerized Provider Order Entry Systems

Computerized provider order entry (CPOE) systems assist health care organizations in developing and maintaining evidence-based order sets and prompt medical and APN providers with alerts and reminders. Organizations that deploy CPOE systems realize benefits in terms of automated data capture and more detailed and accurate information about performance metrics and attribution of these measures to particular clinicians, including APNs, than previously available with traditional hospital information systems.

Because CPOE systems are typically integrated with existing information systems within a health care setting (e.g., admitting-discharge-transfer [ADT] systems; pharmacy, laboratory, and electronic medical records systems) and are customized by individual organizations, a tremendous effort is required when initially implementing CPOE systems. In addition, APNs working in such settings will likely find themselves engaged in development of standard order sets, which require interdisciplinary collaboration and consensus building among multiple stakeholders before they can be adopted for use. Once the CPOE system is in place, the APN will be involved in ongoing maintenance of it, which is required to monitor the effectiveness and efficiency of standardized order sets and their continued alignment with current best practice literature.

Electronic Medical Record

An electronic medical record (EMR) is a medical record in digital format. The two primary categories of the EMR are the "born digital" record and the scanned/imaged record. The born digital record is information captured in an electronic format originally entered into a database, transcribed from an electronic tablet or notebook personal computer (PC), or in some other manner captured electronically from its inception. The information is then transferred to a server or other host environment, where it is stored. The second category consists of records originally produced in a paper or other hardcopy form (e.g., x-ray film, photographs) that have been scanned or imaged and converted to a digital form. It is not unusual for health care organizations implementing an EMR System to have a blend of both types of digital records, although scanned and imaged records are typically more costly to implement and sustain.

Box 25-4   OUTCOME ASSESSMENT WEBSITE RESOURCES*

Resource and Information Available	Website
Agency for Healthcare Research and Quality (AHRQ)	
• Reports from evidence-based practice centers; outcomes and effectivenes`s trials	www.ahrq.gov
• Outcome measures	www.qualitymeasures.ahrq.org
• Consumer Assessment of Healthcare Providers and Systems (AHPS)	
• Consumer Assessment of Health Plans	
• National Quality Measures Clearinghouse	
• Funding opportunities	
American Health Information Management Association (AHIMA)	www.ahima.org
• Documentation guidelines	
• Search engine for quality management topics; professional measurement tools; research	
Centers for Medicare & Medicaid Services (CMS) (Formerly Health Care Financing Administration [HCFA])	www.cms.hhs.gov
• Laws and regulations	
• Quality initiatives	
• Data collection instruments (Outcome and Assessment Information Set [OASIS]; Minimum Data Set [MDS 3.0])	
Center for Evaluative Clinical Sciences, Dartmouth College	www.dartmouth.edu/~cecs/
• Atlas of Health Care	
• Centers for Medicare & Medicaid Services database	
Centers for Disease Control and Prevention (CDC)	www.cdc.gov
• Search engine for health topics	
• Databases for health statistics	
• Funding opportunities	
Cochrane Library of Clinical Trials	www.cochrane.org
• Systematic reviews of evidence	
• Search engine for evidence-based reviews	
Foundation for Accountability (FACCT)	www.facct.org
• Quality measures	
• Clearinghouse for health care information	
Health Resources and Services Administration (HRSA)	www.hrsa.org
• Health interest area information for HIV/AIDS; primary health care; maternal/child health; health professions; rural health	
• Center for Quality: quality activities; providers' guide to quality	www.hrsa.org/quality
Institute for Healthcare Improvement (IHI)	www.ihi.org
• Continuous improvement newsletter	
• Search engine for quality; patient safety	
• Quality improvement methods, measures, tools, and resources	www.qualityhealthcare.org
• White papers on CQI, system redesign	
Institute for Safe Medication Practices (ISMP)	www.ismp.org
• Bibliography	
• Medication safety pathways	
• Organizational self-assessment for medication safety practices	

*These resources can be located by using most search engines. Google (www.google.com) is particularly helpful for identifying additional sites.
AIDS, Acquired immunodeficiency syndrome; *ANA,* American Nurses Association; *APN,* advanced practice nurse; *CQI,* continuous quality improvement; *HIV,* human immunodeficiency virus.

Continued

Box 25-4   OUTCOME ASSESSMENT WEBSITE RESOURCES*—CONT'D

Resource and Information Available	Website
Institute of Medicine (IOM) • Reports for health-related reviews of evidence • Best practices and quality improvement projects underway • Topic-related information	www.iom.edu
The Joint Commission • Search engine for quality of health care organizations • Glossary of terms • Performance measurement standards • Core measures for evidence-based assessment of performance	www.jointcommission.org
Medical Outcomes Trust • Outcomes assessment instruments, including the SF-36 & SF-12 Health Survey	www.outcomes-trust.org
Medscape from WebMD • Updates on health issues information • Search engine of selected health care journals • Resources for APN prescribing law and billing for services	www.medscape.com/ nurses home
MedWeb, Emory University Health Sciences Center Library • Search engine for evidence-based medicine; practice guidelines; databases	www.medweb.emory. edu/medweb
National Center for Nursing Quality, University of Kansas • ANA National Database for Nursing Quality Indicators (NDNQI) • Bibliography of nursing quality articles • Abstracts of research	www.nursingquality.org
National Committee for Quality Assurance (NCQA) • Quality performance databases: Healthcare Effectiveness Data and Information Set (HEDIS); Quality Compass • Publications related to measurement of quality (for purchase)	www.ncqa.org
National Guideline Clearinghouse (NGC) • Evidence-based practice guidelines	www.guideline.gov
National Institutes of Health (NIH) • Specialty-focused Institutes' reports • Search engine for health topics; clinical trials • Funding opportunities	www.nih.org
National Library of Medicine (NLM) • Reference databases: PubMed/ MEDLINE; MeSH • Funding opportunities	www.nlm.nih.gov
National Patient Safety Foundation (NPSF) • Bibliography of safety-related articles • Fact sheets	www.npsf.org
ZYNX Health Incorporated • Bibliography of evidence-based medicine and nursing articles • ZynxEvidence: Referential articles of evidence-based medical and nursing practice • ZynxCare: interdisciplinary plans of care (for purchase)	www.zynx.com

*These resources can be located by using most search engines. Google (www.google.com) is particularly helpful for identifying additional sites.
AIDS, Acquired immunodeficiency syndrome; *ANA,* American Nurses Association; *APN,* advanced practice nurse; *CQI,* continuous quality improvement; *HIV,* human immunodeficiency virus.

In health informatics, an EMR is considered to be one of several types of electronic "health" records, but confusion between the two terms still exists. The term *electronic health record* has become expanded to include *practice management systems,* which support medical office functions for physicians and APN providers working in primary care settings. As of 2006, adoption of EMRs and other HIT, such as CPOE systems, has been minimal in the United States. Fewer than 10% of American hospitals have implemented HIT, and only 6% of primary care physicians use electronic health records (Cutler, Feldman, & Horowitz, 2005). As of 2005, one of the largest national EMR projects is the National Health Service's (NHS) in the United Kingdom. The goal of the NHS is to have 60,000,000 patients with a centralized electronic medical record by 2010.

In the United States, the Department of Veterans Affairs (VA) has the largest nationwide health information system that includes an EMR, known as the *Veterans Health Information Systems and Technology Architecture* or *VISTA.* Health care providers can review and update a patient's EMR at any of the VA's over 1000 health care facilities. The VA's computerized system further includes the ability to place orders, including medications, special procedures, x-ray examinations, patient care nursing orders, diets, and laboratory tests.

In spite of numerous advantages, there are major barriers to widespread EMR adoption. One of the biggest is startup costs compared with financial return from better charge capture and more efficient record keeping and management. The majority of small physician offices can afford neither the capital outlay to implement EMR software and supporting hardware nor the loss of productivity that accompanies this transition for about a year (retrieved June 29, 2007, from *www.hhs.gov/healthit/ahic/materials/05_07/ehr/recs.doc).* In addition, most EMR systems use templates that are customized by the vendor to the individual institution, because every health care setting, whether it is an acute care hospital, an LTC facility, or a medical practice, has distinct requirements. In spite of these challenges, the need to manage large volumes of patient data means that APNs will likely find themselves engaged in the customization of electronic documentation systems. APNs are in key positions to account for workflow issues of the interdisciplinary team, identify the type of electronic information needed to care for specific populations, understand data capture requirements to evaluate practice outcomes, meet regulatory requirements or collect registry information, and understand the need for elimination of duplication and redundancy in the documentation process. Familiarity with their institution's data sources will help APNs access critical data needed for outcomes evaluation. In addition, the APN competencies of expert coaching and guidance, consultation, collaboration, and clinical, professional, and systems leadership will be critical to supporting successful implementation of an EMR System.

Integrated Data Management Systems

Integrated data management systems are vital components to evaluating outcomes, improving quality, and ensuring efficient and effective care. APNs require information from clinical documentation systems such as the EMR, as well as ancillary and specialty information systems, to create a holistic view of their population of interest or to gain a systems perspective before offering strategies for improvement. Data may be needed from multiple sources, such as laboratory, pharmacy, radiology, materials management, risk management, infection control, quality management, surgery scheduling, financial/cost accounting, outpatient services, clinics, patient relations, and home health, to name a few. Unfortunately, no single database or health care information system houses all data on a single platform, despite numerous attempts by large hospital information system vendors to promise such a system.

For the foreseeable future, data must be extracted from multiple systems and knitted together. This requires APNs to be knowledgeable about the various information systems used in their settings and to become skilled in querying information from each source. Although few APNs will become proficient "report writers" in each of the disparate systems across their organization, they can become proficient in terms of how to define their population of interest, how to specify the data elements they need, how the data display should be organized, and how the output should appear. This is discussed in greater detail later in the Strategies for Designing Quality Improvement and Outcome Evaluation Plans for Advanced Practice Nursing section.

When the APN identifies the need for frequent reports or requires access to a more integrated view of the patient's care, he or she should communicate this need to the organization's IT department and request an "automated" approach to accessing this information. Several strategies exist for data integration between information systems. The first involves "interfacing" selected data variables from one information system into another. Typically this is done to address a very specific need or problem. For example, selected laboratory values can be interfaced into a system that creates automated alerts to staff when potentially unsafe patient care situations arise (e.g., patients with elevated international normalized ratios [INRs] who are taking heparin or diabetics with hypoglycemia). In another example, selected data variables may be extracted from the risk management system (e.g., history of fall, injury, or loss of personal property during a previous care encounter) into the nursing documentation system so that bedside caregivers are alerted to the patient's history and can intervene to prevent injury or dissatisfaction.

The challenge with interfacing data between systems is that it requires the upfront identification of a specific "limited data set" (in other words, not everything from one system can be brought over into another) and it is costly to implement and maintain. A large number of data variables associated in an interface between two systems will require a significant amount of time and effort to program and test the interface by the affected technology vendors before "going live." In addition, the data and information needs of the end users will change over time; thus ongoing interface modifications must be made to accommodate these changes.

Clinical Data Repository

The creation of a clinical data repository (CDR) is a growing area of interest to many leaders in hospital and other health care systems. A CDR is a real-time database that consolidates data from a variety of clinical sources to present a unified view of a single patient. It is optimized to allow clinicians to retrieve data for a single patient rather than to identify a population of patients with common characteristics or to facilitate the management of a specific clinical department. Typical data types that are often found within a CDR include clinical laboratory test results; patient demographics; pharmacy information; radiology reports and images; pathology reports; hospital ADT dates; ICD-9 codes; discharge summaries; and progress notes. The APN managing chronic disease populations within an IDN, for example, would be able to use a CDR to rapidly track and monitor patients over time and across settings to ensure maximum compliance

with best practices for any given patient or group of patients within the APN's practice.

Clinical Data Warehouse

In contrast to a CDR, a clinical data warehouse is a database that supports analytic queries on clinical data across patients. Typically, a warehouse integrates data from over 20 clinical electronic sources and organizes the data by topic or clinical indicator. Sources may include laboratory, radiology, pathology, and operative reports; discharge summaries; demographics; diagnostic and procedure codes; charge or cost information; and more. Patient identities whose records match search criteria are generally protected. Knowledgeable end users, with appropriate authorizations can obtain direct access to the clinical data warehouse to perform searches, although, typically, designated analysts are available to conduct ad hoc queries. Some data warehouses may also have the ability to search on specific text information within a database, depending upon how the digital EMR is designed. Regularly scheduled reports can typically be generated. APNs will find this type of information helpful when evaluating outcomes on populations or conducting research on evidence-based practice patterns; however, very few health care institutions currently have this type of integrated information system available.

Organizational and social issues associated with the selection and adoption of all these new technologies include restructuring workflows, dealing with physician and nursing staff resistance to change, lack of typing skills, and generalized technology aversion and training. This is particularly true of older nurses and APNs who have had little to no prior computer experience and who tend to be fearful of changing their practice patterns and embracing new toolsets. In addition, successful adoption of new technology is more likely to occur when there is a collaborative environment that fosters effective change management and communication among physicians, pharmacists, nursing, administrative leadership, and IT project managers. Exemplifying this need is the highly publicized HIT implementation fiasco at Cedars Sinai Medical Center in Los Angeles, in which physicians revolted and forced the administration to abort a $34 million CPOE system. In the press release describing the CPOE implementation failure, Chief Nurse Linda Burnes Bolton was quoted as attributing the failure "First and foremost, to [the failure to manage] change" (Connolly, 2005).

STRATEGIES FOR DESIGNING QUALITY IMPROVEMENT AND OUTCOME EVALUATION PLANS FOR ADVANCED PRACTICE NURSING

Much of health care practice in today's economic market is data driven, with APNs assuming greater responsibility for collecting and using clinical, economic, and quality outcomes data. In particular, interdisciplinary QI teams are increasingly charged with improving care delivery outcomes or redesigning workflow processes for greater effectiveness or efficiency. Because APNs routinely monitor and maintain clinical care delivery systems, they are in an ideal position to plan QI initiatives by leading or actively participating in interdisciplinary QI teams. As clinical experts, APNs influence practice patterns and develop meaningful standards, practice protocols, clinical guidelines, health care programs, and health care policies that promote teamwork, improve clinical outcomes, and reduce costs. Moreover, APNs' pattern recognition skills facilitate the identification of system inefficiencies, barriers to continuity of care, and other ineffective ways of delivering health care services. These in turn become opportunities for APNs to influence processes and outcomes positively—at both the individual patient and system levels.

With these opportunities comes the responsibility to be knowledgeable in outcome evaluation. In the remainder of this chapter, the author proposes a stepwise approach to develop and implement an outcome evaluation plan that demonstrates an APN's value and contribution to the health care setting. Although the term *outcome evaluation* is used throughout this section, these steps can be applied to impact analysis, outcomes measurement, performance evaluation, process improvement, program evaluation, or clinical research.

Phases of Preparing a Plan for Data Analysis

There are three phases in this organizing framework to develop an effective outcome evaluation plan. The first of these involves defining the core questions that need to be answered. The second focuses on determining the data required to answer the questions. The third is directed at interpreting the data and acting on the results. Several steps within each of these phases are described to promote successful completion of the phase. Box 25-5 lists the phases and related steps in developing and conducting an outcomes evaluation. A description of each step follows.

Define the Core Questions.   The demand for data-based information to objectively quantify the contributions of APNs has increased significantly over the past 10 years. Before any useful data can be gathered, however, the questions foremost in key stakeholders' minds must be understood and described. These questions serve as the focus and foundation for the development of an effective outcome evaluation plan. In formulating the core questions, the APN must ensure that the questions clarify the APN's role within the organization, define the population targeted, identify the relevant stakeholders, and articulate the priority program goals and interventions to be evaluated. Once these foundational aspects have been established, the APN can formulate an approach to the outcome evaluation plan and determine whether and to what degree the APN's contributions are independent or value-added.

Clarify Purpose of the Advanced Practice Nurse's Role.   In developing an outcome evaluation plan, APNs often are required to revisit the purposes of their employment, their organization's mission, and the goals for their position. If the purposes of their roles are unclear, APNs may need to identify and discuss reasonable and appropriate expectations with administrators and collaborators. It is not possible to decide what outcomes to measure without clarity about the APN's clinical populations and their accountability for the structures and processes of care. Because an APN's role usually changes over time because of improved technology, changes in patient population, care management mandates, or organizational change, the desired outcomes for an individual APN may also shift. Therefore APNs must have an accurate understanding of their employer's expectations at the time the outcome evaluation process begins. In some cases, employers may not recognize the APN's full range of services or potential benefit to the organization. If that occurs, the APN may need to take the lead in identifying specific processes and areas of focus within the setting and set appropriate goals and performance objectives to meet these.

An APN's role may also change as a direct result of performance improvement and outcome evaluation studies. Findings may indicate that APN interventions are better suited to other points of care across the continuum of services than originally envisioned, or they may reveal that care may be delivered more efficiently by other providers. As an example, Lamb

Box 25-5   SUMMARY OF OUTCOME EVALUATION PLANNING PROCESS

PHASE I: DEFINE THE CORE QUESTIONS

I-1. Clarify the purpose of the APN's role.
- Review organization's mission, vision, and goals.
- Clarify role expectations.
- Confirm clinical and reporting accountability.

I-2. Define the target population.
- Identify differences in patient characteristics within target population.
- Clarify relationships between APN role behaviors and population needs and outcomes.
- Compare target group with other groups monitored through QI activities.
- Assess level of risk, complexity, and resource use of subpopulations within target group.

I-3. Identify the stakeholders.
- Facilitate participation by and input from key stakeholders.
- Isolate APN interventions and actions from those of other care providers.
- Secure early buy-in from stakeholders.

I-4. Articulate program goals and interventions.
- Review literature for supportive evidence.
- Consider resources needed to implement and maintain the intervention.
- Formulate specific questions.
- Implement practice change or quality improvement strategy.

PHASE II: DEFINE THE DATA ELEMENTS

II-1. Identify selection criteria for the population of interest.
- Clarify inclusion and exclusion criteria.
- Identify electronic data sources of information about the target population.

II-2. Establish performance and outcome indicators.
- Identify measures to determine evidence of APN impact.

- Ensure alignment between program goals, proposed interventions, and outcome indicators.
- Consider the use of national databases for comparison and benchmarking purposes.

II-3. Identify and evaluate data elements, collection instruments, and procedures.
- Evaluate ease of collecting data and compare with need.
- Identify data resources available.
- Link use of intermediate outcome indicators to target goals and outcome achievement.
- Summarize the outcome evaluation plan.

PHASE III: DERIVE MEANING FROM DATA AND ACT ON RESULTS

III-1. Analyze data and interpret findings.
- Seek assistance from others as needed.
- Select data analysis and reporting procedures.

III-2. Present and disseminate findings.
- Prepare reports according to audience and stakeholder needs and interests.
- Select software programs and other resources to support presentation approach.

III-3. Identify improvement opportunities.
- Work with stakeholders to identify most appropriate opportunity for improvement.
- Select most-effective tools to facilitate performance improvement planning process.
- Conduct pilot studies to assess new program feasibility, cost, and resource needs.

III-4. Formulate a plan for implementation and reevaluation.
- Summarize goals of performance improvement plan.
- Identify proposed interventions, responsible persons, and target dates for completion.
- Select indicators and measures based on goals and interventions identified.
- Provide educational programs to support intervention, as needed.

APN, Advanced practice nurse; QI, quality improvement.

and colleagues (1996) evaluated the effectiveness of hospital-based APN case management on HF patients and found that readmission rates were higher than expected. In light of these findings, the APN case management intervention was shifted to the patient's home and provided within 24 to 48 hours of discharge. Subsequent assessment of this change in APN intervention on care delivery outcome determined that readmission rates declined significantly and that patients' adherence to their therapeutic regimen improved. Eventually, non-APN case managers assumed responsibility for the case management intervention and similar results were seen. This confirmation of comparable impact allowed the APNs to shift their attention to other high-risk populations. Conversely, findings may support the effectiveness and efficiency of the APN intervention, which could lead to program growth and expansion to other populations or points of care. In all cases, outcome evaluation and APN role definition and scope of practice go hand in hand.

Define the Target Population for Study.
Once the APN's role has been clarified, the APN defines the population targeted for evaluation. APNs use a range of activities to manage heterogeneous clinical populations; therefore when designing an outcome evaluation plan, it is necessary to focus on specific aspects of their practice with a particular patient group. This focus helps create a more manageable outcome evaluation plan and limits the impact of extraneous variables that could interfere with the interpretation of findings. Aspects of APN activities used with the target population need to be identified and included in the design. Whenever possible, the target population should be comparable to other groups monitored through quality improvement initiatives at either the organizational or department level so that the vested interests of the organization's commitment to improving care and APN's activities are aligned. The decision to target subpopulations of patients may be based on a desire to evaluate patients who are high-risk, are complex, or tend to use more services than others.

Other factors to consider when defining a target population include patient satisfaction and financial performance. For example, when a large pediatric medical group hires a pediatric nurse practitioner (PNP) to provide routine physical examinations and vaccinations, parent satisfaction is likely to be an important component of the outcome evaluation plan. Patient factors such insurance provider, age, ethnicity, or co-morbid conditions also may be used to define the target population at risk for adverse outcome.

Finally, some populations are targeted because of the need for organizations to determine their level of compliance with national care delivery guidelines, best practice standards, or regulatory requirements. Frequently, APNs are involved in the care of several populations of interest and, as such, must prioritize which populations warrant first review and evaluation. APNs must be sensitive to the resource requirements of any outcome study, working closely with information systems, QI, and medical records staff

for the support required to conduct the review. A tool developed by Mahn and Heller (1998) at Carondelet Healthcare Systems in Tucson, Arizona, provides one example of an approach to prioritizing performance improvement initiatives within larger health care systems (Figure 25-5). The weighted scoring method used in this tool provides an objective approach to obtain input from other departments and stakeholders and identify and prioritize target populations for outcome evaluation.

Identify the Stakeholders.
APNs must identify the structures and processes of care for which they share accountability. Although APNs are rarely the only or the primary stakeholder in the provision of care to the populations they serve, often they serve as "the glue" that holds the team together. As such, they often move the team, the health care agency, and/or the system toward a shared vision of desired outcome. Creating this vision is not an isolated APN activity; APNs must also facilitate the contributions, ideas, and creativity of professionals who participate in the care of the target population. Stakeholders most commonly involved are physicians, physician assistants, other APNs, other nurses, pharmacists, administrators, and other members of the health care team. In some cases, APNs will need to include stakeholders from outside their immediate practice settings. For example, a community-based APN serving fragile elderly patients with chronic diseases may need to include stakeholders from managed care payers and insurers, primary care clinics, physicians' offices, skilled nursing facilities, home health care agencies, and hospitals. Although including all stakeholders in the development of an outcome evaluation plan may not be feasible or desirable, attention to the impact of primary stakeholders on care delivery outcomes will aid understanding and measurement of processes and outcomes that are interdependent with APN practice.

Typically, APNs are only one component of a greater whole, so they cannot receive full credit for the positive results. Therefore APNs must articulate APN-specific inputs and interventions that contribute to the team effect so that the value of an APN to the organization can be documented and demonstrated. The need to carve out additional measures of role effectiveness results in a more complex outcomes plan, requiring multiple measurement methodologies, instruments, and analysis techniques. For instance, part of an outcome evaluation plan may use

Prioritization Tool for Performance Improvement Initiatives

Proposed Population or Process: _____

	Low 1 Point	Medium 2 Points	High 3 Points
Cost	<$5,000 ❏	$5,000 - $10,000 ❏	>$10,000 ❏
Annual Volume	<50 cases ❏	50-150 cases ❏	>150 cases ❏
Risk	<1/1000 deaths ❏	<1/100 deaths ❏	>1/100 deaths ❏
Problem Prone	Minor problems infrequently reported ❏	Minor to moderate problems reported occasionally ❏	Steady stream of minor to major problems reported ❏
Regional Variation	Process of care delivery generally consistent ❏	Normal or expected variation exists ❏	Process of care delivery highly variable ❏
Improvement Opportunity	Few if any opportunities to improve exist ❏	Minor to moderate opportunities to improve exist ❏	Significant opportunities to improve exist
National Guidelines	No guidelines exist and rarely discussed in the literature ❏	Topic widely discussed in the literature ❏	Guidelines exist and are recognized nationally ❏
Controversial Therapy	Process or procedure is widely accepted nationwide ❏	The literature suggests alternative approaches may be of value ❏	Process or procedure has widely accepted alternatives ❏
Market Interest	Little if any focus exists in the community ❏	Process or procedure is of general concern in the community ❏	Process of major concern to the community ❏
Physician/Staff Interest	Very few professional staff would agree this area is important ❏	Selected professional staff would agree this area is important ❏	There are many staff who would agree this area is important ❏
Total Number of Points			
	____ x 1 = [ ]	____ x 2 = [ ]	____ x 3 = [ ]
Note: *Lowest possible score is 10. Highest possible score is 30.* **TOTAL SCORE**			

FIGURE **25-5:** Prioritization tool for performance improvement initiatives. (From Mahn, V.A., & Heller, C.J. [1998]. *Prioritization of target populations for care management and process improvement activities.* Copyright 1998-2007 by ACS MIDAS+, Tucson, AZ.)

quantitative methods to capture specific outcomes of treatment (e.g., average number of clinic visits per year, total costs, and number of diabetic patients with a normal HbA_{1c} level within 2 months of diagnosis). Another part of the plan may employ a qualitative approach, using verbal or written feedback from physician and dietitian colleagues about APN effectiveness facilitating development of new patient care guidelines to manage the diabetic population.

Once the plan for an evaluation study has been shared with stakeholders, buy-in to any proposed change must be obtained in order to proceed. APNs not only will be change recipients as a result of the outcome evaluation but also will serve as change implementers and change strategists for others and their organization. Involving stakeholders early in the process of change, using some of the CQI techniques described in Table 25-1, will facilitate ongoing communication, reduce resistance to change, and promote adoption of recommended changes.

Articulate Program Goals and Interventions. The easiest way to demonstrate positive outcomes of care is to do the right things, at the right times, for the right patients, in the right ways. Thereafter, the task of measurement becomes an artful assembly of necessary data and information that reflects the outcomes and processes associated with the intervention. Determining which interventions to implement for a given population and which to include in an outcome evaluation plan may be based in part on the resources required to accomplish the interventions and maintain them in practice. To begin, APNs should engage in a comprehensive literature review to examine all standards of care, regulatory requirements, national guidelines, and established or emerging evidence-based best practices that are relevant to their clinical population. Box 25-4 identifies relevant sites that can aid the literature search.

Using information from literature and experience, APNs can identify appropriate interventions for managing populations. For example, interventions may include attention to early detection and diagnostic modalities, timeliness of interventions, drug appropriateness, or patient education. The organization's needs and any political agendas should also be considered. APNs should limit the number of evaluated interventions to keep the project scope manageable. Committing to too many interventions or unrealistic data collection activities may result in "project

scope creep." This unplanned expansion of project activities can overwhelm available resources and undermine or stall performance improvement and outcome evaluation initiatives.

Once the program goals and interventions are defined, the APN can begin to formulate specific questions of interest to stakeholders. Sketching out some basic questions serves as a useful exercise for establishing the outcome evaluation plan. The following are some sample questions:

- How cost-effective is this program?
- How satisfied are patients with the services they received?
- How closely does the health care team adhere to best practice standards?
- How many patients experienced complications of care?
- What patient safety issues associated with this population should we examine?
- What can be done to reduce resource utilization for this population?
- What do we need to do differently to become a center of excellence for this population?
- How has the APN contributed to the training and development of other staff?

Once the core questions have been formulated, the APN can design the data collection methodology that will be used to answer key questions. Typically, this step occurs simultaneously with the actual implementation of the practice change or quality improvement strategy. In the event that a pre-intervention baseline of performance measurement needs to be established, the implementation of the improvement strategy would be deferred until after the baseline measurement has been established.

Define the Data Elements. After APNs clarify the program goals, identify the key interventions to evaluate in the outcome evaluation plan, and determine the core questions to be answered, they are ready to define the outcome indicators and the data elements they will use to measure the intervention's success. This phase in the outcome evaluation plan often poses the greatest challenge for APNs, particularly for those who have had little or no exposure to QI principles and management information systems—both of which support outcome evaluation. There are three steps in this phase. First, APNs decide how they will qualify patients or encounters of care for inclusion in the outcome evaluation; second, they identify which indicators they will use to answer the study's core questions; and third, they determine which data elements will be collected for each indicator chosen for the study. APNs with limited expertise in these areas may wish to seek assistance from other health care professionals with experience in CQI principles, Six Sigma theory (Marash et al., 2003), health care statistics, nursing informatics, program evaluation, or nursing research.

Identify Selection Criteria for the Population of Interest. Although this may seem like an obvious first step, it is important to consider what patient characteristics will be included in the evaluation. Identifying electronic data sources that contain information about the target population is generally the most efficient way to begin. For example, NPs who practice in a physician's office or clinic may be able to retrieve a list of all patients seen within a given time frame. This is possible because the NP's provider number, which identifies his or her patients in the claims database and generates the bill for services rendered, can be used to define the population of interest. The NP could further reduce this list to patients seen for a specific diagnosis or symptom through the use of ICD-9 codes, Current Procedural Terminology, 4th edition (CPT-4) codes, and/ or Ambulatory Payment Classifications (APC) codes. In behavioral health settings, the use of the *Diagnostic and Statistical Manual of Mental Disorders,* Version 4 (DSM-IV) codes are generally more useful.

In contrast, CNSs who practice in acute care environments may have a more difficult time obtaining a list of patients whose care they managed or influenced, because CNSs do not typically bill directly for services. In this scenario, the population may be identified by non-electronic data sources, such as a log or referral list. If the CNS's influence extends to a general clinical population, specified DRG or ICD-9 diagnostic or procedure codes can be used to obtain a patient list. This information is generally available from hospital information systems.

Such specificity in identifying the target population is important because these inclusion criteria become the calculation denominator for specific indicators that are used to monitor the effectiveness of APN intervention. For example, if one indicator being evaluated is the impact the APN makes on evaluating patients with left ventricular systolic dysfunction, examining all patients discharged from the hospital does not make sense. Examining a specific population of patients served or influenced by the APN (e.g., patients discharged with heart failure, as identified by a specific DRG or an array of ICD-9 codes) may be more useful. Additional inclusion or exclusion criteria may be applied to the population to ensure greater homogeneity. In some cases, filtering the population by either a primary or secondary ICD-9 diagnosis or procedure code may also create a more clinically homogeneous population. Because ICD-9 codes are typically more diagnostically specific than DRG classification, this additional process may further refine the description of the population. APNs should consult with experts in medical records coding to determine the most reliable and valid ways of isolating a specific clinical population of patients for their outcome evaluation.

Establish Performance and Outcome Indicators. Once the patient population is defined, APNs and colleagues specify measures of performance that will be used to draw conclusions about how well the population was managed or the degree to which favorable outcomes were achieved. In general, measures are classified into three types—proportion measures (e.g., mortality rates, readmission rates, complication rates), ratio measures (e.g., falls per 1000 patient days, central line infections per 1000 line days, restraint episodes per psychiatric patient days), and continuous variable measures (e.g., median time to initial antibiotic, average length of stay). Some measures are direct counts of a particular phenomenon within a given time period, such as number of allergic reactions in patients receiving antibiotics. Others are sums, such as total costs of care for a given population or total patient days. The type of measure selected is less important than how well it answers the core questions of the study (although, ultimately, the type of measure will determine the approach required for data analysis and presentation to stakeholders). The best approach is to create a draft list of indicators and obtain feedback from stakeholders about how well the indicators address their core questions and concerns. Only after stakeholder buy-in is secured should the APN formally establish the indicators for the evaluation plan. Otherwise, in the eyes of the stakeholders, the APN runs the risk of conducting an outcome evaluation study that fails.

Alignment between program goals, interventions, and performance and outcome indicators is another important consideration when designing the outcome evaluation plan. This process ensures that the findings of the outcome evaluation can be traced back to APN practice. For example, if ALOS is selected as one outcome indicator for a population of AMI patients under the direction of a hospital-based CNS, this variable should be linked in theory and in practice to an intervention for which the CNS has or shares accountability—such as discharge planning or management of complications. Measures that reflect the sub-processes of other providers, such as time from first incision for patients undergoing angioplasty to the time the wire crosses the lesion in the coronary artery, may be of interest to invasive cardiologists and other stakeholders from the cardiac catheterization laboratory; however, they may have little to do with the APN's direct practice role.

Often, APNs are lured into coordinating data collection for other providers as part of the performance monitoring process. APNs may agree to perform these data coordination or data collection activities, but they must be careful not to become overburdened with tasks that diminish their own clinical effectiveness or assessment of intervention effect. If this happens, APNs should examine other potential resources within the organization so they can continue to perform and provide service to the institution. Staying focused on the interventions and specific program goals for which they are responsible will assist APNs to formulate a meaningful and manageable outcome evaluation plan.

As decisions are made about which sources to use for measurement of interventions and outcomes, APNs may wish to consider data available from national comparative database services. Subscribing to such services provides access to definitions of measurement and to benchmark or comparison data that may be helpful to evaluate levels of performance. As noted earlier, use of such benchmarking indicators can assist with building a consistent set of core APN-sensitive indicators necessary to strengthen assessment of APN effect across providers and settings. Table 25-2 provides selected web-based resources of national comparison and benchmark data.

Identify and Evaluate Data Elements, Collection Instruments, and Procedures.
Box 25-6 lists a "minimum set" of data elements commonly available in most HIT systems, although this list is rapidly expanding as HIT systems become more integrated with the EMR and other ancillary and financial systems. To ensure an efficient data collection process, APNs should evaluate the effort to collect each individual data element compared with

the overall usefulness of the indicator. Indicators that require extensive, resource-intense data collection efforts may need to be eliminated in favor of indicators that adequately reflect the core questions of the study but are much less expensive to collect. If, for example, a rate or proportion measure is selected, then the specific definitions for the numerator and the denominator of the measure must be provided. Inclusion and exclusion criteria should be stated, and the data elements required to construct the indicator's numerator and denominator should be listed. Finally, the specific data source for each data element needs to be identified, as was illustrated in Figure 25-4.

Table 25-3 illustrates an analysis of the data required for a single indicator that examines the percentage of pneumonia patients who receive antibiotics within 8 hours of arrival at an acute care hospital. In this illustration, the indicator is dissected into its component parts so that each component can be carefully reviewed.

Data that are available through electronic sources are considered easier to obtain, even if the APN lacks the specialized knowledge necessary for running such reports. Running queries and reports may or may not become an essential part of the APN's role. In most cases, expert resources are available within health care systems to assist APNs in retrieving the information. Data available only through specialized or resource-intensive instruments, such as phone surveys, home follow-up visits, or comprehensive chart reviews, are considered difficult to obtain and should be carefully evaluated before making a final decision to include them in the outcome evaluation plan.

When collecting patient identifiable data, APNs should be cognizant of the restrictions on their use. The Health Insurance Portability and Accountability Act of 1996 (PL 104-191, 104th Congress), commonly referred to as *HIPAA*, includes significant restrictions on the manner in which identifiable patient information may be used for research and QI activities. Typically, information used for quality improvement and outcome evaluations is less restrictive. In some circumstances, particularly if they are contracted in a fee-for-service arrangement with the health care agency, APNs may be required to sign a Business Associate Agreement with the health care provider. For more information about HIPAA regulations and impact on evaluation activities, APNs should refer to their organization's policies and procedures.

Setting and Description	Website
ACUTE CARE HOSPITALS	
MEDPAR UB-92 (Uniform Billing): Billing information sent to state intermediaries and available through MEDPAR. This information is free and available to download from CMS website. A limitation of this information is that it is 18 to 24 months old by the time it is released.	http://cms.hhs.gov/researchers/statsdata.asp
Hospital Compare: This CMS website contains summary level data for the CMS Seventh Scope of Work initiatives for acute MI, HF, pneumonia, and surgical care.	www.hospitalcompare.hhs.gov
TJC ORYX®: Receives data from hospitals related to acute MI, HF, pneumonia, surgical care, children's asthma, hospital-based inpatient psychiatric services, and pregnancy-related conditions. National comparison data are available through performance measurement systems listed with TJC for ORYX®.	www.jointcommission.org/
Proprietary Software Vendors: A wide variety of for-profit vendor services exist for the provision of comparison data. Comparative data pool may vary in size, and hospital participation may be limited to selected states or hospital specialties (e.g., academic teaching facilities, behavioral health hospitals). See TJC website for a full listing.	www.jointcommission.org/
California Nursing Outcomes Coalition Report: Statewide database linking patient outcomes to hospital nursing care. Benchmark data currently available for patient falls.	www.nursingworld.org/snas/ca/calnoc/intro.htm
MANAGED CARE AND EMPLOYER	
Milliman USA, Healthcare Management Guidelines: A set of utilization criteria that provide benchmark data for hospital ALOS for various managed care markets.	www.milliman.com
HEDIS: A set of standardized measures used by purchasers and consumers to compare performance of managed health care plan. HEDIS is sponsored by the NCQA.	www.ncqa.org/Programs/HEDIS/
LONG-TERM CARE	
MDS: Provides data for quality improvement, benchmarking, and shared best practices for Medicare-certified long-term care facilities. The MDS Version 2.0 contains a core set of screening elements that can be used for a comprehensive assessment of residents at time of arrival and at various points in time during their stay. The CMS is responsible for oversight of this data set.	http://cms.hhs.gov/medicaid/mds20/man-form.asp
HOME HEALTH CARE	
OASIS: Used by home health agencies for quality improvement and client assessment. The CMS is responsible for oversight of this data set.	http://cms.hhs.gov/providers/hha/
PUBLIC HEALTH	
Minnesota and Washington Departments of Health: Uses the Omaha System (Monsen & Martin, 2002a, 2002b) to assist public health departments with organizing, documenting, analyzing, and disseminating data to the public. Public data are available for population characteristics, nursing interventions, and client outcomes using the KBS scale.	www.co.washington.mn.us/pubhlth/pubhlth.html

ALOS, Average length of stay; *CMS*, Centers for Medicare & Medicaid Services; *HEDIS*, Healthcare Effectiveness Data and Information Set; *HF*, heart failure; *KBS*, knowledge, behavior, and status; *MDS*, Minimum Data Set; *MEDPAR*, Medicare Provider Analysis and Review; *MI*, myocardial infarction; *NCQA*, National Committee For Quality Assurance; *OASIS*, Outcome and Assessment Information Set; *QIOs*, quality improvement organizations; *TJC*, The Joint Commission.

Box 25-6 Data Elements Typically Available from Hospital Information Systems

- Admission date and time
- Admitting physician
- Primary ICD-9 diagnosis
- Secondary ICD-9 diagnoses
- Diagnosis status not present on admission
- Attending physician
- Medical record number
- Reason for admission
- Total charges
- Social Security number
- Admit status
- Total cost
- Date of birth
- Emergency admit

- Insurance carrier
- Primary ICD-9 procedure
- Secondary ICD-9 procedures
- Gender
- Discharge date
- Insurance type
- Patient type
- Discharge time
- Insurance plan
- Financial class
- Discharge disposition
- DRG number and description
- Home zip code
- Primary care physician

DRG, Diagnosis-related group; ICD-9, International Classification of Diseases, 9th revision.

Table 25-3 Anatomy of a Sample Process Indicator Used in Performance Improvement Studies

Indicator	Percentage of patients admitted to hospital with pneumonia who receive initial antibiotic within 8 hours of arrival
Numerator Definition	Patients who receive any antibiotic, regardless of route, type, or dose, within 8 hours of arrival to the hospital
Denominator Definition	All patients admitted to the hospital with a working diagnosis of pneumonia **Inclusion criteria:** • Patients admitted as inpatients • Patients with a working diagnosis of pneumonia on arrival • Patients 18 years of age and older • Patients with a principal ICD-9 diagnosis code of pneumonia **OR** • Patients with a principal ICD-9 diagnosis of respiratory failure **AND** a secondary ICD-9 diagnosis code of pneumonia **OR** • Patients with a principle ICD-9 diagnosis of sepsis **AND** a secondary ICD-9 diagnosis code of pneumonia **Exclusion criteria:** • Patients admitted from other acute care hospitals • Patients admitted for comfort care only

Required Data Elements	Data Source
• Encounter type (inpatient, outpatient, ED, short-stay) • Age on day of discharge • Working diagnosis on arrival • Admission source	Hospital ADT system
• Final discharge diagnosis	Hospital DAB system
• Time of arrival to hospital • Working diagnosis on arrival • Admission for treatment or comfort care only	Chart review: Allowable data sources include ED record, progress notes, physician orders
• Administration of any antibiotic	Pharmacy drug system
• Initial time of initial antibiotic administration	Chart review: Allowable data sources include medication record, physician orders, ED record

ADT, Admit, discharge, transfer; *DAB*, discharge abstract; *ED*, emergency department; *ICD-9*, International Classification of Diseases, 9th revision.

Other types of information, such as the time when a specific medication was administered or length of time waiting in the emergency department (ED), must be abstracted from a careful review of the medical record. Still other types of information may be found in specialized information systems (e.g., surgery, pharmacy, risk management, cost accounting). If specific laboratory or radiology results are required (e.g., lipid level or confirmation of pneumonia on admission), however, access to medical records may be required. Clinical documentation systems, if available, may also house data elements common to the medical record, such as the NYHA classification for heart failure, diagnostic results, and disease history. Nursing departments may collect patient acuity data, information on CQI team activities, and other unit-based quality monitoring reports. APNs can avoid duplication of effort and data collection redundancy by becoming familiar with the many sources of data and information available in their respective organizations.

In some cases, questions about the effective management of clinical populations can be answered only through longitudinal studies. For example, for a diabetic population, clinical outcomes such as reduced hospitalization, improved functioning, reduced evidence of retinopathy, and reduced limb amputations may be sound but they are typically too long-range to be useful for performance improvement or outcome evaluation activities. The link between APN practice and the outcomes may be difficult to assess over long periods, making intermediate outcomes assessment more desirable for a short-term evaluation.

The usefulness of intermediate outcomes measures will be most evident if they clearly indicate progress toward some desired endpoint or outcome. Case management literature provides a framework to identify intermediate outcomes of nursing care that may be applicable to APN practice. The Second Council for Case Management Accountability (Case Management Society of America) and the State of the Science Papers from the Council's annual meeting identify intermediate outcomes as improved patient adherence to therapeutic regimen, increased patient and family involvement in treatment plan, education and empowerment that lead to higher levels of self management, and improved access to services (Braden, Lamb, & Koithan, 2002).

Only after all the indicators within the plan are evaluated will the APN have a full appreciation of the scope of the outcome evaluation project and the resources required for successful completion. Once the indicators and the individual data elements have been finalized and the sources of data have been secured, APNs should summarize the outcome evaluation plan in a concise document that describes the plan. Table 25-4 illustrates a high-level outcome evaluation plan for an APN case manager charged with evaluating the effectiveness of a case management program for heart failure patients. Specific interventions and key process steps are listed for each program goal. For clarity, the indicators that reflect the relative success of the interventions are listed alongside the goals and the interventions. Finally, specific sources of data, timelines, and accountability for data collection and analysis are included to highlight the full scope of the outcome evaluation plan. Data collection should then take place over a designated time period that is sufficient to capture the outcomes and processes being influenced by the APN intervention. For example, if changes in practice are likely to reflect more desirable trends in the immediate future (e.g., changes in the care delivery process to ensure more timely and complete discharge instructions are provided to heart failure patients at discharge), a 30- to 120-day period may be sufficient. Other outcomes, such as reduction in amputation rates in diabetics who are managed in a disease management program, will require longitudinal analysis.

Derive Meaning from Data and Act on Results. The final phase of the outcome evaluation process involves evaluation and dissemination of the findings and identification of opportunities for improvement. In these final steps, results are transformed into meaningful information that can be used to improve quality, cost, and patient satisfaction, as well as evaluate the contributions of the APN. The final step involves formulating a plan to implement and re-evaluate changes that occur as a result of the study.

Analyze Data and Interpret Findings. Typically, data analysis is the responsibility of the APN, although the inclusion of other peer reviewers is useful, especially when the APN has a vested interest in the outcomes. Including others helps eliminate any perceived bias during the final data analysis and reporting phases. In some cases, the APN may wish to enlist the support and guidance of a statistician or a doctorally prepared nurse researcher to ensure the end product is methodologically sound and contains the information necessary to convince others.

Table 25-4   Sample Institutional Outcome Evaluation Planning Grid: Program for Heart Failure Patients

Goal	Interventions	Key Process Steps	Indicators	Data Source	Data Collection	Data Analysis	Time Frame
Reduce number of admissions and acute care utilization by 5%-10%	1. Identify patients in capitated groups	—Review all patients admitted with CHF during past 12 months —Mail out SF-36 survey	—Number of inpatient days/year —Mean number of acute care days/quarter —Number of ED visits/year	QA/UR system	Director of UR	CHF CM QA Medical Director PI Director	Quarterly
			—Number of returned SF-36 surveys/total	SF-36 software	Case manager	APN	Quarterly
				Care management log	Clerk		
		—Phone interview to patients with physical score <50	—Number with scores <50/total received —Hours/case/month —Number of patients declined CM service —Number of high-risk patients currently taking ACE inhibitor	Care management log	APN	APN	Monthly
	2. Patient and family education and monitoring	—Schedule home visits for patients taking more than eight medications	—Number of home visits/month —Number of patients/zip code	Care management log	APN	APN	Monthly
		—CHF video	—Pretest/posttest improvement scores on CHF video	Care management log	APN	APN	Quarterly
		—Assess KBS scores on admission and at 6-month intervals	—Mean improvement of Omaha KBS scores	Care management log	APN	APN	Biannually

Continued

Table 25–4 Sample Institutional Outcome Evaluation Planning Grid: Program for Heart Failure Patients—cont'd

Goal	Interventions	Key Process Steps	Indicators	Data Source	Data Collection	Data Analysis	Time Frame
Decrease overall cost of care by 10%	1. Daily rounds in critical care triage	—Establish triage criteria with critical care committee	—Number of critical care bed days/total days —Mean critical care cost/patient —Mean telemetry care cost/patient	QA/UR system	Finance department	Director, Critical Care	Quarterly
	2. Home health referrals for patients who meet criteria	—Meet with home health liaison daily to review referrals	—Mean home health cost/case —Readmit rate 31 days after discharge from home health	CMS-1500 QA/UR System	Finance department	Director, Home Health	Quarterly
	3. Establish CQI team to review opportunities to reduce radiology and pharmacy costs	—Secure membership for CQI team —Identify team facilitator —Develop mission statement —Schedule monthly meeting	—Mean cost per admission —Mean pharmacy cost/admission —Mean radiology cost/admission —Total CQI team meeting expenses/year	Cost accounting system CQI meeting minutes	Finance department Team facilitator	Director, Pharmacy Director, Radiology	Biannually

ACE, Angiotensin-converting enzyme; *CHF,* congestive heart failure; *CM,* case manager; *CQI,* continuous quality improvement; *ED,* emergency department; *KBS,* knowledge, behavior, and status; *PI,* performance improvement; *QA,* quality assurance; *UR,* utilization review.

Comparing pre-intervention with post-intervention performance data is one effective way to evaluate the degree of change resulting from APN interventions. Pre-intervention performance data are commonly collected retrospectively and then compared with data collected either during or after an APN intervention. Retrospective data are generally available for measures constructed from electronic data sources. When electronic data are insufficient to provide adequate baseline information, APNs may elect to collect more detailed data from non-computerized medical records. Although this approach generally requires more effort, time, and planning, it may be warranted when specific processes of care are altered as part of the APN's intervention. For example, a certified registered nurse anesthetist (CRNA) evaluating the frequency of intraoperative hypotensive episodes may have to review medical records because this phenomenon is not contained in common electronic source data. In some cases, a baseline study must be conducted before the APN intervention to ensure that appropriate baseline data are available for comparison. For example, an NP who is implementing changes in clinic protocols to reduce waiting times for prenatal patients undergoing glucose tolerance testing may have to conduct a pre-intervention time-and-motion study to establish a baseline against which to compare post-intervention results.

Although baseline information is useful for evaluating outcomes, not everything measured by APNs will have suitable baseline data for comparison. In these cases, performance can be evaluated against a known standard of care or benchmark, especially when an area of practice is supported by evidence-based practice. When no best practice standard of performance is known, APNs may use comparative data provided by a national database if the measures used for comparison are the same as those contained within the national database.

Present and Disseminate Findings. Effective communication of data-based findings, conclusions, and recommendations for future practice is an essential component of the outcome evaluation process. How the findings are presented depends on the audience. Non-clinical audiences with a business focus, such as boards of directors or operations teams, will require briefings that summarize pertinent findings, draw conclusions, and provide reasonable options or recommendations for consideration. Clinical audiences generally require additional detail about how the evaluation was conducted and a more extensive discussion of the clinical and statistical strengths of the evidence. Clinical audiences are becoming more sophisticated in their understanding of data analysis techniques and their assessment of the applicability of evidence to practice.

One of the most effective methods for demonstrating change over time is statistical process control (SPC) analysis, which examines process variation and its source. SPC uses control charts, which visually display performance data against upper and lower control limits reflective of normal variation in a system. Performance data lying outside these upper and lower limits and clusters of data within limits indicate the existence of some special cause of variation requiring exploration (Melum, Bartleson, Panzer, & Ron, 1995). Control charts document processes over time, eliminating the need to rely on isolated "snapshots" of performance—which may or may not capture the true picture of process variation. Figure 25-6 contains an example of a control chart displaying the time until antibiotics were initially administered to patients treated for pneumonia in an ED. Data for the control chart were used to detect meaningful changes that occurred as a result of an APN's implementation of standard protocols for management of patients with pneumonia. The longitudinal display of data provides a more accurate and informative representation of APN impact than would be evident by simply comparing average time before and after the intervention. A detailed discussion of these data analysis techniques is beyond the scope of this chapter, although a basic knowledge of control charts is useful for most situations (Wheeler, 1993).

The APN may be responsible for packaging the study's findings to present to stakeholders. Assistance from the facility's media department may be required. Findings should be disseminated using visual graphs and summary documents to facilitate rapid review and comprehension of information. Microsoft PowerPoint and Excel programs are useful for this process. For APNs who wish to produce their own control charts, one low-cost and user-friendly tool that is used in conjunction with Microsoft Excel (QI Macros) is available for purchase at *www.quantum-i.com*. This software includes tutorials on producing a variety of quality improvement tools and control charts suitable for proportion, ratio, and continuous variable data. Findings are commonly presented in committee meetings and formal presentations, although the APN should also consider posters, newsletters, white

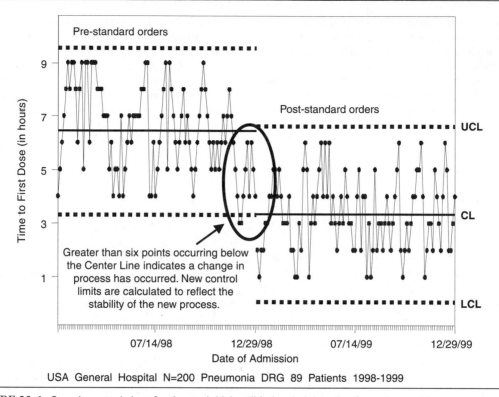

FIGURE **25-6:** Sample control chart for time to initial antibiotic administration for patients with pneumonia treated in an emergency department. *UCL,* Upper control limit; *CL,* center line; *LCL,* lower control limit. (Copyright 2007 by ACS MIDAS+, Tucson, AZ.)

papers, articles, and bulk e-mail communications as additional ways to disseminate information.

Identify Improvement Opportunities. Once the outcome evaluation findings have been interpreted and assembled for presentation, the APN begins to work closely with stakeholders to evaluate the effectiveness of the practice change or quality improvement strategy, as well as to identify additional opportunities for improvement or potential leverage points to further impact outcomes. Leverage points are specific aspects of care delivery processes, technology resources, or points in time that can be altered to achieve greater efficiency or effectiveness within the health care system. For example, the APN working in an acute care hospital may identify opportunities to improve performance in teaching discharge patients with heart failure and approach this by leveraging the hospital's decision to participate in the American Heart Association's *Get With The Guidelines Program,* a national demonstra-

tion of best practice performance for the treatment of AMI and HF (*www.americanheart.org/presenter.jhtml? identifier=3045578,* retrieved September 8, 2007). During this third step, the APN assists team members to develop a shared vision of which intervention(s) to adopt and why. Bringing stakeholders together to review existing processes of care and isolate any process failures or barriers that have contributed to suboptimal performance is useful. Tools for this purpose include flow charting; cause-and-effect (Ishikawa) diagrams; failure modes and effects analysis; strengths, weaknesses, opportunities, and threats (SWOT) analysis, and formal brainstorming techniques. The reader is referred to Powell (2000) for additional reading on these and other quality improvement tools.

The process to identify opportunities for improvement is similar to any work redesign initiative. The APN should identify champions and potential opponents of change. Careful specification of program components and delegating responsibility for project-related activities are also part of the process. Change theory can serve as a useful foundation for APNs responsible for preparing stakeholders and overcoming their resistance to new care delivery practices (see Chapter 9). Issues such as level of difficulty with deploying the intervention should be addressed, as well as projected costs and the human and technology resources required to implement and sustain the plan (The University of York, 1999). Consider how much time the APN will be engaged in the project and how this may affect other areas of practice. A staged pilot-testing approach is useful for new or large-scale projects. As noted earlier, these smaller-scale versions help identify potential implementation problems and determine whether the intervention can achieve the desired effect. As an example, if one of the goals of a performance improvement plan is the timely administration of initial antibiotics to pneumonia patients in an acute care setting, interventions might include using a risk appraisal tool or instituting fast-tracking of admission orders to the pharmacy department. These interventions might be pilot-tested on one shift in the ED for 2 to 3 weeks before deploying the strategy across the hospital or using it on all shifts.

Formulate a Plan for Implementation and Reevaluation. Once the findings have been shared and the goals of the performance improvement initiative are established, the APN should document and distribute the results to all stakeholders. Each goal should specify the primary intervention or interventions that will be deployed to reach the goal, along with who is accountable for the actions required and the target dates for completion. When the interventions, accountabilities, and timelines are established, the APN can use the identified indicators/measures to reevaluate the outcome. This reevaluation then becomes the basis for future outcome evaluation plans. Once performance in a particular area is stabilized, the APN may elect to discontinue monitoring a given area of performance or periodically revisit performance through intermittent monitoring.

For interventions that focus on change in practice patterns or processes of care, the APN may be called upon to provide educational programs for other providers and disciplines affected by the new process or change. For example, an APN overseeing a QI project geared toward the management of a diabetic population in a community clinic may need to provide an educational program about the appropriate and timely screening, diagnostics, treatment, and referrals required for the diabetic population. The educational content of these sessions should focus on the standards of practice expected for the population and the strategies, tools, and supports available (e.g., revised documentation systems, flow sheets, computerized alerts) to assist in the adoption of the care delivery standard. Providers also should be informed about the measures that will be used to monitor performance. In some cases, this action will alter performance in and of itself simply because the providers know they are being observed and their performance is being monitored. This reaction, called the *Hawthorne effect*, is troublesome for process measurement. The program should continue for a sufficient period to ensure that the novelty of the intervention has worn off and the changes in behaviors are a true reflection of intervention effect.

SUMMARY

This chapter illustrates the interconnectivity among outcomes measurement, systems thinking, performance improvement, and information technologies with every aspect of APN practice. Effective outcomes measurement and management require APNs to work collaboratively with others, to plan and organize processes of care and assessment of quality in highly complex health services environments, and to effectively manage change within their sponsoring organizations. Because reimbursement decisions are driven by evidence of both organizational and individual provider performance, APNs lacking reliable and valid data to substantiate their impact will struggle for equitable reimbursement for their services— and possibly employment.

Decisions made solely on the basis of physician-derived outcome indicators seriously limit the understanding of APN impact on patient care. Currently, the majority of managed care organizations that list APNs as primary care providers evaluate them according to physician standards (Mason, Cohen, O'Donnell, Baxter, & Chase, 1997). In such situations, the magnitude of APN contributions to care is often lost because managed care organizations and national regulatory initiatives often attribute all outcomes to the principal attending or admitting physician billing for services (Mason et al., 1999). In complex health care environments in which multiple providers work within an increasingly interdisciplinary model, the issue of provider attribution will continue to be a challenge for both physicians and APNs.

Some will argue that this invisibility of APNs in the health care system threatens the recognition of APNs as important providers of health care services. But this challenge also presents an opportunity for APNs willing to spearhead performance improvement initiatives in their institutions. It may be that APNs who successfully steward safer care environments, improve clinical performance, and achieve greater efficiencies in caregiving processes will demonstrate their value more than they have ever been able to do to date. APNs who develop robust and ongoing outcome evaluation plans place themselves in the strongest positions to demonstrate their impact on outcomes of care delivery. In so doing, they also render advanced practice nursing visible to patients, other providers, administrators, payers, and communities.

REFERENCES

American Association of Colleges of Nursing (AACN). (2006). *Essentials of doctoral education for advanced nursing practice.* Washington, DC: Author.

Berry, P., & Dahl, J. (2000). The new JCAHO pain standards: Implications for pain management nurses. *Pain Management Nursing, 1*(1), 3-12.

Braden, C.J., Lamb, G., & Koithan, M. (2002). State of the science: Involvement/participation, empowerment and knowledge outcome indicators of case management. Little Rock, AR: Case Management Society of America.

Brooten, D., Younblut, J.M., Deatrick, J., Naylor, M., & York, R. (2003). Patient problems, advanced practice nurse (APN) interventions, time and contacts among five patient groups. *Journal of Nursing Scholarship, 35*(1), 73-79.

Centers for Medicare and Medicaid Services (CMS). (November 21, 2007). U.S. Department of Health and Human Services report to Congress: Plan to implement a Medicare hospital value-based purchasing program. Retrieved December 1, 2007, from www. cms.gov/.

Connolly, C. (March 21, 2005). Cedars-Sinai doctors cling to pen and paper, *The Washington Post.* Retrieved August 3, 2007, from www.washingtonpost.com.

Cutler, D.M., Feldman, N.E., & Horowitz, J.R. (2005). U.S. adoption of computerized physician order entry systems. *Health Affairs, 24*(6), 1654–1663.

Institute of Medicine (IOM). (2001). *Crossing the quality chasm: A new health system for the 21st century.* Washington, DC: National Academies Press.

Institute of Medicine (IOM). (2003). Health professions education: A bridge to quality. Washington, D.C.: National Academies Press.

Lamb, G., Mahn, V., & Dahl, R. (1996). Goals of an effective delivery system for the chronically ill. *Managed Care Quarterly, 43*(3), 46-53.

Mahn, V.A., & Heller, C.J. (1998). *Prioritization of target populations for care management and process improvement activities.* Available from ACS MIDAS+, Tucson, AZ.

Mahn-DiNicola, V. (2004). Changing competencies in health care professions: Will your nurses be ready? *Nurse Leader, 2,* 38-43.

Marash, S., Berman, P., & Flynn, M. (2003). *Fusion management: Harnessing the power of Six Sigma, Lean, ISO 9001:2000, Malcolm Baldrige, TQM, and other quality breakthroughs of the past century.* Fairfax, VA: QSU Publishing Company.

Mason, D J., Alexander, J.M., Huffaker, J., Reilly, P.A., Sigmund, E.C., & Cohen, S.S. (1999). Nurse practitioners' experiences with managed care organizations in New York and Connecticut. *Nursing Outlook, 47,* 201-208.

Mason, D.J., Cohen, S.S., O'Donnell, J.P., Baxter, K., & Chase, A.B. (1997). Managed care organizations' arrangements with nurse practitioners. *Nursing Economic$, 15,* 306-314.

Masys, D.R. (2002). Effects of current and future information technologies on the health care workforce. *Health Affairs, 21*(5), 33-41.

Melum, M.M., Bartleson, J.D., Panzer, R., & Ron, A. (1995). *Total quality outcomes management: A guide to interpreting outcomes measurement and TQM to improve health.* Methuen, MA: GOAL/QPC.

Monsen, K.A., & Martin, K.S. (2002a). Developing an outcomes management program in a public health department. *Outcomes Management, 6,* 62-66.

Monsen, K.A., & Martin, K.S. (2002b). Using an outcomes management program in a public health department. *Outcomes Management, 6,* 120-124.

Papenhausen, J.L. (1996). Discovering and achieving client outcomes. In E.L. Cohen (Ed.), *Nurse case management in the 21st century* (pp. 257-268). St. Louis: Mosby.

Perez-Wilson, M. (1997). Six Sigma strategies: Creating excellence in the workplace. *Quality Digest, 17*(12), 27-31.

Powell, S.K. (2000). *Advanced case management: Outcomes and beyond.* Philadelphia: Lippincott.

Shortell, S.M., Bennett, C.L., & Byck, G.R. (1998). Assessing the impact of continuous quality improvement on clinical practice: What it will take to accelerate progress. *The Milbank Quarterly, 76*(4), 593-624.

The University of York. (1999). *Effective health care: Getting evidence into practice.* Retrieved September 26, 2003, from www.york.ac.uk/inst/crd/ehc51.pdf.

Ward, M.D., & Rieve, J.A. (1997). The role of case management in disease management. In W.E. Todd & D. Nash (Eds.), Disease management: A systems approach to improving patient outcomes (pp. 235-259). Chicago: American Hospital Publishing.

Wheeler, D.J. (1993). *Understanding variation: The key to managing chaos.* Knoxville, TN: SPC Press.

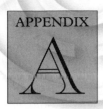

APPENDIX

Sample Employment Contract

EMPLOYMENT AGREEMENT (the "Agreement") made as of May 1, 2008, by and between EMPLOYER, INC., a (your state) corporation with its principal place of business in (your city, state) ("EMPLOYER") and EMPLOYEE, an individual resident of (your city, state) (the "Employee").

1. **Purpose and Employment.** The purpose of this Agreement is to define the relationship between EMPLOYER and Employee. EMPLOYER hereby employs Employee, and Employee hereby accepts employment by EMPLOYER, upon all of the terms and conditions of this Agreement.

2. **Duties**

   2.1 Employee shall serve EMPLOYER by providing women's health services to EMPLOYER's clients, and shall further perform such similar duties as may be assigned to Employee from time to time by EMPLOYER. EMPLOYER anticipates that it will schedule Employee to work approximately sixteen (16) hours per week, with additional hours added according to practice demands and both parties' mutual consent.

   2.2 Employee shall (i) devote Employee's attention and best efforts to the duties hereunder, including the promotion of the success of the business of EMPLOYER; (ii) perform such duties in a reasonable, prompt, honest, and faithful manner. Only by mutual consent will (1) Employee accept work as a NP for another entity, and (2) EMPLOYER hire an additional NP; (iii) not participate actively in any other business during the term of Employee's employment under this Agreement without EMPLOYER's consent.

   2.3 Employee acknowledges that Employee owes full loyalty to EMPLOYER, and shall not engage in any activity or enter into any transaction that would constitute a conflict of interest with the duties and loyalties owed to EMPLOYER.

   2.4 EMPLOYER is employing Employee based on Employee's representations that she is a licensed and certified R.N., M.S., and F.N.P. Employee shall, upon EMPLOYER's request, provide proof of such professional certifications. At Employee's sole expense, Employee shall also take any and all such steps (including, without limitation, timely acquisition of continuing education units) as are necessary to maintain said professional license throughout the term of this Agreement (and any extensions thereto).

3. **Contract at Will**

   3.1 The term of Employee's employment under this Agreement will commence on May 1, 2008 (the "Commencement Date") and continue through April 30, 2009 (the "Initial Term"). Either party may terminate this contract by giving written notice of no less than sixty days to the other of a desire to terminate. This agreement will automatically extend for twelve (12) month periods commencing on the first anniversary of the Commencement Date and each subsequent anniversary thereof. Unless either party gives written notice to the other of a desire not to extend the term of this Agreement at least sixty (60) days before the end of the Initial Term or any extension, the Agreement will automatically be extended for successive additional twelve (12) month periods commencing on the first anniversary of the Commencement Date and each subsequent anniversary thereof.

   3.2 Employee's employment under this Agreement may be terminated prior to the end of the Initial Term or any extension thereof as provided below:

   (a) upon the death of Employee, this Agreement will automatically terminate, and the only obligation EMPLOYER will have under this Agreement will be to pay Employee's personal representative, administrator or executor Employee's unpaid base salary through the date of Employee's death;

(b) EMPLOYER may terminate Employee's employment hereunder at any time without notice for cause. Upon such termination for cause, the only obligation EMPLOYER will have under this Agreement will be to pay Employee's unpaid base salary through the date of termination. For purposes of this Agreement, "for cause" shall mean:
 (i) Employee's disability;
 (ii) Breach of conduct as defined in the employee policy manual;
 (iii) any other conduct by Employee generally recognized under applicable laws as cause for termination;
 (iv) a sale of all or substantially all of the assets of Company;
 (v) a staff reduction or reorganization resulting in the elimination or substantial redefinition of Employee's position with EMPLOYER or
 (vi) a termination or substantial curtailment of the business of EMPLOYER within the area or division in which Employee works.

For purposes of this Agreement, "disability" shall mean any physical or mental condition that prevents Employee, after EMPLOYER has made such accommodations as may be required by law, from performing Employee's full duties to EMPLOYER for any cumulative period of three (3) months during any six (6) month period.

    3.3 Notwithstanding the above, before terminating the employment of Employee for any of causes (iii) through (vi) above, EMPLOYER shall give Employee ten (10) days' written notice and an opportunity to cure, except that if the nature of Employee's conduct is such that EMPLOYER may be materially harmed if it so postpones terminating Employee's employment, then EMPLOYER need not give Employee an opportunity to cure and may terminate Employee's employment immediately.

4. **Compensation.** Employee shall be compensated at the rate of $35 per hour, payable weekly or in accordance with Company's payroll policies. EMPLOYER shall withhold state and federal taxes to the extent required by applicable law. Hourly compensation shall be subject to review at 6 months and then annually thereafter.

5. **Employee Benefit Plans; Fringe Benefits.** Employee shall be entitled to benefits as per EMPLOYER stated policies that hold for any other EMPLOYER employee.

6. **Expenses.** If EMPLOYER requires Employee to incur any travel, entertainment, or similar expenditures for the benefit of the Practice during the term hereof, it will reimburse Employee for such expenditures on the basis of vouchers submitted by Employee that have been approved by Employee's supervisor. Employee is responsible for all expenses of her professional liability insurance. During the term of this Agreement (plus extensions thereto), Employee shall maintain professional liability insurance coverage and with coverage equal to or greater that of the other Nurse Practitioner.

7. **Property of Company.** All records, files, client lists, or plans, developed or created by Employee during the term of this Agreement, individually or in conjunction with others, which may directly or indirectly relate to the practice of EMPLOYER or any of its affiliates shall be the property of EMPLOYER.

8. **Restrictive Covenants**
   8.1 Nondisclosure. Employee acknowledges, covenants and agrees that:
 (a) During employment by EMPLOYER under this Agreement, Employee has and will come to have knowledge and information with respect to confidential plans, projects, practice methods, operations, techniques, clients, client lists, employees, financial condition, policies, and accounts of EMPLOYER and its affiliates with respect to their practice ("Confidential Information"),
 (b) During the term of Employee's employment and for one (1) year, Employee will not divulge, furnish, or make accessible to anyone (other than in the regular course of Employee's performance of services for the benefit of EMPLOYER, its successors, assigns, and affiliates) any knowledge or information with respect to any Confidential Information, and
 (c) All organizational or administrative papers and records, including all memoranda, notes, plans, data, or other documents, and any and all copies thereof, whether made by Employee or not, reasonably related to EMPLOYER's practices are the sole and exclusive property of EMPLOYER. Employee shall not remove from the Practice's premises any such written information concerning the Practice's business.

8.2 Solicitation. Employee agrees that at all times during the term of employment under this Agreement and for a period of twelve (12) months after the termination of employment with EMPLOYER under this Agreement or otherwise, Employee will not, directly or indirectly, for or on behalf of any other practice solicit, divert, take away, or accept the medical records of any of the clients of EMPLOYER that were served by EMPLOYER during the term of employment or any prospective clients of EMPLOYER that EMPLOYER actively served within one (1) year prior to the termination of this Agreement for the purpose of selling the services provided by EMPLOYER during the term hereof to any such client or prospective client. Employee further agrees that Employee will not, within the foregoing period of time, directly or indirectly, attempt or seek to cause any of the foregoing clients of EMPLOYER to refrain from seeking care from EMPLOYER.

8.3 Interference with Employees. Employee agrees that during employment under this Agreement and for a period of twelve (12) months after the termination of Employee's employment with EMPLOYER under this Agreement or otherwise, Employee will not, directly or indirectly, for or on behalf of any other practice request or induce any other employee of EMPLOYER or its affiliates to terminate employment of such persons with EMPLOYER or its affiliates.

8.4 Remedy for Breach. The parties recognize that the services to be rendered under this Agreement by Employee are special, unique, and of an extraordinary character, and that in the event of a breach of this Agreement by Employee or EMPLOYER, then either party shall be entitled to institute and prosecute proceedings in any court of competent jurisdiction, either in law or in equity, to obtain damages, or to enforce the specific performance of any terms, conditions, obligations and requirements of this Agreement, or to enjoin the party who breached the Agreement from continuing those actions which cause a breach of this Agreement, or to take any or all of the foregoing actions. Nothing herein contained shall be construed to prevent the pursuit of any other remedy, judicial or otherwise, in case of any breach of this Agreement by either party.

8.5 Effect of Termination. Expiration of the term of Employee's employment under this Agreement or termination of Employee's employment either by EMPLOYER or Employee shall in no way limit or restrict Employee's obligations under this Section 8 which shall remain in full force and effect for the remaining periods set forth in such Section.

9. **Paragraph Headings.** Paragraph headings contained in this Agreement are for convenience only and shall in no manner be construed as a part of this Agreement.

10. **Amendment.** This Agreement may be amended or modified only in writing signed by both parties.

11. **Counterparts.** This Agreement may be executed in two or more counterparts each of which shall be deemed to be an original but all of which together shall constitute one and the same instrument.

12. **Waiver.** The failure of either party hereto in any one or more incidences to insist upon the performance of any of the terms or conditions of this Agreement, or to exercise any rights or privileges conferred in this Agreement, or the waiver of any breach of any of the terms of this Agreement shall not be construed as waiving any such terms, and the same shall continue to remain in full force and effect as if no such forbearance or waiver had occurred.

13. **Applicable Law.** This Agreement shall be construed according to the laws of the State of (your state).

14. **Severability.** In the event any term of this Agreement shall be held invalid or unenforceable by any court of competent jurisdiction, such holding shall not invalidate or render unenforceable any other term contained in this Agreement.

15. **Entire Agreement.** This Agreement embodies the entire understanding of the parties with respect to Employee's employment with EMPLOYER and incorporates any previous agreement, written or oral, relating to such employment.

16. **Assignment and Successors**

    16.1 Employee's rights under this Agreement shall not be assignable by Employee.

    16.2 This Agreement may be assigned by EMPLOYER and shall inure to the benefit of and be binding upon EMPLOYER, its successors and assigns.

17. **Mediation.** If a dispute arises under this Agreement that the parties are unable to resolve through direct negotiations, the parties agree to engage jointly the services of a professional mediator and to participate

in good faith in such mediation. If the dispute is not resolved as a result of such mediation within thirty (30) days after such mediation is commenced or such longer period to which the parties may agree, each party shall be free to pursue any legal or equitable action as it considers appropriate.

IN WITNESS WHEREOF, EMPLOYER has hereunto caused its corporate name to be signed and sealed, and Employee has hereunto set her hand, all being done in duplicate originals, with one original being delivered to each party as of the day and year first above written.
EMPLOYER, INC.

By: _____
Date: _____
EMPLOYER

Date: _____
Employee

Sample Collaborative Practice Agreement

It is the intent of this document to authorize the nurse practitioner(s) at the _____ clinic(s) to practice under these protocols without direct supervision, as specified in the Medical Practice Act, Texas Civil Statutes, Article 4495b, section 3.06(d)(5) and (6). This document sets forth guidelines for collaboration between the supervising physician(s) and the nurse practitioner(s).

Development, Revision, and Review

The protocols are developed collaboratively by the nurse practitioners, delegating medical director, and supervising physicians. These protocols will be reviewed annually and revised as necessary.

Approval

The protocols will be approved annually on the initial approval date by the nurse practitioners, medical director, and supervising physicians. The *Statement of Approval* will be signed by all the above parties recognizing the collegial relationship between the parties and their intention to follow these protocols. Signature on the Statement of Approval implies approval of all the policies, protocols, and procedures in this document. Nurse practitioners and physicians who join the staff mid-year or who cover the practice also signify approval of the protocols. It is the task of the medical director to see that the written approval of all the above parties is obtained.

Setting

The nurse practitioners will operate under these protocols at the (Name of Institution) clinics listed below:

Clinic 1: (name and address)
Clinic 2: (name and address)

Supervision

The nurse practitioners are authorized to practice under the protocols established in this document without the direct (on-site) supervision or approval of the supervising physicians. Consultation with the supervising physicians or their designated back-up is available at all times, either on-site or by telephone when consultation is needed for any reason.

Consultation

The nurse practitioners are responsible for providing health services to clients of the (Name of Clinic or Agency). The nurse practitioners will provide health promotion, screening, safety instructions, and management of acute episodic illness and stable chronic diseases. Referrals will be made as needed to other health care providers. Physician consultation will be sought for all of the following situations and any others deemed appropriate. Whenever a physician is consulted, a notation to that effect, including the physician's name, must be recorded in the patient's medical record. Consultation will occur:

- Whenever situations arise that go beyond the intent of the protocols or the competence, scope of practice, or experience of the nurse practitioners.
- Whenever the patient's condition fails to respond to the management plan within an appropriate time frame, based on the provider's clinical judgment.
- For any uncommon, unfamiliar, or unstable patient condition.
- For any patient condition that does not fit the commonly accepted diagnostic pattern for a disease/condition.
- For any unexplained physical examination or historical finding or abnormal diagnostic finding.
- Whenever a patient requests.
- For all emergency situations after initial stabilizing care has been initiated.

Medical Records

The nurse practitioners are responsible for the complete, legible documentation of all patient encounters using the SOAP format.

Education and Training

The nurse practitioners must possess a valid Texas license as a Registered Nurse and be recognized by the Texas Board of Nurse Examiners as a Nurse Practitioner.

Evaluation of Clinical Care

Evaluation of the nurse practitioners will be provided in the following ways:

- A minimum of a monthly review by the supervising physicians of a minimum of 10% of patient charts.
- A written record of the review is to be kept.
- Annual evaluation by the supervising physicians based on written criteria.
- Informal evaluation during consultations and case review.
- Periodic chart review a part of chart audits by the Quality Assurance Committee.

Practice Guidelines

The nurse practitioners are authorized to diagnose and treat common medical conditions under the following current guidelines (including, but not limited to): Barker, L.R., Burton, J.R., & Zieve, P.D. (1999). *Principles of Ambulatory Medicine* (5th ed.), Philadelphia: Williams & Wilkins or comparable current edition of medical references available on-site at the respective clinics.

OR

Other published, accepted sources of medical information, as agreed upon by the collaborating parties and/or identified below:

- OSHA guidelines
- CDC guidelines for immunizations
- Uphold, C.R., & Graham, M.V. (1998). *Clinical Guidelines in Family Practice* (3rd ed.). Gainesville, FL: Barmarrae Books, Inc.

Drug Prescriptions

Nurse practitioners at this facility shall be authorized to prescribe dangerous drugs (excluding controlled substances) as authorized by the Texas Board of Nurse Examiners (BNE) under Rule 222, Advanced Practice Nurses Limited Prescriptive Authority and the Texas Board of Medical Examiners (BME) under Rules 193.2-193.4 and 193.8, Delegation of Prescriptive Authority. Authority shall be delegated by the Medical Director of the Methodist Health Care Ministries, and supervision of prescribing activity shall be conducted by the Medical Director and supervising physicians as indicated in the Rules. It is the responsibility of the nurse practitioners to obtain prescription ID numbers from the appropriate Board. The Medical Director shall inform the BME, in writing, of his intent to delegate prescriptive authority as required in the Rules. References for prescriptions will be the current Physician's Desk Reference and/or the Nurse Practitioner/Physician Monthly or Quarterly Prescribing Guide. Additionally, there may be limitations placed on prescriptions to an approved formulary for the MHCM.

Collaborating Parties: Statement of Approval

We, the undersigned, agree to the terms of this Collaborative Practice Agreement as set forth in this document.

_____ Medical Director
_____ Supervising Physician
_____ Supervising Physician
_____ Supervising Physician
_____ Nurse Practitioner
_____ Nurse Practitioner
_____ Nurse Practitioner

Approval Date _____
Renewal Date _____
Renewal Date_____

NOTE: This is an example of a broad collaborative practice agreement. Permission is given to download, copy or modify. Each state will have different board of nursing or public health code rules and regulations that will need to be identified in the wording.

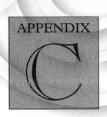

Sample Query Letter

March 15, 2008

Mr. John Andrews, CEO
Mayberry Health Clinic, PC
1111 Twin Forks Avenue
Littleton, GA 00012

Dear Mr. Andrews,

I will be moving to the area in a few months and am inquiring about the possibility of a position as a family nurse practitioner in your health care facility. It appears that your agency has the attitude and holistic perspective that matches what I am looking for in a practice environment.

Over my 20 years as a family nurse practitioner, I have provided primary care to newborns, children, adolescents, and adults in rural Tennessee. I have worked with underserved populations in a rural health clinic, in a community hospital outpatient clinic, and in private practice. I have also been a guest lecturer and primary care preceptor for nurse practitioner students in the local university's graduate nursing program. I thoroughly enjoy providing prevention-oriented care to improve patients' health care outcomes using an evidence-based approach. In addition, during my 15 years as a baccalaureate-prepared registered nurse, I provided care in hospital, extended-care, and home health facilities.

I have attached a résumé with more details regarding my education and experience. I can be easily reached by e-mail or by phone. I look forward to hearing from you soon as I complete arrangements for my move to Littleton.

Sincerely,

Jane Doe, MSN, FNP-BC
123 North Street
Cason, TN 12345
800-222-1222
tarzansjane@google.com

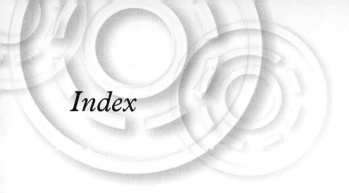

Index

A

---

b indicates boxed material, *e* indicates examplars, *f* indicates illustrations, and *t* indicates tables.